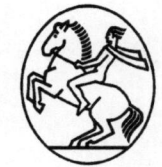

New Trends in Management of Cerebro-Vascular Malformations

Proceedings of the International Conference
Verona, Italy, June 8–12, 1992

Edited by
A. Pasqualin and R. Da Pian

In collaboration with
R. Scienza

Springer-Verlag Wien New York

Alberto Pasqualin, M.D.
Renato Da Pian, M.D.
Department of Neurosurgery, Verona City Hospital, Verona, Italy

This publication was supported by an educational grant from The Upjohn Company and Bayropharm

Typesetting: Thomson Press, New Delhi, India

Printed on acid-free and chlorine-free bleached paper

With 268 partly coloured Figures

Library of Congress Cataloging-in-Publication Data.

New trends in management of cerebro-vascular malformations : proceedings of the international conference, Verona, Italy, June 8-12, 1992 / edited by A. Pasqualin and R. Da Pian : in collaboration with R. Scienza.
p. cm.
"International Conference "New Trends in Management of Cerebro-vascular Malformations" — Pref. ISBN-13: 978-3-7091-9332-7
ISBN-13: 978-3-7091-9332-7   1. Intracranial aneurysms—Congresses. 2. Subarachnoid hemorrhage—Congresses.
I. Pasqualin, A. (Alberto), 1951- . II. Da Pian, R. (Renato), 1928- . III. Scienza, R.
IV. International Conference "New Trends in Management of Cerebro-vascular Malformations" (1992 : Verona, Italy).
[DNLM: 1. Cerebral Arteriovenous Malformations—therapy—congresses. 2. Cerebral Aneurysm—therapy—congresses. WL 355 1994]
RD594.2.N494 1992. 616.8'1—dc20. DNLM/DLC 94-7680

ISBN-13: 978-3-7091-9332-7   e-ISBN-13: 978-3-7091-9330-3
DOI: 10.1007/978-3-7091-9330-3

Foreword

Every so often a gathering of minds and experience occurs that results in an all encompassing overview in depth of such a vast subject as Cerebro-Vascular Malformations, as occurred in Verona in June 1992 and which warrants publication. Professors Da Pian and Pasqualin deserve high compliment and it is a measure of the respect in which they are held that virtually all those most knowledgeable around the world attended, presented their work and thoughts and contributed to intense discussion.

Ljunggren's opening historical survey set the stage and must be the most comprehensive yet published.

Subarachnoid hemorrhage from aneurysm rupture still constitutes, I dare say, the most difficult problem for neurosurgeons, in relief of the brain injury and arterial reaction and the technical perfection of aneurysm obliteration, even for small, as well as large and giant sacs. Very large high flow AVMs can be as demanding too. The bulk of the conference was devoted to subarachnoid hemorrhage, aneurysms and AVMs which were discussed under about 14 headings each. But vein of Galen malformations, dural AVMs, cavernous angiomas and venous angiomas (renamed developmental venous anomalies) came under scrutiny, not always with consensus.

Trends are perceptible such as fibrinolysis of subarachnoid clot, non surgery for Galenic and dural malformations, the benignity of venous angioma, but there is still much variation in approach, pharmacologically, technically and with such as the evolving endovascular and radiosurgical stories, used alone or in conjunction.

Of the more than 200 presentations, just about 100 have been selected for publication but these best survey the gamut of the conference

March 1994   Charles G. Drake, OC. M.D. FRCS (C)

Preface

The management of cerebral aneurysms and arteriovenous malformations (AVMs) still poses considerable problems and is still the subject of controversy. In spite of dramatic advances in surgical techniques, endovascular therapy and anesthesia, the largest lesions – as well as those located in deep areas of the brain – remain a challenge for the neurosurgeon. When dealing with aneurysms, the initial subarachnoid hemorrhage can be devastating – creating difficulties in management – and cerebral vasopasm has still to be solved. The hemodynamic consequences of the occlusion of large AVMs are difficult to predict and combined or alternative treatments may be preferable to surgical removal of these lesions. For less common malformations – such as dural fistulas, cavernomas and venous angiomas – the indications for treatment have still to be established.

In order to discuss these problems, the International Conference "New Trends in Management of Cerebro-Vascular Malformations" was held in Verona, Italy, from June 8 to 12, 1992; Prof. Renato Da Pian was the President of the meeting, and Prof. Charles C. Drake was the Honored Guest. During the Conference, the major international experts discussed in depth the various aspects of this pathology, including diagnosis, pathophysiology, pharmacology, surgery, embolization and endovascular occlusion, radiosurgery, anesthesia and perioperative care.

This book contains the proceedings of that Conference, which – as a whole – represent an update of the achievements made in the management of cerebro-vascular malformations, with particular attention paid to the hemodynamics of subarachnoid hemorrhage and intracranial AVMs, and to the new possibilities of interventional neuroradiology.

Our gratitude goes to the many contributors to this book and to all those who participated in the Conference.

We are indebted to The Upjohn Company and Bayropharm for support in the publication of this book. We also want to express our gratitude to Mrs. Giuliana Rossi Pasqualin for her skilfull assistance.

March 1994   The Editors

Contents

Endovascular Approaches to Vasospasm

Anesthesia and Temporary Clipping in Aneurysm Surgery

Surgery of Giant Aneurysms

Surgery of Posterior Circulation Aneurysms

Endovascular Treatment of Aneurysms

Severe Subarachnoid Hemorrhage, Unruptured and Intracavernous Aneurysms, Aneurysm Rests

Intracranial Arteriovenous Malformations

Classification of Cerebral AVMs

Hemodynamics of Cerebral AVMs and Perioperative Management

Surgery of Deep-Seated and Posterior Fossa AVMs

Introduction

History and Epidemiology of SAH and Cerebrovascular Malformations

B. Ljunggren, S. Sharma, and **H. Fodstad***

Division of Neurosurgery, Department of Surgery, Faculty of Medicine and Health Sciences, Al Ain, United Arab Emirates University and Tawam Hospital, United Arab Emirates

Summary

Intracranial aneurysms and the results of rupture of such treacherous lesions, i.e., subarachnoid hemorrhage (SAH), were first recognized in the early 19th century. With the introduction of cerebral arteriography in 1927 by Egas Moniz and Almeida Lima the stage was set for consideration of surgical obliteration of intracranial aneurysms. Epidemiological studies have shown varying incidence rates of aneurysmal SAH from one geographical area to another. Interestingly, aneurysmal SAH seems to be very rare amongst nomadic bedouins whereas the incidence of this dreadful condition is high or >20/100.000/year among their "opposite", the nomadic Laplandish ethnic group of the Ural-Altaic family. Attempts to approach ruptured intracranial aneurysms in the anterior circulation were made by several pioneers in the 1930s to 1960s but turned out most hazardous and many a pioneer neurosurgeon experienced more of operative disasters than of successful surgery. It was learnt that by delaying surgery the operative outcome could be improved but in the waiting period many patients died or became disabled due to early rebleeds and/or SAH-induced cerebral ischemic deterioration of delayed onset. Visualization of cerebral anteriovenous malformations, AVMs, was greatly improved by Lysholm and consequently surgical treatment of AVMs was first developed by Olivecrona, who in 1936 reported four successful resections of cerebral AVMs; as of May 1948 his operative mortality was below 10%. With the introduction of the counterbalanced operating microscope, a wide range of microsurgical instruments for cerebrovascular surgery, improved neuroanaesthesia, and concentration of such demanding cases – as those with a cerebral AVM or a ruptured intracranial aneurysm – to specially geared major referral centres with an accumulated experience and organization to handle such cases, operative results have improved considerably. In parallel, timing of the surgical intervention has swung in favour of attempts to perform surgery as soon as possible. In the last decade endovascular coil occlusion of ruptured aneurysms has evolved rapidly and may with future improvements become the method of choice instead of open surgery with 'external' clipping of the ruptured sac. Endovascular embolization techniques and radiosurgery represent recent advances in the treatment of cerebral AVMs although direct surgical excision is still recommended for most cases. The evolution of surgery for aneurysms and AVMs are depicted chronologically with emphasis on some historical landmarks.

Keywords: Circle of Willis; intracranial aneurysms; intracranial arteriovenous malformations (AVMs); history; conservative management; excision; carotid ligation; late aneurysm surgery; early aneurysm surgery; endovascular embolization techniques; radiosurgery; pioneers.

Introduction

The English physician Thomas Sydenham three centuries ago observed: "No investigator can point out the origin of Medicine – mysterious as the source of the Nile[80]". The stages of development regarding our knowledge and management of subarachnoid hemorrhage (SAH) and cerebrovascular malformations such as aneurysms and AVMs is not terribly diffuse; on the contrary the historical landmarks can be quite well located and defined. Some of the landmarks are as follows.

Description of the Cerebral Arterial Supply in 1664

In 1650 a young woman by the name of Anne Green was sentenced to death by hanging. The official execution took place at Cattle Yard in Oxford on 14th December and the body was cut down after 30 minutes and transported to the anatomy theatre of the University for a customary autopsy. However, when young Drs. William Petty and Thomas Willis opened the coffin they were appalled by finding that the poor young woman showed faint signs of still being alive and instead of performing a post-mortem they started immediate resuscitation with an ultimate rewarding result[57]. Anne Green's life was saved and she recovered without cerebral ischemic complications. Fourteen years later, in 1664, Thomas Willis published his famous *Cerebri Anatome: cui accessit Nervorum Descriptio et Usus*[92] with his description of the circle of arteries at the base of the brain, concluding that "... there may be a manifold way for the blood to go into diverse

*Present address: Bayville, Long Island, New York, U.S.A.

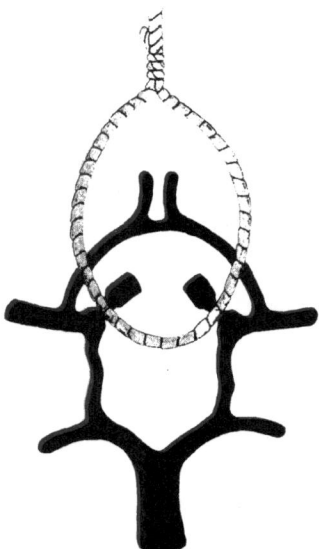

Fig. 1. Thomas Willis's greatest contribution to medicine was his description in 1664 of the circle of arteries at the base of the brain: "...there may be a manifold way for the blood to go into diverse regions of the brain that if by chance one or two should be stopped there might easily be found another passage instead of them"

regions of the brain that if by chance one or two should be stopped there might easily be found another passage instead of them"[92] (Fig. 1).

The Classical Description of an Aneurysmal SAH in 1813

One and a half century later, in 1813, another English physician, John Blackall, published a brilliantly clear report[5] of a previously healthy young lady, who had suddenly and without any apparent cause suffered from headache of the most excruciating kind associated with violent vomiting and intolerance to light. She spent many days in intolerable agony before her death. Blackall was curious to find the cause of her apoplexy and on autopsy was able to demonstrate a major hemorrhage under the membranes covering the brain with breakthrough into the ventricular system. Furthermore, he was able to trace the origin of the hemorrhage to a ruptured aneurysmal sac in the posterior part of Thomas Willis' circle, on the top of the basilar artery. He also made the important observation that the extravasated blood extended further down the meninges around the spinal cord.

Diagnosis and Recognition of SAH

In the 19th century there had been several independent reports of cases of hemorrhage from identifiable aneurysms at different locations in the circle of Willis described in publications by various workers in Europe like Serres (1819)[75], Bright (1831)[8], Jennings (1833)[44], Brinton (1852)[9], Gull (1859)[38], and Bramwell (1886)[6]. The latter author described that the *extravasation of blood* resulting from rupture of an intracranial aneurysm ensues under the arachnoid i.e., is located in the *subarachnoid* space. Bramwell also emphasized that subarachnoid hemorrhage does not inevitably lead to death witin 48 hours which had been stated by a previous author.

The Norwegian physician Edvard Bull in 1877 reported the case of a teenage girl who was treated by him for meningeal apoplexy with oculomotor palsy[10]. He attributed the condition to be due to rupture of a right internal carotid artery (ICA) aneurysm with pressure on the oculomotor nerve. In spite of clinical improvement in the patient's condition he had warned the possibility of a second hemorrhage. Unfortunately, the girl bled a month later and postmortem revealed an aneurysm at the predicted location. Bull postulated that ligation of the carotid artery in the neck might have prevented further hemorrhage. This procedure had been known for almost 300 years. In fact, carotid ligation was first used by Parè in 1585 to control bleeding following stabbing and Astley Cooper used it in 1805 to treat an extracranial carotid aneurysm. In Denmark, Gundelach Möller ligated the left common carotid artery in a patient with a carotico-cavernous fistula in 1832 and his countryman David Withusen repeated the procedure in a Swedish lady with the same affliction in 1864[52]. Edvard Bull should, however, be credited for being the first to suggest the method to prevent fatal aneurysm rebleeds. His and Blackall's case descriptions from the previous century certainly testify them to have been far ahead of their time.

Heinrich Quincke, German physiologist, internist and first pulmonary surgeon, all in one person, invented the concept of lumbar puncture (Lp), which he first described in 1872. In 1914, he summarized his knowledge and experience with Lp over the past 32 years, pointing to the diagnostic and therapeutic value of his important innovation[66]. Then, after a couple of years, an Austrian mathematician, Johann Radon, prepared the ground for computerised tomography (CT) by presenting the necessary mathematical formula[67], that was a prerequisite for CT, although his published results went completely unobserved by the scientific world over the next fifty years.

In 1920, the British neurologist Charles Symonds, Harvey Cushing's first scholar in Boston, suggested that a patient upon which Cushing planned to operate for a suspected pituitary tumor, instead was suffering from an intracranial aneurysm. The Chief scoffed at the suggestion. It turned out that Symonds was right and the patient died on the day of surgery itself. Cushing took immediate and appropriate action and released Symonds from all ward duties so that he could put forward further scientific proof to support his correct conclusions. The resulting study[81], which appeared in 1923, involved a breakthrough for clinical diagnosis of ruptured intracranial aneurysms and SAH in North America and in the next years Symonds extended his studies on SAH[82] and brought the attention of Cushing to this catastrophic condition[15]. Then, following successful pituitary secretion studies, a 26-year-old Scot by the name of Norman McComish Dott was awarded a Rockefeller travelling scholarship in 1923 and worked with Cushing from 1923 to 1924[83].

First Visualization of Intracranial Aneurysm by Arteriogram in 1932

With the introduction of cerebral arteriography in 1927 by Egas Moniz and Almeida Lima in Portugal, the stage was set for visualizing intracranial aneurysms and for possible surgical treatment. In July 1932 these pioneers visualised the very first intracranial aneurysm by arterial contrast injection[56].

The Early Pioneers

Norman Dott (1897–1973)

Amongst the forerunners in the diagnosis and surgical treatment of cerebrovascular malformations, Norman Dott (1897–1973) deserves the honour of being entitled most distinguished pioneer[72, 83]. He enthusiastically adopted the pioneer work of Moniz on cerebral angiography and was the first in the United Kingdom to demonstrate by this method a cerebral arteriovenous malformation five years after his return to Edinburgh from Boston. Three years later, in 1932, he was the first in the United Kingdom to demonstrate an intracranial aneurysm by arteriography. By then he had already performed a bold attack on a ruptured aneurysm in a

patient diagnosed by the clinical presentation only. His own words describe his thoughts and reasoning which led to this most courageous intervention:

"A beloved wife and mother aged 47. As we watched her go, in company with her anguished relatives, we could hardly bear it. This had been a dearly loved lady with everything to live for, who had been in perfect bodily condition except for one minute defect on one of her arteries. Surely, some surgical measure could be devised to meet such devastating minutiae? We answered by carrying out some 'blind' cervical ligations in cases that we could diagnose clinically but this did not always suffice. I observed a series of cases and became familiar with and confident of their diagnosis and I noted that in some there were signs pointing to the site of the responsible aneurysm. Those which bled recurrently in rapid succession died. I watched them die and afterwards noted at autopsy, how accurately one could have exposed the ruptured aneurysms during life, on the clinical facts. These were healthy subjects and it seemed too bad that they should be lost because of a weak spot in a cerebral artery. These considerations led me to attempt operative treatment and I had the privilege of repairing such a leaking aneurysm for a personal friend and benefactor. It required knowledge and confidence in diagnosis, an appreciation of the surgical possibilities, combined into a feeling of rebellion against letting these cases die"[83].

First Direct Operation of Ruptured Aneurysm (MCA) in April 1931 by Dott

The patient, a 53-year-old Edinburgh solicitor and governor of the Royal Hospital for Sick Children in Edinburgh suffered a SAH confirmed by lumbar puncture on 6th April 1931 to be followed by a 2nd bleed on 14th April and a third coma-producing hemorrhage on 20th April. Dott had by then lost other patients with recurrent fatal hemorrhages and discussed the problem with the general practitioner and the patient's wife before he decided "the apparently desperate measure of directly exposing the aneurysm". Dott was fully aware of the extreme technical difficulties he expected to encounter by exposing the aneurysm obscured in surrounding clot and he felt uncertain whether the application of muscle would control it or not. Dott's patient had recovered consciousness after the 3rd bleed although he showed some degree of dysphasia.

Dott was only 33 years old, had been Honorary Surgeon to the Royal Hospital for Sick Children since 1925 and although he had been appointed as Consulting Neurological Surgeon in 1929 it was not until 1931, the year of his operation, that he was to achieve official status at the Edinburgh Royal Infirmary as Associate Neurological Surgeon[72]. He later described his patient as, "an able, middleaged, legal gentleman, who ruled the medical staff as with a rod of iron, sometimes with whips of scorpions". How much easier would it have been to let his illness pursue its accepted course to unavoidable death. Fortunately, Dott had the "feeling of rebellion against letting these cases die".

An eminent and senior Edinburgh surgeon had warned Dott against operating on the Chairman of the hospital, saying that it would not be successful and would damage his career and reputation. Dott replied: "My career and reputation have nothing to do with it. He will die if I don't operate, he might live if I do[72]."

Consequently, the young unestablished surgeon proposed to tell the able lawyer, who was used to ruling his medical staff, Dott himself included, that he appeared to be heading for certain death and that his only chance of escape was an untried operation to be carried out by one of the younger members of his staff. So well did he impart this information to an analytical mind, so well did he impart confidence, that the operation was arranged. His patient was in Hunt and Hess Grade III[43] and subjected to early operation on Day 2 following a 3rd SAH within two weeks.

For this occasion on 22nd April 1931 Dott chose his sister Keith and colleagues Ian Aird and A.B. Wallace. At surgery under ether anaesthesia, a bicoronal scalp flap was incised and then a left frontal bone flap was raised. The left carotid artery was approached sub-frontally and the arachnoid uncovered up to the bifurcation where "a comparatively recent blackish clot ... was gently detached ... with a blunt spoon". The MCA was "literally dug out of blood clot. As this was being done some frank arterial bleeding occurred, this appeared to come from the posterior surface of the middle cerebral artery about 1 cm from its origin." Meanwhile Dr. Wallace had obtained a muscle graft from the lower limb. Dott controlled the hemorrhage by applying muscle "steadily maintained for twelve minutes" and wrapped the aneurysm: "muscle was now carefully packed in such a way as to clothe the middle cerebral artery for its first 2 cms in quite a thick layer of muscle". He then performed a subtemporal decompression before closing the wound. The operation occupied 3 hours and 40 minutes.

This very first directed attack on a ruptured aneurysm turned out most successfully. When enquired of his important patient by Dr. Wallace on the day following surgery Dott could reply: "Oh! he's fine. All he complains of is his leg where you took the muscle from!" Actually, the patient recovered so well that two years later he was fully able to indulge in his previous hobbies of shooting, mountaineering and fishing. Dott was also a keen fisherman and they went fishing together on a number of occasions. Dott's former patient had no signs of further cerebral hemorrhage and died eleven years after his operation of a coronary thrombosis[83].

Norman Dott's Further Contributions

Dott "wrapped" two more patients with "tumortype" aneurysms in 1931 and 1932, respectively. Unfortunately, the first patient rebled fatally within 24 hours whilst the other patient died from pneumonia five days after surgery.

On 27th October 1932 Dott performed his first carotid ligation on 26-year-old Isobel McNeil, a hospital nurse, who had suffered a coma-producing SAH confirmed by Lp and associated with 3rd nerve palsy. He first made bilateral subtemporal decompressions and when these became tense on 23rd October he suspected a further leak from the aneurysm and felt reinforced "to take the comparatively small risk of tying the left internal carotid artery" which was then done under local anaesthesia. Isobel McNeil subsequently was able to return to her nursing duties. Between 1932 and 1936 Dott performed internal carotid ligation in a total of eight patients, in six of whom the aneurysm had been proven by angiography to be on the ICA, in one on the MCA, and in one with unknown site with a good outcome in 63% (5 out of 8 patients alive and well).

Altogether between 1926 and 1936 Dott managed 39 patients with suspected SAH. In 1941, he again successfully operated upon a hospital staff person, a nursing sister with a giant aneurysm which was opened and stuffed with muscle.

Apart from the 1941 case Dott abandoned intracranial operations with muscle wrapping and preferred carotid ligation, this probably being because in the early series his mortality was 67% for intracranial operation whereas it was only 25% for carotid ligation.

This Scottish pioneer lived long enough to see cerebrovascular surgery develop and become a major interest of many talented and skilful neurosurgeons the world over. It always amused him to listen to young enthusiasts describing new approaches and techniques to deal with the too often deadly lesions to which he had devoted so much of his life. Dott never denied fear and his own words appear most valuable for present and future physicians involved in the management of cerebrovascular malformations:

"Surgical capacity is an attitude of mind, manual dexterity is a small but important adjunct. Sometimes courage is required. Courage implies an appreciation of risk – in fact it implies fear under control. He who knows no fear is not courageous but reckless"[72].

Walter Dandy (1886–1946)

The American pioneer Walter Dandy, who often was not content with existing procedures and who wasted no efforts to break new ground to find solutions to life saving procedures in hopeless situations[31], also showed an early interest in the surgical treatment of cerebrovascular malformations. He made his first operation for an intracranial aneurysm in 1928, when, persuaded by Fuller Albright, he performed a carotid ligation in a patient with an ICA-PCoA aneurysm causing a 3rd nerve palsy[2,16]. The patient did not survive but Dandy's interest had been aroused.

In 1935 and 1939 Dandy published articles in Annals of Surgery on "The treatment of carotid cavernous arteriovenous aneurysms[17] and "The treatment of internal carotid aneurysms within the cavernous sinus and the cranial chamber"[19].

The first paper was based on eight cases of carotid cavernous arteriovenous aneurysms and Dandy concluded that three conditions clearly define the syndrome i.e., "exophthalmos, pulsations of the protruding eye, and subjective roar which to the observer is a systolic murmur on ausculation". By establishing a successful procedure for ligating intracranially the internal carotid artery he made yet another contribution to the advancement of surgery of cerebrovascular malformations.

In his 1939 paper Dandy reported on the favorable treatment of three cases of intracranial aneurysms located "in the intracavernous portion of the internal carotid artery or just as the carotid artery enters the cranial chamber". His approach had been a trapping procedure with ligation in the neck and intracranial occlusion by a silver clip.

First Clipping of Intracranial Aneurysm in March 1937 by Dandy

Dandy added immeasurably to cerebrovascular surgery when he occluded the neck of an ICA aneurysm at the take-off of the posterior communicating artery (PCoA) by using a McKenzie silver clip on 22nd March 1937[18]. This clip was a modification of the silver clip described for brain-tumor surgery in 1910 by Cushing "for the occlusion of vessels inaccessible to the ligature"[14]. In 1944 he offered another major impetus to the surgical treatment of intracranial aneurysms when he published his next last major publication, the classical monograph "Intracranial Arterial Aneurysms"[20]. His monograph was based on a study of 108 patients with 138 aneurysms verified by either necropsy or operation or both. Concerned by the toxic effects and the thromboembolic complications associated with the use of contrast media of the era, he never used angiography and, in his series only four aneurysms had been visualized prior to operation by angiography performed by his referring colleagues.

Since 1937 Dandy had continued to perform direct surgical attacks with occlusion of aneurysm necks in a few more cases of aneurysms originating from the ICA. In four instances he had experienced rupture of the aneurysm while trying to perform a neck clipping and had then went on to perform a trapping, usually with clips on the carotid artery on either side of the torn aneurysm base. All four patients with aneurysms originating from the middle cerebral artery (MCA) died following surgery and Dandy concluded[18] that "such aneurysms are always so intimately connected with the main trunk of the artery that it may not be possible to cure them without sacrificing this artery, and such a result would be worse than death, and there is therefore probably less likelihood of curing an MCA aneurysm, at least in leaving a useful citizen". He was also concerned about aneurysms originating from the anterior communicating artery (ACoA), and remarked that "since both of the anterior cerebral arteries lie very close together, the risk of operative treatment is very great". When considering posterior circulation aneurysm he cautiously stated: "I know of no successful outcome from an operative attack upon such an aneurysm, but for those on the vertebral and posterior cerebellar arteries, which afford good exposure, cures will certainly come in time".

Some Early Scandinavian Pioneers

In 1885, Victor Horsley exposed a suspected middle fossa tumor that instead turned out to represent an aneurysm. He then ligated the carotid artery and according to William Keen the patient was in "extremely good health" five years later[39,46,89]. The Norwegian pioneer neurosurgeon Vilhelm Magnus (1871–1929), who had been trained by Horsley, whom he held in high esteem, in May 1927 reported a successful outcome following ligation of the internal carotid artery in a similar patient: a 69-year-old man suffering from intractable trigeminal neuralgia[29]. As Magnus detached the dura in the middle cranial fossa to explore the Gasserian ganglion, he "came on a tumor about the size of a chestnut with a smooth surface and glistening like mother of pearl". During his further attempts at detaching the dura, a hole was torn and the contents of the "tumor" poured out. Then there was "a great gush of blood, that could not be stopped by tamponade". In the subsequent paper on his aneurysm case, Magnus declared that "the patient stood the operation very well" and remarked that "he could not have been given a better birth-day gift, as he had completed his sixty-ninth year on the day of surgery"[55].

Two future neuroscience pioneers were born in 1891 on the island of Gotland in the Baltic and both completed high school education at the only available high school in the town of Visby in 1911[53]. Both did their medical studies at the Upsala University on the mainland in Sweden. Following graduation both moved to Stockholm where Herbert Olivecrona (1891–1980) established the foundation of Swedish neurosurgery and his friend Erik Lysholm (1891–1947) won a world-wide reputation for his many technical innovations in radiology. He was the absolute prerequisite for Olivecrona's successes and made many genial inventions like "the Lysholm grid," a scanning density type of device to improve the quality of x-ray images and "the Lysholm skull table", without which the further development of pneumography and cerebral angiography would not have been possible. Forced by Olivecrona to absolute perfection Lysholm's diagnostic neuroradiology became unmatched.

Lysholm was explicitly manodepressive to his disposition and in his prime, during manic phases, he generously sprinkled ideas, impulses and projects to anyone who listened. With time the phases of depression came more often and of longer duration and finally he isolated himself completely from the surrounding world although by then the value of his contributions was well realized all over the world and had put Olivecrona's department on the world map.

It was not due to epoch-making discoveries that Olivecrona's clinic became the Mecca to which so many scholars went on a pilgrimage. The international reputation of the clinic was founded by resolute and practical applications of methods already launched elsewhere and by the exemplary organization which Olivecrona had founded in collaboration with Lysholm.

Under hardships and primitive working conditions during a long succession of years the clinic at the Serafimer Hospital successively developed to the ideal prototype for a modern neurosurgical department to which so many young men in thirst for more knowledge came flocking, colourful personalities who later were to lay the foundation for neurosurgery in their home countries.

By then Vilhelm Magnus had already established neurosurgery in Norway. On the 26th and 30th of September 1913 he made an exploratory craniectomy over the left motor cortex in a 39-year-old lady with frequent Jacksonian seizures in her right limbs and first stage papilledema[54]. Magnus found a large arterio-venous "angioma" and performed a decompressive craniectomy including removal of a piece of dura measuring 6 × 6 cm for decompressive purposes, but refrained from any attempts to remove the malformation. He had no difficulties in orienting himself on the brain surface and decided that an attempt to remove the malformation, which included large pathological vessels in the Rolandic fissure, would be too hazardous, considering the risk of creating motor deficits. Instead, the patient received radium therapy on four occasions in 1914 (dose not given). The patient had altogether five epileptic seizures in 1914–1916. She was then free from seizures and in 1921, Magnus concluded that "in this case radiotherapy was more lenient than the knife". As in so many other matters, his thoughts in this case demonstrate how far ahead of his time he was.

Unlike Walter Dandy, Olivecrona had the privilege of access to Lysholm, who performed cerebral angiographies of ever increasing quality and was able to visualize cerebral aneurysms and arteriovenous malformations (AVM), which Olivecrona could then deal with surgically. Olivecrona's first excision of a large posterior fossa AVM was in 1932. In the same year he explored a suspected posterior fossa tumor in a 50-year-old man who turned out to harbour a large thrombosed PICA aneurysm which he successfully "trapped" and excised[58]. In 1936 Olivecrona reported four successful cases of AVM resection[4]. In 1948, Olivecrona and Riives reported 42 more case.[61] They described the standard technique of ligating feeding arteries first, then dissecting around the lesion , and finally ligating the veins. As of May 1948 Olivecrona's mortality was only 9.3%.

Then, in 1951, one of Olivecrona's scholars, Lars Leksell, coined the provocative concept of "radiosurgery", a technique by which narrow beams of ionizing radiation are focused to targets within the brain[47]. Leksell, developed the cobalt 60 gamma unit which was specially designed to be included in his stereotactic system[48]. The ^{60}Co gamma unit at the Karolinska Hospital in Stockholm was first used to irradiate cerebral AVMs in 1970[78,79]. In the next two decades the use of Leksell's ingenious innovation, the gammaknife, was increasingly adopted elsewhere and this completely new way of thinking doubtless came to represent a revolution in the treatment of many intracranial disorders, and especially certain types of cerebral AVMs.

Towards a More Aggressive Surgical Approach

In the early 1950s radiologists got access to less toxic contrast media and with improved techniques were able to provide better visualization of major intracranial arteries and aneurysms. This drew the interest of a few neurosurgeons to the possibilities of operative approaches to occlude intracranial aneurysms. In the United Kingdom, Murray Falconer showed an early interest in the surgical treatment of these treacherous lesions[25]. He originally attempted to trap aneurysms by isolation of the parent artery, wrapping the aneurysm with muscle or use the old technique of carotid ligation. He avoided clipping because "the placing of a clip across the neck of an aneurysm is apt to tear it and cause bleeding". Then, with improved vascular clips he soon learnt that intracranial aneurysms could be occluded without surgical catastrophes and subsequently he clipped the neck whenever possible.

In 1953, Falconer published a study of 250 forensic cases of sudden death due to ruptured intracranial aneurysms[22] in an attempt to learn the natural history of the disease and to prove the benefit of active surgical intervention. He found that in 66% of the cases "the fatal attack seemed to have come like a bolt from the blue". Falconer concluded that percutaneous cerebral arteriography should be performed in all patients who have had but a single and mild attack of SAH, since "rebleeds are frequent and carry a very high mortality".

In the United States, Wallace Hamby at the same time was interested in aneurysm surgery and showed that MCA and ACoA aneurysms were not prohibitory[39]. In Sweden, Olof Sjöquist, an early advocator of the use of thread ligature in occlusion of aneurysms, in 1953 published a report "17 cases of basal brain aneurysm treated by thread ligature of the stalk" with 12% operative mortality, 53% morbidity and 35% good recovery (6 patients returning to full working capacity)[74].

Sjöquist emphasized the risk to induce arterial spasm by manipulating the main arteries which had to be weighed against the risks of repeat bleeds "which very often takes place within a few days of the first leak."

In 1953, Olivecrona and his scholar Gösta Norlén, published a paper[59] comprising a series of 63 patients who had been subjected to a direct surgical attack in the "free interval quiescent period". It had been possible to ligate the aneurysm neck in 76% of the patients. In 15 patients operated upon "in the acute stage", that is between a few hours and up to 3 weeks after hemorrhage the mortality rate was 53% and the success rate 40%.

Further Establishment of Surgical Procedures

Spasm of the intracranial arteries appearing several days after aneurysm rupture and SAH was first described in the early 1950s[24]. Later in mid 1950s it was suggested that subarachnoid blood clot may "maintain narrowing of cerebral arteries and cause serious ischemia and this might be an indication for early surgery in an attempt to free the main vessels, quite apart from treatment of the aneurysm itself". The limitations in therapy regarding timing for the operative occlusion of ruptured aneurysms were certainly not conceptual but purely technical at this time when neurosurgeons were faced with all the threats of imminent recurrent hemorrhages as well as delayed onset cerebral vasospasm with SAH-induced ischemic cerebral dysfunction at worst leading to focal brain infarction(s). These complications took a heavy toll from the victims who had survived the first ictus while awaiting surgery.

In the late 1950s and early 1960s Pool[64] and Hunt[42] advocated operation in the acute phase in patients in good clinical grade and in 1965 Norlén declared that he had become convinced that patients in good clinical grade could be operated upon in the first days after rupture to prevent the disastrous effects of rebleeds[60].

In 1957, Olivecrona and Ladenheim published another classic in cerebrovascular surgery. Congenital Arteriovenous Aneurysms of the Carotid and Vertebral Arterial Systems[62]. In his Hunterian lecture for the Royal College of Surgeons of England in the same year John Gillingham reported five patients whom he had operated for aneurysms in the posterior circulation; three had died and one had survived in a vegetative state[35]. By 1960 there were not many published reports on the surgical treatment of basilar or other posterior fossa aneurysms. At this stage the available clips for aneurysm occlusion were usually those designed by Olivecrona, Mayfield and Scoville. Surgery of posterior circulation aneurysms was further taken up by Drake, Yasargil and Sugita, who amongst others published increasingly encouraging results.

Since 1960s the need for improved aneurysm clips was realized and a large variety of clips were designed and made available[69]. The results of aneurysm clipping in the late stage after bleed-usually performed 12–14 days after ictus by an experienced surgeon-showed a remarkable improvement with significantly lowered surgical morbidity and mortality. However, still in the late 1970s early operation was considered most hazardous and not safe for any patient irrespective of clinical grade. With a *general policy of delayed operation* the Danish Aneurysm Study Group reported an *overall morbidity and mortality rate* of 73% in 1076 *patients* who were *alive upon hospital admission*[71]. Thus, despite major advances up until the 1980s the overall outcome was not much improved although expert neurosurgeons were able to approach and successfully clip aneurysms at most locations.

The 1970s – Dawn of a New Era

Computerized Tomography

In 1979 the South African physicist Allan Macleod Cormack and the British engineer Godfrey Newhold Hounsfield were awarded the Nobel Prize for inventing computerized tomography (CT)[32]. Neither of Cormack or Hounsfield had any background in physiology or medicine, neither held a doctorate and their names were new and not well known to radiologists. Nevertheless, their independent works came to revolutionize clinical medicine and represented a great step forward in the diagnosis and understanding of SAH pathophysiology as well.

At the Groote Schur Hospital in Capetown the law required the presence of a physicist to monitor the use of radioactive material and when the hospital lost its resident physicist in 1956, Cormack accepted a temporary appointment. While overseeing the treatment of patients with radiotherapy he became aware of the difficulties posed by weakening of the x-ray beam when it enters the patient's body and the need to measure that differential quantitatively. He began to consider the possibilities of taking a series of radiographs from several different angles and then comparing them. He continued to work on his composite imaging idea and

developed a more workable mathematical formula on a sabbatical leave. In 1963 he applied his formula to a new set of pictures taken of a nonsymmetrical construction of plastic and aluminium, using a computer to complete the calculations[12]. Although his results were successful he was unable to find radiologists who would share his vision and like Johann Radon's 1917 paper[67] his published results sank without a trace.

Four years after Cormack's publications, Hounsfield independently began his exploration of the problem as a result of his work in pattern recognition studies. Hounsfield had joined EMI company of His Master's Voice in 1951 and his great contribution was to measure the attenuation of a highly collimated beam of x-rays passing through a thin horizontal slice of a patient's head from successive directions and then to recreate a display from the resulting data by means of a computer. Although he was not a mathematician, he deviced a practical method of doing it that proved to be consistent with the rigorous mathematical theory buried in the paper of Johann Radon. Hounsfield's mathematical model was less elegant than Cormack's but equally accurate with sufficient computer time. His experiments with test objects quickly attracted interest from British radiologists and the first clinical CT scanner was installed in a Wimbledon hospital in 1971. This machine, designed for brain scans only, rotated an x-ray tube and detector around the head one degree at a time, projecting and recording 180 images. Hounsfield published the results obtained from this prototype in 1973[41]. Much of the credit to EMI's successes belonged to its chairman, Jo¹ Powell, who was a steadfast champion of Hounsfiel⸛ s invention. That he succeeded in persuading the EMI board to support the project was in part due to the company's excellent financial condition after a decade during which it dominated the popular-music market with the Beatles and other recording artists. By 1979 there were more than 12 CT scan manufacturers and more than 2.000 CT scanners in operation. Hounsfield was the actual inventor of the clinical instrument, but Cormack's model, published ten years earlier, would have been equally successful had anyone acted on his proposals.

Fisher and coworkers took an early advantage of CT and in 1980 were able to demonstrate that there is a direct relationship between the amount and distribution of CT-visualised subarachnoid blood and later development of cerebral vasospasm and/or delayed ischemic dysfunction (DID)[26]. These authors found that when subarachnoid blood was not detected or was diffusely distributed on CT, severe vasospasm was almost never encountered. In the presence of subarachnoid blood clots or layers of blood in fissures and vertical cisterns, severe spasm followed almost invariably and there was a close correlation between the site of the major subarachnoid clots and the location of severe vasospasm. It gradually became recognized that vasospasm or DID is a complex phenomenon involving release of many vasoconstrictive substances that appear in CSF after SAH such as serotonin, prostaglandins, oxyhemoglobin, etc. Early operation within a few days of hemorrhage appeared increasingly desirable.

The Microscope

The birth place of cerebrovascular microsurgery was the University of Vermont School of Medicine where Gazi Yasargil performed a series of experimental small vessel anastomoses under the microscope followed by its routine use in neurosurgery in Zürich[36]. Subsequently the use of balanced operation microscopes was quickly adopted by aneurysm surgeons who gained improved knowledge of microsurgical anatomy and became equipped with an armament of new microsurgical instruments. This made it feasible, in the mid 1970s, to adopt the desirable early surgical intervention to occlude ruptured aneurysms before fatal rebleeds and to evacuate as much CT-visualized clot and blood-contaminated CSF as possible to reduce delayed cerebral ischemic complications[49].

Early Diagnosis and Timing of Surgical Intervention

With the introduction of CT and microneurosurgical techniques a new era took place and renewed attempts to operate victims of aneurysmal SAH in the acute stage were made. In the early 1980s operation in the acute stage was, however, still met with considerable scepticism. In the next decade the attitude towards early surgical intervention was increasingly adopted by experienced aneurysm surgeons who also advocated early operative timing for posterior circulation aneurysms in good grade patients. Also, ultraearly surgery in devastated patients suspected of harboring a ruptured aneurysm with space-occupying intracerebral hemorrhage was proposed[7]. Increasingly, in the 1980s, studies focused on analysis of unfavorable outcome despite early operation[50,73] and effects of early operation upon overall outcome were published[51,74,87]. It is now

apparent that with microneurosurgical techniques the experienced aneurysm surgeon can obtain similar morbidity and mortality rates as with delayed operation just a decade ago.

In patients with SAH who had Lp before CT and within 12 hours after the bleed, severe clinical deterioration occurred in 13%[21]. In a series of 100 consecutive patients who were suspected of aneurysmal rupture, fifteen had a non-aneurysmal hematoma and eight of these were located in the cerebellum[85]. A third of patients with a ruptured aneurysm harbour an associated intracerebral hematoma, and even in individuals without neurological signs other than neck stiffness 10% may have a hematoma of at least 30 mm[40]. Neck stiffness takes three to 12 hours to develop and is an unreliable test to diagnose SAH. For a long time Quincke's brilliant invention was the mainstay for diagnosis but should now be replaced by CT, which gives important diagnostic information on the source of hemorrhage and reveals complications that may require emergency treatment such as hydrocephalus or lifethreatening hematomas. Early CT also serves as a baseline against which future changes can be measured. On the day of SAH, intracranial blood is detected by CT in about 95% of patients. This proportion declines to 90% after one day, 80% after five days, and 50% after one week[1].

It may be concluded that referral systems for patients who have suffered a subarachnoid hemorrhage should be organized so that such patients are admitted without delay. Ideally, patients with suspected SAH should be considered as emergency cases and immediately admitted to centers with clockround CT scanning facilities and access to cerebrovascular neurosurgical expertise.

Epidemiology

Over 50% of non-traumatic SAH is caused by ruptured intracranial aneurysms[70]. The ratio of ruptured to non-ruptured (incidental) aneurysms found at necropsy is approximately 1:1[30]. Early reports estimating the incidence of intracranial aneurysms were derived from general autopsy series and in 25 reports between 1890 through 1973 the reported incidence varied from 0.2 to 7.9%[30]. In epidemiological studies from the United States the incidence of aneurysmal SAH has been reported at approximately 10/100,000/year[33,63]. The natural history of intracranial AVMs is difficult to assess[90,91]. The incidence of aneurysmal SAH is higher in females (12.2/100,000/year) than in males (7.6/100,000/year)[27].

These aforementioned figures correlate with reports from Great Britain with 6–11/100,000/year[13], the Netherlands with 8–10/100,000/year[34,86], and Estonia with 8.7/100,000/year[84]. A high incidence has been reported from Finland with 16–24/100,000/year and Lapland with 30/100,000/year[27]. A low incidence of aneurysmal SAH has been reported from the Middle East countries, India and China[11,68]. This may be related to a combination of inadequate health care, environmental factors and a true low incidence[3]. In conclusion, the incidence appears to show some variations from one geographical area to another and it is likely that in certain subpopulations there may be common factors of race, inheritance and/or environmental factors that increase the predisposition to intracranial aneurysm formation[27].

Concluding Remarks

When looking back on the history of SAH it is obvious that major achievements that paved the way to an improved management were made in the previous century and first half of this century by many outstanding individual pioneers. Still in the midst of this century the surgical outcome, however, was extremely gloomy and the pathophysiology of SAH was poorly understood. Before the introduction of microneurosurgery, operation could not be attempted in the acute stage without disastrous results and it is today known that with a policy of delayed surgery, the overall outcome is not markedly improved as compared to the natural history of this dreadful disease. Great expectations followed the introduction of antifibrinolytic drugs (AFD) 25 years ago and it was hoped for that such drugs should prevent rebleeds in the waiting period for planned delayed aneurysm repair[28]. Treatment with AFD however turned out to be of no benefit because ischemic complications were enhanced, thereby neutralizing any positive effects in delaying or preventing rebleeds.

The *limitations* in an optimal *early timing for surgical intervention to prevent fatal aneurysm rebleeds* were *not conceptual* – the first advocators for early surgery expressed their opinion in the 1960s – *but purely technical*. The introduction of the operation microscope and computerized tomography in the 1970s represented a major break-through in improved management. With subsequent microneurosurgical advancements it

has been shown that aneurysms at all locations, also at such considered as "no man's land" a century ago, can be surgically approached. Furthermore, such surgery can now (1992) be undertaken in the acute stage by specially trained and well experienced aneurysm surgeons working in centers with adequate technical equipment and resources. Early operation may also be performed in obtunded patients so that disastrous rebleeds may be prevented. The intense search for specific antispasmodic agents in the 1960s and 1970s were not advantageous. With the introduction of calcium channel blockers in combination with early operation and intraoperative washout of clots and blood-contaminated CSF from the basal cisterns, SAH-induced cerebral ischemic dysfunction of delayed on-set has been significantly reduced although the exact pathophysiology of this phenomenon remains to be clarified.

Despite recent, major improvements in the surgical management of ruptured aneurysms less than 50% of all victims who are alive upon admission to well-equipped neurosurgical centers with a policy of early operation may be expected to make a good neurological recovery[51]. In addition a significant number of individuals who recover without neurological deficits do show persistent problems relating to emotional adjustment, energy resources and social competency that will interfere with their reintegration[77].

Hope for further improvements may depend upon further development of endovascular techniques[37] to achieve occlusion of ruptured intracranial aneurysms and endoscopic techniques to approach the cisternal systems and evacuate extravasated blood and blood-contaminated CSF combined with cisternal irrigation with thrombolytic agents such as t-PA.

The old marriage between the cerebrovascular surgeon and the radiologist was not so intimate in the first half period (1932–1962) but then accelerated and became more and more intense towards the end of the second half period (1962–1992) of the matrimony. This meeting in Romantic Verona on New Trends in this Old Marriage will certainly shed light on the future prospects for the alliance. Maybe the bold aneurysm and AVM clipping man may be at risk to become reduced to an endoscopic cisternal lavageur living in polygamy with a decisive innovative endovascular occlusionist and an equally demanding ^{60}Co gamma beam radiotherapist who fight for the honour to perform the risky stroke to occlude the ruptured aneurysm or symptomatic AVM.

When summarizing the history it appears that the individuals who are to be credited the title of Great Pioneers are Thomas Willis, John Blackall, William Gull, Edvard Bull, Norman Dott, Walter Dandy, John Gillingham, Herbert Olivecrona, Murray Falconer, Gösta Norlén, Charles Drake, Gazi Yaşargil, and Kenichiro Sugita. The events in the last 328 years since Willis described his circle of arteries may be summarized in the words (1775) of pioneer neurosurgeon Percivall Pott (1714–1788)[65]:

> "Many and great are the improvements which the chirurgic art has received within these last fifty years; and much thanks are due to those who have contributed to them; but when we reflect how much still remains to be done, it should rather excite our industry than inflame our vanity".

Acknowledgments

This work, supported by the Thorsten Westerström Foundation in Sweden, is dedicated to HH Shaikh Nahyan Bin Mubarak Al-Nahyan, Minister of Higher Education and Supreme Chancellor of the United Arab Emirates University for kind and much appreciated support to neurosurgical activities at the Faculty of Medicine and Tawam Hospital in Al Ain, United Arab Emirates.

References

1. Adams HP, Kassell NF, Torner JC, Sahs AL (1983) CT and clinical correlations in recent aneurysmal subarachnoid hemorrhage: a preliminary report of the Cooperative Aneurysm Study. Neurology 33: 981–988
2. Albright F (1929) The syndrome produced by aneurysm at or near the function of the internal carotid artery and the circle of Willis. Johns Hopkins Hosp Bull 44: 215–245
3. Al-Mefty O, Al-Rodhan N, Fox JL (1988) The low incidence of cerebral aneurysms in the Middle East: a myth? Neurosurgery 22: 951–954
4. Bergstrand H, Olivecrona H, Tönnis W (1936) Gefässmissbildungen und Gefässgeschwülste des Gehirns. Thieme, Leipzig, p 181
5. Blackall J (1813) Observations on the nature and cure of dropsies, 5th Ed. Longman, London, pp 132–135
6. Bramwell B (1886) Clinical and pathological memoranda. IV. Case of aneurism of the right internal carotid cartery. Edin Med J 32: 97–101
7. Brandt L, Sonesson B, Ljunggren B, Säveland H (1987) Ruptured middle cerebral artery aneurysm with intracerebral hemorrhage in younger patients appearing moribund: emergency operation? Neurosurgery 20: 925–929
8. Bright R (1831) Reports of medical cases, Vol 2, Part 1. Longman, London, pp 226–267 and 613–614
9. Brinton W (1852) Report on cases of cerebral aneurism. Trans Path Soc London 3: 46–49
10. Bull E (1877) Acute brain aneurisma-oculomotor palsy-meningeal apoplexia. Norwegian Magazine of Medicine 7: 890–895
11. Cho S, Ngan H, Ong GB (1979) Intracranial aneurysms causing subarachnoid hemorrhage in the Chinese. Surg Neurol 12: 319–321
12. Cormack AM (1963) Representation of a function by its line integrals, with some radiological applications. J Appl Phys 34: 2722–2727; 35: 2908–2913
13. Crawford MD, Sarner M (1965) Ruptured intracranial aneurysm. Community study. Lancet ii: 1254–1257
14. Cushing H (1911) The control of bleeding in operations for brain tumors. With the description of silver clips for the occlusion of vessels inaccessible to the ligature. Ann Surg 54: 1–19
15. Cushing H (1923) Contributions to the study of intracranial aneurysms. Guys Hosp Rec 73: 159–163
16. Dandy WE (1928) Arteriovenous aneurysms of the brain. Arch Surg 17: 190–243
17. Dandy WE (1935) The treatment of carotid-cavernous arterio-venous aneurysms. Ann Surg 102: 916–920
18. Dandy WE (1938) Intracranial aneurysm of internal carotid artery, cured by operation. Ann Surg 107: 654–657
19. Dandy WE (1939) The treatment of internal carotid aneurysms within the cavernous sinus and the cranial chamber. Report of three cases. Ann Surg 109: 689–709
20. Dandy WE (1944) Intracranial arterial aneurysms. Comstock, New York Cornell University, pp 1–147
21. Duffy GP (1982) Lumbar puncture in spontaneous subarachnoid haemorrhage. BMJ 285: 1163–1164
22. Dinning TAR, Falconer MA (1953) Sudden or unexpected natural death due to ruptured intracranial aneurysm; survey of 250 forensic cases. Lancet ii: 799–801
23. Dott NM (1932–1933) Intracranial aneurysms. Cerebral arterioradiography: surgical treatment. Trans Med Chir Soc Edinb 1933: 219–234
24. Ecker A, Riemenschneider PA (1951) Artheriographic demonstration of spasm of the intracranial arteries with special reference to saccular arterial aneurisms. J Neurosurg 8: 660–667
25. Falconer MA (1950) Surgical treatment of spontaneous subarachnoid haemorrhage. Preliminary report. BMJ 1: 809–813
26. Fisher CM, Kistler JP, Davis JM (1980) Relation of cerebral vasospasm to subarachnoid hemorrhage visualized by computerized tomographic scanning. Neurosurgery 6: 1–9
27. Fodstad H, Forssell Å, Ängquist KA, Norrgård O, Lindberg M (1990) Epidemiology of aneurysmal subarachnoid hemorrhage in Northern Sweden. In: Sugita K, Shibuya M (eds) Intracranial aneurysms and arteriovenous malformations. Nagoya University Press, Nagoya, pp 3–9
28. Fodstad H, Ljunggren B (1990) Antifibrinolytic drugs in subarachnoid hemorrhage. In: Sawaya R (ed) Fibrinolysis and the central nervous system. Hanley and Belfus, Philadelphia, pp 257–273
29. Fodstad H, Ljunggren B, Kristiansen K (1990) Vilhelm Magnus – pioneer neurosurgeon. J Neurosurg 73: 317–330
30. Fox JL (1983) Intracranial aneurysms, vol 1. Springer, Berlin Heidelberg New York Tokyo, pp 15–18
31. Fox WL (1984) Dandy of Johns Hopkins. Williams and Wilkins, Baltimore
32. Fox, Meldrum, Rezak (1990) Noble laureates in medicine and physiology. Garland, New York, pp 104–107; Hounsfield, pp 269–272
33. Garroway WM, Whisnant JP, Furlan AJ, et al (1979) The declining incidence of stroke. N Engl J Med 300: 449–452
34. Giel B (1965) Notes on the epidemiology of the spontaneous subarachnoid hemorrhages. J Psychiatry Neurol Neurochir 68: 265–271
35. Gillingham FJ (1958) The management of ruptured intracranial aneurysm. Hunterian lecture for the Royal College of Surgeons of England 1957. Ann Roy Coll Surg Engl 23: 89–117
36. Goldring S (1985) The need to trace our roots in difficult times. The 1985 AANS Presidential Address. J Neurosurg 63: 485–491

37. Guglielmi G, Vinuela F, Dion J, Duckwiler G (1991) Electro-thrombosis of saccular aneurysms via endovascular approach. J Neurosurg 75: 8–14

38. Gull W (1859) Cases of aneurism of the cerebral vessels. Guys Hosp Rep 5: 281–304

39. Hamby WB (1952) Intracranial aneurysms. Thomas, Springfield

40. Hillman J (1986) Should computed tomography scanning replace lumbar puncture in the diagnostic process in suspected sub-arachnoid hemorrhage? Surg Neurol 26: 547–550

41. Hounsfield GN (1973) Computerised transverse axial scanning (tomography). Br J Radiol 46: 1016–1022 and 1023–1047

42. Hunt WE, Meagher JN, Barnes JE (1962) The management of intracranial aneurysm. J Neurosurg 19: 34–40

43. Hunt WE, Hess RM (1968) Surgical risk as related to time of intervention in the repair of intracranial aneurysms. J Neurosurg 28: 14–19

44. Jennings EA (1833) Case of aneurism of the basilar artery, sud-denly giving way, and occasioning death by pressure on the medulla oblongata. Transactions of the Provincial Medical and Surgical Association 1: 270–276

45. Johnson RJ, Potter JM, Reid RG (1958) Arterial spasm in subarachnoid haemorrhage: mechanical considerations. J Neurol Neurosurg Psychiatry 21: 68

46. Keen WW (1890) Intracranial lesions. Med News NY 57: 443

47. Leksell L (1951) The stereotaxic method and radiosurgery of the brain. Acta Chir Scand 102: 316–319

48. Leksell L (1971) A note on the treatment of acoustic tumours. Acta Chir Scand 137: 763–765

49. Ljunggren B, Brandt L, Kågström E, Sundbärg G (1981) Results of early operation for ruptured aneurysms. J Neurosurg 54: 473–479

50. Ljunggren B, Saveland H, Brandt L (1983) Causes of unfavor-able outcome after early aneurysm surgery. Neurosurgery 13: 629–633

51. Ljunggren B, Säveland H, Brandt L, Zygmunt S (1985) Early operation and overall outcome in aneurysmal subarachnoid hemorrhage. J Neurosurg 62: 547–55

52. Ljunggren B, Fodstad H, Kristiansen K, Søgaard S, Törmä T (1987) When Nordic neurosurgery was still in its infancy. Br J Neurosurg 1: 207–233

53. Ljunggren B (1993) Herbert Olivecrona–founder of Swedish neurosurgery. J Neurosurg, 78: 142–149

54. Magnus V (1921) Bidrag til hjernechirurgiens klinik og resultater. Supplement to Norsk Magazin for Laegevidenskaben, September 1921 (in Norwegian). Merkur bok Kristiania, pp 9, 101–102. See also (1990) Correspondence in Neurosurgery 27: 1027

55. Magnus V (1927) Aneurysm of the internal carotid artery. JAMA 88: 1712–1713

56. Moniz E (1933) Anevrysme intra-cranien de la carotide inferne droite rendu visible par l'arteriographie cerebrale. Rev Oto-Neuro-Ophtal 11: 746–748

57. Newes from the Dead or A True and Exact Narration of the miraculous deliverance of Anne Green (1651) Written by a Scholler in Oxford. Oxford: Printed by Leonard Lichfield for Tho Robinson. See also: Hughes JT (1982) Miraculous deliver-ance of Anne Green: an Oxford case of resuscitation in the seven-teenth century. BMJ 285: 1792–1793

58. Norlén G (1952) The pathology, diagnosis and treatment of intra-cranial saccular aneurysms. Proc Soc Roy Soc Med (London) 45: 291–302

59. Norlén G, Olivecrona H (1953) The treatment of aneurysms of the circle of Willis. J Neurosurg 10: 634–650

60. Norlén G (1965) Some aspects of the surgical treatment of intra-cranial aneurysms. Neurol Med Chir (Tokyo) 7: 14–27

61. Olivecrona H, Riives J (1948) Arteriovenous aneurysms of the brain: their diagnosis and treatment. Arch Neurol Psychiatry 59: 567–602

62. Olivecrona H, Ladenheim J (1957) Congenital arteriovenous aneurysms of the carotid and vertebral arterial systems. Springer, Berlin Göttingen Heidelberg

63. Phillips LH, Whisnant JP, O'Fallon WM, *et al* (1980) The un-changing pattern of subarachnoid haemorrhage in a community. Neurology 30: 1034–1040

64. Pool JL (1959) Early treatment of ruptured intracranial aneu-rysms of the circle of Willis with special clip techniques. Bull NY Acad Med 35: 357–369

65. Pott P (1775) Chirurgical observations relative to the cataract, polypus of the nose, the cancer of the scrotum, the different kinds of ruptures, and the mortification of the toes and feet. London, pp x–xi

66. Quincke H (1914) Über die therapeutischen Leistungen der Lumbalpunktion. Therapeutische Monatshefte 28: 469–480

67. Radon, J (1917) Über die Bestimmung von Funktionen durch ihre Integralwerte langs gewisser Mannigfaltigkeiten. Berichte der Sächsischen Akademie der Wissenschaften 67: 262–277

68. Ramamurthi B (1969) Incidence of intracranial aneurysms in India. J Neurosurg 30: 154–157

69. Romner B, Olsson M, Ljunggren B, Holtås S, Säveland H, Brandt L, Persson B (1989) Magnetic resonance imaging and aneurysm clips. J Neurosurg 70: 426–431

70. Romy M, Werner A, Wildi E (1973) De la fréquence des anévrysmes artériels intra-craniens et de leur rupture, d'apres une série d'autopsies de routine. Neurochirurgie 19: 611–626

71. Rosenörn J, Eskesen V, Schmidt K, *et al* (1987) Clinical features and outcome in 1076 patients with ruptured intracranial sac-cular aneurysms: a prospective consecutive study. Br J Neurosurg 1: 33–46

72. Rush Ch, Shaw JF (1990). With sharp compassion. Norman Dott, freeman surgeon of Edinburgh. University Press, Aberdeen, pp 198–203

73. Säveland H, Ljunggren B, Brandt L, Messeter K (1986) Delayed ischemic deterioration in patients with early aneurysm operation and intravenous nimodipine. Neurosurgery 18: 146–150

74. Säveland H, Hillman J, Brandt L, Edner G, Jakobsson KE, Algers G (1992) Overall outcome in aneurysmal subarachnoid hemorrhage: a prospective study from neurosurgical units in Sweden during a 1-year period. J Neurosurg 76: 729–734

75. Serres ERA (1819) Annuaire Méd-Chir d Hopital de Paris 1: 314–316

76. Sjöquist O (1953) Intracranial ligature of saccular aneurysms. Technical considerations. In: Proceedings of the 5th Inter-national Congress of Neurology Lisboa, pp 108–115

77. Sonesson B (1992) Neurobehavioural functioning and adjust-ment after subarachnoid haemorrhage. A long-term assessment of cognitive and psychological sequelae. Academical thesis, Uni-versity of Lund, Sweden

78. Steiner L, Leksell L, Greitz T, Forster DMC, Backlund E-O (1972) Stereotaxic radiosurgery for cerebral arteriovenous mal-formations. Report of a case. Acta Chir Scand 138: 459–464

79. Steiner L, Leksell L, Forster DMC, Greitz T, Backlund E-O (1974) Stereotactic radiosurgery in intracranial arteriovenous malformations. Acta Neurochir (Wien) [Suppl] 21: 195–209

80. Strauss MB (1968) Familiar Medical Quotations. Little Brown, Boston, p 213

81. Symonds CP (1923) Contributions to the clinical study of intra-cranial aneurysms. Guys Hosp Rec 72: 139–158

82. Symonds CP (1924–25) Spontaneous subarachnoid haemorr-hage. QJ Med 18: 93

83. Todd NV, Howie JE, Miller JD (1990) Norman Dott's contribution to aneurysm surgery. J Neurol Neurosurg Psychiatry 53: 455–458
84. Tomberg T (1977) Spontannoe subarachnoidalnoe krovoizilijanie (Russian). Tartu
85. Van Gijn J, Van Dongen KJ (1980) Computed tomography in the diagnosis of subarachnoid haemorrhage and ruptured aneurysms. Clin Neurol Neurosurg 82: 11–24
86. Van der Werff AJM (1972) Clinical aspects of subarachnoid hemorrhage and the significance of vasospasm. J Psychiatry Neurol Neurochir 75: 411–415
87. Vapalahti M, Ljunggren B, Säveland H, Herniesniemi J, Brandt L, Tapaninaho A (1984) Early aneurysm operation and outcome in two remote Scandinavian populations. J Neurosurg 60: 1160–1162
88. Vermeulen M, van Gijn J (1990) The diagnosis of subarachnoid haemorrhage. J Neurol Neurosurg Psychiatry 53: 365–372
89. Wilkins RH (1982) Partial carotid artery ligation in the treatment of intracranial aneurysms. In: Hopkins LN, Long DM (eds) Clinical management of intracranial aneurysms. Raven, New York, pp 39–47
90. Wilkins RH (1985) Natural history of intracranial vascular malformations: a review. Neurosurgery 16:421–430
91. Wilkins RH (1990) Natural history of arteriovenous malformations of the brain. In: Barrow DL (ed) Intracranial vascular malformations. AANS, Park Ridge, pp 31–44
92. Willis T (1664) Cerebri Anatome: cui accessit Nervorum Descriptio et Usus.

Correspondence: Bengt Ljunggren M.D., Division of Neurosurgery Department of Surgery, Faculty of Medicine and Health Sciences, P.O. Box 17666, Al Ain, United Arab Emirates.

Clinical Usefulness of Magnetic Resonance Angiography in Neurosurgical Practice

R. McKenzie, I. Awad[2], M. Magdinec, and T. Masaryk[1]

[1]Departments of Neurological Surgery and Neuroradiology, Cleveland Clinic Foundation, Cleveland, Ohio, U.S.A., and [2]Yale Cerebrovascular Center, Yale University School of Medicine, New Haven, Connecticut, U.S.A.

Summary

The potential role of magnetic resonance angiography (MRA) in clinical neurosurgical practice was retrospectively evaluated in 150 patients in an attempt to define clinical situations in which it aided in diagnosis, helped guide treatment options and/or possibly eliminated the need for conventional angiography. Two patient populations were studied, those with nonvascular pathology ($n = 42$) and those with vascular neurologic disease ($n = 108$). In the nonvascular category, MRA provided useful clinical information in 55% of patients effectively replacing catheter angiography in 76% of cases. MRA provided excellent depiction of tumor and vessel relationships and with MRI reliably ruled out the question of tumor versus aneurysm whenever that question was raised. The vascular neurologic disease group was subdivided into aneurysms, vascular malformations and occlusive vascular disease. In these groups the MRA visualized 90% (18 of 20) of aneurysms, 100% (11 of 11) of vascular malformations, 100% (31 of 31) of cases of known occlusive vascular disease, and reliably excluded occlusive vascular disease in 63% (19 of 30) of cases. MRA had relatively short imaging time, 10 to 20 minutes for intracranial vessels and 6 to 13 minutes for extracranial vessels. However, the technical constraints of MRA limited its usefulness in the surgical management of vascular neurologic diseases. This was in part due to insufficient spatial resolution or dynamic blood flow information necessary for surgical decisions. In the setting of vascular malformations, MRA added little useful information beyond conventional MRI, and did not reliably distinguish different lesion types. Flow information, steal and shunts within vascular malformations were not reliably assessed, and hematoma or thrombosis within the lesions introduced significant artifactual information on MRA. Nevertheless, technical advances may gradually eliminate these shortcomings in the future.

Keywords: MRA; angiography; vascular lesions.

Introduction

The effects of blood flow in magnetic resonance imaging (MRI) are related to two aspects of the imaging process: the radiofrequency pulse sequence used to create the signal and the magnetic imaging gradients used to anatomically localize the signal. The effects of blood flow (i.e. flight of protons) relative to the timing of the radiofrequency pulses are collectively called the time-of-flight (TOF) effects[2,3,10,23]. The TOF effects are capable of increasing or decreasing signal from flowing blood in vascular structures. Increased vascular signal is referred to as "flow related enhancement" (seen commonly in gradient echo imaging of the spine), while decreased signal is referred to as "signal void" (seen with spin echo imaging of the brain). Blood flow relative to the application of signal localizing magnetic field gradients produces so-called "spin-phase phenomena"[1-3,10,23].

Pulse sequences and the imaging gradients may be manipulated independently to enhance vascular signal without the administration of exogenous contrast agents. This has resulted in the technique of visualizing extracranial and intracranial vasculature known as magnetic resonance angiography (MRA). MRA methods have utilized both TOF techniques and phase contrast (PC) techniques. The TOF techniques are characterized by rapid image acquisition and are less susceptible to artifacts produced by fast flow[2,3,6,8,13,15,16,19-24]. However, they rely heavily on computer postprocessing which may introduce other artifacts and may limit vascular contrast[1,3,22,26]. The PC techniques provide high vascular contrast and are sensitive to even very slow flow[3,5,8,10,18]. They are quite effective in imaging vessels with slow flow such as venous structures. Additionally, PC techniques can simultaneously provide flow velocity and vascular flow rate information. However, PC MRA is quite time consuming and may be more prone to artifacts in the presence of fast (arterial) flow lesions.

A variety of MRA signal acquisition and postprocessing techniques are now available in clinical practice. These have undergone preliminary evaluation as to sensitivity, specificity and precision of imaging a variety of vascular lesions[1-3,5-28]. However, the clinical usefulness of MRA in neurosurgical practice and decision-making has not been evaluated critically. In this report, we analyze the potential role of MRA in clinical decision-making during the evaluation of patients for possible neurosurgical intervention.

Patients and Methods and MRA Techniques

One hundred and fifty consecutive cases evaluated for possible neurosurgical intervention underwent MRA *in addition to* other diagnostic studies as per routine clinical indications. These included 42 cases with nonvascular neurologic pathology where vascular information was necessary (i.e. possible major arterial compromise or dural sinus occlusion by a tumor, carotid siphon imaging before transsphenoidal surgery, etc....), and 108 cases with potentially surgical cerebrovascular lesions.

In an effort to implement such studies without significantly prolonging examination time, two dimensional (2D) and three dimensional (3D) TOF studies were used[3,15-17,19-21,23]. The 3D TOF MRA was used for suspected arterial (fast flow) lesions while 2D TOF techniques were employed for suspected lesions involving the dural sinus. All MR studies were performed on 1.5 T magnet with 10 mT/m gradient capability (Siemens, Magnetom SP 63). All studies used a transmit/receive head coil. Conventional spin echo studies typically included coronal T_1 (500/17/2), and axial T_2 (2000/17-90/1) acquisitions. The 3D TOF MRA used a fast imaging with steady precession (FISP) pulse sequence (40/7/1) with a 15° flip angle and first order flow compensation gradients in the read and slice select direction. The technique of 2D TOF MRA used sequential fast low angle shot (FLASH) pulse sequence (30/9/1) with a 30° flip angle and first order flow compensation in two directions. Appropriately placed spatial presaturation pulses were implemented to selectively enhance venous or arterial flow. Both 2D and 3D acquisitions were subsequently postprocessed online using a maximum intensity pro-

jection (MIP) algorithm, to render an angiographic display at any desired obliquity or angle. When necessary the native MRA images could also be reviewed to evaluate specific lesions. Imaging time with the above TOF techniques was relatively short, 10-20 minutes for intracranial vessels and 6.5-13 minutes for extracranial vessels. In the case of vascular structures with low flow where there may have been a question about the technical performance of the above TOF MRA methodology, the technique of PC MRA was used more recently to supplement the TOF studies[18]. This study typically required significantly longer imaging time (45-60 minutes). We sought to answer three questions using a "question driven technology assessment" as suggested by Caplan[4]: 1) did MRA visualize the lesion? 2) did MRA add clinically useful information? 3) did or could MRA replace conventional catheter angiography? In order to answer these three questions we subdivided our patient population into two separate diagnostic categories, the nonvascular neurologic disease group and the vascular neurologic disease group.

Results

The nonvascular neurologic disease group included 42 patients. Of these the MRA added clinically useful information in 55% of patients and provided enough vascular information so as to replace conventional angiography in 76% of cases. Sinus patency or occlusion was easily demonstrated by MRA (Fig. 1a, b). We found that the MRA provided excellent vessel tumor relationships, including deviations and/or compromise of major arteries and veins while also reliably ruling out (in conjunction with MRI) the question of tumor versus aneurysm whenever that question was raised.

The various vascular neurologic disease groups were divided into aneurysms, vascular malformations, and occlusive cerebrovascular disease. The cerebral aneurysm

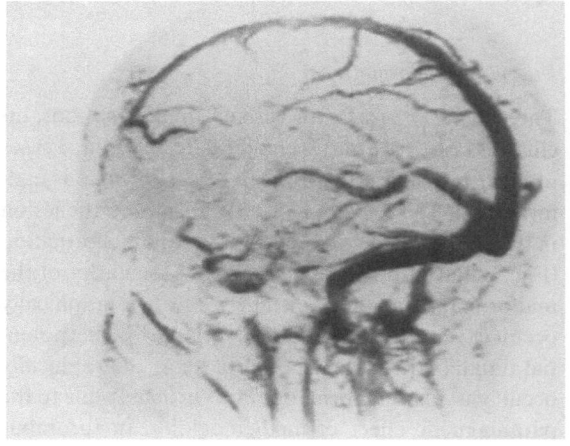
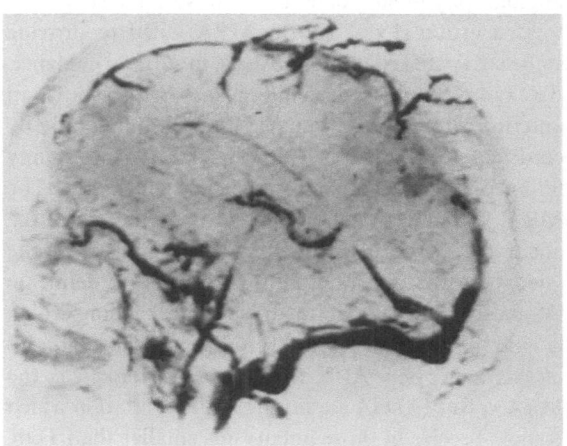

a　　　　　　　　　　　　　　　　　　　　　b

Fig. 1. (a) MRA venous phase imaging in a patient with pseudotumor cerebri excluding major dural venous sinus occlusion. (b) MRA venogram of another case with posterior parasagittal meningioma, demonstrating occlusion of a segment of the superior sagittal sinus and prominent cerebral venous collaterals

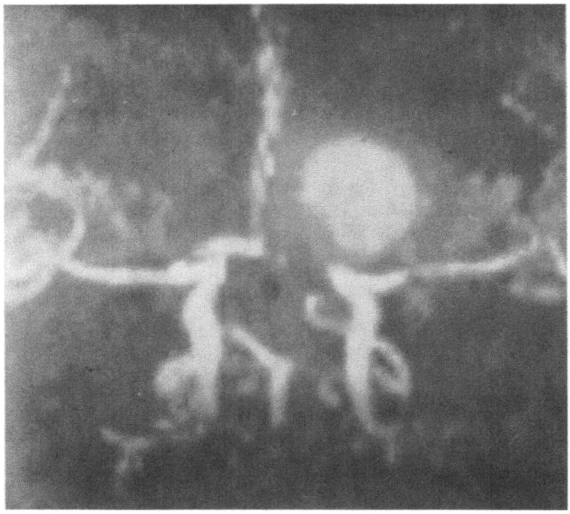
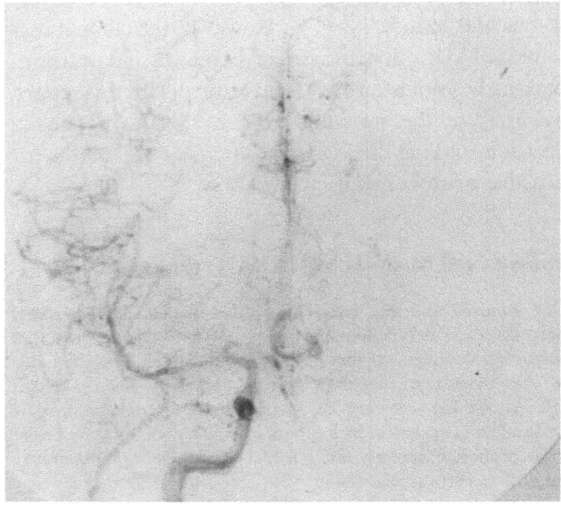

a   b

Fig. 2. (a) MRA revealing giant cerebral aneurysm with partial thrombosis, probably arising from a nonvisualized segment of the left anterior cerebral artery. Left internal carotid artery injection showed total occlusion of the left anterior cerebral artery, and no aneurysmal filling whatsoever (not shown). (b) Anteroposterior view of the right (contralateral) internal carotid artery arteriographic injection showing filling of both distal anterior cerebral arteries, the left recurrent artery of Heubner, and a subtle minimal filling of a portion of the aneurysm neck. In this study, the MRA and conventional angiography provided complementary information not available from each study alone. Each information was invaluable in the final surgical strategy of patient management

group comprised 20 patients of which MRA visualized 90% of the aneurysms present. Aneurysms as small as 3 to 4 mm· were visualized and the parent artery of origin was visualized in a majority of cases as has been reported elsewhere[18,20]. In the nonsurgical candidates, the MRA could have replaced conventional catheter angiography in 86% of cases. However, in a surgically treated group (13 of 20) the MRA failed to provide sufficient spatial resolution to assist in surgical guidance. An example of this is seen in Fig. 2a, b, which shows an anterior cerebral artery aneurysm neck filling only by contralateral carotid IADSA injection without any filling of the aneurysm by ipsilateral injection. The MRA, while accurately depicting the true size of the aneurysm, failed to show that the majority of the aneurysm was thrombosed. It also failed to delineate the pattern of residual aneurysmal neck filling which is vital information essential to the surgical treatment of this aneurysm. Also, not to be overlooked is the MRA versus IADSA aneurysmal size correlation which is most precise in those aneurysms smaller than 1 cm. When aneurysms larger than 1 cm in size are present, their size is often misrepresented by the MRA (interpreted as smaller than true size) which is probably secondary to their blood flow effects (slow flow) or

paramagnetic effects of thrombosis within the aneurysm. In addition, although there are numerous aneurysm clips that are MR compatible, these still show significant postoperative artifact when visualized in the MRI. These artifacts significantly diminish the quality of the MRA thus rendering the MRA useless as a postoperative study to insure proper aneurysmal clipping.

Vascular Malformations

There were 11 cases with vascular malformations, including 7 cases of arteriovenous malformations, 3 cases of cavernous malformations, and 1 case of venous malformation. The MRA adequately visualized the lesion in the 8 cases of angiographically evident malformation (Fig. 3), but also showed abnormal vascularity of the malformation in the 3 instances of angiographically occult cavernous malformation (Fig. 4a, b). This potential pitfall (MRA visualization of an angiographically occult vascular malformation) was probably due to the paramagnetic effect of methemoglobin in thrombus resulting in high signal structures misrepresented as flow-related enhancement on the post-processed MRA. The use of PC MRA may avoid this pitfall because it is a subtraction technique (analogous to DSA) which

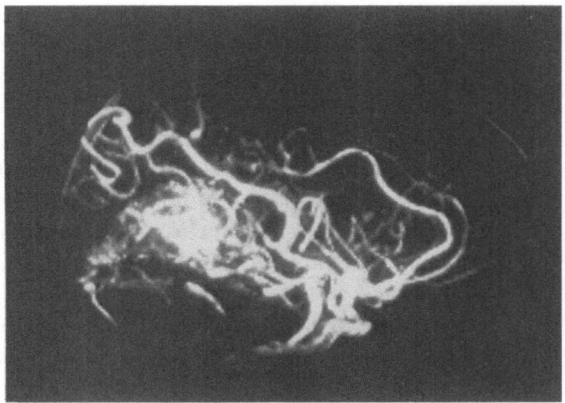

Fig. 3. AVMs were well visualized by MRA; however, MRA was not necessary for diagnosis since all AVMs were seen on MRI. In addition, MRA failed to provide sufficient spatial resolution or dynamic blood flow information

eliminates stationary background signal prior to computer post-processing[18], but this may falsely exclude visualization of slow flow areas within the malformation.

MRI/MRA was felt to provide clinically useful information not available from conventional MRI in only 2 of the 11 (18%) cases, mostly because MRI alone was able to visualize every lesion and provide general characteristics necessary for diagnosis. MRA in conjunction with conventional imaging could have replaced conventional catheter angiography in 4 of the 5 (80%)

cases treated expectantly. MRA did not provide sufficient spatial resolution or dynamic flow information required for surgical planning in any of the 6 cases treated by embolization and/or surgery.

Occlusive Cerebrovascular Disease

There were 61 cases with known or suspected occlusive vascular lesions. Among 31 cases with known occlusive vascular pathology (26 extracranial carotid, 2 intracranial carotid, and 3 vertebrobasilar), MRA visualized the occlusive lesion in every instance. The MRA reliably excluded occlusive pathology in 19 of 30 (63%) cases when there was non present. Of 56 cases treated medically, MRA could have replaced conventional angiography in 42 (75%) cases. However, among 5 cases treated surgically, the MRA proved inadequate information in 4 of these cases, secondary to insufficient spatial resolution. Generally, the MRA and intra-arterial catheter angiography showed excellent correlation (Fig. 5a, b) in visualizing the degree of stenosis. However, slight overestimation of stenos is by MRA was common in extremely tight stenoses, probably secondary to signal loss from turbulent blood flow, or saturation effect in the presence of slow flow (which may even mimic occlusion). In no case did MRA diagnose a "surgical lesion" which proved insignificant on angiography. However, among significant preocclusive stenoses, MRA tended to distort the fine spatial

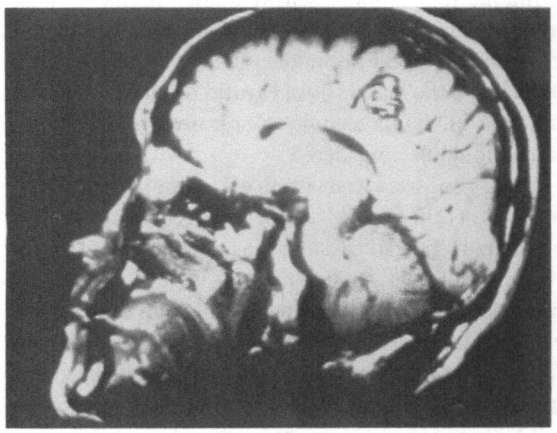

a

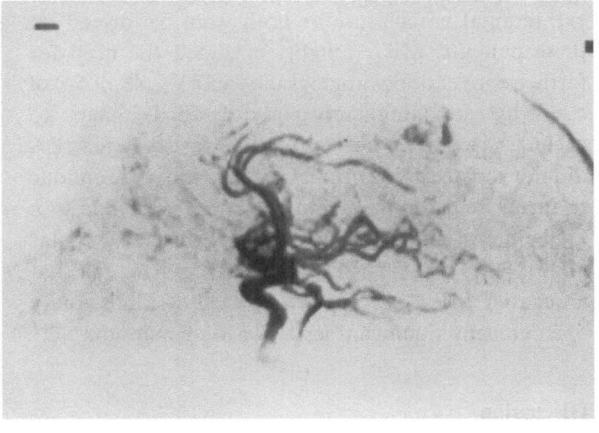

b

Fig. 4. (a) T_1 weighted MRI image revealing a mesial hemispheric vascular malformation, with signal characteristics consistent with cavernous malformation. Conventional catheter angiography did not visualize the malformation (not shown). (b) TOF MRA of the same case erroneously "visualizing" this angiographically occult malformation, and falsely suggesting that it may be an arteriovenous malformation with feeders from the anterior cerebral artery and cortical venous drainage

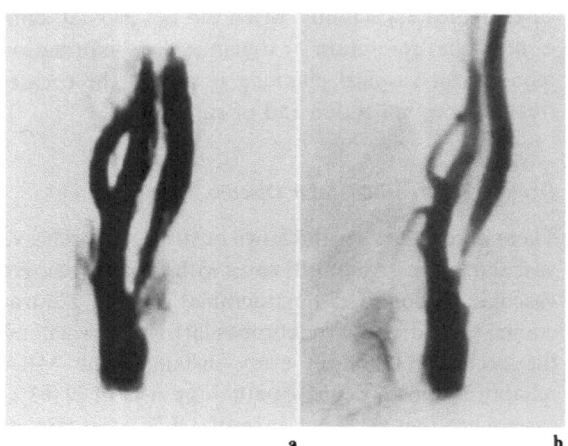

a   **b**

Fig. 5. (a) MRA of the left extracranial carotid bifurcation revealing severe stenosis at the origin of the internal carotid artery and no significant disease of the common or external carotid arteries. (b) Intraarterial conventional catheter digital subtraction angiogram with accurate visualization of the same pathology

details of the vascular lesion (ulceration, luminal thrombosis, luminal webs, etc.). A newer MRA technique (black blood) may be more sensitive and specific to high grade preocclusive stenosis and thus may be more suitable for their study[5].

A question of rule out vascular pathology was asked in 54 patients in whom the MRI showed no evidence of tumor, trauma, vessel or parenchymal changes associated with vascular pathology. Of these patients, a vascular lesion was found in 20% (11 of 54). Depending upon symptomatology, MRA of the intracranial or extracranial vasculature or both were performed on these patients. MRA reliably excluded the need for further conventional angiography in 83% (45 of 54) of cases by providing sufficiently detailed images to exclude vascular pathology. Of the 9 cases where MRA did not replace conventional angiography, 5 were due to insufficient spatial resolution and 4 were due to a high index of clinical suspicion (where we felt a vascular abnormality was very likely) in which case we felt that a negative MRA did not totally exclude a possibility of a clinically significant lesion or tandem lesion.

Discussion

The concept of clinical usefulness includes information about sensitivity and specificity of a diagnostic modality, spatial resolution and fidelity, and the overall ability of the technique to guide decision-making in individual clinical scenarios. This last characteristic is probably the most important clinically, but one of the least investigated in clinical research. A "question driven technology assessment" methodology was suggested by Caplan to attempt to define clinical usefulness in specific clinical situations[4]. In this study, we applied this methodology to a wide spectrum of pathologies encountered in neurosurgical practice where vascular information was essential to diagnosis, therapeutic options, or surgical strategy.

Among cases with nonvascular pathology, MRA provided a great deal of useful vascular information, including tumor-vessel relationships and patency or compromise of dural venous sinuses. In conjunction with MRI, MRA could successfully distinguish between giant aneurysm and tumor. In a large number of such cases where angiographic information was desirable, MRA could have satisfactorily replaced conventional angiography. At our center, we currently use MRA to examine vessel-tumor relationships, to visualize the carotid siphon in sellar lesions, and to examine dural venous sinus patency. Rarely is conventional catheter angiography still necessary in such instances.

MRA is an excellent screening modality (for cases with low suspicion) of vascular pathology. It depicts with good accuracy the severity of extracranial carotid stenosis. The stenoses that are more high grade may be overestimated by 3D TOF MRA, thus leading one to believe that segment of vessel may be occluded when in actuality there is a high grade stenosis present[15,17]. This may be alleviated by the "black blood" MRA technique that is more sensitive and specific to high grade stenosis and vascular occlusion when compared to the "bright blood" techniques used at our institution[5]. However, if the diagnosis of carotid occlusion is entertained, a 2D TOF technique or conventional angiogram should be considered.

Aneurysms were well visualized in our patient population as in others[16,20,24]. Ninety percent of all patients with aneurysm were visualized as was the parent artery of origin; however, aneurysm necks were inconsistently visualized. Aneurysms as small as 3–4 mm were visualized and good IADSA MRA aneurysmal size correlation was found with those smaller than 1 cm. Giant aneurysms were generally overestimated in size by MRA secondary to their intraluminal thrombus that may have been present or underestimated due to the presence of slow moving blood within the aneurysm due to lack of flow related enhancement. Nevertheless, the spin-echo MRI often accurately defined both the aneurysm lumen and mural thrombus. Other studies report that MRA sensitivities up to 95% in detecting aneurysms when used in conjunction with individual image slices and spin echo MRI[20]. It has been suggested that MRA may be used as a diagnostic or screening test for those patients at particular risk of extracranial carotid stenosis or harboring unruptured aneurysms (i.e. family history of aneurysms, polycystic kidney disease, fibromuscular disease, and coarctation)[20]. It has also been used for serial follow-up in patients who have undergone aneurysmal balloon occlusion[24]. Sensitivity may be less at the carotid siphon, which is more susceptible to artifacts on MRA than the remaining intracranial vasculature. This may be secondary to the signal dropout within the siphon; however, it has been suggested that if the cephalocaudal height at a carotid siphon is small, then vessel loops tend to merge on MRA thus making the distinction between aneurysmal dilatation in normal vasculature very difficult[20].

Among cases with cerebral vascular malformations, MRA showed excellent sensitivity of visualizing the lesion. However, MRA contributed little beyond conventional MRI to lesion detection and specific characteristics. A potential pitfall of TOF MRA was the possibility of "visualizing" an angiographically occult vascular malformation because of high signal thrombus "masquerading" as flow-related enhancement. In cases where medical or expectant therapy was entertained, MRI (alone or with MRA) was sufficient for clinical management.

In instances where invasive therapeutic intervention was entertained, MRA did not provide sufficient spatial resolution and dynamic flow information so as to guide endovascular or surgical therapy. Also, it is our opinion that MRA alone does not provide sufficient spatial fidelity to guide radiosurgical therapeutic planning. It is possible that newer MRA technical advances, including PC MRA techniques and other innovations in image acquisition and postprocessing may overcome some of these technical limitations of MRA. Such specialized MRA techniques may allow in the future the quantification of nidus volume, and/or blood flow in vascular malformations without resorting to catheter angiography[6].

As the quality of MRA technology has advanced so has the quality of imaging. The future needs of TOF MRA include shorter exam times, shorter echo times, higher special resolution, improved postprocessing procedures, functional (i.e. physiologic) examinations which have only recently begun, and prospective clini-

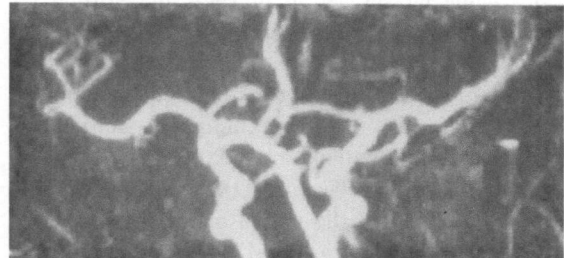

Fig. 6. MRA using rectangular field of view. Sequencing will decrease imaging time (in this case 3,5 minutes) while still maintaining excellent image quality

cal trials to better define accuracy. To shorten examination times, we have recently implemented rectangular field of view sequences which allow for the use of fewer phasing coding steps while still maintaining excellent image quality (i.e. spatial resolution) (Fig. 6). As echo times shorten (with new gradient systems and acquisition schemes) there is less phase dispersion and therefore increased signal which will eliminate artifacts from areas of turbulent flow[9,25,27]. Improvements in postprocessing procedures will also enhance vascular contrast. Vessel tracking is a post-processing technique which connects high signal vascular voxels on the basis of operator selected seed points and local backward signal[12]. The use of magnetization transfer contrast (MTC) and fat saturation pulses improve vascular contrast (Fig. 7a, b)[7]. MTC suppresses "bound" brain

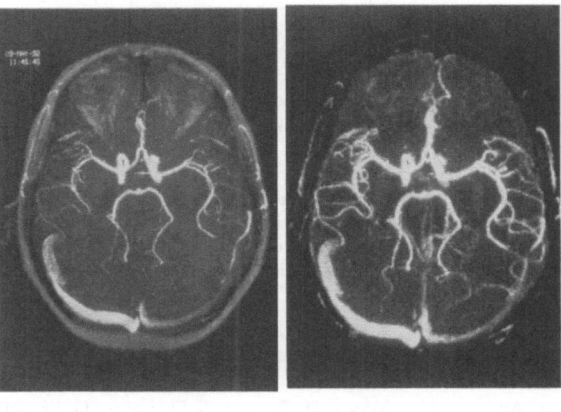

a   b

Fig. 7. (a) Standard MRA. (b) MRA with MTC (magnetization trans for contrast) and fat saturation. Note the improvement of vascular signal by suppression of bound brain water by MTC and suppression of fat signal by fat saturation. Thus vascular signal is improved by suppression of background signal water while fat saturation prevents the normal fat signal from appearing on standard MR angiogram. Vascular signal may also be enhanced by acquisition techniques such as specialized radiofrequency pulses. For example, the tone pulse technique maximizes vascular signal by spatially modulating flip angle to minimize saturation effect in 3-D TOF MRA[14]. This is especially helpful in the region of the smaller distal vessels. The combination of MTC and tone pulses is especially dramatic when reconstructed using a 512 image matrix.

The experience presented here and the published literature allows the clinician to understand the advantages and potential pitfalls of MRA. In most situations where lesion recognition is sufficient for management decisions, MRA could effectively be expected to replace catheter angiography. MRA is also quite useful in cases of low or moderate clinical suspicion to rule out vascular pathology (screening). Additionally, MRA is a useful guide to conservative therapy and serial follow-up while adding no risk and only a short amount of time to the MRI imaging time. Shortcomings, however, do exist. Currently the technical constraints of MRA include insufficient spatial resolution or dynamic flow information, thereby diminishing its usefulness for surgical guidance. Erroneous information may also be seen in low flow states and with hemorrhage. In conclusion, although MRA cannot replace conventional catheter angiography (at this time) for surgical guidance and planning, it is helpful in the diagnosis and exclusion of both vascular and nonvascular neurologic diseases.

Acknowledgements

This work was previously presented in modified form at the International Conference on Stroke in Geneva, Switzerland on May 30, 1991, the 17th International Joint Conference on Stroke and Cerebral Circulation in Phoenix, Arizona on January 30, 1992, the American Association of Neurological Surgeons in San Francisco, California on April 16, 1992, and at the New Trends in Cerebrovascular Research Conference in Verona, Italy on June 8, 1992, and has been accepted for publication in modified form in Neurological Research.

References

1. Anderson CM, Saloner D, Tsuruda JS, Shapeero LG, Lee RE (1990) Artifacts in maximum-intensity-projection display of MR angiograms. AJR 154: 623–629

2. Axel A, Shimakawa A, MacFall J (1986) A time-of-flight method of measuring flow velocity by magnetic resonance imaging. Magn Reson Imaging 4: 199–205

3. Bradley WG, Waluch V (1985) Blood flow: magnetic resonance imaging. Radiology 154: 443–450

4. Caplan LR (1991) Question-driven technology assessment: SPECT as an example. Neurology 41: 187–191

5. Edelman RR, Mattle HP, Wallner B (1990) Extracranial carotid arteries: evaluation with "black blood" MR angiography. Radiology 177: 45–50

6. Edelman RR, Wendtz KU, Mattle HP, O'Reilly GV, Candia G, Liu C, Zhao B, Kjellberg RN, Davis KR (1989) Intracerebral arteriovenous malformations: evaluations with selective MR angiography and venography. Neuroradiology 173: 831–837

7. Edelman RR, Ahn SS, Chien D, Wei L, Goldmann A, Mantello M, Kramer J, Kleefield J (1992) Improved time-of-flight MR angiography of the brain with magnetization transfer contrast. Radiology 184: 395–399

8. Haacke EM, Masaryk TJ (1989) The salient features of MR angiography. Radiology 173: 611–612

9. Jackson JI, Nishimora DG, Macovski A (1992) Twisting radial lines with application to robust magnetic resonance imaging of irregular flow. Mag Reson Med 25: 128–140

10. Kaufman L, Crooks LE, Sheldon PE (1982) Evaluation of NMR imaging for detection and quantification of obstructions in vessels. Invest Radiol 17: 554–560

11. Kido DK, Barsotti JB, Rice LZ (1991) Evaluation of the carotid artery bifurcation: comparison of magnetic resonance angiography and digital subtraction arch aortography. Neuroradiology 33: 48–51

12. Lin W, Haacke EM, Masaryk TJ, Smith AS (1993) An automated version of local maximum intensity projection using vessel tracking. JMRI, in press

13. Litt AW, Eidelman EM, Pinto RS (1991) Diagnosis of carotid artery stenosis: comparison of 2DFT time-of-flight MR angiography with contrast angiography in 50 patients. AJNR 12: 149–154

14. Laub G, Purdy De (1992) Variable-tip-angle slab selection for improved three-dimensional MR angiography. Presented at the 10th Meeting of the Society of Magnetic Resonance Imaging, New York, April 25–29

15. Masaryk TJ, Modic MT, Ruggieri PM, Ross JS, Laub G, Lenz GW, Tkach JA, Haacke EM, Selman WR, Harik SI (1989) Three-dimensional (volume) gradient-echo imaging of the carotid bifurcation: preliminary clinical experience. Radiology 171: 801–806

16. Masaryk TJ, Modic MT, Ross JS, Ruggieri PM, Laub GA, Lenz GW, Haache EM, Wiznitzer M, Harik SI (1989) Intracranial circulation: preliminary clinical results with three-dimensional (volume) MR angiography. Radiology 171: 793–799

17. Masaryk AM, Ross JS, DiCello MC (1991) 3DFT MR angiography of the carotid bifurcation: potential and limitations as a screening examination. Radiology 179: 797–804

18. Pernicone JR, Siebert JE, Potchen EJ (1990) Three-dimensional phase-contrast MR angiography in the head and neck: preliminary report. AJNR 155: 167–176

19. Ross JS, Masaryk TJ, Modic MT, Harik SI, Wiznitzer M, Selman WR (1989) Magnetic resonance angiography of the extracranial carotid arteries and intracranial vessels: a review. Neurology 39: 1369–1376

20. Ross JS, Masaryk TJ, Modic MT (1990) Intracranial aneurysms: evaluation by MR angiography. AJNR 11: 449–456

21. Ross JS, Masaryk TJ, Ruggieri PM (1991) Magnetic resonance angiography of the carotid bifurcation. Top Magn Reson Imaging 3: 12–22

22. Riles TS, Eidelman EM, Litt AW, Pinto RS, Oldford F, Schwartzenberg GW (1992) Comparison of magnetic resonance

angiography, conventional angiography, and duplex scanning. Stroke 23: 341–346

23. Ruggieri PM, Laub GA, Masaryk TJ, Modic MT (1989) Intracranial circulation: pulse-sequence considerations in three-dimensional (volume) MR angiography. Radiology 171: 785–791

24. Sevick RJ, Tsuruda JS, Schmalbrock P (1990) Three-dimensional time-of-flight MR angiography in the evaluation of cerebral aneurysms. J Comput Assist Tomogr 14: 874–881

25. Tkach J, Ruggieri PM, Dillinger JJ, Ross JS, Modic MT, Masaryk TJ (1992) 2D and 3D time-of-flight magnetic resonance angiography using a specialized gradient head coil. JMRI, in press

26. Tomai LA, Panzer RJ, Phelps CE, Kido DK (1988) Noninvasive carotid artery imaging with magnetic resonance imaging: what is the challenge region for equal efficacy with invasive angiography? Med Decis Making 8: 339

27. Urchuk SN, Plewes DB (1992) Mechanism of flow-induced signal loss in MR angiography. JMRI 2: 453–562

28. Wiznitzer M, Ruggieri PM, Masaryk TJ (1990) Diagnosis of cerebrovascular disease in sickle cell anemia by magnetic resonance angiography. J Pediatr 117: 551–555

Correspondence: Issam A. Awad, M.D., M.Sc., F.A.C.S., Section of Neurological Surgery, Yale University School of Medicine, 333 Cedar Street, TMP 405, P.O. Box 3333, New Haven, Connecticut 06510, U.S.A.

Intracranial Aneurysms and Subarachnoid Hemorrhage

Research in Cerebral Vasospasm

New Evidence Pointing to Oxyhemoglobin as the Cause of Vasospasm

R.L. Macdonald and **B.K.A. Weir**

Department of Neurosurgery, University of Alberta, Edmonton, Canada, and Section of Neurosurgery, University of Chicago, Illinois, U.S.A.

Summary

Experiments were conducted in monkeys to determine which substances in blood may cause cerebral vasospasm following subarachnoid hemorrhage (SAH), and to examine the mechanism of action of these substances. In the first experiment, monkeys were given intrathecal injections, twice a day for 6 days, with one of the following solutions: mock cerebrospinal fluid (CSF); oxyhemoglobin (OxyHb); methemoglobin; bilirubin; supernatant fluid from an incubated mixture of autologous blood and mock CSF ($n = 8$ in each group). Comparison of cerebral angiograms taken before and after the injections showed significant vasospasm only in the groups which had received OxyHb and supernatant fluid (mean reduction in middle cerebral artery diameter, $27\% \pm 5\%$ and $26\% \pm 7\%$, $p < 0.05$, respectively). These data suggest that OxyHb is an important cause of cerebral vasospasm following SAH. In the second experiment, monkeys were randomly assigned to have subarachnoid placement of one of the following: agarose gel alone ($n = 2$); agarose plus OxyHb ($n = 3$); agarose plus OxyHb plus intrathecal administration of superoxide dismutase and catalase ($n = 6$); agarose plus OxyHb plus intrathecal administration of placebo ($n = 6$). Vasospasm was assessed by comparing angiograms taken before and 7 days after placement of subarachnoid compounds. Agarose-OxyHb gel alone caused significant reduction in middle cerebral artery diameter ($41\% \pm 8\%$, $p < 0.005$, paired t-test) which was associated with ultrastructural damage to smooth muscle. Treatment with superoxide dismutase plus catalase or with placebo attenuated vasospasm, although significant narrowing persisted in both groups ($27\% \pm 12\%$ and $26\% \pm 13\%$, $p < 0.05$, paired t-test, respectively). The failure of superoxide dismutase and catalase to prevent OxyHb-induced vasospasm suggests free-radical mediated mechanisms may not be important in its genesis. However, only one combination of doses of enzymes was administered and other dose schedules might be efficacious.

Keywords: Free radicals; oxyhemoglobin; subarachnoid hemorrhage; vasospasm.

Introduction

Cerebral vasospasm following subarachnoid hemorrhage (SAH) is probably caused by a compound or compounds released from subarachnoid clot, although the identity of these compounds has not been conclusively established[3,4,8,17,20]. There is evidence, largely from studies performed in vitro, that oxyhemoglobin (OxyHb) is an important spasmogen.

Questions remain regarding the role of hemoglobin (Hb) in the genesis of vasospasm. It is unclear whether Hb can cause arterial narrowing lasting for days since most experiments have studied its effect in vitro[8,17,18]. Other issues are whether Hb is the only chemical responsible for vasospasm, or whether it interacts in some way with other spasmogens, such as bilirubin[3,20]. The importance of the oxidation state of the iron in the heme molecule is also uncertain. If Hb, and specifically, OxyHb, is important in vasospasm, the mechanism by which it produces vasospasm is unknown. One theory is that OxyHb causes vasospasm through a free radical-mediated mechanism[15].

We have given intrathecal injections of OxyHb, methemoglobin (MetHb), and bilirubin to monkeys for a week[9]. Vasospasm was assessed angiographically and by microscopic examination of the affected arteries. Effects of these substances were compared to vasoactivity of substances released into supernatant fluid of blood incubated ex vivo. In a second experiment, vasospasm was produced in monkeys using a gel composed of agarose and OxyHb, which slowly released pure OxyHb into the subarachnoid space near cerebral arteries[10]. The contribution of free radical reactions to OxyHb-induced vasospasm was assessed by treating spasm with free radical scavenging enzymes, superoxide dismutase (SOD) and catalase. This work has been reported in detail[9,10].

Materials and Methods

First Experiment[9]

Forty cynomolgus monkeys (Macaca fascicularis) were randomly divided into 5 equal groups. On day 0, animals underwent baseline cerebral angiography, microsurgical opening of the basal cisterns, and placement of an Ommaya reservoir with a catheter along the right middle cerebral artery (MCA) for intrathecal injections. Animals were given intrathecal injections twice a day on days 1 to 6 with one of the following solutions: OxyHb; MetHb; bilirubin; supernatant fluid of an incubated blood-mock cerebrospinal fluid (CSF) mixture; mock CSF alone. Details of experimental procedures have been published[9]. All animals injected with Hb-containing solutions received the same total dose of Hb, equal to the amount found in 5 ml of monkey blood. Previous experiments with the monkey model of SAH showed 3 to 5 ml clotted arterial blood caused vasospasm when placed in the subarachnoid space[5]. The total amount of bilirubin injected was equal to that which would be produced by complete metabolism of the Hb. On day 7, angiography was repeated and the cerebral arteries were removed and evaluated by scanning and transmission electron microscopy.

Second Experiment[10]

Seventeen monkeys were randomly divided into 4 groups. On day 0, animals underwent baseline cerebral angiography, right craniectomy, and arachnoid dissection by previously reported methods[5,10]. Each animal had subarachnoid placement of one of the following next to exposed cerebral arteries of the right side of the circle of Willis: agarose gel in group 1 ($n = 2$) or agarose gel plus OxyHb in groups 2, 3, and 4 ($n = 3, 6$, and 6, respectively). Each animal had 350 mg OxyHb placed in the subarachnoid space, an amount contained in 3 ml monkey blood. Preliminary experiments showed that OxyHb-

agarose gel released OxyHb at a rate similar to lysing subarachnoid erythrocytes. In groups 3 and 4, intrathecal catheters were placed along the right sylvian fissure and connected to osmotic pumps anchored in the subcutaneous tissue over the dorsal thorax. Group 3 received 5×10^5U catalase and 5×10^5U human recombinant copper/zinc SOD (Chiron Corporation, Emeryville, California) administered continuously over 7 days by osmotic pump. Group 4 had intrathecal catheters and subcutaneous pumps filled with placebo consisting of inactivated SOD plus additional protein to account for protein in catalase. Earlier experiments in vitro and in vivo showed that the pumps continuously released high levels of enzymes into the fluid adjacent to the catheter. Vasospasm was assessed by comparing baseline angiography with angiography done 7 days later, and by transmission electron microscopy of cerebral arteries removed following day 7 angiography.

Results

First Experiment[9]

Cerebral Vasospasm

Significant reduction in vessel caliber between day 0 and day 7 developed in the right intradural cerebral arteries in animals injected with supernatant fluid (mean reduction, $24\% \pm 5\%$) and OxyHb (mean reduction, $21\% \pm 4\%$) (Table 1). There were no significant

Table 1. *First Experiment: Per Cent Change in Right Cerebral Artery Diameters Between Angiograms Taken Before and After 6 Days of Intrathecal Injections of the Various Solutions, by Group*[a]

Artery	Supernatant fluid	Mock CSF	Oxyhemoglobin	Methemoglobin	Bilirubin
C3	-22 ± 2[c]	7 ± 8	-19 ± 2[b]	5 ± 7	-10 ± 5
C4	-17 ± 6[b]	2 ± 3	-18 ± 5[c]	-1 ± 5	-11 ± 4
ACA	-31 ± 10[c]	-3 ± 3	-20 ± 6[b]	-9 ± 5	-14 ± 6
MCA	-26 ± 7[b]	2 ± 6	-27 ± 5[c]	3 ± 6	-13 ± 6

[a] Values are expressed as per cent change in means $\pm$ the standard error of the means. *C3* extradural internal carotid artery; *C4* intradural internal carotid artery; *ACA* precommunicating segment of the anterior cerebral artery; *MCA* sphenoidal segment of the middle cerebral artery; *CSF* cerebrospinal fluid.
[b] $p < 0.05$.
[c] $p < 0.005$.

Table 2. *Second Experiment: Per Cent Change in Right Cerebral Artery Diameters Between Angiograms Taken Before and 7 Days After Subarachnoid Placement of the Various Gels, by Group*[a]

Artery	Agarose alone	Agarose + OxyHb	Agarose + OxyHb + treatment	Agarose + OxyHb + placebo
C3	1 ± 5	3 ± 10	-28 ± 8[c]	-24 ± 15[b]
C4	0 ± 4	-33 ± 9	-29 ± 11[c]	-16 ± 12[b]
ACA	-7 ± 5	-30 ± 10	-24 ± 4[b]	-19 ± 11
MCA	2 ± 3	-41 ± 8[c]	-27 ± 12[c]	-26 ± 13[b]

[a] Values are expressed as percentage of change in means $\pm$ the standard error of the means. *C3* extradural internal carotid artery; *C4* intradural internal carotid artery; *ACA* precommunicating segment of the anterior cerebral artery; *MCA* sphenoidal segment of the middle cerebral artery; *OxyHb* oxyhemoglobin.
[b] $p < 0.05$.
[c] $p < 0.005$.

changes in vessel caliber in the groups receiving bilirubin, MetHb, and mock CSF, although mild arterial narrowing occurred in the bilirubin-treated animals (mean reduction, $12\% \pm 2\%$).

Pathology

Scanning electron microscopy showed convolution of the endothelium and tunica intima, narrowing of the lumen and thickening of the vessel wall in right MCA's of animals which had received supernatant fluid or OxyHb. Right MCA's from animals injected with bilirubin showed mild convolutional changes and vessel wall thickening. Transmission electron microscopy revealed smooth muscle cell contraction, vacuolation, and necrosis in arteries from monkeys treated with

supernatant fluid and OxyHb. Pathologic changes were less severe in arteries from animals treated with bilirubin. Arteries from animals injected with MetHb and Elliott's solution B were normal. One monkey injected with OxyHb had a cerebral infarction in the right MCA territory. This monkey had a 50% reduction in right MCA diameter on angiography; volume depletion probably contributed to development of infarction.

Second Experiment[10]

Cerebral Vasospasm

At day 7, analysis of variance between groups showed right MCA diameter was significantly different from

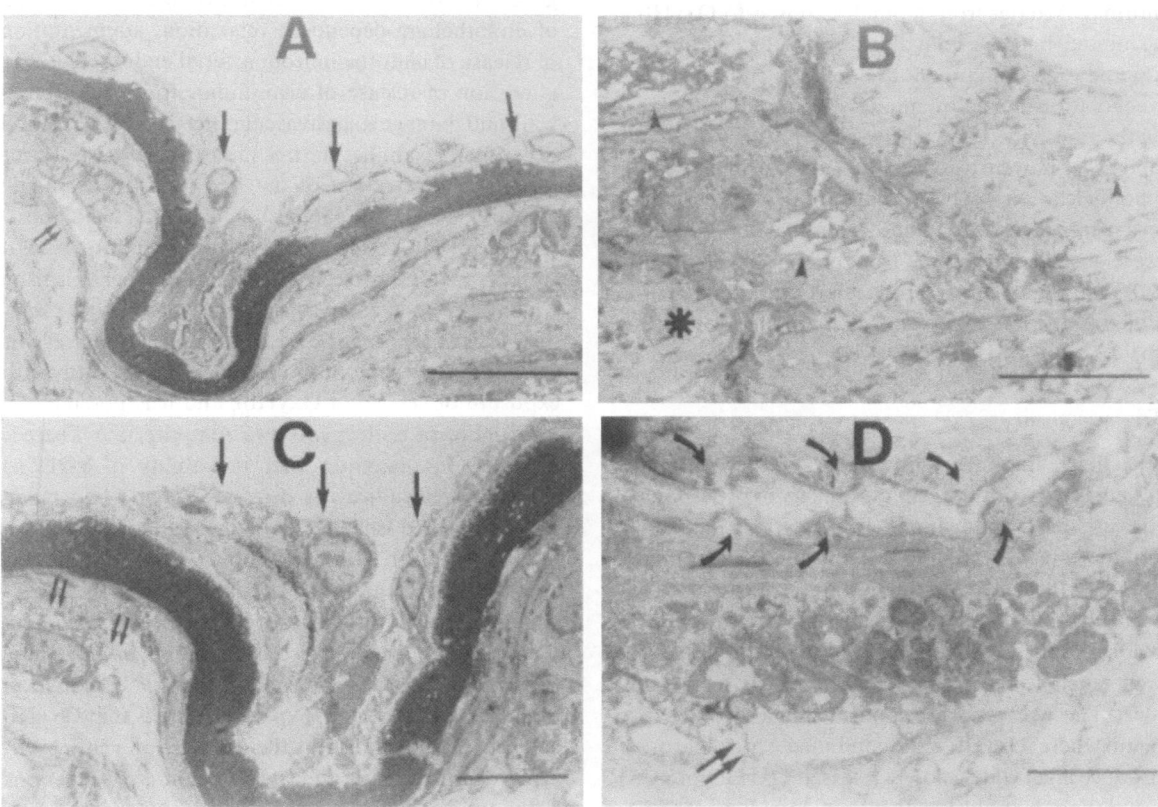

Fig. 1. Electron photomicrographs of anterior cerebral arteries from monkeys exposed to oxyhemoglobin (OxyHb)-agarose gel. (A) After exposure to subarachnoid OxyHb-agarose gel, there is vacuolation of endothelial cells (arrows), convolution of internal elastic lamina, and contraction and vacuolation of smooth muscle cells (double arrows, scale bar = 10 μm). (B) Medial smooth muscle shows contraction and vacuolation after exposure to OxyHb-agarose gel. Most vacuoles represent swollen mitochondria (arrowheads). One smooth muscle cell has decreased electron density (asterisk), indicative of necrosis (scale bar = 5 μm). (C) Similar changes with endothelial cell vacuolation (arrows), folding of the internal elastic lamina, and smooth muscle cell contraction and vacuolation (double arrows) are seen after placement of subarachnoid OxyHb-agarose and treatment with superoxide dismutase and catalase (scale bar = 5 μm). (D) Swollen mitochondria and vacuolation within contracted smooth muscle cell (double arrow) after exposure to OxyHb-agarose gel and treatment with placebo. Folding of the cell membrane, a feature of smooth muscle contraction, is visible (curved arrows, scale bar = 2 μm)

the agarose gel alone group in all three groups exposed to OxyHb, although there were no pairwise differences (p < 0.05, analysis of variance, Table 2). Comparisons within groups between baseline and day 7 showed monkeys exposed to agarose gel alone did not develop significant vasospasm. In the group with placement of OxyHb-agarose gel only, there was significant reduction in caliber of the right MCA (41% ± 8%, p < 0.005, paired t-test). In animals treated with SOD and catalase, there was significant vasospasm of the right MCA (27% ± 12%, p < 0.005, paired t-test). Similar vasospasm developed after administration of placebo (reduction in right MCA; 26% ± 13%, p < 0.05, paired t-test).

Pathology

On transmission electron microscopy, the anterior cerebral arteries of animals exposed to agarose were normal. Arteries from animals exposed to OxyHb gel exhibited marked convolution of tunica intima and internal elastic lamina as well as endothelial cell vacuolation and desquamation. In smooth muscle cells of the tunica media, extensive contraction, vacuolation, and necrosis were present (Fig. 1). Occasional polymorphonuclear leucocytes and macrophages were present in superficial areas of tunica adventitia. Similar changes were observed in arteries from animals given intrathecal SOD plus catalase or placebo. No differences were noted in the frequency or severity of changes between the 3 groups exposed to OxyHb.

Discussion

The first experiment shows that of the compounds tested, OxyHb is the agent most likely to be responsible for vasospasm following SAH. The arterial narrowing produced by OxyHb and supernatant fluid from incubated erythrocytes was angiographically and morphologically similar to spasm caused by the presence of whole blood in the subarachnoid space[5,19]. Bilirubin was much less active while MetHb was essentially inert. These results were confirmed in a second experiment where OxyHb was combined with agarose to produce a gel which slowly released OxyHb into CSF, simulating hemolysis of subarachnoid erythrocytes after SAH. The vasospasm which developed differed only in severity from that produced by whole blood in the monkey subarachnoid space[5,19]. There seems little doubt that OxyHb is the major cause of cerebral vasospasm[8]. This conclusion is consistent with a large number of studies which show that OxyHb produces prolonged arterial contraction and is released into the

CSF during the time vasospasm develops[8]. Studies in vitro and in vivo have found erythrocytes to be necessary for the development of vasospasm, and generally point to OxyHb as the spasmogenic compound released as red blood cells hemolyze[4,8,11,17].

The monkey model of surgical placement of formed clot developed at the University of Alberta causes a 50% reduction in right MCA diameter, a greater degree of vasospasm than observed in these experiments[5,19]. Although the bulk of arterial narrowing seems to be due to OxyHb, it is likely that OxyHb acts synergistically with other vasoactive agents, such as lipid peroxides, amphiphiles, or other chemicals, in the production of vasospasm[3,15,20].

The pathogenesis of OxyHb-induced vasospasm may involve autoxidation to MetHb with subsequent generation of oxygen-derived free radicals[15], inhibition of endothelium-dependent relaxation, augmentation of release of endothelin from arterial endothelial cells, alteration of release of eicosanoids from the arterial wall, and damage to perivascular nerves[8,9]. The second experiment examines the free radical hypothesis. Intrathecal administration of the free radical scavenging enzymes, SOD and catalase, failed to alleviate vasospasm due to OxyHb. These results, therefore, do not support a role for free radicals in the mechanism by which OxyHb causes vasospasm. Only one dose regimen of each agent, however, was tried (although it was administered continuously starting simultaneously with exposure of vessels to OxyHb), and it is possible the dose of one or both agents was inappropriate. There is evidence, for example, that the ability of SOD to scavenge free radicals is dose-dependent. Too much SOD worsened ischemic damage to the myocardium in rabbits[14]. Little is known about what combinations and ratios of the naturally occurring free-radical scavenging enzymes would best remove free radicals and there are few previous studies of the use of these enzymes against vasospasm[13]. Another explanation for lack of efficacy of SOD plus catalase is that OxyHb clogged the adventitia of the arteries, preventing enzymes from reaching the site of free radical reactions in the tunica media.

These results conflict with evidence both in vitro and in vivo that OxyHb causes smooth muscle contraction and vasospasm through generation of injurious oxygen free radicals[8,12,15]. An inhibitor of iron-dependent lipid peroxidation, U74006F, significantly diminished vasospasm after SAH in monkeys[19]. Lipid peroxidation is a process by which free radicals may damage cells[6].

There are reports of beneficial effects of 1,2-bis(nicotinamide)-propane, a free-radical scavenger, on vasospasm in dogs and humans[1,13,15]. Ohue investigated effects of SOD plus catalase on vasospasm in a double-hemorrhage dog model[13]. Treatment "slightly reduced" basilar artery narrowing but had no effect on levels of malondialdehyde, a marker for lipid peroxidation, in CSF.

These results add to previous reports of failure of SOD and catalase to alleviate processes which are thought to be due to free radicals. There are, for example, conflicting data on the effects of anti-free radical therapy for cerebral ischemia[7,16] and following ischemia and reperfusion in the heart[2,14]. Limited knowledge about appropriate doses, as well as about the particular free radicals which are involved, necessitates further work before the problem will be fully understood.

These studies shows that OxyHb causes vasospasm in monkeys. The spontaneous oxidation product, Met-Hb, is inactive. Metabolism of the heme group of Hb to bilirubin produces a less vasoactive agent. The pathogenesis of vasospasm likely involves the slow and prolonged release of high concentrations of OxyHb from hemolysing subarachnoid erythrocytes. There are several possible mechanisms by which OxyHb may cause vascular contraction, although these experiments suggest free radical mechanisms may not be critical to development of or may not be the sole pathogenetic process in cerebral vasospasm. Further work, however, is necessary before the biochemistry by which increased extracellular concentrations of OxyHb affect the configuration of intracellular contractile proteins will be elucidated.

Acknowledgements

This work was presented in part at the 59th and 60th Annual Meetings of the American Association of Neurologic Surgeons, 1991, and 1992. Dr. Macdonald was a fellow of the Alberta Heritage Foundation for Medical Research. This work was supported in part by grants to Dr. Weir from the National Institutes of Health and the Medical Research Council of Canada and to Dr. Cook from the Alberta Heart and Stroke Foundation.

References

1. Asano T, Sasaki T, Koide T, Takakura K, Sano K (1984) Experimental evaluation of the beneficial effect of an antioxidant on cerebral vasospasm. Neurol Res 6: 49–53
2. Downey JM (1990) Free radicals and their involvement during long-term myocardial ischemia and reperfusion. Ann Rev Physiol 52: 487–504
3. Duff TA, Feilbach JA, Yusuf Q, Scott G (1988) Bilirubin and the induction of intracranial arterial spasm. J Neurosurg 69: 593–598
4. Duff TA, Louie J, Feilbach JA, Scott G (1988) Erythrocytes are essential for development of cerebral vasculopathy resulting from subarachnoid hemorrhage in cats. Stroke 19: 68–72
5. Findlay JM, Weir BKA, Steinke D, Tanabe T, Gordon P, Grace M (1988) Effect of intrathecal thrombolytic therapy on subarachnoid clot and chronic vasospasm in a primate model of SAH. J Neurosurg 69: 723–735
6. Halliwell B, Gutteridge JMC (1986) Oxygen free radicals and iron in relation to biology and medicine: some problems and concepts. Arch Biochem Biophys 246: 501–514
7. Imaizumi S, Woolworth V, Fishman RA, Chan PH (1990) Liposome-entrapped superoxide dismutase reduces cerebral infarction in cerebral ischemia in rats. Stroke 21: 1312–1317
8. Macdonald RL, Weir BKA (1991) A review of hemoglobin and the pathogenesis of cerebral vasospasm. Stroke 22: 971–982
9. Macdonald RL, Weir BKA, Saito K, Kanamaru K, Findlay JM, Grace M, Runzer T, Mielke B (1991) Etiology of cerebral vasospasm in primates. J Neurosurg 75: 415–424
10. Macdonald RL, Weir BKA, Runzer TD, Grace MGA, Poznansky MJ (1992) Effect of intrathecal superoxide dismutase and catalase on oxyhemoglobin-induced vasospasm in monkeys. Neurosurgery 30: 529–539
11. Mayberg MR, Okada T, Bark DH (1990) The role of hemoglobin in arterial narrowing after subarachnoid hemorrhage. J Neurosurg 72: 634–640
12. Nakagomi T, Yamakawa K, Tsubaki S, Sasaki T, Saito I, Takakura K (1990) Effect of a new free radical scavenger, MCI-186, on experimental cerebral vasospasm. In: Sano K, Takakura K, Kassell NF, Sasaki T (eds) Cerebral vasospasm. University of Tokyo Press, pp 141–142
13. Ohue S, Sakaki S, Nakamura H, Kohno K, Matsuoka K (1990) Free radical reaction and biological defense mechanism in the pathogenesis of prolonged vasospasm. In: Sano K, Takakura K, Kassell NF, Sasaki T (eds) Cerebral vasospasm. University of Tokyo Press, Tokyo, pp 137–138
14. Omar BA, Gad NM, Jordan MC, Striplin SP, Russell WJ, Downey JM, McCord JM (1990) Cardioprotection by Cu, Zn-superoxide dismutase is lost at high doses in the reoxygenated heart. Free Radical Biol Med 9: 465–471
15. Sano K (1988) Cerebral vasospasm as a deficiency syndrome. In: Wilkins RH (ed) Cerebral vasospasm. Raven, New York, pp 285–295
16. Schurer L, Grogaard B, Gerdin B, Arfors KE (1990) Superoxide dismutase does not prevent delayed hypoperfusion after incomplete cerebral ischaemia in the rat. Acta Neurochir (Wien) 103: 163–170
17. Sonobe M, Suzuki J (1978) Vasospasmogenic substance produced following subarachnoid haemorrhage, and its fate. Acta Neurochir (Wien) 44: 97–106
18. Steele JA, Stockbridge N, Maljkovic G, Weir B (1991) Free radicals mediate actions of oxyhemoglobin on cerebrovascular smooth muscle cells. Circ Res 68: 416–423
19. Steinke DE, Weir BKA, Findlay JM, Tanabe T, Grace M, Krushelnycky BW (1989) A trial of the 21-aminosteroid U74006F in a primate model of chronic cerebral vasospasm. Neurosurgery 24: 179–186
20. White RP, Macleod RM, Muhlbauer MS (1987) Evaluation of the role of hemoglobin in cerebrospinal fluid plays in producing contractions of cerebral arteries. Surg Neurol 27: 237–242

Correspondence: R.L. Macdonald, M.D., Section of Neurosurgery, University of Chicago Medical Center MC 3026, 5841 South Maryland Ave., Chicago, Illinois 60637, U.S.A.

Recent Advances in Research of Cerebral Vasospasm – Possible Participation of Endothelin in the Genesis of Vasospasm

T. Sasaki, S. Itoh, and **M. Nishikibe**[1]

Departments of Neurosurgery, University of Tokyo, and [1]Tsukuba Research Institute, Banyu Pharmaceutical Co., Japan

Summary

We presented the following results of our experimental studies performed for testifying the possibility that ET-1 may participates in the genesis of cerebral vasospasm: (1) ET-1 induced strong, long-lasting contractions in major cerebral arteries in vitro, (2) cerebral arteries exposed to SAH were more sensitive to low concentrations of ET-1 than normal control arteries, (3) intrathecal injection of ET-1 produced not only angiographic vasospasm but also sustained decrease in rCBF, (4) intrathecal injection of the novel ET_A receptor antagonist attenuated significantly the degree of angiographic vasospasm on Day 7. These results suggest that ET-1 synthesized in cerebral arteries contributes to the pathogenesis of vasospasm, together with the impairment of endothelium-related relaxation.

Keywords: Subarachnoid hemorrhage; cerebral vasospasm; endothelin; endothelium.

Introduction

Cerebral vasospasm following subarachnoid hemorrhage (SAH) is a significant cause of cerebral ischemia and infarction[7]. Although many vasoactive agents have been reported to be causative factors of vasospasm, its pathogenesis remains obscure.

The vascular endothelium has been generally regarded as a homogeneous cell lining of blood vessels, serving as separation of the intravascular from the extravascular space. Over the last 15 years, it has become apparent that vascular endothelial cells undertake several important functional roles to maintain adequate circulation of blood, including physical and metabolic barrier properties, regulation of vascular tone, and antithrombogenic properties[3]. Of these, endothelium-dependent relaxing factor (EDRF) and endothelin are two recent major discoveries.

Endothelial cells in major arteries are well known to be injured following SAH[21]. On the basis of such observations, we have directed our attention to the role of the endothelial injury in the pathogenesis of vasospasm as an alternative or supplementary hypothesis to the role of vasoactive substances from the subarachnoid blood clot. And, previous studies of ours have demonstrated increased permeability in the major cerebral arteries[18,19], decreased synthesis of PGI_2[17], and impairment of endothelium-dependent relaxation after SAH[12].

On the other hand, De May and Vanhoutte[1] have recently reported vasoconstriction dependent on or enhanced by the endothelium, and in 1988 Yanagisawa et al.[23] isolated a novel vasoconstrictor peptide, endothelin, from the supernatant of porcine aorta endothelium culture. The human endothelin family consists of three distinct isopeptides (endothelin-1,-2,-3)[6]. Endothelin-1 (ET-1) is produced by vascular endothelial cells, and ET-3 is possibly a neural form of ET. ET-1 has been reported to be one of the most potent vasoconstrictors ever known[23]. In addition, the local production of ET-1 in cerebral arteries exposed to SAH could be increased, because the amounts of substances such as thrombin[23] and oxyhemoglobin[8], which stimulate the synthesis of ET-1, are icreased in the cerebrospinal fluid (CSF) or in the subarachnoid blood clots after SAH. Therefore, ET-1 synthesized in cerebral arteries could also contribute to the pathogenesis of vasospasm, together with impairment of endothelium-related relaxation.

In this article, we present the results of our experimental studies performed for testifying the possibility that ET-1 may participate in the genesis of cerebral vasospasm.

Vasocontractile Activity of ET-1 in Cerebral Arteries

In vitro Study

Vasocontractile activity of ET-1 in cerebral arteries was evaluated using an isometric tension recording method[13,14]. As shown in Fig. 1, ET-1 at concentrations of 10^{-12} M to 10^{-7} M elicited dose-dependent contractions of canine, rabbit, and monkey cerebral arteries. The maximum contractile responses were much stronger than those induced by 40 mM KCl. Characteristically, those contractions induced by ET-1 were long-lasting. In monkey cerebral arteries, nearly 70% of the initial contraction was still noted even 12

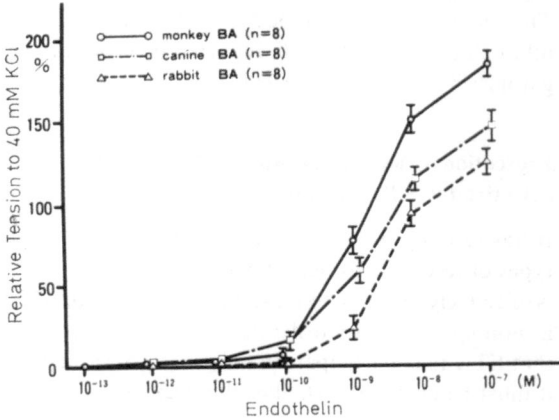

Fig. 1. Contraction-response curves to ET-1 for monkey, canine, and rabbit basilar arteries. *BA* basilar artery (see[14])

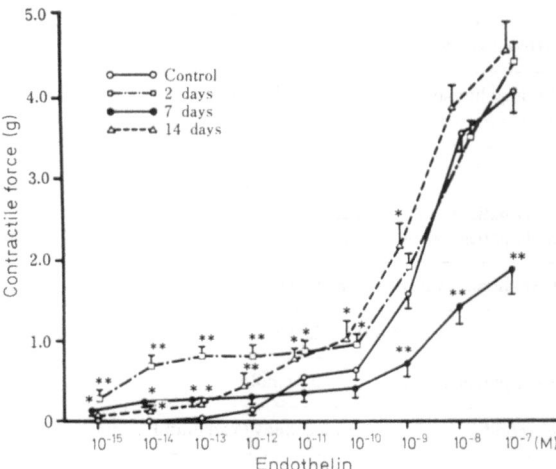

Fig. 2. Effect of SAH on the ET-1-induced contraction of canine basilar arteries (see[14]), $*p < 0.05$, $**p < 0.01$

hours after ET-1 administration. Nicardipine (10^{-8} M) reversed the contraction induced by 10^{-8} M ET-1; however, it took more than 1 hour for the basilar artery to relax to baseline after treatment with the calcium-channel blocking agent. Further more, the increased tone did not quickly return to the resting level after repeated washing with fresh Krebs solution. Those indicate the strong binding of ET-1 to the receptor.

We have also examined whether the sensitivity to ET-1 is altered in cerebral arteries exposed to SAH[14]. As shown in Fig. 2. we have revealed the increased sensitivity to low concentrations of ET-1 in cerebral arteries exposed to SAH.

In vivo Study

It was evaluated whether intracisternal injection of ET-1 induces long-lasting contraction of cerebral artery[4]. Adult mongrel dogs, weighing 8.5 to 12 kg, were anesthetized with pentobarbital (25 mg/kg and supplemental doses as needed). Endotracheal intubation was done and respiration was maintained in the normocapneic state under spontaneous, or, if necessary, controlled ventilation. The right vertebral artery was catheterized for angiography. The femoral artery was also catheterized for the recording of systemic blood pressure and pulse rate. ET-1 dissolved in 2 ml of 10 mM phosphate buffer was injected intracisternally after withdrawing 2 ml of the cerebrospinal fluid. The dose of intracisternally injected ET-1 is 0.2, 0.6, 1.2 or 2.0×10^{-12} mol/kg. Angiograms were obtained before and after the injection of ET-1 at predetermined time intervals (before, 15, 30 min, 1, 2, 24 and 48 h after the injection).

An intracisternal injection of $0.6 - 1.2 \times 10^{-12}$ mol/kg of ET-1 caused biphasic contraction of the basilar artery lasting for more than 24 hours (Fig. 3). The initial phase of the contraction accompanied remarkable changes in vital signs such as an acute rise of blood pressure, bradycardia and respiratory arrest. An intracisternal injection of 2.0×10^{-12} mol/kg of ET-1 also induced acute contraction of the basilar artery. However, all of the dogs which received an intracisternal injection of 2.0×10^{-12} mol/kg of ET-1 died from sustained respiratory insufficiency. In all dogs receiving an intracisternal injection of 0.2×10^{-12} mol/kg of ET-1, neither vasocontractions nor changes in vital signs were observed.

These results indicate that ET-1 induces strong and long-lasting contractions of cerebral arteries. However,

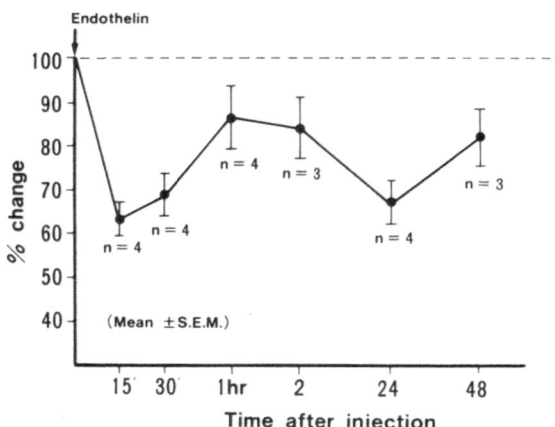

Fig. 3. Changes in the diameter of the basilar artery in dogs receiving intracisternal injection of 0.6 or 1.2×10^{-12} mol/kg of ET-1 (see[4])

the concentration of ET-1 could vary within limited narrow range even under pathological conditions.

Effect of Intracisternal Injection of ET-1 on Regional Cerebral Blood Flow

The effect of ET-1 on regional cerebral blood flow (rCBF) was investigated in adult mongrel cats[11]. Animals were anesthetized with halothane and intubated. ET-1 was injected into the cisterna magna and rCBF was measured by the hydrogen clearance method before and every 30 minutes for 180 minutes after the injection. ET-1 (10^{-11} mol and 10^{-9} mol) induced a sustained decrease in rCBF (Fig. 4) and an increase in arterial pressure. The effects of ET-1 on rCBF and arterial pressure were mediated, at least in part, by Ca^{2+}, because pretreatment with intracisternally injected nicardipine (0.5 mg) prevented the changes. Cerebral angiograms obtained before and after ET-1 injection demonstrated severe constriction of the basilar artery, but constriction of

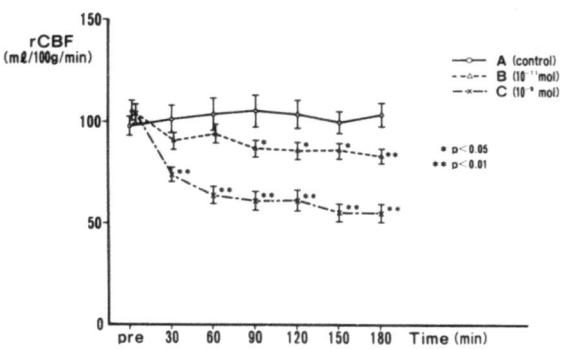

Fig. 4. rCBF before and after intracisternal injection of ET-1

the internal carotid and middle cerebral arteries was mild. Since the rCBF measured was in the territory of the middle cerebral artery, the decrease in blood flow was probably not solely due to the major artery constriction. Other mechanisms such as arteriole constriction may also occur.

Concentration of ET-1 in Plasma, CSF, and Cerebral Artery

The contents of ET-1 in plasma and bloody CSF from patients with SAH were measured by enzyme-immunoassay. The contents of ET-1 in plasma were 1–5 pg/ml, and those in patients with vasospasm were slightly higher than those in patients without vasospasm. The contents of ET-1 in bloody CSF were below 0.5 pg/ml in all patients. The data reported by other investigators[9,20,22] are shown in Table 1.

Prevention of Vasospasm with an Antagonist Selective for ET_A Receptor

It has recently been reported that there are two subtypes of receptors for endothelin; ET_A receptor which is selectively sensitive to ET-1, and ET_B receptor which is non-specific[16]. In order to testify the hypothesis that ET-1 may participate in the genesis of vasospasm, it must be evaluated whether the occurrence of vasospasm is prevented with the antagonist selective for ET_A receptor. As an antagonist selective for ET_A receptor, named BQ-123[5], was supplied by Banyu Pharmaceutical

Table 1. *Concentration of ET-1 in Plasma, CSF, and Cerebral-Arterial Walls Following SAH*

Plasma: human study (Masaoka H, *et al.*)

	Control	Day 3	Day 7
	1.5 ± 0.5		
SAH patients without spasm		4.5 ± 4.2	4.8 ± 4.7
SAH patients with spasm		9.1 ± 3.2	12.0 ± 4.3 pg/ml

CSF: human study (Sato S, *et al.*)

	Day 0-1	Day 6
SAH patients	0.4	2.2 pmol/l

Cerebral arterial walls: animal study (Yamaura I, *et al.*)

	pre-SAH	Day 2	Day 7
SAH dogs	112.9 ± 7.0	180.4 ± 24.7	115.0 ± 24.0 pg/mg protein

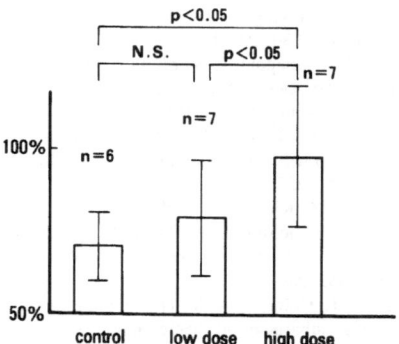

Fig. 5. Effect of intracisternal ET_A receptor antagonist on cerebral vasospasms on day 7 of SAH. The caliber of basilar artery before producing SAH was taken as 100%

Co., Ltd., we investigated the effect of the ET_A receptor antagonist on chronic cerebral vasospasm in the canine two-haemorrhage model. Adult mongrel dogs weighing 8 to 14 kg were anesthetized with intravenous pentobarbital sodium (25 mg/kg). After endotracheal intubation, arterial CO_2 tension was kept at 40 ± 5 torr by adjusting the ventilator or by adding intravenous pentobarbital sodium. Vertebral artery was catheterized for angiography. Experimental SAH was produced by two successive injections 2 days apart, each of 0.4 ml/kg of fresh arterial blood into the cisterna magna after withdrawing 0.2 ml/kg of CSF.

Two days prior to the first SAH, cisterna magna was catheterized with two silicon tubes; one connected with a subcutaneously implanted micro-osmotic pump containing the ET_A receptor antagonist, BQ-123, and the other for producing SAH. The rate of intracisternal injection of BQ-123 was 10^{-6} mol/day for the low-dose group and 5×10^{-6} mol/day for the high-dose group.

On Day 7 after the first SAH, vertebral angiography was performed and the animal was sacrificed.

The caliber of basilar artery before producing SAH was taken as 100%. In control SAH dogs, it decreased to $70.7 \pm 10.2\%$ on Day 7 after the first SAH. In SAH dogs treated with BQ-123, the caliber on Day 7 was $79.3 \pm 17.5\%$ in the low-dose group and $97.6 \pm 20.7\%$ in the high-dose group (Fig. 5). Thus, angiographic vasospasm on Day 7 was significantly attenuated in the high-dose group.

Discussion

As originally reported[23], ET-1 induced strong, long-lasting contractions in major cerebral arteries in vitro.

In addition, the increased tone did not quickly retrun to the resting level after repeated washing with fresh Krebs solution. It indicates strong binding of ET-1 to the ET_A receptor. Further-more, intrathecal injection of ET-1 produced not only angiographic vasospasm but also a sustained decrease in rCBF. Considering these features, it is reasonable to assume that ET-1 may play some important roles in the genesis of vasospasm.

To be a candidate as the real spasmogen, however, the concentration of ET-1 in subarachnoid cisterns or in the vessel wall must be sufficiently elevated during the periods when vasospasm occurs. In our clinical studies measuring the level of plasma ET-1, the level in patients with vasospasm was higher than that in patients without vasospasm. These our results were consistent with previously reported results[9]. The level of ET-1 in bloody CSF has also been reported to be increased between Day 4 and Day 6 after SAH[20]. Thus, the concentrations of ET-1 in both plasma and CSF were increased following SAH. However, those increased concentrations do not appear to be enough high to induce strong, long-lasting contractions of cerebral arteries. Based on the results in both in vitro[13,14] and in vivo[4] experiments in which the vasocontractile activity was evaluated, 10 to 100 times more higher concentrations of ET-1 must be present to induce strong, long-lasting contractions.

Then, we examined whether the sensitivity to ET-1 is altered in cerebral arteries exposed to SAH, and revealed the increased sensitivity to low concentrations of ET-1[14]. However, such augmented contractions induced by low concentrations of ET-1 appear to be still weak for explaining the severe vasospasm.

As ET-1 is presumably acting like a local hormone, the level of ET-1 in cerebral arterial wall is more important than those in plasma and in CSF. Yamaura, et al.[22] have recently measured the level of ET-1 in cerebral arterial wall, and reported that it was 112.9 pg/mg protein prior to SAH, 180.4 on Day 2, and 115 on Day 7. Thus, the level of ET-1 on Day 2 was significantly increased. The results lend support to the idea that ET-1 acts as a trigger in the early stage of vasospasm, although it is not clear whether this increased level of ET-1 is sufficiently high to induce strong vasospasm.

What is the mechansim for the increase of ET-1 in cerebral arterial wall exposed to SAH? Not only vascular endothelial cells but also vascular smooth muscle cells[15] and macrophages[2] synthesize ET-1. Macrophages are frequently observed in the adventitia of cerebral arteries after SAH.

It has also been demonstrated that thrombin[23], oxyhemoglobin[8], and hemodynamic shear stress[24] stimulate the synthesis of ET-1. The hemodynamic shear stress along the luminal side of endothelial cells might be increased in cerebral arteries after SAH, and this may stimulate the synthesis of ET-1 in endothelial cells.

Following SAH, large quantities of thrombin and oxyhemoglobin are present in the blood clots surrounding cerebral arteries. These substances may stimulate the synthesis of ET-1 in smooth muscle cells and macrophages.

Prevention of experimental vasospasm has recently been evaluated with monoclonal antiboby against ET-1[22] or an inhibitor of ET converting enzyme; phosphoramidon[10]. However, the results are controversial. As neither antibody against ET-1 nor phosphoramidon blocks the ET receptor on the membrane of vascular smooth muscle cells, it could be better evaluated with receptor antagonists selective for ET-1 whether ET-1 may participate in the genesis of vasospasm.

There are two subtypes of receptors for endothelin: ET_A receptor which is selectively sensitive to ET-1, and ET_B receptor which is non-specific[16]. Therefore, it must be evaluated whether the occurrence of vasospasm can be prevented with the antagonist selective for ET_A receptor for clarifying the role of ET-1 in the genesis of vasospasm.

Our experimental results in the canine two-hemorrhage model demonstrated that intrathecal injection of the novel ET_A receptor antagonist attenuated significantly the degree of angiographic vasospasm on Day 7. These results strongly suggest the participation of ET-1 in the genesis of vasospasm.

Conclusion

ET-1 synthesized in cerebral arteries contributes to the pathogenesis of vasospasm, together with the impairment of endothelium-related relaxation.

References

1. De May JG, Vanhoutte PM (1982) Heterogeneous behavior of the canine arterial and venous wall. Circ Res 51: 439–447
2. Ehrenreich H, Anderson RW, *et al* (1990) Endothelins, peptides with potent vasoactive properties, are produced by human macrophages. J Exp Med 172: 1741–1748
3. Gerlach E, Nees S, Becker BF (1985) The vascular endothelium: a survey of some newly evolving biochemical and physiological features. Basic Res Cardiol 80: 459–474
4. Ide K, Yamakawa K, Nakagomi T, *et al* (1989) The role of endothelin in the pathogenesis of vasospasm following subarachnoid hemorrhage. Neurol Res 11: 101–104
5. Ihara M, Noguchi K, Saeki T, *et al* (1991) Biological profiles of highly potent novel endothelin antagonists selective for the ET_A receptor. Life Sci 50: 247–255.
6. Inoue A, Yanagisawa M, Kimura S, *et al* (1989) The human endothelin family: three structurally and pharmacologically distinct isopeptides predicted by three separate genes. Proc Natl Acad Sci (USA) 86: 2863–2867
7. Kassell NF, Sasaki T, Colohan ART, *et al* (1985) Cerebral vasospasm following subarachnoid hemorrhage. Stroke 16: 562–572
8. Machi T, Stewart D, Kassell NF, *et al* (1990) Hemoglobin enhances the release of endothelin from cultured bovine endothelial cells. In: Sano K, *et al* (eds) Cerebral Vasospasm-Proceedings of the IVth International Conference on Cerebral Vasospasm. University of Tokyo Press, Tokyo, pp 262–265
9. Masaoka H, Suzuki R, Hirata Y, *et al* (1989) Raised plasma endothelin in aneurysmal subarachnoid haemorrhage. Lancet 9: 1402
10. Matsumura Y, Ikegawa R, Suzuki Y, *et al* (1991) Phosphoramidon prevents cerebral vasospasm following subarachnoid hemorrhage in dogs: the relationship to endothelin-1 levels in the cerebrospinal fluid. Life Sci 49: 841–848
11. Morimoto T, Hanamura T, Sasaki T, *et al* (1991) Effect of intracisternal injection of endothelin-1 on regional cerebral blood flow in cats. Neurol Med Chir (Tokyo) 31: 635–640
12. Nakagomi T, Kassell NF, Sasaki T, *et al* (1987) Impairment of endothelium-dependent vasodilation induced by acetylcholine and adenosine triphosphate following experimental subarachnoid hemorrhage. Stroke 18: 482–489
13. Nakagomi T, Ide K, Yamakawa K, *et al* (1989) Pharmacological effect of endothelin, an endothelium-derived vasoconstrictive peptide, on canine basilar arteries. Neurol Med Chir (Tokyo) 29: 967– 974
14. Nakagomi T, Yamakawa K, Ide K, *et al* (1990) Role of endothelin-1 in experimental cerebral vasospasm. In: Sano K, *et al* (eds) Cerebral Vasospasm-Proceedings of the IVth International Conference on Cerebral Vasospasm. University of Tokyo Press, Tokyo, pp 242–245
15. Resink TJ, Hahn AWA, Scott-Burden T, *et al* (1990) Inducible endothelin mRNA expression and peptide secretion in cultured human vascular smooth muscle cells. Biochem Biophys Res Commun 168: 1303– 1310
16. Sakurai T, Yanagisawa M, Takuwa Y, *et al* (1990) Cloning of a cDNA encoding a non-isopeptide-selective subtype of the endothelin receptor. Nature 348: 732–735
17. Sasaki T, Murota S, Wakai S, *et al* (1981) Evaluation of prostaglandin biosynthetic activity in canine basilar artery following subarachnoid blood injection. J Neurosurg 55: 771–778
18. Sasaki T, Kassell NF, Yamashita M, *et al* (1985) Barrier disruption in the major cerebral arteries following experimental subarachnoid hemorrhage. J Neurosurg 63: 433–440
19. Sasaki T, Kassell NF, Zuccarello M, *et al* (1986) Barrier disruption in the major cerebral arteries during the acute stage after experimental subarachnoid hemorrhage. Neurosurgery 19: 177–184
20. Sato S, Ishihara N, Yunoki K, *et al* (1990) The changes of endothelin concentrations in CSF following subarachnoid hemorrhage. In: Sano K, *et al* (eds) Cerebral Vasospasm-Proceedings of the IVth International Conference on Cerebral Vasospasm. University of Tokyo Press, Tokyo, pp 269–271

21. Someda K, Morita K, Kawamura Y, *et al* (1979) Intimal change following subarachnoid hemorrhage resulting in prolonged arterial luminal narrowing. Neurol Med Chir (Tokyo) 19: 83–93

22. Yamaura I, Tani E, Maeda Y, *et al* (1992) Endothelin-1 of canine basilar artery in vasospasm. J Neurosurg 76: 99–105

23. Yanagisawa M, Kurihara H, Kimura S, *et al* (1988) A novel potent vasoconstrictor peptide produced by vascular endothelial cells. Nature 332: 411–415

24. Yoshizumi M, Kurihara H, Sugiyama T, *et al* (1989) Hemodynamic shear stress stimulates endothelin production by cultures endothelial cells. Biochem Biophys Res Commun 161: 859–864

Correspondence: Tomio Sasaki, M.D., Department of Neurosurgery, University of Tokyo, 7-3-1, Hongo, Bunkyo-ku, Tokyo 113, Japan.

Cerebral Blood Flow in Middle Cerebral Ischaemia is Increased by Calcitonin Gene-Related Peptide

W.A.S. Taylor, S.G.C. Sydserff, and **B.A. Bell**

Department of Neurosurgery, Atkinson Morley's Hospital, Wimbledon, London, U.K.

Summary

This study investigates the effect of an intravenous infusion of calcitonin gene related peptide (CGRP), an endogenous vasodilatory neuropeptide, on cerebral blood flow (CBF) in anaesthetised rats before and after an ischaemic insult.

Anaesthetised male Wistar rats were ventilated at normocapnia, and CBF was measured by hydrogen clearance. A dose-response curve for CGRP was established by infusing 40, 80, 100, and 120 ng/kg/min intravenously. No change in CBF occurred until a dose of 120 ng/kg/min was reached, when mean arterial pressure fell from 96.4 ± 3.0 mm Hg to 85.1 ± 2.4 mm Hg (t = 3.00, p < 0.01), and CBF fell from 91.5 ± 3.0 ml/100g/min to 81.9 ± 1.8 ml/100g/min (t = 2.92, p < 0.01). Middle cerebral artery (MCA) occlusion was produced using an intraluminal filament, and a dose of 100 ng/kg/min was given to rats undergoing MCA occlusion. Groups of ten rats were infused with either CGRP or normal saline, and in the CGRP group CBF was significantly higher (85.9 ± 2.9 ml/100g/min) when compared to the control group (63.7 ± 2.1 ml/100g/min; t = 6.26, p < 0.001). This difference was maintained throughout the period of ischaemia in both the ischaemic and non-ischaemic hemispheres.

These findings suggest that CGRP when given intravenously has a different effect on CBF in the normal and the insulted cerebral circulation and may suggest that it is more likely to influence CBF following a pathological insult such as ischaemia.

Keywords: Calcitonin gene-related peptide; cerebral blood flow; cerebral ischaemia.

Introduction

Calcitonin gene-related peptide (CGRP) is an endogenous neuropeptide which is found throughout the mammalian central nervous system[9] and within nerves of the trigemino-cerebrovascular system[3]. It is a potent vasodilator of cerebral and other blood vessels in vitro and in vivo[3,7,8] and has been shown to have a selective effect on carotid vessels when given intravenously[4,6]. It is this selectivity which has raised interest in a possible therapeutic role in cerebral ischaemia. This study investigates the effect of CGRP on CBF in the normal brain in the anaesthetised rat. It also evaluates the effect of pre-treating an area of focal ischaemia with an infusion of CGRP.

Methods

Male Wistar rats weighing 300–400 g were anaesthetised with fentanyl (0.24 mg/kg), fluanisone (0.75 mg/kg) and midazolam (0.38 mg/kg) i.p., a tracheostomy was performed and they were then paralysed with gallamine (20 mg/kg) i.p. and ventilated. One femoral artery and vein were cannulated to allow continuous arterial blood pressure and heart rate monitoring, arterial blood sampling and administration of drugs and fluids. Middle cerebral artery (MCA) occlusion was produced by an intraluminal filament which produces a proximal MCA occlusion[5]. CBF was measured using the hydrogen clearance technique[1] from four 0.125 mm diameter platinum electrodes placed to a depth of 1 mm in the cortex via burrholes. These were at standardised sites, lateral to the bregma suture and 6 mm posterior to this 4 mm from the superior aspect of the skull. The currents generated by hydrogen gas administered at a concentration of 20% by volume via the tracheostomy were amplified and graphically displayed using computer software developed in our laboratory. The desaturation curves were analysed by fitting the curve to a single exponential and the portion of the curve analysed was from 60–120 seconds after stopping hydrogen administration. Human alpha CGRP was supplied by Celltech Ltd and stored in aliquots at −40 °C and prior to use was dissolved in 1% bovine serum albumin in 0.9% NaCl solution.

In the first series of experiments four groups of ten rats were used and one hour after electrode placement CBF was measured during the next hour whilst 0.9% NaCl solution was given intravenously. After this period CGRP was given in doses of 40, 80, 100 and 120 ng/kg/min by continuous infusion and CBF measured during the subsequent hour. In the second series of experiments two groups of ten rats were used, one group of controls and one group which were infused with 100 ng/kg/min of CGRP as opposed to 0.9% NaCl solution in the controls. These infusions were started after electrode placement but prior to carotid dissection. Once this had been completed and one hour had passed from electrode placement CBF was measured and then MCA occlusion was carried out. CBF was measured immediately after occlusion and at one hourly intervals for a four hour period of occlusion.

CBF and physiological data was collected from all experimental groups and compared using paired and unpaired t-tests. Confidence limits were set at 95%.

Table 1. *Physiological Data*

Dose of CGRP (ng/kg/min)	pH	pO_2	pCO_2	MAP	HR
Control	7.31 ± 0.01	22.21 ± 1.59	4.81 ± 0.08	104.39 ± 2.42	421.60 ± 3.17
After 40	7.28 ± 0.01	22.86 ± 1.53	4.74 ± 0.08	106.50 ± 2.33	416.43 ± 2.99
Control	7.32 ± 0.01	20.99 ± 1.52	4.88 ± 0.07	102.74 ± 2.32	421.33 ± 3.07
After 80	7.33 ± 0.01	21.88 ± 1.32	4.65 ± 0.06	103.85 ± 2.01	420.49 ± 2.62
Control	7.33 ± 0.01	22.31 ± 1.39	4.87 ± 0.14	99.57 ± 2.29	431.43 ± 3.27
After 100	7.34 ± 0.01	18.41 ± 1.26	4.55 ± 0.12	98.62 ± 2.08	426.67 ± 3.01
Control	7.34 ± 0.01	22.07 ± 1.66	4.81 ± 0.13	$96.40 \pm 2.95*$	402.96 ± 3.76
After 120	7.35 ± 0.01	22.43 ± 1.32	4.57 ± 0.11	$85.07 \pm 2.36*$	407.32 ± 3.05

All results mean $\pm$ SEM. *HR* heart rate, *MAP* mean arterial pressure, pCO_2 partial pressure of CO_2 in arterial blood, pO_2 partial pressure of O_2 in arterial blood.
* = $p < 0.05$.

Results

In the first series of experiments there was no change in CBF or physiological parameters in rats infused with 40, 80 or 100 ng/kg/min of CGRP (Tables 1 and 2). However when an infusion of 120 ng/kg/min of CGRP was given there was a significant fall in CBF from 91.47 ± 2.55 ml/100g/min to 81.88 ± 2.07 ml/100g/min ($t = 2.92$, $p < 0.01$). This was associated with a fall in mean arterial pressure (MAP) from 96.40 ± 2.95 mm Hg to 85.07 ± 2.36 mm Hg ($t = 3.00$, $p < 0.005$).

In the second series of experiments physiological parameters were maintained within normal physiological limits throughout the experiments (Table 3). There was a significant difference in the CBF recorded prior to MCA occlusion but after preliminary carotid dissection, with a higher CBF in those treated with CGRP (85.9 ± 2.9 ml/100g/min) compared to the controls (63.7 ± 2.1 ml/100g/min, $t = 6.25$, $p < 0.001$). How-

Table 2. *Cerebral Blood Flow Data*

	CBF (mls/100g/min)
Control	103.26 ± 3.69
After 40 ng/kg/min CGRP	98.37 ± 3.45
Control	90.72 ± 2.35
After 80 ng/kg/min CGRP	87.83 ± 1.83
Control	95.08 ± 3.05
After 100 ng/kg/min CGRP	97.85 ± 2.66
Control	$91.47 \pm 2.55*$
After 120 ng/kg/min CGRP	$81.88 \pm 2.07*$

* $p < 0.05$.

ever, when the CBF in the controls is compared to that of the controls in the first group of experiments it is significantly lower suggesting that carotid surgery causes a fall in CBF. Following MCA occlusion, CBF fell at all electrode sites with the largest fall at the

Table 3. *Physiological Data*

		Pre-occlusion	Post-occlusion	+ 1 Hour	+ 2 Hours	+ 3 Hours
pH	controls	7.32 ± 0.01	7.31 ± 0.01	7.32 ± 0.01	7.34 ± 0.01	$7.35 \pm 0.02*$
	100 ng/kg/min CGRP	7.29 ± 0.01	7.30 ± 0.01	7.32 ± 0.02	7.33 ± 0.02	$7.30 \pm 0.01*$
pO_2	controls	18.64 ± 1.01	14.90 ± 0.96	14.21 ± 0.06	14.23 ± 0.61	14.45 ± 2.42
(kPa)	100 ng/kg/min CGRP	20.10 ± 1.15	17.65 ± 0.78	17.64 ± 1.55	17.03 ± 1.61	17.90 ± 1.45
pCO_2	controls	4.86 ± 0.11	5.03 ± 0.13	4.82 ± 0.09	4.66 ± 0.11	$4.51 \pm 0.12*$
(kPa)	100 ng/kg/min CGRP	4.95 ± 0.08	5.01 ± 0.17	4.64 ± 0.11	4.65 ± 0.17	$5.03 \pm 0.11*$
MAP	controls	92.56 ± 1.80	92.81 ± 2.71	96.36 ± 2.68	96.00 ± 3.83	91.75 ± 3.82
(mmHg)	100 ng/kg/min CGRP	89.57 ± 1.57	89.30 ± 2.25	87.11 ± 2.51	92.67 ± 2.51	92.17 ± 2.21
HR	controls	422.50 ± 2.50	418.18 ± 3.25	418.18 ± 3.25	418.00 ± 4.67	420.00 ± 8.16
(bts/min)	100 ng/kg/min CGRP	421.43 ± 1.42	416.00 ± 2.67	413.33 ± 3.355	415.00 ± 2.94	413.33 ± 6.67

* $p < 0.05$ (unpaired t-test).

Table 4. *CBF Data*

		Pre-occlusion	Post-occlusion	+ 1 Hour	+ 2 Hours	+ 3 Hours
Left ant. electrode	controls	74.21 ± 4.59*	08.62 ± 2.82	10.13 ± 2.13	12.26 ± 3.14	20.12 ± 5.59
	100 ng/kg/min CGRP	99.42 ± 4.96*	16.70 ± 3.38	10.65 ± 2.26	17.56 ± 3.33	29.63 ± 4.56
Left post. electrode	controls	57.61 ± 4.12*	18.08 ± 4.29	13.54 ± 4.56[#]	17.83 ± 4.92	15.36 ± 5.51[#]
	100 ng/kg/min CGRP	82.14 ± 4.75*	29.87 ± 4.56	30.30 ± 4.84[#]	32.20 ± 4.92	35.36 ± 5.03[#]
Right ant. electrode	controls	67.68 ± 5.41[#]	44.70 ± 5.69[#]	45.26 ± 6.66	43.15 ± 6.52	48.75 ± 9.46
	100 ng/kg/min CGRP	87.67 ± 5.18[#]	65.20 ± 6.03[#]	61.95 ± 7.06	58.74 ± 6.52	60.32 ± 7.72
Right post. electrode	controls	57.20 ± 2.53*	43.79 ± 3.88	37.06 ± 2.20	39.09 ± 3.29[#]	37.60 ± 9.72[#]
	100 ng/kg/min CGRP	91.22 ± 1.40*	45.95 ± 4.11	46.69 ± 2.33	49.80 ± 3.49[#]	68.05 ± 6.87[#]

* $p < 0.05$, [#]$p < 0.01$ (unpaired t-test).

anterior electrode in the lesioned hemisphere. The trend for higher CBF in the CGRP treated group was maintained at all electrode sites with the most significant differences observed at the posterior electrode site of the lesioned hemisphere (Table 4).

Discussion

The findings in the first series of experiments would appear to conflict with previous findings that an infusion of CGRP increases carotid blood flow[4,6], with the expectation that CBF would also be increased. Our findings indicate that although carotid blood flow may be increased this is not associated with an increase in CBF. The increased flow may be diverted into the external carotid circulation as part of an autoregulatory response and this is supported by the observation in man that marked facial flushing occurs during infusion of CGRP[6]. However, when a dose which produced systemic hypotension is used, there appears to be a loss of the normal autoregulatory response as there is a corresponding fall in CBF. This observation may be important if the peptide is used clinically for ischaemia because a dose which produces hypotension may adversely affect cerebral perfusion which could be deleterious.

In the second group of experiments preliminary carotid surgery appears to cause a fall in CBF, a finding previously observed following carotid arteriotomy in the rat[2]. This fall in CBF is reduced in those animals treated with CGRP suggesting that whatever factors cause a fall in CBF following carotid surgery they are reversed by an infusion of CGRP. This effect was continued throughout a four hour period of experimental ischaemia. Although this data is encouraging in suggesting that CBF during ischaemia is influenced by CGRP it does not follow that CGRP will influence CBF in a clinical situation as the effect observed experimentally may simply reflect an effect on the fall in CBF produced by carotid surgery.

However, despite these limitations this study shows that the action of CGRP on CBF differs between a normal and an insulted cerebral circulation and this does not rule out its potential use as a therapeutic agent for cerebral ischaemia.

References

1. Aukland K, Bower BF, Berliner RW (1987) Measurement of local blood flow with hydrogen gas. Circ Res 14: 164–187
2. Bell BA, Foubister GC, Neto NGF, Miller JD (1985) Effect of experimental common carotid arteriotomy on cerebral blood flow in rats. Neurosurgery 16: 322–326
3. Edvinsson L, Ekman R, Jansen I, Mc Culloch J, Uddman R (1986) Calcitonin gene related peptide and cerebral blood vessels: distribution and vasomotor effects. J Cereb Blood Flow Metab 7: 720–728
4. Gardiner SM, Compton AM, Bennett T (1986) Regional haemodynamic effects of calcitonin gene related peptide. Am J Physiol 246: R1–6
5. Longa EZ, Weinstein PR, Carlson S, Cummins R (1989) Reversible middle cerebral artery occlusion without craniectomy in rats. Stroke 20: 84–91
6. Mac Donald NJ, Butters L, O' Shaughnessy D, Riddel AJ, Rubin PC (1989) A comparison of the effects of human alpha calcitonin gene related peptide and glycerol trinitrate on regional blood velocity in man. Br J Pharm 28: 257–261
7. Mc Culloch J, Udman R, Kingman TA, Edvinsson L (1986) Calcitonin gene related peptide: functional role in cerebrovascular regulation. Proc Natl Acad Sci USA 83: 5731–5735
8. Mejia JA, Pernow J, Van Holst H, Rudehill A, Lundberg JM (1988) Effects of neuropeptide Y, calcitonin gene related peptide, substance P and capsaicin on cerebral arteries in man and animals. J Neurosurg 69: 913–918
9. Wimalawansa SJ, Emson PC, MacIntyre I (1987) Regional distribution of calcitonin gene related peptide and its specific binding sites in rats with particular reference to the nervous system. Neuroendocrinology 46: 131–136

Correspondence: Mr. W.A.S. Taylor, Department of Neurosurgery, Atkinson Morley's Hospital, Copse Hill, Wimbledon, London SW20 One, U.K.

Anticoagulation Factors, Protein C, Protein S, and Antithrombin III in Subarachnoid Haemorrhage Patients

K. Kanamaru[1], S. Waga[1], K. Tanaka[1], M. Sakakura[2], and A. Morikawa[3]

Departments of Neurosurgery, [1] Mie University School of Medicine, [2] Yamada Red Cross Hospital, and [3] Chusei Sogo Hospital, Japan

Summary

This study evaluated the clinical value of consecutive activity measurements of anticoagulation factors, protein C, protein S, and antithrombin III in plasma from patients with subarachnoid haemorrhage (SAH). Sequential plasma samples were obtained from 22 patients on the following days; 0–3, 5, 8, 14, and 20 after SAH. Then protein C, protein S, and antithrombin III levels were measured using an electroimmunoassay, and vasospasm on angiograms and clinical state of the patients determined. The time courses of 3 factors were classified into 5 groups as following; A) 3 factors abruptly decreased on Days 5 to 8, then increased (N = 2), B) 3 factors continuously increased (11), C) 3 factors under normal range (1), D) 3 factors within normal range (4), and E) 3 factors continuously decreased (4). When clinical outcome was compared to the patient group, the patients in Group B had a significantly better outcome than those in Group E (p < 0.01). Ten of the 11 patients in Group B had an excellent outcome without vasospasm. Three of the 4 in Group D had a favorable outcome. All 4 patients in Group E had a poor outcome due to delayed neurological deficit (DND). The patient in Group C had low anticoagulation factors and a mild DND. Temporary deficiencies of 3 factors occurred in a patient of Group A at the time of DND.

Keywords: Protein C; protein S, antithrombin III; subarachnoid haemorrhage.

Introduction

Recently, activation of coagulation system has been reported in SAH patients[5,8,9]. It was remarkable that the patients with vasospasm had a significantly higher amount of immunocomplexes in serum than those without vasospasm (VSP)[5,8,9]. In extreme disseminated intravascular coagulation (DIC) has been reported as a complication of aneurysmal SAH[11]. In DIC patients anticoagulation factors, such as protein C, protein S, and antithrombin III levels are very low in plasma[3]. The deficiencies of plasma protein C, protein S, and antithrombin III have been demonstrated in the patients with arterial thrombosis[1,7]. Moreover, it has been observed that cerebral arterial thrombosis was associated with a partial temporary plasma protein C deficiency[2]. In the present study we report a decrease in plasma anticoagulation factors in SAH patients and discuss its significance in the pathogenesis of delayed neurological deficit (DND).

Clinical Material and Methods

The series included 22 patients who ranged in age from 27 to 80 years. There were 16 women and 6 men, and mean age was 58 years. The presence of cerebral vasospasm was identified by the occurrence of DND or cerebral infarction. Outcome was defined as following: excellent, no neurological deficits; good, focal neurological deficit without limitation of activity; disabled, partial or total disability; or dead.

Blood samples were obtained on the following days; 0–3, 5, 8, 14, and 20 after SAH. The plasma was prepared and stored at $-20\,^\circ$C. Plasma protein C and protein S antigens were measured by the Laurell rocket electrophoresis method[1]. Antithrombin III activity was measured by chromogenic substrate method. Normal protein C, protein S, and antithrombin III activities were assumed to be in the ranges of 69–134%, 66–134%, and 79–121%, respectively.

Results

Fourteen of the 22 patients had an excellent outcome (63.6%) and 3 patients had a good outcome (13.6%). Three of the 4 patients who died presented severe vasospasm (13.6%). Vasospasm was demonstrated in 9 patients (40.9%). Biochemical and hemostatic tests were performed on the following days; 0–3, 5, 8, 14, and 20, and those were all within normal range. The patients were classified into 5 groups according to courses of 3 factors as following; A) 3 factors decreased on 5–8 days after SAH, then increased, B) 3 factors continuously increased, C) 3 factors under normal range, D) 3 factors within normal range and E) 3 factors continuously decreased. The most common type was Group B ($N = 11$), in which all the patients had a favorable outcome. Three of the 4 patients in Group D had a favorable outcome and normal levels of anticoagulation factors were maintained during the time of observation. The patient in Group C had an excellent outcome, although he had a mild vasospasm on Day 13. All the patients in Group E died due to heart failure. Interestingly, vasospasm occurred in one case of Group A on Day 5 when 3 anticoagulation factors decreased. In Groups A and E clinical condition of the patients was poor when 3 factors were low. When clinical outcome was compared to the patient group, the patients in Group B had a significantly better outcome than those in Group E ($p < 0.01$).

These results suggest that the decrease in anticoagulation factors may play a role in pathogenesis of DND and that low anticoagulation factors might precede the onset of DND and high anticoagulation factors precede favorable outcome after SAH.

Discussion

Activation of coagulation system has been demonstrated in SAH patients[5,8,9,11]. A satisfactory explanation for this event may be the inflammatory process developed in SAH[5,8,9,11]. Activation of coagulation system in SAH may cause the decrease in protein C, protein S, and antithrombin III.

Both protein C and protein S are vitamine K-dependent plasma proteins that together have an anticoagulant function. The enzymatically active form of protein C inhibits the clotting cascade at the levels of factors V and VIII, and protein S as a cofactor in these reactions. Initially protein C activation occurrs on the surface of the vascular endothelium. Because thrombomodulin, a surface protein of the vascular endothelium, forms a complex with thrombin and activates protein C in a Ca^{2+}-dependent reaction. In brain parenchymal vessels thrombomodulin was not demonstrated histochemically[6]. On the other hand, thrombomodulin was present in large cerebral arteries, such as carotid and basilar arteries. Lack of activation system of protein C on the surface of endothelium in brain parenchymal vessels may cause a multiple cerebral microthrombosis in symptomatic cerebral vasospasm[12]. In addition, extensive endothelial cell damages have been demonstrated in spastic cerebral arteries[10]. Endothelial cell damage may also accelerate cerebral thrombosis.

Antithrombin III inactivates thrombin, and factors Xa, IXa, XIa, and XIIa by binding with the target enzyme to form a proteolytically inactive complex. It was suggested that antithrombin III levels decrease with time in poor grade patients with SAH[4]. In addition, antithrombin III might have a significant ability to reverse delayed vasospasm in experimental model of SAH[13]. Decrease in plasma antithrombin III may deteriorate vasospasm.

References

1. Coller BS, Owen J, Jesty J, Horowitz D, Reitman MJ, Spear J, Yeh T, Comp PC (1987) Deficiency of plasma protein S, protein C, or antithrombin III and arterial thrombosis. Arteriosclerosis 7: 456–462
2. Dusser A, Boyer-Neumann C, Wolf M (1988) Temporary protein C deficiency associated with cerebral arterial thrombosis in childhood. J Pediatr 113: 849–851
3. Griffin JH, Mosher DF, Zimmerman TS, Kleiss AJ (1982) Protein C, an antithrombotic protein, is reduced in hospitalized patients with intravascular coagulation. Blood 60: 261–264
4. Kamada K, Takeuchi S, Koike T, Tanaka R, Arai H, Miyakawa T, Sasaki O (1989) Blood coagulation-fibrinolytic changes in patients with severe subarachnoid haemorrhage (in Japanese). Surg Cereb Stroke 17: 111–116
5. Kasuya H, Shimizu T (1989) Activated complement components C3a and C4a in cerebrospinal fluid and plasma following subarachnoid haemorrhage. J Neurosurg 71: 741–746
6. Maruyama I, Bell CE, Majerus PW (1985) Thrombomodulin is found on endothelium of arteries, veins, capillaries, and lymphatics, and on syncytiotrophoblast of human placenta. J Cell Biol 101: 363–371
7. Meada TW, Cooper J, Miller GJ, Howarth DJ, Stirling Y (1991) Antithrombin III and arterial disease. Lancet 337: 850–851
8. Østergaard JR, Kristensen BØ, Svehag SE, Teisner B, Miletic T (1987) Immune complexes and complement activation following rupture of intracranial saccular aneurysms. J Neurosurg 66: 891–897
9. Pelletieri L, Nilsson B, Carlsson CA, Nilsson U (1986) Serum immunocomplexes in patients with subarachnoid haemorrhage. Neurosurgery 19: 767–771
10. Sasaki T, Kassell NF, Yamashita M, Fujiwara S, Zuccarello M (1985) Barrier disruption in the major cerebral arteries following experimental subarachnoid haemorrhage. J Neurosurg 63: 433–440
11. Spallone A, Mariani G, Rosa G, Corrao D (1983) Disseminated intravascular coagulation as a complication of ruptured intracranial aneurysms. J Neurosurg 59: 142–145
12. Suzuki S, Suzuki M, Iwabuchi T, Kamata Y (1983) Role of multiple cerebral microthrombosis in symptomatic cerebral vasospasm: with a case report. Neurosurgery 13: 199–203
13. Vollmer DG, Hongo K, Kessell NF, Ogawa H, Tsukahara T, Lehman RM (1989) Effect of intracisternal antithrombin III on subarachnoid haemorrhage-induced arterial narrowing. J Neurosurg 70: 599–604

Correspondence: Kenji Kanamaru, M.D., Department of Neurosurgery, Mie University School of Medicine, Tsu, Mie 514, Japan.

A Study on Cisternal CSF Levels of Endothelin-1 After Subarachnoid Haemorrhage

P. Gaetani, G. Grignani[1], G. Spanu, and **R. Rodriguez y Baena**

Department of Surgery, Neurosurgery, IRCCS Policlinico S. Matteo and [1]Institute of Patologia Medica I, University of Pavia, Italy

Summary

The aim of the present study was to verify the presence of ET-1 in CSF collected nearby an intracranial aneurysm and to discuss the relationship of cisternal CSF levels of ET-1 with different clinical aspects of the disease (vasospasm grading, Hunt and Hess grading at admission, CT classification of subarachnoid clot deposition, timing of surgery). 55 selected patients with diagnosis of intracranial aneurysms are considered. The control group is represented by 12 patients bearing an unruptured intracranial aneurysm. In all 55 patients a positivity for ET-1 was found; 12 patients were operated on for unruptured aneurysms; twenty-four patients were operated on between day 1 and 4 from last SAH episode and 19 patients were treated with delayed surgery: no statistical difference was found within the three subgroups. No statistical difference in mean cisternal CSF level of ET-1 was found on the basis of CT classification or classification of vasospasm. Mean ET-1 CSF level is significantly higher (p < .05) in patients with high clinical grade at admission (Hunt and Hess 2 and 3) if compared to unruptured aneurysms and Hunt and Hess 1 subgroup. The results of the present study suggest that the rupture of an intracranial aneurysm "per se" does not influence the release of ET-1 in cisternal CSF and that occurrence of vasospasm is not significantly related with cisternal CSF levels of the polipeptide.

Keywords: Endothelin-1 (ET-1); vasospasm; subarachnoid haemorrhage; cisternal CSF levels.

Introduction

Recent experimental works have suggested that specific endothelium deriving factors are involved in the regulation of arterial tone in cerebral arteries[10,23]. Several studies have shown that the endothelium dependent vasodilatory effect due to prostacyclin and EDRF, is significantly reduced after the aneurysm rupture, while, more recently, the class of potent vasoconstrictor polipeptides named endothelins, has been claimed as a possible important vasoconstrictor agent involved in the pathogenesis of vasospasm following subarachnoid haemorrhage (SAH)[2,31].

A lot of experimental work has been done with special regards for aneurysmal subarachnoid haemorrhage (SAH) and the possible involvement of ET-1 in the pathogenesis of arterial vasospasm[2,13,15,20,22,30]. ET-1 elicits a dose-dependent contraction of cerebral artery strips "in vitro" and when injected intracisternally leads to a characteristic biphasic vasospastic response of basilar artery in dogs[15].

However, data available in literature about levels of ET in CSF and plasma of patients with SAH are controversial regarding the possible relationship with arterial vasospasm occurrence. Some authors[16,19] found a direct correlation between a significant peak in plasma level of ET-1 and the occurrence of symptomatic vasospasm; in other series[5] no correlation was found between CSF levels of ET and vasospasm, although a higher plasma level of ET-1 at 8–14 days after SAH was found and related to a possible "stress response" in patients presenting vasospasm[5]. These data cast the doubt whether determination of CSF levels of ET may represent a predictive factor of the clinical outcome, mainly regarding vasospasm occurrence.

In order to verify in a large clinical series the amount of ET-1 in CSF after the aneurysm rupture, we measured in 55 patients with diagnosis of intracranial aneurysm cisternal CSF levels of endothelin 1 and we look for any possible correlation with different clinical patterns of the disease: cisternal CSF is strictly in contact with the arterial branches which display vasospasm and has been considered a reliable mirror of the neurochemical SAH-related patterns[21], more than ventricular or lumbar CSF.

Materials and Methods

Clinical Material

Fifty-five selected patients with diagnosis of intracranial aneurysms are considered. The control group is represented by 12 patients bearing an unruptured intracranial aneurysm which was diagnosed during angiographic studies performed for other reasons (previous episodes of transient cerebral ischemia). For ethical reasons it was not possible to obtain "pure" control cisternal CSF samples and we have to consider these cases as the best control group. Forty-three patients with diagnosis of aneurysmal SAH were included and classified according to the following parameters: timing of surgery, CT classification at diagnosis according to Fisher *et al.*[4] and Hunt and Hess grading at admission[11].

Vasospasm Assessment

Vasospasm was assessed by angiographic study and trans-cranial doppler (TCD) serial measurements. Patients operated on day 1–4 from last SAH episode had angiographic study at admission, prior to surgery, while patients operated on after day 10 from last SAH episode had angiography never before day 8 after the haemorrhage; moreover, all the patients were studied with serial TCD measurements every second day after SAH in order to verify the occurrence of vasospasm during the time of maximal expectation. According to previous experiences reported by other authors[1,7] we have considered the mean velocities found in MCA and ICA because there is a significant correlation between vasospasm intensity and flow velocity measured by TCD in these territories. Combining the data of the angiographic study (according to Fisher's criteria, see[3]) and TCD the following groups were considered: vasospasm (VSP) = 0 for patients with unruptured aneurysm; VSP = 1 when minimal changes and/or mean flow velocity between 80 and 100 cm/s during the first two weeks after SAH; VSP = 2 for ACA and/or MCA diameter at least 1 mm wide and/or mean flow velocity between 100 and 120 cm/s; VSP = 3 for ACA and/or MCA diameter of 0.5 mm and/or mean flow velocity between 120 and 160 cm/s; VSP = 4 for ACA and/or MCA diameter < 0.5 mm and/or mean flow velocity > 160 cm/s.

CSF samples were obtained at surgery by cisternal puncture before the aneurysm exclusion from the subarachnoid cistern nearest to the aneurysm. All patients undergoing early surgery were treated with osmotic agents (mannitol 20%), and clonidine, when required. Patients undergoing delayed surgery were treated with tranexamic acid (6 g/day i.v.) and osmotic agents until surgery.

Radioimmunoassay

All CSF samples were rapidly frozen in vials after centrifugation and stored at −80°C until analysis. The radioimmunoassay was performed on CSF after protein extraction[28]. ET-1 was measured according to Kraus *et al.*[14] using a kit from Peninsula Laboratories, Belmont, CA (Cat. RIK 6901). The kit is 125I labelled and utilizes a rabbit antiserum specific for endothelin (125I-ET-1 from pig), and goat antirabbit IgG serum. Results are expressed in pg/ml of CSF.

Statistical Analysis

Statistical evaluation among groups was performed using the ANOVA and Student's t Test for unpaired data; statistical significance was accepted for p < .05.

Results

In all 55 patients a positivity for ET-1 was found. Four patients presented clinical evidence of arterial vasospasm with angiographical demonstration of high degree of arterial narrowing: because of statistical reasons we have cumulated these cases with 6 patients classified with VSP grade 3 according to grading of Fisher *et al.*[23] and TCD mean velocity > 120 cm/s, although only mild and transient neurological deficits were recorded in these patients.

Twelve patients were operated on for unruptured aneurysms and were classified as CT 0, Hunt and Hess 0 and Vasospasm 0. The ET-1 mean cisternal CSF level was 7.39 ± 1.39 (range 2.4–18.3); twenty-four patients were operated on between day 1 and 4 from last SAH episode: mean cisternal CSF level of ET-1 was 8.56 ± 1.22 pg/ml, without any statistical difference if compared to control cases. In 19 patients treated with delayed surgery the mean ET-1 CSF level was 7.16 ± 1.06 pg/ml: no statistical difference was found with the other two subgroups (Fig. 1).

Figure 2 shows that there is no statistical difference in mean cisternal CSF level of ET-1 according to CT classification. Figure 3 shows that mean ET-1 CSF level is significantly higher (p < 5.0) in patients with high clinical grade at admission (Hunt and Hess 2 and 3) if compared to unruptured aneurysms and Hunt and Hess 1 subgroup.

Regarding the classification of vasospasm, we have found no statistical correlation between the degree of arterial narrowing and or peaked TCD velocities in MCA territory and the mean cisternal CSF level of ET-1 (Fig. 4).

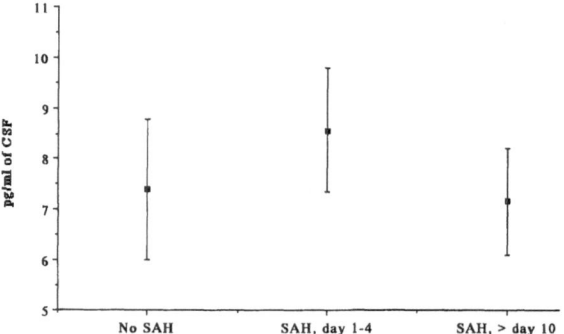

Fig. 1. Graph representation of the cisternal CSF levels of endothelin-1 (mean ± S.E.M.) in subgroups of patients operated for intracranial aneurysm and classified by timing of surgery. Statistical analysis (Anova and Student's t-test for unpaired data) showed no significant differences

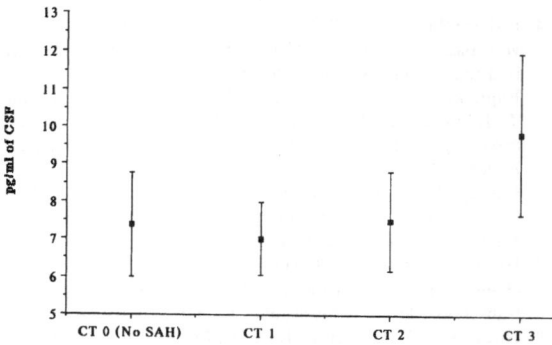

Fig. 2. Graph representation of the cisternal CSF levels of endothelin-1 (mean ± S.E.M.) in subgroups of patients operated for intracranial aneurysm and classified by the amount of subarachnoid blood deposition as shown in CT scan. Statistical analysis (Anova and Student's t-test for unpaired data) showed no significant differences

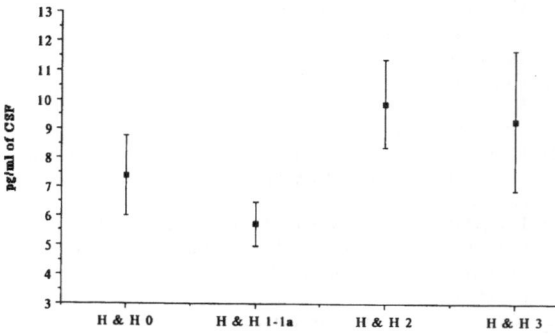

Fig. 3. Graph representation of the cisternal CSF levels of endothelin-1 (mean ± S.E.M.) in subgroups of patients operated for intracranial aneurysm and classified by Hunt and Hess grading at admission. Statistical analysis (Anova and Student's t-test for unpaired data) showed that CSF levels are significantly higher (p < .05) in patients presenting in Hunt and Hess grade 2 and 3 when compared to Hunt and Hess grade 0 and 1

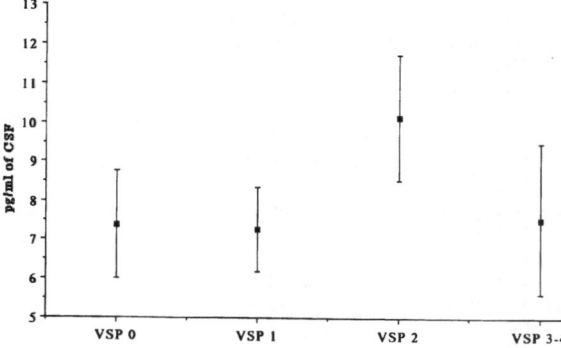

Fig. 4. Graph representation of the cisternal CSF levels of endothelin-1 (mean ± S.E.M.) in subgroups of patients operated for intracranial aneurysm and classified by the degree of arterial vasospasm. Statistical analysis (Anova and Student's t-test for unpaired data) showed no significant differences

Discussion

Since the discovery of ET-1, a possible role in the pathogenesis of arterial vasospasm has been suggested[31]. Many experimental designs "in vitro" and "in vivo" have confirmed the potent vasoconstrictor effect of ET-1 on major arteries in most systemic vascular beds. Recently it has been evident that the endothelial damage occurring after SAH may lead to platelet adhesion and thrombus formation[6,10,23,26]: these events may enhance the local accumulation of factors which in turn stimulate the production of pro-ET-1. On the other hand, ET-1 has been shown to induce a long-lasting vasoconstrictor effect on basilar artery of cats[17], in adult mongrel dogs[4] and a significant reduction of regional CBF in cats[18] after intracisternal administration. However, to date no data about the normal range of ET-1 in CSF and its circulation are available.

Previously reported values of ET-1 CSF levels widely vary because of the different methods used in CSF sampling[14,19,29]. Fujimori et al.[5] did not found any correlation between serial levels of ET obtained in CSF collected through a catheter placed in basal cisterns or in the lateral ventricle. The availability of a "normal range" of ET in CSF was not achieved until now because of the different methods used in deproteinization and different characteristics of CSF samples considered[5,9]. Endothelin does not penetrate across the endothelium and may act only from the adventitial site, as reported in other studies[17,27]. In this, the CSF sampling from the subarachnoid cisterns by a direct puncture before the aneurysm exposure and clipping procedure, allows to detect a level of ET-1, slightly affected by the "stress response" due to surgical procedures[8,24] and to avoid questionable interpretations of data obtained with long-lasting placement of a cisternal catheter in the subarachnoid space[24].

The aim of the present study was to verify the presence of ET-1 in CSF collected nearby an intracranial aneurysm: in contrast with data obtained by other authors, we have found that levels of ET-1 are -in control cases-quite similar to those observed in patients with diagnosis of SAH (Fig. 1) and that there was no significant difference among ET-1 levels in CT classified subgroups according to the amount of subarachnoidal blood deposition (Fig. 2). Only if we consider the clinical classification of patients at admission (Hunt and Hess grading system), we observed a marked increase of ET-1 cisternal CSF levels in patients in grade 2 and 3 when compared to control cases and patients with minimal signs (grade 0 and 1) (Fig. 3). These results suggest that there is no close relationship between cisternal CSF level of the polipeptide and the aneurysm bleeding.

The second remark concerns VSP occurrence: there is no significant correlation between cisternal CSF levels of ET-1 and the classification of vasospasm, nor any difference between levels in control patients and patients with SAH (Fig. 4). On the other hand, if we consider biological characteristics of ET-1 and its role as a local autacoid whose expression may be transiently induced by the accumulation of thrombin, B-TGF, shear stress and other factors after the aneurysm rupture[27,31], measurements of cisternal CSF levels may not reflect events related to a local factor like the proliferative angiopathy characteristic of post-hemorrhagic vasospasm. Thereafter, ET-1 has been demonstrated to activate the phospholipase A2 enzymatic pathway via a G protein and the consequent release of metabolites that in some series have been correlated with the occurrence of symptomatic vasospasm, such as for leukotrienes[21] and lipid hydroperoxides[25]. Thus, ET might at least in part indirectly participate to mechanisms involved in the pathogenesis of arterial vasospasm.

The results of the present study suggest that the rupture of an intracranial aneurysm "per se" does not influence ET-1 release in cisternal CSF; however, considering that values of ET-1 in cisternal CSF of patients operated on either in the acute and in the delayed phase did not significantly differ from levels measured in control cases, we cannot exclude that the presence of the abnormal wall of the aneurysm "per se" may exert a some influence on cisternal CSF level of ET-1.

Acknowledgements

This research was granted by the Italian Ministry for University and Scientific Research, Rome, 1991.

References

1. Aaslid R, Huber P, Nornes H (1984) Evaluation of cerebrovascular spasm with transcranial Doppler ultrasound. J Neurosurg 60: 37–41
2. Asano T, Ikegaki I, Suzuki Y, Satoh S-I, Shibuya M (1989) Endothelin and the production of cerebral vasospasm in dogs. Biochem Biophys Res Comm 159: 1345–1351
3. Fisher CM, Robertson GH, Ojemann RG (1977) Cerebral vasospasm with ruptured saccular aneurysm – the clinical manifestations. Neurosurgery 1: 245–248
4. Fisher CM, Kistler JP, Davis JM (1980) Relation of cerebral vasospasm to subarachnoid hemorrhage visualized by computerized tomographic scanning. Neurosurgery 6: 1–9
5. Fujimori A, Yanagisawa M, Saito A, Goto K, Masaki T, Mima T, Takakura K, Shigeno T (1991) Endothelin in plasma and cerebrospinal fluid of patients with subarachnoid haemorrhage. Lancet 336: 633
6. Furchgott RF, Zawadzki JV (1980) The obligatory role of endothelial cells in the relaxation of arterial smooth muscle by acetylcholine. Nature 288: 346–358
7. Harders AG, Gilsbach JM (1987) Time course of blood velocity changes related to vasospasm in the circle of Willis measured by transcranial Doppler ultrasound. J Neurosurg 66: 718–728
8. Hirata Y, Itoh K, Ando K, Endo M, Marumo F (1989) Plasma endothelin levels during surgery. N Engl J Med 321: 1686
9. Hoffmann Am Keiser HR, Grossmann E, Godstein DS, Gold PW, Kling M (1989) Endothelin concentrations in cerebrospinal fluid in depressive patients. Lancet ii: 1519
10. Hongo K, Kassell NF, Nakagomi T (1988) Subarachnoid haemorrhage inhibition of endothelium derived relaxing factor in rabbit basilar artery. J Neurosurg 69: 247–253
11. Hunt WE, Hess RM (1968) Surgical risk as related to time of intervention in the repair of intracranial aneurysms. J Neurosurg 28: 14–19
12. Kobayashi H, Hayashi M, Kobayashi S, Kabuto M, Handa Y, Kawano H (1990) Effect of endothelin on the canine basilar artery. Neurosurgery 27: 357–361
13. Kobayashi H, Hayashi M, Kobayashi S, Kabuto M, Handa Y, Kawano H, Ide H (1991) Cerebral vasospasm and vasoconstriction caused by endothelin. Neurosurgery 28: 673–679
14. Kraus GE, Bucholz RD, Yoon K-W, Knuepfer MM, Smith KR (1991) Cerebrospinal fluid endothelin-1 and endothelin-3 levels in normal and neurosurgical patients: a clinical study and literature review. Surg Neurol 35: 20–29
15. Ide K, Yamakawa K, Nakagomi T, Sasaki T, Saito I, Kurihara H, Yosizumi M, Yazaki Y, Takakura K (1989) The role of endothelin in the pathogenesis of vasospasm following subarachnoid haemorrhage. Neurol Res 11: 101–104
16. Masaoka H, Suzuki R, Hirata Y, Emori T, Marumo F, Hirakawa K (1989) Raised plasma endothelin in aneurysmal subarachnoid haemorrhage. Lancet ii: 1402
17. Mima T, Yanagisawa M, Shigeno T, Saito A, Goto K, Takakura K, Masaki T (1989) Endothelin acts in feline and canine cerebral artteries from the adventitial side. Stroke 20: 1553–1556
18. Morimoto T, Yoshimoto S, Sasaki T, Saito I, Takakura K (1990) Effect of intracisternal injection of endothelin-1 on regional cerebral blood flow in cats. In: Sano K, Takakura K, Kassell NF, Sasaki T (eds) Cerebral vasospasm. University Tokyo Press, Tokyo, pp 256–258
19. Nakagomi T, Kassell NF, Sasaki T, Fujiwara S, Lehman RM, Joshita H, Nazar GB, Torner JC (1987) Effect of subarachnoid haemorrhage on endothelium-dependent vasodilatation. J Neurosurg 66: 915–923
20. Nakagomi T, Yamakawa K, Ide K, Sasaki T, Saito I, Takakura K (1990) Role of endothelin-1 in experimental cerebral vasospasm. In: Sano K, Takakura K, Kassell NF, Sasaki T, (eds) Cerebral vasospasm. University Tokyo Press, Tokyo, pp 242–245
21. Paoletti P, Gaetani P, Grignani G (1988) CSF leukotrience C4 following subarachnoid haemorrhage. J Neurosurg 69: 488–493
22. Papadopoulos SM, Gilbert LL, Webb RC, D'Amato CJ (1990) Characterization of contractile responses to endothelin in human cerebral arteries: implications for cerebral vasospasm. Neurosurgery 26: 810–815
23. Rubanyi GM, Vanhoutte PM (1985) Hypoxia releases a vaso-

constrictor substance from the canine vascular endothelium. J Physiol 364: 45–56

24. Saito T, Yanagisawa M, Miyauchi T, Suzuki N, Matsumoto H, Jujino M, Masaki T (1989) Endothelin in human circulating blood: effects of major surgical stress. Jpn J Pharmacol 49 [Suppl]: 215

25. Sano K, Asano T, Tanishima T, Sasaki T (1980) Lipid peroxidation as a cause of cerebral vasospasm. Neurol Res 2: 253–272

26. Sasaki T, Murota S, Wakai S (1981) Evaluation of prostaglandin biosynthetic activity in canine basilar artery following subarachnoid injection of blood. J Neurosurg 55: 771–778

27. Shigeno T, Mima T (1990) A new vasoconstrictor peptide, endothelin: profiles as vasoconstrictor and neuropeptide. Cerebrovasc Brain Metab Rev 2: 227–239

28. Suzuki N, Matsumoto H, Kitada C, Masaki T, Fujino M (1989) A sensitive sandwich-enzyme immunoassay for human endothelin. J Immunol Meth 118: 245–250

29. Suzuki H, Sato S, Suzuki Y, Takekoshi K, Ishihara N, Shimoda S (1990) Increased endothelin concentration in CSF in patients with subarachnoid hemorrhage. Acta Neurol Scand 81: 553–554

30. Suzuki R, Masaoka H, Isotani E, Hirakawa K, Hirata Y (1990) "In vivo" effect of endothelin-1 on the basilar artery of rabbits. In: Sano K, Takakura K, Kassell NF, Sasaki T (eds) Cerebral vasospasm. University Tokyo Press, Tokyo, pp 259–261

31. Yanagisawa M, Kurihara H, Kimura S, Tomobe Y, Kobayashi M, Mitsui Y, Yakazi Y, Goto K, Masaki T (1988) A novel potent vasoconstrictor peptide produced by vascular endothelial cells. Nature 332: 411–415

Correspondence: Paolo Gaetani, M.D., Department of Surgery, Neurosurgery, IRCCS Policlinico S.Matteo, I-27100 Pavia, Italy.

Early Blood-Brain Barrier Changes After Experimental Subarachnoid Haemorrhage: a Quantitative and Electron Microscopy Study

D. d'Avella, A. Germano', and F. Tomasello

Neurosurgical Clinic, University of Messina, Italy

Summary

Basic mechanisms underlying blood-brain barrier (BBB) responses to SAH are still to be defined in details. In a rat model of SAH, we assessed BBB changes by means of the quantitative (14C)-a-amino-isobutyric acid (AIB) technique and electron microscopy. Studies of the transendothelial passage of endogenous albumin and IgG permitted comparative quantitative isotopical and qualitative morphological data. Experiments were carried out on the 2nd day post SAH. Compared with sham-operated and mock cerebrospinal fluid injection controls, animals receiving SAH showed a marked increase in Ki for AIB in both cerebral cortices and cerebellar gray matter, averaging 1.3–1.5 times control values, but not in subcortical gray matter or brain stem. Electron microscopy observations disclosed a functional response of the microvascular endothelium, occurring without opening of tight junctions, and resulting in a conspicuous transport of endogenous protein across the intact endothelia. The present study indicates that SAH induces well-defined early changes in BBB function, possibly involved in the pathogenesis of the post-SAH cerebral dysfunction in humans. Results reported here have also potential clinical implications for the management of aneurysm patients.

Keywords: Subarachnoid haemorrhage; blood-brain barrier; experimental models.

Introduction

The trend towards early operation in the management of patients with ruptured intracranial aneurysms[1] has created the need for a detailed understanding of the pathomechanisms operational at the acute stage of subarachnoid haemorrhage (SAH). Early changes in blood-brain barrier (BBB) function have been suspected to be a major causative factors responsible for the post-SAH cerebral dysfunction. An impairment of BBB following SAH has been demonstrated in humans and has been correlated with the development of delayed cerebral ischemia and with a poor clinical outcome[2]. However, only a few laboratory studies have examined the relationship between SAH and changes in BBB function. Results of these investigations have been controversial: some authors reported BBB permeability to be decreased[3,4], others increased[5], and others unchanged[6]. These discrepancies may have originated from limitations inherent to the experimental design or the time window chosen for assessment of the BBB status. The present study was designed to determine the magnitude of subacute changes in BBB function induced by experimental SAH. Permeability changes were assessed by means of the quantitative (14C)-a-aminoisobutyric acid (AIB) technique, as well as electron microscopic (EM) examination of brain microvasculature and observations of endogenous protein leakage.

Methods and Materials

Induction of SAH

Studies employed male Sprague-Dawley albino rats, 250–300 g body weight. Under light halothane anesthesia SAH was induced by administration of autologous blood into the subarachnoid space via the cisterna magna. Details of the procedure were published earlier[7]. Briefly, the atlantoccipital membrane was exposed through an occipital midline incision. For simulation of SAH, 0.4 ml of autologous arterial blood was injected into the cisternal space via a 30 gauge needle over a period of approximately 30 s. Control rats received an intracisternal injection of the same amount of mock CSF.

14C-a-Aminoisobutyric Acid Transport Studies

Six blood-injected, six control, and six sham operated uninjected animals were employed in AIB permeability studies, that were performed two days after the cisternal injections. Under light halothane anesthesia catheters were inserted into femoral artery and vein. Blood pressure, heart rate, body temperature, blood glucose and blood gas concentrations were intermittently monitored throughout the experiments.

Capillary permeability was determined using the method of Blasberg et al.[8] and with standard techniques originated in our laboratory[9]. Seventy-five Ci/kg of (14C) -AIB (Amersham Corp., Arlington Heights, IL, USA) was injected intravenously as a bolus. During the following 20 minutes timed arterial plasma samples were obtained for calculation of the (14C) concentration-time integral. Animals were then killed, and the brains rapidly removed. Measurements of brain isotope concentration were obtained from loci in the frontal, somato-sensory, temporal and occipital cortices, caudate-putamen and thalamus, cerebellar gray matter, and brain stem. Radioactivity in blood and brain was determined by liquid scintillation counting. The blood-to-brain transfer constant for the AIB (Ki) was determined for each locus from the tissue (14C) concentration, and the arterial plasma (14C) concentration-time integral, according to the operational Blasberg's equation.

Morphological Studies

To assess the cerebrovascular permeability two circulating large molecular weight proteins were used. Both proteins, endogenous albumin and endogenous blood-borne IgG, are normally excluded from brain parenchyma by the integrity of the blood-brain barrier[10]. With the aid of the immunocytochemistry IgG and albumin can be visualized. Four rats were injected with blood according to the procedure previously described. At the time of sacrifice, the animals were given an overdose of pentobarbital, and perfused transcardially and fixed with a solution of 2.5% of glutaraldehyde and 4% of paraformaldehyde in 0.1 M of phosphate buffer. Brains were serially sectioned with vibratome at 40 m. The tissue was processed according to the cobalt-glucose oxidase method[11], for the visualization of the horse-radish peroxidase (HRP) reaction products. Brain sections processed for the visualization of IgG were immersed in 10% NRS with 10% Triton X for 1 hour, followed by a 30 min washed in 1% NRS in phosphate buffer saline. The tissue was incubated in byotinyleted rabbit anti-rat IgG (Vector) in a phosphate buffer saline with 1% NGS 1:250 for 30 min at room temperature. All tissue was then washed in phosphate buffer saline and immersed in a byotinelated horseradish-peroxidase complex (ABC Vector) for 45 min. Following several washes in phosphate buffer saline, followed by Tris-HCl buffer, the tissue was reacted for the visualization of the HRP reaction products with the use of the diaminobenzidine.

Brain sections processed for the visualization of the albumin were immersed in 10% NRS in 10% Triton X for 60 min, then were incubated in goat anti-rat albumin kit 1:10000 in 1% NRS overnight in refrigerator. After several washes in 1% NRS in PBS for 30 min, brain sections were incubated in byotinelated rabbit anti-goat IgG in 1% NRS in PBS for 1 hour, then rinsed in PBS and incubated in byotinelated horse-radish peroxidase complex (ABC Vector) for 45 min. Following several washes in phosphate buffer saline, followed by Tris HCl buffer, the tissue was then reacted for the visualization of the HRP reactions products with the use of the diaminobenzidine. Following processing brain sections were prepared for the examination at either light or electron microscopy. Section for LM examination were mounted on glass slides, cleared and coverslipped. The EM sections were osmicated, dehydrated and flat embedded in Medcast resin. Thin sections were cut on a diamond knife, viewed, and photographed on a transmission electron microscope.

Results

AIB Transport

Values of the transfer constant, Ki for AIB, obtained from various brain loci in control animals are consistent

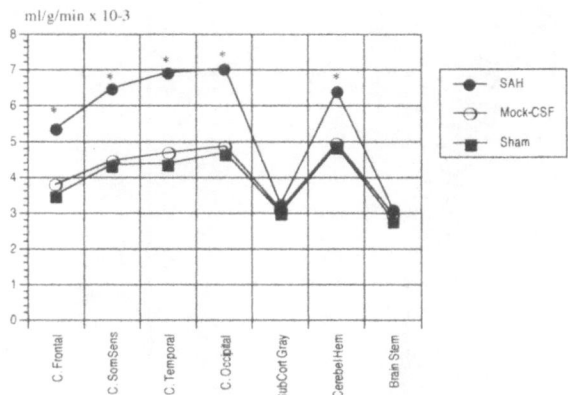

Fig. 1. Transfer constant of Ki for 14C-AIB, *p < 0.05

with those described by others[6,10,12]. In mock CSF-injected animals there was no appreciable increase in AIB transfer constants as compared to control rats. In blood-injected rats Ki for AIB values were significantly elevated (p < 0.05), as compared to controls, in several brain regions. These regions included the frontal, parietal, temporal and occipital cortices, as well as cerebellar gray matter (Fig. 1). This increase ranged from 1.3 times the normal Ki value for the cerebellar cortex, to 1.5 times the normal Ki value for the cerebral cortices. In each instance the increase over the normal value was highly significant.

Morphological Observations

Light microscopy examination revealed spotty staining with horseradish peroxidase reaction product most remarkable in specimens taken from the cerebral and cerebellar cortices. In these areas, electron microscopic observations focused at the level of the cerebral microvasculature revealed antibodies targeted against rat albumin and IgG within the endothelium of the intraparenchymal vessels and a well-demarcated permeation into the basal lamina of the capillaries. The presence of conspicuous immunoreactivity throughout the endothelium suggested movement of albumin and IgG from the blood to the brain front via transendothelial passage. Presumably due to their different molecular weights, the passage of albumin across the BBB was more clearly identifiable than the IgG. This widespread and consistent response of the cerebral microvasculature was identified within vascular beds that failed to reveal any evidence of mechanical rupture or damage. No ultrastructurally visible tearing of endothelial mem-

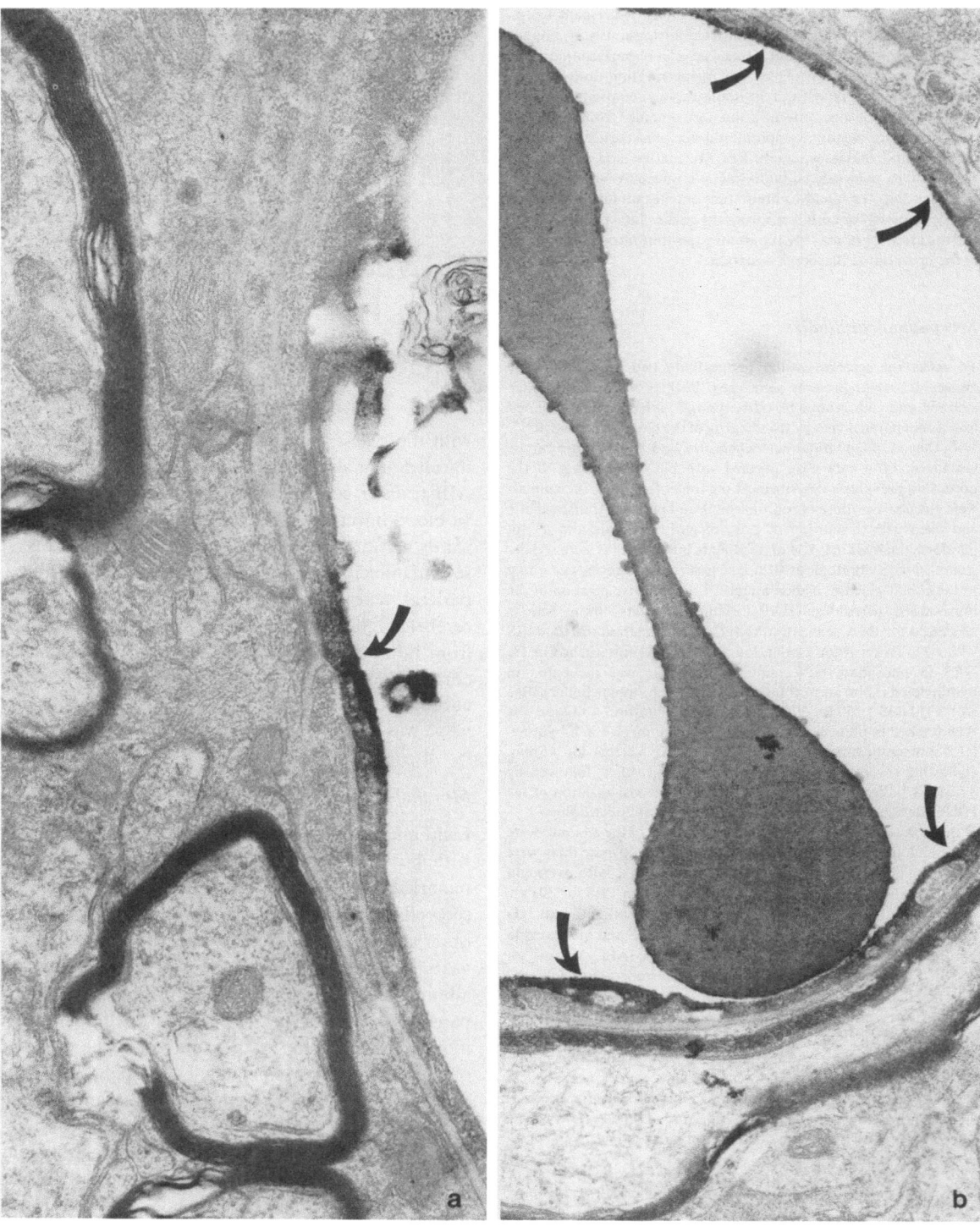

Fig. 2.(a) Forty-eight hours after autologous blood infusion, antibodies targeted against rat albumin reveal albumin immunoreactivity (curved arrow) within the endothelium of an intraparenchimal vessel. The presence of immunoreactivity within the endothelium suggest movement of albumin from the blood to the brain. X 45,000; (b) Forty-eight hours after blood infusion, an intraparenchimal capillary reveals conspicuous albumin immunoreactivity (curved arrow) throughout the endothelium, again suggesting that albumin is moving from the blood to brain front. X 36,000

branes nor frank endothelial destruction was observed, and vascular tight junction appeared intact (Fig. 2a, b).

Discussion

The purpose of this investigation was to quantify the sub-acute effects of SAH on rat brain capillary permeability. The major observations deriving from the present study are as follows:

1. There are regional alterations in the permeability of the rat's BBB to AIB consequent upon release of autologous arterial blood into the subarachnoid space;

2. Electron microscopic observations disclose a functional response of the microvascular endothelium, occurring without opening of tight junctions and resulting in a conspicuous transport of endogenous proteins across the intact endothelia;

3. Barrier alterations occur with a wide range of molecular size species, from a small aminoacid (AIB, MW 140) to large plasma proteins (albumin, MW 70.000, IgG, MW 140.000), although there seems to be some limitation to the permeation of larger molecular weight IgG's.

The findings in the present study substantiate the previously reported increased BBB permeability following SAH and suggest that BBB dysfunction is operational on the 2nd day after the haemorrhage. We chose a 2-days interval in an attempt to correlate BBB changes with increased vasoactive eicosanoids CSF levels seen in our laboratories within two days after the haemorrhage[7].

Although the significant difference in species does not allow direct extrapolation to humans of the present results, we speculate that the permeability changes in the BBB observed at the level of the cerebral microvasculature could be involved in the pathogenesis of the post-SAH cerebral dysfunction in humans.

References

1. Saveland H, Hillman J, Brandt L, Edner G, Jakobsson K, Algers G (1992) Overall outcome in aneurysmal subarachnoid haemorrhage. A prospective study from neurosurgical units in Sweden during a 1-year period. J Neurosurg 76: 729–734
2. Doczi T (1985) The pathogenic and prognostic significance of blood-brain barrier damage at the acute stage of aneurysmal subarachnoid haemorrhage. Clinical and experimental studies. Acta Neurochir (Wien) 77: 110–132
3. Peterson EW, Cardoso ER (1983) The blood-brain barrier following experimental subarachnoid haemorrhage. J Neurosurg 58: 338–344
4. Peterson EW, Cardoso ER (1983) The blood-brain barrier following experimental subarachnoid hemorrhage: response to mercuric chloride infusion. J Neurosurg 58: 345–351
5. Doczi T, Joo F, Adam G, Bozoky B, Szerdahelyi P (1986) Blood-brain barrier damage during the acute stage of subarachnoid hemorrhage, as exemplified by a new animal model. Neurosurgery 18: 733–739
6. Todd NV, Picozzi P, Crockard HA, Ross-Russel R (1986) Duration of ischemia influences the development and resolution of ischemic brain edema. Stroke 17: 466–471
7. d'Avella D, Germano' A, Santoro G, Costa G, Zuccarello M, Caputi AP, Hayes RL, Tomasello F (1990) Effect of experimental subarachnoid haemorrhage on CSF eicosanoids in the rat. J Neurotrauma 7: 121–129
8. Blasberg RG, Fenstermacher JD, Patlak CS (1983) Transport of alpha-aminoisobutyric acid across brain capillary and cellular membranes. J Cereb Blood Flow Metab 3: 8–32
9. Germano' A, d'Avella D, Cicciarello R, Hayes RL, Tomasello F (1992) Blood-brain barrier permeability changes after experimental subarachnoid haemorrhage. Neurosurgery 30: 882–886
10. Ellison MD, Povlishock JT, Hayes RL (1986) Examination of the blood-to-brain transfer of a-aminoisobutyric acid and horseradish peroxidase: regional alterations in blood-brain barrier function following acute hypertension. J Cereb Blood Flow Metab 6: 471–480
11. Ito U, Ohno K, Nakamura R, Suganuma F, Inaba Y (1979) Edema during ischemia and restoration of blood flow. Measurement of water, sodium, potassium content and plasma protein permeability. Stroke 10: 542–547
12. Gross P, Teasdale G, Graham D, Angerson W, Harper A (1982) Intra-arterial histamine increases blood-to-brain transport in rats. Am J Physiol 243: H307–H317

Correspondence: Domenico d'Avella, M.D., Clinica Neurochirurgica, Policlinico, I-98100 Messina, Italy.

Prevention of Experimental Vasospasm with Intermittent Intracisternal rtPA

T. Sasaki[1], K. Takakura[1], T. Wakamatsu[2], and T. Tsuboi[3]

[1]Department of Neurosurgery, University of Tokyo, [2]Department of Neurosurgery, University of Kyorin, and [3]Daiichi Pharmaceutical Co., Japan

Summary

Effect of intermittent intrathecal injection of rtPA(TD-2061) on subarachnoid clot lysis and angiographic vasospasm was evaluated in canine double SAH model. Animals were divided into 5 groups; SAH control dogs, SAH dogs treated with physiological saline, SAH dogs treated with vehicle, SAH dogs treated with rtPA(5kIU/0.5 ml/kg), and SAH dogs treated with rtPA(25kIU/0.5ml/kg). Measurement of tPA activities in CSF following the intracisternal injection of rtPA revealed that thrombolytic activities of rtPA lasted for about 2 h after the injection. In SAH dogs treated with 25kIU/kg of rtPA, the amount or residual subarachnoid clot on Day 7 was significantly less than in SAH control dogs. Intracisternal injection of either 5kIU/kg or 25 kIU/kg of rtPA reduced the degree of vasospasm significantly. These results indicated that four times intermittent infusion of 5-25kIU/kg of rtPA into the cisterna magna was effective in reducing the severity of vasospasm.

Keywords: Subarachnoid haemorrhage; cerebral vasospasm; thrombolytic therapy; plasminogen activator.

Introduction

Cerebral vasospasm following aneurysmal subarachnoid hemorrhage (SAH) is the leading cause of death and disability after aneurysm rupture[6]. Although the pathogenesis of vasospasm has not been clearly understood, there is little doubt that subarachnoid blood is related to the development of vasospasm[5].

Removal of subarachnoid clot prior to the onset of vasospasm is a theoretically attractive approach. Recently, a powerful fibrinolytic agent, recombinant tissue plasminogen activator (rtPA), has been produced, and efficacy of intracisternal rtPA to prevent vasospasm has been evaluated[1-3,11,13]. These investigators have reported that intrathecal fibrinolytic therapy with rtPA appears effective in reducing vasospasm. However, local bleeding complications occurred in some patients after a single injection of high dose of rtPA[4,9]. Lower dose regimens with interval administration should be evaluated.

The present experimental study in canine SAH model was undertaken to determine the satety and efficacy dose of rtPA in the intermittent intracisternal administration.

Materials and Methods

Adult mongrel dogs, weighing 9 to 16 kg, were anesthetized with pentobarbital (25 mg/kg and supplemental doses as needed). Endotracheal intubation was done and respiration was maintained in the normocapneic state under spontaneous, or, if necessary, controlled ventilation. The head was fixed in a stereotactic frame. The right vertebral artery was cathetelized for angiography.

The animals were divided into 5 groups as shown in Table 1. After the control angiography, a silicon catheter was placed in the cisterna magna. This catheter was used for the aspiration of cerebrospinal fluid (CSF) and the cisternal injection of fresh autologous blood or rtPA.

The CSF (0.2 mg/kg) was aspirated, and SAH was produced by two successive injection of fresh autologous blood (0.4 ml/kg) given 48 hours apart.

Physiological saline, vehicle, 5000 international unit (5 kIU)/0.5 ml/kg of rtPA, or 25 kIU/0.5 ml/kg of rtPA was injected four times via the cisternal catheter at 3 h, 12 h, 24 h and 36 h after the 2nd SAH. The rtPA (TD-2061; Daiichi Pharmaceutical Co., Ltd.) was dissolved in distilled water and diluted with physiological saline. The pH of the rtPA solution was then adjusted to around 7.4 with sodium bicarbonate solution.

Serial CSF samples were obtained before and after rtPA administration. The tPA activities were measured with an assay of fibrin clot lysis time.

Table 1. *Experiment Groups*

SAH untreated (control)	n = 11
SAH treated	
Physiological saline	n = 7
Vehicle (solution for dissolving tPA)	n = 5
tPA (5k IU/0.5 ml/kg)	n = 6
tPA (25k IU/0.5 ml/kg)	n = 9

The animals were divided into 5 experimental groups.

On Day 7, animals were perfusion-fixed after angiography. The brains were removed and photographed. Based on the amount of remaining subarachnoid blood clot, the effect of intrathecal rtPA on subarachnoid clot-lysis was evaluated.

Results

Cisternal tPA Activities

The results of serial assays of cisternal tPA activities following the last injection of rtPA on Day 4 are presented in Fig. 1. Cisternal tPA activities prior to the last injection of rtPA(pre 2) were significantly higher than those before induction of SAH(pre 1). This is presumably due to the effects of prior injection of rtPA 12 hours before the last injection. In dogs receiving 5 kIU/kg or 25 kIU/kg, cisternal activities of tPA increased significantly one hour after the last injection of rtPA. Two hours after the rtPA injection activities of cisternal tPA returned to the same level as pre 2.

In dogs receiving vehicle, no such increase of cisternal tPA activities was observed.

Effect of Intrathecal rtPA on Subarachnoid Clot-Lysis

The amount of remaining subarachnoid clots was compared between four experimental groups (Table 2).

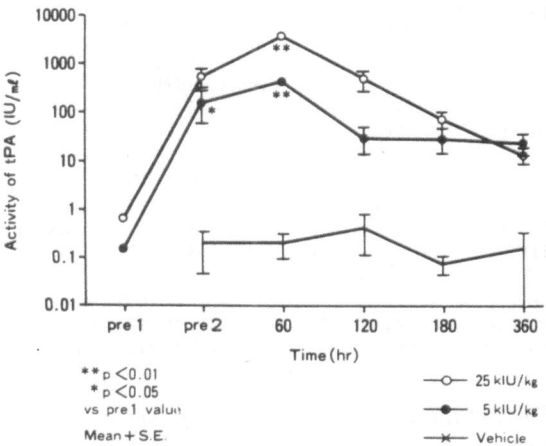

Fig. 1. tPA activity in CSF following intracisternal injection of TD2061 (rtPA) in canine SAH model. The effective increase of tPA activity in CSF was observed for about 2 hours following intrathecal injection of TD2061

Compared to control SAH dogs, no statistical difference was observed in dogs treated with neither physiological saline nor vehicle. In dogs receiving 25 kIU/kg of rtPA the amount of subarachnoid clots was significantly less than those in control SAH dogs (Fig. 2).

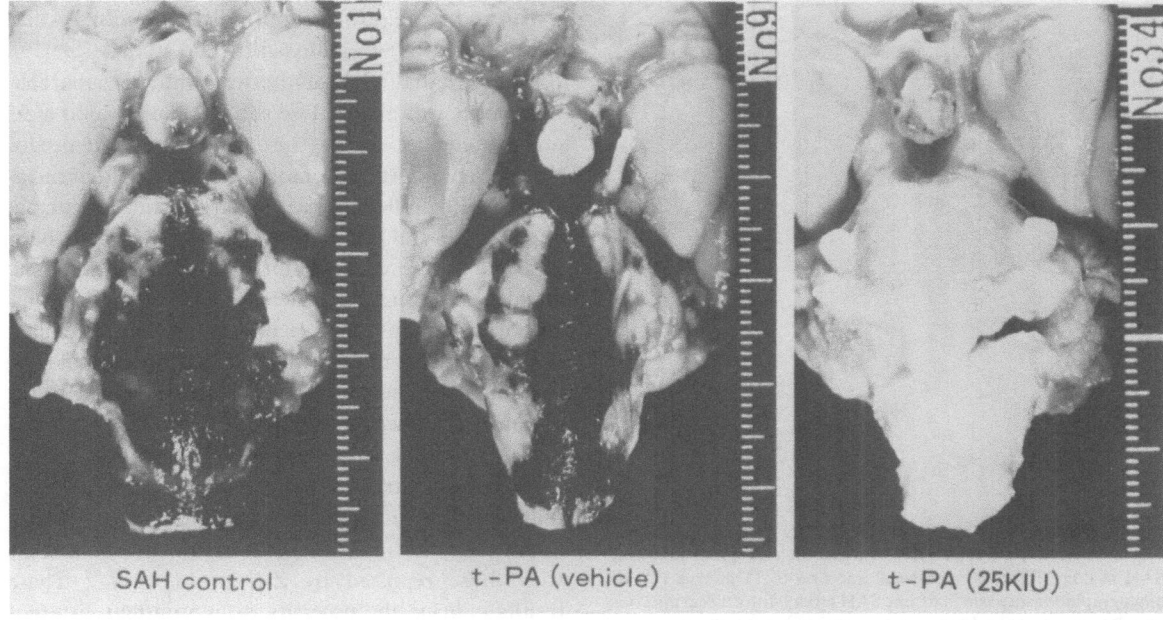

Fig. 2. Photographs of perfused brains on Day 7. Left: a SAH control dog. Center: a SAH dog treated with vehicle, Right: a SAH dog treated with rtPA (25kIU/0.5 ml/kg). No residual subarachnoid clot was observed in a dog treated with rtPA (25kIU/0.5 ml/kg)

Table 2. *Effect of Intrathecal Injection of TD2061 on Blood Clot-lysis in Canine SAH Model*

Groups	Amount of clots					
	Total	⧻	⧾	+	−	X^2test
Control	6	3	3	0	0	
Saline	7	2	1	2	2	N.S.
Vehicle	5	2	1	1	1	N.S.
TD2061 25 kIU/kg	9	0	1	3	5	p < 0.01

In SAH dogs treated with 25 kIU/kg of rtPA, the amount of residual subarachnoid clot was significantly less than in SAH controlled dogs.

Effect of Intrathecal rtPA on Angiographic Vasospasm

Changes of vessel caliber of the basilar artery on Day 7 in each experimental group were shown in Fig. 3. The vessel calibers of the basilar arteries on angiograms prior to the induction of 1st SAH were taken as 100%. In the control SAH group there was a 31% reduction of the vessel calibers on Day 7. The reduction of vessel calibers in dogs treated with physiological saline, vehicle, 5 kIU/kg of rtPA, and 25 kIU/kg of rtPA was 34%, 35%, 23% and 13%, respectively. Between SAH control dogs and SAH dogs treated with physiological

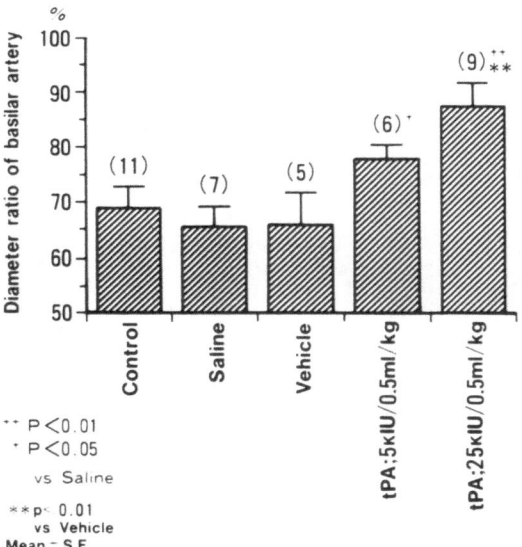

** P < 0.01
* P < 0.05
    vs Saline

** p < 0.01
    vs Vehicle
Mean ± S.E.

Fig. 3. Protective effect of TD2061 (tPA) on vasospasm following SAH in dogs. Effect of intrathecal injection of TD2061 (rtPA) on angiographic vasospasm in canine SAH model. Intrathecal injection of rtPA (25kIU/0.5 ml/kg) significantly decreased the degree of angiographic vasospasm on Day 7, compared to the injection of either vehicle or physiological saline

saline or vehicle, there was no statistical difference in the severity of vasospasm. In SAH dogs treated with 5 kIU/kg or rtPA, the degree of vasospasm appeared to be less than in SAH control dogs. However, there was no statistical difference. Compared to SAH dogs treated with physiological saline, the reduction of vessel caliber was significantly less in SAH dogs treated with 5 kIU/kg of rtPA. Intrathecal injection of 25 kIU/kg of rtPA reduced the degree of vasospasm on Day 7 significantly, compared to SAH dogs treated with either physiological saline or vehicle.

Discussion

The pathogenesis of vasospasm following SAH has not been clearly understood. However, a close association between vasospasm and the amount of subarachnoid blood clots has been demonstrated[5], and extensive removal of subarachnoid blood clots during early aneurysm surgery has been advocated for the prevention of vasospasm[10,12], while several authors[10,12] have reported encouraging results, mechanical removal of clotted blood at the acute stage of SAH is difficult and even hazardous.

An alternative approach for the removal of clotted blood is the use of fibrinolytic agents. A number of japanese neurosurgeons[7,14] have suggested the efficacy of cisternal irrigation therapy with urokinase. Recently, a new and more powerful fibrinolytic agent, rtPA has been produced. Several experimental studies[1,2,3,11,13] have shown that rtPA administered into the subarachnoid space was able to lyse subarachnoid blood clots and prevent vasospasm. The experimental evidence for the efficacy of rtPA promoted clinical trials of intrathecal rtPA following early surgery for aneurysm clipping. Several preliminary results[4,8,9,15] have been reported to be effective for preventing vasospasm, while there is some risk of local bleeding complications. The occurrence of local bleeding complications tended to be in patients treated with a single injection of high dose of rtPA. Then, lower dose regimens with interval administration were evaluated.

The present serial assays of tPA activities in CSF following the intracisternal injection of rtPA revealed that thrombolytic activities of rtPA lasted for about 2 hours after the injection. Our results are consistent with those reported by Zabramski, *et al.*[15] These results indicate the necessity of intermittent cisternal injection of rtPA in the case the low dose of rtPA will be administered.

The present experimental studies also demonstrated that four times intermittent infusion of 5–25 kIU/kg of rtPA into the cisterna magna was effective in reducing the severity of vasospasm. Safety and efficacy of this protocol should be evaluated in clinical trials.

References

1. Findlay JM, Weir BKA, Steinke D, Tanabe T, Gordon P, Grace M (1988) Effect of intrathecal thrombolytic therapy on subarachnoid clot and chronic vasospasm in a primate model of SAH. J Neurosurg 69: 723–735
2. Findlay JM, Weir BKA, Gordon P, Grace M, Baughman R (1989) Safety and efficacy of intrathecal thrombolytic therapy in a primate model of cerebral vasospasm. Neurosurgery 24: 491–498
3. Findlay JM, Weir BKA, Kanamaru K, Grace M, Baughman R (1990) The effect of timing of intrathecal fibrinolytic therapy on cerebral vasospasm in a primate model of subarachnoid hemorrhage. Neurosurgery 26: 201–206
4. Findlay JM, Weir BK, Kassell NF, Disney LB, Grace MGA (1991) Intracisternal recombinant tissue plasminogen activator after aneurysmal subarachnoid hemorrhage. J Neurosurg 75: 181–188
5. Fisher CM, Kistler JP, David JM (1980) Relation of cerebral vasospasm to subarachnoid hemorrhage visualized by computerized tomographic scanning. Neurosurgery 6: 1–9
6. Kassell NF, Sasaki T, Colohan ART, Nazar G (1985) Cerebral vasospasm following aneurysmal subarachnoid hemorrhage. Stroke 16: 562–572
7. Kodama N, Sasaki T, Kawakami M, Sato M, Yamanobe K, Watanabe Z, Yamao N (1990) Prevention of vasospasm; Cisternal irrigation therapy with urokinase and ascorbic acid. In: Sano K, et al (eds) Cerebral vasospasm. University of Tokyo Press, Tokyo, pp 292–296
8. Mizoi K, Yoshimoto T, Fujiwara S, et al (1991) Prevention of vasospasm by clot removal and intrathecal bolus injection of tissue-type plasminogen activator: preliminary report. Neurosurgery 28: 807–813
9. Öhman J, Servo A, Heiskanen O (1991) Effect of intrathecal fibrinolytic therapy on clot lysis and vasospasm in patients with aneurysmal subarachnoid hemorrhage. J Neurosurg 75: 197–201
10. Saito I, Sano K (1980) Vasospasm after aneurysm rupture: incidence, onset, and course. In: Wilkins RH(ed) Cerebral arterial spasm. Williams and Wilkins, Baltimore, pp 294–301
11. Seifert V, Eisert WG, Stolke D, Goetz C (1989) Efficacy of single intracisternal bolus injection of recombinant tissue plasminogen activator to prevent delayed cerebral vasospasm after experimental subarachnoid hemorrhage. Neurosurgery 25: 590–598
12. Taneda M (1982) Effect of early operation for ruptured aneurysms on prevention of delayed ischemic symptoms. J Neurosurg 57: 622–628
13. Yamakawa K, Nakagomi T, Sasaki T, Saito I, Takakura K (1991) Effect of single intracisternal bolus injection of tissue plasminogen activator on experimental vasospasm after subarachnoid hemorrhage. Surgery for Cerebral Stroke (Japanese) 19: 312–317
14. Yoshida Y, Hayashi T, Amoh M, Ahagon A, Kusuno K, Uno T, Ogino T, Kobayashi H, Shibata N, Ueki S (1983) Post-operative intrathecal irrigation with plasminogen activator (urokinase) after early stage operation on ruptured cerebral aneurysm. Neurol Med Chir (Tokyo) 23: 659–666
15. Zabramski JM, Spetzler RF, Lee KS, Papadopoulos SM, Bovill E, Zimmerman RS, Bederson JB (1991) Phase I trial of tissue plasminogen activator for the prevention of vasospasm in patients with aneurysmal subarachnoid hemorrhage. J Neurosurg 75: 189–196

Correspondence: Tomio Sasaki, M.D., Department of Neurosurgery, University of Tokyo and University Hospital, 7-3-1, Hongo, Bunkyoku, Tokyo 113, Japan.

Cerebral Hemodynamics After SAH

Cerebral Blood Flow Assessment Following Subarachnoid Hemorrhage

H. Yonas

Departments of Neurological Surgery and Radiology, University of Pittsburgh, Pittsburgh, U.S.A.

Summary

Quantitative CBF information, especially when coupled with blood pressure and CO_2 challenge, has proven highly useful in guiding day to day management of patients following subarachnoid hemorrhage. As technology continues to improve and become more acessible, clinical management of patients will undoubtedly move toward decisions based on solid physiology, eliminating the use of clinical impressions hastily made at early morning rounds from the foot of the bed.

Keywords: Xe/CT; CBF; vasospasm; SAH; stroke.

Introduction

In this paper I will review CBF physiology, review current CBF methods and present an overview of the types of clinical questions that stable xenon-enhanced computed tomography (Xe/CT) CBF studies are used to answer in the clinical management of SAH patients at the University of Pittsburgh.

Cerebrovascular Haemodynamics

Much of the work leading to an understanding of cerebral ischemia and symptomatic vasospasm following subarachnoid hemorrhage (SAH) has been done using positron emission tomography (PET)[4]. In ischemic tissues compromised perfusion pressure is accompanied by dilation of the arterial supply. Increased blood volume accompanies this autoregulatory attempt to maintain cerebral blood flow (CBF). Mixed cortical CBF values, which normally remain around about $50 \, cc/100 \, g/min$, decline only when the primary and secondary collateral capacity to supply blood is compromised beyond the ability of the arterial vessels to dilate further. The threshold for neurologic symptoms is reached when blood flow values fall to about $20 \, cc/100 \, g/min$. Neurologic dysfunction does not occur before reaching this flow level because initial flow reduction is compensated for by a rise in extraction of essential nutrients, O_2 and glucose from the available blood supply. Once the threshold for neurologic dysfunction is reached, the reversibility of these deficits depends on the depth and duration of the ischemia. Flow values at or near zero are only able to support neuronal survival for a few minutes after which the absence of metabolism occurs.

CBF Techniques

In the past few years a number of new techniques have become available for the clinical study of cerebral perfusion. While each presents advantages, none is as yet ideal.

Positron emission tomography is theoretically the ideal physiological study, but it has limited broad application in clinical management due to limited availability and expense per study. As noted above, PET has provided critical insight into the physiological processes that accompany SAH.

Qualitative CBF measurements using isotopes which bind to the vasculature (iodoamphetamine and HM-PAO) in combination with SPECT imaging have become widely available. By providing multiple planes of flow analysis, flow pattern can be readily assessed. However, there are several disadvantages to this technique: 1) these studies can not be rapidly repeated; usually requiring an interval of approximately 24 hours between studies, 2) each study delivers significant radiation to the entire body, 3) SPECT studies require patient transport to the nuclear medicine department, and 4) patients must remain absolutely still for 15–30 minutes if high resolution images are to be obtained.

Another *qualitative* measure of cerebral perfusion is the transcranial Doppler (TCD) velocity measurement, which provides a comparatively simple and rapidly accessible means for studying cerebral hemodynamics at the bedside. These measurements are primarily made within the major intracranial vessels in and about the Circle of Willis. While velocity measurements have not correlated with either clinical course, CBF values or clinical grade, progressive elevation of TCD's on sequential studies is predictive of compromised CBF and symptomatic vasospasm[1]. TCD change from study to study, although not directly correlated to blood flow, is related to proportional changes in blood flow and therefore should yield important information. Drawbacks to using TCD measurements include: 1) lack of "cranial window" in 10–15% of patients which makes TCD measurements impossible and 2) the inability of TCD to detect spasm in "second order vessels", which in at least 10% of patients is where vasospasm occurs[10]. The later problem may be overcome by more rigorous assessment of the velocity wave form.

Quantitative CBF measurement using Xe^{133} has been available since early 1970's[9]. Arrays of 4–16 scintillation counters placed over each hemisphere provide regional CBF information within and below the cortical mantle. Xe^{133} is most commonly introduced by intravenous bolus and CBF is calculated by analyzing the washout curve using the Kety Schmidt equation assuming a two compartment model. Studies can be repeated after 20 minutes and the smaller arrays can be moved to the bedside. CBF studies using Xe^{133} are, however, limited by poor resolution, insensitivity to focal low flow, and dependence upon normative partition coefficient (lambda values)[13]. Integration of single photon emission computerized tomographic technology (SPECT) and Xe^{133} provides improved CBF localization, but still yields relatively poor resolution, especially within the center of the brain. Xe^{133} CBF studies are associated with a low total body radiation exposure.

Xe/CT CBF has several advantages over the above techniques. Because the Xe/CT CBF calculation integrates tissue specific lambda values it provides more accurate flow information even in the presence of local

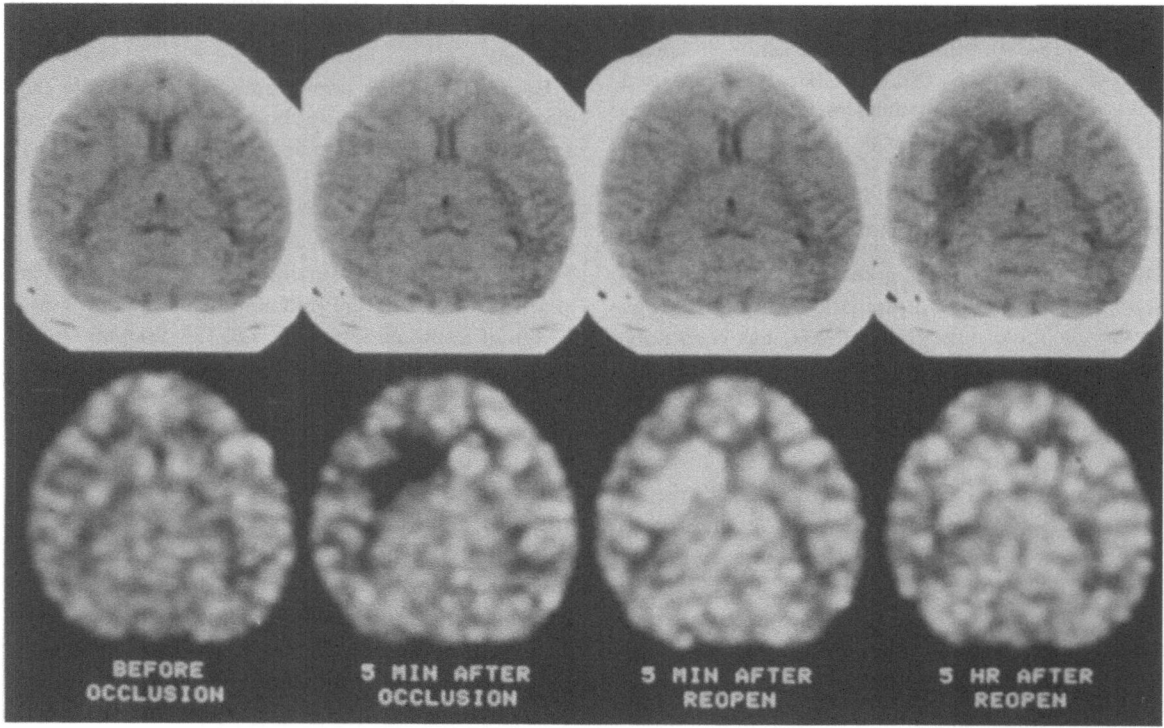

Fig. 1. Clip closure of the lateral striate arteries of the baboon resulted in an abrupt fall in flow to below 5 cc/100 g/min within the ipsilateral caudate and putamen. One hour later, clip removal was followed by absolute hyperemia (CBF > 140 cc/100 g/min). Reperfusion resulted in accelerated CT conversion to low density and CBF fell within 4 hours post reperfusion

pathology. Xe/CT is uniquely able to record very high and very low flow values, both globally or within small central brain regions[5,15] (Fig. 1). CBF data generated using Xe/CT correlates well with Xe[133] as well as other non-clinical quantitative flow techniques. As with CBF studies using Xe[133], stable Xe/CT CBF studies can be repeated within 20 minutes in order to test the effectiveness of proposed therapeutc interventions. However, Xe/CT CBF can only examine 3–4 brain levels/study and studies demand that patients remain still for the 6 minute duration of the complete study. Because of the high resolution associated with current CT technology, motion is a serious problem which is aggravated by the tendency of xenon to induce a mild sensorium alteration. Although xenon is well tolerated by most patients, 5–10% of individuals find the associated sensorial change unpleasant and constant reassurance is required to acquire useful studies in these patients. CBF activation may accompany xenon inhalation, but because these increases are only moderate and are delayed they do not have significant clinical impact[1] or effect the CBF calculation[3]. Although these studies require patient transport to the CT facility, CT imaging is an integral part of the management of most critically ill patients, thus Xe/CT studies add little stress to the critically ill patient. Even though CT is associated with a relatively high radiation dose, a Xe/CT CBF exam is highly focused to highly radiation insensitive structures, with essentially no exposure to the more sensitive organs of the body.

Methods

The Xe/CT CBF imaging protocol at the University of Pittsburg dictates that standard CT images be taken immediately before and during 4.5 minutes of stable xenon inhalation (33% Xe/67% O_2). This data is used to derive high resolution *quantitative* CBF data with direct anatomic reference[5]. In this technique xenon acts similarly to iodine as a radiodense contrast agent. CT enhancement data and the arterial build-up curve of xenon (derived from the measurement of end-tidal xenon) are then used to solve the Kety-Schmidt equation using iterative mathematics. Calculation of flow using Xe/CT assumes a single compartment for flow in each of the 24,000 voxels, measuring $1 \times 1 \times 10\,mm^3$, per CT slice.

To evaluate the use of hypertensive therapy in patients with symptomatic vasospasm double Xe/CT CBF studies in which studies are conducted before and after an induced change in blood pressure are used. Similarly, double CO_2 studies are used evaluate the therapeutic use of hyperventilation.

Results

We have conducted several studies which have proven that Xe/CT CBF is able to record flow values near zero,

even in tissues centrally located within the brain. If near zero flow is maintained for one hour pathological evidence of infarction consistently follows. In a study using baboons the lateral striate artery was occluded and reopened after one hour. This procedure resulted in severe absolute hyperemia and an accelerated conversion of CT to low density (≈ 2 hours post reperfusion)[11]. Ten years of clinical Xe/CT has shown that mixed cortical flow $< 5\,cc/100\,g/min$ results in CT defined infarction. In a study of 14 aneurysm patients, the threshold for irreversible ischemia was defined at $\approx 15\,cc/100\,g/min$ and conversion to CT defined infarction consistently occurred in any region that fell below this threshold (Fig. 2)[17].

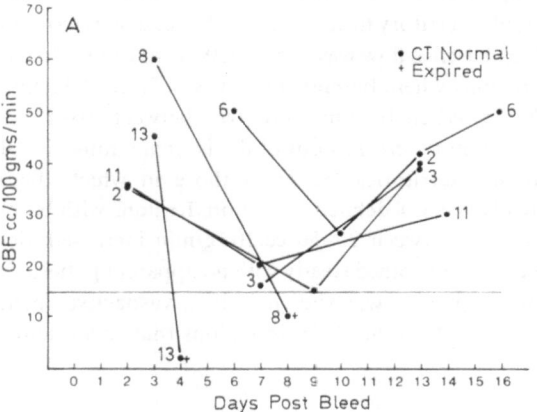

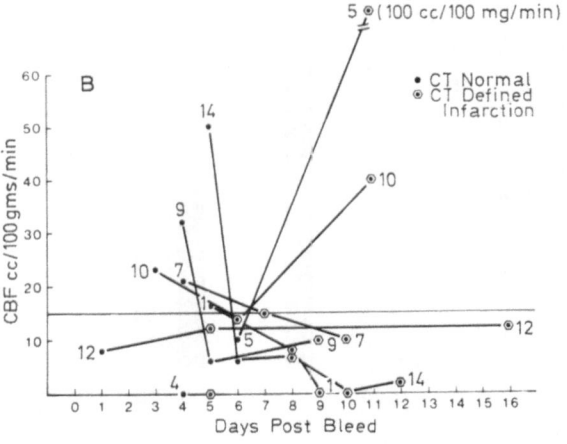

Fig. 2. Patients with symptomatic vasospasm (A) who did not develop CT-defined infarctions and (B) who did develop CT defined infarctions (the numbers represent case numbers and + notes those patients who died). See Yonas H, Sekhar L, Johnson DW, Gur D (1989) Determination of irreversible ischemia by xenon-enhanced computed tomographic monitoring of cerebral blood flow in patients with symptomatic vasospasm. Neurosurgery 24(3): 368–372

Table 1. CO_2 Reactivity

| TEST | CO_2 | | | CO_2 | CBF | | | Percent |
	Pre	Post	Delta CO_2	Reactivity*	Pre	Post	Delta CBF**	Delta CBF#
High to low CO_2	37	28	9 ± 1.53	5.85	43	30	13.9 ± 9.4	51.7 ± 32.9
Low to high CO_2	29	37	8 ± 2.41	3.04	32	39	7.2 ± 11.5	31.5 ± 45.6

t-test, *$p = .011$, **$p = .008$, #$p = .029$.

In a study of 13 SAH patients suspected of having vasospasm, the average of all cortical blood flow resulted in no significant change in global CBF despite blood pressure elevation with dopamine. The inconsistency of CBF response is explained by the fact that CBF tended to go up in low flow areas and go down in high flow areas. When flow was analyzed for each vascular territory flow tended to decrease in regions in which baseline flow was > 50 cc/100 g/min and increase in regions where baseline flow was < 25 cc/100 g/min (Fig. 3). When baseline flow was between 10–25 cc/100 g/min it increased out of the ischemic range in all vascular territories except in those in which there already was CT defined infarction. Regions with baseline flow between 25–50 cc/100 g/min increased, decreased or remained steady with no apparent pattern[18]. Thus dopamine was shown to be a vasoactive agent capable of lowering CBF in regions that retain auto-regulation while being very capable of elevating ischemic levels of flow.

In patients (N = 14) who underwent a CBF study before and after a change in ventilator controlled pCO_2 we observed that CBF change deferentially depended on whether CO_2 was increased or decreased (Table 1). While CO_2 reduction lowered CBF in all but the most injured regions, elevation of CO_2 produced the expected rise in CBF in only 64% of territories. In the remainder of the regions there was either no change or a fall in flow, implying a state of maximal vasodilation and a "steal" response.

Discussion

During the initial hours post SAH the major question in the care of a severely injured patient is viability. The capacity for quantitative CBF methods to rapidly define the absence of cerebral perfusion in all vascular compartments has proved to be a powerful tool for avoiding unnecessary prolongation of family distress as well as the expenditure of vital resources. The measurement of zero flow in the distribution of a deep perforating artery or within the entire brain as recorded by Xe/CT CBF one hour post injury, provides essential insight that the region in question has undergone irreversible ischemic injury[16] (Fig. 1).

While the delayed onset of ischemic symptoms has poorly correlated with angiographic findings, it has consistently correlated with compromised cerebral perfusion. Flow values ranging from 20–25 cc/100 g/min have been reported in individuals with moderate and more reversible clinical deficits while flows less than 12–15 cc/100 g/min are more consistent with severe irreversible ischemic deficits[11] (Fig. 4). The ability to rapidly confirm the presence of an ischemic region is vital in making the diagnosis of symptomatic vasospasm and in guiding clinicians to aggressively improve cerebral perfusion. In a review of our cases, nearly half of the individuals with delayed deficits did not have ischemia due to vasospasm. Instead, deficits were due

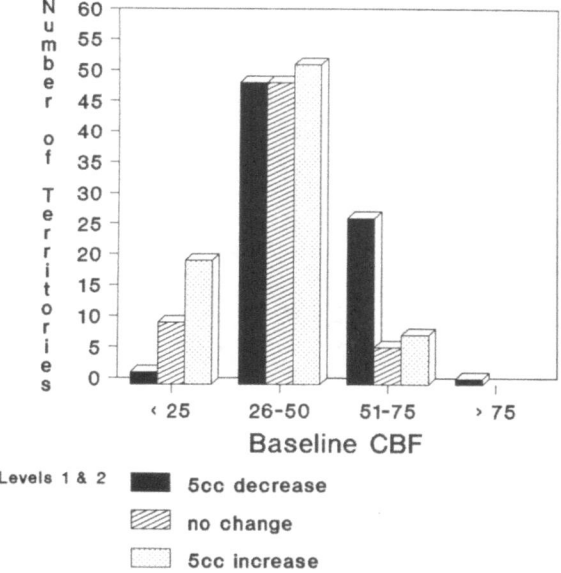

Fig. 3. Territorial CBF response to dopamine administration in patients with subarachnoid hemorrhage

to delayed swelling of small deep infarctions usually secondary to perforator occlusion[14].

Prior to the routine use of selective CNS calcium channel blockade with nimodipine the fall of flow to values near zero was usually abrupt, leaving little warning before the transition to irreversible ischemia. Since the introduction of nimodipine, more moderate flow reductions are often associated with transient symptomatology. This more moderate course has made it easier to identify individuals in ischemic disteess and successfully introduce aggressive therapy to correct the perfusion difficulty.

One method to confirm the need for the treat ischemia entails increasing perfusion pressure. This can be done by elevating blood pressure. Muizelaar was the first to report using Xe^{133} CBF studies prior to and following neosynephrine to provide such information[8]. In contrast to the consistent CBF increase following neosynephrine administration reported by Muizelaar, we have found that dopamine not only elevates CBF in ischemic areas of the brain (regions with flow between 10–25 cc/100 g/min), but can also significantly lower flow in other regions with normal to high perfusion (Fig. 5). The latter responses indicated not only

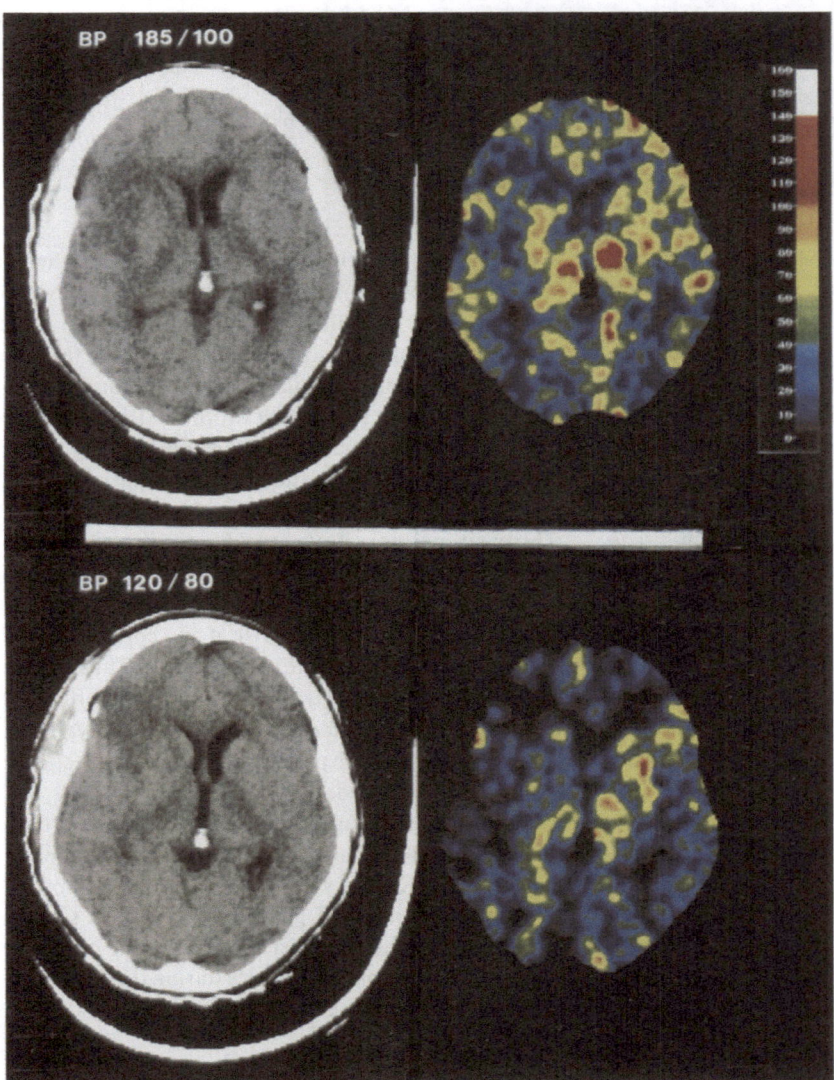

Fig. 4. This 30 year old woman developed left hemiparesis 5 days after subarachnoid hemorrhage despite blood pressure elevation to 150 mmHg. Flow within the left middle cerebral artery territory remained below 20 cc/100 g/min. After blood pressure elevation to 190 mmHg, flow rose to between 25–30 cc/100 g/min and clinical deficit cleared fully

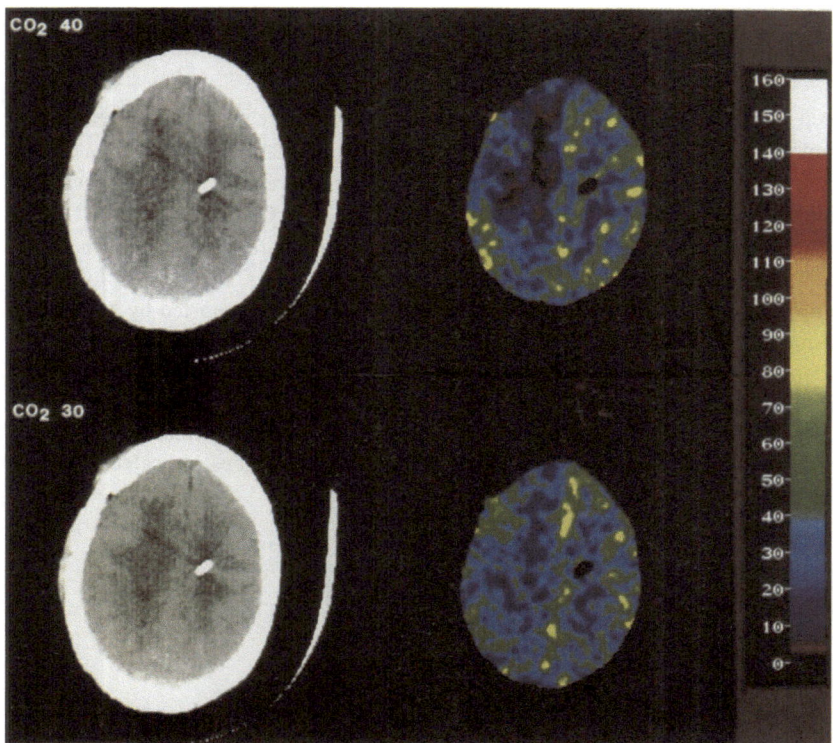

Fig. 5. Ten days after a subarachnoid hemorrhage from a left internal carotid artery aneurysm and 5 days after onset of delayed neurological deficit due to vasospasm, CBF was examined during dopamine elevated blood pressure and again 20 minutes after dopamine withdrawal. Flow was significantly higher in all regions at the lower blood pressure without dopamine

intact autoregulation but a hypersensitivity of the vasculature following subarachnoid hemorrhage to circulating catecholamines. Regions with CT defined infarction consistently had flow values less than 10 cc/100 g/min and tended to remain steady or even fall with blood pressure elevation. Thus only those individuals in whom flow elevated from ischemic to nonischemic levels within defined vascular territories were in need of hypertensive therapy. An equivocal or negative CBF response to dopamine infusion in tissues appearing normal on CT is a useful test confirming the integrity of autoregulation and proves the lack of need for aggressive efforts to improve cerebral perfusion.

Another improtant factor in the diagnosis of SAH is CO_2 reactivity. While CO_2 reactivity has been shown to remain intact except in severely ischemic tissues[12] our work suggests that it is important to discriminate between the CBF response to CO_2 elevation and CO_2 reduction. Volby et al. reported that lowering CO_2 lowers CBF except in near moribund individuals, but our experience suggests greater variability in CBF response and a higher average response to CO_2 lowering. In twelve paired Xe/CT CBF studies we found a 6% reduction in CBF per mmHg drop in CO_2. When

CO_2 was below 30 mmHg, CBF reached ischemic levels in half of the patients. Conversely CO_2 elevaion is a test of the vasodilatory status of the brain. Thus just as in occlusive vascular disease, patients that are already maximally vasodilated can not further vasodilated in response to CO_2 elevation and instead may have lower flow focally (steal response) (Fig. 6). In ventilator dependent grade III and IV patients, CO_2 elevation raised CBF 3% per mmHg CO_2 elevation. Thirty-six percent of all vascular territories demonstrated either steady or *decreased* CBF. Identification of regional steal was useful in identifying vascular territories that remained at risk if any compromise of cerebral perfusion pressure were to occur. Thus neither CO_2 reduction or elevation should be performed cautiously if CBF information is not also available, especially in comatose patients whose clinical response can not be monitored.

The decision to surgically intervene between days 4–10 post SAH remains a major clinical question. As suggested by Knuckey et al., the presence of normal flow has been a useful guide to proceed to surgery irrespective of the day post bleed[7]. At our center 15 patients with normal flow values during this "high risk

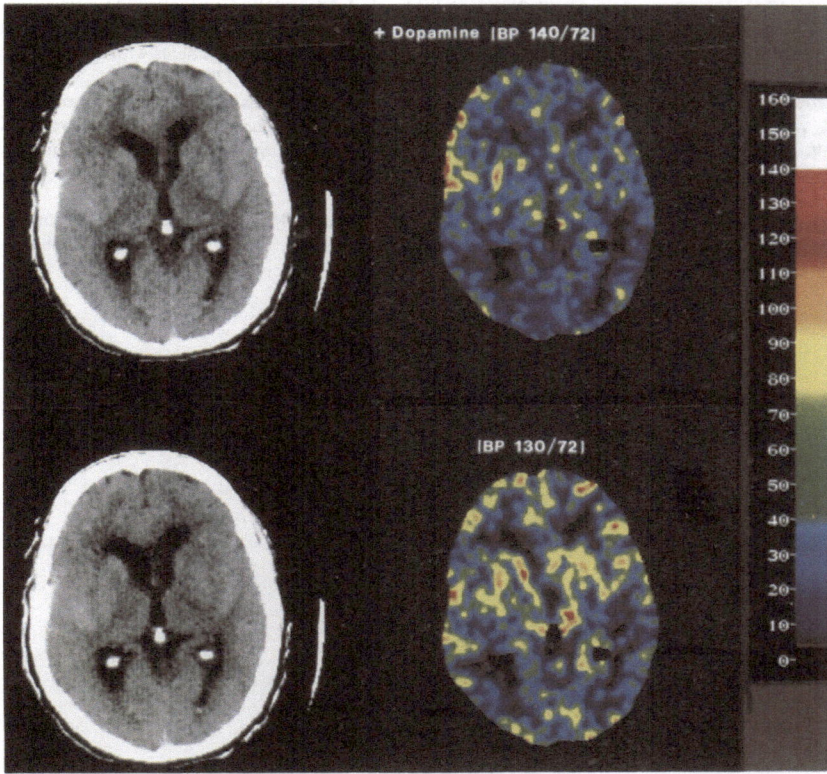

Fig. 6. This 40 year old woman remained comatose and on ventilator support one week after subarachnoid hemorrhage due to a right internal carotid artery aneurysm. The initial CBF study was obtained 20 minutes later at a pCO_2 of 40 mmHg by slowing the ventilator rate. Raising pCO_2 flow steal from the right middle cerebral artery territory

period" sustained no post-operative deficits. Ischemia was then aggressively treated if it later developed. In contrast, patients with regional flow less than 30 cc/100 g/min or an irregular pattern of hot and cold flow consistent with small vessel compromise had a 40% stroke rate. Because only a relatively small percentage of patients today actually develop ischemia secondary to vasospasm, the most rational approach is to operate on individuals with normal CBF values and withhold surgery during days 4–10 in those with reduced flows who may not tolerate brain retraction especially when accompanied by temporary vessel occlusion.

References

1. Darby JM, Yonas H, Pentheny S, Marion D (1989) Intracranial pressure response to stable xenon inhalation in patients with head injury. Surg Neurol 32: 343–345
2. Davis SM, Andrews JT, Lichtenstein M, *et al* (1992) Correlations between cerebral arterial velocities, blood flow, and delayed ischemia after subarachnoid hemorrhage. Stroke 23: 492–497
3. Good WF, Gur G (1991) Xenon enhanced CT of the brain: effect of flow activation on derived cerebral blood flow measurements. AJNR 12: 83–85
4. Grubb RL Jr, Raichle ME, Eichling JO (1977) Effects of subarachnoid haemorrhage on cerebral blood volume, blood flow and oxygen utilization in humans. J Neurosurg 46: 446–453
5. Gur D, Good WF, Wolfson SK, Yonas H, Shabson L (1982) In vivo mapping of local cerebral blood flow by xenon-enhanced computed tomography. Science 215: 1267–1268
6. Hughes RL, Yonas H, Gur D, Lachaw RE (1989) Cerebral blood flow determination within the first 8 hours of cerebral infarction using stable xenon-enhanced computed tomography. Stroke 20: 754–760
7. Knuckey NW, Fox RA, Surveyor I, Stokes BA (1985) Early cerebral blood flow and computerized tomography in predicting ischemia after cerebral aneurysm rupture. J Neurosurg 62: 850–855
8. Muizelaar JP, Becker DP (1986) Induced hypertension for the treatment of cerebral ischemia after subarachnoid haemorrhage. Direct effect on cerebral blood flow. Surg Neurol 25: 317–325
9. Obrist WD, Thompson HK, Wang HS, Wilkinson WE (1975) Regional cerebral blood flow estimated by [133]Xenon inhalation. Stroke 65: 245–255
10. Sekhar LN, Wechsler LR, Yonas H, Luyckx K, Obrist W (1988) Value of transcranial doppler examination in the diagnosis of cerebral vasospasm after subarachnoid hemorrhage. Neurosurgery 22: 813–821
11. Symon L (1978) Disordered cerebrovascular physiology in aneurysmal subarachnoid hemorrhage. Acta Neurochir (Wien) 41: 7–22
12. Volby B, Enevoldsen EM, Jensen FT (1985) Regional CBF, intraventricular pressure, and cerebral metabolism in patients with ruptured intracranial aneurysms. J Neurosurg 62: 48–58

13. Welch KM, Levine SR, Ewing JR (1986) Viewing stroke patho-physiology: an analysis of contemporary methods. Stroke 17: 1071–1077
14. Yonas H (1990) Cerebral blood flow measurements in vasospasm. In: Winn R, Mayberg M (eds) Neurosurgery clinics of North America, Vol 1. Saunders, New York, pp 307–318
15. Yonas H, Gur D, Claassen D, Wolfson SK, Moosy J (1990) Stable xenon-enhanced CT measurement of cerebral blood flow in reversible focal ischemia in baboons. J Neurosurg 73: 266–273
16. Yonas H, Darby JM, Marks EC, Durham SR, Maxwell C (1991) CBF measured by Xe-CT: approach to analysis and normative values. J Cereb Blood Flow Metab 11: 716–725
17. Yonas H, Sekhar L, Johnson DW, Gur D (1989) Determination of irreversible ischemia by xenon-enhanced computed tomographic monitoring of cerebral blood flow in patients with symptomatic vasospasm. Neurosurgery 24: 368–372
18. Yonas H, Snyder R, Marks EC, Johnson DW (1992) Hypertensive therapy in patients with SAH guided by CBF studies. Presented at the Second World Congress of Stroke, Washington, DC, September 1992

Correspondence: Howard Yonas, M.D., Department of Neurosurgery, Montefiore-University Hospital, 3459 Fifth Avenue, Pittsburgh, PA 15213, U.S.A.

Haemodynamic Evaluation of Cerebral Perfusion After Subarachnoid Haemorrhage – a Review

J.D. Pickard[1,2], M. Czosnyka[1], R. Nelson[2], J. Stanley[2], D. Reid[2], R. Coull[2], A.H.J. Lovick[2], and M. Campbell[3]

[1] University of Cambridge Neurosurgery Unit, Addenbrooke's Hospital, Cambridge, [2] Wessex Neurological Centre, Southampton General Hospital, Southampton, and [3] Department of Medical Statistics, University of Southampton, Southampton, U.K.

Summary

The pathophysiology of delayed cerebral ischaemia following aneurysmal subarachnoid haemorrhage is reviewed in the context of the techniques available to study the cerebral circulation in these circumstances. The intravenous [133]Xenon technique has been used to assess cerebrovascular reactivity to a period of brief hypotension and is shown to be a powerful predictor of which patients will develop delayed ischaemia following surgery. The potential of transcranial Doppler to substitute for freely diffusible indicator techniques is discussed.

Keywords: Subarachnoid haemorrhage; cerebral blood flow; cerebral ischaemia; transcranial Doppler.

Introduction

The development of delayed cerebral ischaemia remains a major problem in the surgical management of subarachnoid haemorrhage[19,24]. This occurs despite appreciation of the importance of the pre-operative severity of the patient's condition, his hypertensive status and the timing of surgery, in addition to the proven benefit of hypertensive, hypervolaemic therapy[13,24] and the use of Nimodipine[18]. Several studies have demonstrated a fall in cerebral blood flow (CBF)[8,11,16] following subarachnoid haemorrhage (SAH) and some have suggested that low flows and large falls in CBF are related to poor outcome. There may be some correlation between vasospasm and regional CBF, although experimental work in the monkey indicates that a decrease in vessel calibre of at least 50% is needed to decrease CBF[22]. This is presumably due to vasodilatation of the parenchymal arterioles distal to the stenosis. This phenomenon has been quantified with positron emission tomography: cerebral blood volume increases with increasing vasospasm[8]. In healthy man, normal baseline CBFs fall within a wide range. It is not surprising that a baseline CBF study has little predictve value for the individual patient, although there may be reasonable correlation on a population basis with clinical condition and conscious level. Sequential studies indicate a poor correlation between resting CBF and development of delayed ischaemia in the individual patient and there may be wide regional variations revealed by [133]Xenon, ^{99m}Tc HMPAO-SPET or positron emission tomography. Such results obtained by comparing populations of patients in different clinical grades cannot be used to predict what will happen to an individual patient particularly in the better grades. Cerebrovascular reactivity is a much more robust discriminant between patients than is resting cerebral blood flow alone[4,5,7,10,11,15,17,25]. Studies in man, primates and other species have revealed that autoregulation of cerebral blood flow may be impaired following a recent subarachnoid haemorrhage and that minor additional insults such as moderate hypotension may precipitate cerebral ischaemia in the presence of cerebral vasospasm[24]. Delayed ischaemia is multifactorial in aetiology and a combination of a fall in baseline CBF and impairment of autoregulation of CBF renders the cerebral circulation vulnerable to further insults, for example, vasospasm, hypotension, hyponatraemia, hypovolaemia or hydrocephalus that may complicate SAH. The problem is how best to evaluate the predicitve value of impairment of autoregulation in the pre-operative patient with SAH.

CBF techniques either measure big tube flow (angiography, transcranial Doppler) or true tissue perfusion (non-diffusible and diffusible tracers, "chemical microspheres" such as HMPAO with or without the use of tomography to record regional changes). Big tube flow techniques indicate true blood flow only if arterial diameter remains unchanged. Alternatively, such techniques can only be used to indicate arterial diameter if total blood flow remains unchanged. Hence under conditions of changing diameter (cerebral vasospasm) and tissue perfusion after SAH, it may be very difficult to interpret changes in transcranial Doppler velocity. However, there are also problems with the use of diffusible tracers even when combined with tomographic techniques to avoid the "look-through" phenomenon, whereby areas of ischaemia are not seen by the external counter. Single photon emission computed tomography is difficult to quantify and positron emission tomography is very expensive and logistically very difficult to use with acutely ill patients. However, it is possible to assess cerebrovascular reactivity using the relatively simple intravenous ^{133}Xenon technique.

Method

Wessex CBF Trolley[14]

The Wessex CBF trolley is robust and portable and has been used both in and out of the operating theatre. 60 MBq-Xenon^{133} was injected intravenously, and the subsequent cerebral clearance of ^{133}Xenon measured by scintillation counters. Global or hemisphere CBF may be measured using one or two probes respectively. Analysis of the clearance curve was restricted to a period of 1–3 min after the injection, and the initial slope index used for CBF computation. End-tidal PCO_2 was measured via a catheter in the postnasal space, and a chest probe used to estimate arterial Xenon concentration. This technique may be repeated every 10 min and the results were available within 6 min after the injection of Xenon. The need for a face mask was obviated, and hence minimising the co-operation required from the patient.

Preoperative Assessment of CBF Autoregulation in SAH Patients: the "Stress Test"

In the awake, preoperative SAH patient, hypotension was induced by infusion of trimetaphan, a short-acting ganglion blocker, until mean arterial blood pressure fell to 70% of its baseline value. Patients were sedated with diazepam during the procedure and tilted to 30°

Table 1. *Preoperative Assessment of SAH Patients Using the Stress Test*

	Postoperative ischaemic deficit		Poor outcome
	Immediate	Delayed	
Group A n = 74	31%	9%	12%
Group B n = 29	23%	37%	28%

Group A, patients without significantly impaired autoregulation.
Group B, patients with significant impaired autoregulation.

whilst hypotension was induced. CBF was recorded both before and during hypotension. If global CBF (or hemispherical CBF in later studies) fell by more than 30% from baseline values, the patient was deemed to have significantly impaired autoregulation.

Correlation of Preoperative Cerebrovascular Autoregulation with Delayed Postoperative Cerebral Ischaemia and Outcome Following SAH

One hundred and three patients with proven SAH were studied. The "stress test" was performed prior to clipping of the aneurysm once the surgeon had made the decision to operate on the usual clinical and radiological grounds. The results of the test were withheld from the neurosurgeons.

There were three end points to the trial; immediate ischaemic deficit (present immediately on reversal of anaesthesia), delayed ischaemic deficit, and clinical outcome at 3 months. A bad outcome was defined as severe disability or death.

Retrospective Study of the Correlation Between Impairment of Autoregulation of CBF and Other Factors Following SAH

After the analysis of the previous study in 1985, the stress test became part of the routine clinical management of SAH patients in the Wessex Neurological Centre. Data was collected retrospectively on all the 165 patients who had undergone 196 Stress Tests under the following categories:

Stress test result. Percentage fall in hemispherical or global CBF from baseline during hypotension.

Clinical data. These were obtained from the patient's case notes, and included age, sex, hypotension, smoking, family history of subarachnoid haemorrhage, diastolic blood pressure on admission, World Federation of Neurological societies grade on admission, duration of coma following haemorrhage and drugs administered.

Radiological data. Two independent reports were made on each CT scan and cerebral angiogram, by a neurosurgeon and by a neuroradiologist. The reports were compared and a consensus reached. The amount of subarachnoid blood in the basal cisterns was determined from the CT scan and substantial cisternal blood was defined as either a clot of greater than 2 mm or blood diffusely dispersed throughout the basal cisterns. Previous studies suggested that the amount of cisternal blood is an accurate predictor of subsequent vasospasm and DID[2,6]. The degree of arterial narrowing of the circle of Willis was determined from the angiogram.

Statistics. Multiple regression analysis was used to determine the relationship between the clinical and radiological variables, and the percentage fall in CBF during the stress test.

Results

The mean age of the 165 patients studied was 47 years (range 16–70 years); 57% were female. Preoperative stress tests were carried out between 1 and 95 days following SAH (median 9 days). During the stress test two patients developed transient deficits that had been present earlier during their admission. There were no permanent sequelae.

There was a significant relationship between the fall in CBF during the stress test and the time after SAH. Autoregulation was impaired immediately in many patients following SAH, and remained impaired for 2–3 weeks before starting to return towards normal (multiple regression analysis, $p < 0.05$). Elderly patients had greater degrees of impairment of autoregulation ($p < 0.05$, multiple regression analysis).

In the first "blinded" study of 103 patients, two groups of patients, A or B, were defined on the basis of whether CBF fell by more than 30% (group B) during the period of hypotension. Patients in group B were considered to have significantly impaired autoregulation. The incidence of immediate deficit was the same in the two groups, but the risk of progression or failure to improve was increased from 10.5% in group A to 50% in group B. The incidence of DID was 9% in group A, but 37% in group B. Similarly the risks of a bad outcome were higher in group B at 28% as opposed to 12% in group A. Preliminary analysis of the data demonstrated that the presence of substantial cisternal blood on the CT scan in conjunction with impaired autoregulation significantly increased the risk of DID. Five out of six (83%) patients with both these risk factors developed cerebral ischaemia.

Discussion

A recent study of 3,521 SAH patients from 68 neurosurgical units found no difference in outcome between early surgery (0–3 days) and late surgery (11–14 days)[12]. Hence the neurosurgeon is presented with the task of weighing up the possible risk of precipitating cerebral ischaemia by early surgery to clip the aneurysm against those of delaying surgery and increasing the chances of second haemorrhage for each individual patient. The CBF stress test described here has revealed that even in relatively well patients following SAH, autoregulation of cerebral blood flow may be impaired immediately following the ictus and such impairment may last for two to three weeks. Impaired autoregulation was associated with an increase in delayed ischaemia and a poorer outcome at three months. These results are in agreement with our previous studies[17] and those of other workers. Messeter et al.[15] in a small series of patients found that diminished reactivity to controlled hyperventilation correlated with an increase in delayed ischaemia compared with patients with

intact reactivity. Also in small series of patients[4,10], poorer postoperative results were noticed in patients with global lack of autoregulation. Interstingly, Voldby and colleagues[25] noted a clear association between the presence of vasospasm and impaired autoregulation, and also that the severity of the vasospasm was related to the degree of impairment of autoregulation, although the resting CBF and the neurological condition of the patient may have been normal. He also found that CBF reactivity to hyperventilation was impaired, that these changes were less marked, and a preserved CO_2 response was seen in some patients with impaired autoregulation. Impaired autoregulation or reactivity to hypercapnia is not the sole cause of postoperative delayed ischaemia and subsequent poor outcome, but it will put the patient at increased risk of delayed ischaemia should the circulation be subjected to further insults, e.g. vasospasm, hypotension, hyponatraemia, hypovolaemia or hydrocephalus. Such a hypothesis would explain why patients with a substantial cisternal blood (and thus increased risk of vasospasm) had such a high risk of developing delayed ischaemia in our study. The use of the Stress Test suggests caution in some good grade patients and encourages earlier surgery in apparently poorer grade patients.

Transcranial Doppler

There remains considerable controversy over the value of sequential studies of the mean cerebral artery velocity measured with TCD and their prognostic value[1,9,20,21,23]. However, recent studies have suggested that it is possible to estimate whether hemisphere autoregulation is intact or not[3,16,17] and more substantial clinical series examining this technique in patients with subarachnoid haemorrhage are awaited.

Acknowledgement

The authors are very grateful to the Chest Heart and Stroke Association for their support.

References

1. Aaslid R, Huber P, Nornes H (1984) Evaluation of cerebrovascular spasm with transcranial ultrasound, J Neurosurg 60: 37–41
2. Bell B, Kendall B, Symon L (1980) Computed tomography in aneurysmal subarachnoid haemorrhage. J Neurol Neurosurg Psychiatry 43: 522–524
3. Czosnyka M, Pickard JD, Whitehouse H, Piechnik S (1992) The

hyperaemic response to a transient reduction in cerebral perfusion pressure – a modelling study. Acta Neurochir (Wien) 115: 90–97

4. Dernbach P, Little JR, Jones SC, Ebrahim Z (1988) Altered cerebral autoregulation and CO_2 reactivity after aneurysmal subarachnoid haemorrhage. Neurosurgery 22: 822–826

5. Farrar JK, Gamache FW, Ferguson GG, Drake CG (1981) Effects of profound hypotension on cerebral blood flow during surgery for intracranial aneurysms. J Neurosurg 55: 857–864

6. Fisher CM, Kistler JP, David JM (1980) Relation of cerebral vasospasm to subarachnoid haemorrhage visualised by computed tomographic scanning. Neurosurgery 6: 1–9

7. Geraud G, Tremaulet M, Gueii A, Beo A (1984) The prognostic value of non-invasive cerebral blood flow treatment in subarachnoid haemorrhage. Stroke 15: 301–305

8. Grubb RL Jr, Raichle ME, Eichling JO, Gado MH (1977) Effects of subarachnoid haemorrhage on cerebral blood volume, blood flow and oxygen utilization in humans. J Neurosurg 46: 446–453

9. Harders AG, Gilsbach JM (1987) Time course of blood velocity changes related to vasospasm in the circle of Willis measured by transcranial Doppler ultrasound. J Neurosurg 66: 718–728

10. Heilbrun MP, Olesen J, Lassen N (1972) Regional cerebral blood flow studies in subarachnoid haemorrhage. J Neurosurg 37: 36–44

11. Ishii R (1979) Regional cerebral blood flow in patients with ruptured intracranial aneurysms. J Neurosurg 50: 587–594

12. Kassell NF, Torner JC, Haley EC, *et al* (1990) The International Cooperative Study on the timing of aneurysm surgery I. Overall management results. J Neurosurg 73: 18–36

13. Kosnik E, Hunt W (1970) Postoperative hypertension in the management of intracranial arterial aneurysms. J Neurosurg 45: 148–154

14. Lovick AHJ, Pickard JD, Goldard BA (1982) Prediction of late ischaemic complications after cerebral aneurysm surgery – use of a mobile microcomputer system for the measurement of pre-, intra – and post-operative cerebral blood flow. Acta Neurochir (Wien) 63: 37–49

15. Messeter K, Brandt L, Ljunngren B, *et al* (1987) Prediction and prevention of delayed ischaemic dysfunction after aneurysmal SAH and early operation. Neurosurgery 20: 548–553

16. Meyer CHA, Lowe D, Meyer M, *et al* (1983) Progressive change in cerebral blood flow during the first three weeks after subarachnoid haemorrhage. Neurosurgery 12: 58–76

17. Nelson RJ, Perry S, Hames TK, Pickard JD (1990) Transcranial Doppler ultrasound studies of cerebral autoregulation and subarachnoid haemorrhage in the rabbit. J Neurosurg 73: 601–610

18. Nelson RJ, Czosnyka M, Pickard JD, *et al* (1993) Experimental aspects of cerebrospinal haemodynamics: the relationship between blood flow velocity waveform and cerebral autoregulation. Neurosurgery, in press

19. Pickard JD, Mathieson M, Patterson J, Wyper D (1980) Prediction of late ischaemic complications after cerebral aneurysm surgery by the intraoperative measurement of CBF. J Neurosurg 53: 305–308

20. Pickard JD, Murray GD, Illingworth R, *et al* (1989) Effect of nimodipine on cerebral infarction and outcome after aneurysmal subarachnoid haemorrhage: British aneurysm nimodipine trial. BMJ 298: 636–642

21. Pickard JD, Nelson R, Martin JL (1992) Pathophysiology of aneurysmal subarachnoid haemorrhage. In: Teasdale GM, Miller JD (eds) Current neurosurgery. Churchill Livingstone, Edinburgh, pp 1–38

22. Romner B, Ljunngren B, Brandt L, *et al* (1990) Correlation of transcranial Doppler sonography findings with timing of aneurysm surgery. J Neurosurg 73: 72–76

23. Sekhar L, Wechsler LR, Yonas H, *et al* (1988) Value of transcranial Doppler examination in the diagnosis of cerebral vasospasm after subarachnoid haemorrhage. Neurosurgery 22: 813–821

24. Simeone FA, Trepper PJ, Brown DJ (1972) Cerebral blood flow evaluation of prolonged experimental vasospasm. J Neurosurg 37: 302–311

25. Sloan MA, Haley EC, Kassell NF, *et al* (1989) Sensitivity and specificity of transcranial Doppler ultrasonography in the diagnosis of vasospasm following subarachnoid haemorrhage. Neurology 39: 1514–1518

26. Symon L (1978) Disordered cerebrovascular physiology in aneurysmal subarachnoid haemorrhage. Acta Neurochir (Wien) 41: 7–22

27. Voldby B, Enevoldsen EM, Jensen FT (1985) Cerebrovascular reactivity in patients with ruptured intracranial aneurysms. J Neurosurg 62: 59–67

Correspondence: J.D. Pickard, M.D., Academic Neurosurgery Unit, University of Cambridge, Addenbrooke's Hospital, Box 167, Cambridge CB2, QQ, U.K.

Transcranial Doppler Evaluation of Cerebral Perfusion After SAH

B. Romner

Department of Neurosurgery, University Hospital, Lund, Sweden

Summary

Transcranial Doppler sonography (TCD) flow velocities and cerebral blood flow (CBF) measurements were evaluated in 14 patients who has suffered a major aneurysmal subarachnoid hemorrhage (SAH). Cerebrovascular reactivity to hypocapnia was evaluated simultaneously by the two methods. Measurements were performed under general anesthesia preoperatively, within 72 hours after the bleed, during normocapnia and hypocapnia. There was poor correlation between absolute values of hemispheric CBF and corresponding TCD mean flow velocity. Controlled hyperventilation was associated with a significant decrease in CBF as well as TCD flow velocity ($p < 0.001$). In terms of reactivity indices the correlation was poor and not significant ($r = 0.33$, $p = 0.09$). Further 21 patients were subjected to repeated assessment of TCD flow velocities during the first 12 hours after SAH. In 19 patients, recordings were performed following the first SAH, and in two after early rebleeds. Flow velocities did not indicate an early phase of arterial narrowing in any case. Following the first TCD recording, flow velocities were evaluated repeatedly in the 19 survivors. Increased flow velocities suggesting arterial vasospasm occured only after a delay of at least 4 days. Additional 36 patients with a proven first SAH from a ruptured supratentorial aneurysm were subjected to repeated TCD assessments. 18 individuals were operated within 48 hours, while the other 18 had surgery between 49 and 96 hours after SAH. Postoperative flow velocities were significantly lower in patients operated within 48 hours ($p < 0.001$).

The results of the studies favor a referral system which enables early surgical intervention not only to prevent rebleeds but also aimed at reducing delayed ischemic dysfunction.

Keywords: Cerebral blood flow; transcranial Doppler sonography; CO_2-reactivity; subarachnoid hemorrhage.

Introduction

There has been considerable interest in cerebral hemodynamics after recent subarachnoid hemorrhage (SAH) in patients as well as in experimental studies. In 1980, Pickard and coworkers[6] demonstrated that prediction of late ischaemic complications after cerebral aneurysm operation was possible by intra-operative measurement of the cerebral blood flow response to drug-induced hypotension. Patients with impaired autoregulatory capacity after SAH run a much greater risk of suffering late ischaemic deterioration. Patients with normal autoregulatory capacity however, seem to have a low probability of developing this complication.

A study in 1987 of patients undergoing early operation for a ruptured aneurysm, indicated that delayed ischemic deterioration (DID) after uncomplicated early operation may be associated with an early disturbance of cerebral vasoreactivity in terms of impaired CO_2-response[5]. These data suggested that measurement of cerebral vascular response to hyperventilation may be as good as induced hypotension in revealing patients at risk for DID after aneurysmal SAH. However, the disadvantages of the CBF technique including radioactive isotopes, the fact that it is time-consuming, rather expensive, and involves complicated measurements have reduced the use of the CBF technique in daily neurosurgery, although several investigators have suggested that the clinical management of patients suffering from aneurysmal SAH should be guided by serial measurements of CBF.

For the direct detection of intracranial arterial narrowing, i.e. vasospasm, cerebral angiography was for many years the only proper diagnostic tool. However, similarly to the CBF technique, the disadvantages of this procedure are the extremely high costs of the equipment, the invasiveness, radiation exposure, and the inability to be performed bedside. Angiography is also associated with definite morbidity and mortality, and over the years extensive research has been conducted to identify non-invasive, more simple procedures for evaluation of intracranial hemodynamics.

With the introduction of non-invasive transcranial Doppler (TCD), by Aaslid et al.[1], a new technical device has been added which allows non-invasive assessment of blood flow velocity and flow direction in large basal cerebral arteries. Information on cerebral hemodynamic changes may be obtained from the amplitude between the systolic and the diastolic flow velocities which also are related to the cerebrovascular resistance.

In a study 1984, Aaslid *et al.*[2] found a clear correlation between the TCD flow velocity and the angiographic diameter of the MCA in SAH patients and suggested that the TCD technique may be used to evaluate vasospasm. Comparing the blood velocity recordings with concurrent angiograms, they found flow velocities in the middle cerebral artery (MCA) above 120 cm/s when the angiogram revealed spasm in the MCA.

In order to explore the potential benefits of the TCD technique compared with CBF measurements and angiography, the present studies were undertaken.

Clinical Material and Methods

a) Evaluation of Cerebrovascular Reactivity After Subarachnoid Haemorrhage Using CBF and TCD

Fourteen patients (age range 19–63 years, mean 41 years) with rupture of an intracranial aneurysm resulting in a major SAH were studied[7]. Only patients in Hunt and Hess neurological grades I–III were included. In all patients aneurysm surgery was performed within 72 hours after SAH. No patient had arterial hypertension prior to the bleed. In order to prevent delayed ischaemia all patients were treated with intravenous nimodipine infusion, however not started until the measurements had been completed.

Mean hemispheric CBF was determined after intravenous administration of 0.5 GBq of 133-Xe. Clearance of the tracer was monitored by one extracranial scintillation detector over the MCA territory bilaterally, and from the expired air, using a mobile bedside equipment.

TCD was performed using a 2 MHz pulsed transcranial Doppler instrument a depth of 50–60 mm to examine the main trunk of the MCA. Recordings were performed bilaterally, simultaneously with the early portion of the CBF measurement. The CBF and TCD response to controlled hyperventilation (25% increase of minute volume, aiming at > 1.0 kPa reduction in pCO_2) was determined after induction of anesthesia but prior to craniotomy.

b) Transcranial Doppler and Timing of Aneurysm Operation

Twenty-one individuals were subjected to repeated assessment of cerebral blood flow velocities (FV) using transcranial Doppler sonography (TCD) during the first 12 hours after SAH[8].

Additional thirty-six individuals, who had suffered a proven first SAH from a supratentorial aneurysm, were investigated with repeated TCD recordings[9]. Eighteen patients (group A) were subjected to acute surgery within 48 hours after aneurysm rupture, while the other 18 (group B) were operated between 49 and 96 hours after the bleed.

Results

a) CBF, TCD and relevant physiological data (mean $1 \pm SD$) in the anaesthetized patients subjected to normo- and hypocapnia are presented in Table 1.

Table 1

N = 14	Normocapnia	Hypocapnia
Temperature (°C)	36.8 ± 0.1	36.9 ± 0.1
Hemoglobin (g × l⁻¹)	139.5 ± 4.1	137.9 ± 4.0
PaO_2 (kPa)	18.7 ± 1.8	21.6 ± 2.8
(mm Hg)	140.5 ± 13.7	162.4 ± 21.8
$PaCO_2$ (kPa)	5.4 ± 0.2	$3.9 \pm 0.1*$
(mm Hg)	40.2 ± 1.4	$29.5 \pm 1.1*$
pH	7.4 ± 0.02	7.5 ± 0.01
MABP (mm Hg)	73.4 ± 2.5	72.4 ± 3.1
CBF_{dx} (ml × 100 g⁻¹ × min⁻¹)	45.5 ± 3.0	$31.4 \pm 2.0*$
CBF_{sin} (ml × 100 g⁻¹ × min⁻¹)	44.5 ± 2.8	$31.8 \pm 2.1*$
TCD_{dx} (cm/s)	53.9 ± 4.3	$36.6 \pm 3.6*$
TCD_{sin} (cm/s)	53.0 ± 5.4	$35.9 \pm 3.2*$

Body temperature, hemoglobin, PaO_2, $PaCO_2$, pH, MABP, CBF and TCD in 14 anesthezised patients with aneurysmal SAH during normo- and hyperventilation.
* Significant difference between normocapnic and hypocapnic values (p < 0.05). Values are mean ± 1 SD. *MABP* mean arterial blood pressure; *CBF* cerebral blood flow; *TCD* transcranial Doppler.

There was > 1.0 kPa reduction in pCO_2 between the two measurements in all investigated individuals. A poor correlation was found between absolute values of CBF and corresponding MCA flow velocity (Fig. 1). Controlled hyperventilation was accompanied by a significant (p < 0.001) decrease in CBF (mean 30% change) as well as TCD mean flow velocity (mean 32% change). Figure 2 demonstrates the individual CBF and TCD responses to hyperventilation, where the expected direction of change is demonstrated with both methods. Figure 3 shows the individual values for CBF (a) and TCD (b) plotted against pCO_2. A linear

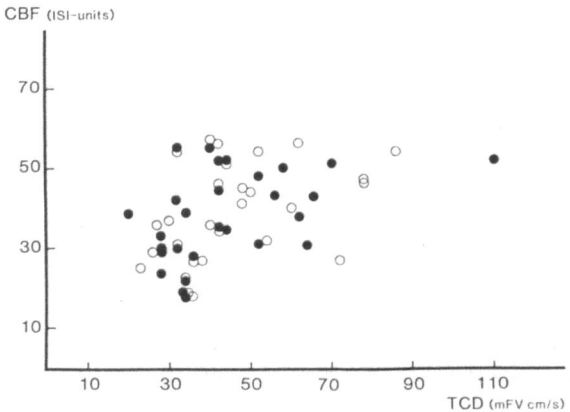

Fig. 1. Absolute CBF and TCD values in 14 patients after aneurysmal SAH during normo- and hypocapnia. ● Left side; ○ right side

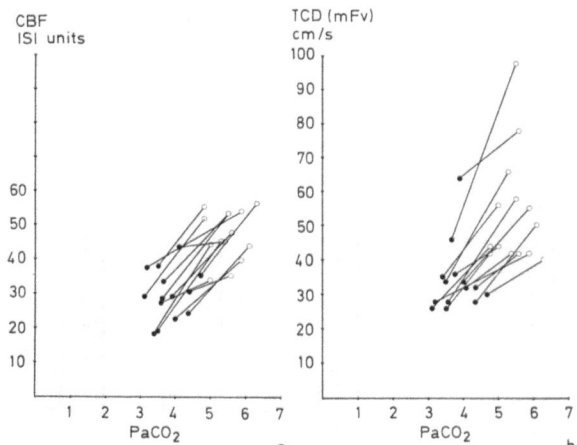

Fig. 2. Individual changes of CBF(a) and TCD(b) to hypocapnia in 14 patients after aneurysmal SAH. Both methods demonstrated significant changes (p < 0.001) between normo- and hypocapnia. ○ Normocapnia; ● hypocapnia

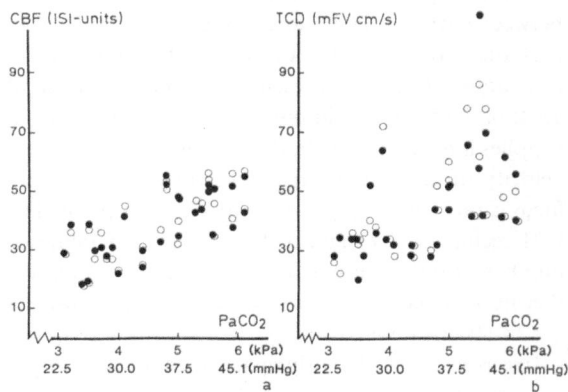

Fig. 3. CBF change (a) plotted against pCO_2 change (r = 0.70). TCD change (b) plotted against pCO_2 change (r = 0.52). ● Left side; ○ right side

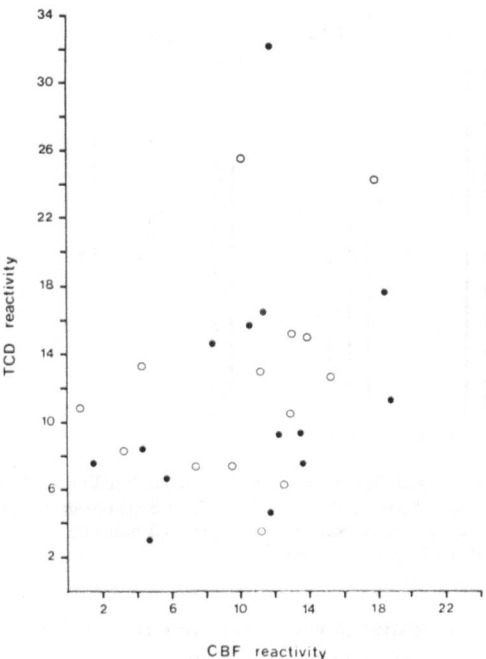

Fig. 4. CBF reactivity (% change of CBF/kPa change pCO_2) compared with TCD reactivity (% change TCD flow velocity/kPa change pCO_2) in 14 patients after aneurysmal SAH. The correlation between the two methods was poor (r = 0.33, p = 0.09). ● left side; ○ right side

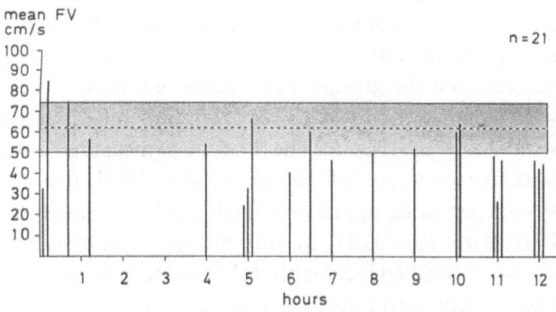

Fig. 5. Early transcranial Doppler measurements after SAH in 21 patients. Mean middle cerebral artery (MCA) flow velocities within or below normal range (shadowed area)

relationship was found between CBF and pCO_2 (r = 0.70). The corresponding relationship for TCD and pCO_2 was less striking (r = 0.52). In these patients with recent SAH, CBF was better correlated to changes in pCO_2 than MCA flow velocity. A quantitative comparison between the individual reactivity indices, measured by CBF and TCD, respectively, revealed a wide scatter and poor correlation (r = 0.33, p = 0.09) as seen in Fig. 4.

b) As shown in Fig. 5, flow velocities within the first 12 hours after SAH were below the normal range in 12 patients (57%), within the normal range in eight (38%)

and slightly above in only one patient (case 2). No patient showed increased flow velocities of the type seen in patients with cerebral vasospasm (> 120 cm/s). Angiography performed within 24 hours after the bleed showed no evidence of vessel narrowing in any of the 18 patients undergoing four-vessel angiography. Following the first assessment, flow velocities were repeatedly measured in the survivors. No increased flow

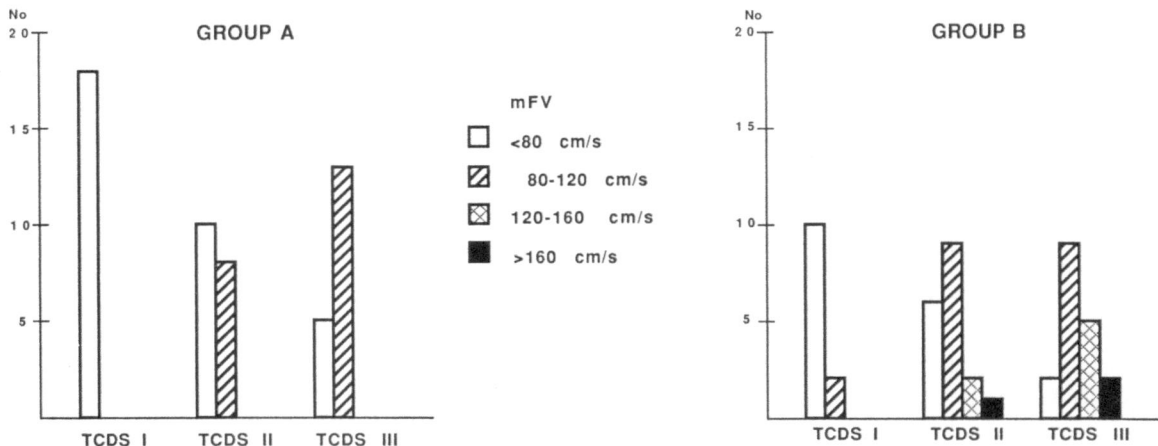

Fig. 6. Transcranial Doppler mean flow velocities (mFV) in the MCA of 36 patients: 18 operated on within 48 hours after SAH (group A) and 18 operated between 49 and 96 hours after SAH (group B). *TCDS-I* TCD performed < 72 hours post-SAH. (Due to delay in referral, assessment could not be performed in 6 group B patients). *TCDS-II* TCD performed 5 to 7 days post-SAH. *TCDS-III* TCD performed between 10 and 12 days post-SAH

velocities indicative of vasospasm were recorded until after a delay of at least 4 days. In case 2, a TCD evaluation 6 minutes after an early MCA aneurysmal rebleed showed flow velocities in the upper normal range in both MCA's. In case 1, TCD measurements were performed within minutes after an early rebleed.

In the first 72 hours post-SAH, no increased flow velocities suggestive of acutely disturbed hemodynamics ("acute vasospasm") were recorded. There was no significant difference in preoperative flow velocities between the groups. Postoperative flow velocities were significantly lower ($p < 0.01$) in patients operated within 48 hours (Fig. 6). The third TCD measurements, obtained between day 10 and 12 after SAH, demonstrated persisting significantly higher velocities in group B patients ($p < 0.01$). In this group, 11 individuals showed a marked increase in MCA velocity bilaterally. Five patients had velocities of more than 120 cm/s, and in another 2 patients the velocities exceeded 170 cm/s, indicating severe vasospasm. These 2 patients developed cerebral ischemia and later died from cerebral infarction.

Discussion

In the present study, controlled hyperventilation was associated with a significant decrease in CBF as well as TCD flow velocity in all 14 individuals. However, when comparing individual reactivity indices between the two simultaneously studied techniques no significant correlation could be established.

In this respect, the fundamental principal differences between CBF and TCD should be considered. The fact that the target area for the two different modes of measurements may represent anatomically different areas of the brain is of importance. The Doppler signal supplies information on both blood flow direction and velocity in individual large intracranial arteries and focuses on a single large artery at a certain point. The CBF technique gives a mean flow value for an unknown number of blood vessels of different calibre and, furthermore, the cerebral area covered by the detector can not be strictly defined.

Irrespective of the principal ifferences, a major prerequisite for a detection of blood flow changes with both methods is calibre changes in the arteries. A change in MCA velocity, if the blood pressure is unchanged, may indicate either a change in peripheral flow or a calibre change in the MCA, or both.

Which of the methods is more appropriate in determining cerebral vasoreactivity remains to be proven. Providing that cerebral vasoreactivity and autoregulation is not uniformly disturbed in several SAH patients, the present discrepancy between the two methods might be explained. The TCD and CBF methods both provide useful information on cerebrovascular events which, however, are not directly interchangeable, but, in many respects might complement each other.

The optimum timing of surgical intervention for ruptured intracranial aneurysms remains a controversial issue. The leading cause of morbidity and mortality following aneurysmal subarachnoid hemorrhage (SAH) is delayed cerebral ischemia resulting from SAH-induced disturbances in cerebral hemodynamics ("cerebral vasospasm"). It has been argued that operative occlusion of ruptured aneurysm must be delayed in order to avoid additional operative trauma to a brain supposed to suffer from disturbed hemodynamics in the acute phase after extravasation of blood in the subarachnoid spaces ("acute vasospasm")[3]. Whether such "acute vasospasm" at all occurs as a regular phenomenon in humans who have suffered from rupture of an intracranial aneurysm is, however, not proven. On the contrary, angiographical examinations in the acute stage after SAH do not support the existence of an acute phase of large vessel narrowing[10].

In the present study, early MCA flow recordings did not indicate any increased flow velocities, instead did the curve profile show a pattern indicating a severely increased intracranial pressure (ICP). This is in agreement with results obtained by Grote and Hassler[4], who studied 6 patients during a recurrent bleed. Three patients were recorded with TCD immediately before, during and after a rebleed. The flow patterns during the bleed reflected an abrupt rise in ICP, but did not indicate any proximal arterial narrowing. In the other 3 patients the aneurysm bled during angiography, but no signs of vascular narrowing were seen.

Our early TCD results favor the assumption of restored flow velocity patterns in surviving patients and do not indicate that there exists an acute phase of vasospasm. The flow pattern in the patients recorded within minutes after a rebleed, only reflected an abrupt rise in ICP.

The present results indicate aneurysm surgery without unnecessary delay, not only with the aim to prevent rebleeds but also to evacuate accummulated blood in the subarachnoid cisterns to prevent delayed subarachnoid blood induced disturbances in cerebral hemodynamics.

References

1. Aaslid R, Markwalder TM, Nornes H (1982) Noninvasive transcranial Doppler ultrasound recording of flow velocity in basal cerebral arteries. J Neurosurg 57: 769–774
2. Aaslid R, Huber P, Nornes H (1984) Evaluation of cerebrovascular spasm with transcranial Doppler ultrasound. J Neurosurg 60: 37–41
3. Adams HP Jr, Kasell NF, Torner JC, Haley EC Jr (1987) Predicting cerebral ischemia after subarachnoid hemorrhage: influences of clinical condition, CT results, and antifibrinolytic therapy. A report of the Cooperative Aneurysm Study. Neurology 37: 1586–1591
4. Grote E, Hassler W (1988) The critical first minutes after subarachnoid hemorrhage. Neurosurgery 22: 654–661
5. Messeter K, Brandt L, Ljunggren B, Svendgaard NA, Algotsson L, Romner B, Ryding E (1987) Prediction and prevention of delayed ischemic dysfunction after aneurysmal subarachnoid hemorrhage and early operation. Neurosurgery 20: 548–553
6. Pickard JD, Matheson M, Patterson J, Wyper D (1980) Prediction of late ischemic complications after cerebral aneurysm surgery by the intraoperative measurement of cerebral blood flow. J Neurosurg 53: 305–308
7. Romner B, Brandt L, Berntman L, Algotsson L, Ljunggren B, Messeter K (1991) Simultaneous transcranial Doppler sonography and cerebral blood flow measurements of cerebrovascular CO_2-reactivity in patients with aneurysmal subarachnoid haemorrhage. Br J Neurosurg 5: 31–37
8. Romner B, Ljunggren B, Brandt L, Säveland H (1989) Transcranial Doppler sonography within 12 hours after subarachnoid hemorrhage. J Neurosurg 70: 732–736
9. Romner B, Ljunggren B, Brandt L, Säveland H (1990) Correlation of transcranial Doppler sonography findings with timing of aneurysm surgery. J Neurosurg 73: 72–76
10. Wilkins RH (1976) Aneurysm rupture during angiography: does acute vasospasm occur? Surg Neurol 5: 299–303

Correspondence: Bertil Romner, M.D., Ph.D., Department of Neurosurgery, University Hospital, S-22185 Lund, Sweden.

Combined Transcranial Doppler Sonography and rCBF Measurements in the Early Stage of Subarachnoid Hemorrhage

A. Pasqualin, A. Talacchi, F. Chioffi, G. Pavesi, and **R. Da Pian**

Department of Neurosurgery, City Hospital, Verona, Italy

Summary

Thirty-nine patients in grade I–III (Hunt and Hess classification) – admitted to our Department within 3 days from aneurysmal subarachnoid hemorrhage (SAH) and submitted to i.v. nimodipine treatment – were evaluated with sequential transcranial Doppler (TCD) and rCBF measurements – at 1 to 3 day intervals – for the first 20 days after SAH. TCD velocities were significantly higher in patients with consistent/thick subarachnoid depositions than in patients with absent/thin depositions, especially after 9 days from SAH. In the early stage of SAH average hemispheric flow was significantly lower in patients with consistent/thick depositions (p < 0.01); the lowest values of hemispheric flow were observed at 10–12 days after SAH in both groups, with a non-significant difference. Patients with consistent/thick depositions ($n = 30$) showed a significantly higher incidence of hemispheric hypoperfusion (67% vs 22%, p < 0.05) and hemispheric asymmetry (47% vs 11%, p = 0.05) than patients with absent/thin depositions, with a non-significantly higher incidence of regional hypoperfusion in the former group. Patients with TCD velocities over 120 cm/sec showed a significantly higher incidence of hemispheric hypoperfusion (82% vs 36%, p < 0.01) and regional hypoperfusion (71% vs 32%, p < 0.01) than patients with lower TCD velocities, with a trend to a higher incidence of hemispheric asymmetry, angiographical spasm, ischemic deterioration and CT infarction in the former group. In conclusion, cerebral vasospasm appears to be a secondary phenomenon established on an early hypoperfused cerebral tissue; consequently a combination of serial TCD and rCBF recordings constitutes an helpful atraumatic approach to evaluate patients with ruptured aneurysms during the early stage of SAH.

Keywords: Transcranial Doppler sonography; rCBF; subarachnoid hemorrhage; vasospasm.

Introduction

Cerebral vasospasm still constitutes the most severe complication related to subarachnoid hemorrhage (SAH). The arterial narrowing observed on angiography may develop on a cerebral tissue that is frequently hypoperfused in the early stage of SAH, thus leading to further hypoperfusion and to ischemic symptoms.

The aim of this study has been to investigate cerebral hemodynamics in patients with freshly ruptured aneurysms – on the basis of sequential recordings of transcranial Doppler (TCD) and regional cerebral blood flow (rCBF) – in order to define the influence of cerebral vasospasm and early cerebral hypoperfusion on the delayed neurological deterioration.

Clinical Material and Methods

Between July 1989 and December 1991, 39 patients with ruptured aneurysms were prospectively submitted to the following protocol of study: a) admission 0–3 days after SAH, and clinical grade I to III (Hunt and Hess classification); b) aneurysm documented on angiography; c) intravenous nimodipine infusion (2 mg/h) until day 14 after SAH, followed by oral administration (360 mg/die).

25 patients were female, 14 patients were male. Age ranged between 26 and 78 years; the mean age was 50.2 years, and the most involved decade was 40–49 years (46% of cases). 5 patients were in grade I (13%), 18 in grade II (46%), 16 in grade III (41%). Aneurysmal location is presented in Table 1. 12 patients were submitted to an early operation (within 3 days from SAH) and 27 to a delayed operation.

In each patient, sequential recordings of TCD and rCBF – at 1 – to 3 day intervals – were made for the first 20 days from SAH. Time-mean velocities recorded on the middle cerebral and anterior cerebral arteries have been considered significantly increased when higher than 120 cm/sec. Hemispheric CBF – determined with Cerebrograph 32C by 133-Xe inhalation and reported in initial slope index (ISI) units, according to Obrist[22] – has been considered reduced (= hemispheric hypoperfusion) when significantly different from values of a standard control population. Regional hypoperfu-

Table 1. *Aneurysmal Location*

	n	%
Int. carotid	11	28%
Middle cerebral	10	26%
Ant. communic.	8	21%
Ant. cerebral	5	13%
Post. circul.	1	2%
Multiple	4	10%

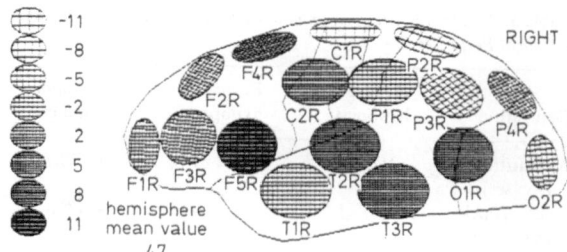

Fig. 1. Regional hypoperfusion in C1 and P2 detectors (right hemisphere); less perfused areas are represented with a larger grid; ISI (%) (relative to hemispheric mean)

Table 2. *Clinical Outcome in Relation to Adopted Policy*

	Complete recovery	Disability: moderate	severe	death
Early surgery (11 cases)	7 (64%)	3 (27%)	1 (9%)	—
Delayed policy (28 cases)	14 (50%)	6 (22%)	4 (14%)	4 (14%)
Total (39 cases)	21 (54%)	9 (23%)	5 (13%)	4 (10%)

sion has been considered to occur when values for 2 or more adjacent detectors were significantly different from the control population (Fig. 1), or showed a significant reduction from the hemispheric mean, if the hemisphere itself was globally hypoperfused. Hemispheric asymmetry has been considered to occur when mean hemispheric CBF values were significantly different from the values of the controlateral hemisphere. A regional hypoperfusion (RH) index has been adopted in order to assess the severity of hypoperfusion during each study period: this index was expressed by the ratio between the number of hypoperfused areas and the number of patients evaluated, according to the following formula:

$$RH\ index = \frac{(n)\ areas\ of\ regional\ hypoperfusion}{(n)\ patients\ evaluated}.$$

Data achieved from TCD and rCBF have been related to amount of subarachnoid deposition on CT scan[23], grade on admission (according to Hunt and Hess classification), angiographical spasm, development of ischemic deterioration, and incidence of CT infarction.

Results

Clinical outcome is presented in Table 2, in the overall series and in relation to the adopted policy.

TCD velocities were significantly higher in patients with consistent/thick subarachnoid depositions than in patients with absent/thin depositions, especially after 9 days from SAH (Fig. 2).

In the early stage of SAH average hemispheric flow was significantly lower in patients with consistent/thick

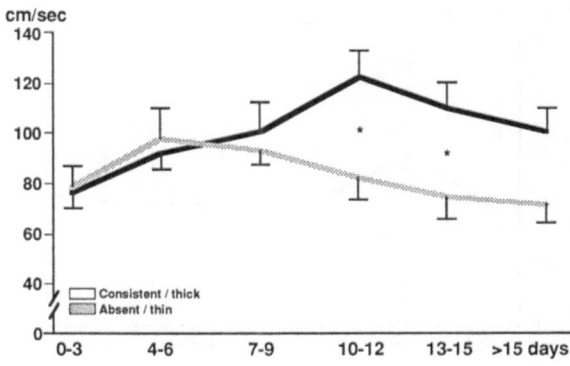

Fig. 2. Time-course of mean flow velocity (highest recorded value for each patient) according to amount of subarachnoid blood deposition (vertical bars indicate the standard error of the mean; * = p < 0.05)

depositions (p < 0.01); from 4 to 9 days after SAH hemispheric flow was stable around 40 ml/100 g/min (ISI values) in patients with consistent/thick depositions, and around 50 ml/100 g/min in patients with absent/thin depositions; the lowest values of hemispheric flow were observed at 10–12 days after SAH in both groups (with a non-significant difference) (Fig. 3). When considering the lowest regional flow values, the difference between patients with absent-thin and consistent-thick depositions remained significant for each study period (Fig. 4). As regards the RH index, it was lowest at 4–6 days from SAH, with a secondary decrease at 13–15 days from SAH (Fig. 5).

As opposed to patients with absent/thin depositions (n = 9), patients with consistent/thick depositions (n = 30) showed – during the period of the study – a signifi-

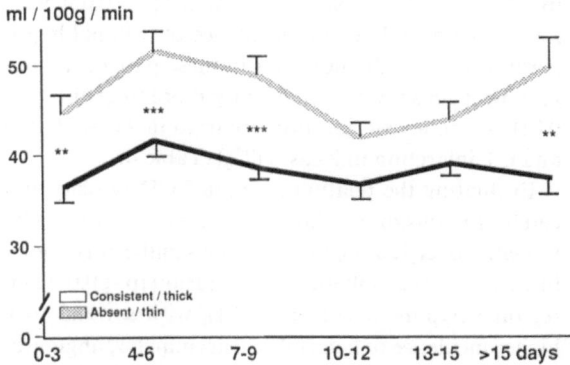

Fig. 3. Time-course of average hemispheric flow (ISI values), according to amount of subarachnoid blood deposition (vertical bars indicate the standard error of the mean; ** = p < 0.01; *** = p < 0.001)

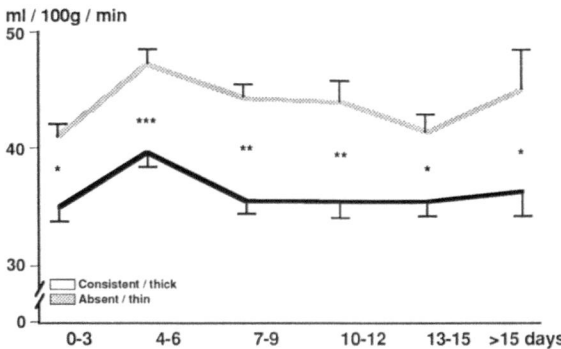

Fig. 4. Time-course of lowest regional flow values (ISI parameter), according to amount of subarachnoid blood deposition (vertical bars indicate the standard error of the mean; $* = p < 0.05$; $** \ p < 0.01$; $*** \ p < 0.001$)

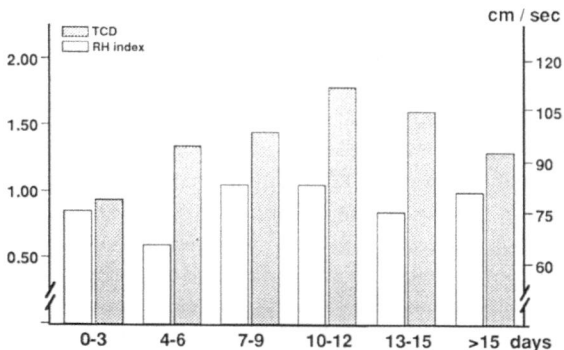

Fig. 5. Time-course of RH index and mean TCD velocity (RH index values are represented in the left column, TCD values in the right column)

Table 3. *Relation Between Amount of Cisternal Blood Deposition and Cerebral Perfusion*

Deposition	Hemisph. hypoperf.	Regional hypoperf.	Hemisph. asymmetry
Absent/thin (9 cases)	2 (22%)	2 (22%)	1 (11%)
Consist/thick (30 cases)	20 (67%)	17 (57%)	14 (47%)
Signif.	$p < 0.05$	N.S.	$p = 0.05$

Table 4. *Relation Between Amount of Cisternal Blood Deposition and Clinical/Instrumental Data*

Deposition	Vessel narrow.	Ischemic deterior.	CT infarct
Absent/thin (9 cases)	1 (11%)	—	—
Consist/thick (30 cases)	20 (67%)	9 (30%)	2 (7%)
Signif.	$p < 0.01$	N.S.	N.S.

Table 5. *Relation Between TCD Flow Velocity and Cerebral Perfusion*

Mean velocity	Hemisph. hypoperf.	Regional hypoperf.	Hemisph. asymmetry
< 120 cm/s (22 cases)	8 (36%)	7 (32%)	6 (27%)
> 120 cm/s (17 cases)	14 (82%)	12 (71%)	9 (53%)
Signif.	$p < 0.01$	$p = 0.01$	N.S.

Table 6. *Relation Between TCD Flow Velocity and Clinical/Instrumental Data*

Mean velocity	Vessel narrow.	Ischemic deter.	CT infarct
< 120 cm/s (22 cases)	9 (41%)	4 (18%)	—
> 120 cm/s (17 cases)	12 (71%)	5 (29%)	2 (12%)
Signif.	N.S.	N.S.	N.S.

cantly higher incidence of hemispheric hypoperfusion ($p < 0.05$) and hemispheric asymmetry ($p = 0.05$), with a non-significantly higher incidence of regional hypoperfusion (Table 3); moreover in these patients angiographical spasm was significantly more frequent ($p < 0.01$), ischemic deterioration occurred in 9 cases (30%) and CT infarction in 2 cases (7%) (Table 4).

Evaluating the relation between TCD velocity and cerebral perfusion or clinical data, patiens with TCD velocities over 120 cm/sec showed a significantly higher incidence of hemispheric hypoperfusion ($p < 0.01$) and regional hypoperfusion ($p = 0.01$), with a trend to a higher incidence of hemispheric asymmetry, angiographical spasm, ischemic deterioration and CT infarction, when compared to patients with lower TCD velocities (Tables 5 and 6). Considering only patients with consistent/thick depositions, when TCD velocities over

120 cm/sec were observed the incidence of hemispheric and regional hypoperfusion increased significantly (Table 7), as well as the incidence of vessel narrowing (Table 8).

Patients with ischemic deterioration (n = 9) showed a significantly higher incidence of regional hypoperfu-

Table 7. *Relation Between TCD Flow Velocity and Cerebral Perfusion, in Patients with Consistent/Thick Depositions*

Mean velocity	Hemisph. hypoperf.	Regional hypoperf.	Hemisph. asymmetry
< 120 cm/s (15 cases)	6 (40%)	8 (53%)	5 (33%)
> 120 cm/s (15 cases)	14 (93%)	14 (93%)	9 (60%)
Signif.	p < 0.01	p = 0.01	N.S.

Table 8. *Relation Between TCD Flow Velocity and Clinical/Instrumental Data, in Patients with Consistent/Thick Depositions*

Mean velocity	Vessel narrow.	Ischemic deter.	CT infarct
< 120 cm/s (15 cases)	8 (53%)	4 (26%)	—
> 120 cm/s (15 cases)	13 (86%)	5 (33%)	2 (13%)
Signif.	p = 0.05	N.S.	N.S.

Table 9. *Relation Between Ischemic Deterioration and Cerebral Perfusion or Elevated TCD Velocity*

	Hemishp. hypoperf.	Regional hypoperf.	Hemisph. asymmetry	TCD velocity > 120 cm/s
No ischemic deterioration (30 cases)	16 (53%)	11 (37%)	8 (27%)	12 (40%)
Ischemic deterioration (9 cases)	6 (67%)	8 (89%)	7 (78%)	5 (55%)
Signif.	N.S.	p < 0.01	p < 0.01	N.S.

sion (p < 0.01) and hemispheric asymmetry (p < 0.01) when compared to patients without deterioration (n = 30), while the difference in incidence of hemispheric hypoperfusion and high TCD velocities was not significant (Table 9).

Discussion

According to the equation $V = Q(\pi r^2)^{-1}$, flow velocity is inversely proportional to the square radius of the vessel (V = flow velocity, Q = CBF, and r = vessel radius); therefore TCD recording is a sensitive tool to monitor the development and the resolution of cerebral vasospasm[1,10,15,25,27,29]. Furthermore, in our study high TCD velocities were significantly related to an increased risk of regional and hemispheric hypoperfusion; this indicates TCD velocity as an important parameter for the evaluation of cerebral hemodynamics in patients with SAH. The inverse relation between velocity and vessel radius is true only if we consider CBF as constant; however, during the first two weeks after SAH, CBF may change (globally and/or regionally) according to intracranial pressure, vasospasm and several other factors[13,14,18,19,29,31], as shown also by our experience. Moreover, TCD sonography may provide false negatives, since it cannot study distal and convexity branches, which may be so constricted as to produce clinical symptoms[10,20,29]; on the contrary rCBF measurements give information about tissue perfusion, on a more distal territory than the one investigated by TCD[8]. Indeed, also in our study patients with angiographical spasm and reduced CBF have not always shown high TCD velocity values. Consequently, a more correct evaluation of vasospasm should result from a combination of TCD and rCBF measurements.

According to previous reports, patients with SAH – especially those with severe hemorrhage on CT scan[13] and with a worse clinical grade on admission[3,5,8] – present an early global reduction of flow, that cannot be attributed to vasospasm[8]. The pathogenesis of this early hypoperfusion may be related to metabolic depression[7,9,12,19] and/or increased intracranial pressure[21]. Our data show that CBF is already reduced in the early stage of SAH (0–3 days), when angiographical spasm or high TCD velocities are never observed; in the subacute period CBF decreases again (with the lowest values recorded on days 10–12 after SAH) exhibiting a chronological relation with the highest TCD velocities and thus supporting a strict dependency from cerebral vasospasm. A comprehensive view of these data suggest a "dualistic" interpretation of cerebral hemodynamics in patients with SAH: on one hand global early CBF reduction, on the other hand subsequent development of cerebral vasospasm and regional hypoperfusion, well detected by TCD and rCBF measurements.

In our series of patients, autoregulation or vasoreactivity to CO_2 have not been evaluated; other authors consider these tests as a valuable adjunct to the evaluation of cerebral hemodynamics in the early stage of SAH[4,5,11,16,17,24,31], particularly to predict the risk of delayed ischemia in the individual patient.

The time-course of mean flow velocity or average hemispheric flow is affected by the amount of subarachnoid deposition on CT scan; patients with consistent/thick depositions show a significantly higher incidence of hemispheric hypoperfusion and hemispheric asymmetry. It has already been demostrated that patients with consistent or thick cisternal hemorrhages show a higher incidence of angiographical spasm, ischemic deterioration, and CT infarction[6,23]. The present data add further value to the prognostic role of early CT scan in the hemodynamic evaluation of patients with SAH.

As for surgical timing, our data have not disclosed significant hemodynamic differences between patients submitted to early surgery and patients submitted to a delayed approach, probably due to the small groups considered. From our experience, in patients who do not undergo an early operation (within three days from SAH) the following complementary parameters should be balanced, in order to decide for surgery in the subacute stage (notoriously the most risky period): 1) the amount of cisternal deposition; 2) the mean flow velocity on the middle cerebral artery; 3) hemispheric and regional cerebral perfusion. When one (or more) of these factors results unfavourable (consistent/thick depositions, mean TCD velocity over 120 cm/sec, regional hypoperfusion or hemispheric asymmetry), surgery is delayed to a chronic stage (after 14 days from SAH). Other authors have considered rCBF or TCD recordings as valuable guidelines for timing of surgery[2,26,28].

In conclusion, since cerebral vasospasm appears to be a secondary phenomenon established on an early hypoperfused cerebral tissue, the combination of serial TCD and rCBF recordings should be considered an helpful atraumatic approach to conveniently "frame" patients with SAH, offering also indications about timing of surgery in each patient. Moreover, this combined approach can better evaluate the efficacy of treatments aimed to improve cerebral hemodynamics and to relieve cerebral vasospasm.

References

1. Aaslid R, Huber P, Nornes H (1984) Evaluation of cerebrovascular spasm with transcranial Doppler ultrasound. J Neurosurg 60: 37–41
2. Brawanski A, Gaaab MR, Bockhorn J, Haubitz I (1982) A traumatic rCBF measurement: an aid in the timing of surgery and the management of spasm following SAH. Acta Neurochir (Wien) 63: 43–51
3. Brawanski A, Maximilian VA (1985) Utility of non invasive rCBF measurements in the clinical management of patients with subarachnoid hemorrhage. In: Hartman A, Hoyer S (eds) Cerebral blood flow and metabolism measurement. Springer, Berlin Heidelberg New York Tokyo, pp 165–171
4. Dernbach PD, Little JR, Jones SC, Ebrahim ZY (1988) Altered cerebral autoregulation and CO_2 reactivity after aneurysmal subarachnoid hemorrhage. Neurosurgery 22: 822–826
5. Farrar JK, Ferguson GG, Drake CG, Peerless SJ (1985) Xenon-133 CBF measurements in the clinical management of patients with subarachnoid haemorrhage. In: Hartmann A, Hoyer S (eds) Cerebral blood flow and metabolism measurement. Springer, Berlin Heidelberg New York Tokyo, pp 161–165
6. Fisher CM, Kistler JP, Davis JM (1980) Relation of cerebral vasospasm to subarachnoid hemorrhage visualized by computerized tomographic scanning. Neurosurgery 6: 1–9
7. Gelmers HJ, Becks JWF, Journee HL (1979) Regional cerebral blood flow in patients with subarachnoid haemorrhage. Acta Neurochir (Wien) 47: 245–251
8. Geraud G, Guell A, Andrieu P, Tremoulet M, Bes A (1985) The prognostic value of atraumatic CBF measurement in subarachnoid hemmorhage. In: Hartmann A, Hoyer S (eds) Cerebral blood flow and metabolism measurement. Springer, Berlin Heidelberg New York Tokyo, pp 153–159
9. Grubb RL, Raichle ME, Eichling JO, Gado MH (1977) Effects of subarachnoid hemorrhage on cerebral blood flow, blood volume and oxygen utilization in humans. J Neurosurg 46: 453–466
10. Harders AG, Gilsbach JM (1987) Time course of blood velocities changes related to vasospasm in the circle of Willis measured by transcranial Doppler ultrasound. J Neurosurg 66: 718–728
11. Hassler W, Chioffi F (1988) CO_2 reactivity of cerebral vasospasm after aneurysmal subarachnoid hemorrhage. Acta Neurochir (Wien) 98: 167–175
12. Hino A, Mizukawa N, Tenjin H, Imahori Y, Takemoto S, Yano I, Nakahashi H, Hirakawa K (1989) Postoperative hemodynamic and metabolic changes in patients with subarachnoid hemorrhage. Stroke 20: 1504–1510
13. Knuckney NW, Fox RA, Surveyor I, Stokes BAR (1985) Early cerebral blood flow and computerized tomography in predicting ischemia after cerebral aneurysm rupture. J Neurosurg 62: 850–855
14. Kontos HA (1989) Validity of cerebral arterial blood flow calculations from velocity measurements. Stroke 20: 1–3
15. Lindegaard KF, Nornes H, Bakke SJ, Sorteberg W, Nakstad P (1989) Cerebral vasospasm: diagnosis by means of angiography and blood velocity measurements. Acta Neurochir (Wien) 100: 12–24
16. Lovick AHJ, Pickard JD, Goddard BA (1982) Prediction of late ischaemic complications after cerebral aneurysm surgery – use of a mobile microcomputer system for the measurement of pre-, intra- and post-operative cerebral blood flow. Acta Neurochir (Wien) 63: 37–49
17. Messeter K, Brandt L, Ljunnggren B, Svendgaard NA, Algotsson L, Romner R, Ryding E (1987) Prediction and prevention of delayed ischaemic dysfunction after aneurysmal subarachnoid hemorrhage and early operation. Neurosurgery 20: 548–553
18. Meyer CHA, Lowe D, Meyer M, Richardson PL, Neil-Dwyer G (1983) Progressive change in cerebral blood flow during the first three weeks after subarachnoid hemorrhage. Neurosurgery 12: 58–76
19. Mickey BM, Vorstrup S, Voldby B, Lindewald H, Harmsen A, Lassen NA (1984) Serial measurement of regional cerebral blood flow in patients with SAH using Xe-133 inhalation and emission computerized tomography. J Neurosurg 60: 916–922
20. Newell DW, Grady MS, Eskridge JM, Winn HR (1990) Distribution of angiographic vasospasm after subarachnoid hemorrhage: implications for diagnosis by transcranial Doppler ultrasonography. Neurosurgery 27: 574–577
21. Nornes H (1973) The role of intracranial pressure in the arrest

of hemorrhage in patients with ruptured intracranial aneurysm. J Neurosurg 39: 226–234

22. Obrist WD, Thompson HK, Wang HS, Wilkinson WE (1975) Regional cerebral blood flow estimated by Xe-133 inhalation. Stroke 6: 245–256

23. Pasqualin A, Rosta L, Da Pian R, Cavazzani P, Scienza R (1984) The role of computed tomography in the management of vasospasm following subarachnoid hemorrhage. Neurosurgery 15: 344–353

24. Pickard JD, Matheson M, Patterson J, Wyper D (1980) Prediction of late ischemic complications after cerebral aneurysm surgery by the intraoperative measurement of cerebral blood flow. J Neurosurg 53: 305–308

25. Romner B, Ljunggren B, Brandt L, Saveland H (1989) Transcranial Doppler sonography within 12 hours after subarachnoid hemorrhage. J Neurosurg 70: 732–736

26. Romner B, Ljunggren B, Brandt L, Saveland H (1990) Correlation of transcranial Doppler sonography findings with timing of aneurysm surgery. J Neurosurg 73: 72–76

27. Seiler RW, Grolimund P, Aaslid R, Huber P, Nornes H (1986) Cerebral vasospasm evaluated by transcranial ultrasound correlated with clinical grade and CT-visualized subarachnoid hemorrhage. J Neurosurg 64: 594–600

28. Seiler RW, Reulen HJ, Huber P, Grolimund P, Ebeling U, Steiger HJ (1988) Outcome of aneurysmal subarachnoid hemorrhage in a hospital population: a prospective study including early operation, intravenous nimodipine, and transcranial Doppler ultrasound. Neurosurgery 23: 598–604

29. Sekhar LN, Wechsler LR, Yonas H, Luyckx K, Obrist W (1988) The value of transcranial Doppler examination in the diagnosis of vasospasm after subarachnoid hemorrhage. Neurosurgery 22: 813–821

30. Voldby B, Enevoldsen EM, Jensen FT (1985) Cerebrovascular reactivity in patients with ruptured intracranial aneurysms. J Neurosurg 62: 59–67

31. Yonas H, Sekhar L, Johnson DW, Gur D (1989) Determination of irreversible ischemia by Xenon-enhanced computed tomographic monitoring of cerebral blood flow in patients with symptomatic vasospasm. Neurosurgery 24: 368–372

Correspondence: A. Pasqualin, M.D., Department of Neurosurgery, City Hospital, I-37126 Verona, Italy.

Pharmacological Treatment of Vasospasm

Principles of Pharmaceutical Therapy for Vasospasm Following Subarachnoid Hemorrhage

E.C. Haley

Departments of Neurology and Neurological Surgery, University of Virginia School of Medicine, Charlottesville, Virginia, U.S.A.

Summary

An ideal drug therapy for delayed cerebral vasospasm following aneurysmal subarachnoid hemorrhage requires a detailed understanding of the fundamental biochemistry and pathophysiology of this disorder. Unfortunately, key elements of the vasospasm enigma, such as the identity of the primary spasmogen, remain unknown. Nevertheless, advances in the treatment of vasospasm have occurred using several basic strategies. These include removal or dissolution of the subarachnoid clot, pharmacological prevention of the arterial narrowing, dilation of the narrowed arteries (mechanically or chemically), augmentation of collateral flow, and pharmacological protection of cellular homeostasis in the ischemic environment. Several recently developed treatments also take advantage of the differential characteristics of the cerebral vis-a-vis the systemic vascular beds. Development of an effective therapeutic agent must take into consideration the time course of the arterial narrowing, the method of drug delivery, its pharmacokinetics and pharmacodynamics, interactions with other therapies, and the risk/benefit ratio.

Keywords: Cerebral vasospasm; subarachnoid hemorrhage; cerebral aneurysm.

Introduction

A decade ago, the major cause of combined death and disability in patients with aneurysmal subarachnoid hemorrhage (SAH) who survived long enough to be referred for definitive treatment was cerebral infarction secondary to the effects of delayed cerebral vasospasm[15]. The narrowing of large arteries visible on appropriately timed cerebral arteriograms, though poorly understood, was recognized as a common phenomenon, occurring in as many as 60–80% of SAH patients[26]. Most of the initial attempts at therapy for this condition were uniformly unsuccessful[27,28]. Moreover, it seemed that design of an ideal treatment must await a more detailed understanding of the underlying pathophysiology. Although much evidence now implicates oxy-

hemoglobin released from degenerating red blood cells in the subarachnoid clot as a major contributor to the process[16], numerous other substances have been implicated[14], as well, and their relative importance in this complex biochemical environment remains to be fully determined.

Despite the many unknowns surrounding the vasospasm enigma, therapeutic advances have been occurring with remarkable speed. The calcium antagonist, nimodipine, has been approved for use in the United States, and has been incorporated into standard practice in many areas worldwide. Other promising agents are in Phase III clinical trials. This discussion will review some of the basic strategies being employed to develop new treatments and examines some of the problems that must be addressed during the testing of new pharmaceutical agents for cerebral vasospasm.

Management Strategies

Investigators have adopted several approaches to the problem of treatment for vasospam. These proposals reflect the evolution of our understanding of the pathophysiology to date, and do not preclude more novel approaches in the future.

Clot Removal

As investigators began to appreciate the association between the amount and distribution of subarachnoid clot and the subsequent development of vasospasm, some neurosurgeons (particularly in Japan) began to advocate early surgery for aneurysm clipping and vigorous attempts at removal of as much of the subarachnoid clot as was technically feasible[17,21]. While uncontrolled studies suggested benefit from this approach, the results of the International Cooperative Study on the Timing of Aneurysm Surgery suggested that although the approach seemed safe when compared to a strategy of surgery after the first week, it did not result in a reduced incidence of vasospasm and overall outcome was not improved[23]. Recently, however, experimental and uncontrolled clinical studies suggest that early surgery combined with the intracisternal administration of the thrombolytic agent, tissue plasminogen activator (TPA), is effective in preventing the arterial narrowing[4,5]. Further studies of this approach are ongoing.

Prophylaxis Against Arterial Narrowing

While development of a specific antagonist to the primary spasmogen would be desirable, progress has been made using other strategies. Recently, it was shown in a large, randomized, placebo-controlled trial (NICSAH) in North America that the continuous infusion of high doses of intravenous nicardipine was effective in reducing both the incidence and severity of angiographically demonstrated vasospasm as well as the incidence of ischemic symptoms following aneurysmal SAH[6,8]. Nicardipine, a dihydropyridine calcium antagonist similar pharmacologically to nimodipine, presumably works by blocking calcium-dependent vasoconstriction of cerebral arteries exposed to subarachnoid clot. The very high doses of nicardipine needed to produce this effect probably accounts for why similar observations have not been made with the use of oral nimodipine.

Experimental evidence also implicates a role for products of lipid peroxidation and generation of oxygen free radicals in the pathogenesis of vasospasm. The 21-aminosteroid, tirilazad mesylate, is a powerful inhibitor of lipid peroxidation in experimental models and has been shown to ameliorate experimental vasospasm due to SAH in several species [13,24,29]. The excellent safety profile of this compound has facilitated its progress into Phase III efficacy testing in humans.

Other cerebral vasodilators take advantage of the unique characteristics of the cerebrovascular circulation in an attempt to produce desired therapeutic effects without inducing potentially detrimental hypotension. A familiar example is the relative cerebroselectivity of the calcium antagonists, nimodipine and nicardipine, for vascular smooth muscle of cerebral vessels compared to systemic vessels[25]. Interest has developed in

calcitonin gene-related peptide (CGRP), a naturally occurring vasodilator substance found in nerve terminals innervating cerebral vessels[11,12]. Similarly, a favorable clinical report has appeared regarding the use of a novel intracellular calcium inhibitor, AT877, which has relative cerebrovascular specificity due to its selective specificity for several protein kinases in cerebral vessels[22].

Dilation of Narrowed Arteries

While topical application of many agents directly on spastic blood vessels at the time of surgery can be shown to have salutary effects, it is well known that the effects are usually transient and ineffective in preventing ischemic sequelae. Many drugs have been tried systemically, and even by local arterial infusion, but without sustained benefit[27,28]. Mechanical dilatation of the narrowed segments is now technically feasible with superselective catheters equipped with specially designed balloons[18]. Superselective infusions with intra-arterial papaverine can also result in improvement in vessel caliber in selected patients. The duration of the benefit with both of these techniques is still uncertain, but has, in some instances, been reported to be long lasting. Obviously, since the technical expertise required to perform these procedures will limit the availability of this treatment, the search for an agent that could be administered systemically should continue.

Augmentation of Collateral Blood Flow

The disruption of the normal physiological mechanisms governing the autoregulation of cerebral blood flow in SAH patients affords the opportunity to improve flow to ischemic zones by manipulating perfusion pressure. Pharmacologically-induced hypertension, frequently combined with intentional hypervolemia to increase cardiac output, has become standard therapy for vasospasm in most neurosurgical centers in North America. While no randomized trials exist to prove the benefits of this approach, clinical experience and a meta-analysis of the reported series suggest the treatment is effective in reversing ischemic deficits from vasospasm[2].

Augmentation of collateral flow by dilating small cerebral resistance vessels may also account for the apparent benefits of calcium antagonists[20] and other cerebral vasodilators.

Brain Protection

Increasing knowledge with respect to the pathophysiology of ischemic cell death has led to several lines of investigation aimed at developing brain protecting agents. Some experimental evidence supports the notion that prevention of a toxic influx of calcium into ischemic neurons might partially explain the benefits of calcium entry blockers in SAH[10]. The 21-aminosteroids might also work in this way by blocking lipid peroxidation of cell membranes[9].

Therapeutic Dilemmas in Drug Development

Regardless of which strategy is chosen to combat the problem of vasospasm, the program for therapeutic drug development must take into account several issues unique to SAH patients:

Time Course of Vasospasm

The characteristic time course of the delayed arterial narrowing will influence the selection of different strategies. For example, therapies designed to prevent vasospasm would not be appropriately employed in patients admitted after day 5 from the hemorrhage, when, presumably, most of the pathophysiological processes that result in the narrowing have already been set into motion. In fact, study of most prophylactic regimens has required that treatment be started within 48–72 hours of the initial hemorrhage. Similarly, rescue therapies designed to reverse ischemic neurological deficits once they occur must be delivered in a timely manner (within a few hours, at the most) before irreversible brain infarction occurs.

Interactions with Other Therapies

Development of new therapeutic agents must not overlook advances already made, and must take into account the realities of current neurosurgical practice. Although there are no randomized trials proving the efficacy of intentional hypervolemia and induced hypertension, the anecdotal evidence seems persuasive, and the therapy is now commonly employed in the United States in up to 70% of patients. New therapeutic agents that have hypotensive side effects must either be compatible with commonly used vasopressor agents, or must be deliverable in such a way that the dosage can be readily titrated if therapeutic hypertension is deemed necessary. Many other drugs, including anti-convulsants, histamine blockers, steroids, and others are also commonly administered[15]. Potential drug interactions must, therefore, be carefully considered when a new agent is introduced.

Method of Drug Delivery

It is now well known that patients with aneurysmal subarachnoid hemorrhage have a systemic illness. The primary central nervous system injury frequently results in widespread autonomic dysfunction leading to alterations in blood pressure (either hypotension or hypertension), cardiopulmonary disorders including arrhythmias[19] and pulmonary edema, and gastrointestinal dysfunction (e.g., ileus and abnormal liver function tests). Other poorly understood phenomena such as coagulopathies may also occur. These complicating features make delivery of a therapeutic pharmacologic agent for vasospasm a difficult task. While oral agents may be appropriate for some patients, the problems imposed by sicker SAH patients make intravenously administered drugs preferable. The problem is further compounded by the blood brain barrier, which rules out systemic administration of some otherwise promising agents. Intrathecal administration, with its own attendant problems, must sometimes be considered. Occasionally, selective intraarterial administration must be utilized to avoid prohibitive systemic adverse effects.

Pharmacokinetics and Pharmacodynamics

The pharmacokinetics of a therapeutic agent are determined by its absorption, distribution, metabolism, and elimination. While drug blood levels are the most common way to study these phenomena, one must keep in mind that brain tissue or cerebrospinal fluid drug levels may sometimes be more relevant to the study of agents for vasospasm. Additionally, consideration must also be given to the pharmacodynamics and duration of biological activity of specific agents. For example, while measured levels of tissue plasminogen activator (TPA) in blood or cerebrospinal fluid may clear rapidly after administration, it is known that once TPA binds to fibrin clot, its lytic activity may last for several hours[3]. Similar considerations may also pertain to agents binding to specific receptor sites in the brain.

Another vexing problem that arises in the development of pharmacologic agents for vasospasm is the problem of dose-response testing. The disease under study is highly variable, and thus, the efficacy or response to a specific agent is hard to measure. Moreover, as the experience with nimodipine suggests, utilization of surrogate endpoints, such as the incidence of angiographic vasospasm, may potentially be flawed. Nevertheless, care must be taken not to discard potentially effective treatments for lack of testing of an adequate dose, nor must the possibility of reducing adverse side effects while preserving efficacy by administering the lowest effective dose be ignored.

Risk/Benefit Ratio

Virtually all pharmacological therapies are associated with risks. On the other hand, ischemia from delayed cerebral vasospasm is a potentially permanently disabling or fatal complication. Thus, there is a rationale for entertaining the idea of testing riskier therapies, such as intrathecal fibrinolytic therapy. Identification of prognostic factors that would confer high risk for development of ischemic symptoms might aid in the selection of patients for the riskier therapies[1], but most clinicians would still require that substantial benefit be demonstrated before widespread use of a risky treatment could be advocated. Safer treatments with lesser degrees of proven benefit might be acceptable by clinicians for a broader group of patients, but cost considerations might need to be included in these situations, as well.

Conclusions

Much remains to be accomplished in preventing death and disability from delayed cerebral vasospasm following subarachnoid hemorrhage. Yet, clinicians should be encouraged by the progress that has already been made, especially in the last decade. Of the 906 patients randomized in the NICSAH trial from 1987 through 1989, vasospasm was reported as the primary cause of death or disability in only 9.7% at the 3 month follow-up. This represents nearly a one third reduction when compared to the North American results in the Timing of Surgery Study (1980–1983)[7]. Moreover, vasospasm in the NICSAH trial was no longer the leading cause of death and disability, having been exceeded by the rates from direct effects of the initial hemorrhage. Further advances, such as the ones to be described in these proceedings, are anxiously awaited.

References

1. Adams HP, Kassell NF, Torner JC, Haley EC (1987) Predicting cerebral ischemia after aneurysmal subarachnoid haemorrhage: Influences of clinical condition, CT results, and antifibrinolytic therapy. A report of the Cooperative Aneurysm Study. Neurology 37: 1586–1591
2. Dorsch NWC (1990) Incidence, effects and treatment of ischaemia following aneurysm rupture. In: Sano K, *et al* (eds) Cerebral vasospasm. Proceedings of the IVth International Conference on Cerebral Vasospasm. University of Tokyo Press, Tokyo, pp 495–498
3. Eisenberg PR, Sherman LA, Tiefenbrunn AJ, Ludbrook PA, Sobel BE, Jaffe AS (1987) Sustained fibrinolysis after administration of t-PA despite its short half-life in the circulation. Thromb Haemost 57: 35–40
4. Findlay JM, Weir BKA, Kassell NF, Disney LB, Grace MGA (1991) Intracisternal recombinant tissue plasminogen activator after aneurysmal subarachnoid hemorrhage. J Neurosurg 75: 181–188
5. Findlay JM, Weir BKA, Steinke D, Tanabe T, Gordon P, Grace M (1988) Effect of intrathecal thrombolytic therapy on subarachnoid clot and chronic vasospasm in a primate model of SAH. J Neurosurg 69: 723–735
6. Haley EC, Kassell NF, Torner JC, Kongable G (1991) Nicardipine ameliorates angiographic vasospasm following subarachnoid hemorrhage (SAH). Neurology 41 [Suppl] 1: 346 (abstract)
7. Haley EC, Kassell NF, Torner JC, and the Participants (1992) The International Cooperative Study on the timing of aneurysm surgery: the North American experience. Stroke 23: 205–214
8. Haley EC, Torner JC, Kassell NF, the Participants (1990) Cooperative randomized study of nicardipine in subarachnoid hemorrhage: Preliminary report. In: Sano K, *et al* (eds) Cerebral vasospasm. Proceedings of the IVth International Conference on Cerebral Vasospasm. University of Tokyo Press, Tokyo, pp 519–525
9. Hall ED, Braughler JM (1989) Central nervous system trauma and stroke II. Physiological and pharmacological evidence for involvement of oxygen radicals and lipid peroxidation. Free Radic Biol Med 6: 303–313
10. Harris RJ, Branston NM, Symon L, Bayhan M, Watson A (1982) The effects of a calcium antagonist, nimodipine, upon physiological responses of the cerebral vasculature and its possible influence upon focal cerebral ischemia. Stroke 13: 759–766
11. Hongo K, Tsukahara T, Kassell NF, Ogawa H (1989) Effect of subarachnoid hemorrhage on calcitonin gene-related peptide-induced relaxation in rabbit basilar artery. Stroke 20: 100–104
12. Johnston FG, Bell BA, Robertson IJA, Miller JD, Haliburn DO, Shaughnessy DO, Ladlre SA (1990) Effect of calcitonin-gene-related peptide on postoperative neurological deficits after subarachnoid haemorrhage. Lancet 335: 869–872
13. Kanamaru K, Weir BKA, Findlay JM, Grace M, Mac Donald RL (1990) A dosage study of the effect of the 21-aminosteroid U-74006F on chronic cerebral vasospasm in a primate model. Neurosurgery 27: 29–38
14. Kassell NF, Sasaki T, Colohan ART, Nazar G (1985) Cerebral vasospasm following aneurysmal subarachnoid hemorrhage. Stroke 16: 562–572
15. Kassell NF, Torner JC, Haley EC, Jane JA, Adams HP, Kongable GL, the Participants (1992) The International Cooperative Study on the timing of aneurysm surgery. J Neurosurg 73: 18–36
16. Macdonald RL, Weir BKA (1991) A review of hemoglobin and the pathogenesis of cerebral vasospasm. Stroke 22: 971–982

17. Mizukami M, Kawasi T, Usani T, Tazawa T (1982) Prevention of vasospasm by early operation with removal of subarachnoid blood. Neurosurgery 10: 301–307

18. Newell DW, Eskridge JM, Mayberg MR, Grady MS, Winn HR (1989) Angioplasty for the treatment of symptomatic vasospasm following subarachnoid hemorrhage. Neurosurgery 71: 654–660

19. Oppenheimer SM, Hachinski VC (1992) The cardiac consequences of stroke. In: Barnett HJM, Hachinski VC (eds) Cerebral ischemia: treatment and prevention. Neurologic Clinics, Vol 10 (1). Saunders, Philadelphia, pp 167–176

20. Robinson MJ, Teasdale GM (1990) Calcium antagonists in the management of subarachnoid hemorrhage. Cerebrovasc Brain Metab Rev 2: 205–226

21. Sano K, Saito I (1980) Early operation and washout of blood clots for prevention of cerebral vasospasm. In: Wilkins RH (ed) Cerebral arterial spasm. Proceedings of the Second International Workshop. Williams and Wilkins, Baltimore, pp 510–513

22. Shibuya M, Suzuki Y, Sugita K, Saito I, Sasaki T, Takakura K, Nagata I, Kikuchi H, Takemae T, Hidaka H, Nakashima M (1992) Effect of AT877 on cerebral vasospasm after aneurysmal subarachnoid hemorrhage. J Neurosurg 76: 571–577

23. Torner JC, Kassell NF, Haley EC (1990) The timing of surgery and vasospasm. In: Mayberg M (ed) Cerebral vasospasm. Neurosurgical Clinics, Vol 1. Saunders, Philadelphia, pp 335–347

24. Vollmer DG, Kassell NF, Hongo K, Ogawa H, Tsukahara T (1989) Effect of the non-glucocorticoid 21-aminosteroid U74006F on delayed experimental cerebral vasospasm. Surg Neurol 31: 190–194

25. Weir B (1984) Calcium antagonists, cerebral ischemia and vasospasm. Can J Neurol Sci 11: 239–246

26. Weir B, Grace M, Hanson J, Rothberg C (1978) Time course of vasospasm in man. J Neurosurg 48: 173–178

27. Wilkins RH (1980) Attempted prevention or treatment of intracranial arterial spasm: a survey. Neurosurgery 6: 198–210

28 Wilkins RH (1986) Attempts at prevention or treatment of intracranial arterial spasm: an update. Neurosurgery 18: 808–825

29. Zuccarello M, Varsch JT, Schmitt G, Woodward J, Anderson DK (1989) Effect of the 21-aminosteroid U-74,006F on cerebral vasospasm following subarachnoid hemorrhage. J Neurosurg 71: 98–104

Correspondence: E. Clark Haley, Jr., M.D., Department of Neurology, Box 394, University of Virginia, Health Sciences Center, Charlottesville, Virginia 22908, U.S.A.

A Calcium Antagonist in Aneurysmal SAH

L. Brandt and **H. Säveland**

Department of Neurosurgery, University Hospital of Lund, Lund, Sweden

Summary

In a prospective study, with participation of five of the six neuro-surgical centers in Sweden, all patients with a verified aneurysmal SAH were included. A uniform management protocol including ultra-early referral, earliest possible surgery and aggressive anti-ischemic treatment, was adopted. A total of 325 patients were admitted during the study period, 69% within 24 hours after hemorr-hage. The distribution according to Hunt and Hess on admission was: Grade I 43 patients (13%), Grade II 119(37%), Grade III 53(16%), Grade IV 76(23%), and Grade V 34(11%). Nimodipine was administered to 269 of the 325 patients; intravenously in 218, orally in 15, and intravenously followed by orally in 36. At follow up exami-nation 3 to 6 months after SAH, 183 patients (56%) were classified as having made a good neurological recovery, 73 patients (23%) suffered some morbidity, and 69 (21%) were dead. Of the 145 patients with supratentorial aneurysms who were preoperatively in Hunt and Hess Grade I–III, and who were operated within 72 hours, 81% made a good recovery. In 5.8% of the patients, morbidity and mortality could be ascribed to delayed ischemia. It is concluded that, among patients in all clinical grades and aneurysm locations, almost 6 out of 10 SAH victims referred to a neurosurgical unit, can be saved to a normal life.

Keywords: Subarachnoid hemorrhage; vasospasm; delayed ischemia; calcium antagonist; nimodipine; overall outcome.

Background

In 1947, at a meeting in Sidney, Graeme Robertson was the first to ascribe late deterioration in patients suffer-ing aneurysmal subarachnoid haemorrhage (SAH) to a consequence of cerebral ischemia[25]. He also proposed that this delayed ischemia, transient or permanent, prob-ably was due to spasm of the arteries of sufficient dur-ation to produce cerebral dysfunction and/or damage. Furthermore, he observed that the cerebral changes promoted by ischemia "may be remote from the ter-ritory of the artery bearing the aneurysm" and also that "this mechanism is far more common than realized".

The second report that suggested direct intracranial arterial narrowing as the underlying factor for the delayed deterioration in SAH appeared in 1951, when Ecker and Riemenschneider[9] using angiography, first demonstrated arterial spasm of intracranial arteries after rupture of an aneurysm.

Gradually, the phenomenon of cerebral arterial narrowing after SAH became accepted by clinicians as being most significant. However, it was not until the mid 60'ies that Kågström and co-workers[16] demon-strated that this radiographic arterial narrowing after aneurysmal SAH is a time dependent phenomenon, which is very rarely seen immediately after aneurysm rupture.

Constriction of arteries has been considered one of the physiological mechanisms for the acute control of haemorrhage since the time of John Hunter. *Delayed* arterial spasm, however, remains one of the least understood of the physiological mechanisms in bleed-ing and haemostasis. From early   k it was recognized that cerebral arteries may constrict in response to mechanical as well as electrical stimulation, topical application of blood and also from a variety of chemical compounds as well as room-air and water[17].

During the decades after the establishment of cerebral vasospasm as an important clinical reality, numerous approaches to the prevention and treatment of this phenomenon have been suggested, and there have been many attempts to elucidate the pathophysiology behind this phenomenon. Among the most visible hypothesis, advanced to explain cerebral vasospasm, are those implicating vasoconstrictive agents, such as serotonin, catecholamines and the prostaglandines, and the list has grown parallel to the discovery of new vasoactive agents in post-hemorrhagic cerebrospinal fluid (CSF)[33]. The basic concept arose that the initial deposition of blood in the subarachnoid spaces around the circle of Willis induces the delayed constriction of these arteries, perhaps owing to a factor or factors liberated from the clotted blood, and that the arterial constriction then leeds to subsequent cerebral ischemia and infarction.

However, still much confusion exists concerning the nature, etiology and pathogenesis of the intracranial arterial narrowing seen angiographically, and called vasospasm. There is also little evidence to link brief transitory constriction of a cerebral artery, which can be produced in the laboratory, with the complex series of clinical and radiographic events that occur in patients after rupture of an intracranial aneurysm. A number of hypothesis have been offered to explain the typical latency of the arterial constriction and the concept that a substance may be released by the lysis of blood was proposed with initial confirmatory evidence.

Among other mechanisms suggested to explain for the delayed arterial narrowing are denervation hypersensitivity, morphological vascular changes, immunreactions as well as brain stem reflexes. When discussing the syndrome of delayed cerebral ischemia after aneurysm rupture, it must be emphasized that this clinical complication most probably results from an interaction of several mechanisms and not exclusively to "vasospasm". Increased intracranial pressure (ICP), drop in systemic blood pressure, hypoxia, hypovolemia, electrolyte disturbances etc. may interact with the arterial narrowing to cause cerebral ischemia.

So far, no single mediator or mechanism has convincingly been proven to be the most important for the delayed arterial constriction and, furthermore, no antagonist of a single mediator candidate has been demonstrated to be therapeutically effective.

Calcium Antagonists

The experimental findings on isolated vessels that calcium antagonists, such as nimodipine, effectively prevent contractions of isolated human cerebral arteries, induced by almost all contractile agents including blood and posthemorrhagic cerebrospinal fluid, made it logical to propose the use of such drugs in the prevention and/or treatment of cerebral vasospasm[1,5,6,8,10,22,27,32].

Calcium is known to be an important link between electrical or chemical stimulation as well as physiological responses in a great variety of contractile and secretory cells. During the 1970'ies, many pharmacological agents blocking transmembrane calcium flux became increasingly used clinically, especially in cardiovascular disorders.

In the cerebrovascular field, much interest has been focused on the dihydropyridines, one of the major groupes of calcium-antagonists, according to the international classification.

Calcium antagonists are generally more potent inhibitors of calcium influx through voltage-dependent than receptor-operated channels. They are also more potent in smooth and cardiac muscle than in skeleton muscle. Thus, in the circulation, they preferentially affect coronary and cerebral vascular smooth muscle cells[2]. This has been documented in several studies both in vitro and in vivo[1,3,4,5,7,15,18,22,31,34].

The detailed mechanisms behind a selective cerebrovascular effect of calcium antagonists have not yet been established, but may be related to a greater dependence on extracellular calcium for contractile activation of cerebral than of peripheral vessels. There is also experimental evidence that calcium influx in cerebral areries to a higher extent takes place through voltage-operated calcium channels, especially in humans[26].

From experiments on rabbit basilar arteries, McCalden and Bevan[20] concluded that K^+ induces contraction by using a single calcium pool, probably of extracellular origin. Noradrenaline (NA) and serotonin (5HT) also primarily utilized extracellular calcium. Skaerby et al.[29] found that in cat middle cerebral artery, both K^+- and noradrenaline-induced contractions were almost exclusively dependent on the presence of calcium in the extracellular medium, and that activation occur through pathways sensitive to calcium antagonists. This is in some contrast with findings in isolated human pial vessels[32] where treatment in a calciumfree medium for 30 mins and exposure to nimodipine markedly reduced K^+-, but to a lesser extent NA- and 5HT-induced contractions. It was suggested that this was due to the amines also using intracellularly stored calcium for their contraction. Available information suggests that the requirement of extracellular versus intracellular calcium for contractile activation of brain arteries is dependent on what agent is used for the activation.

The effects of nimodipine on *cerebral blood flow* was studied by Haws and co-workers[14] in rabbits using the microsphere method. At low doses, which have little effect on systemic blood pressure, nimodpine caused a selective increase in cerebral and myocardial blood flow. Nimodipine increased blood flow in all regions of the brain. There was no change in cerebral O_2 consumption and the increased blood flow was interpreted as the result of a direct vasodilator effect and not secondary to increased cerebral metabolism. In rats,

Mohamed et al.[21] studied the effect of a continuous i.v. infusion of nimodipine on local CBF and local cerebral glucose utilization, using the quantitative autoradiographic techniques. The nimodipine infusion produced only a small reduction in mean arterial blood pressure, and did not alter the rate of glucose utilization in any of the regions examined. By contrast, in 24 regions, CBF was increased significantly by 39–84% from control levels.

A selective action on cerebral vessels may contribute to a beneficial effect of calcium antagonists in cerebral disorders, particularly in the syndrome of "cerebral vasospasm" after subarachnoid haemorrhage, and in cerebral ischemia associated with acute vessels occlusion.

In contrast to occlusive stroke, the complication of cerebral vasospasm and ischemia after SAH mostly developes several days following the first bleed. This very important difference means that after SAH there are unique opportunities for the initiation of treatment before brain damage is already established.

For the support of such use, in vivo experiments in dogs subjected to experimenal SAH by a cisternal injection of autogenous blood[13] were obtained. Intrathecal administration of 4 ml of 10^{-3} M nimodipine promptly and completely reversed vasospasm in all animals studied. However, conflicting experimental results have been obtained by others[11]. In a series of experimental subarachnoid blood deposition in monkeys, Weir and co-workers were neither able to demonstrate any beneficial clinical effect of nimodipine, nor any significant effect on angiographically visible vasospasm[12,19,23].

Although administration of calcium antagonists may be less effective once vasospasm has developed in humans, accumulating clinical evidence occured that such treatment, when started early after haemorrhage, may prevent or reduce symptomatic vasospasm and secondary cerebral ischemia.

Thus, the clinical results in patients are in some contrast to the animal studies on experimental subarachnoid haemorrhage, where nimodipine failed to counteract the development of vasospasm. The reason for this discrepancy may be explained by the fact that delayed ischemic deterioration after SAH from a ruptured intracranial aneurysm appears to be more or less an exclusively human syndrome. At least, there is so far no well controlled reproducible animal model available which completely mimics for the human situation.

In most clinical studies using intravenous nimodipine

in aneurysmal SAH, the incidence of DID leading to permanent deficits or death has been decreased from an average of approximately 15–20% to less than 5%.

Most of the pioneering studies were open, non-randomized and lacking placebo controls. In spite of a very marked reduction of the incidence of DID the results of these studies were, consequently, considered controversial. Subsequently, however, the role of nimodipine in aneurysmal SAH has been studied in 7 prospective, randomized, double-blind, placebo controlled trials using either oral nimodipine or intravenous nimodipine alone or in a sequential regimen of intravenous infusion followed by oral administration[30]. In the majority of the trials, the efficacy parameters were: incidence and severity of persistent ischemic neurologic deficits; overall outcome; mortality. In one study, the incidence of cerebral infarcts was one of the endpoints. In this trial (The British BRANT study[24]) there was a 40% reduction in poor outcomes in the treatment group. Relevant data from these controlled studies will be given elsewhere.

Impact of Early Aneurysm Surgery and Nimodipine on the Total Management Results in a Defined Population

Sweden has six neurosurgical centers. In Lund, we introduced the use of nimodipine in aneurysmal SAH 1982. At that time, deliberate early aneurysm surgery (within 72 h after SAH) in good grade patients had been performed for more than 5 years in our unit. Subsequently during the 1980'ies, the policy of routine early surgery and nimodipine was adopted by the other neurosurgical centers in our country. Today, an early referral system, early aneurysm surgery and nimodipine are well established since several years in swedish neurosurgery.

The impact of this regimen in a defined population, with a uniform management protocol, was evaluated in a prospective, one-year study during 1990[28].

Patient Material and Management Protocol

The participating centers cover 7 million (81%) of Swedens 8.59 million people. All patients with a verified aneurysmal SAH were included in the study. Altogether, 325 patients were admitted alive, the majority within 24 hours after the bleed. The Hunt and Hess grade upon admission were: I 13%, II 37%, III 16%, IV 23% and V 10%. Mean age was 53.5 years (range 9 to 84) and the female/male ratio was 1.7/1.

Nimodipine was administered in 269 of the patients, 254 intravenously and 15 orally.

A clinical follow up was performed 3 to 6 months after discharge from the neurosurgical unit.

The majority of patients (85%) underwent aneurysm surgery, 200 within 72 hours after the bleed. In 49 patients (15%) surgery was not performed due to either high age, poor neurological condition or other medical complicating factors. The remaining patients were operated day 4 or later.

Results and Discussion

In the *total series*, 56% made a good functional recovery (183 individuals), the morbidity was 23% and the mortality 21% (Fig. 1). Outcome in relation to clinical grade on admission and age are given in Figs. 2 and 3, respectively.

Altogether 142 patients had an unfavorable outcome. In 19, this was due to DID (5.8% of the total material).

3–6 Months post SAH
325 Patients arriving alive to a neurosurgical unit
(including 33% poor grade patients)

Good	56%
Morbidity	23%
Mortality	21%

Fig. 1. Total management results

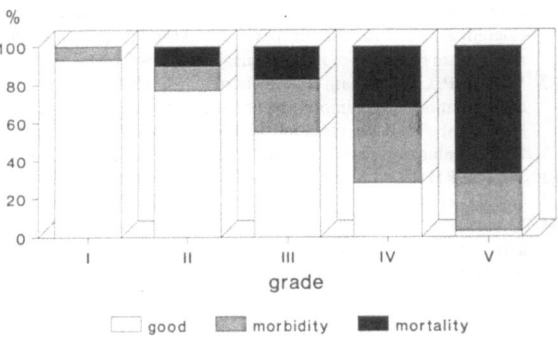

Fig. 2. Outcome in relation to grade on admission

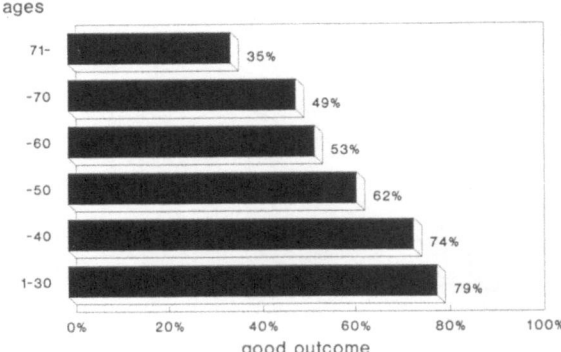

Fig. 3. Outcome in relation to age

Other reasons for an unfavorable outcome were: persistent effects of the initial bleed (65 patients), surgical complications (20 patients), early rebleeding (20 patients), other medical complications (12 patients), hydrocephalus (3 patients) and CNS infection (3 patients).

The *overall management results* in this prospective, one year study are very close to Seilers series presented 1988. The management protocols are also very similar, including *early surgery, nimodipine* administration etc; and the results are most probably close to what is possible to achieve with the present state of the art.

During recent years, an increasing number of poor grade SAH patients are accepted for neurosurgical care. In the present swedish series, this is reflected by the proportion of grade IV and V patients, who constituted no less than 33% of the total patient material.

Further, probably minor, management improvements may be achieved concerning surgical complications, management of elderly as well as poor grade patients etc. However, since almost half of all morbidity and mortality is related to direct effects of the initial bleed, a prerequisit for any major improvements in the overall management results of SAH patients, seems to be detection of *the unruptured aneurysm*.

References

1. Allen GS, Banghart SB (1979) Cerebral arterial spasm, 9. In vitro effects of nifedipine on serotonin-phenylephrine- and potassium-induced contractions of canine basilar and femoral arteries. Neurosurgery 4: 37–42
2. Andersson KE (1986) Pharmacodynamic profiles of different calcium channel blockers. Acta Pharmacol Toxicol 58: II, 31–42
3. Auer LM, Mokry M (1985) Effect of nimodipine and its solvent on superficial cerebral vessels. J Cereb Blood Flow Metab 5: 473–474
4. Bevan JA (1982) Selective action of diltiazem on cerebral vascular smooth muscle in the rabbit: antagonism of extrinsic but not intrinsic maintained tone. Am J Cardiol 49: 519–524
5. Brandt L (1981) Aspects on cerebral vasospasm. A clinical and experimental study. Doctoral Thesis, University of Lund, Sweden
6. Brandt L, Andersson KE, Bengtsson B, Edvinsson L, Ljunggren B, MacKenzie ET (1979) Effects of nifedipine on pial arteriolar calibre: an in vivo study. Surg Neurol 12: 349–352
7. Brandt L, Andersson KE, Edvinsson L, Ljunggren B (1981) Effects of extracellular calcium and calcium antagonists on the contractile responses of isolated human pial and mesenteric arteries. J Cereb Blood Flow Metab 1: 339–347
8. Brandt L, Ljunggren B, Andersson KE, MacKenzie ET, Tamura A, Teasdale G (1982) Effects on feline cortical pial microvasculature of topical application of a calcium antagonist (nifedipine) under normal conditions and in focal ischaemia. J Cereb Blood Flow Metab 3: 44–50
9. Ecker AD, Riemenschneider PA (1951) Arteriographic demon-

stration of spasm of the intracranial arteries: with special reference to saccular arterial aneurisms. J Neurosurg 8: 660–667

10. Edvinsson L, Brandt L, Andersson KE, Bengtsson B (1979) Effect of a calcium antagonist on experimental constriction of human brain vessels: possible efficacy in cerebrovascular spasm. Surg Neurol 11: 327–330

11. Espinosa F, Weir B, Overton T, Castor W, Grace M, Boisvert D (1984) A randomized placebo-controlled double-blind trial for nimodipine after SAH in monkeys. Part I: Clinical and radiological findings. J Neurosurg 60: 1167–1175

12. Espinosa F, Weir B, Shnitka T, Overton T, Boisvert D (1984) A randomized placebo-controlled double-blind trial for nimodipine after SAH in monkeys. Part 2: Pathological findings. J Neurosurg 60: 1176–1185

13. Gioia AE, White RP, Bakiitian B, Robertson JT (1985) Evaluation of the efficacy of intrathecal nimodipine in canine models of chronic cerebral vasospasm. J Neurosurg 62: 721–728

14. Haws CW, Gourley JK, Heistad DD (1983) Effects of nimodipine on cerebral blood flow. J Pharmacol Exp Ter 225: 1, 24–28

15. Högestätt ED, Andersson KE, Edvinsson L (1982) Effects of nifedipine on potassium-induced contraction and noradrenaline release in cerebral and extracranial arteries from rabbit. Acta Physiol Scand 114: 283–296

16. Kågström E, Greitz T, Hanson J, et al (1966) Changes in cerebral blood flow after subarachnoid hemorrhage. Excerpta Medica Foundation Int Congr Series (Amsterdam) 110: 629–33

17. Kapp J, Mahaley MS JR, Odom GL (1968) Cerebral arterial spasm. Part 1: evaluation of experimental variables affecting the diameter of the exposed basilar artery. J Neurosurg 29: 331–338

18. Kazda S, Gardhoff B, Krause HP, Schlossman K (1982) Cerebrovascular effects of the calcium antagonistic dihydropyridine derivative nimodipine in animal experiments. Arzneimittelforschung (Drug Res) 32: 331–338

19. Kreuger C, Weir B, Nosko M, Cook D, Norris S (1985) Nimodipine and chronic vasospasm in monkeys: Part 2. Pharmacological studies of vessels in spasm. Neurosurgery 16(2): 137–140

20. McCalden TA, Beven JA (1981) Sources of activator calcium in rabbit basilar artery. Am J Physiol 241: H129–H133

21. Mohamed AA, Mendelow AD, Teasdale GM, Harper AM, McCulloch J (1985) Effect of the calcium antagonist nimodipine on local cerebral blood flow and metabolic coupling. J Cereb Blood Flow Metab 5: 26–33

22. Müller-Schweinitzer E, Neumann P (1983) In vitro effects of calcium antagonists PN 200–110, nifedipine, and nimodipine on human and canine cerebral arteries. J Cereb Blood Flow Metab 3: 354–361

23. Nosko M, Weir B, Krueger C, Cook D, Norris S, Overton T, Boisvert D (1985) Nimodipine and chronic vasospasm in monkeys: Part 1. Clinical and radiological findings. Neurosurgery 16: 129–136

24. Pickard JD, Murray GD, Illingworth R, Shaw MDM, Teasdale G, Foy PM, Humphrey PRD, Lang DA, Nelson R, Richards P, Sinar J, Bailey S, Skene A (1989) Effect of oral nimodipine on cerebral infarction and outcome after subarachnoid hemorrhage: British aneurysm nimodipine trial. BMJ 298: 636–642

25. Robertson EG (1949) Cerebral lesions due to intracranial aneurysms. Brain 72: 150–185

26. Ryman T, Brandt L, Andersson KE, Mellergård P (1989) Regional and species differences in vascular reactivity to extracellular potassium. Acta Physiol Scand 136: 151–159

27. Salacies M, Maria J, Rico ML, Gonzalez C (1983) Effects of verapamil and manganese on the vasoconstrictor responses to noradrenaline, serotonin and potassium in human and goat cerebral arteries. Biochem Pharmacol 32: 2711–2714

28. Säveland H, Hillman J, Brandt L, Edner G, Jakobsson KE, Algers G (1992) Overall outcome in aneurysmal subarachnoid hemorrhage: a prospective study from neurosurgical units in Sweden during one year. J Neurosurg 76: 729–734

29. Skärby T, Högestätt ED, Andersson KE (1984) Influence of extracellular calcium and nifedipine on 1- and 2-adrenoceptor mediated contractile responses in isolated rat and cat cerebral and mesenteric arteries. Acta Physiol Scand 123: 445–456

30. Tettenborn D, Dycka J (1990) Prevention and treatment of delayed ischemic dysfunction in patients with aneurysmal subarachnoid hemorrhage. Stroke 21(12) [Suppl IV]

31. Towart R (1981) The selective inhibition of serotonin-induced contractions of rabbit cerebral vascular smooth muscle by calcium antagonistic dihydropyridines. An investigation of the mechanism of action of nimodipine. Circ Res 48: 650–657

32. White RP, Cunningham MP, Robertson JT (1982) Effect of the calcium antagonist nimodipine on contractile responses of isolated canine basilar arteries induced by serotonin, prostaglandin F_2, thrombin, and whole blood. Neurosurgery 10(3): 244–248

33. Wilkins RH (1986) Attempts at prevention of treatment of intracranial arterial spasm: an update. Neurosurgery 18: 808–825

34. Yamamoto M, Ohta T, Toda N (1983) Mechanisms of relaxant action of nicardipine, a new Ca^{++}-antagonist, on isolated dog cerebral and mesenteric arteries. Stroke 14: 270–275

Correspondence: Lennart Brandt, M.D., Department of Neurosurgery, University Hospital, S-22185 Lund, Sweden.

Nimodipine and Cerebral Vasospasm: Review of Effects and Mechanisms

N.W.C. Dorsch

Department of Surgery, Westmead Hospital, Sydney, Australia

Summary

One hundred and forty-one patients have been treated with IV nimodipine for symptomatic vasospasm. Treatment was started within three days of onset and continued 7–10 days. Side effects were minor, and serious complications few. Most improved during treatment, and final outcome was GOS 1 105 (74%), GOS 2 8 (6%), GOS 3 13 (9%), and death 15 (11%).

In a literature review the incidence of delayed ischaemic deficit was 32.1% in 30783 reported cases, and the outcome untreated (3306 cases) was death 30.4%, permanent deficit 34.0%, and good result 35.6%. Results appear considerably better with hypervolaemic or hypertensive prophylaxis (2361 cases reported, 17.8% DID) or treatment (1920 cases, 16.9% dead, 28.6% deficit).

Results with calcium antagonists, especially nimodipine, appear even better – in eight studies, DID occurred in 31.7% of control patients and 22.4% of those on nimodipine, a highly significant difference; similarly, outcome of the treated patients was greatly improved. Overall, the incidence of DID with nimodipine pretreatment was 13.5% in 4128 cases, and the combined outcome (762 cases) was: death 16%, permanent deficit 26%, and good outcome 58%. These figures represent a considerable improvement over the variations of HHH treatment, and calcium antagonists are generally easier to administer and safer; also they appear to have no increased risk of rebleeding.

Keywords: Cerebral aneurysm; subarachnoid haemorrhage; cerebral vasospasm; calcium antagonists.

Introduction

Cerebral vasospasm is a major problem after aneurysm haemorrhage. Without specific management angiographic spasm is common, and nearly one-third of patients develop symptomatic vasospasm (delayed ischaemic deficit, DID). Untreated, DID causes death or permanent disability in over half of those affected.

The standard treatment, fluids and induced hypertension, can lower the incidence of DID and improve its outcome, but can be risky, particularly in unoperated cases. Several calcium antagonists have also been used in management of DID.

Experience with nimodipine in treating DID is presented. This is followed by a review of calcium antagonists in vasospasm, with discussion of the possible mechanisms of their action.

Clinical Material and Methods

One hundred and forty-one patients (100 female) of mean age 50 years (range 17–75) have been treated at Westmead or Royal Prince Alfred Hospital in Sydney with nimodipine for symptomatic cerebral vasospasm. 47 (33%) were hypertensive. In the 132 with SAH, ischaemic symptoms developed between one and 18 days after the last known SAH; in the others, it followed an operation for an unruptured aneurysm. The mean overall delay from SAH to DID was 6.5 days; in the 34 unoperated cases the mean delay of 6.7 days (SD 3.4) was similar to that of the 107 postoperative patients (mean 6.4 days, SD 3.4; $t = 0.4$, $p > 0.2$). The clinical grade (Hunt and Hess) of the patients at the time nimodipine treatment was started was: III 67, IV 59, and V 15.

During treatment, patients were kept well hydrated to minimise the risk of hypotension. The nimodipine was given as a central infusion, starting at 7.5–10 µg/kg/h and increasing to 30–45 µg/kg/h. It was continued for at least one week, and for several days after the patient was stable, and then tailed over 1–2 days. Treatment lasted from one (two patients who died soon after starting) to 27 days – mean duration was 6.4 days, SD 3.4.

Results

Hypotension (a fall in mean BP of at least 20 mmHg) was seen in 38 patients. It was more likely in previously hypertensive (18/57 or 38%) than normotensive patients (20/94; $\chi^2 = 3.8$, $p \approx 0.05$). There were altered liver function tests in 55 of the 123 with results available (45%), raised blood sugar in 29% (24/82), and arterial hypoxaemia, usually mild, in 33/110, or 30%.

Five patients developed significant pulmonary oedema, and one each atrial fibrillation, acalculous cholecystitis, and ischaemic colitis. Their relation to the treatment is uncertain. Two with CT infarction before treatment died soon after, one with a haemorrhagic infarct, and the other raised ICP and hydrocephalus. There was one (fatal) rebleed in the 34 unoperated patients.

Table 1. *Effect on Clinical Grade*

Grade	Before	After
I	0	47
II	0	14
III	67	56
IV	59	15
V	15	9*

$\chi^2 = 90$, p < 0.0001.
* Includes some dead.

Table 2. *Effect on GCS*

GCS	Before	After
3	4	6
4–5	6	3
6–7	15	3
8–9	20	4
10–11	19	9
12	15	5
13	29	12
14	23	30
15	10	69

$\chi^2 = 81$, p < 0.0001.

Most patients responded quickly to treatment, improving often within hours. Some, in grade V or deteriorating, continued to do so and died within days. Overall, 117 (83%) of the 141 improved during the treatment course; there were highly significant improvements in both grade and GCS (Tables 1 and 2).

The final outcome, using the Glasgow Outcome Scale (GOS), was assessed at least a month after the end of treatment. It was:

GOS 1: 105,
GOS 2: 8,
GOS 3: 13,
GOS 4: 0,
GOS 5: 15.

In summary, this gives a death rate of 11% (15/141), permanent deficits in 15%, and good outcome in 74% (105).

The cause of death was vasospasm alone in only two, spasm plus the original haemorrhage in four, rebleeding during (one) or after (three) treatment, and intraoperative aneurysm rupture in one; two died from possible complications of treatment as discussed above, one from a pulmonary embolus after treatment, and one from an intracerebral haematoma while on heparin for venous thrombosis. Vasospasm was thus directly a factor in only 40% of deaths, but can be implicated indirectly in other cases, e.g. where a patient rebled while still too disabled for surgery.

For the 21 with permanent deficits, spasm accounted alone for 12, and with other factors for seven; it was not implicated in two (one original ICH, one a previous ischaemic stroke).

Review of Literature on Cerebral Vasospasm

An extensive review of the aneurysm literature since 1960, involving more than 1000 references, has been carried out. An outline of natural history and other management is presented first, as a background for the use of calcium antagonists.

1. Natural History

The overall incidence of angiographic vasospasm, obtained from 216 references, was 13129/30389 or 43.2%. When angiography was carried out around the end of the first week after SAH, it was 67.0% (1808 in 2699 cases), which is probably much closer to the true incidence. Delayed ischaemic deficit or symptomatic vasospasm is considerably less common. Among 30783 reported cases DID occurred in 9882, or 32.1% (271 references).

The outcome of DID was mentioned in 105 reports, and from 3306 patients, death occurred in 1004 (30.4%) and permanent deficits in 1126 cases (34.0%), while 1176 (35.6%) eventually made a good recovery.

2. Fluid and Hypertensive Therapy

Since the first report by Kosnik and Hunt[1] of the use of induced hypertension to treat established DID, many variations of this type of treatment have been introduced. Some have used simply increased fluid loading, others hypertensive treatment with vasopressor drugs, and some the whole spectrum of hypervolaemia, hypertension, and haemodilution, or Triple-H therapy[2]. The reported figures for these variations are not greatly different, and they have been combined.

When HHH therapy or variations have been used for prophylaxis of vasospasm, i.e., administered to all patients as soon as possible after SAH (28 references), the incidence of DID in 2361 cases was 420, or 17.8% – a reduction of nearly half over natural history.

For the treatment of established DID (67 reports), the outcome figures with HHH therapy were: death 325/1920 = 17.9%, permanent deficits 549 or 28.6%, and good outcomes in 1046, or 54.5%. This is again better than without treatment, particularly where death rate is concerned.

3. Nimodipine

A number of well-designed controlled trials of nimodipine have been reported. Combining these with other studies that used historical controls (total eight studies), very significant reductions in DID were seen – in 978 control patients the incidence was 310 (31.7%), and in 702 who received nimodipine there was 22.4% (157) DID ($\chi^2 = 17.3$, p < 0.0001).

In ten more or less controlled studies, which included four of the above, information was available on the outcome of patients. The death rate was 16.6% (192/1159) in controls and 11.8% (115/978) in treated cases ($\chi^2 = 9.6$, p = 0.0002); the incidence of all bad outcomes, death and permanent deficits combined (regardless of cause) was also considerably reduced, with 331/1166 (28.4%) in control patients compared with 181/923 (19.6%) with treatment ($\chi^2 = 21$, p < 0.0001). A meta analysis by Tettenborn and Dycka[3] of seven controlled studies confirmed a highly significant improvement in outcome with nimodipine, and showed a reduction of 42% in the risk of a bad outcome.

3a. Prophylaxis. Forty-seven references mentioned the use of nimodipine for the prevention of DID. From 4128 patients, there was DID in 558 or 13.5%. It has never been tested in a controlled way, but it may be that intravenous use is more effective than oral; DID occurred in 12.2 (418/3421) and 19.8% (140/707) respectively.

3b. Treatment. In reports of patients on prophylactic nimodipine, the outcome of those who developed DID and in whom the nimodipine was continued, was given (31 references, 419 patients). 18% were dead, 32% had permanent disability, and 50% good recovery.

In other cases nimodipine was started de novo after DID developed, ie it was used only for treatment. The 343 cases (6 references) in this category include our own 141 cases. Outcome for this group was better, with 45 deaths (13%), 68 permanent deficits (20%), and 230 (67%) making good recoveries.

4. Other Calcium Antagonists

Nicardipine has been used as prophylaxis in 1045 reported patients (12 references), with an incidence of DID of 24% (247 cases). When it was used as treatment (7 reports, 191 patients) death rate was 12%, deficits 17%, and good outcomes 71%.

In 310 reported cases receiving flunarizine (3 references) there was DID in 15 (5%); 11 out of 13 of these made good recoveries. With diltiazem, the reported incidence of DID (166 patients in 4 reports) was 32%, and the outcome in treatment of DID included 46/68 (68%) good. For verapamil, with only 34 cases in two reports, there was a 15% (five) incidence of DID.

Discussion

It appears that nimodipine is effective in improving the outcome of DID after SAH. The outcome of these 141 patients – dead 11%, permanent deficits in 15% – is vastly better than for untreated DID and a considerable improvement over hypervolaemic and/or hypertensive therapy. In addition, IV nimodipine is simpler to administer and control, and probably safer than hypertension, especially preoperatively.

The hypotension noted in some of our patients treated with nimodipine has been reported by others, and it has also been noted to be more likely in previously hypertensive patients. In our own series, hypotension was severe enough to need support with vasopressors in only six cases – five of these were in the first half of the series, suggesting that experience in fluid maintenance is important.

Other side effects were few, mainly non-clinical disturbances of liver function or glucose metabolism, or possibly systemic hypoxia due to the opening of pulmonary arteriovenous shunts. These patients were often very ill, and receiving many drugs, so that many of these abnormalities may occur in any case. In general, they recover after the drug is stopped.

A few patients continued to deteriorate with treatment. Nimodipine is unlikely to be effective in those deteriorating rapidly or already in grade V. Also, it may carry some risk if there is already extensive infarction or raised ICP.

One concern is that, if calcium antagonists dilate cerebral arteries, they may increase the risk of rebleeding in patients with unclipped aneurysms. In fact, where this complication was mentioned in four more or less controlled studies of nimodipine, there was slightly though not significantly less rebleeding in the treated group (54/448 or 13%) than in controls (80/523, 15%). Overall there were 130 recurrent haemorrhages in 1221 reported cases (11 references), or 11%.

Vasospasm and delayed ischaemia are important complications of aneurysmal SAH. Untreated, more than 20% of patients die or are permanently disabled because of DID. Calculating from the above figures, the prophylactic use of calcium antagonists, continued as treatment when necessary, should reduce the incidence of permanent problems due to vasospasm from 20% to 6%.

Mechanisms of Action of Calcium Antagonists

1) Some of these drugs, especially nimodipine, were developed with specific effects on cerebral arteries. There is laboratory evidence to support this, and angiographic increases in arterial diameter after arterial injection have been shown, but not in every case. Other possible mechanisms include:

2) Improved collateral flow. Topical application of nimodipine has been shown to dilate small pial arteries, and small arteries in general are the most sensitive.

3) Effects at neuronal membrane. It has been shown experimentally and clinically that ischaemic neurones themselves are protected by antagonists against excessive calcium entry, in situations of ischaemic and haemorrhage studies.

4) Intracellular actions have been postulated, both indirect by preventing a too high intracellular calcium, and direct by minimising its effects on mitochondria and other organelles.

5) Rheological effects. An increase in erythrocyte deformability has been shown in the presence of calcium antagonists. In addition, they decrease platelet aggregation, and in SAH patients decrease the platelet production of thromboxanes.

6) Effect on mitogenesis. Studies on the pathophysiology of vasospasm have emphasised the cellular proliferation that occurs, with collagen deposition and wall thickening. This is similar to an accelerated atherogenesis. Calcium antagonists have been shown to inhibit cell proliferation in vascular smooth muscle.

7) Influence on fluid management. It is known that even the so-called cerebral specific drugs do cause some general arterial dilatation, with risk of hypotension. One tends to give more fluids to combat this, which itself is useful against vasospasm.

It is difficult to be sure exactly how these drugs work. Possibly, several different mechanisms may be in operation at different stages of the course of vasospasm, or in different patients. However, there is little doubt that they are effective in preventing vasospasm and in improving outcome after SAH.

References

1. Kosnik EJ, Hunt WE (1976) Postoperative hypertension in the management of patients with intracranial arterial aneurysms. J Neurosurg 45: 148–154
2. Origitano TC, Wascher TM, Reichman OH, Anderson DE (1990) Sustained increased cerebral blood flow with prophylactic hypertensive hypervolemic hemodilution ("Triple-H" therapy) after subarachnoid hemorrhage. Neurosurgery 27: 729–740
3. Tettenborn D, Dycka T (1990) Prevention and treatment of delayed ischemic dysfunction in patients with aneurysmal subarachnoid hemorrhage. Stroke 21 [Suppl] IV: IV85–IV89

Correspondence: N. Dorsch, F.R.A.C.S., Department of Surgery, Westmead Hospital, Westmead, NSW 2145, Australia.

Tirilazad and Aneurysmal Subarachnoid Hemorrhage

N.F. Kassell, E.C. Haley, and **W. Alves**

Departments of Neurosurgery and Neurology, University of Virginia Health Sciences Center, Virginia, U.S.A.

Summary

A randomized double-blind dose-escalation trial of tirilazad mesylate versus placebo was done in patients admitted within 72 hours from SAH. 3 escalating doses of tirilazad were administered (0.6 mg, 2.0 mg, 6.0 mg/kg/day). 245 patients from 12 canadian centers were included in the study: all received concurrent therapy with oral nimodipine, and hypertensive hypervolemic hemodilution therapy as indicated. Out of these patients, 61 received placebo, 51 the 0.6 mg/kg dose, 42 the 2.0 mg/kg dose and 91 the 6.0 mg/kg dose. The group treated with the highest dose presented a significantly higher incidence of thick layers of blood in the subarachnoid space by CT scan.

There were no drug related complications identified in this study, including hepatic dysfunction, thrombophlebitis and CK elevation. There was no significant difference between placebo and the 0.6 mg/kg or the 2 mg/kg doses as regards angiographic vasospasm, transcranial Doppler velocities, and incidence of symptomatic vasospasm. However, there was a statistically significant dose-related improvement in three-month favourable outcome (66% for placebo, 81% for the 0.6 mg/kg dose and 90% for the 2.0 mg/kg dose), and a nonsignificant trend towards reduction in mortality (19% for placebo, 8% for the 0.6 mg/kg dose and 5% for the 2 mg/kg dose).

It is suggested that the mechanism of improvement in favourable outcome is from neuronal protection, owing to the apparently scant influence of tirilazad on vessel narrowing. Two large multi-center Phase III efficacy trials of tirilazad in SAH – currently underway – will help to clarify this point.

Keywords: Tirilazad mesylate; subarachnoid haemorrhage; cerebral vasospasm; transcranial Doppler.

Introduction

Vasospasm is the leading treatable cause and ischemia is the final common pathway in death and disability resulting from aneurysmal subarachnoid haemorrhage. Tirilazad mesylate is a theoretically attractive agent for treating patients with ruptured aneurysms because it has been shown experimentally to prevent cerebral vasospasm[4-7] and to protect against cerebral ischemia[2,3], because it has a rational mechanism of action in decreasing free radical damage[1], and because it is complementary to all other forms of therapy for vasospasm.

We are reporting herein, in a preliminary manner, the results of a Phase II trial of tirilazad in subarachnoid hemorrhage. The purpose of this trial is to evaluate the safety of tirilazad in patients with ruptured aneurysms and to select a dose of tirilazad to be used in definitive Phase III efficacy studies.

Materials and Methods

Study Design

This study is a randomized, double blinded, dose-escalation trial of placebo/vehicle vs. three escalating doses of tirilazad (0.6 mg, 2.0 mg, 6.0 mg/kg per day IV) in patients treated within 72 hours of SAH in twelve Canadian centers (Table 1). The patients included in this study were those admitted in neurological grades I–IV and were treated with study drugs up to ten days following SAH.

Concurrent therapy included the use of oral nimodipine in all patients, and hypertensive, hypervolemic, hemodilution therapy as indicated. Patients were not treated with other steroids.

Outcome measures included clinical safety assessment which focused on adverse medical events and drug related complications, the incidence of angiographic vasospasm, transcranial Doppler measurements, the incidence of symptomatic vasospasm and neurological worsening from vasospasm, functional outcome utilizing the Glasgow Outcome Scale, and death and disability from vasospasm.

Patients eligible for inclusion in the study were those with aneurysmal subarachnoid hemorrhage treated within 72 hours of the ictus and who were 18 years of age or older. All females of child bearing age were required to have a negative pregnancy test. Patients excluded from the trial included those with fusiform, traumatic, or mycotic aneurysms, those with severe complicating illnesses or involved in protocols utilizing other investigational drugs, those patients requiring the use of steroids on a systematic basis, those requiring the use of other calcium antagonists besides nimodipine, and patients with other neurological diseases.

A total of 245 patients were enrolled in the trial of which 61 received placebo and 184 received tirilazad. Of those patients receiving tirilazad, 51 received a dose of 0.6 mg/kg, 42 received a dose of 2.0 mg/kg, and 91 received a dose of 6.0 mg/kg per day. The safety experience at each dose was reviewed by an independent medial monitor prior to proceeding to the next highest dose.

Table 1. *Phase II Dose Escalation Study of Tirilazad in Patients with Subarachnoid Hemorrhage*

Participating Center	Investigator
University of Alberta	Bryce Weir, M.D.
University of Calgary	Francis E. Leblanc, M.D.
McGill University	Ronald Pokrupa M.D.
University of Manitoba	Michael West, M.D.
University of Montreal	Gerard Mohr, M.D.
University of Ottawa	Michael Richard, M.D.
Douglas III, Kingston General Hospital	Francisco Espinosa, M.D.
Dalhousie University	Renn Holness, M.D.
University of Toronto	F. Gentili, M.D.
McMaster University	Robert Hansebout, M.D.
University of Western Ontario	R.F. DelMaestro, M.D., Ph.D.
University Hospital – Saskatchewan	Ashfad Shauib, MBBS

Results

The following results include the safety analysis of the placebo and the tirilazad groups 0.6, 2.0, and 6.0 mg/kg per day. However, the activity analysis was only done on placebo and the lower two tirilazad groups – 0.6 and 2.0 mg/kg per day because the follow-up had not been completed on the patients who received 6.0 mg/ per day.

Adverse medical events and drug related complications were reported by the investigators and tabulated and reviewed at the central registry. More than 60 potential systemic and neurological complications were scrutinized with special attention to cardiac, and hepatic complications and phlebitis, based on pre-clinical and Phase I human studies. There were no drug related complications identified in the study, including hepatic dysfunction, thrombophlebitis, and CK elevation. There was no significant difference in termination of study drug because of serious adverse events in the placebo vs. the three drug-treated groups.

There were no important differences between patients treated with placebo and those treated with 0.6 or 2.0 mg/kg per day tirilazad, with the exception that those patients treated with the highest dose of tirilazad had a significantly higher incidence of thick layers of blood in the subarachnoid space by CT scan. 47% of patients who received placebo had thick layers vs. 45% in the 0.6 mg group and 67% of patients in the 2.0 mg group. Hypertensive hypervolemic therapy was used with equal frequency in all groups.

When placebo was compared to the 0.6 and 2.0 mg/kg per day tirilazad patients, there were no significant differences in moderate or severe angiographic vaso-spasm, transcranial Doppler velocities, incidence of symptomatic vasospasm, and incidence of neurological worsening from vasospasm. There was a non significant trend for patients with tirilazad to have a better neurological status as judged by the NIH Stroke Scale on day 14 following subarachnoid hemorrhage.

The three month functional outcome was assessed by blinded observers who were independent of the management of the patients. The results were shown by favorable outcome, which was defined as good or moderately disabled on the Glasgow Outcome Scale, and crude mortality rates. There was a statistically significant, dose-related improvement in three month favorable outcome in the tirilazad treated patients; 66% of the placebo had favorable outcome vs. 81% in the 0.6 mg group vs. 90% in the 2.0 mg. There was a corresponding non-statistically significant trend toward reduction in mortality at three months; the mortality in the placebo group was 19% vs. 8% in the 0.6 mg group vs. 5% in the 2.0 mg group.

There was a trend for death or disability from vaso-spasm to be lower in patients who received 2.0 mg per day of tirilazad. Furthermore, there was a statistically significant dose related reduction in death or disability from ischemia other than vasospasm at time of three month assessments; in the placebo group, 9% of patients died or were disabled from ischemia, while in the 0.6 to 2.0 mg per day doses of tirilazad the figures were 4% and 0% respectively.

Discussion

In patients with ruptured intracranial aneurysms, tirilazad appears safe in doses up to 6 mg/kg per day for up to ten days following subarachnoid hemorrhage. From these data, the influence of tirilazad on angiographic and symptomatic vasospasm remains uncertain, due to the bias against the effectiveness of the drug because of the increased amount of blood in the subarachnoid space in patients who receive 2 mg/kg per day. Tirilazad produced a dose-related improvement in favorable outcome. Given that there was no difference in angiographic or symptomatic vasospasm noted in the trial, and that death and disability from ischemic causes other than vasospasm was reduced, the proposed mechanism of the improvement in favorable outcome was from neuronal protection. Caution must be exercised in making inferences about activity from safety studies, especially given the preliminary nature of this analysis. Nevertheless, tirilazad remains a promising agent in the management of patients with ruptured aneurysms. Definitive efficacy studies are necessary to prove safety and efficacy. Two large scale, multi-center Phase III efficacy trials of tirilazad in subarachnoid hemorrhage are underway. These studies have the dual hypotheses that tirilazad reduces vasospasm and/or that tirilazad improves outcome in patients with ruptured aneurysms.

References

1. Braughler JM, Pregenzer JF, Chase RL, Duncan LA, Jacobsen EJ, McCall JM (1987) Novel 21-aminosteroids as potent inhibitors of iron-dependent lipid peroxidation. J Biol Chem 262: 10438–10440
2. Hall ED, Pazara KE, Braughler JM (1988) 21-aminosteroid lipid peroxidation inhibitor U74006F protects against cerebral ischemia in gerbils. Stroke 19: 997–1002
3. Hall ED, Yonkers PA (1988) Attenuation of postischemic cerebral hypoperfusion by the 21-aminosteroid U74006F. Stroke 19: 340–344
4. Steinke DE, Weir BK, Findlay JM, Tanabe T, Grace M, Krushelnycky BW (1989) A trial of the 21-aminosteroid U74006F in a primate model of chronic cerebral vasospasm. Neurosurgery 24: 179–186
5. Vollmer DG, Kassell NF, Hongo K, Ogawa H, Tsukahara T (1989) Effect of the nonglucocorticoid 21-aminosteroid U74006F on experimental cerebral vasospasm. Surg Neurol 31: 190–194
6. Zuccarello M, Anderson DK (1989) Protective effect of a novel 21-aminosteroid on the blood-brain barrier following subarachnoid hemorrhage in rats. Stroke 20: 367–371
7. Zuccarello M, Marsch JT, Schmitt G, Woodward J, Anderson DK (1989) Effect of the 21-aminosteroid U74006F on cerebral vasospasm following subarachnoid hemorrhage. J Neurosurg 71: 98–104

Correspondence: N.F. Kassell, M.D., Department of Neurosurgery and Neurology, University of Virginia, Health Sciences Center, Charlottesville, Virginia 22908, U.S.A.

Effect of Calcitonin Gene-Related Peptide on Outcome of Ischaemic Deficits After Subarachnoid Haemorrhage

European CGRP in Subarachnoid Haemorrhage Study Group*

Summary

A randomised multicentre single blind comparison of calcitonin gene-related peptide (CGRP) against standard best management has been conducted in patients suffering ischaemic deficits after surgery for a ruptured intracranial aneurysm. Patients aged 18 to 70 years who developed a focal neurological deficit or had a reduction of two or more points on the Glasgow coma scale (GCS) after surgery, were entered after a CT scan had excluded non-ischaemic causes for their neurological deficits. Informed consent was obtained and pregnancy, uncorrected hypovolaemia, and serious concomitant illness were exclusion criteria. After randomisation, 62 patients were allocated to receive an infusion of 0.6 ug/min of CGRP for a minimum of four hours up to a maximum of 10 days, and 55 patients received standard best management. GCS and haemodynamic parameters were assessed during the patients' hospital stay, and all patients were followed up at three months by an independent investigator, who was blind to their treatment. Outcome was measured on the Glasgow outcome scale, and 16 neurosurgical units contributed patients, 12 centres in the UK and Ireland, and four in the rest of Europe. At three month follow up 66% of those treated with CGRP and 60% of those receiving best management had a good outcome, with the relative risk of a poor outcome in CGRP treated patients being 0.88 (95% confidence interval 0.60 to 1.28). Hypotension was a common side effect of the CGRP infusion. Although a significant beneficial effect has not been demonstrated by the trial, a clinically useful benefit has not been excluded.

Keywords: Subarachnoid haemorrhage; calcitonin gene-related peptide; vasospasm.

*A.M. Aziz, Cork; I.C. Balley, Royal Victoria Hospital, Belfast; M. Barnes, Newcastle General Hospital; J.R. Bartlett, Brook General Hospital, London; B.A. Bell, Atkinson Morley's Hospital, London; I. Bone, Southern General Hospital, Glasgow; G. Braadvedt, Bristol Royal Infirmary; T.F. Buckley, Cork; L. Calandre, Instituto Nacional de la Salud, Madrid; J.P. Castel, Groupe Hospitalier Pellegrin, Bordeaux; U. Choksey, Newcastle General Hospital; J.A. Cozens, Newcastle General Hospital; O.P. Dahl, Regionsykehuset I Trondheim; P.S. Dias, Royal Hallamshire Hospital, Sheffield; D. Dorrance, Brook General Hospital, London; P. Foy, Walton Hospital, Liverpool; R.G. Galvin, Cork; D. Grosset, Western Infirmary, Glasgow; R.W. Gullan, Brook General Hospital, London; D.T. Hope, Queen's Medical Centre, Nottingham; S. Howell, Royal Hallamshire Hospital, Sheffield; P.R.D. Humphrey, Walton Hospital, Liverpool; J. Hutchison, Beaumont Hospital, Dublin; J. Jakubowski, Royal Hallamshire Hospital, Sheffield; D. Jefferson, Queen's Medical Centre, Nottingham; F.G. Johnston, Atkinson Morley's Hospital, London; R. Juul, Regionsykehuset I Trondheim; Y. Kereval, Paris; A. Keshtgar, Cork; J. Lagarrigue, CHR Rangueil, Toulouse; V. Larrue, CHR Rangueil, Toulouse; R.D. Lobato, Instituto Nacional de la Salud, Madrid; J.A. Lyttle, Royal Victorial Hospital, Belfast; J.C. Marks, Cork; B. Martin, Southampton General Hospital; J. Martin, Southampton General Hospital; B. Matthew, Royal Victoria Hospital, Belfast; J. McMahon, Newcastle General Hospital; A.D. Mendelow, Newcastle General Hospital; J.D. Miller, Western General Hospital, Edinburgh; D. Mohan, Derriford Hospital, Plymouth; K. Morris, Walton Hospital, Liverpool; G.D. Murray, Glasgow Royal Infirmary; R.J. Nelson, Frenchay Hospital, Bristol; S.A. O'Laoire, Beaumont Hospital, Dublin; J.-M. Orgogozo, Groupe Hospitalier Pellegrin, Bordeaux; J.D. Pickard, Southampton General Hospital; I.J.A. Robertson, Brook General Hospital, London; M.D.M. Shaw, Walton Hospital, Liverpool; J. Singh, Beaumont Hospital, Dublin; J. Stanley, Southampton General Hospital; G. Stranjalis, Frenchay Hospital, Bristol; S.R. Stapleton, Atkinson Morley's Hospital, London; W.A.S. Taylor, Atkinson Morley's Hospital, London; G.M. Teasdale, Southern General Hospital, Glasgow; B. White, Queen's Medical Centre, Nottingham.

Introduction

After a bleed from a cerebral aneurysm early surgical intervention may increase the incidence of delayed ischaemic deterioration, so that optimum management is a difficult choice between early surgery which prevents re-bleeding but has a high ischaemic morbidity, and late surgery which has a lower ischaemic morbidity, but higher overall management mortality. Many agents had been used to attempt to reduce ischaemic morbidity without convincing evidence of efficacy[1], until 1989 when nimodipine was shown to improve outcome and reduce cerebral ischaemia after subarachnoid haemorrhage (SAH). Death and severe disability still occured in 20% of nimodipine treated patients[2], so the search for other agents to reduce ischaemia after SAH is still pertinent.

The analysis of the structure of the calcitonin gene led to the prediction of the existence of calcitonin gene-related peptides in man[3,4,5]. Two separate genes on chromosome 11 were identified that encode alpha and beta calcitonin gene-related peptide (CGRP)[6,7], and CGRP is widely distributed within the central nervous system and most organs of the body. Within the central nervous system CGRP is predominantly in the alpha form, and is found in high concentrations in the perivascular nerves of blood vessels[8]. CGRP has been shown to be a potent vasodilator and the carotid vascular beds are sensitive to CGRP, with facial flushing, a feeling of fullness in the head, and an increase in internal carotid blood velocity measured by Doppler when it is given to normal volunteers[9]. When CGRP is administered on the intravascular side of the blood-brain barrier, the effect is predominantly on the extracranial vascular bed, and in normal volunteers cerebral blood flow is not increased[10].

The cerebral blood vessels have a network of perivascular sensory fibres in their adventitia that contain substance P and CGRP[11,12]. The cell bodies of these fibres lie in the trigeminal ganglion, and form the trigemino-cerebrovascular system which is activated by the vasoconstriction occuring following SAH, to restore vascular diameter. Experimentally vasoconstriction can be prolonged by trigeminal ganglionectomy, but not by trigeminal nerve section[13], and CGRP fibres are reduced after SAH by up to 50%[13], and in patients who die following SAH there is depletion of CGRP immunoreactivity in brain vessels[14].

CGRP levels in the external jugular vein increase in patients who suffer cerebral vasoconstriction following SAH[15], and the prolonged vasoconstriction occurring after SAH may exhaust the perivascular supply of CGRP and other peptides. Experimentally CGRP can induce relaxation of the basilar artery[13], and following SAH the relaxant response of the basilar artery to CGRP is increased[16]. Cerebrovascular levels of CGRP decline with age[17], and age is a major risk factor for ischaemic complications after SAH. A pilot clinical study in 15 patients following cerebral aneurysm surgery showed an improvement in neurological status in 8 out of 15 patients with ischaemic deterioration[18], and CGRP has been shown to reduce abnormally high middle cerebral artery flow velocities after SAH[19].

The present study is a randomised multicentre single blind trial of the effect of a postoperative infusion of CGRP on outcome at three months following delayed cerebral ischaemia after surgery for a ruptured intracranial aneurysm.

Patients and Methods

Patients who suffered a SAH and underwent aneurysm surgery were entered into the trial if they developed an ischaemic neurological deficit post-operatively. A neurological deficit was defined as a reduction of two or more points on the 14 point Glasgow coma scale (GCS), or a focal neurological deficit, excluding a cranial nerve palsy. The baseline for the development of the deficit was either the pre-surgical neurological status or the best post-operative status. Non-ischaemic causes for the neurological deficit were excluded by a post-operative CT scan of the head prior to entry into the trial. Informed consent was provided for every patient by a responsible relative or by the patient themselves, and ethical committee approval was obtained at each centre.

Patients were excluded if they were pregnant, had uncorrected hypovolaemia, had haematological or biochemical indices significantly outside the normal range, or had evidence of significant cardiac, hepatic, renal, respiratory, or endocrine disease. At least four hours elapsed between the termination of anaesthesia for the intracranial surgery and enrolment into the trial, unless obvious improvement and subsequent deterioration in their neurological state had occurred within those four hours. Patients admitted to a participating neurosurgical unit with a diagnosis of SAH were screened for subsequent eligibility to the trial, and 1556 patients were screened at 19 centres between January 1990 and January 1991. Of these 1556 patients, 271 were excluded because they were outside the age range of 18 to 70 years old, or because pregnancy could not be excluded with certainty. This left 1285 patients, of whom 825 proved to have a cerebral aneurysm, and 722 of these patients proceeded to surgery. Of these 722 patients, 222 developed a postoperative neurological deficit of a reduction of two or more points on the 14 point Glasgow coma scale, or a focal neurological deficit. In 54 of the 222 patients non-ischaemic causes for their deterioration could not be excluded, and 42 were not randomised for reasons ranging from death prior to intended randomisation, to the impracticability of follow up of a foreigner returning after surgery to their home country. Consent was witheld by nine patients, leaving 117 patients who were entered into the study from 16 neurosurgical units, 12 centres in the U.K. and Ireland, and four in the rest of Europe (Table 1). These 117 patients were randomised to receive either an

Table 1. *Patient Recruitment to Trial*

Neurosurgical unit	Patients entered
Liverpool	15
Atkinson Morley's (London)	14
Dublin	14
Bristol	12
Cork	9
Sheffield	9
Belfast	8
Newcastle	8
Glasgow	7
Southampton	5
Nottingham	4
Brook (London)	3
Toulouse	3
Bordeaux	2
Madrid	2
Trondheim	2
Total	117

infusion of CGRP, or standard best management of their neurological deficit without CGRP.

In the treated group CGRP (Celltech Ltd., Slough SL1 4EN) was given by intravenous infusion at a rate of 0.6 micrograms per minute and blood pressure was monitored frequently for the first two hours of the infusion. If systemic hypotension developed the infusion rate was reduced to 0.45 micrograms per minute, and further reduced to 0.3 micrograms per minute if systemic hypotension was still apparent. Of the patients randomised to receive CGRP, treatment was to be for a minimum of four hours and in patients who showed a satisfactory neurological response to the infusion, continued for a minimum of four days and a maximum of 10 days.

Every patient's neurological status was monitored during their stay in the neurosurgical unit. The primary trial endpoint was an independent neurological assessment conducted between three and four calendar months following the date of randomisation by an independent clinician who had not been involved in their management and did not have access to their case records. Recovery was measured on the five point Glasgow outcome scale[20], and the outcome was assessed as either a good outcome (good recovery or moderately disabled on the Glasgow outcome scale) or a bad outcome (severely disabled, vegetative, or dead on the Glasgow outcome scale). The case histories and radiological investigations of every patient entered were reviewed at quarterly intervals to ensure the patient met the inclusion criteria of the trial, by a panel comprising representatives from the contributing centres, and all outcome assessments were reviewed by a panel of the independent assessors.

A total of 117 patients were randomised and entered into a primary analysis. The 99 patients who met all of the protocol entry criteria were entered into a secondary analysis of improvement of GCS at the end of four hours infusion of CGRP, an assessment of ischaemic neurological deficits using the GCS over the 10 day treatment period, and the mortality rate at three months.

Results

Of the 117 patients recruited, 62 received CGRP, and 55 received standard best management, and the two treatment groups were reasonably well matched clinically. There was a preponderance of cigarette smokers

Table 2. *Clinical Characteristics*

		CGRP 62 patients	Best management 55 patients
Mean age (s.d.)		49.1 (11.5)	48.4 (12.1)
Men		23 (37%)	21 (38%)
Cigarette smoking (≥ 10/day)		36 (58%)	22 (40%)
Loss of consciousness		35 (56%)	19 (35%)
GCS on admission			
	< 8	5 (8%)	2 (4%)
	8–12	3 (5%)	9 (16%)
	13–14	53 (87%)	43 (80%)
GCS prior to treatment			
	< 8	7 (12%)	5 (10%)
	8–12	33 (57%)	33 (66%)
	13–14	18 (31%)	12 (24%)

and coma producing haemorrhages in the CGRP group, but patients had slightly better pre-treatment Glasgow coma scores in this group (Table 2). CT scan findings were similar in the two groups of patients (Table 3), as were the timings of surgery and onset of deterioration after the bleed (Table 4). Eighteen patients violated the trial exclusion criteria or did not fulfill the inclusion criteria (Table 5), nine of these patients received CGRP and nine received best management.

Every patient in the best management group had at least one active treatment measure instituted, the most frequent strategy being to maintain normovolaemia (39 of the 55 patients). Plasma expansion to produce a

Table 3. *CT Scan Findings*

	CGRP 62 patients	Best management 55 patients
Intraventricular blood	26 (42%)	21 (39%)
Cisternal blood	49 (79%)	47 (85%)
Hydrocephalus	17 (27%)	15 (28%)
Intracerebral haematoma	13 (21%)	12 (22%)

Table 4. *Timing of Surgery and Onset of Deterioration After Bleed*

		CGRP 62 patients	Best management 55 patients
Time from bleed to surgery	0–2 days	16	16
	3–7 days	26	24
	≥ 8 days	20	15
Time from bleed to deterioration	0–2 days	4	4
	3–7 days	21	26
	≥ 8 days	37	25
Time from surgery to deterioration	0–2 days	35	34
	3–7 days	22	19
	≥ 8 days	5	2

Table 5. *Excluded Patients*

Reason for exclusion	No. of patients
Uncorrected anaemia	10
Non-ischaemic cause for deterioration on CT scan	3
Dopamine given as well as CGRP	2
Untreated infection	1
No post-deterioration CT scan	1
Patient over 70 years old	1
Total	18

Table 6. *Premature Cessation of CGRP Treatment*

Reason for stopping CGRP	No. of patients
Adverse events	19 (31%)
Lack of improvement at 4 hours	17 (27%)
Lack of improvement after 4 hours	4 (6%)
Patient request	1 (2%)
Total	41 (66%)

Table 7. *Outcome at Three Months*

Glasgow outcome score	CGRP 62 patients	Best management 55 patients
Good outcome		
Good recovery	27 (43%)	26 (47%)
Moderately disabled	14 (23%)	7 (13%)
Total	41 (66%)	33 (60%)
Poor outcome		
Severely disabled	9 (14%)	11 (20%)
Vegetative	1 (2%)	0 (0%)
Dead	11 (18%)	11 (20%)
Total	21 (34%)	22 (40%)

degree of hypervolaemia was initiated in 32 patients, and a hypertensive drug was given to 26 patients. Some patients had combinations of more than one active treatment.

Of the 62 patients who received CGRP, 21 (34%) completed treatment with the peptide, and the remaining 41 patients discontinued treatment for the reasons given in Table 6. Outcome at three months is shown in Table 7, and shows a marginal improvement in good outcome (good recovery plus moderately disabled) from 60% to 66% in treated patients, which does not reach statistical significance. The relative risk of a bad outcome in CGRP treated patients is 0.88, but the 95% confidence interval is wide from 0.60 to 1.28. When adjusted by logistic regression for the post-deterioration GCS the relative risk becomes 0.85 (95% confidence interval 0.57 to 1.28), but the difference this adjustment makes relative to the width of the confidence intervals is negligible. The corresponding unadjusted relative risk for the 99 patients fulfilling the protocol completely is 0.85 (95% confidence interval 0.57 to 1.29).

Changes in GCS were assessed for differences between the CGRP and best management groups at four hours by the non-parametric Mann-Whitney test, and none of the changes reached statistical significance. The GCS fell in 16 (26%) patients given CGRP, and in 9 (16%) patients receiving best management (p = 0.26). An analysis of changes in GCS at 10 days, as had originally been intended, was not possible because data was missing for 46 patients, mainly because they had been discharged from hospital by 10 days.

Serious adverse event reporting is likely to be biased in a single blind study, and in 24 patients (39%) who were on CGRP 38 events were reported, and 17 of the events were thought to be related to the treatment. In 16 patients (29%) on best management, 24 serious adverse events were reported, but none were thought to be due to treatment. The 17 adverse events attributed to CGRP affected 14 patients, and eight of the events were hypotension, affecting seven patients and resulting in treatment with CGRP being withdrawn in five.

Discussion

We were unable to show a statistically significant improvement in outcome following post-deterioration infusion of CGRP, but the constraints of trial size and a protocol that would be acceptable to a large number of participating neurosurgeons have limited our conclusions. Only a third of patients randomised to receive CGRP completed treatment, so that two thirds of those analysed in the treatment group had limited exposure to the peptide.

The incidence of systemic hypotension of sufficient severity to warrant cessation of treatment suggests that systemic intravenous infusion of CGRP is not the ideal route of administration. Subarachnoid instillation would seem an attractive route, as it is on the adventitial rather than the endothelial side of the cerebral vessel wall that the peptide is normally found.

A trial of instillation of CGRP into the subarachnoid space at the time of surgery to clip a cerebral aneurysm seems the logical next step, and may well show a more marked protective effect against cerebral ischaemia with a much reduced incidence of systemic hypotension.

Acknowledgement

We are grateful to Celltech Limited, who sponsored this study, and provided the CGRP. This study was first published in the Lancet: European CGRP in Subarachnoid Haemorrhage Study Group: Effect of calcitonin-gene-related peptide in patients with delayed postoperative cerebral ischaemia after aneurysmal subarachnoid haemorrhage. Lancet (1992) 339: 831–834.

References

1. Wilkins RH (1986) Attempts at prevention or treatment of intracranial arterial spasm. An update. Neurosurgery 18: 808–825
2. Pickard JD, Murray GD, Illingworth R, Shaw MDM, Teasdale GM, Foy PM, Humphrey PRD, Lang DA, Nelson R, Richards P, Sinar J, Bailey S, Skene A (1989) Effect of oral nimodipine on cerebral infarction and outcome after subarachnoid haemorrhage: British aneurysm nimodipine trial. BMJ 298: 636–642
3. Amara SG, Jonas V, Rosenfeld MG, Ong ES, Evans RM (1982) Alternative RNA processing in calcitonin gene expression generates mRNAs encoding different polypeptide products. Nature 298: 240–244
4. Rosenfeld MG, Mermod J-J, Amara SG, Swanson LW, Sawchenko P, Rivier J, Vale WW, Evans RM (1983) Production of a novel neuropeptide encoded by the calcitonin gene by tissue-specific RNA processing. Nature 304: 129–135
5. Steenbergh PH, Hoppener JWM, Zandberg J, Van de Ven, WJM, Jansz HS, Lips LJM (1984) Calcitonin gene-related peptide coding sequence is conserved in the human genome and is expressed in medullary thyroid carcinoma. J Clin Endocrinol Metab; 59: 358–360
6. Steenbergh PH, Hoppener JWN, Zandberg J, Lips CJM, Jansz HS (1985) A second human calcitonin/CGRP gene. FEBS Lett 183: 403–407
7. Amara SG, Arriza JL, Leff SE, Swanson LW, Evans RM, Rosenfeld MG (1985) Expression in brain of a messenger RNA encoding a novel neuropeptide homologous to calcitonin generelated peptide. Science 229: 1094–1097
8. Wimalawansa SJ, Emson PC, MacIntyre I (1987) Regional distribution of calcitonin gene-related peptide and its specific binding sites in rats with particular reference to the nervous system. Neuroendocrinology 46: 131–136
9. Salmon P, Fitzgerald D, Lambe R, Darragh A, O'Shaughnessy D, Riddell A, Ney U (1989) A Single rising intravenous dose tolerance and pharmacodynamic study of human calcitonin gene related peptide (CGRP) in healthy male volunteers. Clin Pharm Ther 45: 170
10. Stanley JC, Martin JL, Barron ME, Lovick AHJ, Nelson IJ, Richards HK, Pickard JD (1990) A study of the cardiovascular and cerebrovascular effects of calcitonin gene-related peptide in human volunteers. J Physiol 427: 33
11. Hanko J, Hardebo J, Kahrstrom J, Owman C, Sundler F (1985) Calcitonin gene-related peptide is present in mammalian cerebrovascular nerve fibres and dilates pial and peripheral arteries. Neurosci Lett 57: 91–95
12. Uddman R, Edvinsson L, Ekman R, Kingman T, McCulloch J (1985) Innervation of the feline cerebral vasculature by nerve fibres containing calcitonin gene-related peptide: trigeminal origin and co-existence with substance P. Neurosci Lett 62: 131–136
13. Edvinsson L, Delgado-Zygmunt T, Ekman R, Jansen I, Svendgaard N-Aa, Uddman R (1990) Involvement of perivascular sensory fibers in the pathophysiology of cerebral vasospasm following subarachnoid haemorrhage. J Cereb Blood Flow Metab 10: 602–607
14. Edvinsson L, Ekman R, Jansen I, Kingman TA, McCulloch J, Uddman R (1991) Reduced levels of calcitonin gene-related peptide-like immunoreactivity in human brain vessels after subarachnoid haemorrhage. Neurosci Lett 121: 151–154
15. Juul R, Edvinsson L, Gisvold SE, Ekman R, Brubakk AO, Fredriksen TA (1990) Calcitonin gene-related peptide-LI in subarachnoid haemorrhage in man. Signs of activation of the trigemino-cerebrovascular system? Br J Neurosurg 4: 171–180
16. Hongo K, Tsukahara T, Kassell NF, Ogawa H (1989) Effect of subarachnoid haemorrhage on calcitonin gene-related peptide-induced relaxation in rabbit basilar artery. Stroke 20: 100–104
17. Edvinsson L, Ekman R, Jansen I, Ottosson A, Uddman R (1985) Distribution, concentration and effects of neuropeptide Y, vasoactive intestinal polypeptide, calcitonin gene-related peptide, and substance P in human cerebral blood vessels. J Cereb Blood Flow Metab 5: S 545–546
18. Johnston FG, Bell BA, Robertson IJA, Miller JD, Haliburn C, O'Shaughnessy D, Riddell AJ, O'Laoire SA (1990) The effect of calcitonin gene-related peptide on post-operative neurological deficits following subarachnoid haemorrhage. Lancet 335: 869–872
19. Naylor AR, Robertson IJA, Edwards CRW, Merrick MV, Sellar RJ, O'Shaughnessy D, Miller JD (1991) Cerebral vasospasm following subarachnoid haemorrhage: effect of calcitonin generelated peptide on middle cerebral artery velocities using transcranial Doppler. Surg Neurol 36: 278–280
20. Jennett B, Bond M (1975) Assessment of outcome after severe brain damage: a practical scale. Lancet i: 480–484

Correspondence: B.A. Bell, M.D., Atkins forley's Hospital, Copse Hill, Wimbledon, London SW20 One, England, U.K.

Clinical Effects of Nimodipine in Prevention of Vasospasm After Subarachnoid Hemorrhage

A. Pasqualin, G. Barone, R. Scienza, P. Mortini, B. Cappelletto, C. Licata, and R. Da Pian

Department of Neurosurgery, City Hospital, Verona, Italy

Summary

A retrospective study was undertaken including all patients with a bleeding aneurysm consecutively admitted to our Department within 72 hours from SAH, with Hunt and Hess grades I to IV. The control group consisted of 230 patients admitted from January 1981 to December 1985, and the study group consisted of 196 patients admitted from January 1986 to August 1990, all receiving i.v. nimodipine for the first 14 days of SAH (2 mg/h). Admission clinical grade was very similar in the opposite groups. A consistent or thick subarachnoid hemorrhage was more commonly observed in the study group (84% vs. 71%). Early surgery was adopted in 57% of cases in the study and 61% of cases in the control group. Clinical outcome was significantly better in the nimodipine group, with complete recovery in 71% of patients and a mortality rate of 13% ($p = 0.008$ for complete recovery and $p = 0.0005$ for mortality); considering only patients submitted to early surgery, there was still a significant difference for complete recovery ($p = 0.02$) and mortality ($p = 0.004$) in favour of the nimodipine group. As a whole: a) permanent ischemic disturbances (not associated with other causes of deterioration) were significantly less common in the study than in the control group (4% vs. 13%, $p = 0.001$); b) CT infarction was observed in 9% of nimodipine and 19% of control patients ($p = 0.005$); c) vessel narrowing was observed with the same incidence in the opposite groups (50% in the nimodipine and 52% in the control group). It is concluded that i.v. nimodipine infusion significantly improves the outcome after SAH, and decreases the incidence of ischemic disturbances and CT infarction, although it does not decrease the occurrence of angiographical vessel narrowing; these effects are likely due to vasodilatation of the peripheral resistance vessels and/or to a cerebral metabolic effect.

Keywords: Nimodipine; subarachnoid hemorrhage; vasospasm; early surgery.

Introduction

Cerebral vasospasm remains a fearsome complications of subarachnoid hemorrhage (SAH)[11,29]. In spite of recent therapeutical advances, angiographical vessel narrowing is still present after SAH and the outcome of the patient can be badly affected by this complication. The introduction of calcium antagonists for prevention of this pathology has led to promising results, with significant improvement in outcome in most clinical series[1,17,19,24,25,26].

The aim of this study is to present the results of a unicenter retrospective clinical study on 426 patients with SAH from aneurysmal rupture, 196 treated with nimodipine and 230 not treated: in particular, the incidence of ischemic disturbances, angiographical vessel narrowing and CT infarction has been carefully evaluated in the opposite groups.

Clinical Material and Methods

This study has considered all patients with subarachnoid hemorrhage consecutively admitted to our Department from January 1981 to August 1990. Criteria of inclusion to this study have been: a) admission within 72 hours from SAH, with immediate CT scan; b) clinical grade at admission I to IV (according to Hunt and Hess classification); c) aneurysm diagnosed through an angiographical study. Criteria of exclusion to the study have been: a) life-threatening hematomas; b) severe rebleeding within 12 hours from admission; c) hepatic, renal or cardiac failure; d) severe diabetes.

The study group consisted of 196 patients (77 males and 119 females) admitted to our Department from January 1986 to August 1990 and treated with nimodipine, administered through continuous i.v. infusion (at the dosage of 2 mg/h) until day 14 after subarachnoid hemorrhage, followed by oral administration (360 mg/day) for another 7 days. The control group consisted of 230 patients (92 males and 138 females) admitted from January 1981 to December 1985, not receiving calcium antagonists. The age of the patients ranged between 17 and 79 years (with an average of 51 years) in the nimodipine group, and between 16 and 77 years (with an average of 50 years) in the control group. Admission clinical grade (Hunt and Hess classification) was I or II in 49% of nimodipine and 49% of control patients, III in 35% of nimodipine and 37% of control patients, IV in 16% of nimodipine and 14% of control patients. The opposite groups resulted homogeneous regarding the location of the ruptured aneurysm (Table 1).

The amount of the cisternal blood deposition on early CT scan was divided into 4 grades, according to a previous classification from our group[22]: absent, thin (hardly recognizable), consistent, thick (a large layer of cisternal blood, with cisternal tamponade) (Fig. 1). According to this classification, in the study group 31 patients (16%) presented an absent or thin cisternal deposition and 165 (84%) a

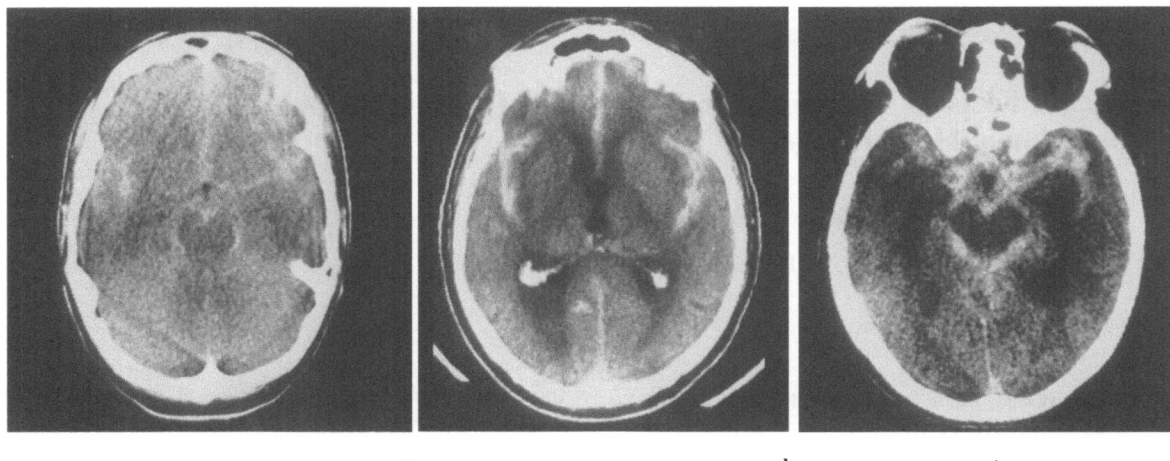

Fig. 1. Degree of subarachnoid blood deposition on early CT scan, according to the classification of Pasqualin *et al.*[22]: (a) thin layer in the basal cisterns, in the frontal interhemispheric fissure and in the rt. insular cistern; (b) consistent layer in the frontal interhemispheric fissure and in both insular cisterns; (c) thick layer (= cisternal tamponade) in the basal cisterns

consistent or thick deposition; in the control group, 66 patients (29%) presented an absent/thin deposition and 164 patients (71%) presented a consistent/thick deposition.

The aneurysm was excluded with an early operation (within 3 days from hemorrhage) in 111 patients treated with nimodipine (57%) and in 141 patients in the control group (61%); the remaining patients of both groups were submitted to a delayed operation, with administration of i.v. tranexamic acid (at the dosage of 6 g/day) in the waiting period. Important risk factors have been summarized in Table 2.

In both groups treatment of ischemic deficit was similar, consisting of hypervolemic therapy, obtained with plasma expanders and colloid gels, with the aim of maintaining central venous pressure around 8–12 cm of H_2O, and in blood transfusions when needed; mannitol was used in patients with severe clinical deterioration; in a few cases, also pharmacologically induced hypertension (with dopamine) was used[21].

In the opposite groups the following end-points were evaluated: a) the clinical outcome according to the Glasgow Outcome Scale[10]; b) the causes of disability and death (with particular attention been paid to vasospasm); c) the incidence of ischemic disturbances (either transient or permanent) and the related clinical outcome; d) the incidence of vessel narrowing, demonstrated on angiography and/or on transcranial Doppler sonography; e) the incidence of CT infarc-

Table 2. *Risk Factors in the Opposite Groups*

	Grades III–IV		Consistent/thick depositions		Early surgery	
Nimodipine (196 cases)	99	(51%)	165	(84%)	111	(57%)
Control (230 cases)	116	(51%)	164	(71%)	141	(61%)
Signif.	N.S.		p = 0.002		N.S.	

tion on delayed CT scan. Regarding end-points c), d) and e), a more detailed evaluation was limited to patients with a consistent or thick cisternal deposition on admission CT scan, i.e. a large-volume SAH, at high risk of vasospasm, according to various authors[5,12,16,22].

The chi-square test was used for statistical analysis.

Results

Comparing the overall outcome in the opposite groups, patients treated with nimodipine showed a significantly higher recovery rate than control patients (71% versus 59%; p = 0.008) and a significantly lower mortality rate (13% versus 27%; p = 0.0005) (Table 3). The best results were observed in patients treated with nimodipine and submitted to early surgery (within 72 hours from hemorrhage), with significantly higher recovery rate (p = 0.02) and significantly lower mortality (p = 0.004) than in control patients also submitted to early surgery (Table 4). The causes of permanent disability and death are presented in Table 5; ischemic

Table 1. *Location of Ruptured Aneurysms*

Nimodipine (n = 196)			Control (n = 230)	
Anter. comm.	92	(47%)	114	(49%)
Middle cer.	42	(21%)	48	(21%)
Int. carotid	36	(18%)	38	(17%)
Carotid bif.	10	(5%)	14	(6%)
Post. circ.	11	(6%)	5	(2%)
Anter. cer.	5	(3%)	11	(5%)
Multiple	32	(16%)	41	(18%)

Table 3. *Overall Results in the Opposite Groups*

	Recovery	Disability: moderate	severe	death
Nimodipine (196 c.)	140 (71%)	19 (10%)	11 (6%)	26 (13%)
Control (230 c.)	135 (59%)	25 (11%)	7 (3%)	63 (27%)
Signif.	p = 0.008	N.S.	N.S.	p = 0.0005

Table 4. *Overall Results in the Opposite Groups, in Relation to Modality of Treatment*

Early surgery	Recovery	Disability	Death
Nimodipine (111 c.)	83 (75%)	14 (12%)	14 (13%)
Control (141 c.)	85 (61%)	16 (11%)	40 (28%)
Signif.	p = 0.02	N.S.	p = 0.004
Delayed policy			
Nimodipine (85 c.)	57 (67%)	16 (10%)	12 (14%)
Control (89 c.)	50 (56%)	16 (18%)	23 (26%)
Signif.	N.S.	N.S.	N.S.

Table 5. *Causes of Permanent Disability and Death*

	Disability: nimodipine (196 cases)	control (230 cases)	Death: nimodipine (196 cases)	control (230 cases)
Rebleeding	2 (1%)	—	6 (3%)	11 (5%)
Ischemic disturb. alone	5 (3%)	17 (7%)	2 (1%)	13 (6%)
Ischemic disturb. associated	5 (3%)	3 (1%)	10 (5%)	23 (10%)
Medical complic.	—	—	6 (3%)	8 (3%)
Effect of initial bleed	8 (4%)	5 (2%)	—	8 (3%)
Edema or hydroc.	5 (3%)	4 (2%)	1 (1%)	—
Surgical trauma	5 (3%)	3 (1%)	1 (1%)	—

disturbances from vasospasm – either alone or associated with other causes of deterioration – largely influenced morbidity and mortality. In particular, ischemic disturbances associated with other causes of deterioration (hydrocephalus or cerebral edema) were observed in both groups with no difference (8% versus 11%); on the opposite, ischemic disturbances not associated with other causes of deterioration were signifi-

Table 6. *Ischemic Disturbances (Transient or Permanent) in the Opposite Groups, and Related Outcome*

Overall	Ischemia	Outcome from ischemia: recovery	disabil.	death
Nimodipine (196 cases)	42 (21%)	20 (48%)	10 (24%)	12 (28%)
Control (230 cases)	82 (36%)	26 (32%)	20 (24%)	36 (44%)
Signif.	p = 0.001	N.S.	N.S.	N.S.
Consistent/Thick Layers only				
Nimodipine (165 cases)	42 (25%)	20 (48%)	10 (24%)	12 (28%)
Control (164 cases)	72 (44%)	21 (29%)	19 (27%)	32 (44%)
Signif.	p = 0.0006	N.S.	N.S.	N.S.

Table 7. *Ischemic Disturbances (Transient or Permanent) and Related Outcome, in Relation to Modality of Treatment*

Early Surgery	Ischemia	Outcome from ischemia: recovery	disability	death
Nimodipine (111 cases)	27 (24%)	12 (44%)	5 (19%)	10 (37%)
Control (141 cases)	53 (38%)	18 (34%)	10 (19%)	25 (47%)
Signif.	p = 0.03	N.S.	N.S.	N.S.
Delayed Policy				
Nimodipine (85 cases)	15 (18%)	8 (53%)	5 (34%)	2 (13%)
Control (89 cases)	29 (33%)	8 (28%)	10 (34%)	11 (38%)
Signif.	p = 0.03	N.S.	N.S.	N.S.

Table 8. *Vessel Narrowing and CT Infarct in the Opposite Groups*

Overall	Vessel narrowing		CT infarct	
Nimodipine (196 cases)	98	(50%)	18	(9%)
Control (230 cases)	119	(52%)	44	(19%)
Signif.	N.S.		p = 0.005	
Consistent/Thick Layers only				
Nimodipine (165 cases)	92	(56%)	18	(11%)
Control (164 cases)	100	(61%)	38	(23%)
Signif.	N.S.		p = 0.004	

cantly less frequent in patients treated with nimodipine (4% versus 13%; p = 0.001).

Considering the opposite groups – regardless of the degree of the cisternal blood deposition – the incidence of ischemic disturbances appeared significantly lower in patients treated with nimodipine than in control patients (21% versus 36%; p = 0.001); the significance increased when patients with consistent or thick cisternal depositions only were considered (25% versus 44%; p = 0.0006) (Table 6). When considering the impact of surgical timing in the opposite groups, the incidence of ischemic disturbances was always significantly lower in nimodipine patients (Table 7).

As shown by Table 8, the incidence of vessel narrowing (on TCD and/or angiography) was not significantly different in the opposite groups; the incidence of CT infarction was significantly lower in the nimodipine group, either considering the overall series (p = 0.005) or patients with a large-volume SAH only (p = 0.004).

Discussion

Cerebral vasospasm constitutes the most frequent cause of death and disability in patients who survive the initial insult of subarachnoid hemorrhage[11].

Based on our results, the overall outcome after SAH is significantly better in patients treated with nimodipine; this observation is in agreement with the various double-blind prospective studies on nimodipine[17,24,26]. The improvement in outcome for patients treated with nimodipine is even more significant when considering patients submitted to surgery in the acute stage; the observation reported previously by Ohman and

Eiskanen[19] is thus confirmed on a larger series of patients.

The incidence of ischemic disturbances has been significantly lower in patients treated with nimodipine; this observation has not been stressed adequately in the previous literature, although various authors have reported a significant decrease in postischemic mortality[1,19,25] and morbidity[24,25] in patients with nimodipine. Besides to the significantly decreased rate of ischemic disturbances, the final outcome of ischemic disturbances has also been better in our patients with nimodipine.

The significant decrease in the incidence of CT infarction in patients submitted to treatment with nimodipine observed in our study has been already pointed out by Pickard *et al.*[26] and observed – without finding a significant difference – by Petruk *et al.*[24]. No significant decrease in the incidence of angiographic vasospasm has been observed in our study group as compared to controls, similarly to other reports[17,24,26]. At this regard, various experimental studies on the monkey[3,4,18] and the dog[32] – regarding prevention of cerebral vasospam with oral administration of nimodipine after experimental subarachnoid hemorrhage – have confirmed the inability of calcium antagonists to prevent angiographical vessel narrowing. Similarly, in two studies in which other calcium antagonists have been administered i.v. in experimental models of SAH (in rabbits and dogs)[23,31] no significant decrease in the incidence of vessel narrowing has been demonstrated.

In the previous experimental studies, the effect of the drug on distal (resistance) vessels has not been evaluated. At this regard, other studies have demonstrated a marked vasodilatory effect of the calcium antagonist on distal arteries[2,9]. The vasodilatation of the most distal cerebral arteries may explain the increase in cerebral blood flow[28] and in doppler flow velocity[20] – as well as the improvement in clinical outcome – observed during treatment with calcium-antagonists.

Trying to explain the improvement in clinical results and the decreased rate of ischemic disturbances, it should be pointed out that treatment with calcium antagonists has shown a protective neuronal effect in focal cerebral ischemia, experimentally induced in the animal[6,8,15,30]. Moreover, in experimental animal models in which global cerebral ischemia has been induced, treatment with calcium antagonists has led to prevention of the post-ischemic hypoperfusion and improvement in the EEG activity[14] and somatosensory evoked responses[7]. In an experimental model of global ischemia in the rabbit, the intracellular calcium overload and the increase in the permeability of the blood brain barrier have been reduced by nimodipine[13]. Calcium antagonists – administered in the ischemic period in a group of primates in which global cerebral ischemia had been induced – have reduced the extent of ischemic parenchymal damage and have improved the clinical outcome[27].

In conclusion, the results of this study – based on a large clinical series coming from a single center – show that i.v. nimodipine prophylaxis significantly improves the overall outcome in patients with SAH from a ruptured aneurysm, and decrease the incidence of ischemic disturbances and CT infarction; however, the inability of nimodipine to prevent vessel narrowing is pointed out. Based on these data, it is suggested that nimodipine exerts either a vasodilatory effect on terminal arteries, or a more generalized metabolic effect, or both, leading to a significantly improved clinical outcome, in particular in patients submitted to early surgery, where the neurological damage may be multi-factorial and not only ischemic.

References

1. Allen GS, Ahn HS, Preziosi TJ, Battye R, Boone SC, Chou SN, Kelly DL, Weir BK, Crabbe RA, Lavik PJ, Rosenbloom SB, Dorsey FC, Ingram CR, Mellits DE, Bertsch LA, Boisvert DP, Hundley MB, Johnson RK, Strom JA, Transou CR (1983) Cerebral arterial spasm. A controlled trial of nimodipine in patients with subarachnoid hemorrhage. N Engl J Med 308: 619–624

2. Auer LM, Oberbauer RW, Schalk HV (1983) Human pial vascular reactions to intracavernous nimodipine-infusion during EC-IC bypass surgery. Stroke 14: 210–213

3. Espinosa F, Weir B, Overton T, Castor W, Grace M, Boisvert D (1984) A randomized placebo-controlled double blind trial of nimodipine after SAH in monkeys. Part 1. Clinical and radiological findings. J Neurosurg 60: 1167–1175

4. Espinosa F, Weir B, Shnitka T, Overton T, Boisvert D (1984) A randomized placebo-controlled double blind trial of nimodipine after SAH in monkeys. Part 2. Pathological findings. J Neurosurg 60: 1176–1185

5. Fisher CM, Kistler JP, Davis JM (1980) Relation of cerebral vasospasm to subarachnoid hemorrhage visualized by computerized tomographic scanning. Neurosurgery 6: 1–9

6. Germano IM, Bartkowski HM, Cassel ME, Pitts LH (1987) The therapeutic value of nimodipine in experimental focal cerebral ischemia. J Neurosurg 67: 81–87

7. Grotta J, Spydell J, Pettigrew C, Ostrow P, Hunter D (1986) The effect of nicardipine on neural function following ischemia. Stroke 17: 213–219

8. Hadley MN, Major MC, Zabramski JM, Spetzler RF, Rigamonti D, Fifield MS, Johnson PC (1989) The efficacy of intravenous nimodipine in the treatment of focal cerebral ischemia in a primate model. Neurosurgery 25: 63–70

9. Haws CW, Heistad DD (1984) Effects of nimodipine on cerebral vasoconstrictor responses. Am J Physiol 247: H170–H176

10. Jennett B, Bond M (1975) Assessment of outcome after severe brain damage: a practical scale. Lancet i: 480–484

11. Kassell NF, Sasaki T, Colohan ART, Nazar G (1985) Cerebral vasospasm following aneurysmal subarachnoid hemorrhage. Stroke 16: 562–572

12. Kassell NF, Torner JC, Haley EC, Jane JA, Adams HP, Kongable GL (1990) The International Cooperative Study on the Timing of Aneurysm Surgery. Part 1: overall management results. J Neurosurg 73: 18–36

13. Lazarewicz JW, Pluta R, Salinska E, Puka M (1989) Beneficial effect of nimodipine on metabolic and functional disturbances in rabbit hippocampus following complete cerebral ischemia. Stroke 20: 70–77

14. Mabe H, Nagai H, Takagi T, Umemura S, Ohno M (1986) Effect of nimodipine on cerebral functional and metabolic recovery following ischemia in the rat brain. Stroke 17: 501–505

15. Meyer FB, Anderson RE, Yaksh TL, Sundt TM (1986) Effect of nimodipine on intracellular brain pH, cortical blood flow, and EEG in experimental focal cerebral ischemia. J Neurosurg 64: 617–626

16. Mizukami M, Takemae T, Tazawa T, Kawase T, Matsuzaki T (1980) Value of computed tomography in the prediction of cerebral vasospasm after aneurysmal rupture. Neurosurgery 7: 583–586

17. Neil-Dwyer G, Mee E, Dorrance D, Lowe D (1987) Early intervention with nimodipine in subarachnoid hemorrhage. Eur Heart J 8K: 41–47

18. Nosko M, Weir B, Krueger C, Cook D, Norris S, Overton T, Boisvert D (1985) Nimodipine and chronic vasospasm in monkeys: Part 1. Clinical and radiological findings. Neurosurgery 16: 129–136

19. Ohman J, Heiskanen O (1988) Effect of nimodipine on the outcome of patients after aneurysmal subarachnoid hemorrhage and surgery. J Neurosurg 69: 683–686

20. Pasqualin A, Acerbi G, Licata C, Caciagli P, Da Pian R (1989) Transcranial Doppler findings in the early stage of subarachnoid hemorrhage: relation to the amount of cisternal blood deposition and modality of treatment. In: Wilkins RH (ed) Cerebral vasospasm. Raven, New York, pp 25–32

21. Pasqualin A, Da Pian R, Scienza R, Formenton A (1982) Terapia ipervolemica ed ipertensiva per il trattamento dei disturbi ischemici susseguenti ad emorragia subaracnoidea. Min Anest 48: 683–685

22. Pasqualin A, Rosta L, Da Pian R, Cavazzani P, Scienza R (1984) The role of computed tomography in the management of vasospasm following subarachnoid hemorrhage. Neurosurgery 15: 344–353

23. Pasqualin A, Vollmer DG, Marron JA, Tsukahara T, Kassell NF, Torner JC (1989) The effect of nicardipine on vasospasm in rabbit basilar artery following subarachnoid hemorrhage. Neurosurgery 29: 183–188

24. Petruk KC, West M, Mohr G, Weir BKA, Benoit BG, Gentili F, Disney LB, Khan MI, Grace.M, Holness RO, Karwon MS, Ford RM, Cameron GS, Tucker WS, Purves GB, Miller JDR, Hunter M, Richard MT, Durity FA, Chan R, Clein LJ, Maroun FB, Godon A (1988) Nimodipine treatment in poor-grade aneurysm patients: results of a multicentric double-blind placebo-controlled trial. J Neurosurg 68: 505–517

25. Philippon J, Grob R, Dagreou F, Guggiari M, Rivierez M, Viars P (1986) Prevention of vasospasm in subarachnoid hemorrhage: a controlled study with nimodipine. Acta Neurochir (Wien) 82: 110–114

26. Pickard JD, Murray GD, Illingworth R, Shaw MDM, Teasdale

GM, Foy PM, Humphrey PRD, Lang DA, Nelson R, Richards P, Sinar J, Bailey S, Skene A (1989) Effect of oral nimodipine on cerebral infarction and outcome after subarachnoid hemorrhage: British aneurysm nimodipine trial. B M J 298: 636–642

27. Steen PA, Gisvold SE, Milde JH, Newberg LA, Scheithauer BW, Lanier WL, Michenfelder JD (1985) Nimodipine improves outcome when given after complete cerebral ischemia in primates. Anesthesiology 62: 406–414

28. Steen PA, Newberg LA, Milde JH, Michenfelder JD (1984) Cerebral blood flow and neurological outcome when nimodipine is given after complete cerebral ischemia in the dog. J Cereb Blood Flow Metab 4: 82–87

29. Sundt TM Jr, Whisnant JP (1977) Subarachnoid hemorrhage from intracranial aneurysms. Surgical management and natural history of disease. N Engl J Med 299: 116–122

30. Uematsu D, Greenberg JH, Hickery WF, Reivich M (1989) Nimodipine attenuates both increase in cytosolic free calcium and histologic damage following focal cerebral ischemia and reperfusion in cats. Stroke 20: 1531–1537

31. Varsos VG, Liszczak TM, Han DH, Kistler JP, Vielma J, Black PMcL, Heros RC, Zervas NT (1983) Delayed cerebral vasospasm is not reversible by aminophylline, nifedipine or papaverine in a "two-hemorrhage" canine model. J Neurosurg 58: 11–17

32. Zabramski J, Spetzler RF, Bonstelle C (1986) Chronic cerebral vasospasm: effect of calcium antagonists. Neurosurgery 18: 129–135

Correspondence: A. Pasqualin, M.D., Department of Neurosurgery, City Hospital, I-37126 Verona, Italy.

Prevention of Cerebral Vasospasm – Cisternal Irrigation Therapy with Urokinase and Ascorbic Acid

N. Kodama, T. Sasaki, K. Yamanobe, M. Sato, and **M. Kawakami**

Department of Neurosurgery, Fukushima Medical School, Fukushima, Japan

Summary

Cisternal irrigation therapy with urokinase and ascorbic acid was applied in 118 cases for preventing vasospasm after aneurysmal subarachnoid hemorrhage (SAH); in other 28 cases only urokinase was used. All of the patients were in Group 3 according to the CT classification by Fisher, and the CT number (Hounsfield number) of the thickest clot was over 60. These CT findings suggested a high chance for occurrence of symptomatic vasospasm. All patients underwent surgery within 72 hours. After clipping the aneurysm, irrigation tubes were placed in the Sylvian fissure (inlet), either on one side or bilaterally, and also in the prechiasmal or prepontine cistern (outlet). Lactated-Ringer's solution with urokinase (60, 120 IU/ml) and ascorbic acid (2, 4 mg/ml) was infused at the rate of 20–60 ml/hours for about 10 days. In the former group with urokinase and ascorbic acid, symptomatic vasospasm was observed in 3 cases (2.5%) and only one of them (0.8%) showed neurological sequelae. In the latter group with only urokinase (30–120 IU/ml), symptomatic vasospasm occurred in three cases (10.7%), transiently. We compared these results with those of 111 control cases without the irrigation therapy, which had the same degree of SAH on the preoperative CT scans. In the control group, symptomatic vasospasm occurred in 38 cases (34.2%).

In conclusion, cisternal irrigation therapy with urokinase and ascorbic acid is effective in preventing symptomatic vasospasm after aneurysmal SAH.

Keywords: Vasospasm; cisternal irrigation; urokinase; ascorbic acid.

Introduction

Cerebral vasospasm is one of the main causes of morbidity and mortality after aneurysmal subarachnoid hemorrhage (SAH). It is now generally considered that cerebral vasospasm is induced by some spasmogenic substances yielded from the clot around cerebral arteries[1,2,11]. In order to prevent vaospasm, removal of this thick clot is carried out in acute surgery of ruptured aneurysms; however, it is difficult to completely prevent vasospasm caused by residual clot.

Our attempt is to add two other means after acute surgery. One is to dissolve and eliminate the residual subarachnoid clot and the other is to change the spasmogenic substance into something harmless. We used urokinase to dissolve the residual clot[16] and also ascorbic acid[5,13] to degenerate oxyhemoglobin (Oxy-Hb), which is thought to be one of the strong spasmogenic substances[11]. Cisternal irrigation therapy with urokinase (UK) and ascorbic acid[6,7] was applied in 118 cases of severe aneurysmal SAH following acute surgery; in other 28 cases only UK was used. In the present study, the results of 111 controlled cases which had the same degree of SAH were compared with those of irrigation therapy, and the efficacy of cisternal irrigation therapy for preventing symptomatic vasospasm was investigated.

Clinical Material and Methods

Irrigation Group with UK and Ascorbic Acid

Cisternal irrigation therapy with UK and ascorbic acid was applied in 118 patients, 46 males and 72 females aged 27–81 (mean 56.5), with severe SAH (Fig. 1). The inclusion criteria were 1) group 3 on preoperative CT scan, according to CT classification by Fisher[4], 2) CT number (Hounsfield number) more than 60 in the highest density area of the SAH, and 3) patients operated on within 72 hours after SAH. Preoperative grade according to the classification by Hunt and Kosnik is given in Table 1.

Surgery was performed as mentioned blow: after removal of subarachnoid clot around the internal carotid artery, outflow of cerebrospinal fluid must be identified by opening Liliequist's membrane. Prepontine clot is aspirated if possible. The space for inserting tube is maintained in Sylvian fissure, and then irrigation tubes are placed deeply to either one side or bilaterally. A drainage tube is put in the chiasmal or prepontine cistern, according to the distribution of SAH (Fig. 2). Hemostasis should be completely confirmed. Continuous ventricular drainage is not usually applied. Thirtysix cases were irrigated bilaterally and 82 cases unilaterally.

Just after surgery, only lactated-Ringer's solution was infused, and then UK and ascorbic acid were added 12 hours after surgery in order to avoid postoperative hemorrhage. Lactated-Ringer's solution with UK (60, 120 IU/ml) and ascorbic acid (2, 4mg/ml) was infused at the rate of 20–60ml/h. The solution for irrigation was adjusted

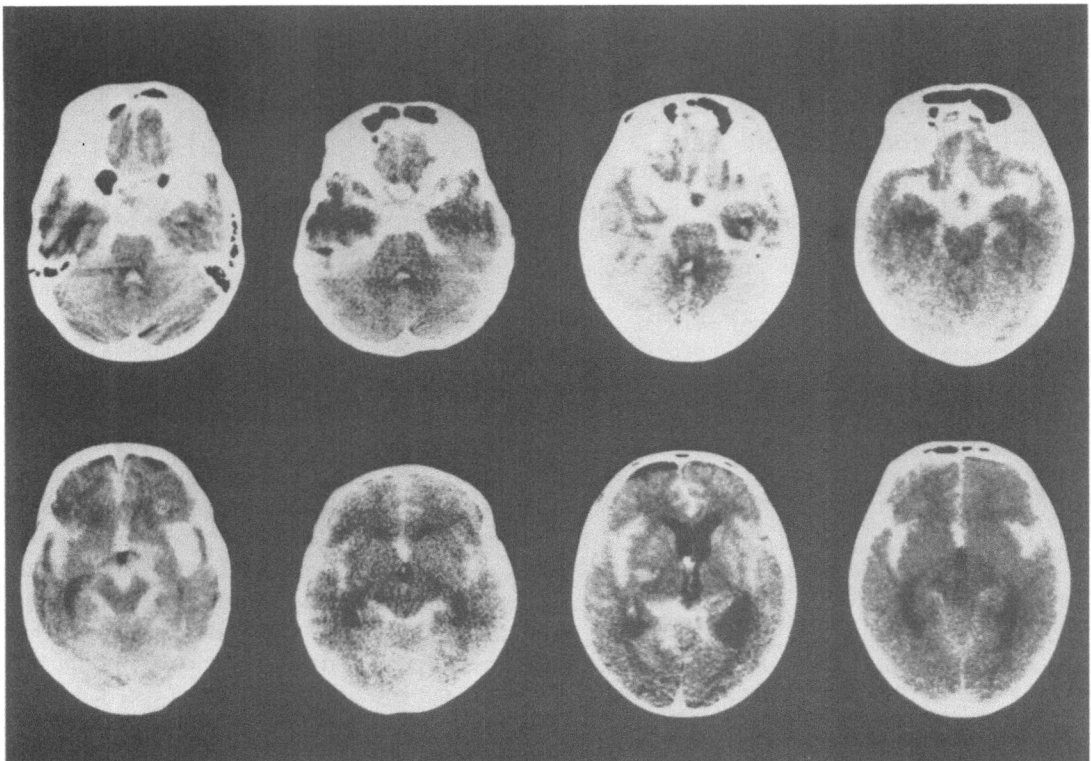

Fig. 1. Preoperative CT scans of 4 representative cases of irrigation group (see text)

Table 1. *Summary of Cases in Each Group*

		Irrigation		Non irrigation
		UK and AsA	UK	
No. of cases		118	28	111
Age (yrs.)		27–81	40–76	34–79
Sex male		46	11	48
female		72	17	63
Grade (H&K)	1	0	2	2
	2	60	10	51
	3	45	12	47
	4	12	4	10
	5	1	0	1

*Grading according to the classification by Hunt and Kosnik.

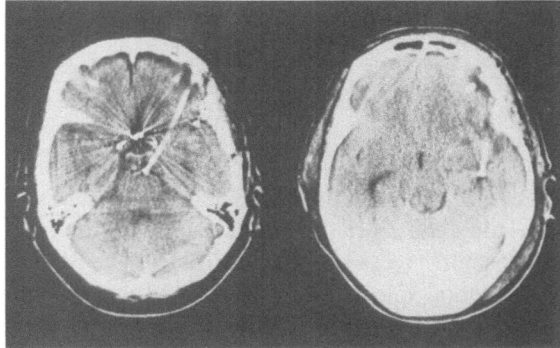

Fig. 2. Positions of irrigation tubes on CT scan

to the almost same pH (7.2–7.6) and osmotic pressure (280–300 mOsm/Kg) as that of normal cerebrospinal fluid. The microdrop was used to control the flow speed and also a microfilter was connected to prevent infection (Fig. 3). The total volume of infused and drained fluid was checked every hour, in order to avoid excessive infusion. The drainage system was usually set at the height of 10 cmH$_2$O (Fig. 3). The red blood cells (RBC), fibrin degradation products (FDP), white blood cells (WBC) and supernatant hemoglobin in the drainage fluid were measured daily.

The end of this therapy was decided by the CT finding of disappearence of high density area in Sylvian fissures and levels of RBC and FDP in the drained fluid below 10,000/mm^3 and 5 mcg/ml respectively.

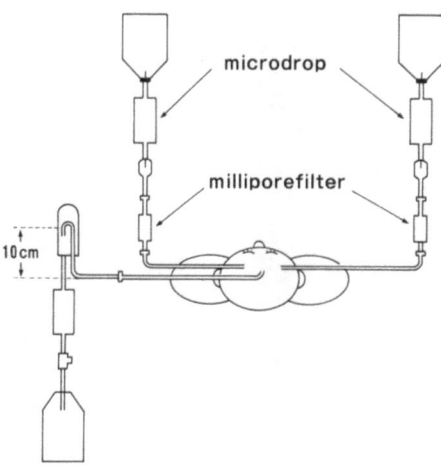

Fig. 3. Cisternal irrigation system

Irrigation Group with Only UK

Twenty eight patients, 11 males and 17 females aged 40–76 (mean 60.5), with severe SAH which had great possibility of vasospasm, received irrigation therapy with only UK. The inclusion criteria were the same as above. Preoperative grade according to the classification of Hunt and Kosnik is given in Table 1.

Cisternal irrigation was carried out only from the unilateral Sylvian fissure even if hematoma existed in bilateral Sylvian fissures. The procedures of surgery and postoperative management were the same as the irrigation group of UK and ascorbic acid.

UK in concentrations of 30,60 and 120 IU/ml was used in 10,9 and 9 cases, respectively at random.

Non-Irrigation Group

A control group of 111 patients, 48 males and 63 females aged 34–79 (mean 54.9), with severe SAH (Fig. 4) took part in this study. The inclusion criteria were the same as those of the irrigation group. A summary of the cases is given in Table 1. In this group, age, sex, operation timing, preoperative grade according to the classification by Hunt and Kosnik and distribution of the site of the aneurysm were almost the same as those of the irrigation group, and some additional therapies were performed: cisternal drainage, ventricular drainage, hypertensive and hypervolemic therapies, etc.

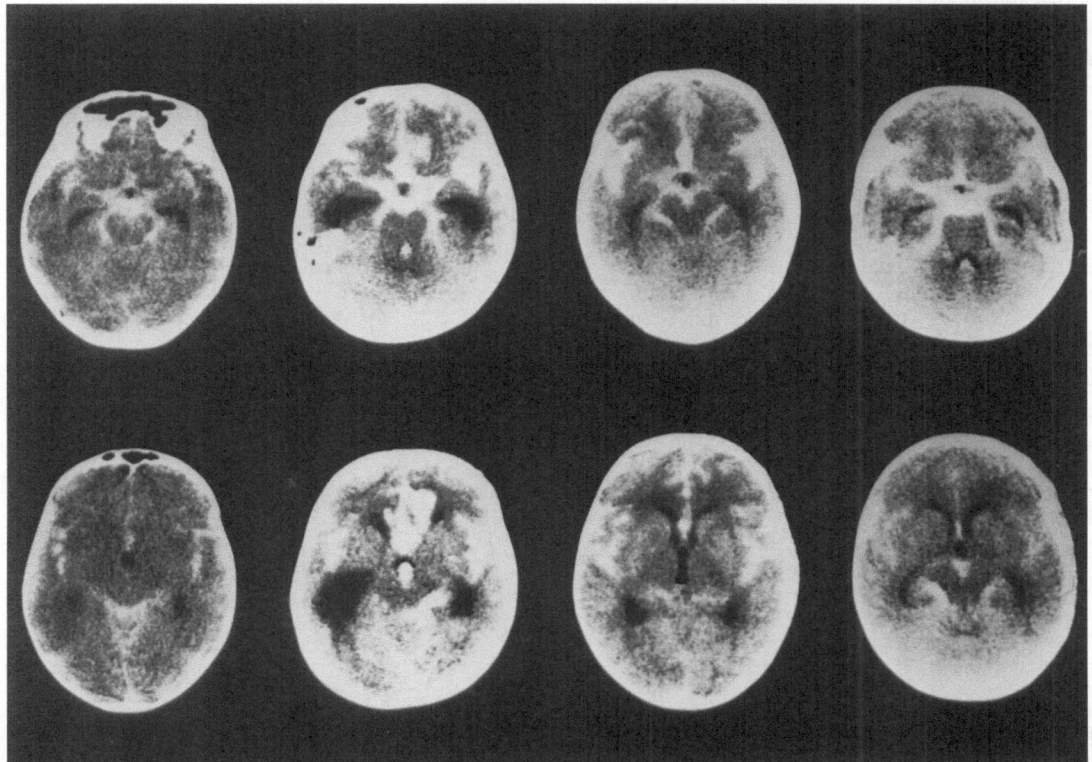

Fig. 4. Preoperative CT scans of 4 representative cases of non irrigation group (see text)

Results

Irrigation Group with UK and Ascorbic Acid

The duration of cisternal irrigation therapy was between 4 and 15 (mean 9.8) days. The outcome assessed at discharge from the hospital was excellent in 58 cases, good in 38, fair in 13, poor in 6; 3 patients died (Table 2). The mortality and morbidity rates were 2.5% and 16.1% respectively.

Among these patients, symptomatic vasospasm occurred in 3 cases at the rate of 2.5% (Table 3). Two of them developed a mild hemiparesis the next day after removal of the irrigation tube. Although CT scan showed a small low density area, both patients recovered completely. The other patient developed a permanent hemiparesis. In this case, as the irrigation tube was not inserted deep enough into the Sylvian fissure (Fig. 5), subarachnoid clot could not be washed out sufficiently. CT scan revealed a new low density area (Fig. 5), and the ADL grade was 3 at discharge from the hospital. The morbidity due to cerebral vasospasm was 0.8%, and the mortality was 0%.

In the irrigation group, 3 patients who had no symptomatic vasospasm died. One of them died of rerupture due to incomplete clipping of the right VA-PICA aneurysm. Another patient who had been receiving hemodialysis before surgery, died of cardiac tamponade due

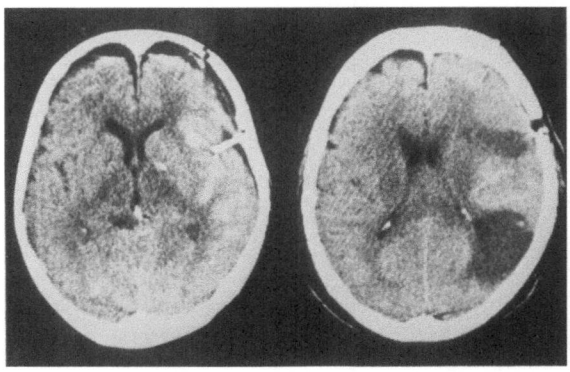

Fig. 5. CT scans of the patient who developed permanent hemiparesis

to aggravated renal failure. The other patient with grade V preoperatively died of pneumonia which complicated delayed consciousness disturbances.

The time course of changes in RBC, FDP, WBC and supernatant hemoglobin levels in drainage fluid are shown in Fig. 6.

Table 2. *Results in the Irrigation Group with Urokinase and Ascorbic acid*

		Irrigation with UK and AsA					
	ADL	1	2	3	4	5	Total
Grade	1	0	0	0	0	0	0
(H&K)	2	40	16	4	0	0	60
	3	17	20	5	2	1	45
	4	1	2	4	4	1	12
	5	0	0	0	0	1	1
	Total	58	38	13	6	3	118
		(2)		(1)			(3)

ADL activity of daily life.

Table 3. *Incidence of Symptomatic Vasospasm in Each Group*

	No. of patients	No. of vasospasm	ADL 1	2	3	4	5
Irrigation with UK and AsA	118	3 (2.5%)	2	0	1	0	0
With UK	28	3 (10.7%)	1	1	1	0	0
Non irrigation	111	38 (34.2%)	7	5	12	5	9

ADL activity of daily life.

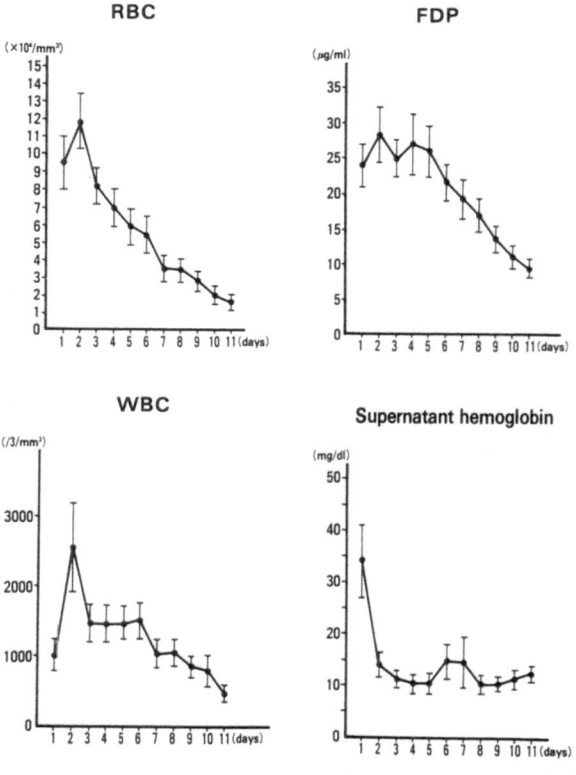

Fig. 6. Time course of changes in red blood cells (*RBC*), fibrin degradation products (*FDP*), white blood cells (*WBC*) and supernatant hemoglobin levels in drainage fluid

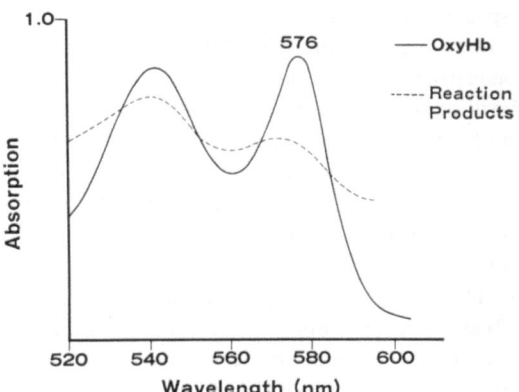

Fig. 7. Absorption spectrum of drainage fluid

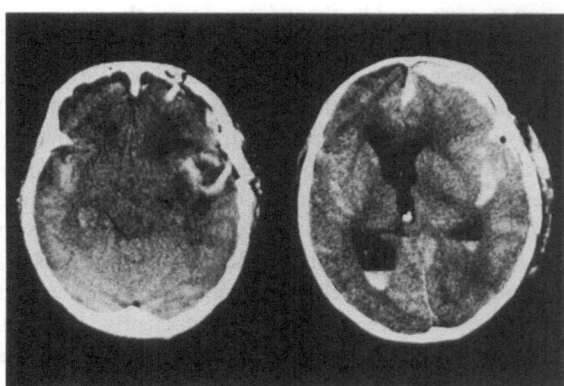

Fig. 8. CT scans of two patients with intracranial hemorrhagic complication

Analysis of the absorption spectrum of drainage fluid revealed a shift of the Oxy-Hb specific 576 nm peak to the short wave-length side, and that spectrum looks like the curve of verdoheme-like products obtained in the previous experiment (Fig. 7).

Complications occurred in 5 patients (4.2%) during irrigation therapy. Two patients (1.7%) had convulsion, 1 patient (0.8%) developed meningitis, and 2 patient (1.7%) bled. In both cases with convulsion, irrigation tubes for outlet were inserted into the subdural space. Although the volume of the drainage fluid was less than that of infused fluid, irrigation was kept for about 1 day. After tubes were pulled out into the epidural space, drainage flow became smooth and symptomatic vasospasm did not occur.

White blood cell proliferation in the drained fluid was found in some cases; however no left deviation of the nucleus nor sign of systemic inflammation were found. Only one case developed meningitis, but the patient recovered completely. Intracranial bleeding occurred in two cases (Fig. 8). These patient did not show the hemorrhagic tendency, and also recovered with no neurological deficits.

Irrigation Group-with Only UK

The irrigation period was 9.6 days on average. Symptomatic vasospasm developed in 1 of 10 cases in the group of 30 IU/ml and in 2 of 9 cases in the group of 60 IU/ml: all of these symptoms were slight and transient. Symptomatic vasospasm was not observed in the group of 120 IU/ml. In all groups, no cases presented permanent symptoms due to vasospasm and no cases developed new low density areas on CT scan (Table 3).

The outcome assessed at 1 month from onset was good in 24 cases; moderate disability was observed in 4 cases (Table 4).

One patient with the complication of a purulent meningitis improved after irrigation of antibiotics in the lateral ventricles, and was discharged without neurological deficit.

The chronological changes of drained blood volume calculated from the red blood cells in drainage fluid are shown in Fig. 9. The highest level was demonstrated in the group of 120 IU/ml. A significant difference in chronological changes in drained blood volume calculated from supernatant hemoglobin in drainage fluid was not observed. Total drained blood volume measured from red blood cells and supernatant hemoglobin in each case was mean 58 ml in the group of 30 IU/ml, mean 106 ml in the group of 60 IU/ml and mean 143 ml in the group of 120 IU/ml. In the three cases of symptomatic vasospasm, the drained blood volume was 49,70 and 98 ml, respectively.

Table 4. *Results in the Irrigation Group with Urokinase*

	ADL	Irrigation with UK					Total
		1	2	3	4	5	
Grade	1	2	0	0	0	0	2
(H&K)	2	4	6	0	0	0	10
	3	3	6	3	0	0	12
	4	0	3	1	0	0	4
	5	0	0	0	0	0	0
	Total	9	15	4	0	0	28
		(1)	(1)	(1)			(3)

ADL activity of daily life.

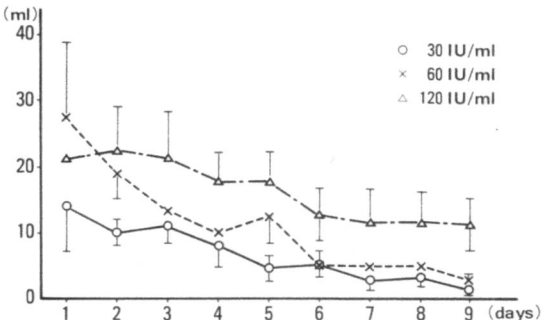

Fig. 9. Blood volume from RBC. Chronological changes of drained blood volume calculated from red blood cells

Table 5. *Results in the Non Irrigation Group*

| | ADL | Non irrigation | | | | | |
		1	2	3	4	5	Total
Grade	1	2	0	0	0	0	2
(H&K)	2	30	11	5	1	4	51
	3	15	10	12	4	6	47
	4	3	1	3	2	1	10
	5	0	0	0	1	0	1
	Total	50	22	20	8	11	111
		(7)	(5)	(12)	(5)	(9)	(38)

ADL activity of daily life.

The highest level of FDP in drained fluid was observed in the group of 120 IU/ml.

Non-Irrigation Group

The outcome of the non irrigation group (Table 5) was excellent in 50 cases, good in 22, fair in 20, poor in 8; 11 cases died. In this group, symptomatic vasospasm occurred in 38 cases out of 111, at the rate of 34.2% (Table 3). The mortality and morbidity rates due to vasospasm were 8.1% and 15.3%.

Discussion

It is now generally considered that subarachnoid clot induces the arterial contraction, although the precise mechanism is not still understood. The best means to prevent vasospasm, therefore, is to remove the clot as much and as early as possible in ultra-early stage surgery. However, complete evacuation of the clot during surgery is technically impossible and dangerous. So we attempted not only to dissolve and eliminate the blood clot nonmechanically, but also to change the spasmogenic substances in the residual clot into

nonspasmogenic ones after surgery. Attention was paid to oxyhemoglobin (Oxy-Hb) which is a strong vasoconstrictor and a source of free radicals.

We already reported the experimental studies on the fibrinolytic agents and the degradation of oxyhemoglobin[5,13,16]. Its summary is as follows: 1) For dissolution of clot, UK was most effective in the concentrations of 60–120 IU/ml, 2) Oxy-Hb was changed to the unknown resolved products by ascorbic acid in vitro. This change was clarified on absorption curve, and 3) ascorbic acid suppressed the ability of Oxy-Hb to constrict the cerebral arteries in vivo and in vitro.

Irrigation therapy with UK was reported by Yoshida[17], Saito[12] and Shiobara[15]. In those reports, however, the results were not satisfactory. This is probably because the UK concentrations and the irrigation systems used by them differed from those we used. Considering that infarction caused by cerebral vasospasm frequently occurs in the territory of middle cerebral artery, and that the clot around the internal carotid artery is relatively easy to remove, we think it is most important to remove the clot around the middle cerebral artery, in particular in the region below the M2 portion. The irrigation tube of the patient who developed a permanent hemiparesis was not inserted deep enough into the Sylvian fissure, and subarachnoid clot could not be washed out sufficiently. For this reason, we make it a rule to insert the tip of the irrigation tube to the periphery of the Sylvian fissure.

Recently some reports using tissue type plasminogen activator[3,8,9,18] (t-PA) demonstrated its efficacy in preventing vasospasm, but there were many hemorrhagic complications. We believe that the single or several times application of high dosage t-PA caused these complications. We chose the low concentrations of UK (30–120 IU/ml) and the continuous irrigation. When we apply a clinical maneuver to a patient, safety is most important.

Intrathecal administration of ascorbic acid for preventing vasospasm was reported by Omoto[10] and Shikinami[14]. Omoto infused 100–200 mg ascorbic acid by a single intrathecal injection, intending to vasodilate. He found this therapy to be effective in 2 of 9 patients, although some patients developed headache, hypertension or tachycardia probably due to drug-induction. With our method, ascorbic acid was used at concentrations of 2–4 mg/ml, and the pH and osmotic pressure of the irrigation fluid were close to those of normal cerebrospinal fluid. No noteworthy complications were associated with our method. Shikinami administered ascorbic acid intrathecally during operation, and repeatedly using Ommaya reservoir. However, a satisfactory result was not achieved with this therapy. He attributed the unsatisfactory results to the failure of ascorbic acid in spreading around arteries. With our method, ascorbic acid seems to spread more widely because subarachnoid clot is eliminated and washed out by irrigation with UK.

Based on the experimental studies, we performed the cisternal irrigation therapy with UK and ascorbic acid following acute surgery of aneurysmal SAH[6,7].

In the irrigation group with UK and ascorbic acid, 3 cases out of 118 (2.5%) developed symptomatic vasospasm, and 1 of them (0.8%) showed neurological sequelae. In the irrigation group with only UK, 3 patients (10.7%) developed mild hemiparesis and deterioration of consciousness due to vasospasm. On the other hand, in the non irrigation group, 38 cases out of 111 (34.2%) developed symptomatic vasospasm and 9 died. These results indicate that UK and ascorbic acid are both effective in preventing symptomatic vasospasm after aneurysmal SAH, and that 120 IU/ml is the most effective concentration of UK to prevent vasospasm.

This therapy caused complications in 6 patients, as mentioned above. In both cases of convulsion, irrigation tubes for outlet were inserted into the subdural space. The irrigation tubes must be inserted into the cistern which has the wider space. During irrigation, white blood cell proliferation in the cerebrospinal fluid was found. This is regarded as chemical meningitis caused by UK or ascorbic acid for the following reasons: 1) no systemic inflammation sign was found, 2) bacterial culture was negative, 3) cell count in drainage fluid decreased rapidly just after irrigation was discontinued. Two infected patients were successfully treated by irrigation with antibiotics. In two patients intracranial bleeding occurred (1 intracerebral and 1 subdural hematoma). These patients suddenly sustained severe headache and the number of red blood cell increased in the drainage fluid. These patients did not show a systemic hemorrhagic tendency in hematological tests. Therefore, the hemorrhagic complication in these patients seems to have been caused by slight injury to the brain and small vessels around irrigation tube. Although one patient was submitted to evacuation of the hematoma, both were discharged from the hospital without neurological deficits. Fortunately, none of these complications caused morbidity or mortality in any patient.

There are, however, some problems in applying this therapy. Although we decide to terminate the irrigation considering the interval from SAH, the CT findings, and the levels of RBC and FDP in the drainage fluid, the duration of this therapy is rather long (mean, 9.8 days). Patients were forced to be bedridden during this period. The greatest energy and care were demanded to the medical staff during the irrigation. However, only 1 patient (0.8%) developed symptomatic vasospasm that caused permanent hemiparesis. Considering this result, the benefit from cisternal irrigation therapy far exceeds its disadvantages.

In conclusion, cisternal irrigation with UK and ascorbic acid is effective in preventing symptomatic vasospasm following acute surgery after aneurysmal SAH.

References

1. Allen GS, Gold LHA, Chou SN, French LA (1974) Cerebral arterial spasm. Part 3: in vivo intracisternal production of spasm by serotonin and blood and its reversal by phenoxybenzamine. J Neurosurg 40: 451–458
2. Boullin DJ, Brandt L, Ljunggren B (1981) Vasoconstrictor activity in cerebrospinal fluid from patients subjected to early surgery for ruptured intracranial aneurysms. J Neurosurg 55: 237–245
3. Findlay JM, Weir BKA, Kassell AF, Disney LB, Grace MGA (1991) Intracisternal recombinant tissue plasminogen activator after aneurysmal subarachnoid hemorrhage. J Neurosurg 75: 181–188
4. Fisher CM, Kistler JR, Davis JM (1980) Relation of cerebral vasospasm to subarachnoid hemorrhage visualized by computerized tomographic scanning. Neurosurgery 6: 1–9
5. Kawakami M, Kodama N, Toda N (1991) Suppression of the cerebral vasospastic actions of oxyhemoglobin by ascorbic acid. Neurosurgery 28: 33–40
6. Kodama N, Sasaki T, Watanabe Z, Yamanobe K, Sato M (1986) Prevention of vasospasm: Cisternal irrigation therapy with urokinase and ascorbic acid. In: Kikuchi H, Fukushima T, Watanabe K (eds) Intracranial aneurysms: surgical timing and techniques. Niigata, Nishimura, pp 228–242
7. Kodama N, Sasaki T, Yamanobe K and Sato M (1988) Prevention of vasospasm: Cisternal irrigation therapy with urokinase and ascorbic acid. In: Wilkins RH (ed) Cerebral vasospasm. Raven, New York pp 415–418
8. Mizoi K, Yoshimoto T, Fujiwara S, Sugawara T, Takahashi A, Koshu K (1991) Prevention of vasospasm by clot removal and intrathecal injection of tissue-type plasminogen activator: preliminary report. Neurosurgery 28: 807–813
9. Öhman J, Servo A, Heiskanen O (1991) Effect of intrathecal fibrinolytic therapy on clot lysis and vasospasm in patients with aneurysmal subarachnoid hemorrhage. J Neurosurg 75: 197–201
10. Ohmoto T, Yoshioka J, Morooka H, Matsumoto Y, Nishimoto A (1980) Effect of ascorbic acid on cerebral vasospasm. In: Wilkins RH (ed) Cerebral arterial spasm. Williams and Wilkins, Baltimore, pp 619–624
11. Osaka K (1977) Prolonged vasospasm produced by the breakdown products of erythrocytes. J Neurosurg 47: 403–411

12. Saito I, Segawa H, Nagayama I, Nihei H (1985) Prevention of postoperative vasospasm by cisternal irrigation. In: Auer LM (ed) Timing of aneurysm surgery. de Greuter Berlin, pp 587–594

13. Sato M (1987) Prevention of cerebral vasospasm: experimental studies on the degradation of oxyhemoglobin by ascorbic acid. Fukushima J Med Sci 33: 55–70

14. Shikinami A (1981) Experimental studies on cerebral vasospasm with special reference to participation of hemoglobin in its pathogenesis. Acta Scholae Medicinalis Universitatis in Gifu 29: 973–1008 (Jpn)

15. Shiobara R, Kawase T, Toya S, Ebato K, Miyahara Y (1985) "Scavengery surgery" for subarachnoid haemorrhage (II) – Continuous ventriculor-cisternal perfusion using artificial cerebrospinal fluid with urokinase. In: Auer LM (ed) Timing of aneurysm surgery. de Gruyter, Berlin, pp 365–372

16. Yamanobe K (1987) Prevention of vasospasm: experimental studies on lysis of the model of subarachnoid clot and intrathecal injection of urokinase. Fukushima Med J 37: 27–39 (Jpn)

17. Yoshida Y, Hayashi T, Amoh M, Awana A, Kusuno K, Uno S, Ogino T, Kobayashi H, Shibata N, Ueki S (1983) Postoperative intrathecal irrigation with plasminogen activator (urokinase) after early stage operation on ruptured cerebral aneurysm. Neurol Med Chir (Tokyo) 23: 659–666 (Jpn)

18. Zabramski JM, Spetzler RF, Lee KS, Papadopoulos SM, Bovill E, Zimmerman RS, Bederson JB (1991) Phase I trial of tissue plasminogen activator for the prevention of vasospasm in patients with aneurysmal subarachnoid hemorrhage. J Neurosurg 75: 189–196

Correspondence: Namio Kodama, M.D., Department of Neurosurgery, Fukushima Medical School, 1, Hikarigaoka, Fukushima, 960–12, Japan.

Intracisternal Recombinant Tissue Plasminogen Activator After Aneurysmal Subarachnoid Hemorrhage: Results of a Preliminary Study

J.M. Findlay, B.K.A. Weir[1], and M.G.A. Grace

Department of Surgery, University of Alberta, Edmonton, Alberta, Canada and [1] Section of Neurosurgery, University of Chicago, Chicago, Illinois, U.S.A.

Summary

Twenty-eight patients undergoing surgery within 48 hours of aneurysm rupture were administered recombinant tissue plasminogen activator (rt-PA) directly into the basal subarachnoid cisterns after minimal surgical clot removal and aneurysm clipping. Preoperatively, 26 patients had thick subarachnoid blood clots on computerized tomography (CT), and two had diffuse thin clots. The rt-PA was given as a single intraoperative injection of 7.5 mg (one patient), 10 mg (twenty-two patients), or 15 mg (five patients).

All patients except one demonstrated partial to complete cisternal clot clearance on CT scans within 24 hours after surgery. The patient who showed on clot reduction was the only patient in this series to develop severe symptomatic vasospasm and was the only fatality due to vasospasm, dying 8 days after rupture. No vasospasm was seen on follow-up cerebral angiography in 12 patients, and mild-to-moderate arterial narrowing was seen in at least one major cerebral artery in 15 patients. Severe angiographic vasospasm was not seen, although the patient who died did not undergo repeat angiography. There was one major complication early in the series which seemed clearly related to treatment, and that was a large extradural hematoma occurring within several hours of craniotomy. Intrathecal fibrinolytic treatment appears effective in clearing subarachnoid clot and reducing vasospasm, and may be associated with acceptable risks if given to patients with large-volume subarachnoid hemorrhages at high risk for severe vasospasm.

Keywords: Subarachnoid hemorrhage; cerebral aneurysm; cerebral vasospasm; plasminogen activator; fibrinolytic treatment.

Introduction

Experimental studies have shown that the fibrinolytic agent, recombinant tissue plasminogen activator (rt-PA), administered into the subarachnoid space, is able to lyse subarachnoid hematoma and reduce vasospasm[2−5,11]. In primates, rt-PA given up to 72 hours after subarachnoid hematoma placement significantly reduced vasospasm compared to control animals[5]. The present study was designed to asses the safety of intracisternal rt-PA in humans after aneurysmal subarach-noid hemorrhage (SAH), and to examine the effect of rt-PA on subarachnoid hematoma and vasospasm.

Methods

No patient in this series had a history of bleeding diathesis, and baseline coagulation screening and liver function tests in all patients were normal.

Surgery for aneurysm clipping was performed within 48 hours after aneurysm rupture in all patients. Although the dose of rt-PA administered ranged from 7.5 to 15 mg, the protocol for the last twenty-one patients consisted of a single 10-mg bolus injection directly into the basal cisterns after aneurysm clipping. The rt-PA is supplied as a lyophilized powder* that, when reconstituted with sterile water, has a concentration of 1 mg rt-PA/ml, pH of 7.3, and osmolarity of 215 mOsm.

Only enough blood clot necessary for exposure and clipping of the aneurysm was removed surgically. In the last twenty-one patients in the series, 15 minutes was allowed to pass after rt-PA administration, followed by vigorous irrigation of the subarachnoid space with approximately 1 liter of warmed saline. Modification of the procedure allowed for dilution and dispersement of enzyme throughout the subarachnoid cisterns and served to reduce the concentration of non-fibrinbound rt-PA from the wound prior to closure. After microscopic inspection of the operative site and pial banks for bleeding, the dura and wound were closed securely. Although a temporary cisternal drain was used early in the series, the last 20 patients did not undergo post-operative cisternal drainage.

All patients had at least one computerized tomography (CT) scan performed within 24 hours of surgery, and scanning was repeated thereafter as necessary. Vasospasm was monitored clinically and with repeat cerebral angiography on or near Day 7 following SAH and, when possible, by daily transcranial Doppler ultrasound (TCD) examination (twenty cases). All patients received nimodipine, 60 mg every 4 hours by mouth or through a nasogastric tube, for 14 to 21 days after surgery. Enough intravenous fluids were administered in each patient to maintain modest hypervolemia, and one patient was treated with induced hypertension.

Renal, hepatic, and coagulation testing was performed pre- and postoperatively in all patients. In addition, systemic fibrinogenolysis

* Tissue-type plasminogen activator manufactured by Genentech, Inc., South San Francisco, California, U.S.A.

was monitored with one or two serum fibrinogen level assays during the first 2 postoperative days in the last six patients. Serum assays for D-dimer, a cross-linked fibrin degradation product, were performed pre- and postoperatively in seven of the last 20 patients treated.

Results

Patient Presentation

There were nine men and nineteen women, with ages ranging from 28 to 84 years (average age 53 ± 16 years). Aneurysm location showed that eleven patients had anterior communicating artery (ACoA) aneurysms, three had internal carotid artery (ICA) aneurysms, seven had posterior communicating artery (PCoA) aneurysms, six had middle cerebral artery (MCA) aneurysms, and one had a basilar artery (BA) aneurysm. Twenty-three patients had one aneurysm, four patients had two aneurysms, and another had three aneurysms. In every patient with multiple aneurysms in was always clear, based upon clinical, radiological and operative findings, that the ruptured aneurysm had been repaired prior to rt-PA administration.

On admission, the patients were classified according to their SAH as follows: one Grade II, seven Grade III, four Grade IVa, fifteen Grade IVb, and one Grade V (World Federation of Neurological Surgeons Scale[1]). Only one patient was alert preoperatively. Admission CT scans classified subarachnoid blood as diffuse and thick in twenty-three cases, localized and thick in three, and diffuse and thin in two. Mean time to surgery was 22.5 ± 11.4 hours, with a range from 8 to 48 hours. There were no significant differences between sexes, time to surgery (> 24 hours vs. $\geqslant 24$ hours), or in aneurysm location.

Complications

There was one major complication that seemed clearly related to rt-PA treatment. This 45-year-old man underwent uneventful clipping of a large right PCoA aneurysm 16 hours postrupture, after which 15 mg of rt-PA was instilled into the basal cisterns. The cisterns were not irrigated, but both ventricular and cisternal drains were inserted. Postoperatively, the patient did not awaken, and an immediate CT scan demonstrated a large right frontal extradural hematoma. This was evacuated, and the following morning the patient underwent removal of residual right subdural and temporal hematomas. He had a prolonged convalescence

and, although he eventually returned home and became independent, he remained with moderate left hemiparesis. In another patient, a thin asymptomatic epidural hematoma was noted beneath the craniotomy and was partially aspirated on the day following surgery.

Dosages of rt-PA used in this study did not result in systemic fibrinolysis. No patient had a prolongation in thrombin or partial thromboplastin time post-operatively. In the 20 patients in whom it was measured, the plasma fibrinogen level did not decrease postoperatively.

Clot Clearance

All patients except one demonstrated clot clearance on CT scans within 24 hours after surgery. Two patients underwent immediate postoperative CT scanning (under anesthesia), and neither study showed significant change in the amount of diffuse thick subarachnoid hematoma compared to their preoperative CT scans; however, scans from both patients 12 hours later showed almost complete resolution of cisternal blood clot. There results suggest that clot lysis mediated by intraoperative rt-PA is not immediate, but occurs over 24 hours. Most often, the overnight reduction in cisternal blood clot was notable.

Vasospasm

Clinical vasospasm was seen in three patients. One of these patients, the only who failed to demonstrate clot clearance, deteriorated from renal, pulmonary, and cardiac failure and became comatose with evidence of severe brain swelling. Although repeat cerebral angiography was not obtained, TCD examinations revealed increased cerebral blood velocities in both MCA's beginning on Day 3 after SAH, reaching values as high as 220 mc/sec (mean value in the left MCA) on Day 5. This patient was declared brain-dead on Day 7 following SAH and died the following day.

The remainder of patients underwent postoperative cerebral angiography. There was no evidence of angiographic vasospasm in 12 of these patients, mild vasospasm ($\leqslant 25\%$ reduction in luminal caliber compared to the preoperative caliber) was seen in 9, and 6 had moderate vasospasm (25% to 50% reduction in luminal caliber). Severe angiographic vasospasm was not observed.

Outcome

Overall outcome has been good in 21 patients. Two patients have sustained moderate disabilities; one due to a postoperative extradural hematoma (discussed above) and one due to perforator occlusion. There have been five deaths, one due to severe vasospasm (discussed above), one due to a gastro-intestinal hemorrhage, and three as a direct effect of the primary SAH.

Discussion

Because of their location within the subarachnoid space, aneurysms have a high propensity for the deposition of large volumes of blood around the basal conducting arteries when they rupture. The progressive lysis of the erythrocytes anmeshed within the clot leads to the release of oxyhemoglobin which is a powerful and long-lasting constrictor of the vascular smooth muscle. This results in the progressive diminution in calibre of the large arteries at the base of the brain which can reach the point three or four days after the hemorrhage of seriously reducing cerebral blood flow. The most powerful predictor of the likelihood of developing delayed ischemia from vasospasm is the volume of subarachnoid clot visible in the CT scan done on the day following the hemorrhage. The degree of vasospasm is a dose related phenomenon affected by the volume of clot and hence concentration of hemoglobin.

There has been speculation over many years that early removal of clot by either mechnaical or pharmacological means might reduce the likelihood of clinically significant vasospasm developing[13,14].

The natural clearance of subarachnoid clot has recently been reviewed[4]. Spinal fluid does not normally contain any significant fibrinolytic activity. Fibrinolysis proceeds slowly over days as plasminogen activators are released from the irritated meninges. Hemolysis of breakdown of the red blood cells also proceeds slowly over a week or two after subarachnoid hemorrhage. We believe that as the erythrocytes break down they release oxyhemoglobin which is a potent and long-lasting spasmogen. This is present in extremely high concentrations adjacent to the adventitia of the cerebral blood vessels because of adjacent clot. The rationale for the use of fibrinolytic agents in the treatment of subarachnoid clot has recently been reviewed[2].

Human studies on the use of cisternal rt-PA following aneurysmal SAH were undertaken on the basis of encouraging preliminary animal experiments. Mizoi *et al.* in Sendai, Japan, used intrathecal rt-PA in patients with thick subarachnoid clot judged to be at high risk from ischemic deficits resulting from vasospasm. They used multiple bolus injections via catheters in the subarachnoid space and ventricles in the days following aneurysm clipping. Their initial experiences with 10 cases showed absence of severe vasospasm or delayed ischemic neurologic deficits[9].

Ohman *et al.* in Helsinki reported on 30 patients treated in a variable dose fashion. One patient in their lowest dose group developed postoperative intracerebral hemorrhage and one patient in the medium group had a postoperative epidural hematoma. There were no deaths attributable to the rt-PA. There was a significant reduction in the degree of residual clot between the middle and highest dose group of rt-Pa. There was also less spasm in the high dose (13 mg rt-PA) as opposed to the low dose (3 mg t-PA)[10].

Another preliminary account of the treatment of 10 patients came from Zabramski and colleagues in Phoenix[15]. They also treated patients in poorer neurologic condition with thick layered clot. They noted oozing from the operative incision in some patients. No bleeding complications were noted in the patients receiving the lower regimen of rt-PA (3 infusions of 0.5 mg rt-PA). By analyzing cisternal CSF they found residual high levels of rt-PA as long as 48 hours after instillation. They found mild to moderate vasospasm 7–8 days after rupture in the patients but no cases of severe diffuse spasm and no delayed ischemic deficits.

Stolke and Seifert[12] have reported 20 patients with thick SAH undergoing aneurysm clipping within 72 hours followed by intraoperative administration of 10 mg rt-PA into the basal cisterns. Although 16 patients developed transcranial Doppler evidence of vasospasm, 5 severe, only one patient demonstrated symptomatic vasospasm, and that patient died. All patients showed a striking reduction of subarachnoid clot following treatment with rt-PA, and there were no complications due to rt-PA treatment.

Another use of rt-PA in the context of recently ruptured aneurysms may be in the rapid dissolution of intraventricular clot by catheter instillation of boluses of rt-PA. Findlay *et al.* demonstrated a dramatic case of early lysis of an intraventricular blood cast[6]. At the University of Alberta an additional nine patients with intraventricular clot have been similarly treated with good effect by this maneuver[8].

Clearly the use of an agent which dissolves fibrin has the potential to cause dangerous postoperative bleeding. It seems obvious that the use of this agent should be restricted to those patients judged to be at high risk of developing delayed ischemic deficits on the basis of severe diffuse spasm. The sooner the rt-PA can be instilled after aneurysm clipping, probably the better. It remains to be established what will be the minimal effective dose to be used in man. Operative technique will obviously have to be meticulous and the use of rt-PA is probably best avoided if there are large, raw brain surfaces which have oozed during surgery. It should also be emphasized that the operating surgeon must be absolutely certain that he has completely clipped the ruptured aneurysm if the patient has more than one aneurysm or if there is doubt as to the adequacy of the clip application. We believe that a tight dural closure should be sought as protection against the development of epidural or scalp bleeding.

The initial experience with rt-PA has been encouraging. In more than 100 patients who were judged to be at very high risk from developing severe diffuse spasm and delayed ischemic infarction, this development has been virtually eliminated. These results, however, were obtained from centres with large volumes of aneurysm patients in which rt-PA was used very cautiously under protocol. It is not clear at this point whether or not the general introduction of this agent would result in an acceptable risk/benefit ratio. We are aware of anecdotal accounts of serious postoperative bleeding associated with the use of this drug. We hope that the prospective, randomized, placebo-controlled trials currently underway will provide a definitive answer to the question, "What is the proper role of fibrinolytic agents following aneurysmal rupture?"

References

1. Drake CG (1988) Report of World Federation of Neurological Surgeons Committee on a universal subarachnoid hemorrhage grading scale. J Neurosurg 68: 985–986
2. Findlay JM, Weir BKA, Steinke D, Tanabe T, Gordon P, Grace M (1988) Effect of intrathecal thrombolytic therapy on subarachnoid clot and chronic vasospasm in a primate model of SAH. J Neurosurg 69: 723–735
3. Findlay JM, Weir BKA, Gordon P, Grace M, Baughman R (1989) Safety and efficacy of intrathecal thrombolytic therapy in a primate model of cerebral vasospasm. Neurosurgery 24: 491–498
4. Findlay JM, Weir BKA, Kanamaru K, Grace M, Gordon P, Baughman R, Howarth A (1989) Intrathecal fibrinolytic therapy after subarachnoid hemorrhage: dosage study in a primate model and review of the literature. Can J Neurol Sci 16: 28–40
5. Findlay JM, Weir BKA, Kanamaru K, Grace M, Baughman R (1990) The effect of timing of intrathecal fibrinolytic therapy on cerebral vasospasm in a primate model of subarachnoid hemorrhage. Neurosurgery 26: 201–206
6. Findlay JM, Weir, BKA, Stollery DE (1991) Lysis of intraventricular hematoma with tissue plasminogen activator. Case report. J Neurosurg 74: 803–807
7. Findlay JM, Macdonald RL, Weir BKA (1991) Current concepts of pathophysiology and management of cerebral vasospasm following aneurysmal subarachnoid hemorrhage. Cerebrovasc Brain Metab Rev 3: 336–361
8. Findlay JM, Weir BKA, Grace MG (1993). Treatment of intraventricular hemorrhage with tissue plasminogen activator. Neurosurgery, in press
9. Mizoi K, Yoshimoto T, Fujiwara S, Sugawara T, Takahashi A, Koshu K (1991) Prevention of vasospasm by clot removal and intrathecal bolus injection of tissue-type plasminogen activator: preliminary report. Neurosurgery 28: 807–813
10. Ohman J, Servo A, Heiskanen O (1991) Effect of intrathecal fibrinolytic therapy on clot lysis and vasospasm in patients with aneurysmal subarachnoid hemorrhage. J Neurosurg 75: 197–201
11. Seifert V, Eisert WG, Stolke D, Goetz C (1989) Efficacy of single intracisternal bolus injection of recombinant tissue plasminogen activator to prevent delayed cerebral vasospasm after experimental subarachnoid hemorrhage. Neurosurgery 25: 590–598
12. Stolke, D, Seifert, V (1992) Single intracisternal bolus of recombinant tissue plasminogen activator in patients with aneurysmal subarachnoid hemorrhage: preliminary assessment of efficacy and safety in an open clinical study. Neurosurgery 30(6): 877–881
13. Weir B (1990) The history of cerebral vasospasm. Neurosurg Clin North Am 1: 265–276
14. Weir B (1990) The effect of clot removal on cerebral vasospasm. Neurosurg Clin North Am 1: 377–385
15. Zabramski JM, Spetzler RF, Lee RS, Papadopoulos SM, Bovill E, Zimmerman RS, Bederson JB (1991) Phase I trial of tissue plasminogen activator for the prevention of vasospasm in patients with aneurysmal subarachnoid hemorrhage. J Neurosurg 75: 189–196

Correspondence: J.M. Findlay, M.D., Neurosurgical Associates, Room 2D 102, Mackenzie Centre, 8440-112 Street, Edmonton, AB, T6G 2B7, Canada.

Intracisternal Therapy with Tissue Plasminogen Activator for the Prevention of Vasospasm in Patients with Aneurysmal Subarachnoid Hemorrhage. A Review

J.M. Zabramski, R.F. Spetzler, S.M. Papadopoulos, and **T. Bovill**[1]

Division of Neurological Surgery, Barrow Neurological Institute, Phoenix, Arizona, and [1]Department of Pathology, University of Vermont, Burlington, Vermont, U.S.A.

Summary

Recent laboratory and clinical studies have suggested that intracisternal administration of recombinant tissue plasminogen activator (rt-PA) can facilitate the normal clearing of blood form the subarachnoid space and prevent or ameliorate delayed cerebral arterial spasm. Results of a Phase I trial and ongoing clinical experience with this form of treatment are reviewed. All patients were at high risk of vasospasm, with poor clinical grade (Hunt and Hess Grade III to V) and CT scan evidence of a large subarachnoid hemorrhage (SAH). Ventriculostomy and surgery for clipping of the ruptured aneurysm was carried out within 48 hours of hemorrhage.

The initial treatment protocol utilized cisternal administration of total doses of rt-PA between 1.5 and 5 mg via a small catheter left in the suprasellar cisterns. Cisternal and ventricular CSF samples were obtained at 8 hour intervals to measure free rt-PA levels. Doses of rt-PA as small as 0.5 mg produced levels of free rt-PA in the range of 10,000 to 17,000 ng/ml with a half-life of rt-PA in the CSF being approximately 2.5 hours. Clinically, 5 mg of rt-PA produced significant oozing from operative incisions and/or ventriculostomy sites in all patients, while doses of 0.5 mg were well tolerated. One patient receiving a dose of 5 mg rt-PA developed a small epidural hematoma that was treated by delayed drainage. Follow-up angiography was carried out 7 to 10 days post hemorrhage to assess the severity of vasospasm: Focal severe spasm of the intracranial segment of the vertebral artery was seen in one patient who underwent clipping of a PICA aneurysm, while the remainder of his angiogram (including the basilar artery) revealed only mild spasm. In the remaining nine patients mild to moderate arterial spasm was documented. No patient in the treatment group had severe diffuse spasm compared to the 50% rate reported in the literature for similar patients.

More recently 10 mg of rt-PA has been placed in the cisterns after clipping of the aneurysm and allowed to remain in place for 20 minutes followed by vigorous irrigation with 1 to 2 liters of saline. Minor bleeding in the form of oozing from the incision line has been noted in 2 patients with this protocol. Follow-up angiography in this group has demonstrated only mild to moderate spasm.

Preliminary evolution of rt-PA appears promising for the prevention and/or amelioration of delayed cerebral vasospasm.

Keywords: Aneurysmal subarchnoid hemorrhage; cerebral arterial vasospasm; recombinant tissue plasminogen activator (rt-PA); intracisternal therapy, prospective clinical trial.

Introduction

Although the etiology and pathophysiology of cerebral vasospasm after aneurysmal subarachnoid hemorrhage (SAH) remain controversial, it is generally accepted that spasmogenic metabolites derived from the degradation of red blood cells during clot lysis play an important role. Recent studies from a number of laboratories have demonstrated that intracisternal fibrinolytic therapy can markedly enhance the clearance of blood from the subarachnoid spaces and reduce the severity of delayed cerebral vasospasm[1,2,4,21]. The most promising of these agents for use in humans appears to be recombinant tissue plasminogen activator (rt-PA)[3,16,26].

This study was undertaken to evaluate the safety and efficacy of intracisternal fibrinolytic therapy with rt-PA for the prevention of delayed cerebral vasopasm in patients with aneurysmal SAH. Data from serial t-PA measurements in ventricular and cisternal cerebrospinal fluid (CSF) were collected to help guide decisions about appropriate dosage-regimens for furture clinical trials.

Clinical Materials and Methods

Patient Population

Fourteen patients (9 females and 5 males) were enrolled in one of three rt-PA protocols. The details of the treatment protocols are summarized in Table 1. Patients ranged from 23 to 83 years of age (mean age, 53 years). All patients were admitted within 48 hours of SAH and were Clinical Grade III or IV (Hunt and Hess)[8]. Admission computed tomography (CT) demonstrated thick layers of blood in the major cisterns and fissures (Grade 3 SAH, Fisher CT Grading Scale) in all patients[5]. Fourteen patients had aneurysms in the

Table 1. *Clinical rt-PA Protocols*

No. 1	single dose of rt-PA (5 mg in 5 ml) via a cisternal catheter 12- to 24-hours after surgery
No. 2	multiple doses of rt-PA (0.5 mg in 5 ml q8h × 3) via a cisternal catheter beginning 12- to 24-hours after surgery
No. 3	single intraoperative dose of rt-PA (10 mg in 10 ml) prior to closure; After allowing the solution to remain in the cisterns for 20 minutes it is flushed out by thorough irrigation with approximately 2 liters of saline irrigation

anterior circulation, and one patient had a posterior inferior cerebellar artery (PICA) aneurysm.

Patients were excluded if they had abnormal coagulation parameters, evidence of active internal bleeding, recent cerebral infarction (within 2 months), recent biopsy of internal organs (within 10 days), or a history of medical illness associated with increased risk of hemorrhage. Patients were also excluded if they were pregnant or if angiography revealed an intracranial vascular malformation. The presence of unclipped intracranial aneurysms was considered an absolute contraindication.

Treatment and Evaluation

The patients' medical and surgical management was dictated by their clinical course with the following restrictions: Ventriculostomy and surgery for clipping of the aneurysm had to be performed within 72 hours of hemorrhage. Routine care in this group of patients included treatment with prophylactic hypervolemic therapy, including placement of a Swan-Ganz catheter.

Pulmonary artery diastolic (PAD) pressure was maintained within 12 to 16 mm Hg using a combination of crystalloids (5% dextrose with lactated Ringer's (D5LR) and/or 0.9% NaCl solution at 150 ml/h) and Plasmanate (100 ml/h as needed, PAD < 12 mm Hg).

Patients were transfused to maintain the level of their hematocrit between 30% and 35%. All patients were treated with nimodipine (60 mg by mouth every 4 hours) for 21 days after hemorrhage. Treatment with rt-PA was initiated only after successful clipping of all aneursysms.

In the first 10 patients, a small Silastic lumbar drain catheter was left in the subarachnoid space and rt-PA was administered 12 to 24 hours after surgery. Patients underwent a postoperative CT scan and coagulation studies. Therapy with rt-PA was withheld if there was evidence of postoperative hematoma or abnormalities in the coagulation profile. In the first version of this protocol (Protocol No. 1), patients received a single

dose of 5 mg of rt-PA between 12 and 18 hours after surgery. Persistent minor bleeding and the results of serial measurements of t-PA in the cisternal CSF in 5 patients led to a reduction in the rt-PA dosage. In version two (Protocol No. 2), a total of 1.5 mg rt-PA was given to five patients in three equally divided dosages of 0.5 mg at 8 hour intervals.

More recently, four patients have received rt-PA using an intraoperative treatment protocol described by Findlay *et al.* (Protocol No. 3). After surgery for clipping of the aneurysm(s), patients received 10 mg of rt-PA in 10 ml of saline solution instilled directly into the basal cisterns and allowed to remain in place for 20 minutes. During this time the rt-PA in solution firmly binds to the firbin contained within the clotted blood within the major fissures and cisterns. The cisterns were then thoroughly irrigated with about 2 liters of saline solution to remove all unbound rt-PA.

Serial ventricular and cisternal CSF samples were obtained after rt-PA administration in the 10 patients enrolled in Protocols No. 1 and No. 2. CSF samples were placed on ice and transported immediately to the laboratory where they were centrifuged. The decant was stored at −70° C. Samples were kept frozen until they were thawed in the central coagulation laboratory immediately before performance of the t-PA assay. The t-PA antigen levels were measured with an enzyme-linked immunosorbent assay (ELISA) based on three murine monoclonal antibodies[7].

Outcome at 3-months was assessed using the Glasgow Outcome Scale (Table 2)[9]. CT scans were repeated 12 to 24 hours after the administration of rt-PA and again 7 to 8 days after aneurysmal rupture to rule out hemorrhagic complications.

The effect of treatment with rt-PA on delayed arterial vasospasm was documented by follow-up angiography

Table 2. *Glasgow Outcome Scale*

Clinical outcome grade	Definition
Good recovery	resumption of normal life with or without minor deficits
Moderate disability	disabled but independent; can travel by public transportation and work in a sheltered environment
Severe disability	conscious but disabled; dependent for daily support by reason of mental and/or physical disability
Persistent vegetative	unresponsive to external environment; speechless
Death	death secondary to brain damage

7 to 9 days after aneurysmal hemorrhage. The severity and distribution of arterial vasospasm were noted. Vasospasm was graded as severe if the angiographic vessel diameter was narrowed to less than 50% of its original diameter, moderate for 30% to 50% narrowing, and mild for less than 30% reduction. Transcranial Doppler (TCD) studies were performed three times a week, and results were correlated with clinical and radiographic findings.

Results

Complications

Overall, there were no serious complications related to intracisternal therapy with rt-PA. There was no evidence of systemic effect on serial coagulation parameters; however, local abnormalities of hemostasis secondary to treatment with rt-PA were apparent in patients who recieved doses of 5 mg to 10 mg of rt-PA. The operative incision oozed in four of five patients in Protocol No. 1 and in two of four patients in Protocol No. 3. The ventriculostomy site also oozed in two patients in Protocol No. 1. One patient in Protocol No. 1 developed a small extra-axial hematoma that was treated by delayed burr-hole drainage. There were no apparent local or systemic effects on coagulation in the five patients receiving the 0.5 mg dosages of rt-PA at 8 hour intervals (total dosage of 1.5 mg).

Evidence of Cerebral Vasospasm

Follow-up angiography 7 to 9 days after hemorrhage revealed mild to moderate vasospasm in 13 of 14 patients (Fig. 1). In the remaining patient, in whom a PICA aneurysm was responsible for hemorrhage, follow-up angiography revealed clinically asymtomatic, severe focal vasospasm that involved the proximal intracranial portion of the vertebral arteries with mild to moderate spasm in the remaining vascular distributions. Serial TCD studies, available in 12 of 14 patients, revealed maximum flow velocities of 110 to 180 cm/c (mean velocity, 138 cm/s) in the middle cerebral artery (MCA) and 90 to 164 cm/sec (mean velocity, 113 cm/s) during the first 2 weeks after SAH.

Clinical Outcome

Outcome was assessed 3 months after hemorrhage in all surviving patients. Eight patients had good outcomes

and were totally independent, while three were independent but had moderate disability. One patient, a 66-years-old man with a long history of poorly controlled hypertension and mild dementia before his hemorrhage, had a poor outcome with severe disability. This patient had evidence of multiple new infarcts on follow-up CT scans, despite normal TCD flow values and only mild to moderate spasm on angiography.

There were two deaths. One patient, a 77-year-old woman, initially did well, but died 9 weeks after hemorrhage from delayed pulmonary complications. There was no evidence of ischemic injury on follow-up CT. The second patient, a 78-year-old woman, died from pneumonia 6 weeks after hemorrhage. Like the patient above with a poor outcome, this woman had a history of severe atherosclerotic vascular disease, previous stroke, and mild dementia. Her neurologic status gradually declined after surgery. Despite evidence of only mild to moderate vasospasm on follow-up angiography and TCD studies, her CT 2 weeks after hemorrhage demonstrated evidence of multiple new infarcts.

Serial t-PA Levels

The results of serial t-PA levels are presented in Table 3 in the four patients who received a single 5 mg dose

Table 3. *Mean tPA Levels.* Single Dosage 5.0 mg

Time (hours)	Cisternal tPA level (ng/ml)	Ventricular tPA level (ng/ml)
0 (base line)	5	2
6	42,000	825
18	1,500	484
24	300	34
36	69	13
48	30	4
72	12	1
96	6	0.5

Table 4. *Mean tPA Levels.* dosage 0.5 mg q8h × 3

Time (hours)	Cisternal tPA level (ng/ml)	Ventricular tPA level (ng/ml)
0 (base line)	3	2
8	11,856	40
16	15,058	48
24	17,377	61
32	561	47
40	46	9
48	24	3

CSF for t-PA levels at 0, 8, and 16 hours were drawn immediately prior to rt-PA administration.

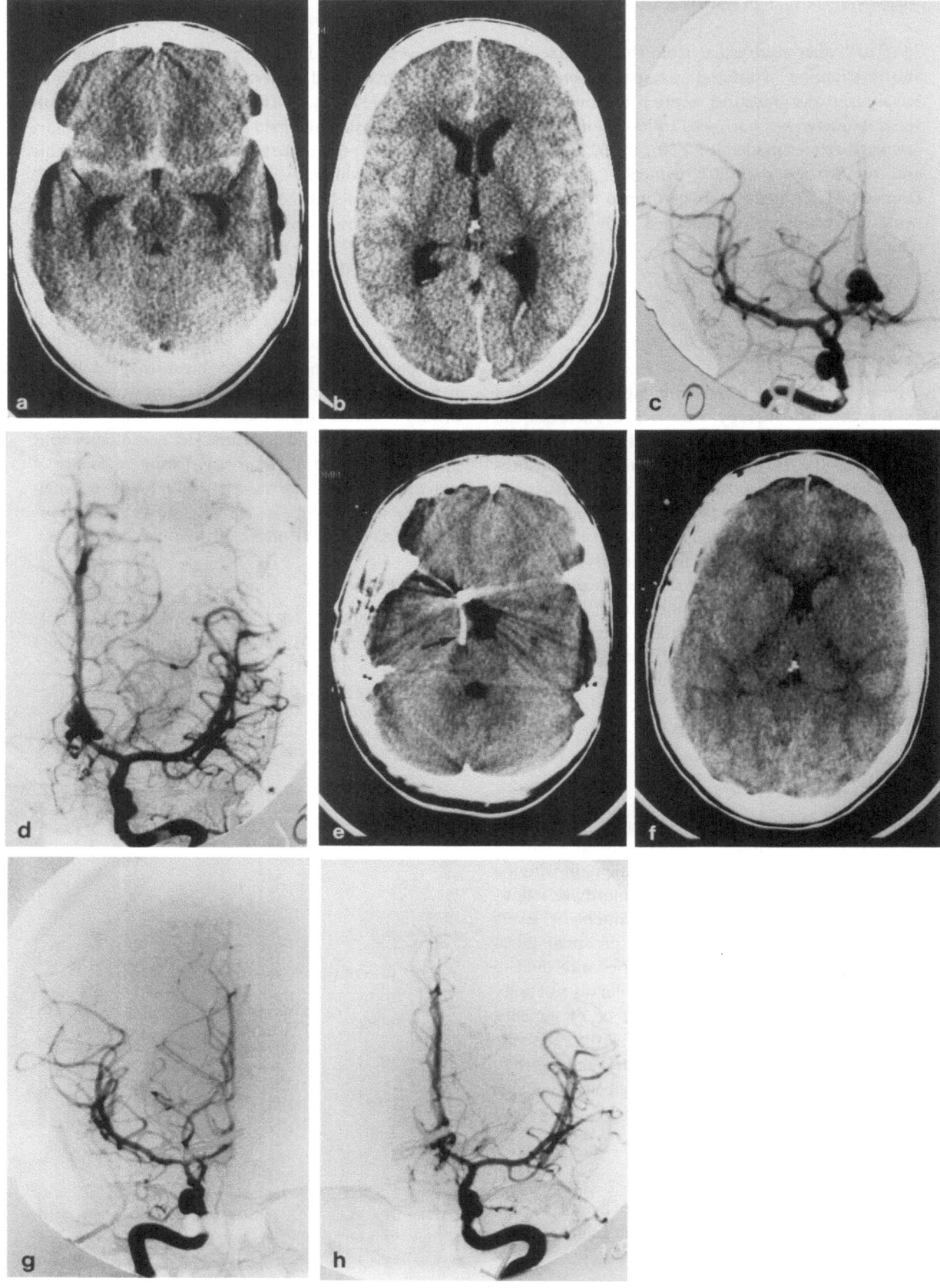

of rt-PA. Table 4 shows the measurements in the five patients who received a total dosage of 1.5 mg (0.5 mg every 8h × 3). CSF levels at 8 and 16 hours in the multiple dose regimen were drawn immediately before rt-PA administration.

Discussion

Despite extensive research, complications related to delayed cerebral vasospasm remain the major cause of morbidity and mortality in patients who survive aneurysmal SAH. The optimal method of treating vasospasm would be to prevent its occurrence. While the exact mechanism(s) responsible for vasospasm is uncertain, there is little doubt that blood in the subarachnoid space is related to its development. In laboratory studies, we have demonstrated a direct relationship between the volume of subarchnoid hemorrhage and the severity angiography vasospasm[25]. Reports in the clinical literature have shown that the severity of SAH visualized on CT soon after aneurysmal rupture is an important indicator for predicting the subsequent risk of clinically symptomatic vasospasm[5,11,13].

In 1977, Osaka[17] suggested that if vasospasm after aneurysmal subarachnoid hemorrhage is produced by the components or breakdown products of blood, then it should be prevented by the early removal of blood from the subarachnoid spaces. In fact, a possible role for the removal of blood from the cerebral cisterns for the prevention of vasopasm was first suggested by Johnson[10] in 1958 and by Pool[19] in 1959.

A number of authors have reported encouraging results from combining early surgical clipping of ruptured aneurysms with aggressive mechanical removal of blood from the basal cisterns[14,20,24]. In laboratory models of SAH, there is clear evidence that early mechanical removal of blood from the subarachnoid spaces can prevent delayed cerebral vasospasm[6,15]. Nevertheless, general clinical experience with attempts at mechanical removal of blood has been disappointing.

Clinically, mechanical removal of clotted blood is usually limited by the operative exposure and can only be accomplished with some bruising of the pial banks and damage to small vessels. A more attractive theoretical alternative for the removal of subarachnoid blood is the use of fibrinolytic agents (e.g., urokinase, rt-PA) to enhance the natural clearing of blood.

The results of laboratory studies with rt-PA for the prevention of vasospasm have been encouraging. Using a primate model, Findlay et al. convincingly demonstrated that treatment with intracisternal rt-PA within 24 to 48 hours of SAH prevented angiographically significant delayed cerebral vasospasm[1,2,4]. In the dog, Seifert et al.[21] have likewise demonstrated that treatment with rt-PA within 48 hours of SAH can prevent angiographic evidence of delayed cerebral vasospasm.

Since its introduction, rt-PA has been extensive clinical use for treatment of acute coronary thrombosis. More recently, attention has been directed at its possible use in treatment of acute stroke. In the perpheral circulation, the pharmacology of rt-PA has been well studied. Its metabolism after intra-arterial or intravenous administration is extremely rapid with a half-life of only 5 to 8 minutes[12]. In contrast, there is little or no clinical information about the safety or metabolism of rt-PA in the CSF cisterns.

The results of the present study demonstrate that rt-PA can be administered in the subrachnoid space with relative safety after the surgical clipping of a ruptured aneurysm. However, the occurrence of local bleeding complications in 80% of patients after dosages of 5 mg in Protocol No. 1 suggests that the initial dosage of rt-PA chosen for evaluation was too high. The results of t-PA levels in the cisternal CSF confirm this impression: t-PA levels averaged 42,000 ng/ml 6 hours after a single 5 mg dose, compared with an effective therapeutic range of 600 to 6,000 ng/ml reported during systemic fibrinolysis[22,23]. Estimates based on the serial measurements made in this study (Table 3) suggest a prolonged half-life in the CSF of 2 to 3 hours.

In Protocol No. 2, interval dosing with 0.5 mg of rt-PA (every 8h × 3) was well tolerated without evidence of local of systemic bleeding complications. Cisternal t-PA levels averaged 11,800 ng/ml 8 hours after the first

Fig. 1. A 23-year old woman who presented with the sudden onset of severe headache, nausea, and confusion. (a, b) Basic head CT scan reveals an extensive Fischer Grade 3 subarachnoid hemorrhage. Note that enlarged temporal horns (straight arrows) consistent with acute hydrocephalus. (c, d) Preoperative angiogram (Day 0) demonstrating a large irregularly shaped anterior communicating artery aneurysm. (e, f) Basic head CT scan 24-hours after completing the administration of rt-PA [three 0.5 mg does of rt-PA via the cisternal catheter (arrow) at 8-hour intervals]. Note the marked clearing of blood from the basal cisterns and intrahemispheric fissure. (g, h) Follow-up angiogram on Day 9 post-hemorrhage revealing mild to moderate cerebral vasospasm

dosage and 17,000 ng/ml after the third dose, suggesting that even further reductions in dosage may be possible. Indeed, Seifert *et al.*[21] recently reported that a single dosage of 0.025 mg or rt-PA effectively cleared blood and prevented delayed cerebral vasospasm in a two-hemorrhage canine model[21]. Unfortunately, t-PA levels in the CSF have not been measured in any of the other published laboratory or clinical studies evaluating intracisternal therapy with rt-PA.

Preliminary results with Protocol No. 3, in which rt-PA was first allowed to bind to fibrin in the subarachnoid spaces and excess (unbound) rt-PA was irrigated out, suggest that this protocol has acceptable risks. Some tendency for oozing from the operative incision site during the first hours after surgery had been noted in about half the patients. This oozing, however, may be related to the spillage of unbound rt-PA outside the dural cavity, particularly during the early phase of irrigation when rt-PA levels are relatively high in the irrigation fluid. Careful irrigation and suction have eliminated this problem in the last two patients. Data are needed on the t-PA levels achieved in the cisternal CSF with this method.

Preliminary experience with rt-PA in this protocol suggests that it may reduce the severity of delayed cerebral vasospasm. Patients were chosen for this protocol on the basis of factors known to be associated with a high risk of clinical and angiographic vasospasm (poor clinical grade and evidence of a large hemorrhage by CT). Follow-up angiography 7 to 9 days after

Table 5. *Angiographic Saverity of Vasospasm*

Degree of vasospasm	Nimodipine (Petruk *et al.*, 1988)	rt-PA + Nimodipine (Zabramski, *et al.*)
Mild	13%	30%
Moderate or severe focal	39%	70%
Severe diffuse	48%	–

Table 6. *Clinical Outcome at 3 Months*

Glasgow outcome score	Nimodipine (Petruk *et al.*, 1988)	rt-p + Nimodipine (Zabramski, *et al.*)
Good	36%	57%
Moderate	10%	22%
Severe	12%	7%
Vegetative	16%	–
Dead	36%	14%

hemorrhage demonstrated mild to moderate angiographic vasospasm in 13 of 14 patients. Severe focal vasospasm was noted in the one remaining patient (Table 5). None of the patients had angiographic evidence of severe diffuse vasospasm. The scale used to measure the severity of angiographic spasm in this protocol is the same as that used by Petruk *et al.*[18] in the Canadian trial of nimodipine given to poor-grade aneurysm patients. Severe diffuse vasospasm was reported in 48% of the patients who received nimodipine and in 56% of the patients in the placebo group (Table 5).

At their 3-months follow-up examination, 57% of our patients had "good" outcomes, 21% were "moderately disabled," and 14% died. These results compare favorably with those reported in the clinical nimodipine trial by Petruk *et al.*[18] (Table 6) in which patients admitted as a Grade III (Hunt and Hess Scale) had a 44% "good" outcome while 28% died. Although no conclusions about the efficacy of rt-PA can be made from such a comparison, it does provide evidence that treatment was not detrimental.

Two patients in our series (14%) developed CT scan evidence of new infarcts that followed a time course consistent with delayed cerebral ischemia. In both of these patients, serial TCDs and the results of angiography revealed only mild to moderate vasospasm. In the absence of evidence of significant vasospasm, the etiology of the ischemic changes seen in these two patients is not clear. Both patients, however, had a history of poorly controlled hypertension and mild dementia before rupture of their aneurysm. These histories suggests that preexisting small vessel disease may have contributed to the ischemic complications.

Conclusion

The results of this preliminary data demonstrate that rt-PA can be administered in the subarachnoid space with relative safety in patients with aneurysmal SAH after definitive surgical clipping of the ruptured aneurysm. The results further suggests that early treatment with rt-PA may reduce the severity of delayed angiographic vasospasm. Certainly further studies are indicated.

References

1. Findlay JM, Weir BKA, Gordon P, Grace M, Baughman R (1989) Safety and efficacy of intrathecal thrombolytic therapy in a primate model of cerebral vasospasm. Neurosurgery 24: 491–498

2. Findlay JM, Weir BKA, Kanamaru K, Grace M, Baugjhman R (1990) The effect of timing of intrathecal fibrinolytic therapy on cerebral vasospasm in a primate model of subarachnoid hemorrhage. Neurosurgery 26: 201–206

3. Findlay JM, Weir BKA, Kassell NF, Disney LB, Grace MGA (1991) Intracisternal recombinant tissue plasminogen activator after aneurysmal subarachnoid hemorrhage. J Neurosurg 75: 181–188

4. Findlay JM, Wier BKA, Steinke D, Tanabe T, Gordon P, Grace M (1988) Effect of intrathecal thrombolytic therapy on subarachnoid clot and chronic vasospasm in a primate model of SAH. J Neurosurg 69: 723–735

5. Fisher CM, Kistler JP, Davis JM (1980) Relation of cerebral vasospasm to subarachnoid hemorrhage by computerized tomographic scanning. Neurosurgery 6: 1–9

6. Handa Y, Weir BKA, Nosko M, Mosewich R, Tsuji T, Grace M (1987) The effect of timing of clot removal on chronic vasospasm in a primate model. J Neurosurg 67: 558–564

7. Holvoet P, Cleemput H, Collen D (1985) Assay of human tissue-type plasminogen activator (t-PA) with an enzyme-linked immunosorbent assay (ELISA) based on three murine monoclonal antibodies to t-PA. Thromb Haemost 54: 684–687

8. Hunt WE, Hess RM (1968) Surgical risk as related to time of intervention in the repair of intracranial aneurysms. J Neurosurg 28: 14–20

9. Jennett B, Bond M (1975) Assessment of outcome after servere brain damage: a practical scale. Lancet i: 480–484

10. Johnson RJ, Potter JM, Reid RG (1958 (Abstract)) Arterial spasm in subarachnoid haemorrhage: mechanical considerations. J Neurol Neurosurg Psychiatry 21: 68

11. Kistler JP, Crowell RM, Davis KR, Heros R, Ojemann RG, Zervas T, Fischer CM (1983) The relation of cerebral vasospasm to the extent and location of subarachnoid blood visualized by CT scan: a prospective study. Neurology 33: 424–436

12. Marder VJ, Sherry S (1988) Thrombolytic therapy: current status. N Engl J Med 318: 1512–1520

13. Mizukami DW, Torner JC, Henderson WG (1978) Computed tomography of ruptured intracranial aneurysms in acute stage. Relationship between vasospasm and high density of CT scan. Brain Nerve 30: 861–866

14. Mizukami M, Kawase T, Usami T, Tazawa T (1982) Prevention of vasospasm by early operation with removal of subarachnoid blood. Neurosurgery 10: 301–307

15. Nosko M, Weir BKA, Lunt A, Grace M, Allen P, Mielke B (1987) Effect of clot removal at 24 hours on chronic vasospasm after SAH in the primate model. J Neurosurg 66: 416–422

16. Ohman J, Servo A, Heiskanen O (1991) Effect of intrathecal fibrinolytic therapy on clot lysis and vasospasm in patients with aneurysmal subarachnoid hemorrhage. J Neurosurg 75: 197–201

17. Osaka K (1977) Prolonged vasospasm produced by the breakdown products of erythrocytes. J Neurosurg 47: 403–411

18. Petruk KC, West M. Mohr G, et al (1988) Nimodipine treatment in poor-grade aneurysm patients. J Neurosurg 68: 505–517

19. Pool JL (1959) Early treatment of ruptured intracranial aneurysms of the circle of Willis with special clip technique. Bull N York Acad M 35: 357–369

20. Satio I, Sano K (1990) Vasospasm after aneurysm rupture; Incidence, onset and course. In: Wilkins RH (ed) Cerebral arterial spasm. Williams and Wilkins, Baltimore, pp 294–301

21. Seifert V, Eisert WG, Stolke D, Goetz C (1989) Efficacy of single intracisternal bolus injection of recombinant tissue plasminogen activator to prevent delayed cerebral vasospasm after experimental subarachnoid hemorrhage. Neurosurgery 25: 590–598

22. Sobel BE, Gross RW, Robinson AK (1984) Thrombolysis, clot selectivity and kinetics. Circulation 70: 160–164

23. Stump DC, Califf RM, Topol EJ, Sigmon K, Thornton D, Masek R, Anderson L, Colleen D (1989) Pharmacodynamics of thrombolysis with recombinant tissue-type plasminogen activator. Correlation with characteristics of and clinical outcomes in patients with acute myocardial infraction. Circulation 80: 1222–1230

24. Taneda M (1982) Effect of early operation for ruptured aneurysms on prevention of delayed ischemic symptoms. J Neurosurg 57: 622–628

25. Zabramski JM, Spetzler RF, Bonstelle C (1986) Chronic cerebral vasospasm: Effect of volume and timing of hemorrhage in a canine model. Neurosurgery 18: 1–6

26. Zabramski JM, Spetzler RF, Lee KS, Papadopoulos SM, Bovill E, Zimmerman RS, Bederson JB (1991) Phase I trial of tissue plasminogen activator for the prevention of vasospasm in patients with aneurysmal subarachnoid hemorrhage. J Neurosurg 75: 189–196

Correspondence: c/o Editorial Office, Joseph M. Zabramski, M.D., Barrow Neurological Institute, 350 West Thomas Road, Phoenix, AZ 85013-4496, U.S.A.

The Use of Dobutamine to Enhance Cardiac Performance and Improve Outcome in Patients Refractory to Hypervolemic Therapy for Cerebral Vasospasm: a Preliminary Study

M.L. Levy, C.H. Rabb, V. Zelman, and **S.L. Giannotta**

Department of Neurosurgery, LAC-USC Medical Center, University of Southern California, School of Medicine, Los Angeles, California, U.S.A.

Summary

We have previously concluded that CVP was an unreliable index of cardiac performance during hypervolemic therapy and that in previously healthy individuals a PAWP of 14 mm Hg was associated with maximal cardiac performance[1]. We describe the use of the Beta-agonist, Dobutamine, in combination with hypervolemic preload enhancement on cardiac performance in a preliminary report of 10 patients who failed to respond to traditional preload enhancement following aneurysmal subarachnoid hemorrhage. All patients had the placement of a flow directed balloon-tipped catheter and measurement of pulmonary artery wedge pressure (PAWP), central venous pressure (CVP), cardiac index (CI), stroke volume index (SVI), total peripheral resistance (TPR), and left ventricular stroke work index (LVSWI) during hyperdynamic therapy. Dobutamine was administered at a rate of 5 to 10 ug/kg/h for a period of up to ten days.

Baseline cardiac function was within normal limits (CI = 3.51 ± .30 l/min M^2). Therapy with dobutamine in the presence of volume loading resulted in a 33% increase in CI, a 10% increase in LVSWI, and a 23% decrease in TPR. The reversal of vasospasm clinically was noted in 80% (8/10) of patients undergoing hyperdynamic treatment.

Keywords: Cerebral vasospasm; cardiac index; pulmonary artery wedge pressure; dobutamine therapy.

Introduction

In order to minimize the cardiac, hematologic and pulmonary sequelae of volume expansion and to maximize cardiac performance during therapy for cerebral vasospasm, we have employed the use of flow-directed balloon-tipped catheters with cardiac output and hemodynamic monitoring.

The current study addresses the treatment of patients with vasospasm who fail to respond to hypervolemic preload enhancement. We evaluated the effect of the beta agonist dobutamine on increasing cardiac output without initiating cerebral, cardiac, and/or pulmonary complications. We also evaluated whether dobutamine may be an effective adjunct in the treatment of patients who fail to respond to hypervolemic preload enhancement.

Materials and Methods

Case Material

During the period from July 1988 until July 1989, 10 patients with aneurysmally-induced subarachnoid hemorrhage and vasospasm refractory to hypervolemic therapy were treated in the intensive care unit at LAC-USC Medical Center or Huntington Memorial Hospital (Table 1). All ten patients had no prior history of cardiac or pulmonary disease. All patients had clinical and/or radiographic evidence of vasospasm which was refractory to hypervolemic therapy.

Patient characteristics are also documented in Table 1. Onset of spasm was typically on day 5 following aneurysmal rupture. Patients in the study were hospitalized for a mean of 18 days. There were no complications secondary to either Swan-Ganz catheter placement or volume expansion in this series.

Treatment Protocol

All patients underwent systemic and pulmonary arterial catheterization, and a 7 fr, 110 cm flow-directed thermodilution pulmonary artery catheter (American-Edward Laboratories) was positioned using a subclavian approach. Baseline cardiac index (CI), stroke volume index (SVI), and left ventricular stroke work index (LVSWI) were calculated as follows:

CI (l/min M^2) = cardiac output: body surface area,

SVI (ml/M^2) = CI: heart rate,

LVSWI (g.m/M^2) = (SVI) × (MAP-WP) × (0.0136).

Following baseline measurements, fluid resuscitation was instituted with 5% albumin at 300 cc/h if the PCWP was less than 10 mm Hg. If the PCWP was greater than 16 mm Hg, mannitol 0.25 g/kg or lasix 40 mg were administered. Cardiac performance curves were then generated for each patient, and their pulmonary artery wedge pressure subsequently maintained at a level where CI and LVSWI

Table 1. *Preliminary Series of 10 Patients Receiving HyperDynamic-Hypervolemic Therapy*

Patient	Age	Sex	Spasm day	Aneurysm	Pre-treatment grade	Post-treatment grade	Response to treatment	Notes
1	13	female	3	acom	3	2	yes	
2	19	female	8	acom	3	3	yes	
3	21	male	4	ICA	3	2	yes	
4	24	female	4	ICA	3	1	yes	
5	26	female	3	cavernous	2	1	yes	calcified
6	31	female	10	ICA	1	1	yes	
7	35	male	7	MCA	1	1	yes	intraoperative rupture
8	36	female	4	multiple	2	1	yes	
9	37	male	5	ICA	2	3	no	
10	54	female	4	multiple	1	3	no	required lobectomy/died

were maximized. Failure of response was defined as no improvement or a decline in neurological status (Hunt and Hess) perioperatively despite hypervolemic management.

Patients who failed volume expansion alone were then given dobutamine 5–10ug/kg/min IV infusion. Infusion rates of dobutamine were predicated upon the maintenance of cardiac performance above that of the patients physiologic baseline as established upon admission to the intensive care unit. Despite the effect of dobutamine in reducing PCWP, patients fluid resuscitation was continued as before with hydroxyethel starch or 5% albumin at 300 cc/h if the PCWP was less than 8 mm Hg. If the PCWP was greater than 16 mm Hg, mannitol 0.25 mg/kg or lasix 40 mg were administered.

Dobutamine treatment was continued based upon patient response. In patients responding to dobutamine treatment, infusions were weaned three to four days following initial response. Infusions were reinitiated with recurrence of ischemic neurologic compromise. In patients failing to respond to dobutamine treatment, infusions were weaned following a ten day course.

Statistical Analysis

In interpreting the relationship between changes in SVI, LVSWI, and CI as PAWP was increased during volume expansion, paired samples were analyzed using the Student's t-test with results being significant at $p < 0.05$ in a two-tailed test.

Results

Patients ranged in age from 13 to 54 years (29.6 ± 11.7 years). There were 3 males and 7 females in the study. There were 3 patients with Grade 1, 3 patients with Grade II, and 4 patients with Grade III Hunt and Hess presentations. There were 4 internal carotid artery (ICA), 2 anterior communicating artery (ACOM), 1 middle cerebral artery (MCA), and 1 cavernous carotid artery (CAV) aneurysm in this series. Two patients had multiple aneurysms. Onset of spasm was typically on day 5 following aneurysmal rupture.

Table 2. *Cardiac Performance Pre and Post-Hyperdynamic Therapy in 10 Patients*

Admission	Baseline	Post-hyperdynamic therapy	Change
PAWP	8.0 mm Hg	8.0 – 16.0 mm Hg	
LVSWI	46.4 g.m/M^2	51.04 g.m/M^2	10%
CI	3.51 L/min M^2	4.66 L/min M^2	33%

Note that hyperdynamic therapy with dobutamine resulted in a 23% decrease in TPR.

Cardiac Parameters

Cardiac response at baseline, and following volume enhancement in conjuction with the institution of dobutamine are detailed in Table 2. Baseline PAWP values were indicative of hypovolemia (8.0 ± 0.9 mm Hg). Baseline cardiac function prior to volume loading was within normal limits (LVSWI $= 46.4 \pm 4.0$ g.m/M^2 and CI $= 3.51 \pm .30$ l/min M^2). Hyperdynamic therapy with dobutamine resulted in a 33% increase in CI, a 10% increase in LVSWI, and a 23% decrease in TPR.

The reversal of vasospasm clinically was noted in 80% (8/10) of patients undergoing hyperdynamic treatment ranging from four to ten days after failure to respond to hypervolemia.

Discussion

Cerebral blood flow has been reported to remain constant despite changes in blood pressure or viscosity when normal autoregulation is present[2]. Favorable results have been reported in patients receiving volume expansion and pressure support with dopamine, or with the continuous infusion of isoproterenol or isoproterenol and aminophyline combination therapy[3-9]. The likely mechanism of reversal of symptomatic vasospasm in these latter studies was resultant from increases in cardiac output secondary to the cardiac stimulant effect of these agents and the copious volume of intravenous volume administered. Our rationale for using dobutamine is that it allows us to maximize the patients cardiac output with only mild to moderate associated increases in blood pressure.

Relationship of Cerebral Blood Flow to the Severity of Vasospasm

It has been well documented in the literature that cerebral blood flow progressively decreases in poor grade patients or those with vasospasm[10-16]. It has also been shown that reductions in CBF occur in the face of increased cerebral blood volume[17]. Rosenstein, *et al.* documented reversal of neurologic deficits associated with increases in cerebral blood flow following hypervolemic therapy using bedside determinations of cerebral blood flow in the management of patients with subarachnoid hemorrhage [18].

Kassell *et al.*[19] in 1982 reported on a protocol of volume expansion, vaso-blockade and pressor agents which resulted in the reversal of neurologic deficits completely in 43 of 58 patients studied. They used Swan-Ganz catheterization to monitor patients cardiac parameters and to avoid potential cardiac and pulmonary complications associated with hypervolemic therapy. They also noted that neurological improvement often occurred in the early stages of fluid replacement prior to any measured elevations in mean arterial pressure.

At our institution, dobutamine is the pressor of choice in the treatment of patients with vasospasm. The use of dobutamine in the post-operative care of patients following cardiothoracic sugery or in the presence of cardiac failure has been widespread for over a decade[20-22]. In addition to markedly increasing cardiac output, dobutamine has also been reported to increase pulsatility[23]. The inotropic effect of dobutamine is balanced by increased coronary blood flow. Thus, cardiac function can be maximized while avoiding ischemic cardiac injury in patients with both normal and compromised cardiac function. Finally dobutamine is not arrhythmiogenic at high infusion rates[24]. Should cardiac function become refractory to dobutamine treatment, cardiac parameters can be enhanced with the simultaneous use of sodium nitroprusside at 85 micrograms per minute. We rely on cardiac index and stroke volume index which can increase up to 120% following the initiation of dobutamine and nipride. This regimen is particularly valuable in patients with ruptured but unsecured aneurysms in the pre-operative state. Reduction in the patients TPR following the initiation of dobutamine with or without nipride is commonplace. We do not advocate the addition of additional agents such as pure alpha agonists or high-dose dopamine.

Relationship of Cerebral Blood Flow to Cardiac Output

Davis and Sundt using an animal model were able to maintain stable arterial blood pressures in an animal model while decreasing cardiac output[25]. They demonstrated a significant decrease in cerebral blood flow despite the maintenance of stable mean arterial pressures thus suggesting a critical link between cardiac output and cerebral blood flow. Keller's data using a stroke model supported this concept demonstrating that increased cardiac output could improve microcirculatory flow without changes in mean arterial pressure or blood viscosity[26].

Pritz *et al.*[27] documented reversal of ischemic neurologic deficits in two patients with subarachnoid hemorrhage-induced vasospasm by maximizing cardiac output with volume expansion. Pritz[28] has further described in detail the use of Swan-Ganz catheterization in the treatment of patients with vasospasm following subarachnoid hemorrhage. The failure to reverse the clinical, neurologic sequalae resultant from vasospasm despite aggressive hypervolemic therapy in the current study, led to the initiation of hyperdynamic therapy with dobutamine. Infusion rates currently range from 5 to 10 µg/kg/min.

Our goal is to enhance cardiac performance without increasing morbidity and/or mortality resultant from such therapy. We recommend that with carefull observation of cardiac parameters in addition to proper fluid management, the complications of fluid overload, congestive heart failure, and cardiac ischemia can be avoided. Hyperdynamic therapy with dobutamine in the presence of volume loading resulted in marked increases in cardiac function in addition to reflexive decreases in TPR. We report on the ability of hyperdynamic-hypervolemic therapy to clinically reverse subarachnoid hemorrhage induced vasospasm in 80%

of patients failing to respond to volume expansion alone.

References

1. Levy ML, Giannotta, SL (1991) Cardiac performance and hypervolemic therapy in the treatment of cerebral vasospasm. J Neurosurg 75: 27–31
2. Muizelaar JP, Becker DP (1986) Induced hypertension for the treatment of cerebral ischemia after subarachnoid hemorrhage. Direct effect on cerebral blood flow. Surg Neurol 25: 317–325
3. Brown D (1951) Treatment of recurrent cardiovascular symptoms and the questions of vasospasm. Med Clin North Am 35: 1457–1474
4. Flamm ES, Ransohoff J (1976) Treatment of cerebral vasospasm by control of cyclic adenosine monophosphate. Surg Neurol 6: 223–226
5. Fleischer AS, Raggio JF, Tindall GT (1977) Aminophylline and isoproterenol in the treatment of cerebral vasospasm. Surg Neurol 8: 117–121
6. Fleischer AS, Tindall GT (1980) Cerebral vasospasm following aneurysm rupture: a protocol for therapy and prophylaxis. J Neurosurg 52: 149–152
7. Sundt TM Jr (1975) Management of ischemic complications after subarachnoid hemorrhage. J Neurosurg 43: 418–425
8. Sundt TM Jr (ed) (1990) Surgical techniques for saccular and giant intracranial aneurysms. Williams and Wilkins, Baltimore
9. Sundt TM Jr, Szurzewski J, Sharbrough FW (1977) Physiological considerations important for the management of vasospasm. Surg Neurol 7: 259–267
10. Bergvall U, Steiner L, Forster DMC (1973) Early pattern on cerebral circulatory disturbances following subarachnoid hemorrhage. Neuroradiology 5: 24–32
11. Kuyama H, Ladds A, Branston NM, Nitta M, Symon L (1984) An experimental study of acute subarachnoid hemorrhage in baboons: changes in cerebral blood volume, blood flow, electrical activity and water content. J Neurol Neurosurg Psychiatry 47: 354–364
12. Meyer CHA, Lowe D, Meyer M, Richardson PL, Neil-Dwyer G (1983) Progressive change in cerebral blood flow during the first three weeks after subarachnoid hemorrhage. Neurosurgery 12: 58–76
13. Mickey B, Vorstrup S, Voldby B, Lindewald H, Harmsen A, Lassen NA (1984) Serial measurement of regional cerebral blood flow in Patients with SAH using ^{133}Xe inhalation and emission computerized tomography. J Neurosurg 60: 916–922
14. Pickard JD, Boisvert DPJ, Graham DI, Fitch W (1979) Late effects of subarachnoid hemorrhage on the response of the primate cerebral circulation to drug-induced changes in arterial blood pressure. J Neurol Neurosurg Psychiatry 42: 899–903
15. Pitts LH, Macpherson P, Wyper DJ, Jennett WB (1977) Cerebral blood flow, angiographic cerebral vasospasm and subarachnoid hemorrhage. Acta Neurol Scand 56 [Suppl] 64: 334–335
16. Solomon RA, Post KD, McMurtry JG III (1984) Depression of circulating blood volume in patients after subarachnoid hemorrhage: implications for the management of symptomatic vasospasm. Neurosurgery 15: 354–361
17. Grubb RL Jr, Raichle ME, Eichling JO, Mokhtar HG (1977) Effects of subarachnoid hemorrhage on cerebral blood volume, blood flow, and oxygen utilization in humans. J Neurosurg 46: 446–453
18. Rosenstein J, Suzuki M, Symon L, Redmond S, (1984) Clinical use of a portable bedside cerebral blood flow machine in the management of aneurysmal subarachnoid hemorrhage. Neurosurgery 15: 519–525
19. Kassell NF, Peerless SJ, Durward QJ, Beck DW, Drake CG, Adams HP (1982) with intravascular volume expansion and induced arterial hypertension. Neurosurgery 11: 337–343
20. DiSesa V, Brown E, Mudge Jr. GH, Collins Jr JJ, Cohn LH (1982) Hemodynamic comparison of dopamine and dobutamine in the postoperative volume-loaded, pressure-loaded, and normal ventricle. J Thorac Cardiovasc Surg 83: 256–263
21. Sibbald WJ, Calvin J, Drieoger HH (1984) Right and left ventricular pre-load and diastolic ventricular compliance: implications for therapy in critically ill patients, In: Shoemaker WC, Thompson WL, Holbrook PR (eds) Textbook of critical care. Saunders, Philadelphia, pp 367–374
22. Zimpfer M, Khosropour R, Lackner F (1982) Effect of dobutamine on cardiac function in man. Reciprocal roles of heart rate and ventricular stroke volume. Crit Care Med 10: 367–370
23. Benedikter L, Mey T (1981) Onset and magnitude of cardiovascular response to dobutamine and AR-L 115 BS, a new positive inotropic agent with additional vasodilating activity, in normal subjects. Arzneim Forsch/Drug Res 31: 239–242
24. Cardiovascular pharmacology II (1987). In: Jaffe AS (ed) Textbook of advanced cardiac life support. Second edition. American Heart Association, Dallas, pp 115–127
25. Davis DH, Sundt TM Jr (1980) Relationship of cerebral blood flow to cardiac output, mean arterial pressure, blood volume, and alpha and beta blockade in cats. J Neurosurg 52: 745–754
26. Keller TS, McGillicuddy JE, LaBond VA, Kindt GW (1982) Volume expansion in focal cerebral ischemia: the effect of cardiac output on local cerebral blood flow. Clin Neurosurg 29: 40–50
27. Pritz MB, Giannotta SL, Kindt GW, Mc Gillicuddy JE, Prager RL (1978) Treatment of patients with neurological deficits associated with cerebral vasospasm by intravascular volume expansion. Neurosurgery 3: 364–368
28. Pritz MB (1984) Treatment of cerebral vasospasm: usefulness of Swan-Ganz catheter monitoring of volume expansion. Surg Neurol 21: 239–244

Correspondence: Michael L. Levy, M.D., Department of Neurosurgery, LAC/USC Medical Center, 1200 State Street, Box 239, Los Angeles, CA 90033, U.S.A.

Single Intracisternal Injection of Recombinant Tissue Type Plasminogen Activator for Prevention of Cerebral Vasospasm

K. Kanamaru[1], S. Waga[1], S. Niwa[1], M. Sakakura[2], H. Sakaida[2], A. Morikawa[3], K. Murao[3], Y. Yamamoto[4], Y. Morooka[5], T. Sakakura[5], M. Okada[6], and M. Furuno[6]

Departments of Neurosurgery, [1] Mie University School of Medicine, [2] Yamado Red Cross Hospital, [3] Chusei Sogo Hospital, [4] Matsusaka Chuou Hospital, [5] Matsusaka Saiseikai Hospital, [6] Kuwana Municipal Hospital, Japan

Summary

We attempted to compare the clinical efficacy of three modalities evacuating clots from basal cisterns as following; simple cisternal drainage (D, N = 14), ventricular or cisternal irrigation combined with cisternal drainage (I, 13), and single intracisternal injection of recombinant tissue type plasminogen activator (rt-PA) with cisternal drainage (T, 26). The patients undergoing surgery within 48 hours of aneurysm rupture were randomly assigned into three groups. Delayed neurological deficit was significantly less frequent in T than D group (15.4% vs. 57.1%, p < 0.01). There was no significant difference between I and T groups. According to Glasgow Outcome Scale, T group had a significantly better outcome than D group (p < 0.01). Severe disability was more common in D group than T group (p < 0.01). In T group, 2 of 7 deaths were due to severe vasospasm (7.7%). The complication in T group was epidural hematoma occurring in 2 patients. Our results suggest that intraoperative injection of rt-PA with cisternal drainage is effective in reducing vasospasm and improving outcome of the patients with SAH.

Keywords: Subarachnoid hemorrhage; intrathecal thrombolytic therapy; cisternal drainage; cisternal irrigation.

Introduction

Vasospasm is recognized as the leading cause of death and permanent neurological disability after aneurysmal subarachnoid hemorrhage (SAH) and surgery. The location and amount of blood deposition around the large conducting arteries that course through the basal subarachnoid cisterns affect the incidence and severity of cerebral vasospasm after SAH. Surgical removal of subarachnoid blood clots at the acute stage of SAH is difficult and may be even dangerous in some cases. Recently, intrathecal thrombolytic therapy has been studied both in primates and humans[1-3,6-9]. Most of the reports demonstrated salutary effect of recombinant tissue type plasminogen activator (rt-PA) for the prevention of cerebral vasospasm (VSP) after SAH. How-

ever, few reports have shown the effect of rt-PA in comparison with other cisternal lavage methods. In the present study we attempt to compare the clinical efficacy of three modalities evacuating clots from basal cisterns in patients with aneurysmal SAH.

Clinical Material and Methods

Fifty three patients undergoing surgery within 48 hours of aneurysm rupture were randomly assigned into three groups as following; simple cisternal drainage (D), ventricular or cisternal irrigation combined with cisternal drainage (I), and single intracisternal injection of rt-PA with cisternal drainage (T). Preoperative clinical grade of the patients according to Hunt and Hess[5] is shown in Table 1. The patients classified in grade II were most common in each group. Computed tomography scan (CT) grading at the onset according to Fisher[4] is shown in Table 2. The patients in Fisher group III were most common in each group. The patients with intracerebral hematoma included in Fisher group IV were 1 (7.1%), 4 (30.8%), and 6 (23.1%) in D, I, and T groups respectively (Table 2). Simple cisternal drainage was employed in 14 patients and continued until Day 20 after SAH. Ventricular or cisternal irrigation with cisternal drainage was employed in 13 patients according to the method described by Kodama et al.[6] The irrigation tube was placed in the anterior horn of the lateral ventricle or in the basal cisterns and the drainage tube was in the basal cisterns. The Hartmann solution (pH 8) containing vitamin C and E was used to irrigate at 1000 ml/day. In twenty six patients, rt-PA was given as a single intraoperative injection of 8 mg, and postoperative cisternal drainage was employed for 7 days. The presence of VSP was identified by occurrence of delayed neurological

Table 1. *Preoperative Clinical Grade**

	I	II	III	IV	V	Total
Cisternal drainage	2	8	4			14
Irrigation/drainage		9	1	2	1	13
rt-PA	3	17	3	3		26

*Clinical grading according to the system of Hunt and Hess[5].

Table 2. *Preoperative CT Grade**

	I	II	III	IV	Total
Cisternal Drainage		1	12	1	14
Irrigation/Drainage			9	4	13
rt-PA		3	17	6	26

*CT computed tomography scan grade according to Fisher[4].

deficit (DND) or cerebral infarction. Outcome of the patients was defined after 3 months following surgery according to Glasgow Outcome Scale.

Results

Delayed neurological deficits occurred in 4 of 26 cases in T group (15.4%), 3 of 13 in I group (23.1%), and 8 of 14 in D group (57.1%). There was a significant difference between T and D groups (p < 0.01). There was a trend DND being more common in D than I group; however, the difference was not significant. When Glasgow Outcome Scale of the patients was compared, 14 cases in T group had good outcome (53.5%), 6 in I group (46.2%), and 5 in D group (35.7%); there was a significant difference between T and D groups (p < 0.01) (Table 3). Furthermore, 1 case in T group was defined as severe disability (3.8%), 3 in I group (23.1%), and 5 in D group (35.7%); there was a significant difference between T and D groups (p < 0.01) (Table 3). While the patients in T group had a better outcome than D group, there was no significant difference between T and I groups. Seven patients in T group died due to the following reasons; 1) intraoperative premature rupture of aneurysm (N = 1, 3.8%), 2) preoperative condition already poor because of large intracerebral hematoma (4,15.4%), and 3) severe VSP (2, 7.7%). Two patients in D group (14.3%) and one in I group (7.7%) died due to severe VSP. One patient in I group was vegetative (7.7%). Although we cannot explain the high mortality in T group, this might be due to inadequate use of rt-PA in patients who had suffered from intracerebral hematoma. The initial CT scan in 4 of the 7 succumbed patients were classified as Fisher group IV.

Table 3. *Glasgow Outcome Scale*

	GR	MD	SD	VS	D	Total
Cisternal Drainage	5	2	5	0	2	14
Irrigation/Drainage	6	2	3	1	1	13
rt-PA	14	4	1	0	7	26

GR good recovery; *MD* moderate disability; *SD* severe disability; *VS* vegetative state; *D* death.

Discussion

Recombinant tissue type plasminogen activator has been effective in prevention of cerebral vasospasm both in primates and humans[1-3,7-9]. Findlay and Weir have demonstrated extensive evidence that extravasated blood in subarachnoid space is an important initiation factor of chronic vasospasm and that early removal of blood, within 48 hours of SAH, could prevent vasospasm in a primate model[1,3]. The same authors advocated intrathecall thrombolytic therapy in the early stage of SAH[2]. This method includes intraoperative injection of 10 mg of rt-PA into the basal cisterns; 15 minutes were allowed to pass after injection, followed by vigorous irrigation of the subarachnoid space with 1 or 2 liters of warmed saline. Our method strictly adhered to it.

In our experimental study, red blood cells in clots showed a morphological change after 48 hours of incubation at 37° C and then cell membrane was disrupted. After disruption of red blood cell membrane, oxyhemoglobin might come out and contract the smooth muscle cells. Hemolyzed red blood cells caused a sustained contraction in the canine basilar arteries. This evidence supports the idea that intrathecal thrombolytic therapy should be done by 48 hours after SAH.

Our results suggest that rt-PA may be more effective in prevention of vasospasm than the drainage and irrigation methods. The problems of irrigation methods. include 1) possible infection, 2) irrigation does not cover the large subarachnoid space of brain and SAH tends to be partially resolved, and 3) irrigation and drainage system may be troublesome.

In our series the patients classified into Fisher group IV had poor outcome even after rt-PA injection. The possible reasons were 1) incomplete surgical removal of intraparenchymal hematoma, 2) initial brain damage had already been extensive, and 3) rt-PA could not reach the hematoma isolated from cerebrospinal fluid pathway. Although the number of the cases is small, our results suggest that the patients with intracerebral hematoma might not be good candidate for rt-PA therapy. The strict indication for rt-PA therapy remains to be solved in forthcoming studies.

References

1. Findlay JM, Weir BKA, Kanamaru K, Grace M, Baughman R (1990) The effect of timing of intrathecal fibrinolytic therapy on

cerebral vasospasm in a primate model of subarachnoid hemorrhage. Neurosurgery 26: 201–206

2. Findlay JM, Weir BKA, Kassell NF, Disney LB, Grace M (1991) Intracisternal recombinant tissue plasminogen activator after aneurysmal subarachnoid hemorrhage. J Neurosurg 75: 181–188

3. Findlay JM, Weir BKA, Steinke D, Tanabe T, Gordon P, Grace M (1988) Effect of intrathecal thrombolytic therapy on subarachnoid clot and chronic vasospasm in a primate model of SAH. J Neurosurg 69: 723–735

4. Fisher CM, Kistler JP, Davis JM (1980) Relation of cerebral vasospasm to subarachnoid hemorrhage visualized by computed tomographic scanning. Neurosurgery 6: 1–9

5. Hunt WE, Hess RM (1968) Surgical risk as related to time of intervention in the repair of intracranial aneurysms. J Neurosurg 28: 14–20

6. Kodama N, Sasaki T, Yamanobe K, Sato M (1988) Prevention of vasospasm: cisternal irrigation therapy with urokinase and ascorbic acid. In: Wilkins R (ed) Cerebral vasospasm. Raven, New York, pp 415–418

7. Mizoi K, Yoshimoto T, Fujiwara S, Sugawara T, Takahashi A, Koshu K (1991) Prevention of vasospasm by clot removal and intrathecal bolus injection of tissue-type plasminogen acivator: preliminary report. Neurosurgery 28: 807–813

8. Öhman J, Servo A, Heiskanen O (1991) Effect of intrathecal fibrinolytic therapy of clot lysis and vasospasm in patients with aneurysmal subarachnoid hemorrhage. J Neurosurg 75: 197–201

9. Zabramski JM, Spetzler RF, Lee KS, Papadopoulos SM, Bovill E, Zimmerman RS, Bederson JB (1991) Phase 1 trial of tissue plasminogen activator for the prevention of vasospasm in patients with aneurysmal subarachnoid hemorrhage. J Neurosurg 75: 189–196

Correspondence: Kenji Kanamaru, M.D., Department of Neurosurgry, Mie University School of Medicine, Tsu, Mie 514, Japan.

Endovascular Approaches to Vasospasm

Angioplasty of Cerebral Vasospasm

C.F. Dowd, R.T. Higashida, V.V. Halbach, K.W. Fraser, T.P. Smith, and **G.B. Hieshima**

Departments of Radiology and Neurological Surgery, University of California, San Francisco Medical Center, California, U.S.A.

Summary

Despite recent advances in medical and surgical therapies, intracranial vasospasm secondary to aneurysmal subarachnoid hemorrhage remains a major cause of mortality and morbidity. Recent technological advances in endovascular therapy have allowed patients with symptomatic vasospasm to be treated with intravascular balloon angioplasty techniques. Twenty-eight patients with clinically symptomatic vasospasm unresponsive to medical therapy have undergone angioplasty at our institution. A total of 99 vessels underwent balloon dilatation using a low atmospheric pressure balloon system in these 28 patients. Improved luminal diameter was demonstrated angiographically in all cases. Neurological improvement was demonstrated in 61% of patients, with the most dramatic responses to angioplasty occurring in patients with deficits of recent onset. Complications include two instances of vessel rupture, and an apparent reperfusion hemorrhage 24 hours after angioplasty. Patients presenting with symptomatic vasospasm unresponsive to medical therapy may be treated by balloon angioplasty techniques to augment cerebral perfusion.

Keywords: Vasospasm; angioplasty; subarachnoid hemorrhage; interventional neuroradiology.

Introduction

Because of the devastating consequences of cerebral intracranial arterial vasospasm which appears in 20–30% of patients with aneurysmal subarachnoid hemorrhage (SAH), a number of therapies have been developed to circumvent this difficult problem, including the application of calcium antagonists[2], administration of aminophyline plus nitroprusside and dopamine[9], cisternal irrigation with thrombolytic agents[6,13,18], early surgical removal of subarachnoid thrombus[11], intraarterial papaverine[5], pulsed-dye laser[16], and hypervolemic-hypertensive-hemodilution therapy[14]. That such a large number of potentially beneficial treatments have been devised underscores the relative lack of effectiveness of any single regimen to impact on clinically significant vasospasm which can result in stroke or death. Advances in interventional endovascular techniques have allowed patients with medically refractory symptomatic vasospasm to undergo transvascular balloon angioplasty. We will describe our patient selection, endovascular techniques and results among a group of 28 patients.

Methods and Materials

Our patient population consists of 28 patients ranging in age from 15–73 years. Eleven were male and 17 were female. All patients had subarachnoid hemorrhage with resulting neurological deficits, angiographic demonstration of vasospasm in arteries referable to these deficits, failure of response to conventional pharmacological and medical therapy for vasospasm, and documentation of absence of infarction or intraparenchymal hemorrhage in the vascular distribution of the vasospasm by computerized tomography (CT) or magnetic resonance imaging (MRI).

All patients are initially treated by volume expansion to produce hypervolemia and hemodilution. Pressors are administered if necessary. These maneuvers constitute the "triple H" therapy of hypervolemia, hemodilution and hypertension. If the ruptured aneurysm has not been fully treated either by surgical or endovascular means, it may not be possible to institute such therapy. More recently, transcranial doppler (TCD) has been utilized as a screening techique to provide earlier assessment of the development of hemodynamically significant vasospasm[1].

Ninety-nine vessels underwent intravascular balloon angioplasty in these 28 patients. These vessels included 53 anterior circulation and 46 posterior circulation arteries. Angiograms in 23 of the 28 patients demonstrated diffuse vasospasm involving multiple vascular territories.

A transfemoral percutaneous arterial approach is performed in the endovascular neuroradiology suite. A complete 4 vessel cerebral arteriogram is obtained to document the presence of angiographic vasospasm, involvement of multiple territories, collateral circulation, and to allow correlation with neurological deficits. Unless medical conditions require otherwise, these procedures are performed under local anesthesia to allow continuous neurological monitoring.

Balloon angioplasty is performed in vessels demonstrating both clinical and angiographic evidence for vasospasm, using a silicone microballoon (Interventional Therapeutics Corporation, Inc., South San Francisco, California) designed specifically for such a purpose. This balloon exhibits several properties which make it optimally suited for its purpose[8]. Silicone demonstrates a special conformational structure assisting the balloon to conform to the arterial lumen without generating excessive intraluminal pressures. The balloon is intended for low atmospheric (1.5 atmospheres or below) dilatation, as opposed to other types of angioplasty balloons designed for atherosclerosis which requires significantly higher atmospheric pressures. The balloon is chemically bonded to a 2-French catheter to allow navigation to the specified arterial segment. Two balloon sizes are available, including a smaller balloon with maximum dimensions of 3.5 mm by 12.0 mm, and a larger balloon with maximum dimensions of 7.5 mm by 12.5 mm. The larger balloon is only used for larger diameter vessels including internal carotid and distal vertebral arteries, as over-dilatation a beyond the normal luminal diameter can risk arterial rupture. The ballon has the characteristic of inflating proximally to distally and deflating in reverse order. The balloon is guided through a 7.2-French guiding catheter to the site of the spasm using both gentle inflation-deflation and the use of a 0.010–0.014 inch micro-guide wire (Target Therapeutics, Fremont, California). Dilatation is carried out under full neurological monitoring with anticoagulation, for a period of several seconds prior to deflation of the balloon and advancement to the next affected segment. This process can be observed by using high resolution road mapping digital fluoroscopy techniques following the course of the contrast-filled balloon.

Results

Ninety-nine cerebral arteries underwent balloon angioplasty using these techniques in 28 patients (Figs. 1 and 2). Angiographic evidence of improved luminal diameter was documented in all vessels. Follow-up angiography demonstrated continued arterial patency in those vessels undergoing angioplasty.

Neurological improvement was demonstrated in 17 to 28 patients (60.7%). Generally, noticeable improvement was demonstrated earlier in those patients in whom angioplasty was performed soon after the onset of the neurological deficits (within 24 hours). Eleven patients (39.3%) showed no significant clinical change despite improved luminal diameter angiographically. Generally, these patients represented the poorer neurological grades (Hunt and Hess classification IV and V) and in whom there was a long delay between the onset of neurological deficit and angioplasty.

On long term follow-up, the patients who demonstrated improvement after angioplasty maintained or improved their neurological condition. Two patients (7.1%) remained in poor condition despite therapy. There were 9 deaths among our 28 patients. Two of these were a direct result of technical complications involving rupture of an intracerebral vessel during the course of angioplasty resulting in subarachnoid hemorrhage. An additional patient developed what was considered to be reperfusion hemorrhage 24 hours following angioplasty of a proximal middle cerebral artery, and subsequently died. Six other patients died from unrelated complications of the initial subarachnoid hemorrhage.

Discussion

The pathophysiology of subarachnoid hemorrhage-induced cerebral vasospasm is not well known. Postulated mechanisms include endothelial cell damage, myointimal cellular proliferation, arterial wall inflammatory changes, and reduced elasticity in arterial smooth muscle[7]. Despite the relatively large number of medical and pharmacological therapies which have been devised, the significant morbidity and mortality from cerebral vasospasm has necessitated development of more efficacious therapies.

Dotter and Judkins[4] first described transvascular dilatation for atherosclerotic lesions in 1964. Twenty years later, Zubkov *et al.*[19] published the first report describing their results for transvascular angioplasty for subarachnoid hemorrhage-induced vasospasm using latex microballoons. They reported encouraging results in 33 patients. This pioneering work stimulated our group to pursue and develop this therapeutic modality. A specifically-designed angioplasty balloon made of silicone elastomer was developed especially for subarachnoid hemorrhage-induced vasospasm[8]. This

Fig. 1. 48 year-old woman with subarachnoid haemorrhage (SAH) from an untreated dissecting right vertebral artery aneurysm and clinical deterioration secondary to vasospasm; (a) transaxial noncontrast CT scan confirms the presence of diffuse cisternal SAH. There was no evidence of intraparenchymal haemorrhage or stroke; (b) right vertebral arteriogram, frontal projection, shows the fusiform aneurysm (closed arrow) and severe spasm of the basilar artery (open arrows); (c) left vertebral arteriogram, lateral projection, confirms the presence of spasm involving the distal left vertebral and basilar arteries; (d) left vertebral arteriogram, lateral projection, after balloon nagioplasty. Luminal diameter of the distal left vertebral and basilar arteries is markedly improved. Note presence of the balloon catheter still within the vessel; (e) transcranial Doppler (TCD), right middle cerebral artery, shows markedly elevated velocities (systolic velocity peaks above the scale) within this artery, indicating significant vasospasm; (f) right internal carotid arteriogram, frontal projection, shows spasm involving the supraclinoid internal carotid artery and proximal middle cerebral artery; (g) right internal carotid arteriogram, frontal projection, after balloon angioplasty. Luminal diameter of supraclinoid internal carotid artery is improved (arrows); (h) transcranial Doppler (TCD), right middle cerebral artery, after balloon angioplasty, Significant reduction of velocities indicates hemodynamic effect of angioplasty; (i) right vertebral arteriogram, frontal projection, after occlusion of the fusiform dissecting aneurysm and distal portion of the artery with Guglielmi Detachable Coils (GDC). Note preservation of the posterior inferior cerebellar artery (arrow)

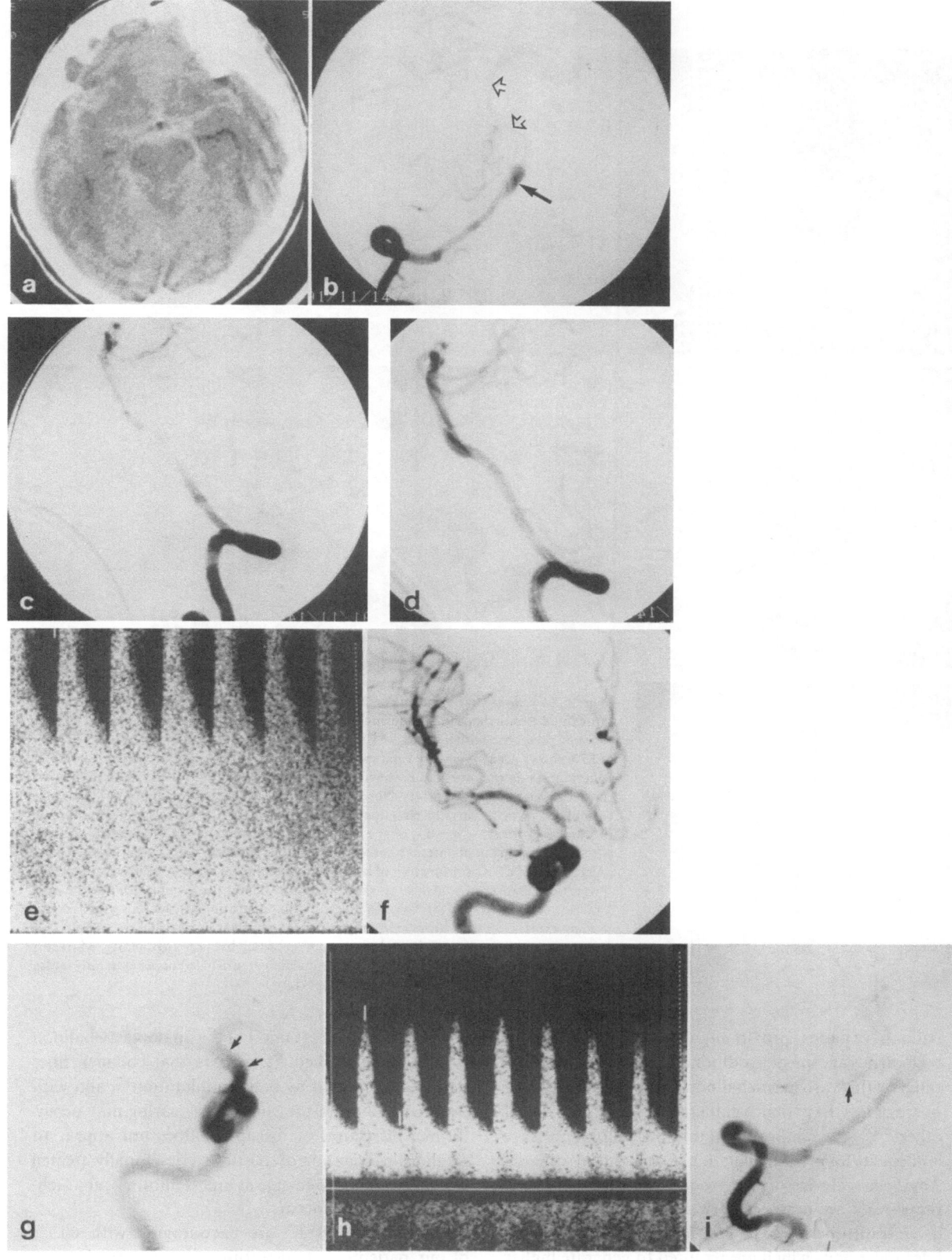

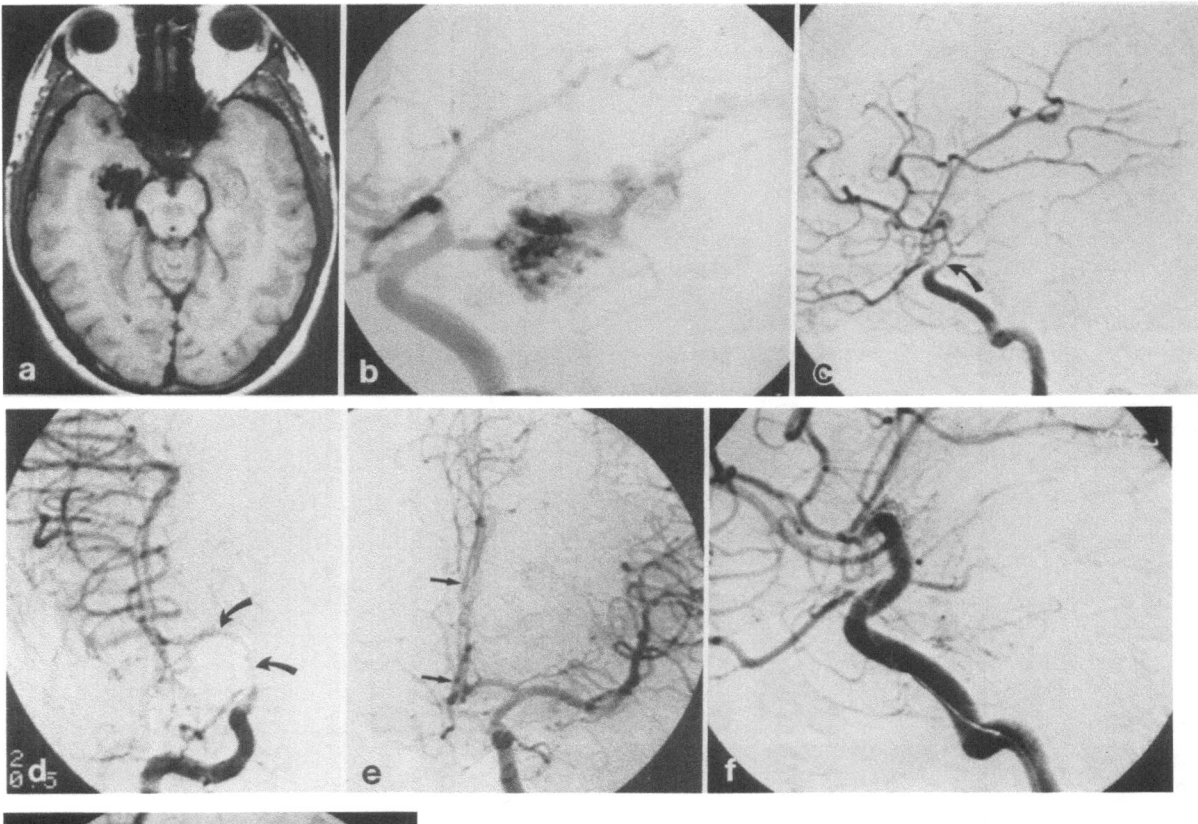

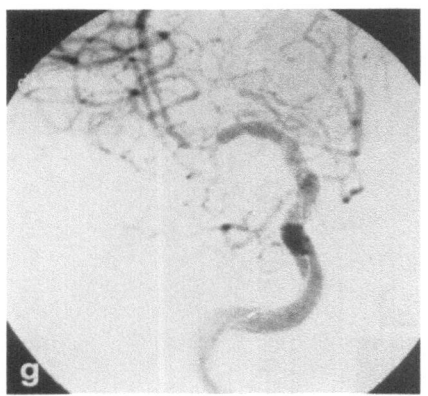

Fig. 2. 34 year-old man with unsual occurrence of focal vasospasm as a result of sub-arachnoid hemorrhage (SAH) during operation for arteriovenous malformation (AVM). Patient presented initially with SAH; (a) transaxial magnetic resonance image (TR 600, TE20) shows AVM involving right medial temporal lobe; (b) right internal carotid (ICA) arteriogram, lateral projection, shows AVM supplied by posterior temporal branch via posterior communicating artery. Note normal caliber of supraclinoid ICA. AVM was fully embolized prior to surgical resection; (c) and (d) right ICA arteriogram, lateral (c) and frontal (d) projections, one day after complete surgical resection of AVM. Note focal vaso-spasm of supraclinoid internal carotid and middle cerebral arteries (arrows). Patient demonstrated no motor function of left upper extremity; (e) left ICA arteriogram, frontal projection, shows no evidence of vasospasm and demonstrates opacification of right anterior cerebral system (arrows) via anterior communicating artery. This angiographic finding explains why left lower extremity motor function was normal; (f) and (g) right ICA arteriogram, lateral (f) and frontal (g) projections, after balloon angioplasty. Markedly improved luminal diameter correlated with immediate return of left upper extremity motor function. Note balloon dilatation catheter in artery

balloon expands proximally-to-distally assisting in balloon advancement. Additionally, the pressures generated by this vasospasm balloon approximate 1 atmosphere or less. Experience gathered by our group[7,8] and others[3,10,12,15] confirms that this low balloon pressure is adequate for arterial dilatation in this clinical scenario. Angioplasty devices which produce higher atmospheric pressures[17] are not necessary and risk vessel rupture, in contradistinction to devices for dilatation of atherosclerotic lesions which are required to generate higher atmospheric pressures.

The mechanism of action of the angioplasty balloon is now being studied. It appears that collagen fiber structure is effected by balloon dilatation[17], and with elevated dilatation pressures, fiber tearing may occur. Intimal dissection or disruption does not appear to result from dilatation of spastic arteries. Finally, treated arteries tend not to re-spasm unless another subarachnoid hemorrhage occurs.

Our clinical results are encouraging with 60.7% of our patients demonstrating clinical improvement. This correlates well with similar studies presented by

Mayberg[10] and Takahashi[15]. The therapeutic challenge remains with those patients experiencing a long duration between onset of symptoms and therapy. Additionally, same patients appear not to respond to angioplasty; the reasons for this are unclear.

Patient selection and timing of the procedure are important. In addition to clinical monitoring after subarachnoid hemorrhage, we have added monitoring of velocity of major cerebral blood vessels with the use of transcranial doppler (TCD)[1]. This allows early assessment of elevated velocities suggesting onset of clinically silent vasospasm and institution of more aggressive medical therapy. We select only patients who develop neurological symptoms referable to vasospasm for angioplasty, as angiographic vasospasm without a corresponding neurological deficit does not warrant the risk of angioplasty. It is important to exclude the presence of recent stroke or parenchymal hemorrhage using cross sectional imaging study to circumvent the possibility of producing reperfusion hemorrhage in a damaged portion of the brain and because dilatation of arteries to this area will not likely improve the patient's condition. Finally, we believe that it is important to perform the procedure as quickly as possible after the development of neurological deficits for optimum efficacy.

While mechanical dilatation is only one therapeutic modality for treatment of subarachnoid hemorrhage induced cerebral vasospasm, this method is effective especially in the earliest stages of vasospasm to improve cerebral perfusion and to limit the possibility of stroke or death.

References

1. Aaslid R, Huber P, Nornes H (1984) Evaluation of cerebrovascular spasm with transcranial Doppler ultrasound. J Neurosurg 60: 37–41
2. Allen GS, Ahn HS, Preziosi TJ et al (1983) Cerebral arterial spasm: a controlled trial of nimodipine in patients with subarachnoid haemorrhage. N Engl J Med 308: 619–624
3. Brothers MF, Holgate RC (1990) Intracranial angioplasty for treatment of vasospasm after subarachnoid hemorrhage: technique and modifications to improve branch access. AJNR 11: 239–248
4. Dotter CT, Judkins MP (1964) Transluminal treatment of arteriosclerotic obstruction: description of a new technique and a preliminary report of its application. Circulation 30: 654–670
5. Eckard DA, Purdy PD, Girson MS, Samson D, Kopitnik T, Batjer H (1992) Intraarterial papaverine for relief of catheter-induced intracranial vasospasm. AJR 158: 883–884
6. Findlay JM, Weir BKA, Kassell NF, Disney LB, Grace MGA (1991) Intracisternal recombinant tissue plasminogen activator after aneurysmal subarachnoid hemorrhage. J Neurosurg 75: 181–188
7. Higashida RT, Halbach VV, Cahan LD, Brant-Zawadzki M, Barnwell S, Dowd C, Hieshima GB (1989) Transluminal angioplasty for treatment of intracranial arterial vasospasm. J Neurosurg 71: 648–653
8. Higashida RT, Halbach VV, Dormandy B, Bell J, Brant-Zawadzki M, Hieshima GB (1990) A new microballoon device for transluminal angioplasty of intracranial arterial vasospasm. AJNR 11: 233–238
9. Levy WJ, Bay JW, Sawhny B, Tank T (1982) Aminophylline plus nitroprusside and dopamine for treatment of cerebral vasospasm. J Neurosurg 56: 646–649
10. Mayberg M, eskridge J, Newell D, Winn HR (1990) Angioplasty for symptomatic vasospasm. In: Sano K, Takakura K, Kassell NF, Sasaki T (eds) Cerebral vasospasm: Proceedings of the IVth International Conference on Cerebral Vasospasm. University of Tokyo Press, Tokyo
11. Mizukami M, Kawase T, Usame T, et al (1982) Prevention of vasospasm by early operation with removal of subarachnoid blood. Neurosurgery 10: 301–307
12. Newell DW, Eskridge JM, Mayberg MR, et al (1989) Angioplasty for the treatment of symptomatic vasospasm following subarachnoid hemorrhage. J Neurosurg 71: 654–660
13. Ohman J, Servo A, Heiskanen O (1991) Effect of intrathecal fibrinolytic therapy on clot lysis and vasospasm in patients with aneurysmal subarachnoid hemorrhage. J Neurosurg 75: 197–201
14. Solomon RA, Fink ME, Lennihan L (1988) Early aneurysm surgery and prophylactic hypervolemic hypertensive therapy for the treatment of aneurysmal subarachnoid hemorrhage. Neurosurgery 23: 699–704
15. Takahashi A, Yoshimoto T, Mizoi K, Sugawara T, Fujii Y (1990) Transluminal balloon angioplasty for vasospasm after subarachnoid hemorrhage. In: Sano K, Takakura K, Kassell NF, Sasaki T (eds) Cerebral vasospasm: Proceedings of the IVth International Conference on Cerebral Vasospasm. University of Tokyo Press, Tokyo
16. Teramura A, MacFarlane R, Owen CJ, de la Torre R, Gregory KW, Birngruber R, Parrish JA, Peterson JW, Zervas NT (1991) Application of the 1-µsec pulsed-dye laser to the treatment of experimental cerebral vasospasm. J Neurosurg 75: 271–276
17. Yamamoto Y, Smith RR, Bernanke DH (1992) Mechanism of action of balloon angioplasty in cerebral vasospasm. Neurosurgery 30: 1–6
18. Zabramski JM, Spetzler RF, Lee S, Papadopoulos SM, Bovill E, Zimmerman RS, Bederson JB(1991) Phase I trial of tissue plasminogen activator for the prevention of vasospasm in patients with aneurysmal subarachnoid hemorrhage. J Neurosurg 75: 189–196
19. Zubkov YN, Nikiforov BM, Shustin VA (1984) Balloon catheter technique for dilatation of constricted cerebral arteries after aneurysmal SAH. Acta Neurochir (Wien) 70: 665–679

Correspondence: Christopher F. Dowd, M.D., Department of Radiology and Neurological Surgery, University of California, San Francisco Medical Center, 505 Parmassus Avenue, Room L-352, San Francisco, California 94143-0628, U.S.A.

Balloon Angioplasty for the Treatment of Symptomatic Vasospasm

J.M. Eskridge, H.R. Winn, D.W. Newell, and **M.A. Alotis**

Department of Neurological Surgery, University of Washington, Seattle, Washington, U.S.A.

Summary

Angioplasty was performed in 45 patients who were symptomatic from vasospasm following subarachnoid hemorrhage. This was done using a micro balloon via a percutaneous transfemoral approach. Two thirds of these patients improved neurologically acutely. One patient died during the procedure secondary to vessel rupture. Long term follow-up has been good without any cases of delayed deterioration. The overall results indicate that angioplasty can offer improvement to patients with ischemic deficits due to vasospasm.

Keywords: Angioplasty; vasospasm; subarachnoid hemorrhage; stroke.

Introduction

Cerebral Vasospasm remains a significant complication of subarachnoid hemorrhage resulting in delayed ischemic deficit in approximately 30 per cent of those who survive the initial aneurysm rupture[3,17]. Two-thirds of the survivors of the aneurysm rupture never regain the quality of life that they had prior to the hemorrhage[17,20,21].

The pathophysiology of vasospasm remains poorly understood. Theories include muscular contraction of the vessel wall, intimal hypertrophy and proliferation, medial necrosis, and increase in vascular tone[2,8,14,15,25,26]. These changes are brought on by vasoconstrictive substances within the surrounding clot[8]. Despite many different pharmacological agents and early surgery to minimize spasm, once a deficit occurs, no entirely effective agent has been found[7,12,16,19,23,27].

Zubkov in 1984 first reported the treatment of vasospasm by angioplasty[28]. Angioplasty involves the mechanical dilation of the narrowed vessel segment by using an inflatable balloon. This is usually inserted via a transfemoral approach. This technique has been used successfully in the dilation of coronary and peripheral vascular arteries[4,5].

Technique

A variety of balloons are available to perform intracranial angioplasty[10]. We have found a silicone microballoon (Interventional Therapeutics Corporation, South San Francisco, California) to be particularly useful when performing this procedure (Fig. 1). This microballoon measures 3 mm in diameter and 12 mm in length when fully inflated. This balloon expands with a low inflation pressure (0.5 atmospheres) and the soft silicone shell is designed to elongate when over-inflated and not increase in diameter. With lower inflation pressures there is less risk of damage to the endothelium[4]. These factors help reduce the risk of vessel rupture. This low pressure balloon has been found to work in the vast majority of cases.

This balloon comes attached to a variable stiffness microcatheter (Target Therapeutics Corporation, San Jose, California). This microcatheter has revolutionized access to the intracranial vasculature[9]. This 150 cm variable stiffness microcatheter allows for transfemoral catheterization which therefore allows for rapid access to all three major intracranial vascular distributions. It is routinely possible to catheterize the proximal segments of the middle and posterior cerebral arteries. Occasionally catheterization of the proximal segments of the anterior cerebral is possible as well. In fact the limiting factor in distal catheterization is not the variable stiffness microcatheter but the balloon size. Once the balloon has passed beyond the proximal segments of the intracranial vessels the balloon size exceeds that of the artery. The balloon should never be inflated in a situation where the balloon size exceeds the vessel diameter because this can result in vessel rupture.

The placement of microcatheters and microballoons into the intracranial circulation requires high resolution

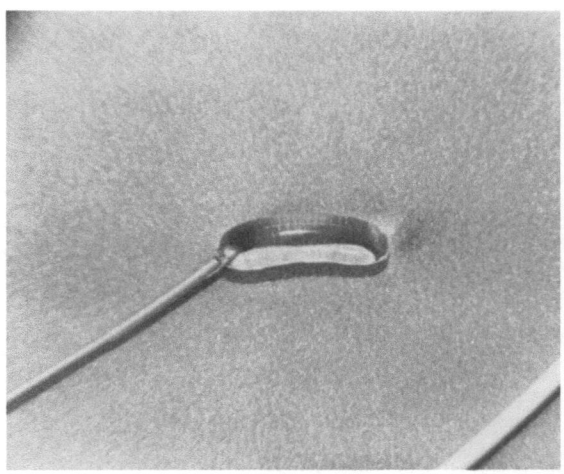

Fig. 1. Low pressure silicone angioplasty balloon (courtesy of Interventional Therapeutics Corporation, South San Francisco, California)

digital fluoroscopic equipment[9] (A 10). Such equipment must have digital road mapping capabilities. With these factors the balloon can be kept out of small side branches that would rupture with balloon inflation. Performing intracranial balloon angioplasty without high resolution fluroscopy and digital road maps carries an unacceptably high risk

If the aneurysm has been previously clipped, which we strongly recommend, heparinization is used during the angioplasty procedure[10] (E19). The heparin is reversed immediately after the procedure with protamine sulfate. It is imperative that the patient remain motionless during the procedure. This improves the safety of the technique. General anesthesia is often used to ensure that the patient remains stationary.

Patient Selection

Our management protocol for patients following subarachnoid hemorrhage includes surgery within 72 hours of aneurysm rupture. All patients undergo four vessel cerebral angiography before and afterwards to confirm clip placement. The patients receive intensive care monitoring via constant arterial blood pressure measurement, intracranial pressure monitoring, and cardiac output assessment using a Swan Ganz catheter. All patients are treated with hypervolemic therapy and calcium channel blockers.

Transcranial Doppler (TCD) has proved useful in diagnosing vasospasm and also in following the development and resolution of spasm over time[1,22]. TCD

has also been useful to document persistent dilation of arteries and to show improvements in blood flow following angioplasty[18]. At our institution base line TCD examinations are performed on all patients. These exams are repeated daily to follow the progression of vasospasm.

Patients are selected for angioplasty if they have a new neurologic deficit despite maximum medical treatment. Other causes of decreased level of consciousness or hemiparesis such as hydrocephalus, intracerebral hemorrhage and mass effect are ruled out by a CT scan. If the transcranial Doppler exam confirms the clinical suspicion of vasospasm, angiography is performed. Angioplasty is performed if there is spasm which could explain the neurologic deterioration and there is no infarction present on the CT scan. When an infarction is present there is concern that angioplasty may lead to re-perfusion hemorrhage in the ischemic vascular bed.

A number of patients have also had single photon emission computerized tomography (SPECT) scans performed immediately before and 24 h following angioplasty to evaluate regional cerebral perfusion. These scans were obtained after the intravenous administration of 25–35 mCi of TC-99M hexamethyl propyleneamine oxine (HM-PAO) or 1.5 mCi of I-123 Idoamphetamine (spectamine). Tomographic acquisition was obtained using a General Electric 400 AT Gamma camera.

Results

Of the 45 patients treated, 31 (68%) improved following angioplasty. Improvement is defined here as a two level increase in coma scale or a two level increase in motor strength within 48 hours of angioplasty (Figs. 2 and 3).

In 37 of 45 patients angioplasty was performed within 18 hours of the onset of symptoms.

All of these patients have sustained their clinical improvement and have continued to do well following angioplasty. Results at one month following the procedure show good outcomes in 33 patients with 24 being normal and nine ambulating with a cane. Poor outcomes were seen 12 patients with five patients being disabled and seven patients having died. Of the seven deaths that occurred four patients were grade five and did not respond to angioplasty and continued to deteriorate. Two patients had aneurysms that had not been clipped prior to angioplasty. In one patient where the aneurysm was not clipped, the patient's poor

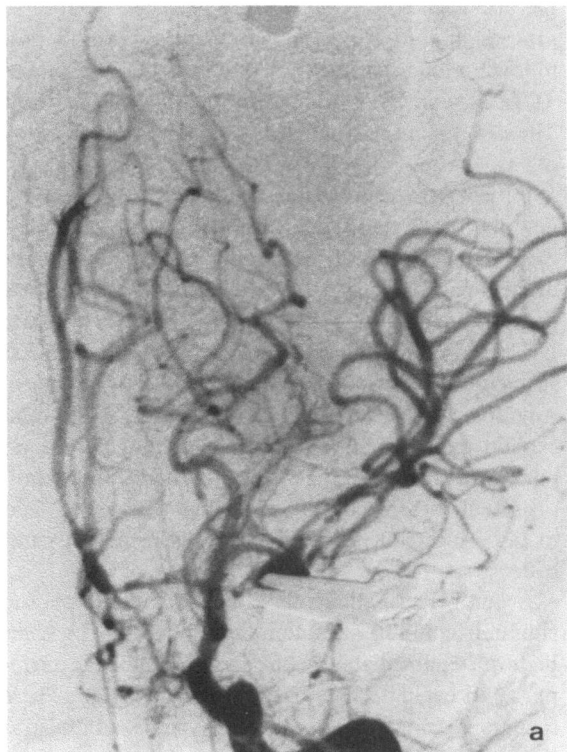 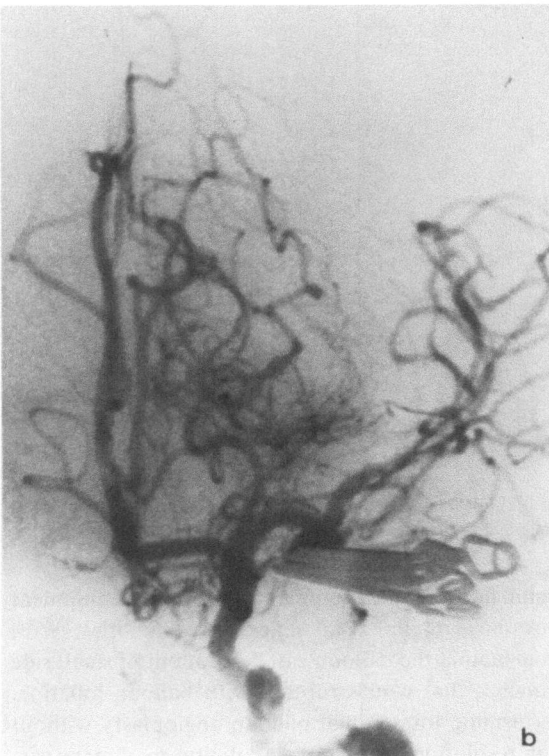

Fig. 2. (a) Left internal carotid angiography reveals severe vasospasm of the middle cerebral artery. The patient was symptomatic with right hemiparesis at the time of the angiogram. (b) Following successful angioplasty the caliber of the middle cerebral artery is now normal. By the following day the patient's hemiparesis had resolved completely

condition did not allow surgery. While waiting for the patient to improve the patient had two more hemorrhages over the next two weeks and died. Another patient had a mycotic aneurysm on the posterior cerebral artery; angioplasty was performed only on the internal carotid arteries. The patient bled again from the unclipped mycotic aneurysm and died a few days later. There was one death due to vessel rupture from the balloon. This occurred at the origin of the anterior cerebral artery.

TCD values in the proximal cerebral arteries and distal internal carotid arteries were decreased following the procedure and in all patients except one. These velocities remained below pre-angioplasty levels during follow-up exams. On a number of occasions vessels other than the dilated vessels showed increasing velocities during the follow-up despite the fact that the velocities in the treated vessels remained low.

SPECT scanning performed before and after balloon angioplasty showed improvement in cerebral perfusion in the majority of patients studied. This improvement in cerebral perfusion also correlated with clinical improvement.

Thirty-two patients have been treated more than one year ago. All these patients are doing well and are stable neurologically. We are not seeing any evidences of long term damage from the vasospasm angioplasty. Three patients have undergone repeat angiography at 18 months following angioplasty and in all cases the dilated vessels remained normal. In only one case did a small branch occlusion occur and that was in a situation where an experimental high pressure balloon was used in a middle cerebral branch and this balloon ruptured. The patient made a full recovery from his hemiparesis following angioplasty, but returned six weeks later with mild right arm weakness due to a small middle cerebral infarct. The patients right arm weakness completely resolved over the next few days. The experimental high pressure balloon that caused this single vessel rupture is no longer used.

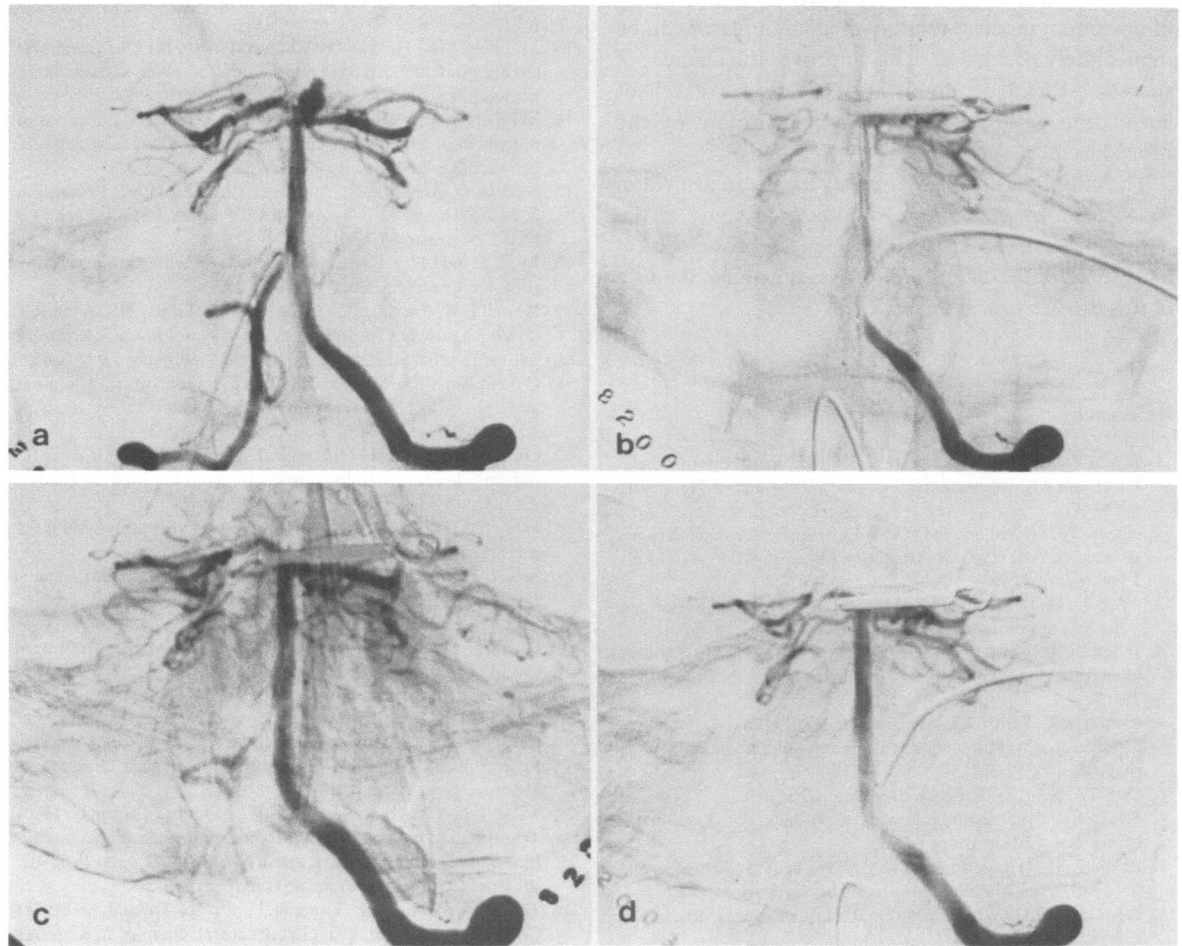

Fig. 3. (a) Lateral arteriogram of the left vertebral artery shows a basilar tip aneurysm. (b) There is severe vasospasm of the basilar artery. The patient was comatose at this point. (c) Following successful angioplasty the caliber of the basilar artery is now normal. The patient recovered and after two weeks was normal neurologically. (d) Repeat arteriogram 18 months later reveals normal vascularity without any evidence of long term damage. The patient continues to work and is doing well

Discussion

Experience with balloon angioplasty for vasospasm is accumulating in many centers and the initial results have been favorable in patients who otherwise have a poor prognosis[10,11,13,18,24]. It is not entirely clear why the procedure works or why the treated arteries do not restenose. There are experimental studies which show that the spasm is not merely muscular contraction but actually a structural change within the vessel wall[6,14,15] One of the most important factors in the success of this procedure is early intervention. The chances of reversing a deficit are greater with earlier treatment. Also vessels are easier to dilate in the early stages of spasm than in the late stages[10]. This may be due to collagen deposition and or fibrosis which increases over time in the vessel wall[6,9,25]. The risk of angioplasty should be lower in the earlier stages of spasm because the vessel is easier to dilate and this should therefore reduce the risk vessel rupture.

TCD and SPECT scanning have also shown improvement in cerebral profusion after angioplasty. Based on these studies and the clinical results this improvement is persistent. The most important role of TCD is in the early detection of vasospasm. Once there is TCD evidence of vasospasm then medical therapy can be instituted. If the patient deteriorates in the face of maximum medical therapy then angioplasty can be immediately performed. This improves the chances of success. SPECT scanning also has shown excellent correlation with clinical improvement following the procedure.

The initial results of angioplasty for the treatment of vasospasm are encouraging. Additional study of the pathogenesis of vasospasm and the effects of angioplasty need to be undertaken to improve our understanding of this disease process.

References

1. Aaslid R, Huber P, Nornes H (1984) Evaluation of cerebrovascular spasm with transcranial Doppler ultrasound. J Neurosurg 60: 37–41
2. Alksne JF, Greenhoot JM (1974) Experimental catecholamine-induced chronic cerebral vasospasm. Myonecrosis in vessel wall. J Neurosurg 41: 440
3. Allcock JM, Drake CG (1965) Ruptured intracranial aneurysms – the role of arterial spasm. J Neurosurg 22: 21
4. Block PC, Myler RK, Stertzer S, Fallon JT (1981) Morphology after transluminal angioplasty in human beings. N Engl J Med 305: 382
5. Clower BR, Smith RR, Haining JL, *et al* (1981) Constrictive endarteropathy following experimental subarachnoid hemorrhage. Stroke 12: 501–508
6. Duff TA, Scott G, Feilbach JA (1986) Ultrastructural evidence of arterial denervation following experimental subarachnoid hemorrhage. J Neurosurg 64: 292
7. Echlin F (1971) Experimental vasospasm, acute and chronic, due to blood in the subarachnoid space. J Neurosurg 35: 646
8. Eskridge JM (1989) Interventional neuroradiology. Radiology 172: 991
9. Eskridge JM, Newell DW, Pendleton GA (1990) Transluminal angioplasty for treatment of vasospasm. Neurosurg Clin N Am 1 (2): 387–399
10. Higashida RT, Halbach VV, Cahan LD, Brant-Zawadzki M, Barnwell S, Dowd C, Hieshima GB (1989) Transluminal angioplasty for treatment of intracranial arterial vasospasm. J Neurosurg 71: 648–653
11. Hunt WE, Hess RM (1968) Surgical risk as related to time of intervention in the repair of intracranial aneurysms. J Neurosurg 28: 14
12. Konishi Y, Sato E, Maemura E, Hara M, Takeuchi K (1990) Percutaneous transluminal angioplasty of vasospasm after subarachnoid hemorrhage. In: Sano K, Takakura K, Kassell NF, Sasaki T (eds) Proc 4th Int Conf Cerebral Vasospasm, Tokyo, p 122
13. Mayberg MR, Houser OW, Sundt TM (1978) Ultrastructural changes in feline arterial endothelium following subarachnoid hemorrhage. J Neurosurg 48: 49
14. Mayberg MR, Okada T, Bark DH (1990) The significance of morphologic changes in cerebral arteries after subarachnoid hemorrhage. J Neurosurg 72: 626–633
15. Mizukami M, Kawase T, Usami T, Tazawa T (1982) Prevention of vasospasm by early operation with removal of subarachnoid blood. Neurosurg 10: 301
16. Mullan S (1975) Conservative management of the recently ruptured aneurysm. Surg Neurol 3: 27
17. Newell DW, Eskridge JM, Mayberg MR, Grady HS, Winn RH (1989) Angioplasty for the treatment of symptomatic vasospasm following subarachnoid hemorrhage. J Neurosurg 71: 654–660
18. Ockenheimer SA, Mathias K (1983) Percutaneous transluminal angioplasty in arteriosclerotic internal carotid artery stenosis. AJNR 4: 791
19. Owada K, Hori S (1977) Cervical sympathectomy for cerebral ischemic lesions; a follow-up study. Tohoku Med J (Sendai) 90: 183
20. Ropper AH, Zervas NT (1984) Outcome 1 year after SAH from cerebral aneurysm. J Neurosurg 60: 909
21. Sah A, Perret GE, Locksley HB, *et al* (1969) Intracranial aneurysms and subarachnoid hemorrhage. Lippincott, Philadelphia
22. Seiler RW, Grolimund P, Aaslid R, Huber P, Nornes H (1986) Cerebral vasospasm evaluated by transcranial Doppler ultrasound correlated with clinical grade and CT visualized subarachnoid hemorrhage. J Neurosurg 64: 594–600
23. Sundt TM Jr (1975) Chemical management of cerebral vasospasm. In: Whisnant JP, Sandoc BA (eds) Cerebral vascular disease. Proceedings of the 9th Princeton Conference. Grune and Stratton, New York, p 77
24. Takahashi A, Mizoi K, Sugawara T, Yoshimoto T, Fujii N (1990) Transluminal balloon angioplasty for symptomatic vasospasm. In: Sano K, Takakura K, Kassell NF, Sasaki T (eds) Proc 4th Int Conf Cerebral Vasospasm, Tokyo, p 109
25. Tanabe Y, Sakata K, Yamada H, Ito T, Takada M (1978) Cerebral vasospasm and ultrastructural changes in cerebral arterial wall. J Neurosurg 49: 229
26. Tanishima T (1980) Cerebral vasospasm: contractile ability of hemoglobin in isolated canine basilar arteries. J Neurosurg 53: 787
27. Wilkins RH (1979) Attempted prevention or treatment of intracranial arterial spasm: a survey. In: Wilkins RH (ed) Cerebral arterial spasm. Williams and Wilkins, Baltimore, p 542
28. Zubkov YN, Nikiforov BM, Shustin VA (1984) Balloon catheter technique for dilatation of constricted cerebral arteries after aneurysmal SAH. Acta Neurochir (Wien) 70: 65

Correspondence: J.M. Eskridge, M.D., Department of Neurological Surgery, University of Washington, Seattle, WA 98195, U.S.A.

Intra-Arterial Papaverine for the Treatment of Cerebral Vasospasm*

G.A. Helm[1], N.F. Kassell[1], N. Simmons[1], C.D. Phillips[2], and W.S. Cail[2]

[1] Department of Neurological Surgery and [2] Department of Radiology, University of Virginia Health Sciences Center, Charlottesville, Virginia, U.S.A.

Summary

Cerebral vasospasm continues to be the leading treatable cause of morbidity and mortality following aneurysmal subarachnoid hemorrhage. In this preliminary anecdotal series of 15 patients who were candidates for balloon angioplasty, vasospasm was treated instead with intra-arterial papaverine. Ten patients had marked angiographic reversal of the arterial narrowing following the papaverine infusion. Five of these patients showed dramatic reversal of profound neurologic deficits following papaverine treatment. Two patients clinically deteriorated five days after the initial successful papaverine infusions. In both, repeat angiograms demonstrated severe recurrent vasospasm which was partially reversed with a second intra-arterial papaverine treatment. Three patients developed focal neurologic deficits during papaverine infusion which spontaneously resolved over several hours after cessation of the intraarterial infusion. Arterial narrowing in the posterior circulation and middle cerebral artery distribution appeared to be more responsive to papaverine infusion than spasm in the anterior cerebral arteries. The infusion of 300 mg of papaverine over one hour seemed to be an adequate and safe dose to effect these angiographic and clinical improvements.

Keywords: Vasospasm; papaverine; subarachnoid hemorrhage.

Introduction

Although significant advances have been made in the treatment of cerebral vasospasm, the arterial narrowing which commonly occurs after subarachnoid hemorrhage is still a leading cause of morbidity and mortality in patients with ruptured aneurysms[5]. Hypertensive hypervolemic hemodilution therapy[4], calcium channel blocking agents[7], and early surgery with clot removal have all contributed to the decreased incidence and severity of vasospasm[3].

Balloon angioplasty has been used with dramatic success in certain patients with vasospasm in the large

cerebral vessels[2], but it is not effective in dilating the distal arteries. In addition, there are significant risks associated with angioplasty, including occlusion or rupture of arteries and displacement of clips on aneurysm necks[6].

In an attempt to find a safer and more comprehensive method for dilating the narrowed vessels, we have utilized an infusion of papaverine into the cerebral arterial system.

Methods and Materials

Clinical Material

Between December 1990 and June 1992, fifteen patients at the University of Virginia who had severe angiographic arterial narrowing following aneurysmal subarachnoid hemorrhage were treated with papaverine infused into the major cerebral arteries in an attempt to reverse the arterial narrowing. All were candidates for ballon angioplasty.

Treatment

A tracker catheter was placed as close to the involved vessels as possible, and papaverine dissolved in normal saline solution was infused for 30–90 minutes. The concentration of papaverine ranged from 100 mg to 300 mg per 100 ml of saline, and the total dose administered ranged from 100 mg to 300 mg. Thirteen patients had infusion into one vessel, and two into two vessels. Two patients had the treatment repeated, both after an interval of five days. The various doses and times of perfusion of papaverine reflects the evolution of the protocol.

The pre- and post-papaverine infusion angiograms were graded by a blinded evaluator at the Central Registry of the Cooperative Aneurysm Study.

Results

Angiographic Arterial Narrowing

Papaverine was infused into a total of 19 arteries on 15 patients on 17 occasions. In ten patients, there was

* Presented in part at the Congress of Neurological Surgeons Orlando, Florida, 1991; and the American Association of Neurological Surgeons, New Orleans, Louisiana, 1991.

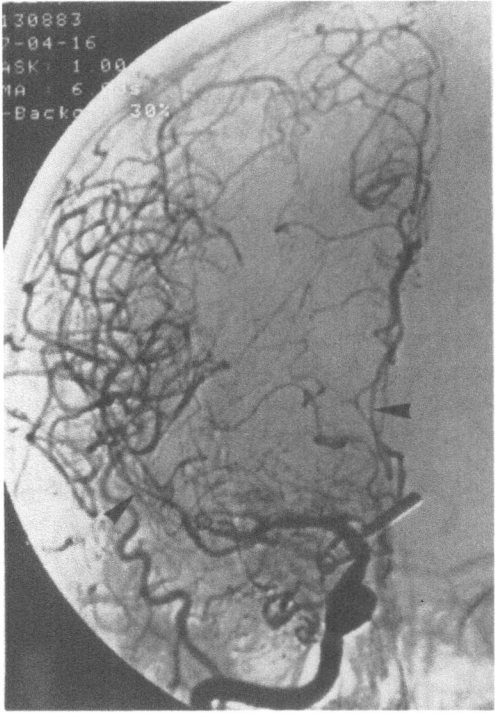

Fig. 1. Pre-papaverine cerebral angiogram. Five days following rupture of a right middle artery aneurysm. a 75 year old female clinically deteriorated. A right cerebral angiogram demonstrated moderate vasospasm in the middle and anterior cerebral arteries (arrowheads). An incidental basilar tip aneurysm was also clipped during her initial surgery

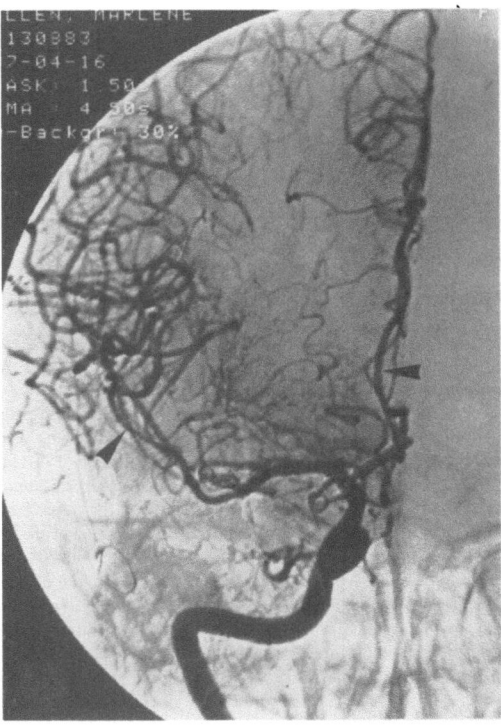

Fig. 2. Post-papaverine cerebral angiogram. Infusion of papaverine (300 mg) into the right internal carotid artery completely reversed the vasospasm in both the middle and anterior cerebral arteries (arrowheads)

dramatic reversal of the angiographic vasospasm. In several patients, the maximal effect was not reached until 90 minutes post-infusion.

Clinical Condition

The clinical condition of the patients pre-versus one hour post-infusion was compared using a modified Glasgow Coma Scale, which uses the worst motor score instead of the best motor score, to evaluate focal cerebral ischemia. Dramatic reversal of profound neurological deficits occurred in five patients and was associated with reversal of severe arterial narrowing in the appropriate vascular distribution.

Toxicity

None of the patient exhibited material reductions in systemic arterial pressure, nor were there any other adverse systemic events related to administration of

papaverine. One patient developed decreased mental status and hemiparesis during the treatment, but she returned to baseline after several hours. The etiology of this deterioration remains unclear. Two other patients with mild pre-infusion deficits had transient dilatation of the ipsilateral pupil during papaverine infusion. Papaverine treatment in these patients was discontinued as soon as these findings were noted.

Recurrence of Vasospasm

In two of the patients who had improvement in both clinical and angiographic vasospasm after papaverine infusion, there was recurrence of ischemic symptoms and arterial narrowing five days after the initial treatment. The vasospasm was confirmed angiographically, and papaverine was re-infused into the affected vessels. In each of these cases, there was marked improvement of the angiography spasm after the second infusion.

Discussion

Papaverine is one of the strongest non-specific vaso-dilator agents[6]. It was one of the first treatments utilized for cerebral vasospasm following subarachnoid hemorrhage. The package insert for papaverine states "papaverine relaxes the smooth musculature of the large blood vessels, including the coronary, cerebral, peripheral, and pulmonary arteries. This action is particularly evident when such vessels are in spasm." This was the foundation upon which we attempted to use papaverine as an alternative to balloon angioplasty.

Papaverine was administered through a tracker catheter inserted as close as possible to the narrowed arteries. The dose of papaverine was selected empirically. The initial attempt was with 100 mg diluted in 100 cc of saline and administered over a 30 minute period. The total dose and duration of administration were progressively increased when no response was seen initially and no adverse effects occurred. In several of the patients, no appreciable change in arterial diameter occurred for 30–60 minutes during infusion, but the fairly dramatic dilatation occurred the last 30 minutes.

The optimal dose and duration of infusion remains to be determined, althouth 300 mg/100 cc infused over 60 minutes appeared to be adequate and safe.

In certain patients, the papaverine treatment was dramatically effective, while in other patients, it was totally ineffective. The reasons for this are unclear. One possibility is that vasospasm, as suggested by Vorkapic et al.[8], has a papaverine-sensitive phase, during which papaverine infusion quickly and completely reversed cerebral vasospasm, and a papaverine-resistant phase when the arterial wall becomes stiff and unresponsive[1]. A second possibility is that the patients who failed to respond to papaverine had an inadequate dose and/or inadequate duration of administration. Obviously, papaverine can only work on vessels where it is delivered by flowing blood and will not be as effective in anterior cerebral artery spasm with a normal middle cerebral artery, where the blood flow preferentially delivers papaverine infused into the internal carotid artery to the middle cerebral artery territory.

Furthermore, uncertainty exists as to the length of duration of the dilatation by papaverine. In at least two patients, the arterial narrowing recurred but was responsive to further papaverine administration. It is possible that multiple intermittent infusions or constant, long-term infusion of papaverine can be utilized in patients with severe arterial narrowing where the effect of the initial treatment is transient.

Intra-arterial papaverine is a theoretically attractive modality for treating severe vasospasm. The results of this preliminary anecdotal series suggest that this approach is at least partially effective. Although there is adequate, suggestive evidence to warrant further investigation, we caution again the widespread adoption of this modality until the safety and efficacy of this approach has been conclusively demonstrated.

References

1. Bevan AJ, Bevan RD (1988) Arterial wall changes in chronic cerebrovasospasm: in vitro and in vivo pharmacological evidence. Ann Rev Pharmacol Toxicol 28: 311–329
2. Brothers MF, Holgate RC (1990) Intracranial angioplasty for treatment of vasospasm after subarachnoid hemorrhage: technique and modifications to improve branch access. AJNR 11: 239–247
3. Handa Y, Weir BKA, Nosko M, Mosewich R, Tsuji T, Grace M (1987) The effect of timing of clot removal on chronic vasospasm in a primate model. J Neurosurg 67: 558–564
4. Kassell NF, Peerless SJ, Durward QJ, Beck DW, Drake CG, Adams HP (1982) Treatment of ischemic deficits from vasospasm with intravascular volume expansion and induced arterial hypertension. Neurosurgery 11: 337–343
5. Kassell NF, Shaffrey ME, Shaffrey CI (1991) Cerebral vasospasm following aneurysmal subarachnoid hemorrhage. In: Apuzzo M (ed) Brain surgery: complication, avoidance, and management. Churchill Livingstone, New York
6. Pal J (1914) Das Papaverine als Gefamittel und Anästhetikum. Dtsch Med Wochenschr 40: 164–168
7. Picard JD, Murray GD, Illinsworth R, Illingsworth R, Shaw MDM, Teasdale GM, Foy PM, Humphrey PRD, Lang DA, Nelson R, Richards R, Sinar J, Bailey S, Skene A (1989) Effect of oral nimodipine on cerebral infarction and outcome after subarachnoid hemorrhage: British aneurysm nimodipine trial. BMJ 298: 636–642
8. Vorkapic P, Bevan RD, Bevan JA (1991) Longitudinal time course of reversible and irreversible components of chronic cerebrovasospasm of the rabbit basilar artery. J Neurosurg 74: 951–955

Correspondence: N.F. Kassell, M.D., Department of Neurological Surgery, Box 212, University of Virginia Health Sciences Center, Charlottesville, Virginia 22908, U.S.A.

Papaverine for the Treatment of Cerebral Vasospasm After Subarachnoid Hemorrhage

T. Tsukahara, Y. Yonekawa, Y. Kaku, and **K. Kazekawa,**

Department of Cerebrovascular Surgery, National Cardiovascular Center, Osaka, Japan

Summary

The present report describes the successful treatment of cerebral vasospasm after subarachnoid hemorrhage (SAH) with super selective intra-arterial infusion of papaverine hydrochloride and the experimental background of this treatment. Since in vitro experiment demonstrated that papaverine is one of the most potent vasodilators of human cerebral arteries following SAH, papaverine was applied clinically as a vasodilator for the spastic arteries after SAH. Thirty-seven vascular territories in 10 patients with symptomatic vasospasm were treated by percutaneous transluminal angioplasty (PTA) and superselective infusion of 0.2% papaverine. Thirty-four of 37 vascular territories were successfully dilated. Superselective intraarterial infusion of papaverine is an alternative method of treatment for symptomatic vasospasm.

Keywords: Cerebral vasospasm; papaverine; angioplasty; subarachnoid hemorrhage.

Introduction

Percutaneous transluminal angioplasty (PTA) for the treatment of cerebral arterial vasospasm has recently been performed in selected cases, with generally favorable results in patients with symptomatic vasospasm refractory to conventional therapy[1]. Angioplasty balloon catheters currently available, however, have limited ability to selectively enter the narrowed branches at a bi- or trifurcation of the major branches, such as the distal middle cerebral artery (MCA), and sharply angled vessels, such as the anterior cerebral artery (ACA). We have treated such peripheral and spastic vessels with intra-arterial infusion of papaverine hydrochloride. Papaverine, a potent vasodilator, has been used for the treatment of clinical and experimental vasospasm by intravenous or intrathecal administration[2,3]. These attempts, however, have not shown sufficient therapeutic effect mainly because of the way of drug administration. The present report describes the successful treatment of cerebral vasospasm after SAH with super selective intra-arterial infusion of papaverine and the experimental background of this treatment.

Materials and Methods

Measurement of Arterial Responses in vitro

Cerebral arterial specimens (cortical branches of the middle cerebral artery with a diameter of 1 mm) were obtained from autopsy cases. The contractile force was recorded isometrically using the force-displacement transducer and displayed on a polygraph. The relaxing effect of papaverine (10^{-8}–10^{-4} M) was measured when the serotonin-elicited contraction reached a plateau. Relaxation was expressed as a percentage of the amplitude of contraction.

Clinical Material and Methods

During a 16-month period between August 1990 and December 1991, we treated 37 vascular territories in ten patients, with patient ages ranging from 35 to 86 years. All cases involved cerebral vasospasm due to subarachnoid hemorrhage following aneurysm rupture, and all had undergone early surgery, i.e., clipping of an aneurysm by Day 2.

Angioplasty of the intracranial vessels was performed in two steps, as follows; a silicone non-detachable balloon 0.9 mm in diameter before inflation (Dow-Corning, Japan) was used for dilatation of the first narrowed segment, for example, the supraclinoid segment of the internal carotid artery and the proximal MCA. A leak silicone balloon or Tracker 18 catheter (Target Therapeutics Inc, San Jose) was then introduced into or just proximal to the site of vasospasm not accessible to the angioplasty balloon catheter, such as the distal MCA or ACA, for super slective infusion of papaverine, 0.5 mg of nicardipine, and occasionally 60000 IU of Urokinase. Papaverine was diluted with normal saline to concentrations of 0.2%, and 1 ml was infused at a rate of 0.1 ml/sec, under monitoring by digital subtraction angiography. Infusion of papaverine was repeated several times until the vessels were dilated to nearly normal caliber size.

Results

In vitro Experiments

Papaverine (10^{-4} M) induced maximal dilatation of all the control and SAH arteries examined. ED50 of

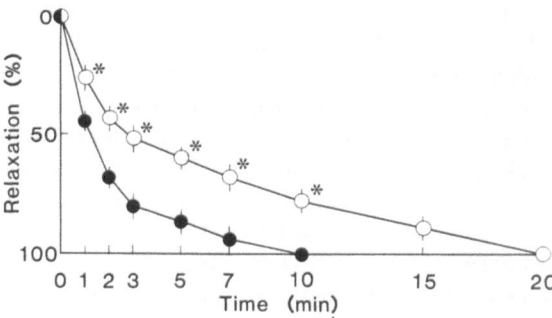

Fig. 1. Time course of relaxing responses to 10^{-4} M papaverine of control (●) and middle cerebral arteries after SAH (○). Values are mean ± SEM for 4 cases in each group. Statistical comparison was performed by Student's t-test for unpaired observations. *Significantly different from control group at $p < 0.01$

papaverine were not statistically different between the control ($3.6 \pm 1.6 \times 10^{-6}$ M, n = 4) and SAH arteries ($4.1 \pm 0.9 \times 10^{-6}$ M, n = 4). As demonstrated in Fig. 1, the relaxing response to papaverine was slower in SAH arteries than that in control arteries.

Clinical Trial

Thirty-four of 37 vascular territories were successfully dilated (Fig. 2), and 8 of 10 patients showed improvement in neurological function after angioplasty. We have experienced no serious side effects due to infusion of papaverine. On follow-up angiography, the dilated vessels exhibited continued patency without evidence of recurrent stenosis.

Discussion

Papaverine is an alkaloid of the opium group well known to cause vasodilatation of cerebral arteries through a direct action on smooth muscle, and it reduces the constriction of smooth muscle produced by a wide variety of stimuli.

Papaverine (10^{-4} M) always induced a maximal amount of vasodilatation of control and spastic arteries following SAH, whereas endothelium-dependent vasodilatation, for example, was markedly disturbed in the arteries after SAH. Although the effective dose of papaverine was not significantly different between

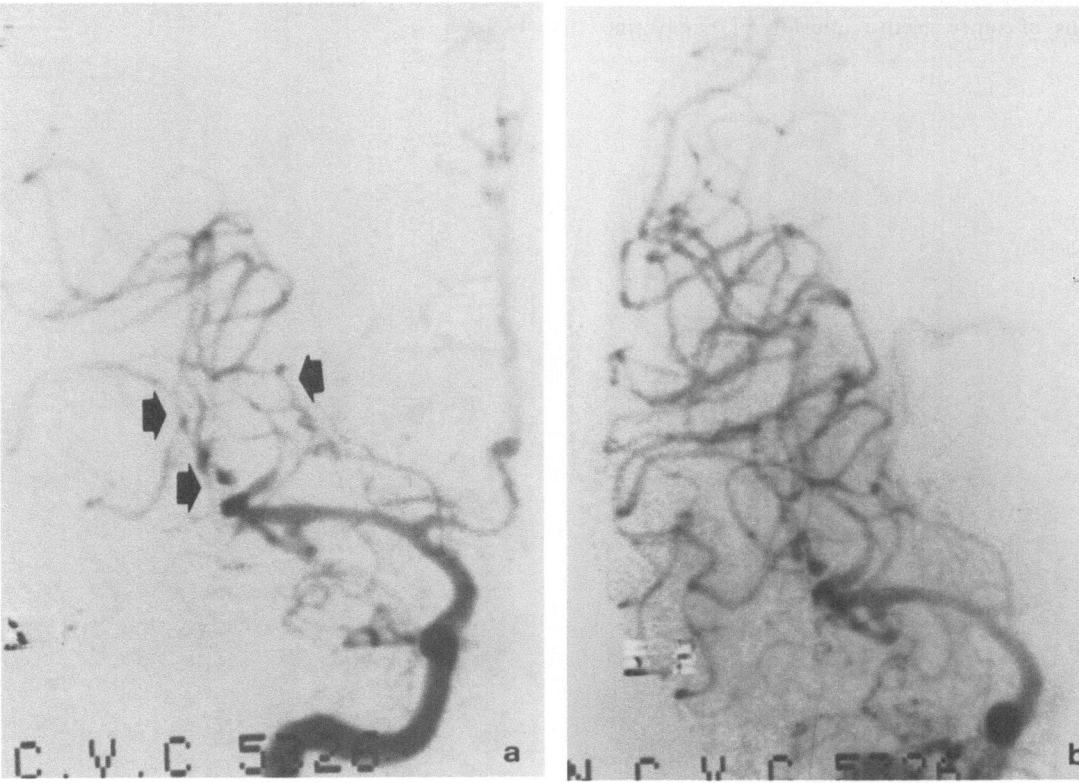

Fig. 2. (a) Right ICA angiogram, AP view, demonstrating severe vasospasm of M2 and M3 (arrows). (b) Angiogram obtained following superselective infusion of papaverine showing return of normal luminal diameter of M2 and M3, with angiographic evidence of improved perfusion

control arteries and SAH arteries, the vasodilating response was slower in SAH arteries; 10^{-4} M papaverine induced 50% dilatation within 1.3 min in control arteries and 2.7 min in SAH arteries. We decided the concentration of papaverine to be used in the clinical trials on the basis of these in vitro data. If the drug is infused at a rate of 0.1 ml/sec into an artery with a diameter of 2 mm and a flow velocity of 100 cm/s, the drug is attenuated 31.4 times in one second by blood flow. Since we used 0.2% papaverine (Ca 30×10^{-4} M papaverine) at a rate of 0.1 ml/s, rough estimation suggests that the target artery received a submaximum (10^{-4} M) dose of papaverine during the infusion. In order to deliver a sufficient concentration of papaverine, it may be essential to infuse papaverine just proximal to the spastic arteries.

Introduction of transluminal angioplasty contributed greatly to progress in the treatment of vasospasm. However, the balloon catheter currently available has limited ability to access distally affected vessels and to access vessel origins that are short and sharply angled, such as the A1 segment of the anterior cerebral artery. We therefore decided to treat such peripheral vessels by means of superselective infusion of papaverine which vasodilating effect is not lost after SAH. Considering these clinical results, it is clear that the pathogenesis of vasospasm, at least its initial stage, is arterial contraction which can be treated with vasodilating agents. Therefore, in order to achieve good results, papaverine should be infused as early as possible before the artery looses the ability to return to normal luminal diameter. In conclusion, superselective intra-arterial infusion of papaverine is an alternative form of treatment for symptomatic vasospasm following SAH.

References

1. Higashida RT, Halback VV, Cahan LD, Brant-Zawadzki M, Barnwell S, Dowd C, Hieshima GB, (1989) Transluminal angioplasty for treatment of intracranial arterial vasospasm. J Neurosurg 71: 648–653
2. Kuwayama A, Zervas NT, Shintani A, Pickren KS (1972) Papaverine hydrochloride and experimental hemorrhagic cerebral arterial spasm. Stroke 3: 27–33
3. Ogata M, Marshall BM, Lougheed WM (1975) Observations on the effect of intrathecal papaverine in experimental vasospasm. J Neurosurg 38: 20–25

Correspondence: Tetsya Tsukahara, M.D., Department of Cerebrovascular Surgery, National Cardovascular Center, Suita 565, Osaka, Japan.

Anesthesia and Temporary Clipping in Aneurysm Surgery

Anesthesia in Aneurysm Surgery

D.J. Stone

Department of Anesthesiology, University of Virginia Health Sciences Center, Charlottesville, Virginia, U.S.A.

Summary

I would like to focus on the actual details of care as provided to patients at the University of Virginia over the past 8 years. Many of these patients have suffered from recent hemorrhage (rather than the detection of an aneurysm or AVM that has not yet bled) and the discussion generally covers the more difficult care of the patient with a recent bleed. Some of what we do is supported by the literature, some has been the result of trial and error with subsequent success, and some is local tradition.

Keywords: Anesthesia; neurosurgical-cerebral aneurysm; neurosurgical A-V malformations; arteries.

Pre-Operative Considerations

Volume Status

The "dried-out" hypovolemic patient prone to anesthetic-induced hypotension appears fairly infrequently in the operating room at the present time. Rather than restricting fluids to control blood pressure, neurosurgeons currently advocate normovolemia or even controlled hypervolemia to prevent vasospasm while employing specific antihypertensive agents and/or early surgery to prevent hypertension-related rebleeding. The vast majority of our patients arrive in the operating room without a central venous or pulmonary artery pressure monitor, and we employ low-tech clinical means of judging the patient's volume status starting with careful observation of the patient for evidence of dehydration and evaluation of vital signs. After empirically administering about 500 ml of crystalloid during the pre-induction period, we have found that the patient's response to a slow, careful induction of anesthesia is the best indicator of volume (and sometimes, cardiac) status. Since it is impossible to "take-back" intravenous drugs once administered, they are given slowly so that response can be observed. Marked respiratory cycling of the arterial pressure wave form also provides a good indicator that significant hypovolemia is present. One of my bioengineer-anesthesia colleagues in Charlottesville is currently working on a minimally invasive measure of intravascular volume that may eventually become an on-line monitor in these patients.

Cardiac Status

Most of our patients are surprisingly free of premorbid cardiac problems although the older patient (who appears to be forming a larger part of our patient population) will have the usual ravages of hypertension, coronary artery disease and congestive heart failure. Most neuroanesthetists and neurosurgeons are familiar with these problems through their experiences with the carotid endarterectomy population. By whatever mechanism, subarachnoid hemorrhage appears to have a cardiovascular impact and produce a form of myocarditis, dysrhythmias, and electrocardiographic changes that mimic those of myocardial ischemia. In our practice, heart failure on the basis of subarachnoid hemorrhage (SAH) related myocarditis has not been a significant problem. At least in the operating room, severe dysrhythmias such as ventricular tachycardia have not really been a problem, either. However, ST-T wave changes, especially in conjunction with slight rises in the myocardial fraction of creatine kinase (CK) have resulted in some real clinical dilemmas. Recently, we took care of a patient who did have electrocardiographic and enzymatic evidence of a small myocardial infarction after her first operation but required another. She was a fairly young woman unlikely to have significant coronary artery disease and did quite well clinically, i.e. did not "look" like someone with a myocardial infarction. Cardiology work-up included a normal coronary angiogram and echocardiogram. For her second operation, we monitored her with a pulmonary artery catheter, which was probably unnecessary, and all went well. Our mistake was measuring cardiac isozymes in the first place as the subendocardial myocarditis present in many of these patients will elevate the enzymes to a level mimicking a myocardial infarction. Of course, an occasional patient will truly have a myocardial infarction after any operation, but even in the very high-risk carotid endarterectomy population, the rate is only a very few percent. The decision to measure CK levels in these patients is not to be taken lightly or decided upon by very junior housestaff people as it may lead to unnecessary and risky interventions such as coronary arteriography, as well as added expense and worry to patient and family.

Interaction with Radiology

Interventional neuroradiology continues to increase its involvement with this group of patients. While some institutions have an anesthetist present at procedures such as embolization, we have not done so up to the present unless a child or extremely uncooperative patient requires general anesthesia. While the need for continuous anesthesia coverage is controversial, the need for the availability of assistance in case of neuroradiological complication/disaster is not and we are quickly available for assistance in airway management and resuscitation. These cases do in fact appear to require expert airway and hemodynamic management in a fair number of instances. Local interest and personnel resources may dictate whether we can attend throughout these procedures. They are often long, boring procedures performed in dark, small underventilated areas to which we must bring our equipment to the despair of the radiology techs, i.e. we have a hard time getting volunteers to go to x-ray at our institution.

One notable problem that we did have was in an aneurysm patient with an intracarotid balloon catheter in place. When transported to the operating room table, she became acutely and densely hemiplegic and aphasic. It was postulated that she suffered an air embolus when the pressure bag was tipped during the move. After 2 days of increasing edema and deterioration, she began a spontaneous recovery and after 5 days, was virtually normal. The lesson here, at least to me, is that the radiologist should be present at all times when a potentially dangerous piece of equipment such as an intracarotid catheter is in place so that such problems can be, hopefully, avoided.

Coagulation

Obviously, the usual evaluation of the coagulation system must be undertaken before these operations. In an occasional patient with a difficult arteriovenous malformation, I have pretreated these patients with DDAVP (desmopressin) 0.3 µg/kg up to 20 µg. This treatment may improve even baseline normal platelet function and reduce blood loss as it has been shown to do after cardiac and Harrington Rod surgery. Because these patients are generally embolized as well, it is difficult to tell what treatment is contributing to what extent. In any case, DDAVP administration may be considered when hemorrhage has been a limiting factor in previous resection attempts. The dose should be given over 10 minutes to avoid hypotension and the theoretical concern of hyponatremia and water retention has not been a clinical problem. An occasional patient will develop an introperative coagulopathy resembling disseminated intravascular coagulation and will require some assortment of platelets, fresh frozen plasma, and even cryoprecipitate until the stimulus is resected.

Monitors

Cardiorespiratory

In addition to the monitors that are standard for any anesthetic, we insert an intra-arterial cannula in all patients to monitor beat to beat changes in blood pressure. The cannula is inserted before the induction of anesthesia in virtually all patients so that the information provided is available at all times during induction. This is necessary to avoid an episode of rupture-provoking hypertension or hypovolemia-related hypotension and later, to provide safe controlled hypotension.

We also employ a monitor of inhaled and exhaled gases that facilitates the determination of anesthetic depth and the presence of venous air embolism. Central venous pressure (CVP) catheters are inserted when the seated position is chosen. However, if after a reasonable length of time a CVP can not be properly placed, I will proceed with the case using a precordial Doppler and end-tidal gas monitoring. Furthermore, the seated position is rarely used at our hospital. Pulmonary artery (PA) catheters are inserted only if necessitated by an underlying cardiorespiratory condition, e.g. the lady described with the possible recent myocardial infarction. These monitors (CVP, PA line) that afford an approximation of intravascular volume are not usually required because given a reasonably normal set of heart, vasculature and kidneys, it is possible to give a "little-extra" fluid and allow the wise physiologists inside the sarcomeres and glomeruli to fine-tune the system. A good indicator of hypovolemia is so-called downward "cycling" of the arterial pressure wave tracing on the oscilloscope. When the patient is hypovolemic, the effects of positive-pressure ventilation on right ventricular preload are magnified with reduction of the amplitude of the pressure wave several beats after mechanical inspiration. The fluid of choice, usually a crystalloid, can be titrated in to diminish or abolish the amount of "cycling" observed. Fluid overload can produce an upward "cycling" of the waveform so that a baseline must be established during apnea.

Neurological

Over the past 8 years, the vast majority of intracranial vascular neurosurgery at our institution has been performed without any special electrophysiological monitoring. In several patients, we have employed compressed spectral analysis of the EEG on the side of the brain contralateral to surgery. This has been employed with the hope of titrating doses of possible brain protective agents (isoflurane, thiopental) to the point of burst suppression. This may be most useful in the highest risk patients who come to the operating room in the worst neurological state and generally have poorer outcomes.

Anesthesia

Induction

Our usual induction of anesthesia consists of the following: A sleep dose of thiopental is administered and mask ventilation of the airway is assured. Propofol or etomidate can be used for this purpose but we have mainly stayed with thiopental, at least in this setting where we are somewhat reluctant to experiment. An intubating dose of a non-depolarizing relaxant is then administered-vecuronium has become our local favorite. A priming dose of 1–2 mg of vecuronium given with the thiopental seems to facilitate mask induction. I also avoid narcotics until the relaxant has begun to take effect in order to avoid the occasional stiff chest wall caused by these drugs. The dose of non-depolarizers is doubled in patients receiving phenytoin or carba-

mazepine as they appear to have a pharmacodynamic resistance to these drugs (with the possible exception of atracurium).

After mask ventilation is felt to be easier due to muscle relaxation, narcotic is administered to stabilize the subsequent hemodynamic response to laryngoscopy and intubation. I use sufentanil 0.5–2.0 µg/kg depending on the blood pressure and the patient's original response to the thiopental. After a minute or two of continued mask ventilation, a small additional dose of thiopental can (or sometimes not) be given and laryngoscopy and intubation performed. In addition to the laryngoscopist (usually a junior level resident), another anesthetist is present (usually me) to observe the blood pressure, give additional drugs, and assist with airway management. We have found that this sequence of anesthetic induction generally provides acceptable hemodynamics even when laryngoscopy is somewhat prolonged by a relatively inexperienced laryngoscopist or by a truly difficult airway.

Brain Exposure

In addition to CSF drainage as chosen and implemented by the surgeons, brain exposure is facilitated by the administration of mannitol, hyperventilation, and anesthetic choice. One hundred grams of mannitol (500 ml of 20% solution) are given both before and after incision. We are not certain of the optimal dose or rate of administration of mannitol. In an occasional patient, rapid mannitol administration appears to cause hypotension, possibly on the basis of vasodilation due to acute hyperosmolarity. Junior house staff must be reminded not to undertake a major laboratory reevaluation of the patient at this time as the results are usually made confusing and worthless by the high levels of mannitol. In difficult cases, we have given another 100 grams of mannitol without apparent adverse results.

The use of hyperventilation in the patient who may have clinical or subclinical vasospasm and then is subjected to controlled hypotension is somewhat controversial in that the risk to areas of focal ischemia is theoretically increased. We believe the benefit of a slack brain overrides this concern and have not noticed much of a clinical problem in spite of warnings in various textbooks of neuroanesthesia. Hyperventilation also increases the theoretical risk of aneurysm rupture via decreasing ICP and, therefore, increasing the pressure gradient across the wall of the aneurysm. We feel this is not of clinical importance (inserting a lumber drain does so also!).

Anesthetic choice really only becomes an issue in difficult cases when the brain is angry and tight. At present, no anesthetic can be said to be "better" than another assuming the basic principles of safe anesthesia are observed. In most cases, I maintain anesthesia with sufentanil, isoflurane, and nitrous oxide, all of which are potential cerebrovasodilators. I have come to use sufentanil in this setting because it has provided the most stable hemodynamics in my experience. When exposure is difficult, I usually respond by turning off the nitrous oxide, rechecking the level of ventilation, and observing the position of the head. A single dose of thiopental in conjunction with discontinuation of the nitrous oxide and substitution of fentanyl for sufentanil may improve the situation. If problems persist, an infusion of lidocaine is begun. A 1 mg/kg bolus followed by 1–2 mg/min produces plasma levels of 2–4 µg/ml and provides about one-third of a MAC (minimum anesthetic concentration). If necessary, isoflurane can be discontinued and replaced with an infusion of thiopental (1–15 mg/min) that results in an anesthetic contribution of approximately 0.5 MAC. Propofol or etomidate can be used for this purpose although large doses of etomidate may result in a delay of resumption of normal neurologic function as well as an inhibition of adrenal steroidogenesis. The use of lidocaine and thiopental infusions with a base of fentanyl (5–15 µg/kg loading dose with or without a 1–4 µg/kg/h infusion) usually quiets the outraged brain. Propofol may provide for quicker awakening of the patient than thiopental, especially when large (> 15 mg/kg of thiopental) doses are required. There is some question that propofol may be epileptogenic but in fact, I use it in infusions for sedation in conscious epilepsy surgery cases.

Anesthetic Maintenance

It is the nature of neurosurgery to consist of a very long, low level stimulus punctuated by major painful stimuli such as head pinning and incision as well as hemodynamic responses to maneuvers such as retraction of various neuroanatomical locations. The measures taken during induction to avoid potentially disastrous hypertension have been described. We generally pin patients at a systolic blood pressure of about 80 mmHg and assure this with a bolus of alfentanil (3–20 µg/kg) or thiopental (1–3 mg/kg) given about 30 seconds before

the stimulus. Anesthesia is then maintained at a mean blood pressure of 60–80 mmHg unless further hypotension is required. Preoperatively, we administer captopril (3 mg/kg) or clonidine (5 µg/kg) orally with a sip of water to facilitate blood pressure control. The use of controlled hypotension has re-entered a phase of some controversy regarding its possible contribution to focal ischemia and simply a lack of need in the era of the microscope and temporary clips. In any case, when hypotension is requested at a mean blood pressure of 40–50 mmHg, an increase in the inspired isoflurane concentration is generally adequate on top of the previously administered oral antihypertensive and sufentanil. Occasionally, a small dose of labetalol (2.5–15 mg IV) is required. Nitroprusside is always available in the room but I have stopped mixing it up for each case as I have used it only a few times in an experience of hundreds of cases.

Brain Protection

Of the anesthetic drugs I usually employ, thiopental and isoflurane are potential brain protective agents. Propofol and etomidate could be used as well; the latter may be particularly useful in the setting of temporary clips when hypotension is to be avoided. The lidocaine infusion used during difficult exposures as well as the routine use of mannitol have the potential for beneficial effects on cerebral ischemia, as well. The alpha-2 agonist clonidine used preoperatively also may contribute to brain protection. Theoretically, nitrous oxide and narcotics have the potential to have an adverse effect in cerebral ischemia but this problem has not yet caused me to abandon these useful drugs.

Our most important measure to provide brain protection may be the use of mild hypothermia until the critical neurosurgical period is finished. We simply provide a cool operating room, unwarmed intravenous fluids (we would warm blood in the uncommon instance it would be needed) and a cooling blanket. The patient is cooled to an esophageal (? brain) temperature of 32–33°C. We have not employed lower temperatures (which generally require more aggressive measures than a cooling blanket). Rewarming is begun after the aneurysm is clipped and may or may not be complete at the end of the operation. If the patient's temperature is less than 35°C, he is brought intubated, paralyzed and ventilated to the intensive care unit. Patients who are warm and who arrived awake in the OR are generally extubated in the operating room and brought to a nearby recovery room until more fully awake. Blood pressure is kept at the desired level with labetalol boluses and rarely, with a nitroprusside infusion. Patients with AVM's (who tend to be more hypertensive post-op than aneurysms in my experience) who are potential candidates for postoperative perfusion pressure breakthrough are left intubated and ventilated to allow a slower, more controlled wake-up period. Hypertension in the intubated patient can also be easily treated with a thiopental bolus, a treatment modality that is not applicable after extubation. Most patients can be neurologically evaluated within 30 minutes after the head dressing is in place.

References

1. Archer DP, Shaw DA, Leblanc RL, Trammer BI (1991) Haemodynamic considerations in the management of patients with subarachnoid hemorrhage. Can J Anaesth 38: 454–470
2. Benzel EC, Hadden TA, Nossaman BD, Lancon J, Kesterson L (1990) Does sufentanil exacerbate marginal neurological dysfunction? J Neurosurg Anesth 2: 50–52
3. Brazenour GA, Chamberlain MJ, Gelb AW (1990) Systemic hypovolemia after subarachnoid hemorrhage. J Neurosurg Anesth 2: 42–49
4. Ghignone M, Calvillo O, Quintin L (1987) Anesthesia and hypertension: the effect of clonidine on perioperative hemodynamics and isoflurane requirements. Anesthesiology 67: 3–10
5. Himes RS, DiFazio CA, Burney RG (1977) Effects of lidocaine on the anesthetic requirements for nitrous oxide and halothane. Anesthesiology 47: 437–440
6. Manninen PH, Gelb AW, Lam AM, Moote CA, Contreras J (1990) Perioperative monitoring of the electrocardiogram during cerebral aneurysm surgery. J Neurosurg Anesth 2: 16–22
7. Mellergard P, Nordstrom CH, Messeter K (1992) Human brain temperature during anesthesia for intracranial operations. J Neurosurg Anesth 4: 85–91
8. Murdoch J, Hall R (1990) Brain protection: physiological and pharmacological considerations. Part I: the physiology of brain injury. Part II: The pharmacology of brain protection. Can J Anesth 37: 663–671, 762–777
9. Pizov R, Ya'ari Y, Perel A (1988) Systolic pressure variation is greater during hemorrhage than during sodium nitroprusside induced hypotension in ventilated dogs. Anesth Analg 67: 170–174
10. Sano T, Drummond JC, Patel PM, Grafe MR, Watson JC, Cole DJ (1992) A comparison of the cerebral protective effects of isoflurane and mild hypothermia in a model of incomplete forebrain ischemia in the rat. Anesthesiology 76: 221–228
11. Stone DJ (1989) Anesthesia for intracranial vascular surgery. In: Sperry RJ, Stirt JA, Stone DJ (eds) Manual of neuroanesthesia. Decker, Philadelphia, pp 131–142
12. Stone DJ, Moscicki JC, DiFazio CA (1992) Thiopental reduces halothane MAC. Anesth Analg 74: 542–546
13. Todd MM, Warner DS (1992) A comfortable hypothesis reevaluated: cerebral metabolic depression and brain protection during ischemia. Anesthesiology 76: 161–164
14. Wijdicks EFM, Ropper AH, Hunnicutt EJ, Richardson GS, Nathanson JA (1991) Atrial natriuretic factor and salt wasting after aneurysmal subarachnoid hemorrhage. Stroke 22: 1519–1524
15. Woodside J, Gasner L, Bedford RF, Sussman MD, Miller ED, Longnecker DE, Epstein RM (1984) Captopril reduces the dose requirement for sodium nitroprusside induced hypotension. Anesthesiology 60: 413–417

Correspondence: David J. Stone, M.D., Department of Anesthesiology, Box 238, University of Virginia Health Sciences Center, Charlottesville, Virginia 22908, U.S.A.

Special Anesthetic Considerations for Management of Cerebral Aneurysm Clipping

W.L. Young[1,2] and J.G. Stone[2]

Departments of [1]Anesthesiology and [2]Neurological Surgery, Columbia University College of Physicians and Surgeons, New York, New York, U.S.A.

Summary

Anesthetic management of cerebral aneurysm clipping includes maintenance of an acceptable transmural pressure to prevent rupture of the aneurysm, especially during surgical manipulation. Systemic hypotension has been widely practiced to achieve this goal. However, increasing use of temporary vascular occlusion requires some modification of the traditional anesthetic management of cerebral aneurysm clipping. In addition, there is a resurgence of interest in use of hypothermic circulatory arrest to clip large and complex lesions. This review addresses some of the evolving issues in the intraoperative management of aneurysm clipping, including cerebral hemodynamic monitoring, induced hypertension and pharmacologic brain protective therapy, and discusses the anesthetic management of hypothermic circulatory arrest.

Electrophysiological monitoring of cerebral function during aneurysm clipping has been advocated by many authors, but there is no clear consensus on the best methods or the reliability of the information gained. Scalp-recorded EEG may be insensitive to ischemic changes occuring in the cortex exposed at surgery and brain regions that fall away from the cranium because of brain relaxation. Subdural electrode recording provide a more sensitive method for detecting ischemia.

Measuring cerebral blood flow by direct means is ideal. Although the 133-Xe method is possible, it is rather cumbersome. Methods with a great deal of potential include laser Doppler and thermal clearance techniques. These methods can provide information about cortical perfusion in the operative field within a small area of brain that should reflect the perfusion territory of interest.

Cerebral autoregulation is impaired or lost during ischemia and cerebral blood flow (CBF) becomes pressure-passive. During temporary vascular occlusion, induced hypertension may reduce cell death in a threatened vascular territory by increasing collateral perfusion pressure and hence flow via collateral inflow channels. Because pharmacologically-induced hypertension and any attendent tachycardia may increase the risk of cardiac ischemia, careful cardiovascular monitoring is essential. Planned surgical occlusion of a major intracranial artery is the ideal setting for application of pharmacologic brain protective therapy. The prototype for pharmacological agents that afford cerebral protection are the barbiturates; no convincing data exist yet for etomidate[77] and propofol[51]. There is accelerating interest in the effects of modest reductions in body temperature in the treatment and prevention of cerebral ischemic injury; it seems reasonable to recommend that the normal temperature decrease seen with induction of anesthesia be allowed to persist (34–35° C) throughout most of the procedure. When the period of greatest risk for neurologic damage has passed and closure is imminent, only then should the heating blankets and humidifiers be called into active play and warming towards 37° C started.

We currently use hypothermic cardiac arrest for selected complex lesions and this technique requires a large multidisciplinary team and careful planning. Monitoring includes pulmonary artery catheter, transesophageal echocardiography, EEG and cerebral blood flow. We utilize a high dose fentanyl anesthetic supplemented with isoflurane and barbiturate infusion titrated to EEG burst-suppression. Spinal drainage is routine. After systemic heparinization, cardiopulmonary bypass is accomplished by the transfemoral route using an active venous return circuit. During cooling we use sodium nitroprusside for peripheral vasodilation and hyperkalemic cardiac arrest after the onset of ventricular fibrillation. When brain temperature reaches 16–18 °C, the circulation is arrested and blood is drained through the venous cannula until the neurovasculature appears relaxed and the aneurysm is then clipped. After rewarming, reversal of anticoagulation and separation from bypass, the thiopental infusion is stopped and the patient is mechanically ventilated overnight and extubated as soon as possible thereafter. Thiopental use has not been associated with difficulties in weaning from cardiopulmonary bypass.

Keywords: Cerebral aneurysm clipping; temporary vascular occlusion; cerebral protection; deep hypothermic circulatory arrest.

Introduction

The management of the patient with subarachnoid hemorrhage has evolved considerably in the past 10 years[59,61]. Anesthetic management of cerebral aneurysm clipping has also undergone significant evolution. This review will address some specific areas of this evolution.

Maintenance of a sufficiently low transmural pressure to prevent rupture of the aneurysm during surgical manipulation had been previously afforded by systemic hypotension. Recently, however, there has been a trend for increasing use of temporary vascular occlusion[6,31], thereby avoiding systemic hypotension in order to secure surgical control of anatomically difficult lesions.

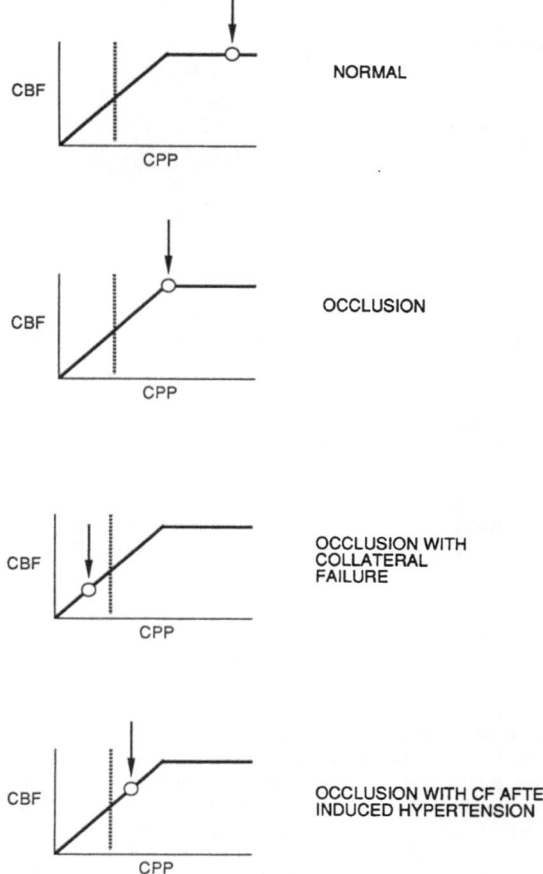

Fig. 1. Induced hypertension model. *Normal*. The arrow indicates the operating point on the autoregulatory curve; in this case, the circulatory bed is in the mid-position in the full range of autoregulation. The lower limit of autoregulation is the knee of the curve. The dotted vertical line represents the ischemic flow threshold. (For the sake of clarity, we have not indicated here whether or not this CBF level is in the penlucida or the penumbra range.) *The case of inflow occlusion*. If a major inflow channel to this vascular territory is interrupted, pressure will drop in the resistive bed. Autoregulatory function now adjusts for this decrease in input pressure by vasodilation of the bed. How much the pressure falls after the major inflow occlusion will be determined by number and calibre of available collateral vascular pathways. In the case labeled "occlusion," there is sufficient collateral perfusion pressure to maintain the operating point above the threshold for ischemia, although the operating point has entered the pressure-passive range (*i.e.*, this bed is maximally vasodilated). *The case of inflow occlusion with collateral failure*. Now we will assume that there is atresia or stenosis of the collateral pathways (high collateral resistance). With occlusion of the major inflow channel, the pressure drops to a much lower level distal to the occlusion. The CBF is lower, because the drop in pressure has exhausted the ability of the resistive bed to compensate by further vasodilation. Now the operating point is below the ischemic threshold. This situation is one that demands treatment. *Augmentation of collateral perfusion pressure*. At this point we increase systemic mean arterial pressure. The pressure transmitted across the collateral pathways, although not sufficient to restore normal pressure in the

This has the potential advantage of preventing ischemic complications in distant brain regions that may not autoregulate normally after subarachnoid hemorrhage (SAH). Furthermore, approximately 10% of intracranial aneurysms are classified as giant aneurysms (> 2.5 cm) which are difficult to clip with conventional surgical techniques. In such difficult settings, either temporary occlusion of parent vessels or clipping under deep hypothermic circulatory arrest are options which may be chosen by the surgeon. These techniques require some modification of the traditional anesthetic management of cerebral aneurysm clipping[11,79]. For example, during temporary vascular occlusion of a major intracranial artery, not only must systemic hypotension be avoided but blood pressure augmentation may be necessary[19,76,78]. General considerations for anesthesia are found in an accompanying article (David Stone, pp. 159–163).

This review will address some of the evolving issues in the intraoperative management of aneurysm clipping—including cerebral hemodynamic monitoring, induced hypertension and pharmacologic brain protective therapy—and discuss the management of hypothermic circulatory arrest.

Induced Hypertension

Cerebral autoregulation is impaired or lost during ischemia and CBF becomes pressure passive. Maintenance of a high collateral perfusion pressure, in concert with optimal viscosity and oxygen delivery, may reduce cell death in a threatened vascular territory. As reviewed by Young and Cole[78], there is ample experimental evidence for this strategy in terms of improvements in cerebral perfusion, electrophysiologic evoked responses, histopathological outcome and neurological outcome.

In a normal vascular bed, a decrease in input pressure elicits vasodilation of its resistance vessels; flow is thereby maintained and, if available, collateral irrigation is recruited. However, with maximal vasodilation, the remaining determinant of vascular resistance will be the length of conduit, if viscosity and pressure remain unchanged. Therefore, the areas furthest from

ischemic bed, is sufficient to raise input pressure to increase CBF just above the ischemic threshold (albeit still on the pressure-passive point on the curve). This small shift above the ischemic threshold may be crucial in determining the final extent of the infarct and the ultimate functional outcome following an ischemic event. (used with permission, *Clinical Neuroscience Lectures*, W. Young © 1991 Cathenart Publishing, Munster, IN)

the driving pressure (watershed regions) will be subject to the lowest effective tissue flows (distal field insufficiency). Blood pressure augmentation is useful to treat or prevent the development of cerebral ischemia when the normal hemodynamic mechanism (vasodilation) of maintaining tissue perfusion has been exhausted. By augmenting systemic perfusion pressure, one can decrease the pressure drop across a collateral pathway to an ischemic area (Fig. 1). Even small increases in CBF may shift a region from the penumbra (destined for infarction) to the penlucida and perhaps to a level of perfusion enabling normal function (Figs. 2 and 3). This has implications for patients with simple hemodynamic ischemia from vascular occlusion. It also applies to the treatment of symptomatic vasospasm from aneurysmal SAH, where an increase in the resistance of the conductance vessels is associated with compensatory peripheral vasodilation of the resistance bed.

Elevation of blood pressure during carotid endarterectomy has been accepted for some time[8,22,24]; many authors recommend keeping blood pressure elevated during the period of temporary occlusion of the carotid artery. Anastomotic cerebral perfusion pressure, as measured in the distal stump of the carotid artery after

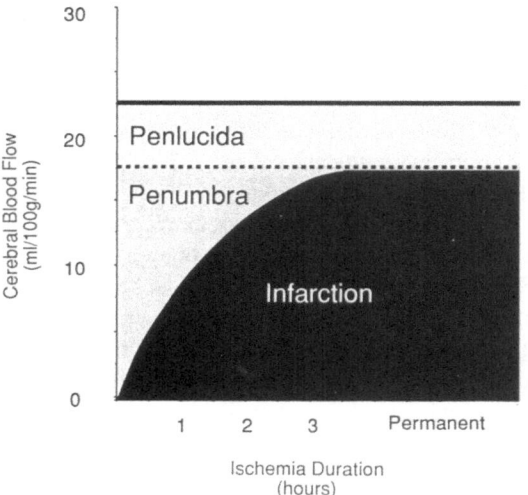

Fig. 2. Influence of degree and duration of ischemia on neuronal viability. Interaction of degree and duration of flow reductions are shown. Tissue receiving flow between approximately 18 and 23 ml/100 g/min is functionally inactive, but function can be restored at any time with reinstituation of increased perfusion (*penlucida*). For tissue perfused at lower levels, the development of infarction is a function of time. If tissue is restored to adequate perfusion before the time limit for infarction, it will recover function (*penumbra*) (adapted from data of Jones *et al.*[33], used with permission, *Clinical Neuroscience Lectures*, W. Young, © 1991 Cathenart Publishing, Munster, IN)

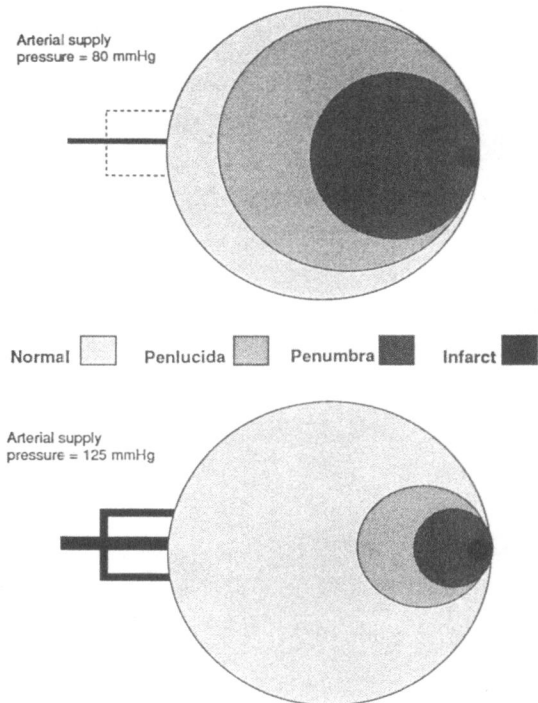

Normal ☐   Penlucida ☐   Penumbra ☐   Infarct ☐

Fig. 3. Effect of induced hypertension on distribution of penumbral tissue. In an underperfused circulatory bed at a normal mean arterial pressure (85 mm Hg in this example), there will be a zone of relative flow reductions. By increasing primary or collateral flow the zones may be shifted to improve neuronal salvage and prevent the original area of irreversible damage from extending (used with permission, *Clinical Neuroscience Lectures*, W. Young, © 1991 Cathenart Publishing, Munster, IN)

clamping, is increased by elevating systemic pressure[22,24], as is cerebral blood flow[8]. Phenylephrine-induced hypertension only minimally increases venous sinus pressure[24].

Induced hypertension has been used in the management of aneurysmal subarachnoid hemorrhage[4,34,44]. But in this circumstance, hypertension is employed in conjunction with hypervolemic-hemodilution; thus, the relative contribution made by increases in perfusion pressure elevation is not well defined. The subject of volume loading for aneurysmal subarachnoid hemorrhage is discussed in detail elsewhere[2,60].

Hazards of induced hypertension include the worsening of ischemic (vasogenic) edema and transforming a pale infarct into a hemorrhagic one. The hypertension must not exceed the limits of cerebral autoregulation in normal brain regions. If blood pressure is used to increase cerebral perfusion pressure (CPP) during brief periods of carotid or intracranial artery occlusion[8,79], these concerns are less important. Because pharmacologically-induced hypertension increases cardiac afterload and the risk of cardiac ischemia, careful cardiovascular monitoring is therefore essential. Phenylephrine is an attractive first choice because it does not increase heart rate.

Cerebral Protective Therapy During Temporary Occlusion

Pharmacologic

Planned surgical occlusion of a major intracranial artery is the ideal setting for application of pharmacologic brain protective therapy. The prototype for pharmacological agents that afford cerebral protection are the barbiturates[55]. The precise mechanism of action whereby barbiturates afford protective effects during cerebral ischemia has not been elucidated. Etomidate[6] and, more recently, propofol[37] are attractive alternatives, but the evidence for cerebral protection is not as compelling as for the barbiturates[51,77].

One of the mechanisms proposed for the salutary effects of barbiturates on focal ischemia has been the redistribution of CBF from normal to ischemic areas[9,46]. Barbiturates are not effective in preventing neurological damage after global cerebral ischemia[1,27]. This may be explained in part by the fact that it is not possible to enhance collateral circulation with a global insult. Other factors contributing to protective effects are their ability to depress $CMRO_2$ and their efficacy as anticonvulsive agents. Excepting cardiopulmonary bypass (CPB), human outcome studies are lacking[74]. Most authors would agree, however, barbiturates are to be recommended in the intraoperative setting of acute temporary focal ischemia.

Pharmacologic protection by thiopental during intracranial vascular occlusion in man has been described anecdotally by several authors during cerebral aneurysm clipping[57,58], during carotid endarterectomy[40] and during extracranial-intracranial shunting procedures[30,66]. There have been no randomized clinical studies documenting the efficacy of such high dose therapy.

Some centers routinely utilize a high-dose barbiturate technique to manage neurovascular procedures intraoperatively[68]. Most applications of barbiturates, however, are as a low single-dose treatment[40].

A perceived disadvantage of using barbiturates is cardiac depression. It does not appear to be a problem in the normovolemic patient with good cardiac function[69,70]. Delayed emergence will result from high-dose administration during neurosurgical or CPB procedures[45,58]. However, the relative "cost" of low doses (300–1000 mg) of barbiturates capable of producing EEG burst-suppression is minimal: a slightly drowsier patient on emergence.

In the case of occlusion during aneurysm clipping, a precise time of potential ischemia is known. A small dose of barbiturate capable of inducing EEG burst-suppression should offer protection during most short occlusion time. However, should occlusion become unexpectedly prolonged or a surgical catastrophe take place, the patient will have maximal drug protection already instituted. For example, during uncontrolled bleeding the surgeons may be forced to place clips blindly in an attempt to stem hemorrhage. In this event, barbiturate therapy would be continued and could be used as a means of or as an adjunct in the induction of mild or moderate temporary arterial blood pressure reduction until bleeding is brought under control. Systemic hypotension, with a vasodilator such as nitroprusside during such a setting of emergent intracranial vascular occlusion to control hemorrhage, invites catastrophe. The distal field of the occluded artery will have little or no opportunity to recruit collateral flow from neighboring (relatively vasodilated) arterial supply regions.

Use of nimodipine is now standard pharmacologic therapy for the aneurysmal subarachnoid hemorrhage patient. However, the prophylactic use of nimodipine in the intraoperative setting has not been systematically addressed, although there is much to recommend it. Preliminary studies suggest a blood-pressure lowering effect during anesthesia[71] that should be carefully weighed against its pharmacologic protective properties.

Hypocapnia

Hypocapnia is widely employed to decrease CBF, and hence cerebral blood volume, in an effort to prevent increases in intracranial pressure during the induction of anesthesia and to achieve intraoperative brain relaxation. The application of hypocapnia in neurosurgical patients is at present undergoing a reassessment and the issues need to be carefully laid out. It is probably true that *routine* application of moderate (23–25 mm Hg) hypocapnia may no longer be necessary for all patients undergoing craniotomy in terms of brain relaxation and, especially, intracranial pressure control. Use of moderate hypocapnia should be restricted to those patients with poorly controlled ICP before induction and those with "tight" brains intraoperatively. We prefer modest 28–32 mm Hg hypocapnia during craniotomy, but some centers use more normocapnic levels. With lumbar CSF pressure monitoring, use of $PaCO_2$ levels of approximately 36 mm Hg in aneurysm and tumor patients has not been associated with complications attributable to increased ICP (Patrick Ravussin, Personal Communication).

The use of hypocapnia, however, may significantly impact the patient with focal or regional cerebral ischemia. The concept that hypocapnia can favorably influence CBF during ischemia is not new[64,65], but not all investigators have been able to demonstrate favorable redistribution[20]. As reviewed by Artru[3], some of the early studies did not support a beneficial effect of hypocapnia, but utilized prolonged, severe ischemic models[39]. In addition, human studies showed trends for improved outcome with hypocapnia but probably lacked sufficient statistical power[5,17]. In the case of induced hypertension in the setting of carotid endarterectomy, there appears to be a distinct improvement in collateral perfusion pressure in the presence of hypocapnia[8,24,41,49,50]. Therefore, it is reasonable to consider hypocapnia as an adjunct to the therapy of regional cerebral ischemia if the clinical circumstances warrant it.

Modest Hypothermia

As discussed in an accompanying article (Young, pp. 159–163), modest reductions in temperature may have a strong neuroprotective effect[12–14], and probably influence neurologic outcome far more than choice of anesthetic drug[53]. The normal temperature decrease seen with induction of anesthesia should be allowed to persist (34–45 °C) throughout most of the procedure with active warming towards 37 °C to anticipate extubation of the trachea.

Monitoring for Cerebral Ischemia During Aneurysm Clipping

It is common to see neurological deficits wax and wane in the SAH patient with changes in systemic blood pressure[34,60]. In the intensive care unit, serial neurological examinations are a reasonable way to assess the need for, or the progress of, treatment of cerebral ischemia. Under anesthesia, however, the endpoint is blurry. It is therefore helpful to use some form of cerebral function monitoring. Unfortunately, the lack of sensitive and reliable means to rapidly assess the status of cerebral perfusion is a practical reality at the present time. What follows is a description of the currently available modalities for assessing CBF in a patient who comes to surgery for aneurysm clipping.

Electrophysiological Monitoring

Electrophysiological monitoring of cerebral function during aneurysm clipping has been advocated by many authors. Nevertheless, in spite of a large experience, there is no clear consensus on methods or reliability[10,16,21,25,26,28,29,32,36,38,42,43,52,54,73,75]. In addition, the sensitivity and specificity of somatosensory evoked potentials versus EEG continues to be debated[35].

Jones et al.[32] reported that the scalp-recorded EEG was not helpful for detecting localized intraoperative ischemic changes associated with vascular clipping and drug-induced hypotension. However, they concluded that the apparent insensitivity of the EEG to cerebral ischemia was probably due to the positioning of their recording electrodes at a distance from the surgical field beyond the area of localized ischemia. To overcome this problem, subdural electrode arrays developed for epilepsy monitoring may be used intraoperatively for EEG monitoring.

The middle cerebral artery (MCA) territory, which includes the lateral surfaces of the frontal and temporal lobes, forms the region at greatest risk for ischemia during temporary occlusion of the vessels in the carotid (anterior) circulation. Cortical electrodes are easily placed on these surfaces after pterional craniotomy, which is most commonly employed for aneurysm surgery on vessels of the anterior circulation. These electrode strips do not interfere with surgical access. It is particularly useful to have a sensitive electrode montage because the majority of EEG monitors currently available for use by anesthesiologists in the operating room have only 2–4 channels. Our experience indicates that localized ischemic changes may be detected using cortical electrodes, even during barbiturate-induced suppression-burst activity[79].

The aforementioned disadvantages of recording the EEG with conventional scalp electrodes during aneurysm surgery are compounded by the application of brain relaxation techniques that improve surgical access to the aneurysm. These include avoidance of cerebral vasodilators and the application of modest hypocapnia, osmotherapy, cerebrospinal fluid drainage and careful head positioning. The result of these maneuvers is to introduce a large air space between the dura and the arachnoid and to increase the distance between the scalp electrodes and the underlying cerebral cortex on the non-dependent side of the head. This causes a substantial attenuation and distortion of the EEG signal. These problems are eliminated by the use of cortical electrodes.

The major potential limitation of electrocorticography is that ischemia may not be detected if it is restricted to subcortical areas or cortical areas at a distance from the recording electrodes. The significance of this problem can only be determined by further studies examining the optimal recording derivations and number and placement of cortical electrodes required for the reliable detecting of ischemia.

Cerebral Hemodynamic Monitoring

Direct monitoring of cerebral perfusion during aneurysm surgery has for the most part been limited to a few experimental series[23,48]. The intraarterial 133-Xe CBF method has been used to monitor for ischemia during carotid endarterectomy, where there is direct access to the exposed carotid artery for isotope administration[72]. As reviewed by Carter[15] and discussed in an accompanying article (Young, pp. 159–163), direct cortical techniques for measuring local cortical CBF (1CoCBF) are relatively easy to use and provide on-line information.

Hypothermic Circulatory Arrest

Although advances in both neurosurgical and anesthetic techniques have considerably improved the surgical treatment of cerebral aneurysms[63], there remains a subset of patients in whom conventional approaches still carry an unacceptable morbidity and mortality. In selected cases, use of hypothermic circulatory arrest to tackle these and related lesions offers the chance of cure for an otherwise untreatable and highly morbid disease process. This idea is not new[18,47]. But recent advances in bypass technology and monitoring methodology have renewed interested in deep hypothermic circulatory arrest, especially with use of femoral-femoral CPB[7,56,67]. Solomon has recently reported our experience with this technique[62]; what follows is a general description of our anesthetic management.

A most daunting problem associated with this form of "high-tech" treatment is operating room logistics, both in terms of personnel and equipment. It requires

careful planning and excellent communication. This is so not only between all the specialists involved in the care of the patient – including anesthesiologist, neurosurgeon, neurologist, cardiac surgeon and cardiologist – but also in communicating with the nursing staff and, for example, with the engineering department to assess the power capabilities of the electrical circuits for the bevy of equipment that is used.

Typically, on a given day we have 2 attending anesthesiologists and a resident, the neurosurgeon and assistant, cardiac surgeon and assistant, 2 scrub nurses and 2 circulating nurses. Added to this, we have several other interested parties present, including perhaps the cardiologist, neurologist, and other curious OR staff and students. The cardiac surgery equipment and CPB system and the neurosurgical assemblage of various cauteries and microscope, coupled with our monitoring equipment and the need for 2 surgical instrument set-ups, strain the capacity of our largest operating rooms. To mesh all these staff and machines into a smoothly functioning unit takes some practice.

A thorough preoperative evaluation of the patient should include evaluation of cardiac disease; peripheral arterial and venous disease, which could contraindicate femoral cannulation; and esophageal disorders that might preclude transesophageal echocardiography (TEE). In particular, aortic valve function is carefully scrutinized. If the aortic valve is insufficient, median sternotomy and left ventricular venting are required for bypass. A history of aneurysm rupture and possible neurologic or cerebral autoregulatory dysfunction will influence blood pressure management intraoperatively.

Midazolam is used (up to 0.07 mg/kg) during pre-induction line placement. Anesthesia is induced with thiopental 4–6 mg/kg and fentanyl 30–50 µg/kg. Tracheal intubation is facilitated with vecuronium 0.3 mg/kg. Ventilation is adjusted to provide a $PaCO_2$ of 26–28 mm Hg isoflurane in oxygen (we avoid nitrous oxide), titrated to control blood pressure in the pre-operative range. If necessary, labetalol and esmolol are used to aggressively treat any intraoperative hypertension in the case of a recently ruptured aneurysm. After induction, a pulmonary artery catheter is inserted. Bladder and continuous spinal drainage catheters* are placed at this time. A transesophageal echocardiography

---

*Although the patient will be fully heparinized, we have had no problems with placement of a subarachnoid catheter. This is presumably related to the fact that it is both placed and removed in a state of normal coagulatory function, *i.e.*, the catheter is immobile during the period in which heparin is given and reversed with protamine.

(TEE) probe is also inserted (1) for assessment of ventricular volume and contractility, (2) to verify the proper position of bypass cannulae and (3) to monitor for ventricular distension during bypass. External defibrillator pads are placed on the chest and back.

The patient is positioned to allow access to the head as well as both inguinal regions and, if necessary, the chest for median sternotomy. The head is locked in rigid pin fixation. For most anterior circulation aneurysms, a standard pterional craniotomy is used; most of the vertebrobasilar lesions are reached through a unilateral suboccipital craniectomy. The head, neck, chest, abdomen and both groins are shaved and sterilely prepared. Temperature probes are placed against the tympanic membrane, nasopharynx, axilla and rectum. Scalp EEG is monitored using a 2-channel compressed spectral array device (Neurotrac, Interspect, Conshohocken PA). A single transcranial Doppler (TCD) probe is affixed to the temporal bone window contralateral to the operative site (Transpect, Medasonics, Fremont, CA). Flow velocities in the contralateral MCA are monitored continuously throughout the procedure. Finally, scintillation detectors for measuring ^{133}Xe CBF are placed.

After dural opening, a cortical temperature probe is placed and a strip of cortical electrodes are placed on the frontal cortex in the middle cerebral artery (or, occasionally, anterior cerebral artery) distribution[79].

During craniotomy and dural opening, platelet-rich plasma and RBCs are harvested for post-bypass reinfusion and volume is replaced with albumin. Mannitol (1 g/kg) is given for brain relaxation. During this period just prior to CPB we institute thiopental loading. While continuously monitoring the raw EEG signal, thiopental is titrated in 100 mg boluses to achieve a 1:5 burst-suppression pattern which is maintained with a continuous infusion. Once cooling begins, the infusion is left constant at the normothermic rate. During circulatory arrest the infusion is interrupted, and then begun again during rewarming at the same rate.

With attention to hemostasis, the aneurysm is dissected free as much as possible during spontaneous circulation. About two hours after the craniotomy begins, CPB is established. The common femoral artery and vein are then cannulated at the inguinal ligament and the position of the venous cannula at the level of the right atrium is confirmed with TEE. After a temperature probe is placed directly into the brain parenchyma, heparin is given.

Arterial and venous Biomedicus centrifugal CPB pumps are used in conjunction with a membrane oxygenator. Fluid loading and a nitroprusside infusion help to maintain bypass flow at 2.5 L/min/m$_2$. Cooling begins after adequate flow is achieved (if flow is inadequate, median sternotomy may be performed and central access to the circulation obtained). Hypothermia is induced by passing extracorporeal perfusate through a Sarns TCM water bath heat exchanger. Ventricular fibrillation often occurs when perfusate temperature decreases below 28 °C; KCl in 20 mEq boluses is given through the right atrial port of the pulmonary artery catheter to achieve asystole. Usually 40–80 mEq is sufficient.

When brain temperature reaches 15 °C, the circulation is arrested and blood is drained through the venous cannula until the neurovasculature appears relaxed. Too much drainage can result in a negative pressure gradient with the consequences of air embolism and perhaps the tearing of small fragile perforating vessels emanating from the aneurysm dome or parent vessels. An occasional beat occurs even during circulatory arrest. This can be a real problem if the cardiac ejection causes significant vascular movement in the operative field. TEE is critical to monitor for LV distension during bypass.

After circulatory arrest, aneurysm clipping may proceed. After the aneurysm is secured, pressure and flow are slowly re-established to test the repair with the perfusate held at brain temperature. Phenylephrine may even be used at this point. If a further period of circulatory arrest is deemed necessary, hypothermic flow is continued at the systemic venous O_2 saturation to the pre-arrest level. We consider a continuous period of 45 minutes to be safe, but shorter periods are usually employed. When the neurosurgeon feels optimal clip placement has been achieved, CPB is resumed and rewarming commences by setting the water bath to 37 °C.

Nitroprusside is used to facilitate rewarming and control arterial vascular resistance. Spontaneous cardiac rhythm usually occurs between 20 and 26 °C. If present, ventricular fibrillation is electrically cardioverted. Inotropes are rarely needed to wean the patient from CPB. After separation from CPB, heparin is reversed with protamine. The pump perfusate is concentrated and transfused after CPB. Only rarely do we need to give exogenous blood.

The patient is transported to the intensive care unit with cardiovascular monitoring. The thiopental infusion is stopped but neither narcotic nor muscle relaxants are reversed. The patients are kept intubated and mechanically ventilated for the first post-operative night and then until clinically appropriate. The uncomplicated patient is extubated the next morning. A rebound hyperthermia is often seen during the first 24 hours. In light of recent evidence concerning temperature and the outcome from cerebral ischemia, strict control of fever seems prudent.

The primary anesthetic goals of this procedure are to provide anesthesia for the safe conduct of CPB and at the same time to tailor the anesthetic management to provide for a high likelihood of cerebral ischemia. Fortunately, most patients we have treated have had generally sound cardiovascular systems, making management of CPB relatively uncomplicated.

The mechanisms of cerebral injury in this setting are similar to those seen when circulatory arrest is used for cardiac lesions, with some modification. The ability of deep hypothermia to afford protection during circulatory arrest is well-documented. As is the case during routine CPB, there is also the possibility of focal cerebral ischemia from various embolic sources including gas, blood products and vascular wall debris. The time of maximal vulnerability for the occurrence seems to be before cooling and after re-warming.

In addition to the above considerations, we are faced with the possibility of focal cerebral ischemia as a result of brain retraction and interruption of small end-arteries by dissection or clip placement. Furthermore, there may be areas of disturbed cerebral autoregulation if the patient has undergone a recent subarachnoid hemorrhage, even if the patient is not overtly symptomatic. If such focal areas of cerebral ischemia exist, a particularly vulnerable period is during rewarming. Nitroprusside accelerates rewarming, but a lower-than-normal systemic cerebral perfusion pressure, coupled with a potential for nitroprusside-induced cerebral vasodilation**, may place at risk ischemic areas dependent on collateral perfusion pressure. The interaction of the period of hypothermic arrest and brain

regions previously damaged from a presenting subarachnoid hemorrhage is unknown. Although most centers maintain relatively low mean arterial pressures during rewarming after routine CPB, it is probably wise to keep cerebral perfusion pressure in the normal range in the patient having suffered a recent hemorrhage and certainly in those patients with evidence of vasospasm or frank ischemia pre-operatively.

Barbiturate use is aimed at affording some modicum of protection for these potential areas of focal cerebral ischemia, both permanent (vessel interruption) and transient (retraction, hypotension). We have encountered no problems with significant systemic cardiovascular depression secondary to thiopental use[69,70]. We monitor the cerebral circulation closely. The EEG is used for thiopental titration and detection of ischemia. The TCD and ^{133}Xe CBF are useful as general monitors of cerebral perfusion and may be useful in the detection of post-circulatory arrest global cerebral hyper- or hypoperfusion. Evoked potentials may be of use in monitoring procedures involving posterior circulation lesions[67].

Acknowledgements

We thank Eugene Ornstein, Ph.D., M.D. for review of and Joyce Ouchi for her assistance in preparation of the manuscript.

References

1. Abramson NS (1986) Randomized clinical study of thiopental loading in comatose survivors of cardiac arrest. N Engl J Med 314: 397–441
2. Archer DP, Shaw DA, Leblanc RL, Tranmer BI (1991) Haemodynamic considerations in the management of patients with subarachnoid haemorrhage (Review article). Can J Anaesth 38: 454–470
3. Artru AA, Merriman HG (1989) Hypocapnia added to hypertension to reverse EEG changes during carotid endarterectomy (Case report). Anesthesiology 70: 1016–1018
4. Awad IA, Carter LP, Spetzler RF, Medina M, Williams Fred W J (1987) Clinical vasospasm after subarachnoid hemorrhage: response to hypervolemic hemodilution and arterial hypertension. Stroke 18: 365–372
5. Baker WH, Rodman JA, Barnes RW, Hoyt JL (1976) An evaluation of hypocarbia and hypercarbia during carotid endarterectomy. Stroke 7: 451–454
6. Batjer HH, Frankfurt AI, Purdy PD, Smith SS, Samson DS (1988) Use of etomidate, temporary arterial occlusion, and intraoperative angiography in surgical treatment of large and giant cerebral aneurysms. J Neurosurg 68: 234–240
7. Baumgartner WA, Silverberg GD, Ream AK, Jamieson SW, Tarabek J, Reitz BA (1983) Reappraisal of cardiopulmonary bypass with deep hypothermia and circulatory arrest for complex neurosurgical operations. Surgery 94: 242–249

**This is controversial; for a lucid discussion of the topic, see Michenfelder JM (1988) Anesthesia and the brain. Churchill Livingstone, New York, pp 155–159. Vasoactive agents may affect different aspects of autoregulatory behavior, as illustrated by recent evidence that nitroprusside impairs the ability of the circulation to maintain CBF when CPP is lowered but not when CPP is increased (Stange K, Lagerkranser M, Sollevi A (1991) Nitroprusside-induced hypotension and cerebrovascular autoregulation in the anesthetized pig. Anesth Analg 73: 745–752)

8. Boysen G, Engell HC, Henriksen H (1972) The effect of induced hypertension on internal carotid artery pressure and regional cerebral blood flow during temporary carotid clamping for endarterectomy. Neurology 22: 1133–1144

9. Branston NM, Hope DT, Symon L (1979) Barbiturates in focal ischemia of primate cortex: effects on blood flow distribution, evoked potential and extracellular potassium. Stroke 10: 647–653

10. Buchthal A, Belopavlovic M, Mooij JJA (1988) Evoked potential monitoring and temporary clipping in cerebral aneurysm surgery. Acta Neurochir (Wien) 93: 28–36

11. Buckland MR, Batjer HH, Giesecke AH (1988) Anesthesia for cerebral aneurysm surgery: use of induced hypertension in patients with symptomatic vasospasm. Anesthesiology 69: 116–119

12. Busto R, Dietrich WD, Globus MY-T, Ginsberg MD (1989) The importance of brain temperature in cerebral ischemic injury. Stroke 20: 1113–1114

13. Busto R, Dietrich WD, Globus My-T, Valdes I, Scheinberg P, Ginsberg MD (1987) Small differences in intraischemic brain temperature critically determine the extent of ischemic neuronal injury. J Cereb Blood Flow Metab 7: 729–738

14. Busto R, Globus MY-T, Dietrich WD, Martinez E, Valdes I, Ginsberg MD (1989) Effect of mild hypothermia on ischemia-induced release of neurotransmitters and free fatty acids in rat brain. Stroke 20: 904–910

15. Carter LP (1991) Surface monitoring of cerebral cortical blood flow. Cerebrovasc Brain Metab Rev 3: 246–261

16. Carter LP, Raudzens PA, Gaines C, Crowell RM (1984) Somatosensory evoked potentials and cortical blood flow during craniotomy far vascular disease. Neurosurgery 15: 22–28

17. Christensen MS, Paulson OB, Olesen J, et al (1973) Cerebral apoplexy (stroke) treated with or without prolonged artificial hyperventilation: 1. cerebral circulation, clinical course, and cause of death. Stroke 4: 568–619

18. Drake CG, Barr HWK, Coles JC, Gergely NF (1964) The use of extracorporeal circulation and profound hypothermia in the treatment of ruptured intracranial aneurysm. J Neurosurg 21: 575–581

19. Drummond JC (1991) Deliberate hypotension for intracranial aneurysm surgery: changing practices (Letter to the editor). Can J Anaesth 38: 935–936

20. Drummond JC, Ruta TS, Cole DJ, Zornow MH, Shapiro HM (1989) The effect of hypocapnia on cerebral blood flow distribution during middle cerebral artery occlusion in the rat. J Neurosurg Anesth 1: 163–164

21. Ducati A, Landi A, Cenzato M, et al (1988) Monitoring of brain function by means of evoked potentials in cerebral aneurysm surgery. Acta Neurochir (Wien) [Suppl] 42: 8–13

22. Ehrenfeld WK, Hamilton FN, Larson CP Jr, Hickey RF, Severinghaus JW (1970) Effect of CO_2 and systemic hypertension on downstream cerebral arterial pressure during carotid endarterectomy. Surgery 67: 87–96

23. Farrar JK, Gamache FW Jr, Ferguson GG, Barker J, Varkey GP, Drake CG (1981) Effects of profound hypotension on cerebral blood flow during surgery for intracranial aneurysms. J Neurosurg 55: 857–864

24. Fourcade HE, Larson CP Jr, Ehrenfield WK, Newton TH (1970) The effects of CO_2 and systemic hypertension on cerebral perfusion pressure during carotid endarterectomy. Anesthesiology 33: 383–390

25. Friedman WA, Chadwick GM, Verhoeven FJS, Mahla M, Day AL (1991) monitoring of somatosensory evoked potentials during surgery for middle cerebral artery aneurysms. Neurosurgery 29: 83–88

26. Friedman WA, Kaplan BL, Day AL, Sypert GW, Curran MT (1987) Evoked potential monitoring during aneurysm operation: onservations after fifty cases. Neurosurgery 20: 678–687

27. Gisvold SE, Safar P, Hendrickx HHL, Rao G, Moossy J, Alexander H (1984) Thiopental treatment after global brain ischemia in pigtailed monkeys. Anesthesiology 60: 88–96

28. Greenberg RP, Fleischer AS (1983) Intraoperative monitoring of brain function with evoked potentials during neurosurgical procedures. Ariz Med 40: 389–392

29. Grundy BL, Nelson PB, Lina A, Heros RC (1982) Monitoring of cortical somatosensory evoked potentials to determine the safety of sacrificing the anterior cerebral artery. Neurosurgery 11: 64–67

30. Hoff JT (1986) Cerebral protection (Review article). J Neurosurg 65: 579–591

31. Jabre A, Symon L (1987) Temporary vascular occlusion during aneurysm surgery. Surg Neurol 27: 47–63

32. Jones TH, Chiappa KH, Young RR, Ojemann RG, Crowell RM (1979) EEG monitoring for induced hypotension for surgery of intracranial aneurysms. Stroke 10: 292–294

33. Jones TH, Morawetz RB, Crowell RM, et al (1981) Thresholds of focal cerebral ischemia in awake monkeys. J Neurosurg 54: 773–782

34. Kassell NF, Peerless SJ, Durward QJ, Beck DW, Drake CG, Adams HP (1982) Treatment of ischemic deficits from vasospasm with intravascular volume expansion and induced arterial hypertension. Neurosurgery 11: 337–343

35. Kearse LA Jr, Brown EN, McPeck K (1992) Somatosensory evoked potentials sensitivity relative to electroencephalography for cerebral ischemia during carotid endarterectomy. Stroke 23: 498–505

36. Kidooka M, Nakasu Y, Watanabe K, Matsuda M, Handa J (1987) Monitoring of somatosensory-evoked potentials during aneurysm surgery. Surg Neurol 27: 69–76

37. Kochs E, Hoffman WE, Werner C, Thomas C, Albrecht RF, Schulte am Esch J (1992) The effects of propofol on brain electrical activity, neurologic outcome, and neuronal damage following incomplete ischemia in rats. Anesthesiology 76: 245–252

38. McPherson RW, Niedermeyer EF, Otenasek RJ, Hanley DF (1983) Correlation of transient neurological deficit and somatosensory evoked potentials after intracranial aneurysm surgery. J Neurosurg 59: 146–149

39. Michenfelder JD, Sundt TM Jr (1973) The effect of $PaCO_2$ on the metabolism of ischemic brain in squirrel monkeys. Anesthesiology 38: 445–453

40. Moffat JA, McDougall MJ, Brunet D, et al (1983) Thiopental bolus during carotid endarterectomy–rational drug therapy? Can Anaesth Soc J 30: 615–622

41. Mohr LL, Smith LL, Hinshaw DB (1976) Blood gas and carotid pressure: Factors in stroke risk. Ann Surg 184: 723–727

42. Momma F, Wang AD, Symon L (1987) Effects of temporary arterial occlusion on somatosensory evoked responses in aneurysm surgery. Surg Neurol 27: 343–352

43. Mooji JJA, Buchthal A, Belopavlovic M (1987) Somatosensory evoked potential monitoring of temporary middle cerebral artery occlusion during aneurysm operation. Neurosurgery 21: 492–496

44. Muizelaar JP, Becker D (1986) Induced hypertension for the treatment of cerebral ischemia after subarachnoid hemorrhage. Surg Neurol 25: 317–325

45. Nussmeier NA, Arlund C, Slogoff S (1986) Neuropsychiatric complications after cardiopulmonary bypass: cerebral protection by a barbiturate. Anesthesiology 64: 165–170

46. Ochiai C, Asano T, Takakura K, Fukuda T, Horizoe H, Morimoto Y (1982) Mechanisms of cerebral protection by pento-

barbital and nizofenone correlated with the course of local cerebral blood flow changes. Stroke 13: 788–795

47. Patterson RH, Ray BS (1962) Profound hypothermia for intracranial surgery: laboratory and clinical experiences with extracorporeal circulation by peripheral cannulation. Ann Surg 156: 377–393

48. Pickard JD, Matheson M, Patterson J, Wyper D (1980) Prediction of late ischemic complications after cerebral aneurysm surgery by the intraoperative measurement of cerebral blood flow. J Neurosurg 53: 305–308

49. Pistolese GR, Citone G, Faraglia V, et al (1971) Effects of hypercapnia on cerebral blood flow during the clamping of the carotid arteries in surgical management of cerebrovascular insufficiency. Neurology 21: 95–100

50. Pistolese GR, Faraglia V, Agnoli A, et al (1972) Cerebral hemispheric "counter-steal" phenomenon during hyperventilation in cerebrovascular diseases. Stroke 3: 456–461

51. Ridenour TR, Warner DS, Todd MM, Gionet TX (1992) Comparative effects of propofol and halothane on outcome from temporary middle cerebral artery occlusion in the rat. Anesthesiology 76: 807–812

52. Rosenstein J, Wang AD-J, Symon L, Suzuki M (1985) Relationship between hemispheric cerebral blood flow, central conduction time, and clinical grade in aneurysmal subarachnoid hemorrhage. J Neurosurg 62: 25–30

53. Sano T, Drummond JC, Patel PM, Grafe MR, Watson JC, Cole DJ (1992) A comparison of the cerebral protective effects of isoflurane and mild hypothermia in a model of incomplete forebrain ischemia in the rat. Anesthesiology 76: 221–228

54. Schramm J, Koht A, Schmidt G, Pechstein U, Taniguchi M, Fahlbusch R (1990) Surgical and electrophysiological observations during clipping of 134 aneurysms with evoked potential monitoring. Neurosurgery 26: 61–70

55. Shapiro HM (1985) Barbiturates in brain ischaemia. Br J Anaesth 57: 82–95

56. Silverberg GD, Reitz BA, Ream AK (1981) Hypothermia and cardiac arrest in the treatment of giant aneurysms of the cerebral circulation and hemangioblastoma of the medulla. J Neurosurg 55: 337–346

57. Smith AL, Hoff JT, Nielsen SL, Larson CP (1974) Barbiturate protection in acute focal cerebral ischemia. Stroke 5: 1–7

58. Sokoll MD, Kassell NF, Davies LR (1982) Large dose thiopental anesthesia for intracranial aneurysm surgery. Neurosurgery 10: 555–562

59. Solomon RA, Fink ME, Lennihan L (1988) Early aneurysm surgery and prophylactic hypervolemic hypertensive therapy for the treatment of aneurysmal subarachnoid hemorrhage. Neurosurgery 23: 699–704

60. Solomon RA, Fink ME, Lennihan L (1988) Prophylactic volume expansion therapy for the prevention of delayed cerebral ischemia after early aneurysm surgery. Arch Neurol 45: 325–332

61. Solomon RA, Onesti ST, Klebanoff L (1991) Relationship between the timing of aneurysm surgery and the development of delayed cerebral ischemia. J Neurosurg 75: 56–61

62. Solomon RA, Smith C, Young WL, Stone JG, Fink M (1991) Deep hypothermic circulatory arrest for the management of complex anterior and posterior circulation aneurysms (Poster no. 1016). Am Assoc Neurolog Surg Ann Mtg

63. Solomon RA, Smith CR, Raps EC, Young WL, Stone JG, Fink

ME (1991) Deep hypothermic circulatory arrest for the management of complex anterior and posterior circulation aneurysms. Neurosurgery 29: 732–738

64. Soloway M, Moriarty G, Fraser JG, White RJ (1971) Effect of delayed hyperventilation on experimental cerebral infarction. Neurology 21: 479–485

65. Soloway M, Nadel W, Albin MS, White RJ (1968) The effect of hyperventilation on subsequent cerebral infarction. Anesthesiology 29: 975–980

66. Spetzler RF, Hadley MN (1989) Protection against cerebral ischemia: The role of barbiturates. Cerebrovasc Brain Metab Rev 1: 212–229

67. Spetzler RF, Hadley MN, Rigamonti D, et al (1988) Aneurysms of the basilar artery treated with circulatory arrest, hypothermia, and barbiturate cerebral protection. J Neurosurg 68: 868–879

68. Spetzler RF, Martin NA, Carter LP, Flom RA, Raudzens PA, Wilkinson E (1987) Surgical management of large AVM's by staged embolization and operative excision. J Neurosurg 67: 17–28

69. Stone JG, Young WL, Khambatta HJ, et al (1991) Effect of massive intraoperative thiopental loading on cardiovascular hemodynamics and myocardial performance (Case report). J Neurosurg Anesth 3: 132–135

70. Stone JG, Young WL, Marans ZS, et al (1993) Cardiac performance preserved despite thiopental loading. Anesthesiology 79: 36–41

71. Stullken EH, Johnston WE, Prough DS, Balestrieri EF, McWhorter JM (1985) Implications of nimodipine prophylaxis on cerebral vasospasm on anesthetic management during intracranial aneurysm clipping. J Neurosurg 62: 200–205

72. Sundt TM, Sharbrough FW, Piepgras DG, Kearns TP, Messick JM, O'Fallon WM (1981) Correlation of cerebral blood flow and electroencephalographic changes during carotid endarterectomy. Mayo Clinic Proc 56: 533–543

73. Symon L, Wang AD, Costa e Silva IE, Gentili F (1984) Perioperative use of somatosensory evoked responses in aneurysm surgery. J Neurosurg 60: 269–275

74. Todd MM, Hindman BJ, Warner DS (1991) Barbiturate protection and cardiac surgery: a different result (Editorial). Anesthesiology 74: 402–405

75. Wang AD, Cone J, Symon L, Costa e Silva IE (1984) Somatosensory evoked potential monitoring during the management of aneurysmal SAH. J Neurosurg 60: 264–268

76. Wasnick JD, Conlay LA (1990) Induced hypertension for cerebral aneurysm surgery in a patient with carotid occlusive disease. Anesth Analg 70: 331–333

77. Watson JC, Drummond JC, Patel PM, Sano T, Akrawi W, U HS (1992) An assessment of the cerebral protective effects of etomidate in a model of incomplete forebrain ischemia in the rat. Neurosurgery 30: 540–544

78. Young WL, Cole DJ (1993) Deliberate hypertension: Rationale and application for augmenting cerebral blood flow. Problems in Anesthesia 7: 140–153

79. Young WL, Solomon RA, Pedley TA, et al (1989) Direct cortical EEG monitoring during temporary vascular occlusion for cerebral aneurysm surgery. Anesthesiology 71: 794–799

Correspondence: William L. Young, M.D., Neuroanesthesia-Room 901, 161 Ft. Washington Ave., New York, NY 10032, U.S.A.

Total Intravenous Anesthesia Using Propofol for Burst Suppression in Cerebral Aneurysm Surgery: Preliminary Report of 44 Cases

N. de Tribolet and **P. Ravussin**[1]

Departments of Neurosurgery and [1]Anesthesiology, Centre Hospitalier Universitaire Vaudois, Lausanne, Switzerland

Summary

Forty-four patients underwent cerebral aneurysm clipping at our institution in 1991, 37 with a ruptured and 7 with an unruptured aneurysm. Preoperatively 30 patients with a ruptured aneurysm were graded I–II according to the World Federation of Neurosurgical Societies (WFNS) and 27 were operated on the first day. All underwent a standard cerebral protective general anesthesia, combining propofol with fentanyl, arterial normotension (mild hypertension with volume loading and/or dopamine during temporary clipping and once the aneurysm was secured), normocarbia or slight hypocarbia, brain relaxation with lumbar drainage, mannitol and propofol, and EEG burst suppression when temporary clipping (≥ 2 min) was required. After clipping, the propofol dose-rate was reduced to allow early recovery and neurological examination in the operating room. In 22 patients temporary clipping was required for a mean duration ($\pm$ SEM) of 7.2 ± 0.6 min (range 2–29); none of these patients deteriorated as compared to their preoperative neurological state. Twenty-six out of the 44 patients had a Glasgow Coma Outcome Score (GOS) of 1, 7 patients had a GOS of 2, 8 of 3, and 3 of 5. 34 patients were extubated in the operating room and 10 later in the ICU. In conclusion, a propofol technique for maintenance and burst suppression in cerebral aneurysm clipping procedures, together with arterial hypertension when indicated, seems to be a worthy alternative to the classical isoflurane-hypertensive technique.

Keywords: Aneurysm clipping; burst suppression; cerebral protection; propofol.

Introduction

During cerebral aneurysm clipping, several anesthetic aims are to be achieved 1) arterial normotension or even hypertension specially when temporary vessel occlusion is applied by the surgeon, 2) normocarbia (at least no deep hypocarbia), 3) a certain degree of brain protection through a decreased $CMRO_2$ when an EEG status of burst suppression is obtained, 4) rapid recovery in the operating room for early postoperative neurological examination and 5) a slack brain in order to decrease the use of brain retractors during surgery. In preference to the "hypertensive" isoflurane technique proposed recently[1], and because of the good results obtained with propofol in neuroanesthesia for tumor resection[2], a total intravenous technique using propofol together with EEG burst suppression was selected for evaluation in 1991 for our neurovascular procedures.

Methods and Material

44 patients underwent aneurysm clipping in 1991 at the CHUV and were all included in the protocol after informed consent and institutional ethical approval. 37 patients had a ruptured aneurysm (5 with 1–3 associated aneurysms), 27 of them were operated on within 24 hours and 10 within the 2nd–6th day after hemorrhage. 7 patients had an unruptured aneurysm of which 4 were giant (sylvian, basilar, and 2 ophthalmic).

Monitoring consisted of arterial blood pressure (via the radial or femoral artery), central venous pressure (PCWP in grade III WFNS patients), SaO_2, $P_{ET}CO_2$, ICP via a lumbar spinal needle (also placed for removal of CSF if a ventricular drain was not in place), and EEG via continuous display of the compressed spectral array (CSA) of a Neurotrac (Interspec, USA) device. The anesthetic technique combined propofol as a continuous infusion for induction titrated to the loss of eyelash reflex (1.8 ± 0.1 mg/kg within 3 min in order to maintain a CCP > 75 mmHg) and maintenance (86 ± 3.5 µg/kg/min aiming for 95% of the CSA activity below 12 Hz), lidocaine 1.5 mg/kg, fentanyl 1.8 ± 0.12 µg/kg/h for induction and maintenance, vecuronium bromide for muscle relaxation, mild hyperventilation to a $PaCO_2$ of 36 mmHg, and mannitol 0.75 g/kg to promote brain relaxation. 4 mg/kg of methylprednisolone were given to all patients as well as 10 mg/kg of prophylactic phenytion, and 1.5 mg/h of nimodipine.

In 22 patients, on 27 occasions, just before and during prolonged temporary clipping of both ACA's, the ICA or the MCA and its branches for 2–37 min (mean 7.2 ± 0.6 min), burst suppression was obtained by increasing the propofol infusion rate and MAP was increased to 100 mmHg with volume and/or dopamine 3–7 µg/kg/min. Once the aneurysm was clipped, circulatory blood volume was increased with colloids and NaCl 0.9% up to a filling pressure of 15 mmHg, and MAP was increased to over 100 mmHg.

Results

Preoperatively 30 patients with a ruptured aneurysm were in grades I and II according to the World Federation of Neurosurgical Societies (WFNS) and remained so on recovery; 5 were in grade III and remained so on recovery. Among them, 8 patients developed symptomatic vasospasm later on, reversed by hypervolemic hypertensive therapy. 2 patients were in grade IV and died 2 and 3 days postoperatively. The 7 patients with an unruptured aneurysm had no post-operative deficit. None of the 22 patients who underwent prolonged temporary clipping (≥ 2 min) were aggravated post-operatively. At the end of surgery 34 patients were extubated in the operating room, 8 patients later in the ICU.

Discussion

Propofol maintains cerebral autoregulation and provokes no cerebrovasodilatation[2,3]. For this reason a total intravenous anesthesia technique with propofol and fentanyl, combining arterial normotension (or even hypertension during temporary clipping), normocarbia or slight hypocarbia, brain relaxation through mannitol and propofol, and the use, when indicated, of burst suppression, appears to be a valuable alternative to the standard deep isoflurane-fentanyl technique specially when the latter is used with arterial hypertension[1].

References

1. Meyer FB, Muzzi DA (1992) Cerebral protection during aneurysm surgery with isoflurane anesthesia. J Neurosurg 76: 541–543
2. Ravussin PA, Tempelhoff R, Modica PA, Berger M (1991) Propofol versus thiopental-isoflurane for neurosurgical anesthesia: comparison of hemodynamics, CSF pressure and recovery. J Neurosurg Anesth 3: 85–95
3. Van Hemelrijck J, Fitch W, Mattheussen M, Van Aken H, Plets C, Lauwers T (1990) Effect of propofol on cerebral circulation and autoregulation in the baboon. Anesth Analg 71: 49–54

Correspondence: Nicolas de Tribolet, M.D., Department of Neurosurgery, Centre Hospitalier Universitaire Vaudois, CH-1011 Lausanne, Switzerland.

Temporary Clipping in Aneurysm Surgery

L. Symon

Gough-Cooper Department of Neurological Surgery, Institute of Neurology, National Hospital for Neurology and Neurosurgery, Queen Square, London, U.K.

Summary

The accumulated experience of aneurysm surgery since the Second World War and most particularly of aneurysm surgery since the advent of the operating microscope is that the key to successful management of these patients is complete obliteration of the aneurysm neck. Careful dissection at open surgery remains the keystone.

Keywords: Aneurysm; temporary clip; collateral circulation.

Introduction

During aneurysm dissection premature rupture of the sac may be inevitable and can lead to considerable difficulty, especially at an early stage of the operation when the aneurysm is not yet adequately exposed[14,17]. Direct pressure or suction may not always be effective in control of the haemorrhage, and hurried dissection can result in serious injury to vital structures. Commonly used techniques to assist control of haemorrhage in these circumstances may involve profound reduction in systemic arterial pressure; an attractive alternative is acute reduction in focal blood pressure by the use of proximal vascular occlusions. In early years compression of the carotid artery in the neck by the anaesthetist might be employed, but with the development of the microscope and modern clips, temporary proximal arterial occlusion is once again available. An early pioneer of the use of temporary clips was Lawrence Pool[23], who reported in 1961 a series of 23 cases in which temporary clips had been used during extensive bifrontal approaches to anterior communicating aneurysms. He reported a mortality rate in this series of only 7.7%, but this initial experience was not repeated in other hands and the technique did not gain general acceptance. Reduction of either focal or systemic perfusion pressure, moreover, carries the risk of damaging ischemia in the territory distal to the occlusion. Scanning electron and transmission microscopy has shown evident arterial and endothelial damage with a potential area of postoperative thrombosis at the site of clamps[1,7,9-13,15,20,24,26,35]. As a result temporary clips, which some have regarded as fairly routine[28,29,30], have been avoided by many except in cases of profound emergency[20].

Others have suggested profound hypotension and suction as adequate in the control of any hemorrhage during dissection[22].

In the dissection of awkward necks, clarity of vision, reduction in tension in the sac, and the capacity to open the sac and evacuate a troublesome clot render more complete occlusion of the aneurysm possible[32]. The hazards of incomplete occlusion of aneurysm necks have been well emphasized[8], with subsequent enlargement of residual aneurysm or even the development of a one-way valve system with progressive expansion and rupture being accepted risks.

Since the late 1970's elective temporary occlusion has been used in a proportion of aneurysmal operations, and this review attempts to determine the impact of such temporary arterial occlusion on clinical outcome.

Clinical Material and Methods

A first study reported in *Surgical Neurology* in 1987 included 66 patients who underwent temporary arterial occlusion of main cerebral branches during surgical treatment of their aneurysm. Since then a further 140 patients have been operated on in 90 of whom temporary vascular occlusion has been used. The age of the patients has varied from the youngest of 8 to the oldest of 79, two-thirds of them presented after recent cerebral subarachnoid haemorrhage. Over 90% of those with recent haemorrhage were operated on in Hunt and Hess Grades 1 through 3[16] and the standard practice in the clinic is to operate as early as possible usually within the first five days of haemorrhage. Ultra early operation within 48 hours is not usually possible in our clinic which is a secondary referral centre and

Table 1. *Preoperative Clinical Grade of Patients Who Presented with Subarachnoid Haemorrhage (from Jabre and Symon 1987)*[18].

Grade	Number of patients
1	18
2	10
3	23
4	4
Total	55

over the years less than 5% of patients have been operated on in the first 48 hours.

In aneurysm surgery the surgeon's experience is often an important factor influencing the results of the operation and the prognosis of the patient. All patients in this review were operated on by the same surgeon (L.S.), providing homogenous data with respect to surgical technique. All aneurysms, except for the pericallosal artery aneurysms, were approached through a standard frontotemporal pterional craniotomy. Aneurysms of the middle cerebral artery were approached through the superior temporal gyrus, and those of the basilar tip by an anterior temporal route[31-34].

Anaesthesia was induced with 5% thiopentone 7 mg/kg after oxygenation. Intubation and artificial ventilation were facilitated by 75–100 mg of succinylcholine and tubocurarine. Anaesthesia was maintained using halothan or isoflurane in a gas mixture of 50% oxygen and 50% nitrous oxide. During dissection of the aneurysm, moderate hypotension to a mean pressure around 70 mmHg was obtained by adjusting the volatile agent, halothane or isoflurane, and adding beta-blockade as necessary. PCO_2 was kept in the range of 30–32 mmHg.

Temporary arterial occlusion was achieved in all cases with a Scoville clip (Down Bros and Phelps Ltd., London, and Codman and Shurtleff Inc., Boston, Massachusetts) a torsion bar spring aneurysm clip, specifically designed for temporary or permanent use[4,25]. Pressure at the blade tip is 75–80 g, with a maximum blade opening of 4–6 mm[27]. The inner surface of the blade is serrated. Where necessary, curved Scoville clips (prepared in The National Hospital by the Instrument Curator); not available commercially were used. In every case anchorage of the clip was ensured by filling the circular tensioning rings of the torsion bar clip with acrylic (Simplex P) after permanent application. The acrylic expands during setting, slightly increasing the closing force of the clip blades and preventing slippage of the clip. No clip has slipped after this manoeuvre, which has been used for some 15 years, and there has been no evidence of electrolytic disruption of the clip. According to Sugita et al.[26], a clip with a blade tip pressure over 80 g should be used for permanent obliteration, whereas a clip with a blade tip pressure under 80 g should be used for temporary occlusion to prevent endothelial damage.

Occlusion time varied from 30 seconds to 45 minutes. Mannitol was rarely used in patients intraoperatively unless considerable fullness of the brain remained after drainage of cerebrospinal fluid, when Mannitol was given in a dose of 40%g to a patient of an average size before or soon after the opening of the dura.

We looked at possible mediators of the safety of temporary vascular occlusion[19] and found by assessing central conduction time from somatosensory evoked response elicited by median nerve stimulation conduction time being measured from the neck peak (C14) to the somatosory cortex (N[20]).

Pre- and postoperative steroid administration was routine to aid the maintenance of the cell membrane and blood-brain barrier; 10% low molecular weight dextran in saline was given for 5 days after each operation to maintain a hematocrit in the range 38–40 in the early part of the series, but because of evidence that such dextran increases plasma viscosity although it undoubtedly decreases blood viscosity, we have changed in the past 4 years to the use of a solution of Haemaccel (Hoechst) for a period of 5 days once again to maintain hematocrit in the low 30s.

The patients were investigated during their hospital stay with regard to neurological deficit of immediate onset, occurring within the first 24 hours after the operation, and of delayed onset, later than the first postoperative day.

The clinical outcome (Table 2) was assessed in a way similar to that used in the international co-operative study on the timing of aneurysm surgery. The period from the time of the operations varied from 6 months to 4.5 years with a mean of 15 months.

Results

Our initial series compared 66 cases in whom temporary vascular occlusion had been used, with 119 cases in which did not. An excellent outcome was achieved in 74.2% of those in whom temporary clipping had been used and 73.1% of those in whom it had not. Since that time temporary clipping has been used with increased frequency and no significant difference in the outcome can be detected although the numbers in poor grade who have not undergone temporary clipping is now small. By the same token the more difficult aneurysms have invariably been subject to temporary clipping.

Electrophysiological assessment showed that postoperative morbidity was observed only when an abnormality in conduction time followed occlusion of major vessels, except in one case of anterior cerebral artery occlusion, where we would now regard somatosensory evoked response monitoring as inadequate. Motor evoked response monitoring however will reveal parameters similar to those of the somatosensory response in the anterior cerebral distribution. In the case of internal carotid or middle cerebral artery occlusion permanent neurological deficit occurred only after abolition of the cortical response. Provided the cortical response recovered quickly and completely within periods of 10 to 20 minutes no abnormal neurological signs beyond those that were present preoperatively could be determined, indeed abolition of the cortical response up to 45 minutes could occur without permanent neurological deficit indicating reversibility of functional suppression of cortical tissue lying in the ischemic penumbra[2]. We have also found and confirmed from a larger series of over 180 cases now that if a cortical response is sustained for over 4 minutes following vascular occlusion even if it then disappears,

Table 2. *Patients with Anterior Communicating Artery Aneurysm*

Age/Sex	Preoperative grade	Time interval between SAH and surgery (days)	Intraoperative aneurysm rupture	Clip location on ACA	Occlusion time	Immediate postoperative deficit	Deficit of delayed onset	Clinical outcome	Follow-up period after surgery
44/F	3	9	yes	A1R dominant	9 min 30 s	deterioration of consciousness, left-sided hemiparesis	decerebrate posture	dead	4 days
33/F	4	7	yes	A1L dominant	4 min	deterioration of consciousness, left-sided hemiparesis	none	dead	3 mo
41/M	1	26	yes	A1 bil	13 min	none	none	excellent	23 mo
47/F	1	7	yes	A1 bil	3 min 4 s	none	none	excellent	18 mo
33/M	2	9	yes	A1 L dominant	4 min	none	none	excellent	15 mo
49/F	1	26	yes	A1 bil / A2 bil	18 min / 6 min	none	none	excellent	14 mo
33/F	3	6	yes	A1 R / A2 R	9 min / 4 min	left-sided hemiparesis	none	excellent	13 mo
42/M	3	5	yes	A1 R dominant	10 min	none	none	good	6 mo
32/M	4	12	no	A1 bil	7 min 20 s	none	none	good	7 mo
41/F	1	7	no	A1 bil	7 min	none	none	excellent	13 mo
59/F	a	—	no	A1 R	4 min 35 s	left-sided hemiparesis	none	excellent	9 mo
60/F	1	11	no	A1 bil	3 min	none	none	excellent	9 mo
47/M	3	9	no	A1 L dominant	5 min	confusion	none	excellent	10 mo
51/F	3	7	no	A1 bil	9 min	none	none	excellent	18 mo
64/F	3	5	no	A1 R dominant	9 min	confusion, left-sided hemiparesis	none	good	7 mo
29/M	3	6	no	A1 R dominant	2 min 40 s	none	none	excellent	8 mo
49/M	3	3	no	A1 bil	10 min	none	none	excellent	14 mo
46/M	2	5	no	A1 R	3 min 50 s	decerebrate posture	none	dead	2 mo
60/M	a	—	no	A1 bil / A2 L	15 min	none	none	excellent	38 mo
40/M	3	11	no	A1 L dominant	4 min 4 s	none	none	excellent	15 mo
55/M	3	37	no	A1 R dominant	40 s	none	none	good	7 mo
48/M	3	30	no	A1 L dominant	30 s	increased left-sided hemiparesis	none	good	50 mo

ACA anterior cerebral artery; *A1* anterior cerebral artery segment proximal to the anterior communicating artery; *A2* anterior cerebral artery segment distal to the anterior communicating artery; *R* right; *L* left; *bil*, bilateral; *SAH*, subarachnoid hemorrhage.
a Symptomatic giant aneurysm without SAH. Patient presented with visual failure.

permanent irrecoverable neurological deficit is unlikely. This period of time may well indicate the necessity for speed in, for example, handling of giant aneurysms when the evoked potential disappears following occlusion. Even if the cortical response disappears the clinical outcome is expected to be good if the N_{20} peak recovers within 20 minutes after recirculation.

Discussion

Our present view is that temporary vascular occlusion of major arteries is safe certainly for a period of 10 minutes. If a monitor of peripheral neural function shows no disturbance after that time the temporary vascular occlusion may be prolonged probably indefinitely. If the evoked cortical response disappears quickly then it is probable that a period of 10 minutes is the maximum that one should allow.

It is particularly important when temporary vascular occlusion is employed and the aneurysm either ruptures or is opened, that the collateral circulation be preserved by vascular occlusion distal to the aneurysm so that exsanguination of the collateral supply does not take place. If this is allowed to occur the perfusion pressure distal to the temporary clips is vastly lowered, the contribution of the lepto-meningeal collateral circulation being allowed to bleed out into the wound. This is of particular importance in the handling of giant aneurysms.

References

1. Acland R (1973) Thrombus formation in microvascular surgery: an experimental study of the effects of surgical trauma. Surgery 73: 766–771
2. Astrup J, Symon L, Branston NM, Lassen NA (1977) Cortical evoked potential and extracellular K^+ and H^+ at critical levels of brain ischemia. Stroke 8: 51–57
3. Barker W F (1966) Peripheral arterial disease. Saunders, Philadelphia, pp46–60
4. Branston NM, Symon L, Crockard HA, Pasztor E (1965) Relationship between the cortical evoked potential and local cortical blood flow following acute middle cerebral artery occlusion in the baboon. Exp Neurol 45: 195–208
5. Cohnheim J (1987) Untersuchungen über die embolischen Processe. Hirschwald, Berlin
6. DePalma RG, Chidi CC, Sternfeld WC, Koletsky S (1977) Pathogenesis and prevention of trauma-provoked atheromas. Surgery 82: 429–437
7. Dodson RF, Tagashira Y, Chu LW-F (1976) Acute ultrastructural changes in the middle cerebral artery due to the injury and ischemia of surgical clamping. Can J Neurol Sci 3: 23–27
8. Drake CG, Vanderlinden RG (1967) The late consequences of incomplete surgical treatment of cerebral aneurysms. J Neurosurg 26: 226–238
9. Dujovny M, Kossovsky N, Laha RK, Leff L, Wackenhut N, Perlin A (1979) Temporary microvascular clips. Neurosurgery 5: 456–463
10. Dujovny M, Osgood CP, Barrionuevo PJ, Perlin A, Kossovsky N (1978) SEM evaluation of endothelial damage following temporary middle cerebral artery occlusion in dogs. J Neurosurg 48: 42–48
11. Dujovny M, Wakenhut N, Kossovsky N, Gomes CW, Laha RK, Leff L, Nelson D (1979) Minimum vascular occlusive force. J Neurosurg 51: 662–668
12. Ebina K, Iwabuchi T, Suzuki S (1982) Histological change in permanently clipped or ligated cerebral arterial wall. Part II: autopsy cases of aneurysmal neck clipping. Acta Neurochir (Wien) 66: 23–42
13. Gertz SD, Rennels ML, Forbes MS, Kawamura J, Sunaga T, Nelso E (1976) Endothelial cell damage by temporary arterial occlusion with surgical clips. Study of the clip site by scanning and transmission electron microscopy. J Neurosurg 45: 514–519
14. Greenberg IM (1984) Cerebral aneurysm rupture during neurosurgery. Neurosurgery 15: 243–245
15. Gregorius FK, Rand RW (1975) Scanning electron microscopic

observations of common carotid artery endothelium in the rat. II: Sutured arteries. Surg Neurol 4: 258–264
16. Hunt WE, Hess RM (1968) Surgical risk as related to time of intervention in the repair of intracranial aneurysms. J Neurosurg 28: 14–19
17. Ljunggren B, Säveland H, Brandt L. Kagström E, Rehncrona S, Nilsson P–E (1983) Temporary clipping during early operation for ruptured aneurysm: preliminary report. Neurosurgery 12: 525–530
18. Jabre A, Symon L (1987) Temporary vascular occlusion during aneurysm surgery. Surg Neurol 27: 47–63
19. Momma F, Wang, A-D, Symon L (1987) Effects of temporary arterial occlusion on somatosensory evoked responses in aneurysm surgery. Surg Neurol 27: 343–354
20. Osgood CP, Dujovny M, Faille R (1976) Early scanning electron microscopic evaluation of microvascular manoeuvres. Angiology 27: 96–105
21. Perneczky A, Koos WT (1982) Special remarks on microsurgical techniques for cerebral aneurysms. Acta Neurochir (Wien) 63: 101–103
22. Pertuiset B (1979) Intraoperative aneurysmal rupture and reduction by coagulation of the sac. In: Pia HW, Langmaid C, Zierski J (eds) Cerebral aneurysms: advances in diagnosis and therapy. Springer, Berlin Heidelberg New York, pp 398–401
23. Pool JL (1961) Aneurysms of the anterior communicating artery, bifrontal craniotomy, and routine use of temporary clips. J Neurosurg 18: 98–112
24. Rosenbaum TJ, Sundt TM Jr (1978) Interrelationship of aneurysm clips and vascular tissue. J Neurosurg 48: 929–934
25. Scoville WB (1966) Miniature torsion bar spring aneurysm clip. J Neurosurg 25: 97
26. Slayback JB, Bowen WW, Hinshaw DB (1976) Intimal injury from arterial clamps. Am J Surg 132: 183–188
27. Sugita K, Hirori T, Iguchi, Mizutani T (1976) Comparative study of the pressure of various aneurysm clips. J Neurosurg 44: 723–727
28. Suzuki J, Kwak R, Okudaira Y (1979) The safe time limit of temporary clamping of cerebral arteries in the direct surgical treatment of intracranial aneurysm under moderate hypothermia. In: Suzuki J (ed) Cerebral aneurysms. Neuron, Sendai, pp 325–329
29. Suzuki J, Yoshimoto T (1979) The effect of mannitol in prolongation of permissible occlusion time of cerebral arteries: clinical data of aneurysm surgery. In: Suzuki J (ed) Cerebral aneurysms. Neuron, Sendai, pp 330–337
30. Suzuki J, Yoshimoto T, Kayama T (1984) Surgical treatment of middle cerebral artery aneurysms. J Neurosurg 61: 17–23
31. Symon L (1982) Perspectives in aneurysm surgery. Acta Neurochir (Wien) 63: 5–13
32. Symon L, Vajda J (1984) Surgical experiences with giant intracranial aneurysms. J Neurosurg 61: 1009–1028
33. Symon L (1982) Surgical approaches to the tentorial hiatus. In: Krayenbühl H (ed) Advances and technical standards in neurosurgery, Vol 9. Springer, Berlin Heidelberg New York, pp 69–112
34. Symon L (1982) Surgical management of middle cerebral artery aneurysms. In: Schmidek HH, Sweet WH (eds) Operative neurosurgical techniques, Vol II. Grune and Stratton, New York, pp 891–908
35. Thurston JB, Buncke JH, Chater NL (1976) A scanning electron microscopy study of micro-arterial damage and repair. Plast Reconstr Surg 57: 197–203

Correspondence: Lindsay Symon, T.D., F.R.C.S., Gough-Cooper Department of Neurological Surgery, Institute of Neurology, The National Hospital, Queen Square, London WC1N 3BG, U.K.

Limits of Temporary Arterial Occlusion

H.H. Batjer and **D.S. Samson**

Department of Neurological Survey, Dallas, Texas, U.S.A.

Summary

A number of clinical circumstances either mandate the use of temporary arterial occlusion as in the reconstruction of complex giant cerebral aneurysms or require that temporary occlusion be considered to minimize the risk of intraoperative hemorrhage during dissection and clipping of routine aneurysms. A variety of temporary clips have proven non-damaging to the vessel wall. However, regional and distal ischemia resulting from this interruption of flow, if prolonged, can give rise to permanent ischemic injury. A number of strategies have been suggested to extend the safe period of temporary occlusion. While barbiturates have been shown to enhance ischemic tolerance in laboratory models, cardiotoxicity with hypotension may minimize collateral potential. Newer agents such as etomidate appear safer systemically, are rapidly reversible, and in burst-suppressive doses appear to eliminate the increased oxygen extraction fraction seen in unprotected ischemic tissue.

In a clinical trial using normotension, normothermia, and burst-suppressive doses of etomidate the 95% confidence level for tolerance of occlusion appeared to be 19 minutes for patients in Grades I and II and 15 minutes for those in Grades III and IV. Patients older than 61 years appeared to tolerate temporary occlusion less well than their younger cohorts. All patients occluded for over 31 minutes developed cerebral infarction. Our current clinical protocol requires that the surgeon attempt to predict the duration of temporary arterial occlusion necessary. When less than 15 minutes of occlusion are anticipated, pharmacologic burst-suppression is used with either etomidate or propofol. For patients in whom anticipated occlusion is between 15 and 20 minutes mild hypothermia is added to the regimen. Deep hypothermia and circulatory arrest are employed for those cases in which temporary occlusion longer than 20 minutes is anticipated.

Keywords: Temporary arterial occlusion; ischemia.

Introduction

The ideal result of an intracranial operation targeting an aneurysm is the complete obliteration of the aneurysmal sac with preservation of all afferent and efferent vasculature. While routine microsurgical technique allows this ideal result in the overwhelming majority of simple aneurysms, several situations make this goal either difficult or impossible to achieve without temporarily interrupting the local circulation. Large and giant aneurysms, particularly if complicated by intramural thrombosis or calcification, often will not permit accurate reconstruction without complete evacuation of the thrombotic mass and clip occlusion of the residual cuff. This procedure obviously involves complete interruption of afferent and efferent flow. Some seemingly straight forward aneurysms are densely adherent to efferent vasculature and/or perforators and by the nature of their thin walls and turgor carry a high risk of intraoperative hemorrhage at the time of final dissection and clipping. In these circumstances temporary arterial occlusion for a brief interval can allow a very straight forward and quite safe surgical procedure to be carried out[16]. While the management of giant aneurysms has been significantly impacted by the availability of long and extremely strong multi-angled and fenestrated clips and the booster clips[23-26], our practice has evolved into the pattern of employing local circulatory arrest for the majority of such lesions[1] with crushing of the neck with forceps if necessary[3]. Following Pool's work[16] a number of manufacturers have successfully developed delicate intracranial arterial clips which have proven non-damaging to the cerebral vasculature[8].

The temporary interruption of flow in virtually all intracranial vessels for short periods is well tolerated. Unfortunately some situations require protracted intervals to successfully evacuate the aneurysm and soften its neck adequately for successful clipping. In these circumstances the ischemic tolerance of brain tissue may be exceeded leading to infarction. A number of strategies designed at ischemic brain protection have been developed approaching the problem from one of three general precepts: 1) increase supply; 2) decrease demand; or 3) elimination of toxic substances. Perhaps the most successful approaches to this problem have been those concerned with decreasing the metabolic requirements of the brain and therefore decreasing demand for blood flow and metabolites. Due to the multiplicity of their pharmacologic actions the barbiturates were studied early on as potential brain protectants. These agents have been shown to protect the brain in numerous animal models of hypoxia and ischemia as well as demonstrating a suggestive benefit in a number of clinical situations[7,10-12,20,22,29]. Unfortunately the cardiac depressant effects of barbiturates at required dosage not infrequently depress mean arterial pressure to levels which may jeopardized collateral flow. The properties of etomidate (Abbott Laboratories, North Chicago, IL) which is an intravenously administered carboxylated imidazole derivative which produces significant depression of cerebral metabolism with minimal cardiac toxicity[4,6,9,13,14,17,27,28] led to its use in our Center during aneurysm procedures. Since roughly 60% of the cerebral metabolic rate is concerned with electrical generation of impulses (a function which may be monitored with the EEG) and approximately 40% of the metabolic rate is concerned with the maintenance of cellular homeostasis, it seems reasonable to assume that the use of a pharmacologic agent such as a barbiturate, etomidate, or propofol should extend the ischemic tolerance of the brain by roughly one half. Early studies of etomidate showed a comparable level of metabolic suppression with the barbiturates as well as a coincident and dramatic decrease in cerebral blood flow resulting in favorable protective properties that met or exceeded those of the barbiturates in comparative studies[27,28]. While remarkable systemic and cardiovascular stability was noted even in high doses of etomidate[14] certain untoward side effects were described. Even with brief use of this agent endogenous cortisol production was found to be substantially decreased[9,15]. In addition some activation of the EEG was noted in patients with pre-operative epilepsy[4]. Nevertheless, the routine practice of using high dose steroids with intracranial procedures common to most units and the rapid reversibility of the anesthetic effect of etomidate made it a very attractive clinical means of enhancing the ischemic tolerance of brain.

Methods

Laboratory Studies

A canine model of incomplete global ischemia was developed using induced severe hypotension with nitroprusside and trimethaphan.

Cerebral blood flow was monitored with global (Kety-Schmidt N_2O washout) and cortical (thermal diffusion probe) techniques. Arterial sampling was derived from the femoral artery and cerebral venous sampling was derived from catheterization of the torcular. The required craniectomy also allowed cortical EEG monitoring and cortical CBF monitoring. A standard general anesthesia was employed with induction by a short acting barbiturate and maintenance with 1.5% inspired isoflurane and 5-10% N_2O. Paralysis was maintained with vecuronium bromide (0.1 mg/kg/hr). The anesthetic technique employed was felt to mimic the clinical setting as close as possible. Following the induction and maintenance of anesthesia and the creation of an appropriate craniectomy with arterial and venous cannulation, a 45-minute period of stabilization was followed by 30 minutes of severe hypotension to approximately 30 mm/Hg. A final 45-minute period of recovery was then observed following the cessation of the hypotensive agents. Three groups of animals were studied: control, low dose etomidate, and high dose etomidate. In the control series, no ischemic protection was employed. In the low dose etomidate group, 1 mg/kg bolus was infused followed by 0.5 mg/kg/min during the study interval. In the high dose etomidate group burst-suppression was induced and maintained with 3 mg/kg bolus followed by 0.1 mg/kg/min with additional supplementation as necessary to maintain burst-suppression[5].

Clinical Studies

As mentioned above, etomidate became routinely employed in our clinical practice. Due to the large volume of aneurysm patients treated at our Center, it seemed possible to investigate the variables associated with the ultimate development of infarction in order to determine the safest and most effective utilization of temporary arterial occlusion. During a two-year period of time, 121 patients were treated by elective temporary arterial occlusion from a group of 234 consecutive aneurysm cases. Twenty-one patients of this initial cohort were excluded for the following reasons: intraoperative aneurysm rupture prior to the establishment of temporary occlusion, operative sacrifice of afferent or efferent arteries, or pre- or post-occlusion performance of an extracranial-intracranial arterial bypass. These exclusions left 100 patients to be studied. Our Institutional technique for the use of temporary arterial occlusion for aneurysm treatment has been previously described[1] with the exception that our current dosage of etomidate to maintain burst-suppressive coma is 1 mg/kg I.V. push followed by 10 micrograms/kg/min. Patient parameters studied included age, clinical grade (Hunt-Hess), presence or absence of subarachnoid hemorrhage, vasospasm, aneurysm size, and vascular territory. The technical parameters studied included the total duration of occlusion, the degree of temporary occlusion, and the use of intermittent versus sustained arrest. All patients were treated using our standard anesthetic technique of etomidate induced burst-suppression during elective circulatory arrest under normotension, normothermia, and normovolemia. Mannitol (1 gm/kg) was administered at the time of skin incision. Temporary occlusion was considered complete if all afferent and efferent vessels were clipped and incomplete if one more efferent vessels was left patent. A separate subcategory was designated for those cases in which only proximal vessel occlusion was used. Post-operative followup evaluations included CT scanning in 100%, angiography in 87%, and MRI in 48%. Clinical followup was obtained to a minimum of 6 months with a mean of 19 months. Outcome parameters measured included final clinical condition and clinical or radiographic evidence of cerebral infarction in the appropriate vascular territory. Simple proximal occlusion was utilized in 39 patients, incomplete trapping was used in 21, and complete trapping in 40 cases.

Results

Laboratory Studies

The initial studies conducted by Frizzell et al. lowered the mean arterial pressure to similar levels in each study group (approximately 30 mm/Hg). The mean cerebral oxygen extraction fraction increased in the control animals tested from 0.23 ± 0.02 to 0.55 ± 0.08 ($p < 0.05$). In the low dose etomidate group the oxygen extraction fraction rose from 0.33 ± 0.02 to 0.53 ± 0.02 ($p < 0.05$). In the high dose etomidate group oxygen extraction fraction did not increase during hypotension. Mean global cerebral blood flow levels decreased in all groups during the hypotensive insult: $52 \pm 12\%$ decrease in the control group, $56\% \pm 13\%$ decrease in the low dose etomidate group, and $60\% \pm 4\%$ decrease in the high dose etomidate group. Global cerebral blood flow levels during hypotension ranged from 21–24 ml/100gm/min. Frizzell et al. concluded that this experiment suggested that burst-suppressive doses of etomidate were required to maintain the cerebral metabolic state during incomplete cerebral ischemia[5]. This study suggests that EEG monitoring is critical to employ during clinical use of cerebral metabolic depressants and that empiric dosage if too low may be completely ineffective.

Clinical Studies

Nineteen patients treated in the above-protocol could be defined as having suffered cerebral infarction following surgery. Eighty-one patients had no clinical or radiographic evidence of ischemia or infarction in the distribution of the arteries occluded intraoperatively. Several parameters were found to be statistically significantly related to the post-operative development of clinical or radiographic cerebral infarction in the anatomical distribution of the arteries temporarily occluded. This correlation with poor ischemic tolerance was noted with advanced patient age, poor preoperative clinical grade, protracted duration of temporary arterial occlusion, and the use of incomplete (as opposed to complete) local arrest. The findings can be summarized as follows:

1. Patients greater than 61 years of age tolerated temporary arterial occlusion poorly developing both clinical and radiographic evidence of ischemia or infarction at time durations shorter than those routinely tolerated in younger patients.

2. Patients in more advanced clinical grades (Hunt and Hess Grades III and IV) demonstrated a higher incidence of ischemic complications than did patients in better clinical grades. Additionally, these complications were found to occur at shorter intervals of temporary occlusion than those tolerated by patients in better neurological condition. The 95% confidence level for the tolerance of temporary occlusion in patients in Grades I and II was 19 minutes; the 95% confidence level for poor grade patients was 15 minutes.

3. All patients undergoing temporary arterial occlusion for greater then 31 minutes had both radiographic and neurologic evidence of infarction in the post-operative period. Patients occluded for time periods between 21 and 30 minutes routinely had both radiographic and clinical evidence of ischemia in the postoperative period although in a number of these cases, neurological recovery was significant. Patients occluded for durations of between 14 and 21 minutes had largely satisfactory clinical and radiographic outcomes although several patients in the 18–20-minute interval developed significant deficits. All patients occluded for less then 14 minutes had no clinical or radiographic sequelae of this iatrogenic ischemic period.

4. The degree of local arterial arrest could be judged as either complete, incomplete, or simple proximal occlusion. These modalities were compared both in the entire patient population and in those occluded for periods greater than 14 minutes. In patients undergoing protracted occlusion (greater than 14 minutes) a strong statistical trend suggested a close relationship between incomplete arrest and the development of post-operative neurological deficit and/or radiographic infarction.

Two additional parameters were found to have suggestive but not statistically significant relationship to the above-mentioned undesirable end-points.

1. Of the specific vascular territories undergoing temporary occlusion, the distribution of perforating arteries appeared to be uniquely sensitive to ischemic injury. While the number of distal basilar artery aneurysms treated in this population was substantially higher than that of middle cerebral aneurysms, a similar sensitivity was suggested for the thalamoperforating vessels and the lenticulostriate arteries.

2. A suggestive but not significant relationship was identified between increasing episodes of temporary occlusion and the post-operative development of ischemia. This finding was weighted by the use of multiple episodes of occlusion in patients treated with incomplete local arrest suggesting that the relative technical inefficiency of incomplete occlusion mandated more extended periods of ischemia to achieve the desired technical result. It should also be noted that our prac-

tice differs from many others in the way we employ temporary occlusion. Patterned after Drake, many Centers employ extremely brief periods of temporary occlusion (1 or 2 minutes) to perform a particular dissection maneuver and then restore flow. This process is then repeated many times during an individual procedure. Our practice on the other hand operates under the unproven assumption that a single episode of protracted ischemia is better tolerated than multiple episodes of brief occlusion. Some experimental documentation would support this concept in order to minimize the reperfusion insult. Due to this characteristic in our clinical practice, we typically occlude the involved circulation and perform as much as possible of the dissection and reconstruction without restoring flow. If it becomes obvious to the surgeon that aneurysmal exclusion cannot be accomplished within a reasonable period of time and irreversible maneuvers have not been performed (wide aneurysmal opening or excision) flow is restored for a period of 10 to 15 minutes.

3. Several factors interestingly failed to demonstrate a significant or suggestive relationship to the outcome measures of the study. No correlation could be found between the patient's sex, the pre-operative presence of subarachnoid hemorrhage, the presence of angiographic vasospasm, or the size of aneurysm and the risk of the development of post-operative neurological or radiographic evidence of infarction.

Additional Laboratories Studies

Hypothermia has been considered and studied for several decades as a means of protecting the brain from a number of insults. Physiologic evidence would suggest that hypothermia decreases the cerebral metabolic rate by a combined effect on electrical generation as well as slowing of homeostatic and enzymatic mechanisms. Therefore it is possible that synergism could potentially exist between pharmacologic metabolic suppression (with EEG burst-suppression) and hypothermia to further diminish the cerebral metabolic rate thus theoretically extending ischemic tolerance. Frizzell *et al.* conducted additional experiments using a canine model of incomplete global ischemia as previously described and studied four groups: control, etomidate, hypothermia (28 °C) and combined etomidate with hypothermia (unpublished data). Under baseline nonischemic conditions, etomidate was found to exert a marked depressant effect on cerebral metabolism (47% reduction) but without lowering brain parenchymal

temperature. Moderate hypothermia (28 °C) was found to have a profound metabolic depressant effect (69% reduction), but the addition of etomidate to this regimen did not further depress cerebral metabolism. In addition, this degree of hypothermia was found to have substantial cardiovascular effects not observed with etomidate alone. In this study, following the production of systemic hypotension and incomplete cerebral ischemia, cortical blood flow decreased to less than 20 ml/100gm/min. Etomidate, hypothermia, or the two combined modalities blunted the rise in oxygen extraction fraction noted in the control group. Therefore in the experimental model utilized in these studies, it was not possible to confirm synergism between pharmacologic and hypothermic brain protection.

Discussion

Despite the limitations of our clinical and laboratory investigations, we feel that several tentative conclusions can be made. First, the use of pharmacologic brain protection with etomidate or propofol is extremely safe for the aneurysm patient and a substantial body of laboratory evidence suggests that cerebral tolerance of iatrogenic ischemic insults will be prolonged utilizing metabolic suppression. Second, despite a lack of supportive literature at present, it is clear that in our unit under our standard neuroanesthetic regimen, the limits of cerebral tolerance for temporary arterial occlusion are between 15 and 20 minutes. It is clear that outliers exist; yet for the population at large, this interval is potentially very significant. Third, the addition of induced of hypothermia to pharmacologic metabolic suppression offers potential synergism. The laboratory studies of Frizzell *et al.* employ 28 °C as the target for a non-circulatory arrest procedure. In practice, however, induced hypothermia below 32 °C seems to induce some degree of coagulopathy as well as a threat to cardiovascular stability. It is certainly possible that the use of surgically induced hypothermia to 32 °C could in fact prove synergistic with pharmacologic metabolic suppression.

The use of deep hypothermia (16 °C) and complete circulatory arrest for the treatment of giant cerebral aneurysms has been known and utilized for sometime[2,18,19]. The early attempts with this technique were not infrequently accompanied by exquisite neurovascular reconstruction only to be complicated by hemorrhagic problems post-operatively. Improvements in the overall systemic safety of circulatory arrest procedures have precipitated a resurgence of interest in this methodology for intracranial aneurysm surgery[21]. In addition to a bloodless field and an empty intracranial circulation which often makes the clipping of formidable lesions very straight-forward, it is clear that the addition of deep hypothermia to the regimen allows circulatory arrest intervals of up to 50 minutes with full neurological recovery. Even massive and thrombotic giant aneurysms can be successfully reconstructed within this time frame.

As a result of our experience, we are currently approaching the aneurysm patient with three strategies for brain protection. For patients in whom we anticipate occlusion times of less than 15 minutes, we routinely employ normothermia, normotension, and EEG burst-suppression with etomidate or propofol. In cases with anticipated occlusion times between 15 and 20 minutes, our neuroanesthesiologists have added mild hypothermia (32–33 °C) to our pharmacologic burst-suppressive regimen. This anesthetic addition has not significantly prolonged the operative procedure and extensive coagulation profiles have not revealed abnormalities with hypothermia to this degree. Additionally, the patients have remained systemically stable without cardiovascular effect. When occlusion times of longer than 20 minutes are anticipated, we are employing the use of deep hypothermia and circulatory arrest to enhance the tolerance of the ischemic interval and expand the spectrum of intracranial aneurysms which can be safely treated.

References

1. Batjer HH, Frankfurt AI, Purdy PD, Smith SS, Samson DS (1988) Use of etomidate, temporary arterial occlusion, and intraoperative angiography in surgical treatment of large and giant cerebral aneurysm. Neurosurg 68: 234–240
2. Baumgartner WA, Silverberg GD, Ream AK, Jamieson SW, Takaber J, Reitz BA (1983) Reappraisal of cardiopulmonary bypass with deep hypothermia and circulatory arrest for complex neurosurgical operations. Surgery 94: 242–249
3. Drake CG (1979) Giant intracranial aneurysms: experience with surgical treatment in 174 patients. Clin Neurosurg 26: 12–95
4. Ebrahim ZY, DeBoer GE, Luders H, Hahn JF, Lesser RP (1986) Effect of etomidate on the electroencephalogram of patients with epilepsy. Anesth Analg 65: 1004–1006
5. Frizzell RT, Meyer YJ, Borchers DJ, Weprin BE, Auen EC, Pogue WR, Reisch JS, Cherrington AD, Batjer HH (1991) The effects of etomidate on cerebral metabolism and blood flow in a canine model for hypoperfusion. J Neurosurg 74: 263–269
6. Ghoneim MM, Yamada T (1977) Etomidate: a clinical and electroencephalographic comparison with thiopental. Anesth Analg 56: 479–485
7. Goldstein A Jr, Wells BA, Keats AS (1966) Increased tolerance to cerebral anoxia by pentobarbital. Arch Int Pharmacodyn Ther 161: 138–143
8. Jabre A, Symon L (1987) Temporary vascular occlusion during aneurysm surgery. Surg Neurol 27: 47–63
9. Kenyon CJ, McNeil LM, Fraser R (1985) Comparison of the effects of etomidate, thiopentone, and propofol on cortisol synthesis. Br J Anaesth 57: 509–511
10. Michenfelder JD, Milde JH (1975) Influence of anesthetics on metabolic, functional and pathological responses to regional cerebral ischemia. Stroke 6: 405–410
11. Michenfelder JD, Milde JH, Sundt TM Jr (1976) Cerebral protection by barbiturate anesthesia. Arch Neurol 33: 345–350
12. Michenfelder JD, Theye RA (1973) Cerebral protection by thiopental during hypoxia. Anesthesiology 39: 510: 517
13. Milde LN, Milde JH (1986) Preservation of cerebral metabolites by etomidate during incomplete cerebral ischemia in dogs. Anesthesiology 65: 272–277
14. Milde LN, Milde JH, Michenfelder JD (1985) Cerebral functional, metabolic, and hemodynamic effects of etomidate in dogs. Anesthesiology 63: 371–377
15. Moore RA, Allen MC, Wood PJ Rees LH, Sear JW (1985) Peri-operative endocrine effects of etomidate. Anaesthesia 40: 124–130
16. Pool JL (1961) Aneurysms of the anterior communicating artery, bifrontal craniotomy, and routine use of temporary clips. J Neurosurg 18: 98–112
17. Renou AM, Vernhiet J, Macrez P, Constant P, Billerey E, Khadaroo MY, Caille FM (1978) Cerebral blood flow and metabolism during etomidate anesthesia in man. Br J Anaesth 50: 1047–1051
18. Silverberg GD, Reitz BA, Ream AK, Taylor G, Enzmann DR (1980) Operative treatment of a giant cerebral artery aneurysm with hypothermia and circulatory arrest: report of a case. Neurosurgery 6: 301–305
19. Silverberg GD, Reitz BA, Ream AK (1981) Hypothermia and cardiac arrest in the treatment of giant aneurysms of the cerebral circulation and hemangioblastoma of the medulla. J Neurosurg 55: 337–346
20. Smith AL, Hoff JT, Nielsen SL, Larson CP (1974) Barbiturate protection in acute focal cerebral ischemia. Stroke 5: 1–7
21. Spetzler RF, Hadley MN, Rigamonti D, Carter LP, Raudzens PA, Shedd SA, Wilkinson E (1988) Aneurysms of the basilar artery treated with circulatory arrest, hypothermia, and barbiturate cerebral protection. J Neurosurg 68: 868–879
22. Steen PA, Michenfelder JD (1978) Cerebral protection with barbiturates. Relation to anesthetic effect. Stroke 9: 140–142
23. Sugita K, Kobayashi S, Inoue T, Banno T (1981) New angled fenestrated clips for fusiform vertebral artery aneurysms. J Neurosurg 54: 346–350
24. Sugita K, Kobayashi S, Inoue T, Takehae T (1984) Characteristics and use of ultra-long aneurysm clips. J Neurosurg 60: 145–150
25. Sugita K, Kobayashi S, Kyoshima K, Takemae T (1982) Fenestrated clips for unusual aneurysms of the carotid artery. J Neurosurg 57: 240–246
26. Sundt TM Jr, Piepgras DG, Marsh WR (1984) Booster clips for giant and thick-based aneurysms. J Neurosurg 60: 751–762
27. Wauquier A (1982) Brain protective properties of etomidate and flunarizine. J Cereb Blood Flow Metab 2 [Suppl 1]: S53–S56
28. Wauquier A, Ashton D, Clincke G (1981) Anti-hypoxic effects of etomidate, thiopental, and methohexital. Arch Int Pharmacodyn Ther 249: 330–334
29. Yatsu FM, Diamond I, Graziano C, Lind Quist P (1972) Experimental brain ischemia: protection from irreversible damage with a rapid acting barbiturate (methohexital). Stroke 3: 726–732

Correspondence: H. Hunt Batjer, M.D., Department of Neurological Surgery, 5323 Harry Hines Blvd., Dallas, Texas 75235-8855, U.S.A.

Deep Hypothermic Circulatory Arrest as an Adjunct to Complex Intracranial Aneurysm Surgery

R.A. Solomon, C.R. Smith, W.L. Young, and J.G. Stone

Departments of Neurosurgery, Cardiac Surgery, and Anesthesiology, Columbia University College of Physicians and Surgeons, Columbia-Presbyterian Medical Center, New York, New York, U.S.A.

Summary

Conventional surgical techniques for clipping of giant intracranial aneurysms carry high operative risks. Therefore, many patients are left untreated, or subjected to alternative treatment. The use of deep hypothermic circulatory arrest as an adjunct for clipping complex giant intracranial aneurysms is being investigated.

Patients are chosen for circulatory arrest on the basis of neuro-radiological studies or failed surgery. Following retraction and aneurysm dissection, the patient is placed on cardio-pulmonary bypass through femoral cannulation. The core temperature is reduced to 18 °C, and complete circulatory arrest is instituted. The dissection is then completed, and the dome can be opened, evacuated, and clipped.

Twenty seven patients with giant intracranial aneurysms have been treated with arrest; 17 were in the posterior circulation, and 10 were in the anterior circulation. The average arrest time was 22 minutes, (9–51). There were 2 deaths due to aortic dissection during bypass. Five patients suffered an intra-operative stroke. Only 2 of these strokes have proved to have caused permanent disability. Two aneurysms were left untreated. One patient underwent proximal ligation of the basilar artery and continues to have filling of the basilar apex aneurysm from the anterior circulation. Overall, 15 patients are neurologically normal and employed full-time. Five patients are independent with mild disability. Only 2 of these patients have disability as a result of operation. Five patients remain in a dependent condition and 4 of these patients are dependent as a result of operation. Two patients died, as mentioned above.

Our experience indicates that in selected centers where the appropriate team of neurosurgeons, cardiac surgeons, and anesthesiologists are available, deep hypothermic circulatory arrest may provide a mechanism to obliterate otherwise unclippable aneurysms with acceptable morbidity.

Keywords: Cerebral aneurysm; circulatory correct; hypothermia; subarachnoid hemorrhage.

Introduction

Surgical clipping of anterior circulation aneurysms less than 1 cm in size can now be performed by appropriately trained neurosurgeons with an intra-operative complication rate of under 2%. This complication rate rises sharply as the aneurysms increase in size and when posterior circulation aneurysms are considered. The complication rate for giant basilar aneurysms can exceed 50% with standard surgical techniques[5]. Giant aneurysm surgery poses a formidable challenge and a large number of neurosurgeons still advise patients against operative intervention unless immediate life-threatening risks are documented.

There has been a recent flurry of interest in the use of interventional neuroradiological techniques to obliterate complex intracranial aneurysms. At first balloons were utilized to obstruct the lumen of the aneurysm, but the failure of this technique gave rise to investigations into platinum coils. Platinum coils have also been shown to have severe limitations, although with improved research these techniques may show promise in the future[8]. Nonetheless, most of the success with endovascular approaches to intracranial aneurysms has been with small aneurysms. The giant intracranial aneurysms continue to pose high risk to both the interventional neuroradiologist and the operating neurosurgeon. Therefore the quest for improved techniques and greater operative safety continues. For these reasons, we have begun to investigate the use of deep hypothermic circulatory arrest as an adjunct for complex intracranial aneurysm surgery.

Although the technique of deep hypothermic circulatory arrest for the treatment of intracranial aneurysms was first reported over 30 years ago[6,9,11–14,21] its incorporation in common neurosurgical practice has been hampered by several factors. Intracranial vascular surgery in the face of full systemic heparinization is difficult. Post bypass coagulopathy has been a serious source of morbidity in the past[6]. The need for cooperation of multiple sub-specialities and the requirements for expensive hi-tech equipment have further limited the availability of this technique.

Recent improvement in techniques and equipment designed for cardiopulmonary bypass have fueled renewed interest in circulatory arrest for the treatment of complex intracranial aneurysms[2,3,15,16,18,19]. From the authors' series of 339 intracranial aneurysms operated on from May 1989 to May 1992, 27 cases were selected for deep hypothermic circulatory arrest. The selection of patients was based on a pre-operative analysis of available studies that suggested extremely high risk for standard surgical intervention, or observation of previously unsuccessful surgery. The significant features of the operative techniques, outcome, and implications for future management of intracranial aneurysms will be discussed.

Methods

A standard pterional craniotomy was utilized for all anterior circulation aneurysms and aneurysms near the basilar apex. The mid-basilar aneurysm in this series was approached via a transpetrosal route[17] anterior to the sigmoid sinus. Vertebral aneurysms were approached via a unilateral suboccipital craniectomy in the supine position. The middle cerebral aneurysm and the carotid bifurcation aneurysms were approached through a dissection of the sylvian fissure. The carotid ophthalmic aneurysms were exposed via the extradural approach of Vinko Dolenc[4].

When circulatory arrest is used as an adjunct for aneurysm surgery, hemostasis must be meticulous, and the aneurysm is dissected as much as possible in its fully arterialized state. Following final aneurysm dissection, heparinization, cardiopulmonary bypass, induced hypothermia, and total circulatory arrest are sequentially instituted.

A transesophageal echo probe was introduced in all patients. Four-chamber and short-axis views of the left ventricle (LV) were studied to assess ventricular volume and contractility under pre-bypass "baseline" loading conditions. Heparin was given after neurosurgical exposure and initial hemostasis are obtained, and after a #25 gauge needle temperature probe is positioned in the brain.

The common femoral artery and vein were exposed and cannulated at the inguinal ligament. The venous cannula tip was positioned in the right atrium, confirmed by transesophageal echo probe. The size and quality of the vessels, design of the extracorporeal circuit, and calculated flow (2.4 l/min/m^2) determined the specific details of cannulation. Usually, #21 French venous and arterial cannulas designed for percutaneous insertion (Biomedicus) were used, with centrifugal pumps on both venous and arterial sides of the circuit, using a parallel circuit venting system in place of a cardiotomy reservoir. The circuit prime was hyperosmolar (315–318 mOsmol/l).

When bypass was begun, cooling was not started until adequacy of flow with peripheral cannulation was confirmed. If flow is < 80% of calculated flow, the cannulation must be satisfactorily revised, or the sternum opened for central cannulation. Cooling was effected by lowering the perfusate temperature as rapidly as possible. Flow was maintained as high as possible, usually requiring sodium nitroprusside infusion and volume expansion. LV volume, as assessed in cross section on short axis by transesophageal echo probe, should be reduced in comparison to pre-bypass. Ventricular fibrillation occurs during cooling when perfusate temperature is 18–28 °C. Up to

80 m Eq of potassium can be given through a central line in 20 m Eq boluses, which appears to induce diastolic arrest. Fibrillation eventually ceases, although an occasional "agonal" beat occurs even during circulatory arrest. Transesophageal echo probe observation is critical to assure that the LV is not distended during fibrillation, which would require immediate LV venting.

Circulation was stopped when brain temperature reaches 16–18 °C, provided that axillary temperature is < 28 °C to minimize the gradient favoring central rewarming from the periphery during arrest. Blood was drained out of the patient through the venous cannula until the neurovasculature appears adequately decompressed, keeping in mind that too much exsanguination carries the risk of air embolism and/or a no-reflow phenomenon in small vessels.

With cessation of arterial circulation, circumferential dissection can easily be achieved. In some instances, giant aneurysms have contained extensive mural thrombus or atherosclerotic walls. During arrest, the dome of the aneurysm can be incised, thrombus removed, and if necessary an aneurysmal endarterectomy can be performed. The neck of the aneurysm is then clipped with single or multiple clips as required. Before rewarming, clip placement is checked by re-instituting pump circulation. If refilling or bleeding is noted within the aneurysm, the pump is again turned off and necessary clip adjustments are made.

When the repair was deemed secure, full flows and normal pressures were restored, and perfusate temperature was gradually increased to a maximum of 40 °C, not to exceed a gradient of 10 °C between perfusate and venous return blood. Nitroprusside was usually required to achieve high flows and more rapid rewarming. During rewarming spontaneous organized rhythm or ventricular fibrillation reappeared at 20–30 °C. The latter was converted with 200 to 400 joules delivered through the external defibrillating pads. When the sum (nasopharyngeal + axillary temperature) equals 70, with axillary > 32 °C, the patient was separated from bypass. Protamine was given and the cannulas removed. Areas of significant endothelial damage were debrided, and each site was closed transversely.

Autologous platelet-rich plasma was returned to the patient, along with red cells spun down from the perfusion circuit (Haemonetics Cell Saver). Brisk diuresis was maintained with loop diuretics to excrete accumulated free water. Inotropic support was rarely necessary.

Example Cases

Case 1: A 48 year old previously healthy female was developing progressive visual loss. An MRI (Fig. 1) revealed a giant bi-lobed partially thrombosed supraclinoid aneurysm which severely compressed the visual apparatus. She then underwent a cerebral angiogram (Fig. 2) which revealed a 3.5 cm carotid ophthalmic aneurysm of the right side. The aneurysm was clipped with the assistance of deep hypothermic circulatory arrest. The post-operative angiogram (Fig. 3) revealed that the aneurysm had been clipped. Post-operatively the patient had gradually improving vision on the right side and no other neurological deficits.

Case 2: A 38 year old man developed progressive numbness and weakness of the right upper extremity. Because of this problem he underwent and MRI scan which demonstrated a giant supraclinoid aneurysm compressing the floor of the third ventricle to the foramen of Monro (Fig. 4). An angiogram was performed and documented a 3.5 cm carotid bifurcation aneurysm on the right side (Fig. 5). The patient was operated on with the assistance of deep hypothermic circulatory arrest and had satisfactory clipping with preservation of the carotid artery. This was confirmed by a post-operative angiogram (Fig. 6). Intra-operatively the patient suffered a small stroke in the

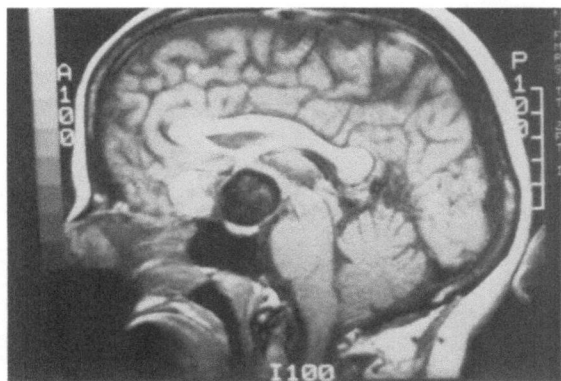

Fig. 1. Sagittal MRI in Case 1 depicting a giant supraclinoid aneurysm

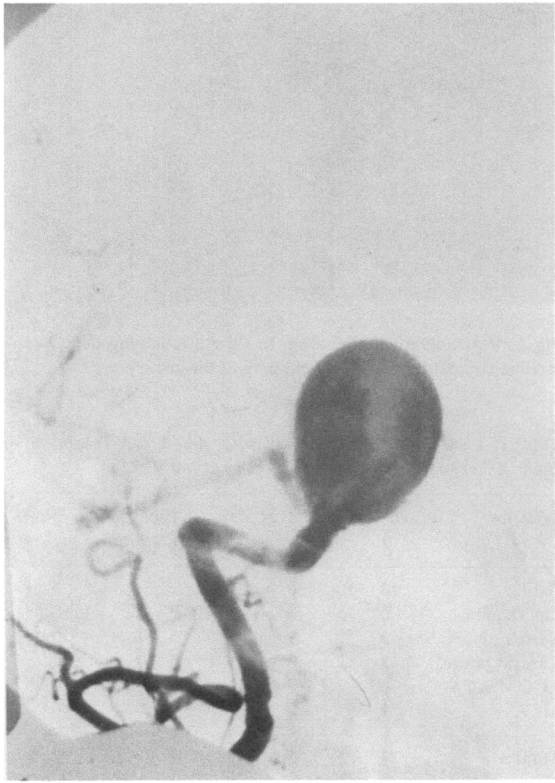

Fig. 2. AP angiogram showing 3.5 cm filling portion of the giant carotid ophthalmic aneurysm

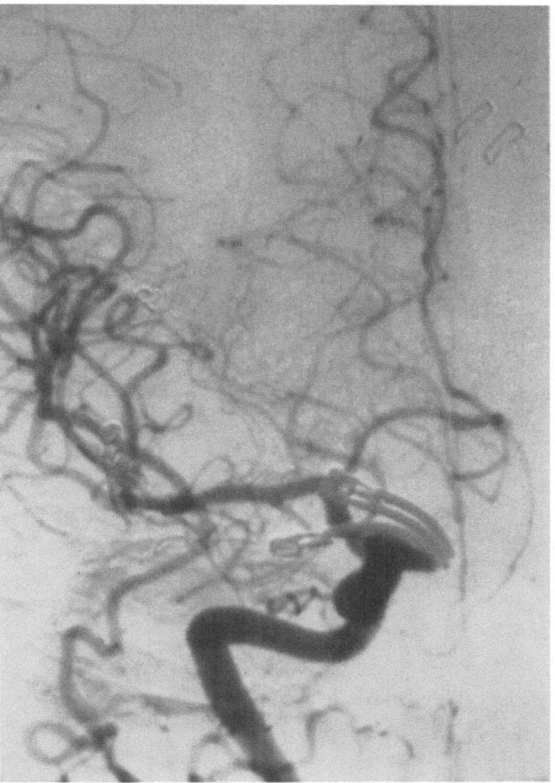

Fig. 3. Post-operative angiogram following clipping under deep hypothermic circulatory arrest

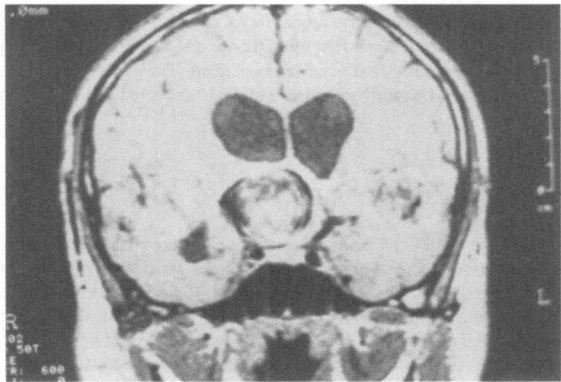

Fig. 4. Case 2: Coronal MRI depicting a giant aneurysm projecting up to region of the foramen of Monro

region of the right caudate nucleus presumably due to perforator injury off the top of the carotid artery. Initially the patient had some mild memory dysfunction but by 6 months was completely normal and had returned to his premorbid full-time employment.

Case 3: A 59 year old man had a subarachnoid hemorrhage referable to a giant basilar apex aneurysm. Initially the patient was Grade I

and an angiogram was performed (Fig. 7a and b). Ten days following the subarachnoid hemorrhage the patient underwent clipping of the aneurysm with the adjunct of deep hypothermic circulatory arrest. The aneurysm was clipped without difficulty but the patient did suffer a small lacunar infarct in the region of the left thalamus presumably related to a perforator injury off the top of the

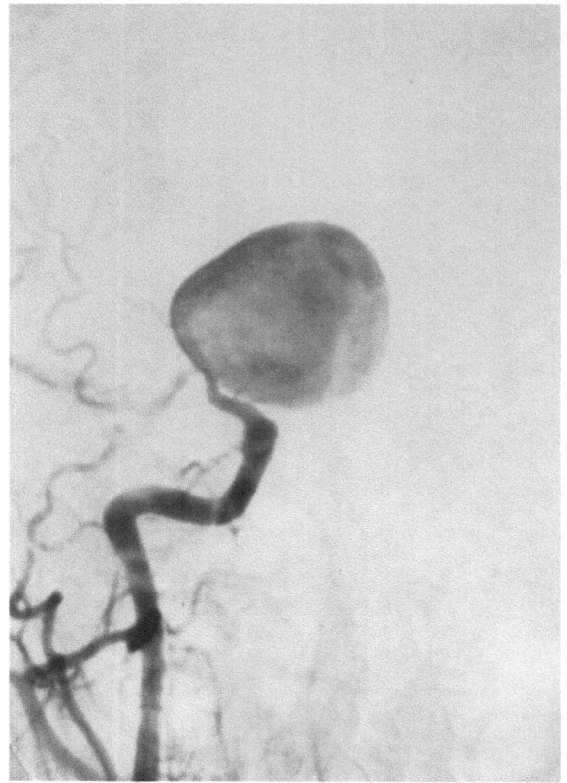

Fig. 5. AP angiogram showing 3.5 cm aneurysm off of the carotid bifurcation region

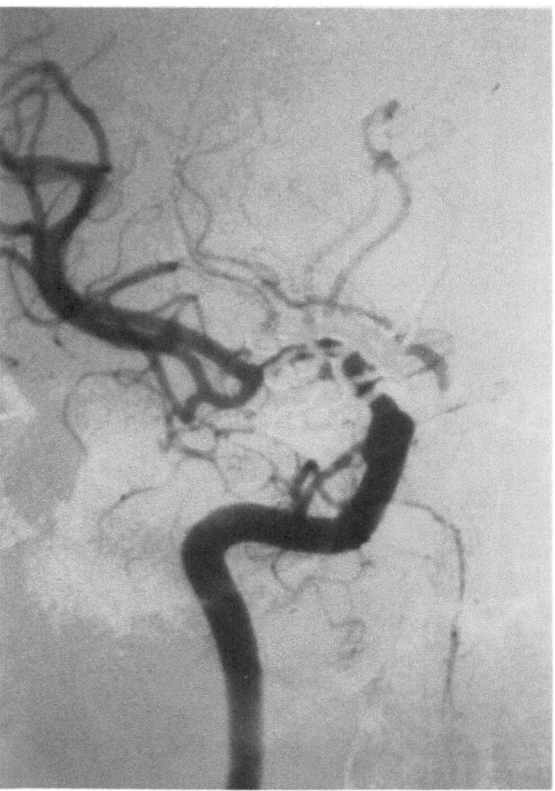

Fig. 6. Post-operative angiogram in Case 2 following deep hypothermic circulatory arrest and clipping of the aneurysm

basilar apex. Post-operative angiography revealed that the aneurysm had been obliterated and that all of the vessels were filling, although there was some residual vasospasm (Fig. 8). The patient has been left with a mild cognitive disorder and has required rehabilitation therapy.

Summary of Clinical Results

Twenty seven patients underwent elective intracranial surgery using the technique of total circulatory arrest under deep hypothermia with barbiturate anesthesia. There were 12 male and 15 female patients with an age range from 17–74. All patients had giant intracranial aneurysms (< 2.5 cm), 14 basilar, 5 carotid ophthalmic, 3 vertebral, 2 carotid bifurcations, 2 anterior communicating artery, and 1 middle cerebral artery.

The giant aneurysm patients treated with deep hypothermic circulatory arrest are outlined in Table 1. Twenty-four of the 27 patients treated with this technique had physical obliteration of the aneurysm by neck clipping, trapping, or proximal ligation. One patient who underwent proximal ligation of a giant basilar aneurysm continues to have retrograde filling of the aneurysm via the posterior communicating arteries. Table 2 indicates the morbidity of the deep hypothermic circulatory arrest procedures. There were 5 strokes caused by the operation; only 2 strokes resulted in devastating neurological outcome. The only other morbidity of note occurred in

Table 1. *Deep Hypothermic Circulatory Arrest for Treatment of Giant Aneurysms – Method of Treatment (1989–1992)*

Location	n	Clip	Trapping	Proximal Ligation	None
Basilar	14	10	0	2	2
Ophthalmic	5	5	0	0	0
Vertebral	3	1	2	0	0
Carotid bifurc.	2	2	0	0	0
ACOM/ACA	2	2	0	0	0
MCA	1	1	0	0	0
Total	27	21	2	2	2

2 patients both elderly and atherosclerotic females who experienced intra-operative aortic dissection from the groin catheterization. Both of these patients expired intra-operatively despite successful clipping of their aneurysms. Table 2 indicates the final outcome of the 27 patients treated with deep hypothermic circulatory arrest for their giant aneurysms. Again, these results include both operative morbidity and complications present pre-operatively attributable to the presence of the aneurysm. Twenty of the 27 patients had a good or excellent result while the others remained in a dependent neurologic condition or died.

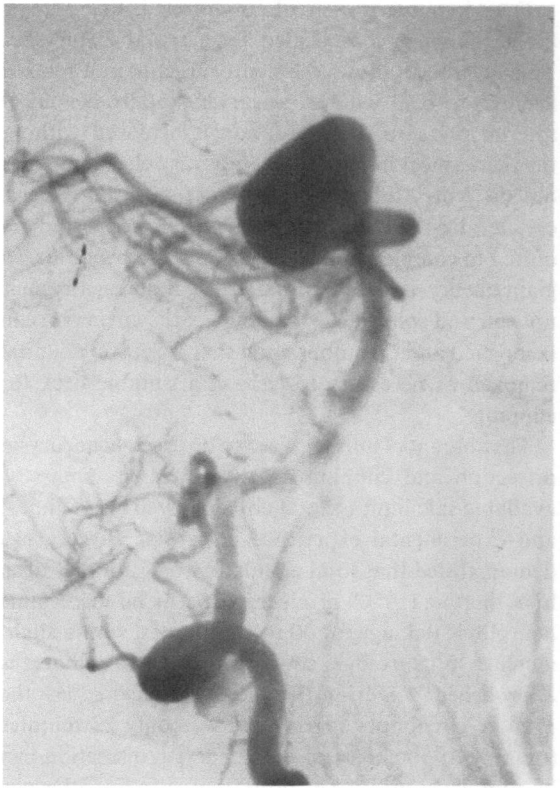
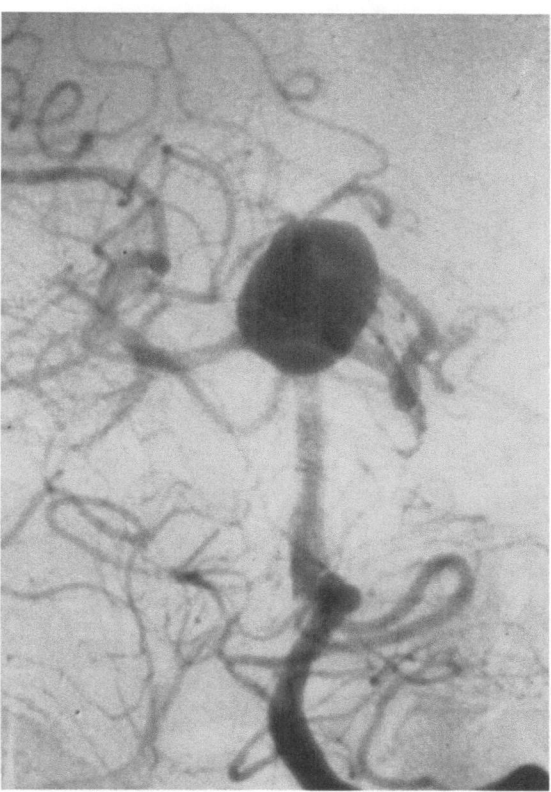

a   b

Fig. 7. Angiogram for Case 3: (a) Lateral angiogram showing 2.5 cm basilar apex aneurysm projecting posteriorly into the interpeduncular fossa; (b) AP angiogram confirming the presence of the giant basilar aneurysm

Table 2. *Deep Hypothermic Circulatory Arrest*

Morbidity		Outcome	
Stroke	5	Excellent	15
ICH[a]	1	Good	5
DVT[b]	3	Poor	5
Groin infection	5	Dead	2
Subdural hygroma	4		
Aortic Dissection	2		

[a] Intracerebral haemorrhage.
[b] Deep venous thrombosis.

Discussion

Surgeons who operate on giant intracranial aneurysms have realized the technical challenges inherent to their attempted repair in the fully arterialized state. Techniques such as systemic hypotension and temporary clipping have conventionally been used to reduce the turgor in giant aneurysms and facilitate safe clipping of the aneurysm neck[5,7,10]. Systemic hypotension has been abandoned by most neurosurgeons because of the possible side-effects in normothermic individuals. Patients who have had a recent SAH have severe disturbances of cerebral autoregulation, and respond unfavorably, often disastrously, to the institution of hypotension, both in terms of cerebral circulation and possible side-effects to other organ systems.

Recently, temporary clips have been extensively utilized to overcome many technical obstacles associated with giant aneurysm surgery[1,10,22]. Temporary clipping has proved especially useful for giant carotid aneurysms where the operative exposure is usually broad enough to permit placement of several clips simultaneously, and collateral circulation around the occluded carotid is usually not an issue. However, prolonged temporary occlusion can be unforgiving when the occluded vessel supplies numerous small perforators such as the carotid bifurcation, the M1 segment of middle cerebral artery, and the anterior communicating artery. These arterial segments supply perforating

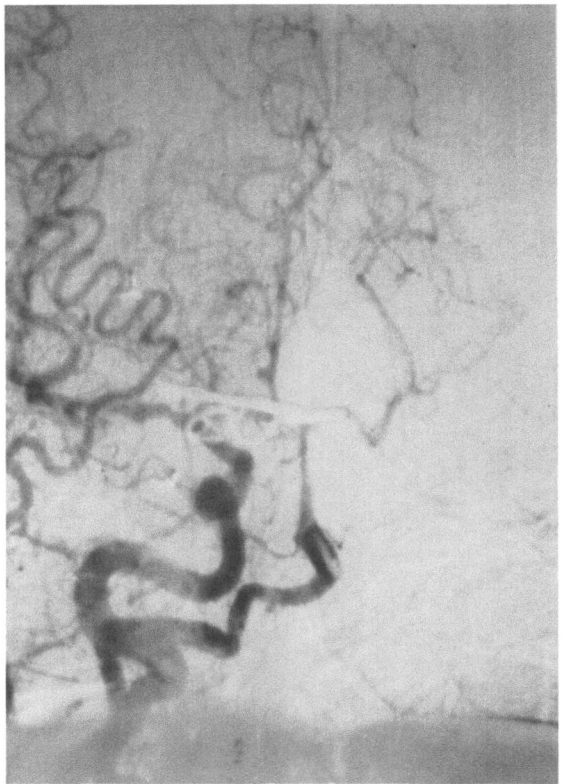

Fig. 8. Post-operative angiogram following clipping of the aneurysm. Note post-operative vasospasm in the basilar circulation

Deep hypothermic circulatory arrest is the ultimate aid in clipping complicated intracranial aneurysms. This technique allows the neurosurgeon, in a relaxed fashion, to deal with an aneurysm totally devoid of arterial pressure. This situation is achieved without the mechanical intrusion of temporary clips and without the worry that perforator vessels will not receive collateral circulation during a prolonged period required to complete a dissection and clip a broad-based giant aneurysm. During total arrest, if the aneurysm is not soft and collapsible, the dome of the aneurysm can be opened and thrombus and atherosclerotic material removed as necessary to fashion a suitable neck for clipping.

The amount of time required to do the final aneurysm dissection and clipping usually is far less than the available safe limit of total circulatory arrest. Clinical and experimental experience in cardiac surgery has demonstrated that total circulatory arrest under deep hypothermia (18 °C) produces virtually no discernible neurologic damage for 30 to 45 minutes, with a slight increase in neurologic consequences as 60 minutes is approached[16]. During the present clinical series, the average circulatory arrest time was only 22 minutes (range 6 to 51). Most of the aneurysm dissection can be completed prior to institution of deep hypothermic circulatory arrest. The final stages of aneurysm clip placement can usually be achieved in a relatively short period of time between 15 and 30 minutes, well within a window of safety in terms of ischemic damage to major organ systems.

This report, combined with other recent publications, justifies renewed interest in deep hypothermic circulatory arrest as an aid for clipping complex giant intracranial aneurysms. The future indications for this technique remain to be elucidated.

vessels without significant collateral circulation. Cessation of flow for more than a few minutes can lead to cerebral infarction. Furthermore, total isolation of the basilar apex via temporary occlusion of the proximal basilar artery and both P1 segments may be disastrous if there is prolonged ischemia to the thalamoperforates and mid-brain penetrating vessels arising from the top of the basilar artery.

The other difficulty that arises with temporary clips is the physical limitation of applying multiple clips into a confined exposure. Attempts to achieve both temporary occlusion of the parent vessel and definitive clipping of the aneurysm neck are often impossible. This issue is most apparent with basilar aneurysms where space is usually the limiting factor. Therefore, although temporary clipping is certainly useful for a large number of intracranial aneurysms, this technique does not provide a definitive solution to the clipping of giant basilar aneurysms and rare giant aneurysms in other locations.

References

1. Batjer HH, Frankfurt AI, Purdy PD, Smith SS, Samson DS (1988) Use of etomidate, temporary arterial occlusion, and intra-operative angiography in surgical treatment of large and giant cerebral aneurysms. J Neurosurg 68: 234–240
2. Baumgartner WA, Silverberg GD, Ream AK, Jamieson SW, Tarabek J, Reitz BA (1983) Reappraisal of cardiopulmonary bypass with deep hypothermia and circulatory arrest for complex neurosurgical operations. Surgery 94: 242–249
3. Chyatte D, Elefteriades J, Kim B (1989) Profound hypothermia and circulatory arrest for aneurysm surgery. Case report. J Neurosurg 70: 489–491
4. Dolenc VV (1985) A combined epi- and subdural direct approach to carotid-ophthalmic artery aneurysms. J Neurosurg 62: 667–672

5. Drake CG (1979) Giant intracranial aneurysms: experience with surgical treatment in 174 patients. Clin Neurosurg 26: 12–95
6. Drake CG, Barr WK, Coles JC, Gergely NF (1964) The use of extracorporeal circulation and profound hypothermia in the treatment of ruptured intracranial aneurysm. J Neurosurg 21: 575–581
7. Heros RC, Nelson PB, Ojemann RG, Crowell RM, DeBrun G (1983) Large and giant paraclinoid aneurysms: surgical techniques, complications, and results. Neurosurgery 12: 153–163
8. Hilal SK, Solomon RA (1992) Endovascular treatment of aneurysms with coils. Letter to the editor. J Neurosurg 76: 337–338
9. Housepian EM, Bowman FO, Gissen AJ (1964) Elective circulatory arrest in intracranial surgery. J Neurosurg 26: 594–597
10. Jabre A, Symon L (1987) Temporary vascular occlusion during aneurysm surgery. Surg Neurol 27: 47–63
11. McMurtry JG, Housepian EM, Bowman FO, Matteo RS (1974) Surgical treatment of basilar artery aneurysms: elective circulatory arrest with thoracotomy in 12 cases. J Neurosurg 40: 486–494
12. Michenfelder JD, Kirklin JW, Uilhein A, Svien HJ, MacCarty CS (1964) Clinical experience with a closed-chest method of producing hypothermia and total circulatory arrest in neurosurgery. Ann Surg 159: 125–131
13. Michenfelder JD, MacCarty CS, Theye RA (1964) Physiologic studies following closed-chest technique of profound hypothermia in neurosurgery. Anesthesiology 25: 131–136
14. Patterson RH, Ray BS (1962) Profound hypothermia for intracranial surgery; laboratory and clinical experience with extracorporeal circulation by peripheral cannulation. Ann Surg 156: 377–393
15. Silverberg GD, Reitz BA, Ream AK (1981) Hypothermia and cardiac arrest in the treatment of giant aneurysms of the cerebral circulation and hemangioblastoma of the medulla. J Neurosurg 55: 337–346
16. Solomon RA, Smith CR, Raps EC, Young WL, JG Stone, Fink ME (1991) Deep hypothermic circulatory arrest for the management of complex anterior and posterior circulation aneurysms. Neurosurgery 29: 732–738
17. Solomon RA, Stein BM (1988) Surgical approaches to aneurysms of the vertebral and basilar arteries. Neurosurgery 23: 203–208
18. Spetzler RF, Hadley MN, Rigamonti D, Carter LP, Raudzens PA, Shedd SA, Wilkinson E (1988) Aneurysms of the basilar artery treated with circulatory arrest, hypothermia, and barbiturate cerebral protection. J Neurosurg 68: 868–879
19. Sundt TM, Pluth JR, Gronert Ga (1972) Excision of giant basilar aneurysm under profound hypothermia: report of a case. Mayo Clin Proc 47: 631–634
20. Uihlein A, MacCarty CS, Michenfelder JD, Terry HR, Daw EF (1966) Deep hypothermia and surgical treatment of intracranial aneurysms: a 5 year study. JAMA 195: 127–129
21. Woodhall B, Sealy WC, Hall KD, Floyd WL (1960) Craniotomy under conditions of quinidine-protected cardioplegia and profound hypothermia. Ann Surg 152: 37–44
22. Young WL, Solomon RA, Pedley TA, Ross L, Schwartz AE, Ornstein E, Matteo RS, Ostapkovich N (1989) Direct cortical EEG monitoring during temporary vascular occlusion for cerebral aneurysm surgery. Anesthesiology 71: 794–799

Correspondence: Robert A. Solomon, M.D., The Neurological Institute, Room 439. 710 West 168th Street, New York, NY 10032, U.S.A.

Surgery of Giant Aneurysms

Clipping Techniques for Partially Thrombosed Giant Aneurysms

K. Sugita, M. Shibuya, M. Negoro, and **Y. Suzuki**

Department of Neurosurgery, Nagoya University School of Medicine, Turumai, Showa, Nagoya, Japan

Summary

Surgery for partially thrombosed giant and large aneurysms is technically more difficult than for nonthrombosed aneurysms. Treatment strategies consisting of intravascular embolization, direct clipping and bypass surgery must be made according to the location, size and degree of thrombosis of the aneurysms and collateral flow. Among 64 giant and large aneurysms 27 were partially thrombosed. Direct clipping was performed in 18, combined interventional and direct surgery in 3 and interventional surgery alone in 6 patients. Surgical results were good in 24, poor in two with death in one patients. Good indications for intravascular surgery are aneurysms in the intracavernous carotid artery, vertebral artery, basilar tip and those unruptured aneurysms with less mass effect in elderly patients. For direct clipping, parent artery is trapped after heparinization and aneurysm is opened at a place more than 5 mm away from the parent artery in order to obtain enough space for multiple clips. After thrombectomy best fitting clips were selected from over 80 different shapes of Sugita clips. Large clips of over 21 mm, fenestrated clips and booster clips were most frequently used. Three to six clips were needed to occlude the wide and thick neck of each aneurysm. Direct clipping with aneurysmectomy was the most preferable procedure from the point of decompression and complete cure for the ruptured, partially thrombosed giant and large aneurysms with mass effects.

Keywords: Giant aneurysms; partial thrombosis; direct surgery; endovascular occlusion.

Introduction

In the past 15 years a total of 64 giant and large aneurysms were operated on. Twenty seven of these aneurysms were partially thrombosed. The treatments of partially thrombosed aneurysms are different from those of non-thrombosed aneurysms. They were treated by either interventional surgery, direct clipping or their combination.

Clinical Material and Methods

Surgery of Partially Thrombosed Giant Aneurysms

Partially thrombosed giant aneurysms were operated on with clipping in 18 cases, combined intravascular surgery and direct clipping in 3 cases and intravascular surgery alone in 6 cases. In elderly patients with unruptured aneurysms, interventional occlusion of the parent artery or the aneurysm was tried before a direct clipping was performed. Balloon occlusion of the parent artery was most satisfactory in patients with the intracavernous carotid and vertebral aneurysms who had sufficient collateral flow. Successful intraaneurysmal occlusion was done in 2 cases, one with a balloon and the other with platinum coils. High flow bypass surgery using saphenous vein graft was performed in two cases with insufficient collateral flow.

In all patients who underwent direct clipping, preoperative balloon occlusion tests of the carotid or vertebral arteries were performed. During direct surgery, the proximal and the distal portions of the parent artery were exposed for temporary occlusion, which was performed in all cases except one. The mean total trapping time was 40 minutes. Aneurysmal bodies were isolated from the surrounding tissue as much as possible. Systemic heparinization was performed before trapping and aneurysmectomy. Aneurysmectomy was performed because clipping was possible only after removing atheroma and thombus in all cases except for two cases who had a small atheroma only in the dome side. Aneurysmal incision was made further than 5 mm from the parent artery. Thrombi and atheromas were removed as briefly as possible to reduce the trapping time[13]. Multiple clips (from 3 to 6) were necessary to close the neck of giant aneurysms. The most suitable clips were selected from among 80 different shapes[10-12]. If there was an important artery branching from the neck or the body of the aneurysm, the portion was left as a residual and wrapped with thin sheets of cotton patty. To prevent clots and atheroma in the neck from entering into the parent artery, temporary and multiple aneurysm clips were released one at the time and blood was flashed before removing temporary clips. All of the necks of excised aneurysms were closed with clips except for one case which was closed with sutures. Heparin was reversed with protamine immediately after clipping was completed.

Results

The treatment methods and results of the 27 partially thrombosed giant and large aneurysms were as follows: all of the 6 cavernous aneurysms were trapped without trouble. Three intracranial carotid artery aneurysms were clipped with satisfactory results. Among five aneurysms of the MCA and ACA, 4 cases were clipped and one case was trapped with good results in 4 cases and poor in one. One basilar aneurysm was clipped

Table 1. *Surgical Results of Partially Thombosed Giant Aneurysms*

	No.	Good	Poor	Death
Intracavernous	6	6	0	0
Carotid	3	3	0	0
MCA and ACA	5	4	1	0
Basilar	2	2	0	0
Vertebral	11	9	1	1
Total	27	24	2	1

and another occluded with coils without trouble. Nine vertebral artery aneurysms were trapped, 2 were occluded with a clip and a balloon respectively. The results of the vertebral artery aneurysms were good in 9 cases, and poor in one with death in one. The surgical results of the total cases were good in 24, and poor in two, with death in one.

Discussion

Partially thrombosed giant aneurysms differ from non-thrombosed ones in that the former have less incidence of rupture but often show stronger neurological deficits, which is particularly true in the aneurysms of the carotid and vertebral arteries[5]. Intravascular surgery is indicated in cases with minor neurological deficits in elderly patients. Neurological deficits improved the next day of the embolization in two cases, though little change was found in the size of the mass on postoperative CT scan. Best indication for the intravascular surgery was the carotid aneurysms in the cavernous sinus, though high flow bypass was needed if the collateral flow was insufficient[2,3,7,9]. The intracranial carotid artery aneurysm often showed severe visual disturbances which could hardly recover in spite of decompression by aneurysmectomy. Intravascular embolization was also indicated for the basilar artery aneurysms because the results of direct clipping in this area were poor[1,4,5]. Severe neurological deficits in patients with vertebral artery aneurysms, improved dramatically by aneurysmectomy, though surgery was not easy[13]. Generally, intravascular treatment was superior to direct surgery when only trapping was intended with the exception of the trunk of basilar artery. On the other hand, neck clipping with aneurysmectomy was preferable from the point of decompression and complete cure.

Clipping of partially thrombosed giant aneurysms is different from that of nonthrombosed ones, in that puncture does not collapse the aneurysm and that

aneurysmectomy and thrombectomy are indispensable because atheroma disturbs complete closure of the clips[6]. Generally aneurysmectomy should be performed as far from the parent artery as possible, to have an enough space for placing the clips. However, if the dome of aneurysm is opened, more thrombus than necessary must be removed; on the opposite, if aneurysms are sectioned close to the parent artery, there may not be enough space to manipulate the clips, causing narrowing of the parent artery. It was often difficult to remove hard atheroma and thrombus quickly enough without injuring the wall of the aneurysmal neck. Rough and quick removal of the central portions of the thrombus and very fine maneuver near the aneurysmal wall like thromboendarterectomy of the cervical carotid artery is recommended[13]. Selection of the most appropriate clips for each aneurysm are essential. The necks were closed by clipping rather than by suturing in order to reduce trapping time. The aneurysms were obliterated using 3 to 6 clips. It was sometimes difficult to close the neck completely even by selecting the most adequate combinations of the clips from more than 80 different shapes of Sugita clips[10-12]. Large clips of over 21 mm is length were most frequently used followed by ring and booster clips. Residual necks were wrapped with thin sheet of cottonoid. In our series of 200 aneurysms which had partially been wrapped with cottonoids, we have not encountered foreign body reaction postoperatively. However, care should be taken since development of granuloma around the cottonoids has been reported by several authors[8].

Although surgical results between intravascular embolization and direct clipping show no obvious difference in this series, more and more intravascular surgery will be performed in the future with technical advancement. While direct clipping will continue to be the first choice for early surgery of ruptured aneurysms, except in elderly patients (over 70 years.)

References

1. Aymard A, Gobin P, Hodes J, Bien S, Rufenacht D, Reizine D, George B, Merland J (1991) Endovascular occlusion of vertebral arteries in the treatment of unclippable Vertebrobasilar aneurysms. J Neurosurg 74: 393–398
2. Guglielmi G, Vinuela F, Dion J, Duckwiler G (1991) Electrothrombosis of saccular aneurysms via endovascular approach. J Neurosurg 75: 8–14
3. Higashida R, Halbach V, Dowd C, Barnwell S, Dormandy B, Bell J, Hieshima G (1990) Endovascular detachable ballon embolization therapy of cavernous corotid artery aneurysms: results in 87 cases. J Neurosurg 72: 857–863

4. Higashida R, Halbach V, Cahan L, Hieshima G, Konishi Y (1989) Detachable ballon embolization therapy of posterior circulation intracranial aneurysms: J Neurosurg 71: 512–519

5. Hosobuchi Y (1976) Direct surgical treatment of giant intracranial aneurysms. J Neurosurg 51: 743–756

6. Kyoshima K, Kobayashi S, Wakui K, Ichinose Y, Okudera H (1992) A newly designed puncture needle for suction decompression of giant aneurysms. J Neurosurg 76: 880–882

7. Linskey M, Sekhar L, Horton J, Hirsch W Jr., Yonas H (1991) Aneurysms of the intracavernous carotid artery: a multidisciplinary approach to treatment. J Neurosurg 75: 525–534

8. McFadzean RM, Hadley DM, McIlwain GG (1991) Optochiasmal arachnoiditis following muslin wrapping of ruptured anterior communicating artery aneurysms. J Neurosurg 75: 393–396

9. Serbinenko F, Filatov J, Spallone A, Tchurilov M, Lazarev V (1990) Management of giant intracranial ICA aneurysms with combined extracranial-intracranial anastomosis and endovascular occlusion. J Neurosurg 73: 57–63

10. Sugita K, Kobayashi S, Kyoshima K, Nakagawa F (1982) Fenestrated clips for unusual aneurysms of the carotid artery. J Neurosurg 57: 240–246

11. Sugita K, Kobayashi S, Inoue T, Takemae T (1984) Characterisitics and use of ultra-long aneurysm clips. J Neurosurg 60: 145–150

12. Sugita K (1984) Microneurosurgical atlas. Springer, Berlin Heidelberg New York Tokyo

13. Sugita K, Kobayashi, S, Takemae T, Tanaka Y, Okudera H, Ohsawa M (1988) Giant aneurysms of the vertebral artery. J Neurosurg 68: 960–966

Correspondence: Kenichiro Sugita, M.D., Department of Neurosurgery. Nagoya University School of Medicine, Turumai 65, Showa, Nagoya 466, Japan.

Complication Avoidance for Large and Giant Carotid Ophthalmic Aneurysms

S.L. Giannotta

Department of Neurosurgery, LAC-USC Medical Center, University of Southern California School of Medicine, Los Angeles, California, U.S.A.

Summary

The author describes the management and complications of 35 large and giant aneurysms of the carotid-opthalmic segment. 18 cases were treated with planned carotid occlusion with or without concomitant extracranial to intracranial bypass. There was a 33% major morbidity. 17 cases were treated with direct exposure and clip ligation, resulting in two ischemic injuries causing death (12%). Analysis of the two cases resulting in death revealed inadvertent narrowing of the segment of the parent artery adjacent to clip application. This has resulted in a subtle modification of the so-called "stacking-seating" technique, which is described in the manuscript.

Keywords: Aneurysm; carotid-ophthalmic aneurysm; ECIC bypass; stacking-seating technique.

Introduction

Certain anatomical characteristics of carotid ophthalmic artery aneurysms present the cerebrovascular surgeon with a unique set of management related challenges. Situated at the skull base and partially covered by the overlying anterior clinoid process, such lesions require the need for a powerful high-speed drill directly adjacent to a large pulsating sac. The adjacent optic nerve, frequently compressed to the point of functional compromise, needs to be manipulated – but at the same time protected – throughout the surgical procedure. Unlike other anterior circulation aneurysms, between 25% and 50% of carotid ophthalmic aneurysms may be large or giant, and up to 50% of cases may present in the absence of subarachnoid hemorrhage with minimal symptoms, thereby making surgical decision making even more difficult[1,3-5,9,10,13-15,17]. The necessity of obtaining control of various sources of collateral flow to the area, along with the occasional necessity for a trapping procedure with or without hemispheric revascularization, adds to the complexity of the decision making. Furthermore, the likelihood of the presence of calcium in the aneurysm wall, the need for occasional surgical excursions into the cavernous sinus, and the requirement of specialized equipment such as angle fenestrated clips round out a group of circumstances that are fraught with potential complications.

Such circumstances made the direct approach for large and giant carotid aneurysms so prohibitively dangerous that indirect approaches were embraced initially[8,11]. Common and internal carotid artery ligation with and without bypass were utilized with some element of success[7,16]. As surgical techniques improved and micro-surgical instrumentation advanced, the direct approach for clip ligation assumed a more prominent role[4,5,9,10,13,17,18,20]. However, continual improvement in technique is mandatory to further reduce risk since alternative methods being developed within the interventional radiologic discipline are ready to compete for the high risk patient[6]. An analysis of 35 large and giant carotid ophthalmic aneurysms treated by indirect and direct surgical approaches are analyzed. Technical maneuvers that led to morbidity are discussed along with strategies to maximize effectiveness of the direct approach.

Clinical Series

A total of 35 large and giant carotid ophthalmic aneurysms treated by the author were retrospectively reviewed. Thirteen were large measuring greater than 1.2 cm in diameter but less than 2.5 cm. Twenty-two lesions were giant measuring greater than 2.5 cm in diameter. Visual loss or other visual symptoms were the presenting complaint in 13 cases. An additional

Table 1. *Operative Procedures for 35 Large and Giant Carotid-Ophthalmic Aneurysms*

Clip ligation	17
Carotid clamp (internal)	10
Carotid clamp (internal/bypass)	1
Carotid clamp (common)	3
Trap	4
	35

Table 2. *Complications in 35 Carotid-Ophthalmic Aneurysms Treated by Direct and Indirect Means*

	Clip (17)	Occlusion or trap (18)
Stroke	2 (12%)	4 (22%)
Visual loss	0	2 (11%)
CSF leak	1 (6%)	0

thirteen patients presented with subarachnoid hemorrhage, four with headache, three with stroke from embolism, and two were found totally incidental to another pathological process. Early in the series indirect approaches were emphasized (Table 1). Ten cases were treated by gradual internal carotid artery occlusion using a Kindt clamp. One case was managed with gradual occlusion plus ECIC bypass. Three cases were treated by gradual common carotid artery occlusion, and four cases were treated by an intracranial and extracranial trapping procedure. Of those 18 cases treated with planned occlusion, with or without bypass, there were four cases of cerebral infarction (22%) (Table 2). None of these cases of cerebral infarction resulted in death. It should be noted that during gradual carotid occlusion, volume expansion and support of blood pressure were emphasized making it unlikely that hemodynamic factors were responsible for the ischemic complications. No patients were treated prophylactically with heparin. There were two instances where visual symptoms worsened with carotid occlusion, one of which was due to embolization of the central retinal artery (11%). Postoperative cerebral angiography demonstrated no filling of the aneurysm in any of the cases of planned vessel occlusion.

Direct operative approach with clip ligation was accomplished in 17 cases. There were two strokes both resulting in death of the patient due to inadvertent narrowing or unrecognized occlusion of the internal carotid artery. There was one case of post-operative CSF leak which required a separate operative procedure for management. No worsening of visual symptoms was noted in those cases treated with direct clip ligation.

Discussion

Ischemic Complications

Indirect approaches with planned vessel occlusions and or trapping resulted in a major morbidity of 33%. The putative mechanisms were felt to be related to embolism in the ischemic cases and to expansile thrombosis of the aneurysm with compressive cranial neuropathy in the visual cases. There was no long-standing morbidity with the direct approach, unfortunately, two ischemic complications both resulted in death (12%). An analysis of these two cases reveals a common pathophysiologic mechanism. In both instances, although clip application looked to be ideal from the standpoint of obliteration of the aneurysm and patency of the internal carotid artery, the internal diameter of the parent vessel was markedly compromised. In one case, this was documented belatedly by postoperative angiography. Both cases resulted in occlusion of the parent vessel with major cerebral infarction ending in death of the patient. As a result, two major alterations in technique were devised to improve safety of direct clip occlusion for large and giant carotid ophthalmic aneurysms.

Clip Application

A subtle modification of the so-called "stacking-seating" technique (Fig. 1) has been used for clip obliteration of large proximal carotid aneurysms. Not infrequently, the position of the initially placed clip will be forced by the bulk of the aneurysm to slip further down toward the base possibly compromising the internal diameter of the parent vessel. Although externally the clip seems to be in good position, the aneurysm may continue to fill due to intermittent slight opening of the clip. Complete obliteration of the aneurysm may then be accomplished by a series of clips stacked one on top of the other above the original clip. Although successful in obliterating the aneurysmal sac, such a stacked arrangement may also inadvertently occlude the parent vessel. Once the stacked arrangement has been satisfactorily accomplished, the original clip adjacent to the parent vessel is removed. This maneuver, although seemingly allowing part of the base of the aneurysm to remain unsecured, actually on post-

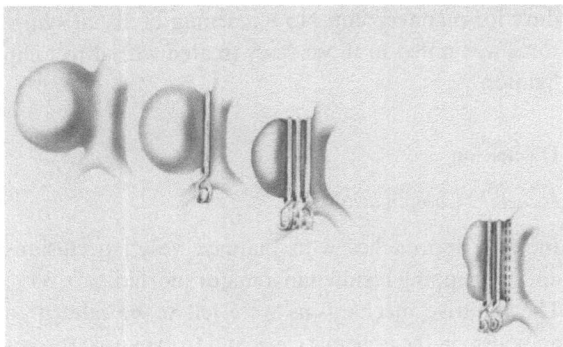

Fig. 1. Artist's rendering of the steps necessary for the "stacking-seating" technique. Once all clips are stabilized in position and the sac is completely collapsed, the most proximal clip is removed and the caliber of the carotid artery is verified by intraoperative angiography

operative angiography will frequently be shown to result in a normal internal diameter of the parent vessel. By stacking a series of clips and allowing several minutes for the clips to settle in place or "seat", removal of the initially placed clip will allow adequate caliber of the parent vessel while maintaining satisfactory position of the stacked clips and thus complete obliteration of the sac (Fig. 2).

Intraoperative Angiography

As a further measure to avoid inadvertant occlusion or narrowing of the carotid artery during direct approaches for complex proximal aneurysms, we have since added intraoperative angiography to our operative routine. The ability to confirm intraoperatively satisfactory occlusion of the lesion, in conjunction with adequate preservation of the parent vessel has dramatically improved the results in management of such complex lesions. Especially in situations where innovative multi-clip strategies are necessary, angiographic feedback has proven indispensible[2,12]. Barrow and colleagues in a series of 60 aneurysm cases in which intraoperative angiography was correlated with post-operative studies, showed excellent agreement suggesting that such technology has adequate resolution to allow reliable decision making[2].

Optic Nerve Injury

Safety of the visual apparatus during direct approaches must be maximized in order for the direct approach to maintain superiority over other indirect strategies. It is our feeling that retraction of the optic nerve and chiasm and removal of the clinoid process, are the two

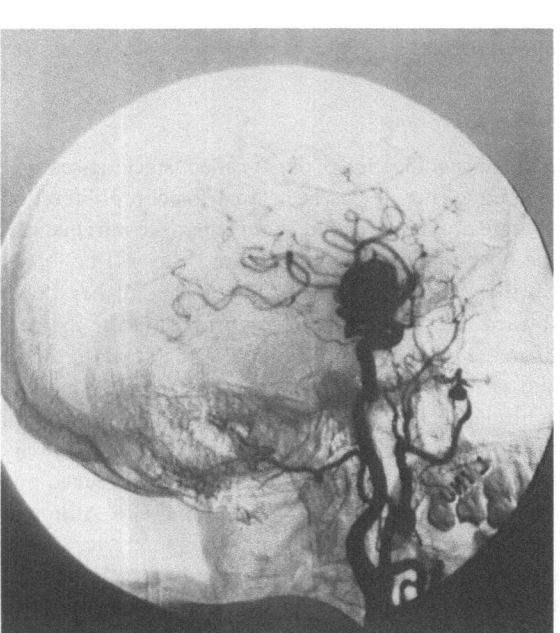

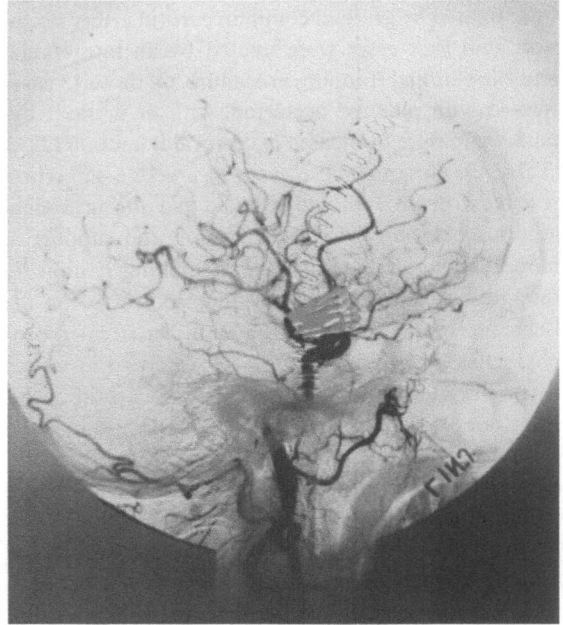

a   b

Fig. 2. (a, b) Pre- and postoperative angiogram of large carotid ophthalmic aneurysn.

maneuvers that most jeopardize vision. Ischemia is the most likely mechanism of optic nerve injury during the former maneuver, with thermal and mechanical trauma being responsible for complications during the latter. We have eschewed continous self-retaining retraction of the optic nerve and have relied upon gentle intermittent retraction to improve safety by reducing prolonged microcirculatory ischemia[19]. Further, we have taken great pains to improve our technique and instrumentation related to removal of the clinoid process and decompression of the optic canal. The key instrument, of course, in this maneuver is the high-speed drill. Important characteristics when considering drill technologies for clinoid removal include: reversibility of direction, adequate torque and power, angled low-profile hand pieces, and an array of cutting and diamond burrs. Since much of microneurosurgery involves the use of diamond burrs near cranial nerves or small vessels, reversibility of the drill mechanism assumes greater priority. A brief loss of control can cause the burr to "run" along a bony surface toward a vulnerable structure. Reversing the direction of rotation can insure that such an excursion will be in a direction away from the optic nerve. Further adjuncts to improve safety include: protection of the shaft of the drill bit, a constant source of cooling irrigation, and foot pedal activation along with a well-balanced and lightweight hand piece such that singlehanded maneuverability is maximized. Most drills available for neurosurgeons are a compromise between micro and macrosurgical uses. It is important to select a technology that is ergonomically suited to microsurgical use. A well balanced handpiece with a foot control will allow maximization of fine motor control. The strategy of clinoid removal is straightforward but it is important to remember that in each case of carotid ophthalmic aneurysm, care should be taken to completely unroof the optic canal, so that intermittant retraction does not further compromise vascular supply.

CSF Leak

We have experienced one case of CSF rhinorrhea following clinoid removal for ophthalmic aneurysm. This can result from several cicumstances. A pneumatized anterior clinoid process may connect with the ethmoid or sphenoid sinuses. With removal of the clinoid an unrecognized breech of the mucosa may occur. An occult fenestration in the greater wing of the sphenoid may be inadvertently entered during removal of the clinoid process. In any event, prophylactic obliteration of all bony surfaces using bone wax and the use of fibrin glue over all exposed mucosal and dural surfaces is recommended to avoid this complication.

Conclusions

Continued alteration in surgical strategies should ultimately improve the results for direct approach to large and giant carotid ophthalmic aneurysms. Strategies to maximize parent vessel internal diameter in conjunction with clip application to completely obliterate the sac should reduce postoperative ischemic complications. Utilization of advanced technologies and careful technique in bony removal of the clinoid process and surrounding structures should enhance safety of the optic pathways. Use of protective anesthetic regimens and employment of intraoperative angiographic imaging should maximize the benefits to clip application over indirect approaches for complex vascular lesions of the proximal internal carotid artery.

References

1. Almeida GM, Shibata MK, Biaco E (1976) Carotid ophthalmic aneurysms. Surg Neurol 5: 41–45
2. Barrow DL, Boyer KL, Joseph GJ (1992) Intraoperative angiography in the management of neurovascular disorders. Neurosurgery 30: 153–159
3. Day AL (1990) Aneurysms of the ophthalmic segment. J Neurosurg 72: 677–691
4. Drake CG, Vanderlinden RG, Amacher AL (1968) Carotid ophthalmic aneurysms. J Neurosurg 29: 24–36
5. Ferguson GG, Drake CG (1981) Carotid-ophthalmic aneurysms: visual abnormalities in 32 patients and the results of treatment. Surg Neurol 16: 1–8
6. Fox AJ, Vinuela F, Pelz DM, Ferguson GG, Drake CG, Debrun G (1987) Use of detachable balloons for proximal artery occlusion in the treatment of unclippable cerebral uneurysms. J Neurosurg 66: 40–46
7. Gelber BR, Sundt Tm Jr (1980) Treatment of intracavernous and giant carotid aneurysms by combined internal carotid ligation and extra- to intracranial bypass. J Neurosurg 52: 1–10
8. Giannotta SL McGillicuddy JE Kindt GW (1979) Gradual carotid artery occlusion in the treatment of inaccessible internal carotid artery aneurysms. Neurosurgery 5: 417–421
9. Guidetti B, LaTorre E (1975) Management of carotid-ophthalmic aneurysms. J Neurosurg 42: 438–442
10. Heros RC, Nelson PB, Ojemann RG, Crowell RM, Debrun G (1983) Large and giant paraclinoid aneurysms: surgical techniques. Neurosurgery 12: 153–163
11. Heros RC, Swearingen B (1987) Common carotid occlusion for unclippable carotid aneurysms: an old but still effective technique. Neurosurgery 21: 288–295
12. Hieshima GB, Reicher MA, Higashida RT, Halbach VV, Cahan LD, Martin NA, Frazee JG, Rand RW, Bentson JR (1987)

Intraoperative digital subtraction neuroangiography: a diagnostic and therapeutic tool. AJNR: 759–767

13. Nutik SL (1988) Ventral paraclinoid carotid aneurysms. J Neurosurg 69: 340–344

14. Pia HW (1978) Classification of aneurysms of the internal carotid system. Acta Neurochir (Wien) 40: 5–31

15. Sengupta RP (1986) Natural history of carotid ophthalmic aneurysms and its influence on surgical management. In: Kikuchi H, Fukushima T, Watanabe K (eds) Intracranial aneurysms. Nishimura, pp 63–99

16. Spetzler RF, Schuster H, Roski RA (1980) Elective extracranial-intracranial arterial bypass in the treatment of inoperable giant aneurysms of the internal carotid artery. J Neurosurg 53: 22–27

17. Sundt TM, Piepgras DG (1979) Surgical approach to giant intracranial aneurysms. Operative experience with 80 cases. J Neurosurg 51: 731–742

18. Sugita K, Kobayashi S, Kyoshima K, Nakagawa F (1982) Fenestrated clips for unusual aneurysms of the carotid artery. J Neurosurg 57: 240–246

19. Sugita K, Kobayashi S, Takemae T, Matsuo K, Yokoo A (1980) Direct retraction method in aneurysm surgery. J Neurosurg 53: 417–419

20. Yasargil MG, Gasser JC, Hodosh RM, Bankin TV (1977) Carotid-ophthalmic aneurysms: direct microsurgical approach. Surg Neurol 8: 155–165

Correspondence: Steven L. Giannotta, M.D., Department of Neurosurgery, University of Southern California School of Medicine, Box 239, 1200 State Street, Los Angeles, California 90033, U.S.A.

Direct Microsurgical Approach to Giant Intracranial Aneurysms. Considerations, Technical Notes and Results in a Series of 47 Cases

R.J. Galzio, G.P. Tassi, D. Lucantoni, and **A. Ricci**

Division of Neurosurgery, "G. Mazzini" Civic Hospital, Teramo, Italy

Summary

A series of 47 giant intracranial aneurysms (GIAs) treated by a direct microsurgical approach is presented. They represent 10.5% of all intracranial aneurysms operated on during the same period (1982–1991). 37 of these GIAs were located on the anterior circulation, 10 in the vertebro – basilar system. A total of 45 patients were operated on, because two patients presented two GIAs each. Clinical presentation was haemorrhagic in 25 patients, not haemorrhagic in 20. In 36 cases the aneurysm was clipped; in 7 it was excluded by trapping; in 1 case it was wrapped; in 1 case only an exploration was performed. In 2 cases an extra-intracranial bypass was performed. Postoperatively 26 patients presented complete recovery; 5 patients presented moderate disability and 4 patients severe disability; 10 patients died.

In our opinion direct microsurgical approach remains the elective treatment of GIAs. Temporary trapping or clipping of the parent vessel under induced hypertension and barbiturate protection, voluntary rupture of the aneurysm and clipping under aspiration, reconstruction of the aneurismal neck by bipolar coagulation, exclusion with multiple and variously shaped clips, are useful intra-operative methods, as well as a large bony resection of the sphenoidal wing and orbital roof, and intermittent brain retraction with microspatulas.

Thrombectomy was easily achieved – in some of our last cases – with the use of the ultrasonic aspirator. Trapping techniques were particularly useful in the treatment of GIAs of the intracavernous carotid and posterior cerebral artery.

Keywords: Giant aneurysms; surgical technique; temporary clipping; thrombectomy.

Introduction

Intracranial aneurysms with a diameter of 2.5 cm or more are – by convention – classified as giant. Giant aneurysms present intrinsic features, which are responsible for their peculiar clinical and radiological presentation and also for their challenging treatment. Our experience with direct surgical approach to this kind of lesions is presented.

Clinical Material

In a 9 years period (1982–1991), 45 patients with 47 giant aneurysms underwent direct intracranial surgery. They represent 10.5% of all patients operated on for intracranial aneurysms during the same period. 37 giant aneurysms were located on the anterior circulation and 10 in the vertebrobasilar system (Table 1). 9 patients presented one or more additional aneurysms: 2 of them harboured two giant aneurysms (Table 2). In our series, both sexes were almost equally represented (23 females and 22 males); the age of patients ranged from 22 to 74 years (mean 51 years). Intracranial haemorrhage was observed in 25 patients, symptoms of expanding mass lesion were observed in 11, ischaemic episodes in 3, headache in 3, seizures in 2; the aneurysm was an incidental discovery in 1 patient. All patients – except 2 with a life – threatening subdural hematoma operated on in emergency after CT scanning – were preoperatively studied by CT scan (without and with contrast enhancement) and transfemoral panangiography. In most of our recent cases MRI was also performed. In some cases an angio-MRI was also performed.

Table 1. *Incidence of Giant Aneurysms (47 GIAs in 45 Patients)*

Location	Hemorrhagic	Non-hemorrhagic
ICA/Siphon		
– ICA/PCoA	7	3
– ICA B.	3	0
– ICA Oph.	3	1
ICA i.c.	1	5
MCA	4	3
ACA	5	2
PCA	0	3
BAC	3	2
VBJ	0	1
VA/PICA	1	0
Total	27	20

ICA internal carotid artery; *PCoA* posterior communicating artery; *ICA B.* bifurcation of the internal carotid artery; *ICA Oph.* origin of the ophtalmic artery from the internal carotid artery; *ICA i.c.* intracavernous internal carotid artery; *MCA* middle cerebral artery; *ACA* anterior cerebral artery; *PCA* posterior cerebral artery; *BAC* basilar artery caput; *VBJ* vertebrobasilar Junction; *VA* vertebral artery; *PICA* posterior inferior cerebellar artery.

Table 2. *Location of Additional Aneurysms (9 Cases)*

Giant aneurysm		Additional aneurysm
ICA/PCoA	(right)	BA/SCA (giant)
ICA/PCoA	(right)	MCA (giant)
MCA	(right)	ICA/PCoA (right)
ICA/PCoA	(right)	MCA (right) + basilar tip
MCA	(left)	MCA (right) + pericallosal artery
MCA	(left)	MCA 1 (right) + MCA2 (left)
ICA/PCoA	(right)	ACoA
VBJ		ACoA
MCA	(right)	BA

Abbreviations see Table 1.

Treatment

Anterior circulation and basilar tip aneurysms were approached by the pterional route; a wide drilling of the sphenoid wing and of the orbital roof was performed in order to obtain a larger working space, with minimal brain retraction. Giant aneurysms of the posterior cerebral artery (3 cases) were approached subtemporally. 10 patients with lesions located on the proximal vertebral artery or vertebro-basilar junction were operated in lateral or prone decubitus, and never in the sitting position. We have treated associated aneurysms, whenever possible, during the same procedure. All patients received mannitol (150 mg/kg in 1 hour) at the beginning of the procedure. Lumbar drainage was rarely used, and never in bleeding aneurysms. Mild hypotension (induced by nitroglicerin or nitroprusside) was employed in the first cases of our series, but actually we use it only if neck dissection appears easy; we prefer, when dissection or neck clipping seems hazardous or troubling, a temporary clipping or trapping of the parent vessel under induced hypertension and barbiturate protection. Obviously, the proximal parent artery is to be exposed and a site where a temporary clip can be applied is to be identified before aneurysmal dissection. Temporary clipping or trapping time ranged between less than 7 minutes – in most or our cases – to a maximum of 22 minutes. Only in cases of giant intracavernous aneurysms, the cervical carotid bifurcation was surgically exposed before craniotomy. Only rarely we have placed definitive clips on the aneurysmal neck at first; in most cases, also if clipping appeared feasible, we preferred to apply one or more clips somewhat distant to the true neck. After clipping or trapping of the parent artery or after initial clipping of the aneurysm, the sac was evacuated by puncture and aspiration or was widely opened and the endoluminal thrombus was evacuated. The ultrasonic aspirator has been useful in shortening the time of thrombectomy. After the evacuation of the sac from blood and/or thrombus, the vessels were inspected and definitive clips were repositioned. Sometimes we used bipolar coagulation to reduce or to create an aneurysmal neck. A great variety of clip modalities has been used: fenestrated or multiple, variously shaped and sized clips, placed in parallel or in tandem along the major axis of the parent vessel prevented narrowing of its diameter and permitted good reconstruction of the circulation.

In 4 cases of intracavernous giant aneurysms we were not able to clip the lesion and we made an intracranial trapping of the internal carotid artery after measuring the distal stump pressure; in 1 case an extra – to intracranial anastomosis was done during the same procedure. All of the 3 cases of posterior cerebral artery lesions were trapped, with excellent outcome. 1 vertebro – basilar junction aneurysm was only wrapped with muscle and 1 global dilatation

of the intracranial carotid was only inspected. We were able to clip 36 out of the 47 giant aneurysms submitted to direct intracranial surgery.

Results

The surgical outcome in our series is graded according to the GOS (Glasgow Outcome Scale)[15]. In the bleeding aneurysms subgroup of 25 patients (with 27 giant aneurysms) we had 6 fatalities and 1 patient remained severely disabled; 18 patients may be regarded as having had satisfactory outcome (which represents 72% of patients in this sub-group) (Table 3). 2 out of the dead patients were operated on acutely, without angiography, because of life-threatening subdural hematoma. Main factors influencing outcome in this subgroup appear to be the preoperative condition, associated pathologies (hypertensive state, atherosclerotic desease, cardiopulmonary or metabolic failure, etc.), and age. Results as related to preoperative Hunt and Hess grade, are presented in Table 4.

Table 3. *Results of Surgery in Giant Aneurysms (47 GIAs in 45 Patients)*

Location	Results of surgery			
	Complete recovery	Moderate disability	Severe disability	Death
Bleeding aneurysms				
Anterior circulation	15	2	1	5
Posterior circulation	1	0	0	1
Non-bleeding aneurysms				
Anterior circulation	7	2	2	3
Posterior circulation	4	1	0	1

Table 4. *Results Related to the Preoperative H-H* Grading (47 GIAs in 45 patients)*

	Results of surgery			
	Complete recovery	Moderate disability	Severe disability	Death
Non-bleeding aneurysms	12	3	2	3
Bleeding aneurysms Grade				
I	9	0	0	3
II	4	1	1	0
III	2	1	0	2
IV	0	0	0	1
V	0	0	0	1

* Preoperative grading according to Hunt and Hess[14].

Early operations for bleeding giant aneurysms are – as it is the case also for smaller bleeding aneurysms – complicated by a higher postoperative mortality (Table 5); however, when the approach does not seems very difficult (at least for cases with lesions located on the anterior circulation) we prefer to submit these patients to early surgery; in our opinion final results are similar to those of standard bleeding aneurysms. In this subgroup of patients we were able to clip the

Table 5. *Results Related to the Operative day Post-SAH (27 GIAs in 25 Patients)*

Operative day post-SAH	Results of surgery			
	Complete recovery	Moderate disability	Severe disability	Death
1–3 days	6	1	0	5
4–7 days	1	0	0	0
8–15 days	4	1	0	1
> 15 days*	4	0	1	1

* Both patients with two GIAs are in this group.

Table 6. *Results Related to the Aneurysm Location (47 GIAs in 45 Patients)*

Aneurysm location	Results of surgery			
	Complete recovery	Moderate disability	Severe disability	Death
ICA siphon	11	1	2	3
ICA i.c.	2	3	0	1
MCA	3	0	0	4
ACA	6	0	1	0
PCA	2	1	0	0
BAC	3	0	0	2
VA/PICA	1	0	0	0
VBJ	1	0	0	0

Patients with two GIAs are considered twice in this table (both harboured a BAC and a MCA GIA). Abbreviations see Table 1.

aneurysmal neck in 24 lesions, while 2 giant aneurysms were trapped and 1 was wrapped (Table 7).

In the non-bleeding subgroup of 20 patients, we obtained satisfactory results in 14 cases (70% of cases); 2 patients presented severe disability and 4 died (Table 3);

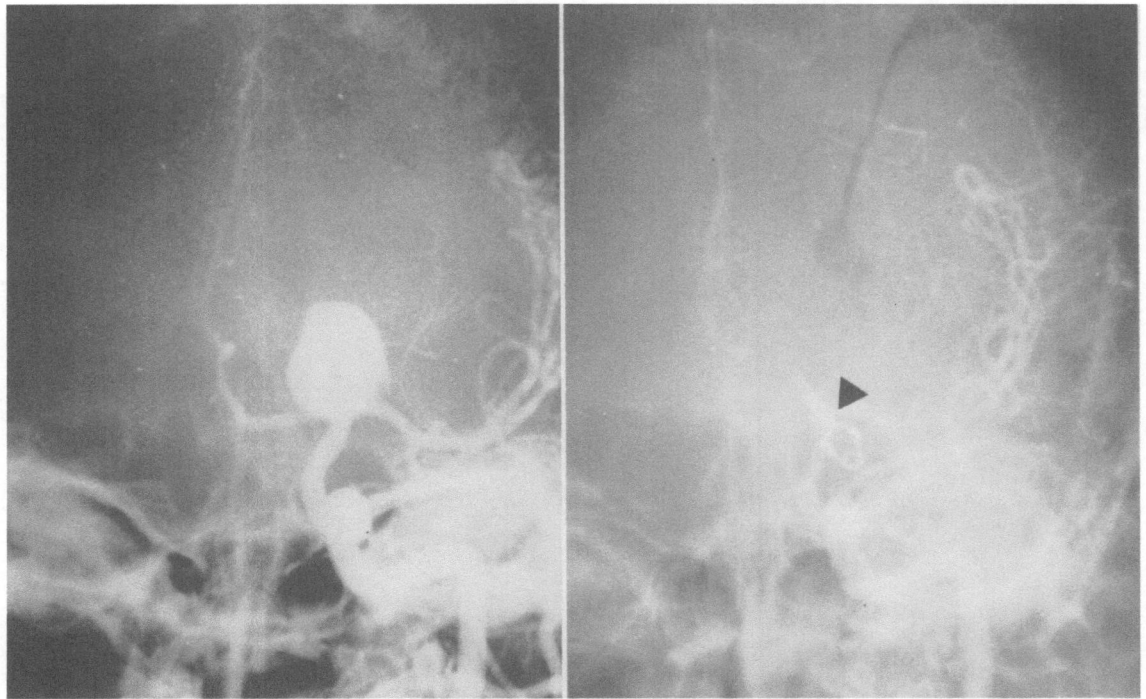

a   b

Fig. 1. Pre-operative (a) and post-operative (b) angiograms of a giant aneurysm of the bifurcation of the left carotid artery. Clipping was obtained with a single clip after reconstruction of a suitable neck with the bipolar coagulation; note the conservation of a large perforator (arrow)

Table 7. *Method of Treatment and Results (47 GIAs in 45 Patients)*

Type of surgery	Results of surgery			
	Complete recovery	Moderate disability	Severe disability	Death
Direct clipping*	21	3	2	8
Trapping	4	1	0	2
Trapping + EC–IC	0	1	0	0
Wrapping	1	0	0	0
EC–IC + exploration	0	0	1	0
Tamponade	1	0	0	0

* Both patients with two GIAs are in this group.
EC–IC extracranial – intracranial bypass.

1 of the fatalities occurred in a patient operated on in a terminal state, because of a giant basilar tip thrombosed lesion embedded into the diencephalon. Also in this subgroup of patients, associated pathologies, age an preoperative condition clearly influenced the final outcome. In this group we were able to clip only 11 lesions. 3 posterior cerebral artery giant aneurysms were trapped, with excellent outcome. 3 intracavernous carotid aneurysms were trapped; in 1 of them an extra-intracranial bypass was done during the same procedure. We were able to clip only one intracavernous lesion, with an unsuspectable very small neck (Fig. 4). In one case of global dilatation of the intracranial carotid artery (early in our series) only an exploration was accomplished. This patient – severely impaired before operation – had been submitted elsewhere to a cervical carotid occlusion and died seven months after the intracranial procedure, during which an extra-intracranial bypass was performed.

In conclusion, we have operated on by a direct surgical approach a total of 45 patients with 47 giant intracranial aneurysms. We were able to clip 35 lesions (which is 77% of lesions) and obtained satisfactory results in 32 patients (71% of cases). 3 patients (7% of cases) presented severe postoperative disability. 10 patients died post-operatively, 4 of them because of causes unrelated to surgery: 2 patients of the haemorrhagic group were admitted in a moribund state and operated on in emergency because of a life-threatening hematoma and 2 patients of the non-haemorrhagic group presented preoperative severe ischaemic brain damage and very limited life expectancy. Therefore we

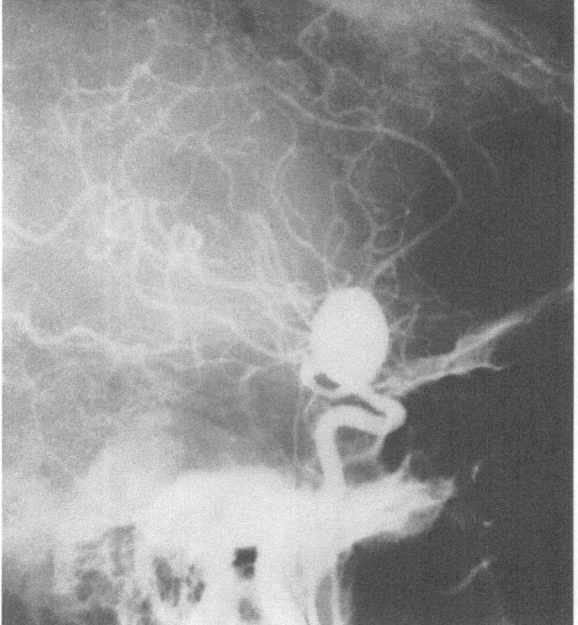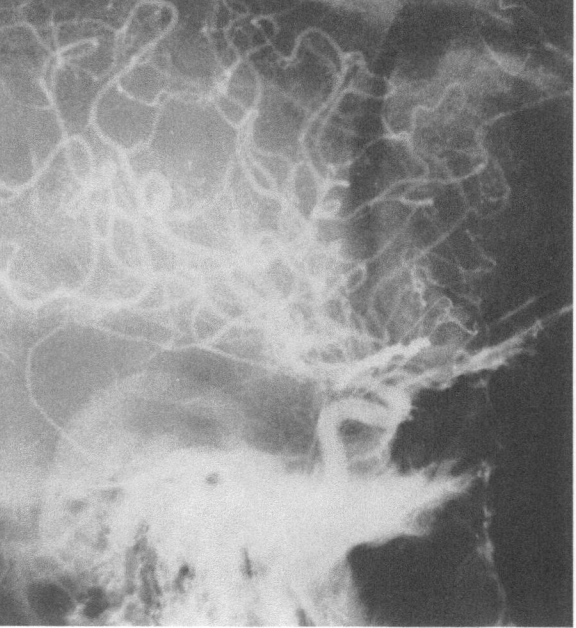

a   b

Fig. 2. Pre-operative (a) and post-operative (b) angiograms of a giant paraclinoid aneurysm. In this case trapping of the parent vessel and aspiration of the intraluminal blood permitted a perfect exclusion of the lesion by a single clip

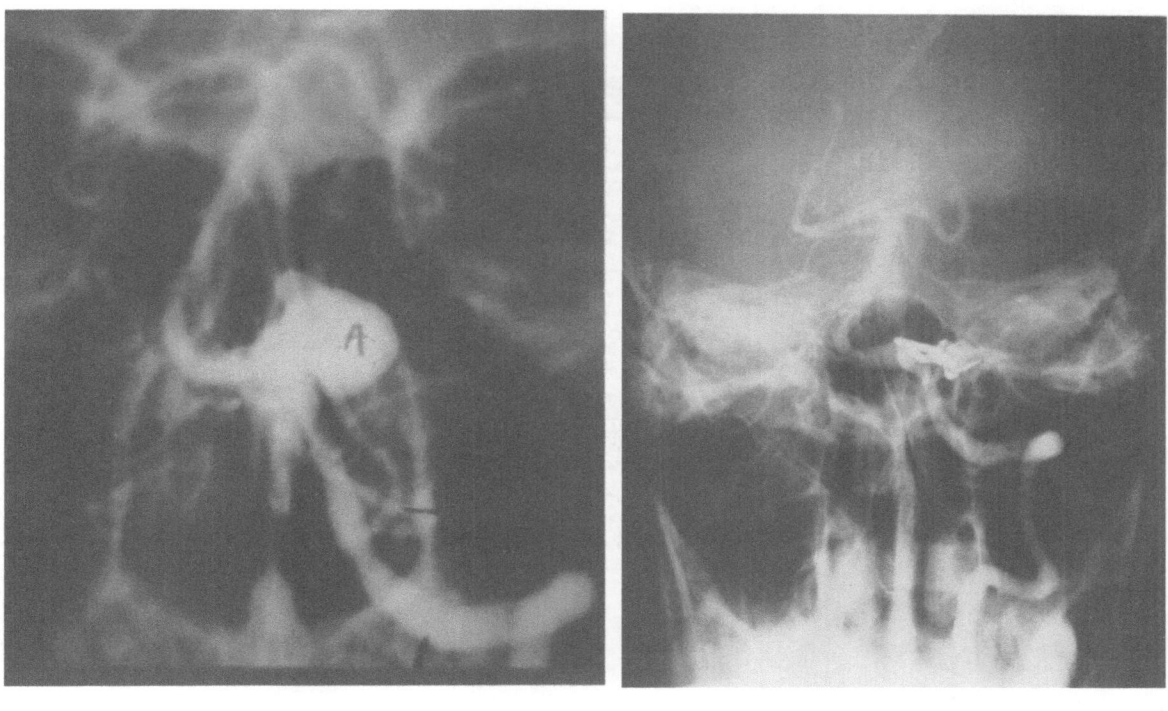

Fig. 3. Pre-operative (a) and post-operative (b) angiograms of a giant left vertebral-PICA aneurysm. This patient was operated on in prone decubitus; the use of two clips disposed in parallel avoided the narrowing of the parent vessel

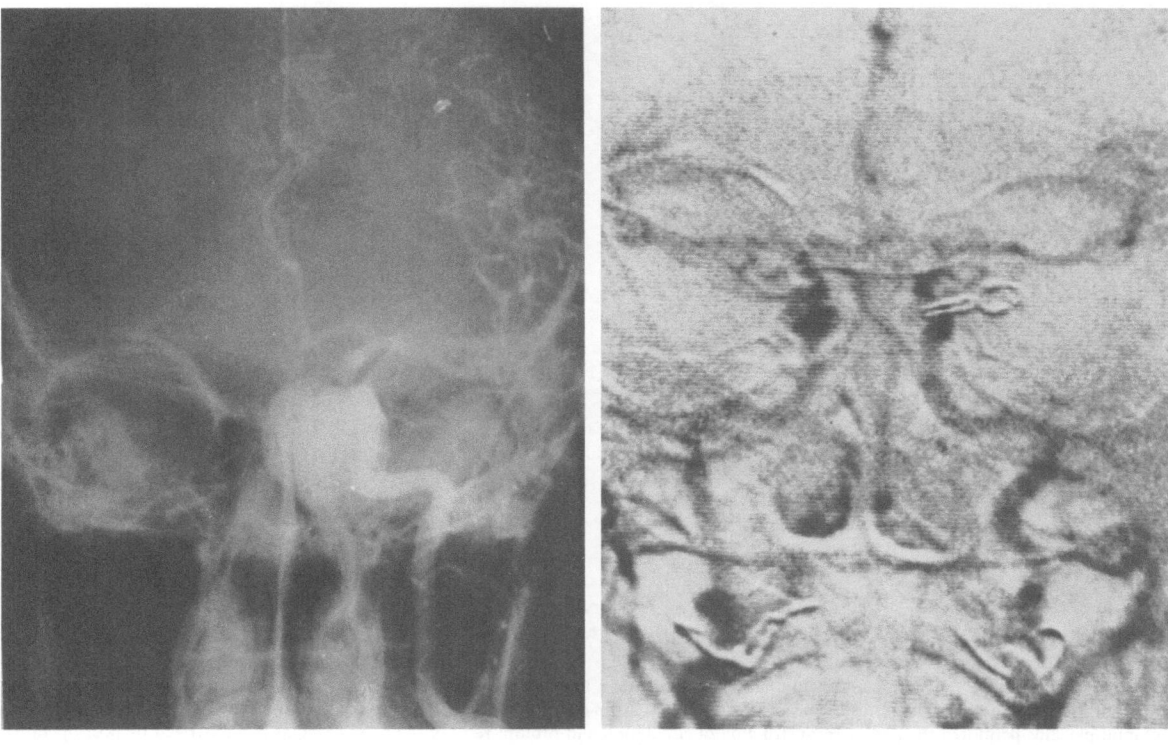

Fig. 4. Pre-operative (a) and post-operative (b) angiograms of a giant intracavernous aneurysm with an unexpectedly small neck which was easily clipped

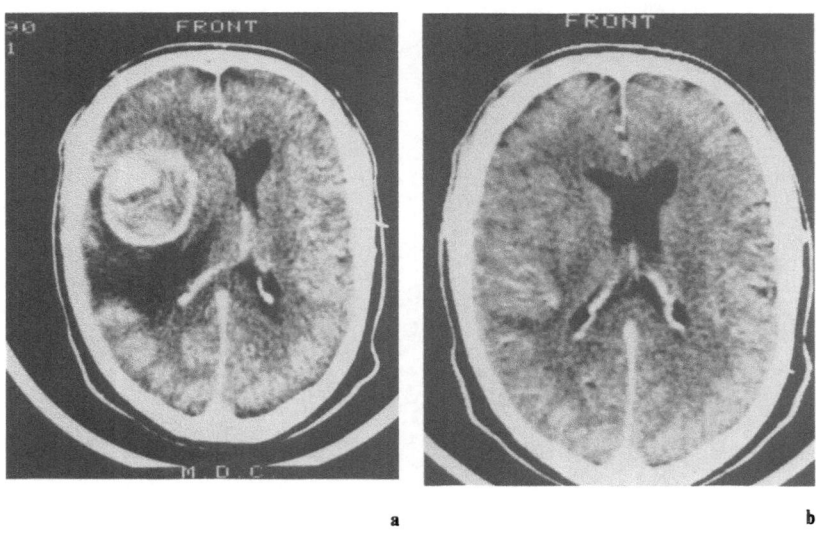

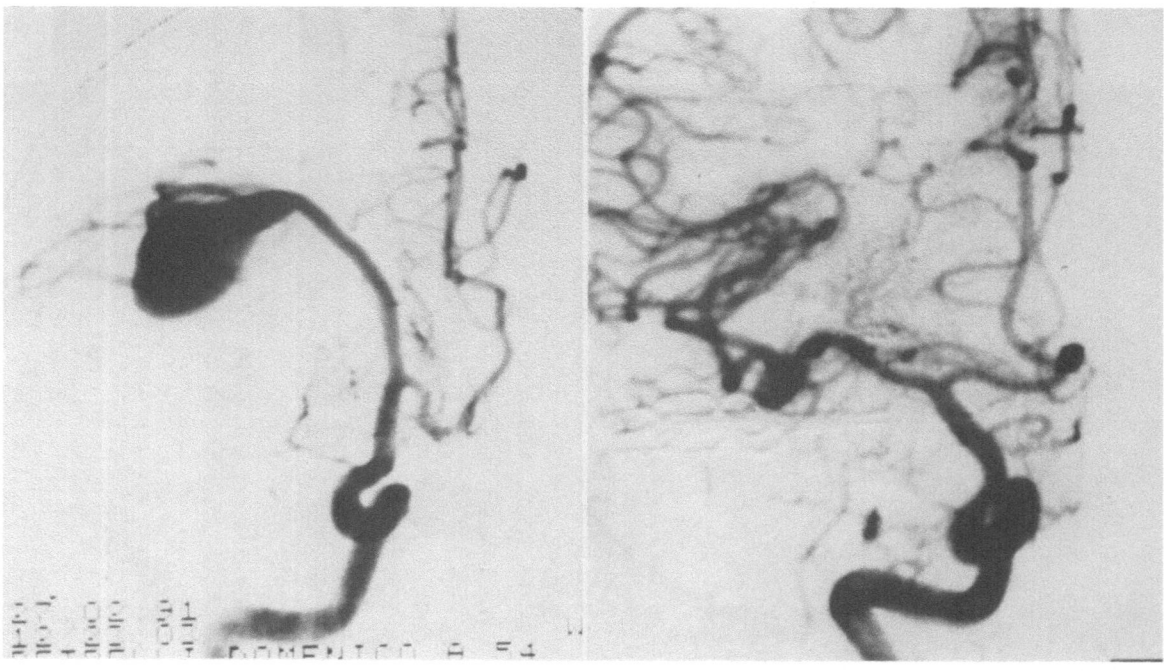

Fig. 5. Pre-operative CT scan (a) and angiogram (c) demonstrate a huge thrombosed aneurysm dislocating brain structures and elevating the right MCA. The use of the ultrasonic aspirator permitted a rapid thrombectomy; temporary trapping of the parent vessel and the use of multiple clips permitted the perfect reconstruction of circulation and prompt relief of the mass effect, as demonstrated by post-operative CT scan (b) and angiogram (d)

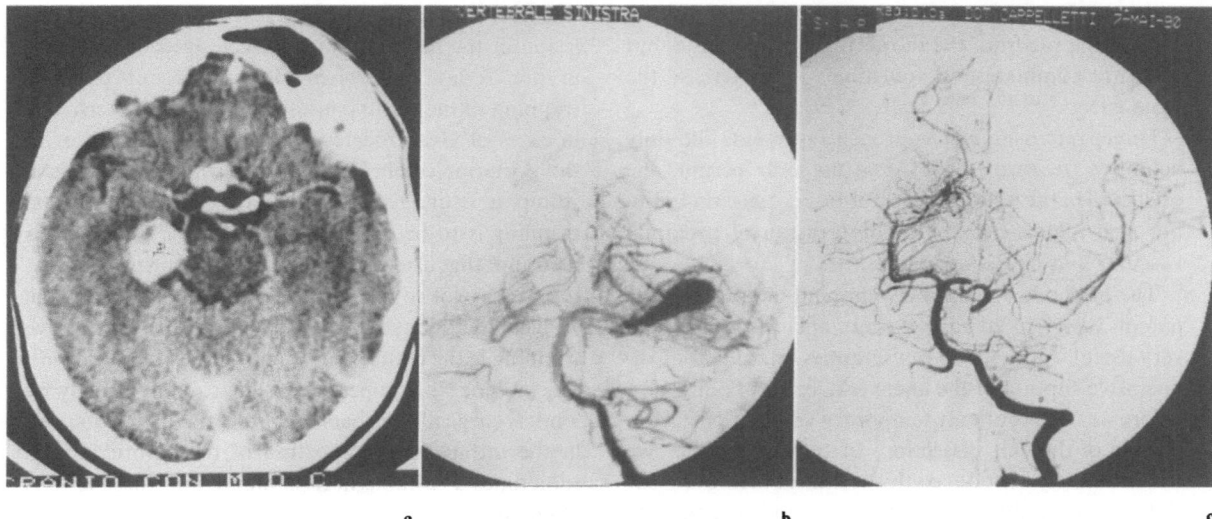

a   b   c

Fig. 6. CT-scan (a) and angiogram (b) demonstrating a huge partially thrombosed giant intracranial aneurysm of the left PCA (P2). Post-operative angiogram (c) after trapping and removal of the aneurysm; it is to be noted that this patient, who had an excellent outcome, had a congenital hypoplasia of the cervical carotid and the intracranial carotid was vascularized directly by the left posterior communicating artery

had a global mortality of 22% (10 cases), but a real post-operative mortality of 13.5% (6 cases).

In our series, a higher postoperative mortality is evident in the group of patients with bleeding aneurysms and a higher postoperative morbidity in the group of patients with non bleeding lesions (Table 3).

The outcome related to the location of the giant aneurysm and to the method of surgical treatment is presented in Tables 6 and 7, respectively.

Discussion

Giant intracranial aneurysms are mainly localized in the basal intracranial arteries, commonly contain a laminated clot of varying consistence and present a large neck; moreover thay may dislocate and distend the parent vessel and proximal arterial branches, incorporating perforating branches in the sac itself. The outer wall of the lesion is almost always fibrous and thick and frequently the wall of the parent artery is rigid and atheromatous; the larger is the aneurysmal sac, the higher is the intraluminal pressure. These characteristic features make direct surgical handling of GIAs difficult and hazardous. On the other hand, the natural course of unoperated giant aneurysms would appear to be grim: GIAs may give rise to chronic cerebral ischaemia due to compression of

major arteries by progressive enlargement of the sac and by occlusion of incorporated perforators or may be responsible for acute vascular occlusion by distal embolization from the intraluminal thrombus. GIAs may directly compress neural structures of high functional or vital importance. Although giant aneurysms were not considered to rupture easily, there is an increasing evidence in more recent reports that haemorrhage occurs unexpectedly often. Up to 80% of patients with GIAs, conservatively treated, die or are severely disabled within a few years after discovery of the aneurysm[1-3,6,13,19,23,29,31].

Cervical carotid ligation was, before the advent of microsurgical techniques, a popular treatment of choice for larger aneurysms of the anterior circulation, specially for those located on the intracranial carotid. It is, however, apparent that cervical carotid occlusion not always prevents further enlargement or rupture of the aneurysms and is gravated by undeniable immediate and late morbidity[4,10,16,18,28]. Hunterian ligation of the parent artery has been also advocated for posterior circulation aneurysms, but this method of treatment has not received wide acceptance because of its intrinsic risks[6,26].

Other alternative methods of treatment have been described for giant aneurysms, but they are not currently useful: intraluminal thrombosis obtained by endovascular or stereotactic methods effectively may esclude the sac from the intracerebral circulation, but does not eliminate and sometimes may increase the mass effect[12,13,19-22,25,26,32].

Direct microsurgical approach represents the only definitive treatment of GIAs: it not only permits the exclusion of the lesion from the intracranial circulation but also allows prompt decompression of proximal vascular and neural structures.

The method of temporary clipping or trapping the parent vessel in handling giant aneurysms appears very useful. At least 3 of our fatalities are due to intraoperative rupture of the aneurysm, early in our series, before we used routinely temporary vascular occlusion in case of difficult dissection. In our series, after we have routinely introduced this technical method, associated with induced hypertension and barbiturate protection before dissection of apparently fragile or hazardous lesions, we have no more had so disastrous eveniences. Severe morbidity is also related to intraoperative rupture of the aneurysm and is reduced if prevention is accomplished by temporary trapping[2,11,17,30,31,33].

The use of multiple clips of various size and shape prevents narrowing of the parent artery and good reconstruction of the perilesional vasculature[2,11,24,31]. Intraluminal decompression of the sac after clipping or trapping of the parent artery or eventually, in cases of easily dissectable aneurysms, during the same procedure of clipping of the aneurysmal neck, permits a better exclusion of the sac itself[1,7,9,11,13,17,24,26,29,31]. The use of ultrasonic aspirator is an important technical adjunct in treating heavily thrombosed lesions, reducing time of thrombectomy and arterial wall damage of the aneurysmal neck[2,31].

In our opinion routine use of prophylactic extra-intracranial bypass before direct exploration of giant aneurysms is not necessary in most cases; in some apparently intractable lesions an unexpectedly small neck may be clipped and in many cases of highly thrombosed lesions a good distal compensatory circulation is present; a massive aneurysm may cause heavy compression of collateral circulation, and when the mass is debulked the perilesional and hemispheric circulation improve, as demonstrated by intraoperative measurement of distal stump pressure[4,13,19,26,31].

We prefer the clinostatic position during surgery of all aneurysms, small or giant, of the posterior circulation, because it favours the use of all possible medical and technical intraoperative supports[8,9].

Direct surgical approach permits clipping of the lesion at the neck in a high percentage of cases (77% in our series), but when clipping is not possible, trapping of the aneurysms appears a good alternative in cases of GIAs located in the carotid siphon or in the posterior cerebral artery; measurements of distal stump pressure is essential if definitive aneurysmal trapping is to be done[2,6,9-11,19,21,24,26-29]. There is no doubt that also intraoperative monitoring of somatosensory evoked responses is of high value during the surgical treatment of GIAs, especially when a definitive trapping is the choice, but we have no experience with this method[31]. It appears possible to treat directly by a microsurgical approach also the aneurysms located in the intracavernous portion of the carotid artery: sometimes a suitable neck is found, and these lesions often may be trapped without problems; GIAs located in the intracavernous carotid are frequently associated with specular controlateral aneurysms and in these cases direct approach of both lesions at the same time may be possible[5,6,10,20,22,24,31].

The results of surgery in our series appear satisfactory: direct occlusion and debulking of the aneurysm was possible, by clipping or trapping, in 42 lesions (89% of cases); 32 patients (71% of cases) had good outcome. Undoubtedly mortality in our series appears high, but most of our fatalities are referred to the first years of our experience and we think that nowadays at least some of them would have been avoided.

In conclusion we believe that, in experienced hands, radical surgery gives good results and is recommended whenever possible, to prevent further haemorrhage but also to promptly relieve mass effect dur to this kind of lesions.

References

1. Ausman JI, Diaz FG, Malik GM, et al (1989) Management of cerebral aneurysms: further facts and additional myths. Surg Neurol 31: 21–35
2. Ausman JI, Diaz FG, Sadasivan B, et al (1990) Giant intracranial aneurysm surgery: the role of microvascular reconstruction. Surg Neurol 34: 8–15
3. Creissard P (1980) Table ronde: les aneurysmes giant. Neurochirurgie 26: 309–331
4. Diaz FG, Ausman JI, Pearce JE (1982) Ischemic complications after combined internal carotid artery occlusion and extracranial-intracranial anastomosis. Neurosurgery 10: 563–570
5. Dolenc V (1983) Direct microsurgical repair of intracavernous vascular lesions. J Neurosurg 58: 690–693
6. Drake CG (1979) Giant intracranial aneurysms: experience with surgical treatment in 174 patients. Clin Neurosurg 26: 12–95
7. Flamm ES (1981) Suction decompression of aneurysms: technical note. J Neurosurg 54: 275–276

8. Galzio R, Lucantoni D, Magliani V, *et al* (1989) La posizione clinostatica nella chirurgia della fossa cranica posteriore. In: Perria C (ed) Atti del XXXVIII Congresso Nazionale della Societa' Italiana di Neurochirurgia. Alghero, 24–27 Maggio 1989. Minerva Medica, Torino, pp 207–16

9. Galzio R, Lucantoni D, Magliani V, *et al* (1991) Gli aneurismi fusiformi giganti del tratto P2 dell' arteria cerebrale posteriore: a proposito di 3 casi trattati mediante approccio chirurgico diretto. In: Iraci G (ed) Atti del XL Congresso della Societa' Italiana di Neurochirurgia. Perugia, 11–14 Settembre 1991. Minerva Medica, Torino, pp 3–16

10. Gelber BR, Sundt TM (1980) Treatment of intracavernous and giant carotid aneurysms by combined internal carotid ligation and extra- to intracranial bypass. J Neurosurg 52: 1–10

11. Heros RC, Nelson PB, Ojemann RG, *et al* (1983) Large and giant paraclinoid aneurysms: surgical techniques, complications and results. Neurosurgery 12: 153–163

12. Hieshima GB, Grinnell VS, Mehringer CM (1981) A detachable balloon for therapeutic transcatheter occlusion. Radiology 138: 227–228

13. Hosobuchi Y (1979) Direct surgical treatment of giant intracranial aneurysms. J Neurosurg 51: 743–756

14. Hunt WE, Hess RM (1968) Surgical risk as related to time of intervention in the repair of intracranial aneurysms. J Neurosurg 28: 14–20

15. Jennett B, Bond M (1975) Assessment of outcome after severe brain damage. Lancet 66: 480–484

16. Matsuda M, Shiino A, Handa J (1985) Rupture of previously unruptured giant carotid aneurysm after superficial temporal – middle cerebral artery bypass and internal carotid occlusion. Neurosurgery 16: 177–184

17. McDermott MW, Durity FA, Bornzny M, *et al* (1989) Temporary vessel occlusion and barbiturate protection in cerebral aneurysm surgery. Neurosurgery 25: 54–62

18. Miller JD, Jaward K, Jennett B (1977) Safety of carotid ligation and its role in the management of intracranial aneurysms. J Neurol Neurosurg Psychiatry 40: 64–72

19. Morley TP, Barr HWK (1969) Giant intracranial aneurysms: diagnosis, course and management. Clin Neurosurg 16: 73–94

20. Mullan S (1984) Intracavernous aneurysms. In: Wilkins RH, Rengachary SS (eds) Neurosurgery. McGraw-Hill, New York, pp 1492–1494

21. Onuma T, Suzuki J (1979) Surgical treatment of giant intracranial aneurysms. J Neurosurg 51: 33–36

22. Pasqualin A, Battaglia R, Scienza R, *et al* (1988) Italian Cooperative study on giant intracranial aneurysms: 3. Modalities of treatment. Acta Neurochir (Wien) [Suppl] 42: 60–64

23. Pasqualin A, Battaglia R, Scienza R, *et al* (1988) Italian cooperative study on giant intracranial aneurysms: 4. Results of treatment. Acta Neurochir (Wien) [Suppl] 42: 65–70

24. Perneczky A, Knosp E, Vorkapic P, *et al* (1985) Direct surgical approach to infraclinoidal aneurysms. Acta Neurochir (Wien) 76: 36–44

25. Scialfa G, Vaghi A, Valsecchi F, *et al* (1982) Neuroradiological treatment of carotid and vertebral fistulas and intracavernous aneurysms. Neuroradiology 24: 13–25

26. Sindou M, Keravel G (1984) Les aneurysmes geants intracraniens. Approaches therapeutiques. Neurochirurgie 30 [Suppl 1]: 1–128

27. Sontag VKH, Yuan RH, Stein BH (1977) Giant intracranial aneurysms: a reveiw of 13 cases. Surg Neurol 8: 81–84

28. Spetzler RF, Schuster H, Roski RA (1980) Elective extracranial-intracranial arterial bypass in the treatment of inoperable giant aneurysms of the internal carotid artery. J Neurosurg 53: 22–27

29. Sundt TM, Piepgras DG (1979) Surgical approach to giant intracranial aneurysms. Operative experience with 80 cases. J Neurosurg 51: 731–742

30. Suzuky J, Yoshimoto T (1979) The effect of mannitol in prolongation of permissible occlusion time of cerebral artery: clinical data of aneurysm surgery. Neurosurg Rev 1: 13–19

31. Symon L, Vajda J (1984) Surgical experience with giant intracranial aneurysms. J Neurosurg 61: 1009–1028

32. Weil SM, Van Loveren HR, Tomsick TA, *et al* (1987) Management of inoperable cerebral aneurysms by the navigational balloon technique. Neurosurg 21: 296–302

33. Yoshimoto T, Suzuky J (1979) Temporary clipping. Prolongation of the time of occlusion by mannitol. In: Pia W, Langmaid G, Ziersky J (eds) Cerebral aneurysms: advances in diagnosis and therapy. Springer, Wien New York, pp 388–392

Correspondence: R. Galzio, M.D., Division of Neurosurgery, City Hospital "G. Mazzini", Villa Mosca, I-64100 Teramo, Italy.

Surgical Treatment of Large and Giant Carotid-ophthalmic Artery Aneurysms

N. Tamaki, K. Ehara, M. Asada, T. Nagashima, K. Fujita, and **K. Taomoto**

Department of Neurosurgery, Kobe University School of Medicine, Kobe, Japan

Summary

Thirty cases of giant and large carotid-ophthalmic aneurysms were treated surgically in our hospital between 1974 and May 1992. Twelve out of these thirty patients had giant or large aneurysms (>20 mm). Seven of twelve patients, all female, were treated by direct clipping utilizing the "trapping-evacuation" technique, which has been devised by the authors. All aneurysms were completely clipped with preservation of patency of the internal carotid artery, which was confirmed by intra- or post-operative angiography. The postoperative outcome was good in six cases and fair in one. The "trapping-evacuation" technique enabled us to completely clip giant and large aneurysms of the paraophthalmic region of the internal carotid artery with greater safety.

Keywords: Giant aneurysm; carotid-ophthalmic aneurysm; "trapping-evacuation" technique.

Introduction

Giant and large aneurysms of the paraophthalmic region of the internal carotid artery (ICA) present a incidence of 37.5% to 47.8% of all aneurysms of this region[6,15]. These aneurysms pose very difficult problems regarding methods of treatment and surgical outcome. Because of difficulties of direct clipping of these aneurysms, indirect methods have been used to treat most giant and large aneurysms of this region. Seven patients with these aneurysms were treated by direct clipping utilizing the "trapping-evacuation" technique, which has been devised by the authors[21]. The surgical technique, surgical outcome and an illustrative case were described in this report.

Material and Methods

Thirty cases of aneurysms of the paraophthalmic region of the ICA were treated surgically in our hospital between 1974 and 1992. There were 18 small aneurysms, and 12 large and giant aneurysms (>2 cm). Seven cases out of 12 large and giant aneurysms of this region were treated by direct clipping utilizing the "trapping-evacuation" technique. All seven patients were female, ranging from 45 to 78 years in age.

Six aneurysms were unruptured. One aneurysm was ruptured. Five aneurysms were located on the right side, and two on the left side.

No patient has any other associated intracranial disease. The largest diameter of each aneurysm was 20 mm in two patients, and >25 mm in five (Table 1). There was good cross-circulation from the contralateral system on cerebral angiograms in all case. Each patient tolerated the balloon Matas test for 20 to 30 minutes. The MR images taken in six patients revealed the completely intradural location in five cases and the partially extradural extension in one. Mural thrombus was not present on CT or MR studies in any case. In all patients eye signs were noted before surgery.

Details of the "Trapping-Evacuation" Technique

The common carotid artery (CCA), external carotid artery (ECA), and internal carotid artery (ICA) are isolated in the neck, and tapes are placed around each artery. A cut-down catheter is introduced into the origin of the ECA through the superior thyroid artery.

A standard frontotemporal craniotomy is then performed via an ipsilateral pterional approach. The carotid and chiasmal cistern are opened and the anterior clinoid process, optic nerve, carotid artery and part of the giant aneurysm are exposed.

Extensive unroofing of the optic canal and removal of the anterior clinoid process are carefully performed with diamond drills. Incision of the dural ring of the optic nerve and gentle mobilization of the optic nerve provide a wider operating field. The anterior part of the cavernous sinus is opened, and bleeding from the sinus is controlled by packing with Oxycel. The ICA is thus exposed proximally in the C3 segment outside the dura propria, at its entry into the dura, as well as in the intradural (C2) segment. The dura around the carotid artery is incised to expose the aneurysm neck. The proximal end of the neck of the giant aneurysm can then be clearly exposed.

The "trapping-evacuation" technique is performed at this stage. First the anerysm is trapped temporarily by occluding the cervical CCA and ECA and the intracranial ICA distal to the neck of the aneurysm. Intra-aneurysmal blood is then aspirated via the catheter placed in the cervical ICA. Approximately 5 to 10 ml of blood is now aspirated with a syringe to collapse the aneurysm. This procedure causes evacuation and collapse of the aneurysm itself, which allows good visualization of the neck in relation to the parent artery, other vessels, and nerves, and permits safer dissection and application of the clips on the aneurysm neck.

In the case of a giant aneurysm with a neck originating from the medial or superior wall of the ICA and projecting medially and superiorly, the C1 and C2 segments of ICA, the anterior carebral

Table 1. *Clinical Summary of Patients with Large or Giant Carotid-ophthalmic Artery Aneurysms*

Case no.	Age (yrs.) Sex	Clinical findings		Associated diseases	Aneurysm			Outcome	Complications
		SAH	Eye signs		Side	Size	Origin		
1	45, F	none	rt, blind	none	rt	large(20 mm)	medial	good	oculomotor palsy(transient)
2	78, F	none	rt, +	none	rt	giant(25 mm)	inferior	good	hemorrhagic infarction, NPH
3	65, F	none	rt, +	none	rt	giant(32 mm)	medial	good	NPH
4	56, F	none	rt, +	none	rt	giant(25 mm)	inferior	good	none
5	51, F	SAH	lt, +	none	lt	large(20 mm)	medial	good	none
6	67, F	none	rt, +	none	rt	giant(25 mm)	medial	fair	hemorrhagic infarction, NPH
7	57, F	none	lt, +	hepatitis leucopenia	lt	giant(28 mm)	inferior	good	none

SAH subarachnoid hemorrhage; + present: *NPH* normal-pressure hydrocephalus.

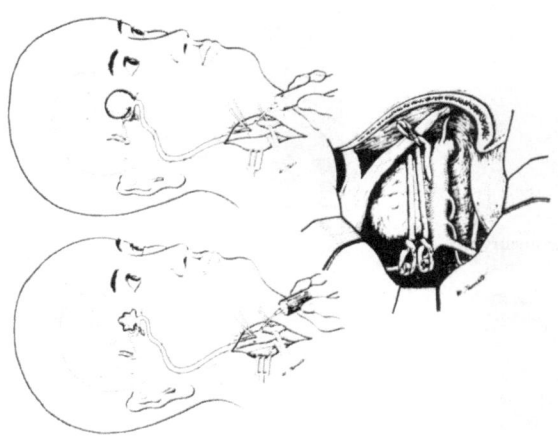

Fig. 1. Diagrams showing the "trapping-evacuation" technique. Left upper: the aneurysm is trapped in the neck and in the intracranial ICA distal to the aneurysm. Right lower: Collapsing the aneurysm by aspiration of the intraneurysmal blood from the catheter in the neck. Right: Clipping the aneurysm with preservation of the parent artery

artery (ACA), and the middle cerebral artery (MCA) may be hidden behind the aneurysm. In such a case, the intradural ICA distal to the aneurysm is exposed by dissection after the cervical ICA is occluded; the "trapping-evacuation" procedure is then performed. This type of giant aneurysm is clipped with a few long straight clips with strong closing power from the distal side of the neck, and with right-angled clips from the proximal side of the neck (Fig. 1).

In the case of a giant aneurysm with a neck originating from the posterior or inferior wall of the ICA, the parent artery is spontaneously reconstructed by the "trapping-evacuation" technique. The giant anerysm is clipped by multiple fenestrated clips in a tendem arrangement with the clips overlapping at their tips.

Illustrative Case Report

Case 7: This 57-year-old right-handed woman began to notice blurred vision on the left side 8 months prior to admission. She

was admitted to our hospital because of progressive worsening of her left vision.

Examination: The abnormal findings on neurological examination consisted of decreased vision, and visual field defects. Cerebral angiography revealed the giant aneurysm (28 mm in diameter) originating from the inferior wall of the paraopthalmic region of the left ICA (Fig. 2). MR imaging demonstrated the complete intradural location of the aneurysm (Fig. 3).

Operation: Direct clipping was performed by means of "trapping-evacuation" technique. The optic nerve was well decompressed at the end of the surgery.

Postoperative Course: After operation vision as well as visual field defects improved markely (Fig. 4). Postoperative angiography demonstrated complete clipping of the aneurysm and preservation of the parent artery (Fig. 5). The patient was discharged without any other neurological deficits.

Discussion

While carotid-ophthalmic aneurysms are not very common among all cerebral aneurysms[7,13,15], a high incidence of giant and large aneurysms of this regin has been reported[6,15]. Because of the technical difficulties in direct surgical treatment of these aneurysms, various conservative alternatives have been performed in treating these aneurysms. Ligation of the parent artery with or without extracranial-intracranial bypass have been reported[2-6,8,11,14,16,18,19]. A technique of thrombosing the aneurysms by copper wire insertion and recently embolization of the aneurysm using detachable balloon have also been performed[9,10]. These indirect methods of treatment are not ideal for the treatment of large and giant aneurysms. The risk of hemmorrhage and optic nerve compression remains. Cerebral ischemia may occur after ligation of the parent artery.

Direct clipping of the aneurysm resolves these complications of the indirect approach. However, a high combined mortality and morbidity rate due to techni-

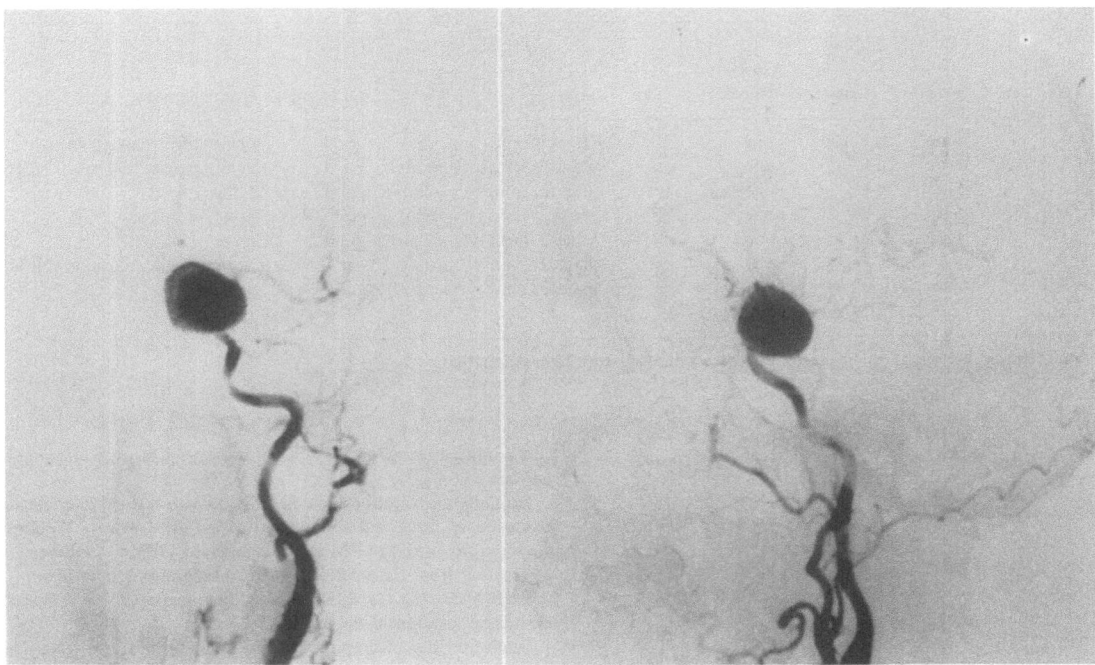

Fig. 2. Left carotid angiograms demonstrating the giant paraophthalmic aneurysm

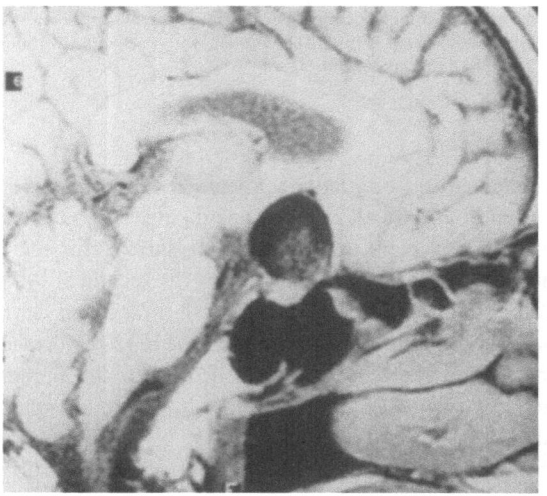
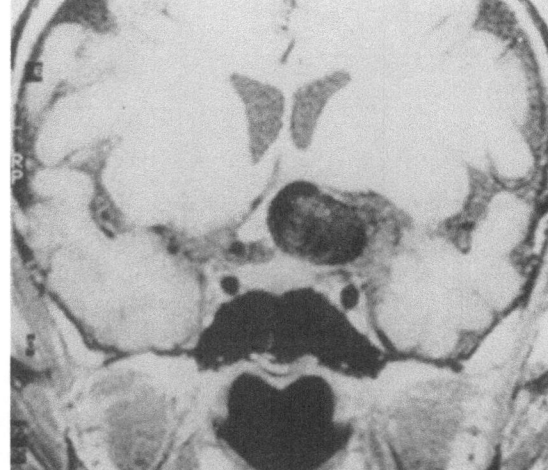

Fig. 3. MR images demonstrating the intradural location

cal problems has been reported[5,7,11]. The "trapping-evacuation" technique provides the useful method in direct surgical treatment of these aneurysms[21]. Similar methods have been reported to collapse the aneurysm during surgery[1,12].

Conclusions

The "trapping-evacuation" technique is of use in the treatment of patients with large and giant aneurysms of the paraopthalmic region of the ICA. This technique facilitated direct clipping of giant aneurysms of this region.

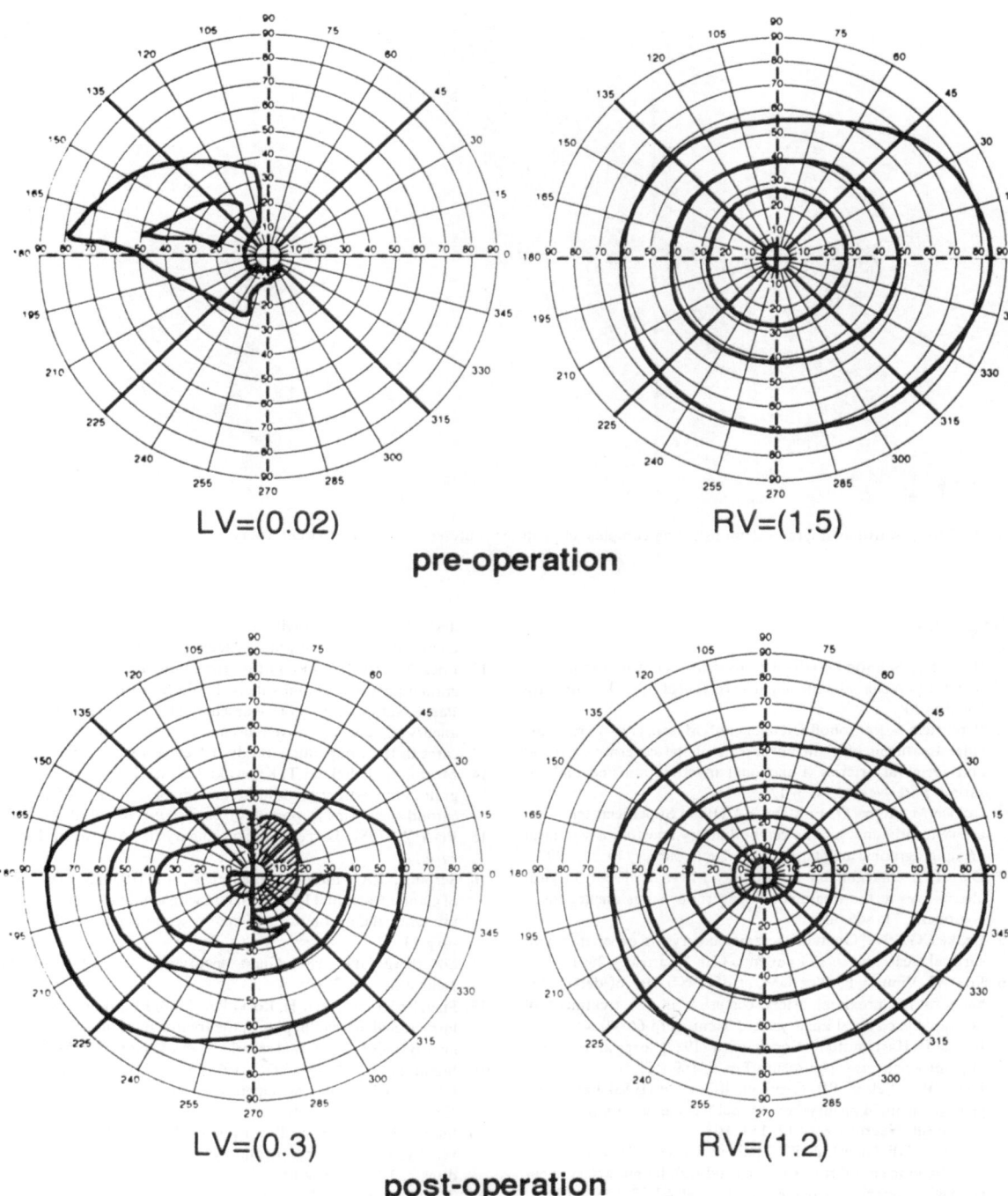

Fig. 4. Pre- and post-operative visual field of the patient demonstrating improvement after surgery

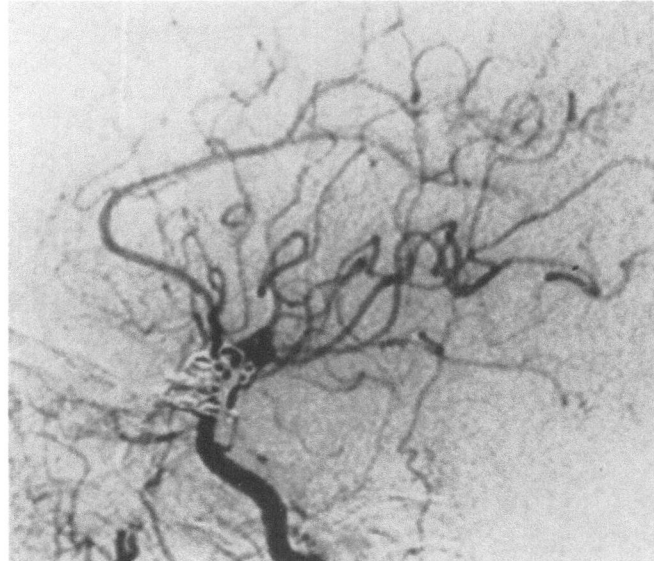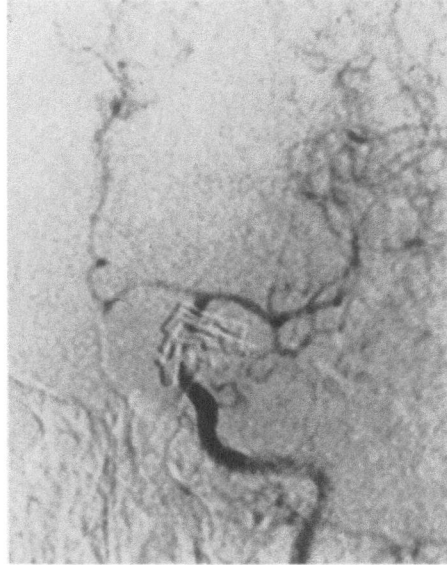

Fig. 5. Postoperative angiograms demonstrating complete clipping with preservation of the parent artery

References

1. Batjer HH, Samson DS (1990) Retrograde suction decompression of giant paraclinoidal aneurysms. Technical note. J Neurosurg 73: 305–306
2. Berenstein A, Ransohoff J, Kupersmith M, *et al* (1984) Transvascular treatment of giant aneurysms of the cavernous carotid and vertebral arteries. Functional investigation and embolization. Surg Neurol 21: 3–12
3. Collice M, Arena O, Fontana RA (1986) Superficial temporal artery to proximal middle cerebral artery anastomosis: clinical and angiographic long term results. Neurosurgery 19: 992–997
4. Diaz FG, Ohaegbulam S, Dujovny M, *et al* (1989) Surgical alternatives in the treatment of cavernous sinus aneurysms. J Neurosurg 71: 846–853
5. Drake CG (1979) Giant intracranial aneurysms: experience with surgical treatment in 174 patients. Clin Neurosurg 26: 12–95
6. Fox AJ, Vinuela F, Plez DM, *et al* (1987) Use of detachable balloons for proximal artery occlusion in the treatment of unclippable cerebral aneurysms. J Neurosurg 66: 40–46
7. Handa H, Hashimoto N, Yonekawa Y (1982) Surgical treatment of giant aneurysms. Neurosurg Rev 5: 169–172
8. Heros RC, Nelson PB, Ojemann RG, *et al* (1983) Large and giant paraclinoid aneurysms: surgical techniques, complications, and result. Neurosurgery 12: 153–163
9. Hieshima GB, Higashida RT, Halbach VV, *et al* (1986) Intravascular balloon embolization of a carotid-ophthalmic artery aneurysm with preservation of the parent vessel. AJNR 7: 196–198
10. Higashida RT, Halbach VV, Hieshima GB, *et al* (1988) Treatment of a giant carotid ophthalmic artery aneurysm by intravascular balloon embolization therapy. Surg Neurol 30: 382–386
11. Hosobuchi Y (1979) Direct surgical treatment of giant intracranial aneurysms. J Neurosurg 51: 743–756
12. Kyoshima K, Kobayashi S, Wakui K, *et al* (1992) A nearly designed puncture needle for suction decompression of giant aneurysms. Technical note. J Neurosurg 76: 880–882
13. Locksley HB (1966) Report on the Cooperative Study of intracranial anerurysms and subarachnoid hemorrhage. Section V, Part I. Natural history of subarachnoid hemorrhage, intracranial aneurysms and arteriovenous malformations. Based on 6368 cases in the Cooperative Study. J Neurosurg 25: 219–239
14. Morimoto T, Sakaki T, Kakizaki T, *et al* (1988) Radial artery graft for an extracranial-intracranial bypass in cases of internal carotid aneurysms. Report of two cases. Surg Neurol 30: 293–297
15. Pia HW (1982) Large and giant aneurysms. Neurosurg Rev 5: 77–81
16. Serbinelp FA, Filtov JM, Spallone A, *et al* (1990) Management of giant intracranial ICA aneurysm with combined extracranial-intracranial anastomosis and endovascular occlusion. J Neurosurg 73: 57–63
17. Silverberg GD (1984) Giant aneurysms: surgical treatment. Neurol Res 6: 57–63
18. Spetzler RF, Schuster H, Roski RA (1980) Elective extracranial-intracranial arterial bypass in the treatment of inoperable giant aneurysms of the internal carotid artery. J Neurosurg 53: 22–27
19. Sundt TM Jr, Piepgras DG (1979) Surgical approach to giant intracranial aneurysms. Operative experience with 80 cases. J Neurosurg 51: 731–742
20. Sundt TM Jr, Piepgras DG, Marsh WR, *et al* (1986) Saphenous vein bypass grafts for giant aneurysms and intracranial occlusive disease. J Neurosurg 65: 439–450
21. Tamaki N, Kim S, Ehara K, *et al* (1991) Giant carotid ophthalmic artery aneurysms: direct clipping utilizing the "trapping-evacuation" technique. J Neurosurg 74: 567–572

Correspondence: Norihiko Tamaki, M.D., Department of Neurosurgery, Kobe University School of Medicine, 7-5-1 Kusunokicho, Chuo-ku, Kobe 650, Japan.

Surgery of Posterior Circulation Aneurysms

Vertebrobasilar Artery Aneurysms: Current Management Techniques

E.S. Flamm and **D. O'Rourke**

Division of Neurosurgery, University of Pennsylvania School of Medicine, Philadelphia, Pennsylvania, U.S.A.

Summary

Basilar artery aneurysms hold a unique place among neurosurgical vascular disorders. Because of their relative rarity and their deep location, many surgical approaches have been advocated. Aneurysms arising from the lower half of the basilar and the vertebral arteries pose unique and difficult challenges because of their location and the infrequency with which they are encountered. Appropriate selection of recent advances in skull base surgery and intravascular techniques can greatly improve the overall management of aneurysms arising from the lower half of the basilar and the vertebral arteries.

We have reviewed our experience with 148 vertebrobasilar aneurysms. These aneurysms represent 14% of a series of 1051 intracranial aneurysms treated by surgery. This paper will address the criteria utilized at our institution for selecting the specific approach to aneurysms of the upper basilar artery. At the present time the pterional exposure is preferred for most aneurysms arising at the upper end of the basilar artery. Other approaches that are used include a subtemporal route, trans-tentorial exposure and utilization of skull base techniques. These will be presented along with details for selection of intravascular approaches. Selected cases required intravascular approaches and profound hypothermnia and cardio-pulmonary bypass.

These combined approaches and utilization of the many options has resulted in an overall favorable result in 78% of patients presenting as Grades 0–3 with an overall morbidity of < 10% and a mortality of 6.9%.

Keywords: Vertebrobasilar aneurysms; surgical approaches; skull base surgery.

Introduction

Aneurysms of the vertebrobasilar arterial complex include those arising from the proximal vertebral and posterior inferior cerebellar artery (PICA), vertebro-basilar junction (VBJ) and basilar trunk as well as those found in the region of the superior cerebellar artery and basilar tip. The surgical approaches to these lesions vary considerably depending on the location, projection and size of the aneurysm. In addition to being uncommon, aneurysms of the lower basilar artery pose a number of difficult surgical problems due to their location. Recent technical advances of both skull base and temporal done surgery can be utilized for these aneurysms to provide a shallow surgical field and reduce the problems of depth, obligatory brain retraction, and lower cranial nerve injury. Electro-physiologic monitoring and other adjunctive measures are now employed to permit the safer visualization and direct manipulation of these unusual lesions. The selective use of more recent endovascular techniques may improve the overall management of these complex aneurysms. This paper reviews our experience with aneurysms of the vertebrobasilar region and empha-sizes the need for a complete armamentarium in their surgical management.

Methods

Patient Population

A total of 148 aneurysms of the vertebrobasilar arterial complex have been treated through 1991. This comprises 14% of a series of 1051 intracranial aneurysms (Table 1). Of these vertebrobasilar aneurysms, 48% arose from the lower basilar trunk, anterior inferior cerebellar artery (AICA), vertebrobasilar junction (VBJ), vertebral-PICA junction, or distal PICA (Table 2). The series includes 100 aneurysms at the distal end of the basilar artery, 26 arising at the origin of the superior cerebellar artery and 74 in the region of the basilar bifurcation (Table 2). The admission grades of all patients with aneurysms of the entire vertebrobasilar arterial complex are shown in Table 3.

Timing and Perioperative Management

The principles applied to all aneurysms are used for basilar aneurysms. Thus in patients who are awake and responsive after SAH or who improve to this level after ventricular drainage, we proceed quickly to surgery within the first 48 hours. With some exceptions such as a particularly threatening aneurysm or a history of more than one recent hemorrhage, surgery is delayed in those patients who are not conscious and able to follow some commands. All patients are managed with a regimen that increases blood volume and maintains maximum perfusion through control of blood pressure, hemodilution and caclium channel blocking agents. The recent addition of trans-

Table 1. *Distribution of Aneurysms*

Location	n	%
Ophthalmic	117	11.1
Post. communicating	249	23.7
Anterior choroidal	50	4.8
Carotid bifurcation	41	3.9
Anterior communicating	198	18.8
Distal anterior cerebral	32	3.0
Middle cerebral	216	20.6
Vertebro-basilar	148	14.1
Total	1051	100.0

Table 2. *Distribution of Vertebro-basilar Aneurysms*

Location	n	%
Basilar tip	74	50.0
Superior cerebellar	26	17.6
Anterior inferior cerebellar	2	1.4
Posterior inferior cerebellar	31	20.9
Vertebro-basilar junction	11	7.4
Other	4	2.7
Total	148	100.0

Table 3. *Admission Grades Vertebrobasilar Aneurysms*

Grade	Lower	Upper
0	2	26
1	34	30
2	1	4
3	9	38
4	2	2
Total	48	100

cranial Doppler monitoring and balloon angioplasty has increased our ability to manage those patients who develop delayed ischemic deficits.

Approaches to the Upper Basilar Artery

In the past 6 years almost all aneurysms in this region have been approached through a right pterional craniotomy. Advantages of this approach are numerous. It is the exposure used for most intracranial aneurysm surgery and thus the entire surgical team is quite familar with it. The exposure requires considerably less brain retraction than the subtemporal approach. This is of particular advantage when operating on the dominant side or in the first few days after SAH when retraction may be difficult. It is done with somewhat more exposure of the temporal lobe than is used for anterior circulation aneurysms. This gives the surgeon the option to utilize a subtemporal approach or a combined pterional and subtemporal exposure if necessary.

Although most aneurysms at the bifurcation of the basilar artery can be approached from the right or non-dominant side, there are certain exceptions. If other aneurysms are to be clipped at the same time, a left sided approach may be indicated. Certain projections of a larger aneurysm may suggest a particular side as being more appropriate. Regardless of the side of origin, aneurysms arising at the superior cerebellar artery can be managed from the right side, even if this requires crossing the basilar artery to place the clip.

Exceptions to this approach are few but should be recognized. A number of authors have commented upon the relationship of the basilar bifurcation of the top of the clivus[43]. This is usually not a problem for aneurysms less than 2 cm in diameter since the exposure is lateral and oblique to the posterior clinoid. Because of this one does not have to come over the top of the clinoid to reach the origin of the aneurysm. If the basilar artery is elongated and the base of the aneurysm is more than a centimeter above the top of the clivus, the pterional approach is more difficult than a subtemporal one and may require even more retraction.

When the situation is unclear preoperatively, the pterional exposure can be modified to allow a conversion of the exposure to a more subtemporal approach if necessary. The exposure can also be improved by the use of spinal drainage. This is utilized in all cases with acute subarachnoid hemorrhage and in younger patients with unruptured aneurysms. In order patients with obvious cerebral atrophy, care must be taken not to over drain the subarachnoid space.

Technical Points

An advantage of the pterional approach is the ability to preserve 3rd nerve function. It is possible to dissect sharply the arachnoid around the 3rd nerve so that it is free from any stretch caused by retraction of the temporal lobe. With a wide opening of the arachnoid, a clearer path for dissecting the aneurysm as well as the ability to avoid injuring the nerve is provided. With attention to this maneuver, postoperative palsy of the oculomotor nerve has been reduced to less than 15% of cases.

A multiple armed self-retaining retractor is necessary because it is often helpful to retract the supraclinoid carotid artery or a loop of the posterior cerebral artery distal to the junction of the posterior communicating artery to improve visualization. This should be done temporarily and should be removed during the case if it is not helpful once the final angle of dissection has been established. Care must be taken to be certain that the carotid artery flow is maintained during the retraction. We have experienced 1 case of carotid occlusion that developed 4 days after surgery presumably related to the retraction of this portion of the artery. An additionl retractor can be used on the edge of the tentorium and avoid the need for sutures or division of the tentorium.

Variations in the skull base can pose unexpected problems. Although it is rarely necessary, the posterior clinoid may have to be drilled away to improve visualization of the neck of the aneurysm. This can be accomplished with a 1 mm diamond burr on a variable speed drill.

Occlusion and division of the posterior communicating artery has been suggested as a means of improving exposure. One should remember that this vessel is not a simple conduit but usually gives rise to a number of small perforating vessels to the chiasm and hypothalamus. For this reason we have avoided sacrificing the PCA in all cases. Similarly great effort should be made to avoid compromise of the proximal posterior cerebral artery. On rare occasions it is necessary to include this vessel in the aneurysm clip. Theoretically supply from the posterior communicating artery should be adequate.

We feel that this places the patient at risk to ischemia in the distribution of both the posterior cerebral artery as well as the perforating branches arising from the P1 segment. Too much cannot be said about the perforating vessels that surround the base of a basilar artery aneurysm. These most often arise from the proximal posterior artery and rarely from the distal basilar artery itself. Care should be taken to separate these from the neck and dome of the aneurysms before the clip is applied. It is not enough to be certain that they are not cought up in the clip. It is equally important that the flow in these small branches is not compromised due to faulty application of the clip which may distort the vessels.

More and more we have resorted to temporary occlusion of the basilar artery prior to making the final dissection. This improves the chances of separating the small perforating vessels from the aneurysm. Furthermore, the vessels can be visualized and dissected better when the dome of the aneurysm is slack when the temporary clip is on.

To improve the safety of temporary clipping, we routinely utilize intraoperative monitoring of brain stem evoked potentials. It is still not clear if it is better to use one application of a temporary clip or to resort to intermittent occlusion and reperfusion. In general we use a single application averaging 8 minutes of occlusion. The clip is applied just proximal to the origins of the superior cerebellar arteries. Careful opening of the arachnoid around the basilar trunk must be done to avoid injury to the small penetrating branches of the basilar artery. Alteration in the evoked potentials is a strong indication to avoid prolonging the occlusion. A single application of a temporary clip also has the advantage of being less disruptive to the conduct of the dissection around the aneurysm since these is less interruption. Removal of a temporary clip from the basilar artery can be difficult if the clip slips beneath the edge of the tentorium. We avoid induced hypotension during temporary occlusion of the basilar artery. No specific pharmacologic regimen aimed at cerebral protection is used. Patients have received mannitol during the opening and they are given corticosteroids, phenytoin and a dihydropyridines calcium channel blocker preoperatively.

Surgical Approaches to Proximal Vertebral/PICA Aneurysms

PICA aneurysms were initially operated upon in the sitting position, but in recent years they have been approached in a lateral recumbent position through a unilateral suboccipital craniectomy[24]. Dandy initially popularized this position for tumors of the posterior fossa and for sectioning of the trigeminal nerve. It is frequently used for a variety of procedures[18,33,40,43,47]. The majority of this group of aneurysms arose at the distal vertebral-PICA junction with a smaller number seen at the proximal vertebral-PICA junction and the distal PICA[24,40]. Two extracranial PICA aneurysms required cervical laminectomy for definitive clipping[21]. PICA aneurysms tend to project antero-superiorly close to the lateral medulla although there is a great deal of variability in the location of both the aneurysm and the parent vessel[34]. The PICA itself can often take part of its origin from the aneurysmal neck[40]. PICA aneurysms and vertebrobasilar junction aneurysms are often associated with anomalies of the vertebral artery (e.g hypoplasia, absence) or anatomic variation of the proximal basilar artery (e.g fenestration)[6,40].

After opening the dura, the cerebellar hemisphere is elevated and the cisterna magna is punctured. The removal of CSF reduces the amount of retraction needed to expose cranial nerves IX, X, and XI. The aneurysm typically has an intimate relationship with the fibers of these nerves. The dissection and clip application must be performed among the branches of the lower cranial nerves. By opening the arachnoid overlying the lower cranial nerves widely, much of the associated morbidity is decreased[24].

A number of modifications have been employed in the surgical management of these aneurysms. Heros performs an extreme lateral bony removal which requires going out to the occipital condyle with removal of the posterolateral arch of C1[18]. This provides for a more inferolateral approach to the region and may be used to treat more rostral aneurysms of the VB junction and lower basilar trunk (see below). Other authors feel that extreme lateral or medial approaches are unnecessary[40]. Lee et al. and others prefer a unilateral suboccipital approach in a modified supine position for proximal vertebral-PICA aneurysms and a bilateral suboccipital (prone) approach for more distal PICA aneurysms[24,33].

Surgical Approaches to Aneurysms of the Distal Vertebral (VB Junction) and Lower Basilar Trunk (AICA)

Most of the aneurysms in this category arose from the region of the confluens of the vertebral and basilar arteries (Table 2). There is an extremely low incidence of aneurysms arising between the AICA and superior cerebellar artery takeoff[40].

We determine the particular surgical approach by the rostral-caudal location of the aneurysm along the clivus, the size of the aneurysm, and its orientation. Most of these lesions are close to the midline near the junction of the lower and mid-third of the clivus. In general, we prefer to approach these aneurysms from the side of the origin of the aneurysm and not from the side to which the dome projects. AICA aneurysms tend to project laterally more often than along an anterior-posterior axis[40]. These aneurysms are often in close proximity to cranial nerves VI, VII and VIII. We use either a lateral suboccipital approach to this region or, in selected cases, a retromastoid transsigmoid approach.

Peerless and Drake have utilized either the unilateral suboccipital approach reviewed above or, more commonly, a subtemporal transtentorial approach to this region; they stress the limitation of working space with either approach[40]. Sugita has utilized a middle subtemporal approach to basilar trunk aneurysms and has experienced a technical limit of 25 mm below the posterior clinoid for this approach (although the junction of the vertebral arteries could be seen in most cases) with the dissection carried out on either side of the trigeminal nerve[49]. The authors emphasize the role of direct retraction of the trigeminal nerve, pons, and aneurysm. Yamaura reports that distal vertebral artery aneurysms are accessible up to 23 mm above the foramen magnum and 16 mm posterior to the clivus with a lateral suboccipital approach[52]. Heros' extreme lateral suboccipital approach provides a trajectory towards this region[18]. Solomon and Stein have utilized a combined supra- and infratentorial approach[26,47]. Although the combined temporal craniotomy and suboccipital craniectomy with division of the sigmoid sinus results in the visualization of the 3rd through 11th cranial nerves, it is a time-consuming operation and requires temporal lobe, cerebellar, and, often, brainstem retraction.

Several authors have sought to reduce the technical problems of retraction and depth of exposure by using other intradural and extradural surgical approaches. Both frontal and lateral approaches have been used to gain safe access to this region. Fujitsu et al. minimize brain retraction by removal of the zygoma which permits an anterolateral approach to the interpeduncular cistern but is best suited to lesions of the upper basilar artery and upper third of the clivus[14]. Archer et al. have successfully treated PICA and proximal basilar artery aneurysms via a transoral, transclival approach with improved access to the clival structures[2]. However, the risks of CSF fistula, infection, and a poor cosmetic result must be considered.

Other modified skull-base methods have been used for a more lateral attack to this region. Kawase et al.[30] describe a subtemporal extradural approach to the lower basilar artery and VBJ which requires bony removal of the anterior pyramidal portion of the petrous bone, ligation of the superior petrosal sinus, and surgical approach anterolaterally between cranial nerves V and VII. Temporal retraction (and potential injury to the vein of Labbe) is reduced with this combined middle and posterior fossa approach ("extended middle fossa approach"), but both injury to the hearing apparatus and cranial nerve palsies are potential morbidities as their report demonstrates. Sen and Sekhar[45] have used a preauricular infratemporal approach combined with an intradural subtemporal approach to a VBJ aneurysm. This exposure also requires the removal of the anterior petrous bone and has been primarily for extradural tumors of the petroclival region; however, wide exposure of all intradural structures along the full course of the clivus can be achieved. The same group[44] has used an extensive transtemporal extradural approach to this region requiring retromastoid and temporal craniectomies. However, the extensive drilling required increases the risk to cranial nerve VII and VIII and the labyrinth. It is important to note that the wide exposure of brainstem vessels often achieved with the removal of tumors is not obtained in aneurysm surgery.

More recently, petrosal bone dissection posterior to the labyrinth has been combined with an extreme lateral dural opening for improved visualization of this region. Canalis et al. have utilized a retrolabyrinthine, transtentorial approach with posterior and middle fossa craniotomies and a presigmoid dural opening for the treatment of petroclival lesions including mid-basilar aneurysms[7]. The middle and inner ear structures are preserved with this direct lateral approach. This is a similar approach to the "petrosal" approach used by A1-Mefty for the treatment of petroclival meningiomas[1].

Retromastoid Transsigmoid Approach

In cases of high vertebrobasilar bifurcation or AICA aneurysms, we now use a retromastoid (retrolabyrinthine) transsigmoid approach similar to that utilized by Giannotta and others[1,7,15]. The particular aneurysms approached in this manner were usually small and located high along the lower vertebrobasilar complex[42]. Interest in combined suboccipital/petrosal approaches to this region was renewed by Hitselberger and House[22] in 1966 in their report on a translabyrinthine transsigmoid approach to the cerebellopontine angle for removal of acoustic neuromas. We use a four by five centimeter U-shaped incision based on the postauricular fold. After a simple mastoidectomy, the vertical portion of VII and the posterior semicircular canal are identified; this represents the anterior extent of the exposure. The sigmoid sinus is skeletonized from the superior petrosal sinus to the jugular bulb. The bone overlying the endolymphatic sac, superior petrosal sinus, and dura anterior to the sigmoid sinus is removed. The dural opening is made 2 cm behind and parallel to the sigmoid sinus and can be modified depending on the individual case. An anteriorly based dural flap is created after the sigmoid sinus is ligated between the superior petrosal sinus and the jugular bulb below. This extends the dural opening 1–2 cm anterior to the sigmoid sinus. Combined with frequent rotation of the patient and the operating table, retraction is reduced and visualization of the basilar artery is improved. After the drainage of CSF, no cerebellar retraction is required to visualize aneurysms in this location.

In spite of the improved exposure provided by this and the other skull-base approaches, it should be stressed that the working space in this region is extremely limited. We have not had to deal with premature rupture of an aneurysm in this location. From our experience, this would be extremely difficult and would likely lead to major neurological deficits if excessive manipulation in this confined space were needed to control the hemorrhage.

Profound Hypothermia and Circulatory Arrest

Two patients in this series required profound hypothermia and cardiopulmonary bypass via a closed chest method in order to achieve definitive surgical clipping. The use of cardiac arrest and extracorporeal circulatory techniques has been described by many authors in the surgical treatment of difficult intracranial aneurysms. Spetzler has utilized hypothermic circulatory arrest via a closed chest method in the treatment of large and giant upper basilar artery aneurysms with good results[48]. He utilizes EEG, SSEP, and BAER and argues for the careful monitoring of the depth of hypothermia (well tolerated at 18–20°), duratin of total circulatory arrest, barbiturate use, and hemostasis/clotting mechanisms. Chyatte has since utilized the open chest method of establishing extracorporeal circulation and cardiac arrest in a patient with a giant vertebral artery aneurysm when systemic hypotension and temporary parent vessel occlusion did not allow for definitive clipping[8]. These authors stress the shorter bypass time, reduced risk of neurologic deficit, coagulopathy, and other systemic bypass-related problems in the direct cannulation of the right atrium and aorta through the chest.

Surgical Adjunctive Methods

Adjunctive methods are of great help in the treatment of lower vertebrobasilar aneurysms. particular problems with this group include intraoperative aneurysm rupture, intraoperative and delayed ischemia, perforator compromise, and inadequate aneurysm treatment. A number of these aneurysms are large and the dissection often requires direct manipulation and protracted periods of temporary vessel occlusion. We routinely utilize evoked potential (EP) monitoring which has permitted temporary vessel occlusions when needed. We have used vascular clips while others have used temporary balloon occlusion in order to achieve better proximal vessel control[46]. Some groups have used cerebral protective agents (etomidate) in order to prolong the safe period of local circulatory arrest by raising the threshold to ischemic brain injury[4]. Total circulatory arrest has been used by this group and others in order to facilitate the clipping of a small subgroup of these aneurysms[8,48]. In general, strategies aimed at cerebral protection have been underutilized in vertebrobasilar aneurysm surgery, which is surprising since periods of ischemia predictably occur both intraoperatively and postoperatively. Other groups utilize intraoperative angiography in order to assess aneurysmal obliteration and parent vessel patency at a time when unsatisfactory results are reversible[4,37].

Intraoperative Monitoring

The goal of intraoperative electrophysiologic monitoring is the accurate assessment of tolerance to reversible surgical maneuvers such as temporary vessel occlusion and retractor placement during aneurysmal dissection and direct clip application. In our experience, loss of either the median nerve SEP or the BAER or both within two minutes of temporary vessel occlusion has suggested poor tolerance and high risk for severe ischemia and postoperative neurologic deficit. Loss of one or both EPs for > 20 minutes has correlated strongly with postoperative neurologic compromise. There have been no false negative neurophysiological findings in our posterior circulation aneurysm series.

Endovascular Treatment of Vertebrobasilar Aneurysms

Intravascular approaches were utilized in the treatment of six aneurysms in this series. Endovascular methods were employed because these lesions were large or giant or had a large, ill-defined neck with or without fusiform dilatation of the parent vessel. The intravascular treatment of choice is selective occlusion of the aneurysmal sac while maintaining patency of the parent vessel. This has been demonstrated with posterior circulation aneurysms by Higashida, Hieshima, and co-workers[19,20]. This group has reported an incidence of vascular perforation as a consequence of all neurointerventional procedures of approximately 1%[17]. Preliminary evidence from other groups suggests that aneurysmal sac obliteration is more difficult in wide-necked aneurysms[16]. If there are technical limitations to aneurysmal sac obliteration, parent vessel occlusion of the vertebral or, less commonly, the basilar artery to induce aneurysmal thrombosis is a reasonable therapeutic alternative[3,23]. Collateral flow must be assessed to determine if the vertebral circulation can be occluded; the competency of the circle of Willis to supply the basilar system must be shown before a basilar occlusion is undertaken.

Aymard *et al.* reported 21 patients with aneurysms along the entire vertebrobasilar complex who underwent endovascular occlusion of the vertebral artery either at the level of C1 or distal to the PICA origin[3]. Thirteen of these patients (62%) had aneurysms > 2.5 cm with 13 (62%) having complete clinical and angiographic cure and six patients (29%) having partial thrombosis of their aneurysms without clinical worsening. Two additional patients (9.5%) died in this series.

Another therapeutic alternative in the treatment of giant aneurysms of the basilar trunk employed by Kashiwagi, Tew, and co-workers is surgical trapping of the involved segment of the basilar artery[27]. Drake initially utilized this technique in two of 13 patients with giant aneurysms in this location with only fair results[9]. The basilar artery is clipped distal to the AICA and proximal to the SCA in order to trap in aneurysm; this has the advantage over parent vessel occlusion in that aneurysmal obliteration and decompression of mass effect can be acheived. Yasargil has noted in autopsy studies that giant basilar trunk aneurysms tend to occur between perforating branches of the basilar artery thus justifying this surgical approach if more direct methods are technically impossible[53].

Results

The results are summarized in Tables 4–8. Definitive surgical clipping was achieved in 98 of the 100 upper basilar artery aneurysms and in 44 of the 48 lower basilar aneurysms Trapping or coating of the aneurysm was performed in 5 cases. In one patient with a giant aneurysm of the basilar tip, no attempt was made to clip the aneurysms after it was exposed. This patient was followed for 10 years with no hemorrhage but progressive enlargement of the aneurysm leading to hydrocephalus. Intravascular adjunctive measures were combined with a surgical approach in 6 cases. Patient outcome in the surgical groups of patients with aneurysms arising from the upper basilar artery is shown in Table 5 and lower half of the basilar and vertebral arteries in Table 6.

The use of these combined surgical approaches and adjunctive techniques has resulted in an excellent or good outcome (able to achieve independent premorbid

Table 4. *Vertebro-basilar Aneurysms Admission Grade Versus Outcome*

Grade	Outcome					
	E	G	F	P	D	T
0	20	3	2	1	2	28
1	46	9	5	1	3	64
2	2	1	1	0	1	5
3	23	9	5	6	4	47
4	0	2	0	0	2	4
Total	91	24	13	8	12	148

E excellent; *G* good; *F* fair; *P* poor; *D* dead; *T* total.

Table 5. *Upper Basilar Aneurysms Admission Grade Versus Outcome*

Grade	Outcome					
	E	G	F	P	D	T
0	18	3	2	1	2	26
1	20	4	3	1	2	30
2	1	1	1	0	1	4
3	16	9	4	5	4	38
4	0	1	0	0	1	2
Total	55	18	10	7	10	100

Table 6. *Lower Basilar Aneurysms Admission Grade Versus Outcome*

Grade	Outcome					
	E	G	F	P	D	T
0	2	0	0	0	0	2
1	26	5	2	0	1	34
2	1	0	0	0	0	1
3	7	0	1	1	0	9
4	0	1	0	0	1	2
Total	36	6	3	1	2	48

status without significant functional disability) in 78% (115/148) of patients (Table 4). In those patients presenting without neurologic deficit (Grades 0, 1, 2), a favorable outcome was achieved in 84% (81 of 97) with 6 deaths, for a mortality rate of 6.2%. In those presenting after a documented hemorrhage with or without neurologic deficit (Grades 1–3), a favorable outcome was achieved in 78% (90/116) with eight deaths, yielding a 6.9% mortality. Neurologic grade on adminission has been shown to correlate with functional clinical outcome by many authors, including the participants of the International Cooperative Study[28].

The outcome of those patients with aneurysms of the lower basilar artery were considerably better than the distal basilar group (Table 6). In these patients 42 of 48

Table 7. *Vertebro-Basilar Aneurysms Overall Outcome*

All grades	148
Excellent or good	115
Favorable outcome	78%
Deaths	12
Mortality rate	8.1%

patients (88%) had a favorable outcome. In those patients presenting without neurologic deficit (grades 0, 1, 2), a favorable outcome was achieved in 92% (34 of 37) with one death, for a mortality rate of 3%. In those presenting after a documented hemorrhage from a lower basilar artery aneurysm with or without neurologic deficit (grades 1–3), a favorable outcome was achieved in 87% (39 of 44) with one death, yielding a 2% mortality.

Surgical Complications

Cranial nerve deficits after vertebrobasilar aneurysm surgery is an often unavoidable neurologic sequela. Most of the cranial nerve palsies in these series were transient as has been in the experience of others[47]. The involved nerves included cranial nerves III, VI and VII and, more commonly, the lower cranial nerves IX–XII. The nerves were left anatomically intact and functional recovery was usually complete within a 6 month interval following operation. There was one case of permanent postoperative deafness after intraoperative VIIIth nerve injury resulting from manipulation of a giant VBJ aneurysm in a patient undergoing reoperation following a second subarachnoid hemorrhage.

Table 8. *Vertebro-Basilar Aneurysms Outcome by Grades*

Grade 0, 1, 2	97
Excellent or good	81
Favorable outcome	84%
Deaths	6
Mortality rate	6.2%
Grade 1–3	116
Excellent or good	90
Favorable outcome	78%
Deaths	8
Mortality rate	6.9%
Grade 3	47
Excellent or good	32
Favorable outcome	68%
Deaths	4
Mortality rate	8.5%

The two mortalities included one patient with a postoperative posterior fossa epidural hematoma and one patient who never regained consciousness following clipping of a VBJ aneurysm.

Discussion

Aneurysms of the posterior circulation pose unique challenges because of their location and the infrequency with which they are encountered. Vertebral and basilar artery aneurysms comprise 15% of all intracranial aneurysms according to some authors[41]; we report an incidence of 14%. However, more recent series indicate that the prevalence of posterior circulation aneurysms may actually be closer to 5–8%[28,29,39]. Aneurysms of the lower basilar and vertebral arteries comprise a smaller fraction of this group. Drake was the first to report success with the management of posterior circulation aneurysms and his group has reported excellent or good results in 85% of 1400 cases of vertebrobasilar artery aneurysms with a surgical mortality of 5.3% and an overall management morbidity of 10%[9–11,40]. Although other authors have reported success in the management of these lesions, the morbidity and mortality in the treatment of posterior circulation aneurysms[28,50,54]. This difference was not seen in the surgical group of the recent International Cooperative Study; however, the number of vegetative outcomes was noticeably higher in the posterior circulation aneurysm group[28]. Basilar artery aneurysm surgery has also been associated with a higher rate of operative vascular complications[25]. Technical limitations in posterior fossa aneurysm surgery account for some of these observed differences.

The region of the lower basilar and vertebral arteries is not felt to have the abundance of perforating vessels seen in the region of the basilar apex. However, microvascular anatomic studies of the pontomedullary junction have shown that perforating vessels are present in this region, most of which occur on the basilar artery below the AICA[36]. Aneurysms in this region present additional challenges for safe visualization and treatment. The working space is small between the pontomedullary region, the anterolateral skull base, and the cranial nerves and there is significant variability in the vertebral artery and PICA course. Traditional surgical approaches often provide a deep operative field, require extensive brain retraction, and necessitate difficult microdissection between fascicles of the lower cranial nerves. Despite these factors, many authors report good success in treating lower vertebrobasilar aneurysms[24,33,47,50,52]. Aneurysms of the posterior inferior cerebellar artery (PICA) tend to be associated with the most favorable outcome. Drake reported a good outcome in 92% of cases of vertebral aneurysms with reduced success with those of the AICA (76%) and VBJ (88%)[11]. In our posterior fossa aneurysm experience, 75% of lower vertebrobasilar aneurysm patients were Grades 0–2 on presentation while only 58% of upper basilar aneurysms patients were without neurologic deficit on presentation, even though 26% of upper basilar aneurysm patients had not bled. This suggests that SAH from a lower vertebrobasilar aneurysm is less likely to produce a poor grade patient than hemorrhage from an upper basilar aneurysm. This may account in part for the high number of favorable outcomes in patients with lower vertebrobasilar aneurysms.

There is a large percentage of giant (> 2.5 cm) aneurysms among those of the vertebrobasilar complex. Drake has reported an incidence of 17% while others have reported an even higher incidence[11,31]. Twenty-five percent of the vertebrobasilar aneurysms in our series were greater than 2.0 cm in diameter. Aneurysmal size is the most predictive factor in surgical outcome[9,11,28,38,50,51]. Many of these large aneurysms have significant intramural thrombus and atherosclerotic, calcified walls which often obscure both perforating and parent vessels. The issues of size and partial thrombosis make postoperative imaging of the adequacy of aneurysm treatment difficult to interpret[5].

The location of these aneurysms and the significant number which are large, irregular, and eccentrically projecting require the use of a full array of surgical and adjunctive techniques. Aneurysms of the vertebral-PICA region are approached commonly via lateral suboccipital craniectomy while aneurysms of the upper basilar artery are commonly approached by either the pterional or subtemporal routes. Aneurysms of the midbasilar artery and VBJ have been approached in a number of ways. This is a continually evolving area and there is no consensus in the surgical management of these rare aneurysms. The suboccipital approach provides a wide operative field which has allowed for adequate proximal vessel control, especially in cases of larger aneurysms. This has been an adequate approach in most cases, but the depth of the operative field, necessary retraction of the cerebellum, and need to perform the microdissection within the cranial nerve fibers must be recognized.

We have been satisfied with the shallow surgical field provided by the retromastoid transsigmoid approach in selected cases of smaller aneurysms located high along the clivus and have in these cases avoided the potential problems associated with temporal lobe, cerebellar, or brainstem retraction. The approach is more lateral and closer to the clivus and allows for definitive clip placement without the need for cerebellar retraction. However, there is very little working room from this angle which may potentially limit adequate proximal vessel control should intraoperative aneurysm rupture occur. Additional disadvantages of this approach include the need for preoperative assessment of the posterior dural venous sinus drainage and the potential for postoperative CSF leak. In our experience, no patient with a patent contralateral sigmoid sinus has had a problem related to inadequate venous drainage following sigmoid sinus ligation. CSF leak is a common problem with this approach since a water tight dural closure is difficult to achieve. In addition to waxing all the mastoid air cells, we utilize temporalis fascia and abdominal fat grafts over the dural defect to help obviate this problem. A subsequent CSF leak was controlled with a lumbar drain in one case and re-exploration has not yet been required for this problem. We have also failed to achieve adequate exposure to this region with this approach in one patient undergoing re-operation with significant dense scar tissue around a giant VBJ aneurysm. This same patient also illustrates the limitations of contemporary techniques. Both the lateral suboccipital and retromastoid transsigmoid approaches resulted in inadequate exposure of the aneurysm; in addition, an intervening intravascular balloon occlusion of the aneurysm did not permanently occlude the aneurysmal sac. Other groups have reported difficulty with balloon occlusion of posterior circulation aneurysms[32].

Although the efficacy of BAER and SSEP monitoring has established in a number of neurosurgical procedures, a firm consensus on its predictive value in vascular surgery of the posterior fossa has not been established. Little et al. reported a 25% false-negative rate in the prediction of postoperative brain stem ischemia in a series of 16 basilar aneurysm patients[35]. Friedman et al. noted a failure of prediction of postoperative sensory or motor deficit in 5 of 8 patients undergoing basilar aneurysm operation[13]. These authors feel this predictive failure demonstrates that the vascular territory at risk, particularly in cases of basilar apex aneurysms, often does not include either the auditory or the somatosensory pathway. We have not experienced such a high false-negative rate in the prediction of either intolerance to ischemia or postoperative neurologic compromise in our posterior fossa aneurysm series, including those aneurysms of the basilar apex and superior cerebellar artery which have not been discussed in this report.

In those cases where a direct surgical approach has not been attempted initially or has failed to achieve successful treatment, endovascular techniques have provided a viable therapeutic alternative. The use of this adjunctive measure should continue to increase as these neurointerventional methods improve, particularly with aneurysms of the posterior fossa. Familiarity with and availability of the full spectrum of management and therapeutic techniques is necessary to safely treat aneurysms of the basilar and vertebral arteries.

References

1. Al-Mefty O, Fox JL, Smith RR (1988) Petrosal approach for petroclival meningiomas. Neurosurgery 22: 510–517
2. Archer DJ, Young S, Uttley D (1987) Basilar aneurysms: a new transclival approach via maxillotomy. J Neurosurg 67: 54–58
3. Aymard A, Gobin YP, Hodes JE, Bien S, Rufenacht D, Reizine D, George B, Merland JJ (1991) Endovascular occlusion of vertebral arteries in the treatment of unclippable vertebrobasilar aneurysms. J Neurosurg 74: 393–398
4. Batjer HH, Frankfurt AI, Purdy PD, Smith SS, Samson DS (1988) Use of etomidate, temporary arterial occlusion, and intraoperative angiography in surgical treatment of large and giant cerebral aneurysms. J Neurosurg 69: 234–240
5. Brothers MF, Fox AJ, Lee DH, Pelz DM, Deveikis JP (1990) MR imaging after surgery for vertebrobasilar aneurysm. AJNR 11: 149–161
6. Campos J, Fox AJ, Vinuela F, Lylyk P, Ferguson GG, Drake CG, Peerless SJ (1987) Saccular aneurysms in basilar artery fenestration. AJNR 8: 233–236
7. Canalis RF, Black K, Martin N, Becker D (1991) Extended retrolabyrinthine transtentorial approach to petroclival lesions. Laryngoscope 101: 6–13
8. Chyatte D, Elefteriades J, Kim B (1989) Profound hypothermia and circulatory arrest for aneurysm surgery. Case report. J Neurosurg 70: 489–491
9. Drake CG (1979) Giant intracranial aneurysms: experience with 174 patients. Clin Neurosurg 26: 12–95
10. Drake CG (1979) The treatment of aneurysms of the posterior circulation. Clin Neurosurg 26: 96–144
11. Drake CG (1981) Progress in cerebrovascular disease. Management of cerebral aneurysm. Stroke 12: 273–283
12. Flamm ES (1981) Suction decompression of aneurysms: technical note. J Neurosurg 54: 275–276
13. Friedman WA, Kaplan BL, Day AL, Sypert GW, Curran MT (1987) Evoked potential monitoring during aneurysm operation: observations after fifty cases. Neurosurgery 20: 678–687
14. Fujitsu K, Kuwabara T (1985) Zygomatic approach for lesions in the interpeduncular cistern. J Neurosurg 62: 340–343
15. Giannotta SL, Maceri D (1988) Retrolabyrinthine transsigmoid approach to basilar trunk and vertebrobasilar artery junction aneurysms. J Neurosurg 69: 461–466
16. Guglielmi G, Vinuela F, Martin N, Duckwiler G, Cantore GP (1992) Endovascular treatment of intracranial saccular aneurysms with detachable coils and electrothrombosis: experience with 39 cases. American Association of Neurological Surgeons, San Francisco, CA, p 165
17. halbach VV, Higashida RT, Dowd CF, Barnwell SL, Hieshima GB (1991) Management of vascular perforations that occur during neurointerventional procedures. AJNR 12: 319–327
18. Heros RC (1986) Lateral suboccipital approach for vertebral and vertebrobasilar artery lesions. J Neurosurg 64: 559–562
19. Hieshima GB, Higashida RT, Wapenski J, Halbach VV, Bentson JR (1987) Intravascular balloon embolization of a large mid-basilar artery aneurysm: case report. J Neurosurg 66: 124–127
20. Higashida RT, Halbach VV, Calan LD, Hieshima GB, Konishi Y (1989) Detachable balloon embolization therapy of posterior circulation intracranial aneurysms. J Neurosurg 71: 512–519
21. Hirschfeld A, Flamm ES (1981) An extracranial aneurysm arising from the posterior inferior cerebellar artery. J Neurosurg 54: 537–539
22. Hitselberger WE, House WF (1966) A combined approach to the cerebellopontine angle: a suboccipital-petrosal approach. Arch Otolaryngol 84: 267–285
23. Hodes JE, Aymard A, Gobin YP, Rufenacht D, Bien S, Reizine D, Gaston A, Merland JJ (1991) Endovascular occlusion of intracranial vessels for curative treatment of unclippable aneurysms: report of 16 cases. J Neurosurg 75: 694–701
24. Hudgins RJ, Day AL, Quisling RG, Rhoton AL Jr., Sypert GW, Garcia-Bengochea F (1983) Aneurysms of the posterior cerebellar artery. J Neurosurg 58: 381–387
25. Karhunen PJ (1991) Neurosurgical vascular complications associated with aneurysm clips evaluated by postmortem angiography. Forensic Sci Int 51: 13–22
26. Kasdon DL, Stein BM (1979) Combined supratentorial and infratentorial exposure for low-lying basilar aneurysms. Neurosurgery 4: 422–426
27. Kashiwagi S, Tew JM Jr., Van Loveren HR, Thomas G (1988) Trapping of giant basilar trunk aneurysms. J Neurosurg 69: 442–445
28. Kassell NF, Torner JC, Haley EC Jr, Jane JA, Adams HP, Kongable GL, and Participants (1990) The International Cooperative Study on the timing of aneurysm surgery. Part 1: overall management results. J Neurosurg 73: 18–36
29. Kassell NF, Torner JC, Jane JA, Haley EC Jr., Adams HP, and Participants (1990) The International Cooperative Study on the timing of aneurysm surgery. Part 2: surgical results. J Neurosurg 73: 37–47
30. Kawase T, Toya S, Shiobara R, Mine T (1985) Transpetrosal approach for aneurysms of the lower basilar artery. J Neurosurg 63: 857–861
31. Kempe LG (1979) Aneurysms of the vertebral artery. In: Pia HW, Langmaid C, Zierski J (eds) Cerebral aneurysms: advances in diagnosis and therapy. Springer, Berlin Heidelberg New York, pp 191–120
32. Kwan ES, Heilman CB, Schucart WA, Klucznik RP (1991) Enlargement of basilar artery aneurysms following balloon occlusion–"water-hammer effect". Report of two cases. J Neurosurg 75: 963–968
33. Lee KS, Gower DJ, Branch CJ Jr., Kelly DL Jr., McWhorter JM, Bell WO (1989) Surgical repair of aneurysms of the posterior inferior cerebellar artery – a clinical series. Surg Neurol 31: 85–91
34. Lister JR, Rhoton AL Jr., Matsushima T, Peace DA (1982) Microsurgical anatomy of the posterior inferior cerebellar artery. Neurosurgery 10: 170–199
35. Little JR, Lesser RP, Luders H (1987) Electrophysiological monitoring during basilar aneurysm operation. Neurosurgery 20: 421–427

36. Mahmood A, Dujovny M, Torche M, Dragovic L, Ausman JI (1991) Microvascular anatomy of foramen caecum medullae oblongatae. J Neurosurg 75: 299–304

37. Martin NA, Bentson J, Vinuela F, Hieshima G, Reicher M, Black K, Dion J, Becker D (1990) Intraoperative digital subtraction angiography and the surgical treatment of intracranial aneurysms and vascular malformations. J Neurosurg 73: 526–533

38. McMurtry JG III, Housepian EM, Bowman FO Jr, Matteo RS (1974) Surgical treatment of basilar artery aneurysms. Elective circulatory arrest with thoracotomy in 12 cases. J Neurosurg 40: 486–494

39. Nishimoto A, et al. (1985) Nationwide Cooperative Study of intracranial aneurysm surgery in Japan. Stroke 16: 48–52

40. Peerless SJ, Drake CG (1988) Surgical Techniques of Posterior Cerebral Aneurysms. In: Schmidek HH, Sweet WH (eds) Operative neurosurgical techniques, 2nd Ed, Vol II. Saunders, pp 973–989

41. Rhoton AL Jr (1977) Congenital and traumatic intracranial aneurysms. CIBA Clin Symp 29: 2–40

42. Rosenberg SI, Flamm ES, Hoffer ME, Schwartz DM (1992) The retrolabyrinthine transsigmoid approach to midbasilar artery aneurysms. Laryngoscope 102: 100–104

43. Samson DS, Batjer H (1990) Intracranial aneurysm surgery: techniques. Futura, Mount Kisoo, NY, pp 165–177

44. Sekhar LN, Estonillo R (1986) Transtemporal approach to the skull base: an anatomical study. Neurosurgery 19: 799–808

45. Sen CH, Sekhar LN (1990) The subtemporal and preauricular approach to intradural structures ventral to the brain stem. J Neurosurg 73: 345–354

46. Shucart WA, Kwan ES, Heilman CB (1990) Temporary balloon occlusion of a proximal vessel as an aid to clipping aneurysms of the basilar and paraclinoid internal carotid arteries: technical note. Neurosurgery 27: 116–119

47. Solomon RA, Stein BM (1988) Surgical approaches to aneurysms of the vertebral and basilar arteries. Neurosurgery 23: 203–207

48. Spetzler RF, Hadley MN, Rigamonti D, Carter LP, Raudzens PA, Shedd SA, Wilkinson E (1988) Aneurysms of the basilar artery treated with circulatory arrest hypohermia, and barbiturate cerebral protection. J Neurosurg 68: 868–879

49. Sugita K, Kobayashi S, Takemae T, Tada T, Tanaka Y (1987) Aneurysms of the basilar artery trunk. J Neurosurg 66: 500–505

50. Sundt TM Jr, Kobayashi S, Fode NC, Whisnant JP (1982) Results and complications of surgical management of 809 intracranial aneurysms in 722 cases. J Neurosurg 56: 753–765

51. Sundt TM Jr, Piepgras DG, Houser OW, Campbell JK (1982) Interpostion saphenous vein grafts for advanced occlusive disease and large aneurysms in the posterior circulation. J Neurosurg 56: 205–215

52. Yamaura A (1988) Diagnosis and treatment of vertebral aneurysms. J Neurosurg 69: 345–349

53. Yaşargil MG (1984) Vertebrobasilar aneurysms. In: Yaşargil MG (ed) Microneurosurgery, Vol 2. Thieme, Stuttgart, pp 232–295

54. Yoshimoto T, Uchida K, Kaneko U, Kayama T, Suzuki J (1979) An analysis of follow-up results of 1000 intracranial saccular aneurysms with definitive surgical treatment. J Neurosurg 50: 152–157

Correspondence: Eugene S. Flamm, M.D., Division of Neurosurgery, University of Pennsylvania School of Medicine, Philadelphia, PA 19104, U.S.A.

The Transsylvian Approach to Basilar Aneurysms

D. Samson and **H. Batjer**

Department of Neurological Surgery, University of Texas Southwestern Medical Center, Dallas, Texas, U.S.A.

Summary

While aneurysms of the distal basilar artery are the most common posterior circulation aneurysms, they are the most difficult to be attacked surgically. The anatomically deep and narrow confines of the interpeduncular cistern and the intimate relationship of the basilar artery to the posterior thalamoperforating branches, the brain stem and diencephalon combine to provide a formidable surgical environment. The pterional transsylvian approach has some unique advantages over the more traditional subtemporal procedure. Perhaps the most important of these is the ease of exposure of the contralateral posterior cerebral artery. Between 1977 and 1991, 201 patients with distal basilar aneurysms have been operated through the transsylvian approach at our Center. We chose this approach for approximately 70% of the distal basilar aneurysms treated during this time period. We feel that this is the preferred approach for most such lesions unless the origin is below the midsellar depth or the aneurysm projects predominantly posteriorly.

Keywords: Basilar aneurysm; transsylvian approach.

Introduction

Aneurysms of the distal basilar circulation represent from 8% to 12% of all intracranial aneurysms brought to neurosurgical attention and from the date of their initial description have been regarded as unique surgical challenges[6]. These have been the last major group of intracranial aneurysms to be treated successfully – a therapeutic triumph reflecting the persistence and ingenuity of Drake, London, Ontario[1,2]. Subsequent to Drake's development of the subtemporal approach, the introduction of both the operating microscope and microvascular dissecting technique into aneurysm surgery in the late 1960s and early 1970s by Yaşargil[10], brought an increased awareness of certain features of cerebral vascular anatomy that has suggested alternatives to the traditional routes of surgical exposure, including exposure of the distal basilar circulation.

One such surgical alternative is the use of the pterional or frontotemporal or sylvian approach to lesions located in and about the interpeduncular sub-arachnoid cistern. This technique, initially described by Yasargil and subsequently modified by a number of his students and other investigators[3,4,7,9], uses the most popular approach to aneurysms of the anterior circle of Willis, extending the exposure deep to the carotid artery to allow visualization of the distal basilar circulation bilaterally.

The transsylvian exposure of the distal basilar artery and its branches offers an unexcelled parasagittal view of the basilar trunk, the origin of both superior cerebellar arteries (SCAs), the basilar bifurcation, and the origins of both posterior cerebral arteries, and the ipsilateral junction of the posterior communicating artery (PComA) and the posterior cerebral artery. Additionally, it provides unimpeded visualization of the critical perforating vessels emanating from the proximal P1 segments bilaterally and from the ipsilateral posterior communicating artery. This approach does not provide an unobstructed view of the posterior aspect of the basilar trunk on basilar bifurcation in the case of bifurcation aneurysms; perforating vessels in these areas must be exposed (as is the case with the subtemporal approach) by manipulation of aneurysms lying in the interpednucular cistern.

Since its initial description in 1977, the pterional approach has been used for a variety of aneurysms of the basilar trunk, superior cerebellar and posterior cerebral arteries, and the basilar bifurcation itself. The principal anatomic deterrent to its routine application to all distal basilar artery aneurysms is the infrequent (15%) interposition of the posterior clinoid process[5,7], which makes visualization of lesions arising below this level somewhat more difficult. Despite a variety of technical maneuvers to deal with this impediment[4,11], the authors believe that any aneurysm whose origin appears radiographically to lie below the level of the mid portion of the sella turcica is presently best approached either from the so-called "half and half" approach or from the more classic subtemporal exposure.

Methods

Patient Positioning

Assuming that both the patient and the surgeon are right-handed, a routine right frontotemporal exposure is used for all aneurysms arising from the basilar trunk, superior cerebellar origin bilaterally, or from the junction of the first (P1) and second (P2) portions of the posterior cerebral arteries. The sole lesions approached from the left side are aneurysms arising from the left posterior communicating-posterior cerebral junction. The patient's head is immobilized in the Mayfield-Keys headholder and is turned some 15°–20° away from the side of the surgical exposure; then, it is tilted so that the maxillary eminence is higher than the area of pterion on the surgical side. In this final position without lessening the degree of lateral rotation or extension, the chin is flexed slightly toward the clavicle on the nonsurgical side in an attempt to bring the floor of the frontal fossa as perpendicular as possible to the long axis of the body.

Incision

A routine curvilinear skin incision is preferred for all pterional approaches, and it is carefully placed to avoid injury either to the frontalis branch of the facial nerve or to the increasingly important superficial temporal artery. The incision extends superiorly immediately anterior to the tragus of the right ear, respecting the course of the superficial temporal artery; then, it curves anteriorly within the hairline to the most anterior aspect of the brow in the midline. Reflecting the scalp and the temporalis muscle as a single layer markedly reduces the incidence of frontalis palsies that are seen when the temporalis facia is cut as a separate layer; in no way does it limit the bony opening or the final surgical approach.

Craniotomy/Craniectomy

A modest sized bone flap is fashioned by using burr holes in the following locations (1) one hole is placed low in the temporal squama; (2) the second is located some 4 cm superior to the squama, immediately posterior to the coronal suture; (3) the third is some 5 cm above the lateral aspect of the brow in the most anterior aspect of the superior temporal line; and (4) the fourth is immediately superior to the zygomatic frontal process at the lateral junction of the frontal fossa and the orbit. The free flap that is formed is removed, and a generous subtemporal craniectomy subsequently is performed with a variety of rongeurs to offer adequate access to the anterior aspect of the temporal lobe.

When the lateral aspect of the sphenoid wing has been generously removed by using small, straight and curved mastoid rongeurs, a radical resection of the entire sphenoid ridge almost to the level of the lateral aspect of the superior orbital fissure is undertaken; the resection should be taken well medially to the origin of the orbital frontal meningeal artery. The dura mater initially is separated on both frontal and temporal lobe aspects of the sphenoid ridge by using a small, slightly curved dissector, and the small meningeal branches of the external carotid artery, which invariably are interrupted during the course of resection, are controlled with bipolar cautery apparatus or with small bits of bone wax.

Microsurgical Exposure

When dural opening has been accomplished, a frontal ventriculostomy is placed and then the inferiolateral aspect of the frontal lobe elevated slightly. The retraction is rapidly and sequentially deepened to expose the optic nerve and prechiasmatic cistern, which is sharply opened from the level of the interhemispheric fissure laterally to the most medial aspect of the Sylvian fissure. The Sylvian fissure is then opened laterally to medially along the course of the horizontal portion of the middle cerebral artery from its bifurcation to its origin from the internal carotid artery. Once the middle cerebral artery can be visualized throughout its entire horizontal course, a very small temporal lobe self-retaining retractor is placed on the anterior aspect of the temporal tip, which is then retracted very gently posteriorly. As Yaşargil first demonstrated, the key to identification and ultimate exposure of the basilar artery via the pterional approach is the posterior communicating artery and its subarachnoid cistern[11]. The leash of perforating arteries that emerge from the superior aspect of the posterior cerebral artery must be respected throughout the exposure. When no posterior communicating artery is present, but rather a large "fetal" posterior cerebral artery emanates from the posterior wall of the carotid artery, the large posterior cerebral artery can be followed posteriorly until the third cranial nerve is visualized; then, once the third cranial nerve is completely liberated from the uncus, gentle dissection immediately inferior to its origin will demonstrate the superior cerebellar artery that can be followed medially to the basilar trunk.

At or about this point, the basilar trunk will be identified deeply in the interpeduncular cistern, running an oblique course from the superior aspect of the right portion of the surgical field toward the inferior corner of the surgical field on the left. Once identified, the basilar artery should be dissected proximally below the level of the origin of the superior cerebellar artery on the surgical side; then, dissection should be carried distally on the contralateral side to provide adequate proximal control of the basilar trunk before exposure of aneurysms of the superior cerebellar origin or of the basilar bifurcation.

Once the basilar-posterior cerebral junction on the right side and the origin of both superior cerebellar arteries have been identified, dissection can be carried across the most anterior aspect of the distal basilar artery to demonstrate the origin of the posterior cerebral artery on the left side. Exposure then should be extended to the superior side of the vessel, with dissection of arachnoid and adherent clot allowing identification of the important and always present perforating branches that emanate from the proximal portion of the P1 segment. Sharp dissection then can be carried across the base of the aneurysm from left to right to identify the right-sided P1 perforators and (again) the aneurysm origin, and also define the ipsilateral site of clip placement. With further gentle dissection using the fine-tip bipolar forceps and occasionally a microdissector, the aneurysm can be tilted slightly anteriorly to inspect the posterior aspect of the bifurcation area to ensure that no crucial perforating branches will be inadvertently occluded at the time of clip placement. In roughly 50% of cases, we employ temporary occlusion of the basilar trunk to facilitate this final step in aneurysm dissection.

Results

In the time period of 1977–1991, 277 aneurysms of this region have been surgically managed at the University of Texas Southwestern Medical Center at Dallas. Two-hundred-one have been operated via the transylvian exposure; the remainder have been operated through the traditional subtemporal approach. In the 201 patients undergoing surgery via the transsylvian approach, a good clinical result (defined as normal neurological function or mild neurological deficit) have been achieved in 83% of patients. Poor results (severe deficit, persistent vegetative state, death) represent the remaining 16%. As is true in all exposures of the distal basilar artery, morbidity and mortality has been primarily related to ischemia and infraction in the distribution of the perforating vessels and P1 segments. Most commonly this has been secondary either to inadvertent perforating artery occlusion by permanent aneurysm clips, or to protracted temporary occlusion of the distal basilar truck and P1 segments during aneurysm dissection and clip application.

Discussion

As stated above, the majority of distal basilar aneurysms treated at our Center are approached through a transsylvian or half-and-half exposure. The easy access of the basilar trunk for proximal control and temporary clipping and the clear exposure of the contralateral posterior cerebral artery are clear advantages of this procedure. For large and giant aneurysms, temporary trapping can facilitate collapse and mobilization of the sac out of the interpeduncular fossa to permit safe clipping. The key to successful basilar surgery by any approach is the preservation of all thalamoperforating vessels. The use of temporary clipping to soften the aneurysm has been extremely helpful in these anterior procedures as considerably better visualization can be achieved posteriorly. The true transsylvian approach

should be avoided in low-lying aneurysms whose necks are below the mid-sellar depth and in those projecting directly posteriorly into the brain stem.

References

1. Drake CG (1961) Bleeding aneurysms of the basilar artery: direct surgical management in four cases. J Neurosurg 18:230–238
2. Drake CG (1973) Management of aneurysms of posterior circulation. In: Youman JR (ed) Neurological surgery, Vol 2. Saunders, Philadelphia pp 787–806
3. Fox JL (1979) Microsurgical exposure of intracranial aneurysms. J Microsurg 1:2–31
4. Fox JL (1981) Microsurgical exposure of intracranial aneurysms. Presented at the annual meeting of the American Association of Neurological Surgeons, Boston, April 5–9
5. Krayenbuhl HA, Yasargil MG (1968) Cerebral angiography. Lippincott, Philadelphia, p 74
6. Locksley HB (1966) The natural history of subarachnoid hemorrhage, intracranial aneurysms and arteriovenous malformations. J Neurosurg 25:219–239
7. Samson DS, Hodosh RM, Clark WK (1978) Microsurgical evaluation of the pterional approach to aneurysms of the distal basilar circulation. Neurosurgery 3:135–141
8. Samson DS, Batjer HH (1990) Distal basilar aneurysms: the pterional approach. In: Samson DS, Batjer HH (ed) Intracranial aneurysm surgery: techniques. Futura, Maint Kisco, NM, pp 121–142
9. Sugita K, Kobayashi S, Shintani A, Matsuga N (1979) Microsurgery for aneurysms of the basilar artery. J Neurosurg 51:615–620
10. Yaşargil MG (1969) Reconstructive and constructive surgery of the cerebral arteries in man: Part C. Aneurysms, arteriovenous malformations and fistulae. In: Yaşargil MG (ed) Microsurgery applied to neurosurgery. Thieme, Stuttgart, pp 140–141
11. Yaşargil MG, Antic J, Laciga R, Jain KK, Hodosh RM, Smith RD (1976) Microsurgical pterional approach to aneurysms of the basilar bifurcation. Surg Neurol 6:83–91

Correspondence: Duke Samson, M.D., Department of Neurological Surgery, University of Texas Southwestern Medical Center, 5323 Harry Hines Blvd., Dallas, Texas 75235-8855, U.S.A.

Transclinoid-Transsellar-Transcavernous Approach to Basilar Tip Aneurysms

V.V. Dolenc, B.P. Prestor, J. Šušteršič and **R. Pregelj**

Department of Neurosurgery, University Hospital Centre, Ljubljana, Slovenia

Summary

A new transclinoid-transsellar-transcavernous (3-T) approach to basilar tip aneurysms is presented. In its initial version this approach was already presented in 1987 by the senior author. In the next few years the 3-T approach was further improved, so that in its present version it offers a much safer and easier method of treating basilar tip aneurysms than the original 3-T approach. The individual steps of the surgical procedure are described in detail. The 3-T approach to basilar tip aneurysms provides the required space around the aneurysm, which is mandatory for safe proximal control as well as for good visualization of the whole aneurysm, and allows for dissection and clipping of the aneurysm. This approach does not exclude the use of any other approaches, on the contrary, it allows for combination of various approaches to different degrees, depending upon the size and position of the basilar tip aneurysm. Final important point to be mentioned is that the 3-T approach no longer requires so extensively practised retraction of the brain during the operation. A series of 47 patients with a basilar tip aneurysm were treated surgically using this approach. The final outcome is as follows: out of 47 patients treated, 33 (70.2%) are symptom-free, 10 (21.3%) have certain symptoms and/or neurological deficits, and 4 (8.5%) died after surgery.

Keywords: Basilar tip aneurysm; vertebrobasilar tree; subarachnoid haemorrhage; surgical technique.

Introduction

Basilar tip aneurysms represent around 50% of aneurysms of the vertebro-basilar system[6,7,16,32,36,39,40]. Usually these aneurysms are solitary, but may also be associated with aneurysms in other locations, as well as with some other malformations, such as persistent primitive hypoglossal artery[1]. The aneurysms at the basilar tip do not show any significant preponderance toward a larger size such as it may be seen in carotid ophthalmic aneurysms. When an aneurysm at the basilar tip is of large or even giant size, it can produce symptoms and signs as a result of compression on the adjacent structures[5,8,12,19,20,27,30,34]. The occurrence of such symptoms and signs, due to compression of the aneurysm on the adjacent structures, is relatively rare, since most of the aneurysms at this location – like most other intracranial aneurysms – are manifested by subarachnoid hemorrhage (SAH).

The prognosis for patients with ruptured basilar tip aneurysm of any size, treated nonsurgically, is generally unfavorable: mortality is more than 50%[42]. The mortality rate for a series of patients operated on for a basilar tip aneurysm before 1966 was as high as that of patients who were not treated surgically[3,26]. Notwithstanding the poor results it should be noted that the operated-on survivors returned to normal life whereas those treated non-surgically did not.

The introduction of microsurgical techniques and new operative approaches has significantly improved the final results of surgical treatment of basilar tip aneurysms[7,10,11,15,18,25,31,40,45]. Additional and special measures – hypotension and hypothermia – represent another important improvement[7,16]. Bypass surgery[24], combined with the ligation of the vertebral or basilar artery, would seem to be a safe, promising and alternative treatment to the direct approach to large and giant basilar tip aneurysms[4,16–18]. Circulatory arrest, hypothermia and appropriate neuroanaesthesia should offer safer operative conditions in this kind of surgery[29,33]. Better knowledge of the anatomical variations of the basilar tip, as well as of the relationships with the brainstem and other nervous structures, has brought further advances[30,38], and understanding of microsurgical anatomy of the region of the tentorial incisura has provided a clear direction for further progress[9,16,18,35,40,44,45]. The larger the volume of the relevant literature, the more polarized the opinions have become – from very sceptical[26,39] to more optimistic – toward the operative treatment of these aneurysms[15–18,38,40,41,43,45].

Two important factors must be taken into consideration, firstly, the extremely difficult location of basilar tip aneurysms and the shortage of space, and secondly, the fact that basilar tip aneurysms constitute a very small percentage of all intracranial aneurysms. These two factors necessitate a rational policy in the treatment of these aneurysms; and hence the rare pathology should be collated in larger neurosurgical centers in order to gain more reliable experience[43]. A very important contribution to the treatment of basilar tip aneurysms was achieved with endovascular occlusion techniques[2,21,22]. Although it has generally been believed that this is the final answer to the treatment of these difficult cases, there remain, however, many situations in which the occlusion of the aneurysm can be performed only partially – or not at all – simply because of the location of the perforators deriving from the so-called neck of the aneurysm. In this case, open surgery and the direct approach is the treatment of choice. The 3-T approach to basilar tip aneurysms is particularly appealing because it does not exclude any of the previous approaches used, and in addition, it combines various approaches whenever necessary, and, most importantly, it provides the necessary operating space[12-14]. The 3-T approach enables a skilled neurosurgeon to perform this demanding surgical procedure without any longer having to resort to brain retraction.

Surgical Technique

The patient is placed in the supine position on the operating table. His head is fixed in the Mayfield tripoint headrest and rotated – in most cases – by about 35 degrees to the left direction[14]. In a few cases, however, where the basilar tip is located to the left of the midline, the patient's head is rotated in the right direction, so that the left pterional area is exposed.

Most basilar aneurysms are located in the midline. The surgeon's approach depends on whether he is right- or left-handed. The skin incision, the retraction of the skin and muscle flaps and formation of the bone flap have been described elsewhere[12-14].

The initial opening of the orbital roof is enlarged and the roof is removed anteriorly and posteriorly in relation to the sphenoid wing, together with the sphenoid wing itself. When the lateral tip of the superior orbital fissure (SOF) is reached, the roof of the orbit is removed posteriorly, so that the dura running through the SOF on its posterior aspect is left completely free and the anterior border of the cavernous sinus (CS),

covered by the dura, is exposed. The next step is dissection of the sphenoid wing on the posterolateral aspect, i.e. on the medial aspect of the SOF. By gentle dissection, the dura covering the cranial nerves III, IV and V1 in the SOF – running from the CS to the orbit on the medial aspect – is peeled off from the bone. This approach enables the sphenoid wing as well as the orbital roof medially to the sphenoid wing to be cut further down in the direction of the anterior clinoid process (ACP) and the optic canal. When the optic canal is reached from the orbital side, i.e. from the peripheral side, further removal of the bony structure should be performed under magnification.

Under magnification, the dural tent covering the cranial nerves III, IV and V1 is cut and then the outer layer of the anterior portion of the CS is peeled off from these nerves. In this manner, the ACP is further visualized from the lateral aspect, and so too is the III. nerve. The ACP should be drilled off from the optic strut by using a diamond drill. It is essential not to use any force while removing the ACP, which should always be hollowed out before removal. Removal of the ACP by force – and in one piece – might easily lead to injury to the nerves III, IV and V1, and to damage of the internal carotid artery (ICA) or the optic nerve (ON). Following the complete removal of the ACP, the optic strut should be meticulously drilled off, so that the ICA and the ON are sufficiently exposed. Next, the lateral and dorsal walls of the optic canal are removed by drilling with a diamond drill. It goes without saying that it is of paramount importance that the drill should not become overheated. In order to prevent overheating of the drill and thus to avoid thermal injury to the ON, it is advisable to restrict the drilling to short periods and to constantly irrigate the drill tip.

Usually no bleeding occurs during the epidural part of the approach. The only locus where venous bleeding may occur is from the very bottom, i.e. behind the anterior loop of the ICA where the tip of the ACP was formerly located. Since the extreme tip of the ACP may in certain patients project into the CS, venous bleeding may result following its removal. This bleeding may easily be stopped by putting a small piece of Surgicel into the cavity. It is also important to perform hemostasis along the nerves III, IV and V1 if there is any minor arterial bleeding. It is better to cover such bleeding points with gelfoam or Surgicel and a small piece of cotton, and to wait, rather than to attempt to perform extensive coagulation, which may cause damage to the nerve(s). On the medial aspect of the optic canal, there exists a danger that the bony sinus wall – either the dorsolateral cells of the ethmoid sinus or the sphenoid sinus – could be opened. If this occurs, the wall should be immediately and meticulously closed, either by bone wax – if the hole is small – or by a piece of muscle and fibrin glue, if the hole is larger than a few millimeters.

The next step is an incision into the dura which is made along the Sylvian fissure down to the dural ring around the ICA. An incision of the arachnoidea is made at the periphery of the Sylvian fissure, and, if possible, medial to the veins running along the Sylvian fissure. An arterial branch is followed into the depth so that the middle cerebral artery (MCA) is found. The MCA is then followed retrogradely toward the bifurcation of the ICA into the anterior cerebral artery (ACA1) and MCA. With gentle retraction, using bipolar forceps and a suction tube, to each side over the cottonoid patties, the MCA is well visualized and then both lobes – temporal and frontal – are separated. Finally, the arachnoidea is cut on both sides of the ICA. Special attention is paid to the lateral aspect of the ICA, to the posterior communicating artery (PCom) and anterior choroidal artery (AChA), and to the IIIrd nerve. The PCom should be visualized in its entire length from the ICA to the posterior cerebral artery (PCA). The PCA should also be dissected at least 1 cm peripherally in the segment of P2. In this way the brainstem is well visualized and so too is the whole segment of the intrathecal IIIrd nerve. The lateral edge of the dural opening, i.e. on the medial aspect of the IIIrd nerve, is fixed with a stay suture. The dural ring is then cut around the ICA, so that the ICA is made free. The diaphragm sellae is now cut in front of the posterior clinoid process (PCP), and the inner aspect of the PCP from the sellar side is exposed. This is only possible when the pituitary body is gently retracted anteriorly and contralaterally. This maneuver usually provokes severe venous bleeding from the ipsilateral CS and also from the intercavernous sinus on the posterior aspect of the sella. This bleeding can easily be stopped by using gelfoam or Surgicel on either side. The PCP is now drilled off from the inside of the sella in the posterior direction (Fig. 1). The closer to the clivus the PCP is, the thinner it is. The drilling of the PCP should be performed meticulously since the IIIrd nerve and the ICA could easily be damaged. Preservation of the dura over the posterior aspect of the dorsum sellae and over the clivus is a good safeguard (though not 100% reliable) for the aneurysm, especially if a jump of the drill should unexpectedly occur. The best way to

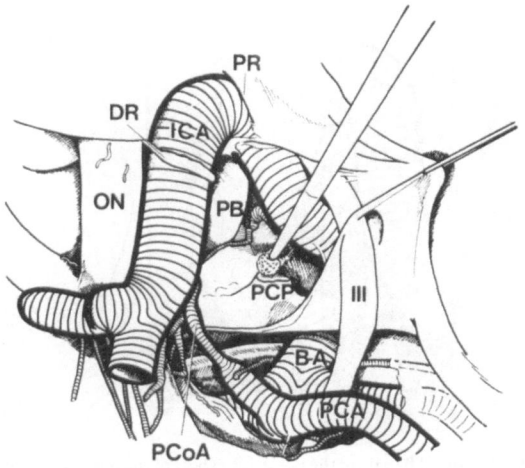

Fig. 1. The anterior loop of the ICA, the pituitary body (*PB*), the horizontal portion of the ICA in the CS, and the PCP are exposed. On the lateral aspect of the PCP the third nerve is entering the lateral wall of the CS and then running along the longitudinal axis of the horizontal segment of the ICA in the CS. The PCP has been drilled off from the sellar side using a high-speed diamond drill. The dura on the posterior aspect of the PCP has been preserved

prevent such a possibly injurious jump is to drill in short intervals and never to force the drill too strongly against the bone. When the PCP is completely removed, additional drilling of the dorsum sellae toward the opposite PCP is usually necessary, and thereafter the drilling is only completed when the floor of the sella can be seen (Fig. 2). In cases where the basilar tip aneurysm is very low and close to the clivus, additional drilling of the upper clivus will be necessary. Once the

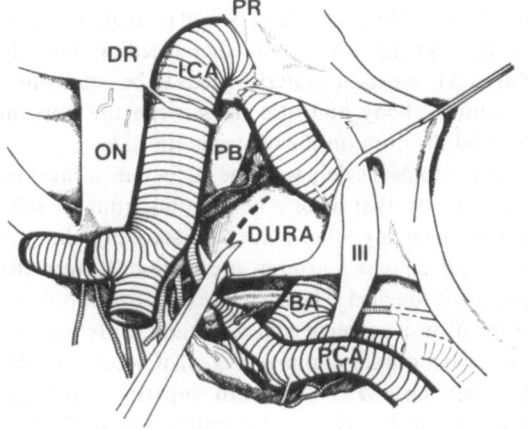

Fig. 2. The PCP has now been completely removed and the dura over the posterior aspect of the PCP has been exposed. The dura is then cut longitudinally, close to or over the midline

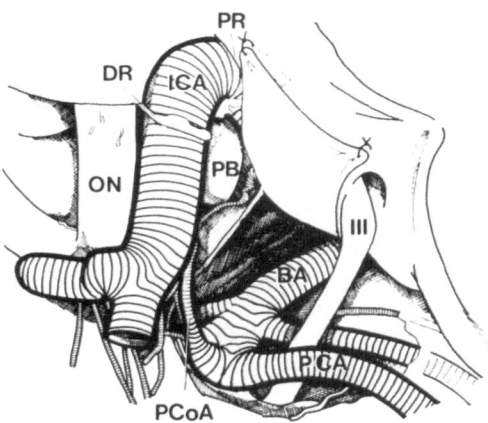

Fig. 3. The dural flap from the posterior aspect of the removed PCP has been reflected in an upward direction and put over the medial aspect of the horizontal segment of the ICA in the CS. The edges of the dural flap are fixed to the dura over the third nerve posteriorly, and to the proximal ring anteriorly

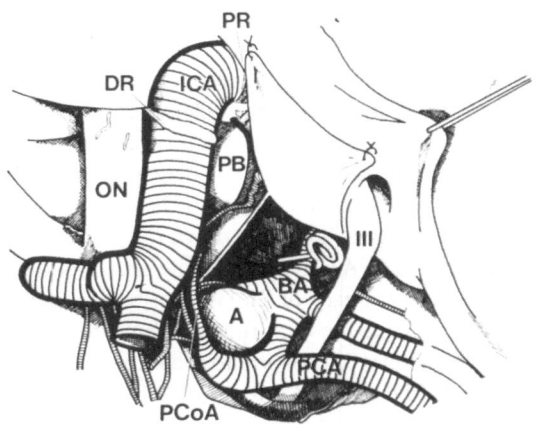

Fig. 4. The aneurysm, and the distal portion of the basilar artery with the branches, as well as a segment of the basilar artery proximally to the superior cerebellar artery, have been exposed, so that a temporary clip can be easily placed on the basilar trunk

drilling has been completed, the dura is cut in a longitudinal direction (Fig. 2), and Surgicel is removed from around the horizontal portion of the ICA in the CS. This will cause further venous bleeding. To stop this bleeding, the edges of the dura from the dorsal side of the dorsum sellae are fixed to the proximal ring and to the dura covering the III. cranial nerve (Fig. 3). If venous bleeding continues, the hemostatic material is again inserted around the ICA, but in much smaller quantities and less compactly than at the initial phase when there was no guard of the dura on the medial aspect of the ICA as there now is after fixation of the dura to the proximal ring and to the dura over the III. cranial nerve (Fig. 3). Thus, a medial CS wall is created against the sella, and this prevents further bleeding. Usually additional hemostatic material needs to be put around the pituitary body and also in between the dorsum sellae and the dura on the contralateral side.

In order to deal safely with the aneurysm, it must be ensured, firstly, that there is no bleeding from the sella or CS, or from any other place; and secondly, that the parent and daughter arteries are exposed before the aneurysm is touched. The basilar artery (BA) should be visualized on a segment which is sufficiently long to allow for temporary clipping (Fig. 4), if necessary, and only when both P1s and both superior cerebellar arteries (SCA), as well as a few millimeters of the BA, are revealed proximal to the origin of both SCAs. In cases in which the perforators are not visible, they should be exposed before the permanent clip is put on

the aneurysm. Sometimes exposure of the perforators from both P1s may prove difficult or even dangerous. In such cases, intermittent temporary occlusion of the BA is practised. The operative solution is to clip the BA for three minutes, close to the origin of the SCAs – preferably distally to this origin – and then to release the temporary clip for at least five minutes. By alternating the temporary clipping with unclipping the BA, the aneurysm can be dissected from all the perfora-

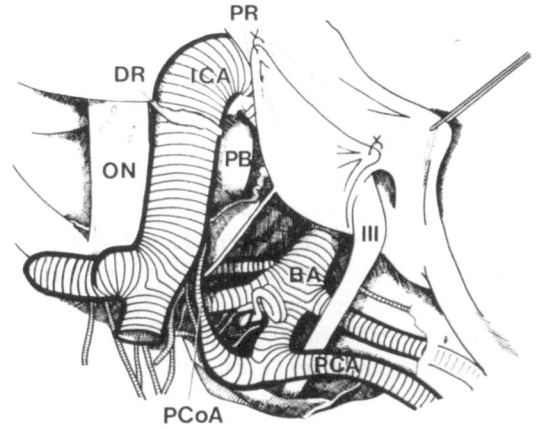

Fig. 5. The final situation is shown after clipping and resection of the basilar tip aneurysm. The perforators originating from the P1 on each side have been preserved. The dura from the posterior aspect of the PCP is covering the horizontal segment of the ICA in the CS and thus prevents bleeding from the CS. The intercavernous sinuses around the pituitary body are plugged with Surgicel. In this manner hemostasis is complete

tors, and then the permanent clipping of the aneurysm can be safely performed (Fig. 5). When the aneurysm is clipped, the dome of the aneurysm should be cut and the blood evacuated. However, removal of the sac of the aneurysm is not advisable in order to avoid damage to perforators to the brainstem. After exclusion of the aneurysm from the circulation, the dura is closed. Usually at the very bottom, i.e. at the former situation of the PCP, this closure is not waterproof, and therefore it requires reinforcement with a piece of muscle, which is placed behind the anterior loop of the ICA and fixed with two-component fibrin glue from the epidural side. The orbital roof is not reconstructed. A drain is inserted epidurally. The bone flap is fixed with separate nylon sutures. Periosteum, temporalis muscle, subcutaneous tissue and skin are sutured in layers.

Results

Among 47 cases operated on for basilar tip aneurysms, 27 were female patients and 20 male. In 31 cases the aneurysms were small, in 13 large, and in 3 giant. All patients presented with subarachnoid hemorrhage, and 10 of them suffered from 2 hemorrhages. Only in one case did the SAH derive from an ACom aneurysm; the basilar tip aneurysm, however, was silent. In 4 cases, multiple (double) aneurysms were recorded. In all cases both aneurysms were clipped at the same time. In 42 cases the clipping of the aneurysm was complete; in 4 it was partial, and combined with wrapping with muslin; and in one case (of a giant aneurysm) it was impossible either to clip or to wrap it, and so the aneurysm was left alone. Morbidity one week postoperatively was relatively high. Of the patients, 23 had paresis of the IIIrd nerve, 4 had hemiparesis, and 2 others were hemiplegic on the contralateral side of the surgical approach. Four patients manifested endocrinological disorders – diabetes insipidus – and 6 were drowsy.

Out of the total number of patients, 4 (8.5%) died – two re-bled (one in whom the aneurysm could not be clipped at all, and one in whom the aneurysm was partially clipped and partially wrapped), one suffered an infarct of the upper brain stem, and one had bleeding in the basal ganglia. In all but one of the cases the IIIrd nerve function recovered. Two patients, who had hemiparesis after surgery, also completely recovered. Two patients with postoperative contralateral hemiplegia improved but did not recover completely; they still have hemiparesis of a spastic character. Three patients

developed epileptic seizures after surgery. Four patients out of six with disorders of consciousness recovered to a great extent, and were able to take care of themselves but remained unable to continue normal work. The outcome one year after surgery in these 47 patients, treated for basilar tip aneurysm by using the 3-T approach, is as follows: 33 (70.2%) remain in normal condition after surgery, 10 (21.3%) have certain symptoms or neurological deficits, and 4 (8.5%) died shortly after surgery.

Discussion

The vital operating space for manipulation with the aneurysm clip holder is provided by the removal of the orbital roof anterior and posterior to the sphenoid wing, of the sphenoid wing itself with the ACP, of the posterior and lateral walls of the optic canal, and of the PCP. The splitting of the Sylvian fissure, with the resection of the PCP, provides a good view down along the lower clivus. Removal of the ACP and slight retraction of the orbital compartments in an anterior direction provides – in conjunction with the space gained by removal of the PCP – a better view upwards, i.e. toward the hypothalamus.

With the tilting of the table and adjustment of the microscope, an upward and downward view is obtained so that the longer segment of the BA is exposed, thus facilitating placement of the temporary clip and dealing with larger aneurysms. If the aneurysm is so large that it is impossible to put a temporary clip proximally, a subtemporal[15-18] or, even better, a transpetrous approach[28] can be used in addition to the 3-T approach. In cases of large aneurysms – and of course in giant ones – this combined 3-T and transpetrosal approach may be the only possible solution. However, using the 3-T approach only, in our practice hitherto we have not been faced with any situation in which a temporary clip could not be placed proximally to the aneurysm on the BA.

We are nevertheless aware that additional measures are required not only because of possible large size of the aneurysm, but all the more so because of the fragility or hardness of the BA which may prove to be sclerotic. In such a case it is possible that the arteriosclerotic plaque may be dislodged and "sent" to the peripheral circulation, and that this may result in a stroke. In such cases it would be far better to insert a catheter with a balloon which could be inflated, thus checking the blood flow through the distal segment of the BA and allowing the surgeon to deal more easily with the aneurysm.

Since giant and large aneurysms, as well as aneurysms with a very broad neck, from which the perforators emerge, are not suitable for endovascular treatment, it is advisable to join forces, so that the neuroradiologist and the neurosurgeon work together. This co-operation is good for two reasons: first, the surgeon does not need to lose his time while placing and removing the temporary clips. Quite simply: the surgeon starts dissecting the aneurysm, the neuroradiologist inflates the balloon, and after 3 minutes the surgeon stops dissecting and the balloon is deflated. In this approach to the operation the periods of the actual dissection are at least 20–30 seconds longer. And secondly, the inflation of the balloon inside the artery does not damage the artery wall, as it may happen with temporary clipping.

We do not, unfortunately, have any experience with extracorporeal circulation and complete stand-still over a certain period of time, which surely enables the surgeon to perform quick and safe dissection of the aneurysm around-and-around, and preservation of all the perforators, as well as complete occlusion of the aneurysm. It goes without saying, however, that by the induced cardiac arrest, maintained by the extracorporeal circulation, neither the temporary clips nor the endovascular occlusion of the BA are necessary. This means that the wall of the BA is not damaged at all.

The 3-T approach is somehow similar to the transoral-transclival approach[23], the difference being that the 3-T approach carries almost no risk of CSF leakage and requires no special measures[29,33].

In several of our patients, monitoring was conducted and no changes on the somatosensory evoked potentials (SEPs) were observed during surgery, not even in cases where contralateral hemiplegia resulted after surgery, nor even in a case where the BA was clipped during surgery for 14 minutes because of rupture of the aneurysm. We must, however, still ask whether today perioperative monitoring in cases of basilar tip aneurysm surgery can really predict diminished or lost function of part of the brainstem. In our opinion, the best way to avoid catastrophic events is to conduct a meticulous and well-planned microsurgical technique throughout the procedure, so that rupture of the aneurysm is avoided rather than treated. Finally, it should be mentioned that the 3-T approach should be well-studied on cadavers before its application on a patient with an "angry" aneurysm at the basilar tip which represents the worst possible location of aneurysm.

References

1. Anderson M (1976) Persistent primitive hypoglossal artery with basilar aneurysm. J Neurol 213: 377–381
2. Aymard A, Gobin YP, Hodes JE, Bien S, Rufenacht D, Reizine D, George B, Merland JJ (1991) Endovascular occlusion of vertebral arteries in the treatment of unclippable vertebrobasilar aneurysms. J Neurosurg 74: 393–398
3. Bartal A, Schiffer J, Weinstein J (1968) A successful case of basilar bifurcation aneurysm surgery. Acta Neurochir (Wien) 19: 163–170
4. Brushan C, Hodges FJ, Posey J (1978) Sucessful surgical treatment of giant aneurysm of the basilar artery: case report. J Neurosurg 49: 124–128
5. Bugiani O, Piola P, Tabaton M (1983) Nontraumatic dissecting aneurysm of the basilar artery. Eur Neurol 22: 256–260
6. Bull JWD (1962) Contributions of radiology to the study of intracranial aneurysm. BMJ 2: 1701–1708
7. Chou SN, Ortiz-Suarez HJ (1974) Surgical treatment of arterial aneurysms of the vertebrobasilar circulation. J Neurosurg 41: 671–680
8. Constans JP, Visot A, Fredy D, Dorland P (1976) Aneurysme geant du tronc basilaire revele par une nevralgie faciale essentielle. Neurochirurgie 22: 493–502
9. Dawson BH (1958) The blood vessels of the human optic chiasm and their relation to those of the hypophysis and hypothalamus. Brain 81: 207–217
10. Dolenc VV (1983) Direct microsurgical repair of intracavernous vascular lesions. J Neurosurg 58: 824–831
11. Dolenc VV (1985) A combined epi- and subdural direct approach to carotidophthalmic artery aneurysms. J Neurosurg 62: 667–672
12. Dolenc VV, Škrap M, Šušteršič J, Škrbec M, Morina A (1987) A transcavernous-transsellar approach to the basilar tip aneurysms. BJN 1: 251–259
13. Dolenc VV (1988) Surgery of vascular lesions of the cavernous sinus. Clin Neurosurg 36: 240–255
14. Dolenc VV (1989) Anatomy and surgery of the cavernous sinus. Springer, Berlin Heidelberg New York Tokyo
15. Drake CG (1961) Bleeding aneurysms of the basilar artery. J Neurosurg 18: 230–238
16. Drake CG (1973) Management of aneurysms of posterior circulation. In: Youmans JR (ed) Neurological surgery, Vol 2. Saunders, Philadelphia, pp 707–806
17. Drake CG (1975) Ligation of the vertebral (unilateral or bilateral) or basilar artery in the treatment of large intracranial aneurysms. J Neurosurg 43: 255–274
18. Drake CG (1978) Treatment of aneurysms of the posterior cranial fossa. In: Progress in neurological surgery, Vol 9. Karger, Basel, pp 122–194
19. Emanuele MA, Dorsch TR, Scarff TB, Lawrence AM (1981) Basilar artery aneurysm simulating pheochromocytoma. Neurology (Ny) 31: 1560
20. Gale AN, Crockard HA (1982) Transient unilateral mydriasis in basilar aneurysm. J Neurol Neurosurg Psychiatry 45: 565
21. Guglielmi G (1990) Balloon embolization of a basilar bifurcation aneurysm. AJNR 11: 653–655
22. Guglielmi G, Vinuela F, Duckwiler G, Dion J, Lylyk P, Berenstein A, Strother C, Graves V, Halbach V, Nichols D, Hopkins N, Ferguson R, Sepetka I (1992) Endovascular treatment of posterior circulation aneurysms by electrothrombosis using electrically detachable coils. J Neurosurg 77: 497–500
23. Hayakawa T, Kamikawa K, Ohnishi T, Yoshimine T (1981) Prevention of postoperative complications after a transoraltransclival approach to basilar aneurysms. Technical note. J Neurosurg 54: 699–703

24. Hopkins LN, Eudny JL, Castellani D (1983) Extracranial–intracranial arterial bypass and basilar artery ligation in the treatment of giant basilar artery aneurysms. Neurosurgery 13: 189–194
25. Ikeda K, Yamashita J, Hashimoto M, Futami K (1991) Orbito-zygomatic temporopolar approach for a high basilar tip aneurysm associated with a short intracranial internal carotid artery: a new surgical approach. Neurosurgery 28: 105–110
26. Jamieson KG (1968) Aneurysms of the vertebrovascular system. Further experience with nine cases. J Neurosurg 28: 544–555
27. Katakura R, Yashimoto T, Suzuki J (1979) A case of giant aneurysm of the basilar artery. Acta Neurochir (Wien) 49: 87–93
28. Kawase T, Toya S, Shiobara S, Mine S (1985) Transpetrosal approach for aneurysms of the lower basilar artery. J Neurosurg 63: 857–861
29. Khambatta HJ, Matteo RS, McMurtry JG, Bowman FO, Jr (1974) Anaesthesia for basilar arterial aneurysms with elective circulatory arrest and moderate hypothermia. Anaesthesiology 41: 512–516
30. Krayenbuhl HA, Yasargil MG (1968) Cerebral angiography. Lippincott, Philadelphia, pp 74
31. Litvak J, Sumners TC, Barron JL, Fisher LS (1981) A successful approach to vertebrobasilar aneurysm. Technical note. J Neurosurg 55: 491–494
32. Logue V (1964) Posterior fossa aneurysms. Clin Neurosurg 11: 183–207
33. McMurty JG, Housepian BM, Bowman FO, Jr, Matteo RS (1974) Surgical treatment of basilar artery aneurysms. Elective circulatory arrest with thoracotomy in 12 cases. J Neurosurg 40: 486–494
34. Nijensohn DE, Saez TJ, Reagan TJ (1974) Clinical significance of basilar artery aneurysms. Neurology 4: 301–305
35. Ono M, Ono M, Rhoton AL, Jr, Barry M (1984) Microsurgical anatomy of the region of the tentorial incisure. J Neurosurg 60: 365–399
36. Pia HW (1979) Classification of vertebro-basilar aneurysms. Acta Neurochir (Wien) 47: 1–30
37. Regli L, de Tribolet N (1991) Tuberothalamic infarct after division of a hypoplastic posterior communicating artery for clipping of a basilar tip aneurysm: case report. Neurosurgery 28: 456–459
38. Samson DS, Hodosh RM, Clark K (1978) Microsurgical evaluation of the pterional approach to aneurysms of the distal basilar circulation. Neurosurgery 3: 135–141
39. Sharr MM, Kelvim FM (1973) Vertebrobasilar aneurysms. Experience with 27 cases. Eur Neurol 10: 129–143
40. Sugita K, Kobayashi S, Shintani A, Mutsuga N (1979) Microneurosurgery for aneurysms of the basilar artery. J Neurosurg 51: 615–620
41. Tiyaworabum S, Wanis A, Schirmer M, Bock WJ (1982) Aneurysms of the vertebro-basilar system: clinical analysis and follow-up result. Acta Neurochir (Wien) 63: 221–229
42. Troupp H (1971) The natural history of aneurysms of the basilar bifurcation. Acta Neurol Scand 47: 350–356
43. Wilson CB, Sang UN (1976) Surgical treatment for aneurysms of the upper basilar artery. J Neurosurg 44: 537–543
44. Yaşargil MG, Fox JL, Ray MW (1975) The operative approach to aneurysms of the anterior communicating artery. In: Krayenbuhl (ed) Advances and technical standards in neurosurgery, Vol 2. Springer, Wien New York, pp 113–170
45. Yaşargil MG, Antič J, Laciga R, Jain KK, Hodosh RM, Smith RD (1976) Microsurgical pterional approach to aneurysms of the basilar bifurcation. Surg Neurol 6: 83–119

Correspondence: V. Dolenc, M.D., Department of Neurosurgery, University Hospital Centre, Zaloska 7, 61105 Ljubljana, Slovenia.

Combined Pterional-Subtemporal Approach to Upper Basilar Artery Aneurysms

R. Da Pian, A. Pasqualin, R. Scienza, G. Pavesi, and **C. Licata**

Department of Neurosurgery, City Hospital, Verona, Italy

Summary

Since 1981 33 patients with bleeding upper basilar artery aneurysms were operated on in our department: 26 aneurysms were located on the basilar bifurcation and 7 at the origin of the superior cerebellar artery. Almost all of the patients were operated on through a combined pterional-subtemporal approach, in order to better expose the aneurysmal neck from different angles and to obtain anatomical details useful for a safe clipping, especially regarding the position of the perforators. A continous lumbar drainage was used in 22 patients (66%) and deep hypotension with sodium nitroprusside was induced in 13 patients (40%). During microsurgical dissection, strong post-hemorrhagic adhesions were found in 18 cases; intraoperative rupture occurred in 5 cases (requiring temporary clipping of the basilar artery in 3 cases). Twenty-nine patients had their aneurysm eventually clipped (with multiple clips applied in 8 cases); 3 aneurysms were explored only and 1 was wrapped. A postoperative third nerve palsy was observed in 24 patients (72%): at follow up the deficit had cleared in 17 patients and had slightly improved or was unchanged in 7. Complete recovery was observed in 17 patients (53%), a moderate disability in 6 (18%), a severe disability in 5 (15%); 5 patients (15%) died (all in preoperative grades III and IV). In conclusion, a combined pterional-subtemporal approach to upper basilar aneurysms allows a better visualization of the aneurysmal neck and of the adjacent vessels; however morbidity and mortality still remain high, especially for patients severely injured by the initial hemorrhage.

Keywords: Basilar artery aneurysms; subarachnoid hemorrhage; microsurgery; combined pterional/subtemporal approach.

Introduction

Aneurysms of the upper basilar artery are relatively rare lesions. Their surgical approach requires to work in a confined place, and yet to get the best possible exposure of the neck and of the adjacent vessels, especially the perforators; moreover, the 3rd nerve is usually in the way, and is very sensitive to surgical trauma.

The aim of this study is to evaluate the merits of a combined pterional-subtemporal approach in the surgical treatment of 33 patients with upper basilar artery aneurysms, all suffering from a pervious subarachnoid hemorrhage.

Materials and Methods

Since 1981, 48 patients with posterior circulation aneurysms were operated on in our Department. Out of these patients, 33 harboured an aneurysm located on the most distal portion of the basilar artery: 26 on the basilar bifurcation and 7 at the origin of the superior cerebellar artery. 16 patients were males, 17 females. Age ranged between 23 and 69 years (average 56.6). All patients presented with subarachnoid hemorrhage (in 8 cases extending to the ventricular system). According to a previous classification from our group[16], in the 18 patients admitted within 3 days of hemorrhage the subarachnoid layer on CT scan was absent or thin in 3 cases (17%), and consistent or thick in 15 cases (83%). Preoperatively, hydrocephalus was present on CT scan in 12 cases. Angiographical data are presented in Table 1, preoperative clinical grade (Hunt and Hess classification) and surgical timing in Table 2. Except for a few early cases, all of the patients were operated on through a combined pterional-subtemporal approach (Fig. 1). Retraction of the temporal lobe was facilitated by hyperventilation, mannitol diuresis and insertion of a lumbar drainage (in 66% of cases). Deep hypotension (with sodium nitroprusside) was used in 13 cases (40%); temporary clipping of the basilar artery was used in 3 cases.

Results

During surgery, strong post-hemorrhagic adhesions were found in 18 cases (55%). A total of 29 aneurysms (88%) were eventually excluded by clip (with multiple clips applied in 8 cases); 4 aneurysms were explored and wrapped. Postoperative complications and additional surgical procedures are presented in Table 3. Clinical outcome was defined on the basis of the Glasgow Outcome Scale[11] (Table 4); moreover, the incidence of postop. 3rd nerve palsy was also evaluated at follow-up (at least 6 months after surgery) (Table 4).

When relating preoperative grade to clinical outcome (Table 5) a significant difference in mortality was found between patients in grades I–II and patients in grades III–IV. When relating intraoperative presence or absence of strong post-hemorrhagic adhesions to clinical outcome, a marked difference in recovery and disability was also observed (Table 6).

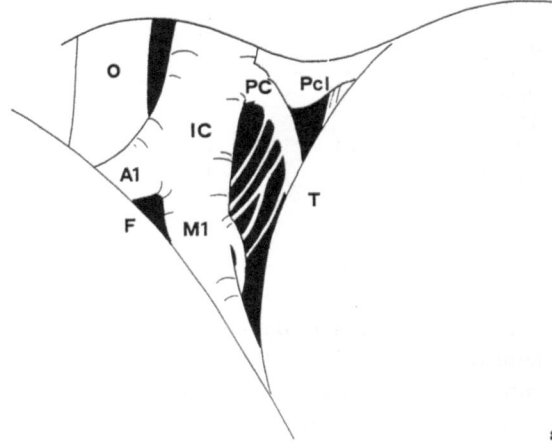

a

Table 1. *Angiographical Data (33 Patients Considered)*

Basilar tip aneurysms (26 Cases)

A) Projection:		B) Size:	
superior	17 (65%)	< 20 mm	22 (85%)
posterior	3 (12%)	≥ 20 mm	2 (15%)
anterior	1 (4%)	C) Associated Aneurysms:	
multiple	5 (19%)	– MCA aneur.	3 (12%)

Superior cerebellar aneurysms (7 cases)

A) Side		B) Size	
right	3 (43%)	< 20 mm	6 (85%)
left	4 (57%)	> 20 mm	1 (15%)

Table 2. *Preoperative Clinical Grade (Hunt and Hess Classification) and Interval from SAH to Surgery*

Prep. grade	n	%	Surg. timing	n	%
I	11	(33%)	0–3 days	2	(6%)
II	9	(28%)	4–9 days	1	(3%)
III	10	(30%)	10–15 days	4	(12%)
IV	3	(9%)	> 15 days	26	(79%)

Discussion

The surgical approach to aneurysms of the upper basilar artery has been evolved from the pioneering work of Drake[5], who introduced the subtemporal route, and of Yaşargil, who adopted the pterional route[29,30]. Each approach has its advantages and its limitations:

a) the subtemporal approach allows to work in a larger space than the pterional approach, but requires retraction of the temporal lobe and dissection below and/or above the 3rd nerve; it is adequate for low-lying basilar tip aneurysms – allowing tentorial section when needed – and permits good visualization of the contro-lateral P1 tract;

b) the pterional approach forces the surgeon to work in a confined space, and often to retract the internal carotid artery in order to approach the aneurysm ade-quately; in a few cases it can require sacrifice of the posterior communicating artery[30]; however it allows a nice visualization of both PCAs and SCAs, it causes

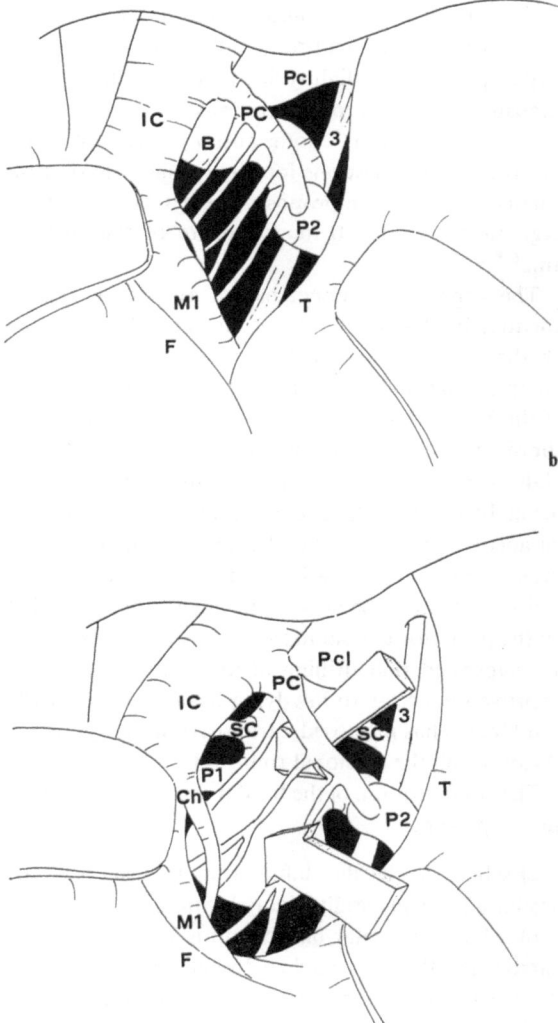

b

c

Fig. 1. Schematic drawing of pterional/sylvian route: (a) wide open-ing of sylvian fissure; (b) exposure of posterior communicating and posterior cerebral arteries (note retraction of frontal and temporal lobes); (c) arrows indicating possible approaches to a basilar tip aneurysm. *O* optic nerve; *F* frontal lobe; *T* temporal lobe; *IC* internal carotid; *A1* anterior cerebral; *M1* middle cerebral; *PC* posterior communicating; *PCl* posterior clinoid; *B* basilar, *P2* posterior cerebral; *3* 3rd nerve, *P1* controlateral posterior cerebral; *SC* superior cerebellar; *Ch* anterior choroidal

Table 3. *Postopcrative Complications and Additional Surgical Procedures*

Postop. complications	n	%	Additional procedures	n	%
Hydrocephalus	12	(36%)	CSF shunt	9	(27%)
Temporal lobe swelling	6	(18%)	Wound revision	3	(9%)
Nuclear ischemia	4	(12%)	Evacuation of epidural hemat.	1	(3%)
Medical complications	4	(12%)	Clip reposition	1	(3%)
Scalp infection	3	(9%)			
Rebleeding	2	(6%)			
Epidural hematoma	1	(3%)			

Table 4. *Clinical Outcome (33 Patients Considered)*

A) Glasgow Outcome Scale (GOS):	
complete recovery	17 (51%)
moderate disability	6 (18%)
severe disability	5 (15%)
death	5 (15%)
B) 3rd nerve palsy:	
occurring postop	24 (72%)
a) transiently	17 (51%)
b) permanently*	7 (21%)

* Minimum follow-up = 6 months.

Table 5. *Clinical Outcome Related to Preoperative Grade (Hunt and Hess Classification)*

Preop. grade	Complete recovery	Disability	Death
I–II (20 cases)	13 (65%)	7 (35%)	—
III (10 cases)	4 (40%)	2 (20%)	4 (40%)
IV (3 cases)	—	2 (66%)	1 (34%)
Significance (grades I–II vs. III–IV)	N.S.	N.S.	p = 0.02

Table 6. *Clinical Outcome Related to Presence of Post-Hemorrhagic Adhesions*

	Complete recovery	Disability	Death
Strong adhesions (18 cases)	7 (38%)	9 (50%)	2 (12%)
No adhesions (15 cases)	10 (67%)	2 (14%)	3 (19%)
Significance	N.S.	N.S.	N.S.

less injury to the 3rd nerve and is excellent for highly-placed basilar tip aneurysms.

In our experience we have been satisfied with a combined pterional-subtemporal approach, that allows alternate views of the aneurysmal area from different angles, thus determining the position of the contro-lateral vessels, as well as of the perforators. With this combined approach, it is sometimes possible to use also an intermediate anterior temporal (temporo-polar) route (Fig. 2)[23], provided that the temporal lobe is very slack (through mannitol administration and lumbar drainage); this anterior temporal route has some advantages over the pterional route, allowing to work in a larger space, with a slightly different angle and a better exposure of the lateroposterior side of the aneurysm and of the perforators[6]. Some authors have considered this route as the best one for highly placed basilar tip aneurysms, and have proposed the detachment of the zygomatic arch for better exposure of the surgical area[6,8,10,15,19,24].

The approach to upper basilar aneurysms can be adequately planned in advance in the individual case on the basis of some anatomical details detected on preop angiography. One important point is the height of the basilar bifurcation in relation to the posterior clinoid process. For aneurysms that are positioned high over the post-clinoid process the pterional route seems better than the subtemporal route; conversely, for aneurysms positioned under the post-clinoid process the subtemporal route is better, because – through the pterional route – the view of the aneurysm is impeded by the posterior clinoid itself. To this regard, Yaşargil has suggested that drilling of this bony process can improve the access to low-lying basilar aneurysms[30], and Dolenc has proposed a transcavernous approach, always using the pterional route[4].

The configuration of the basilar artery bifurcation is also important:

a) when the basilar bifurcation is T-shaped, the basilar apex is generally highly located:

b) when the basilar bifurcation is V-shaped with a narrow (less than 90°) angle between the two P1 tracts, the basilar apex is generally below the edge of the posterior clinoid process[3].

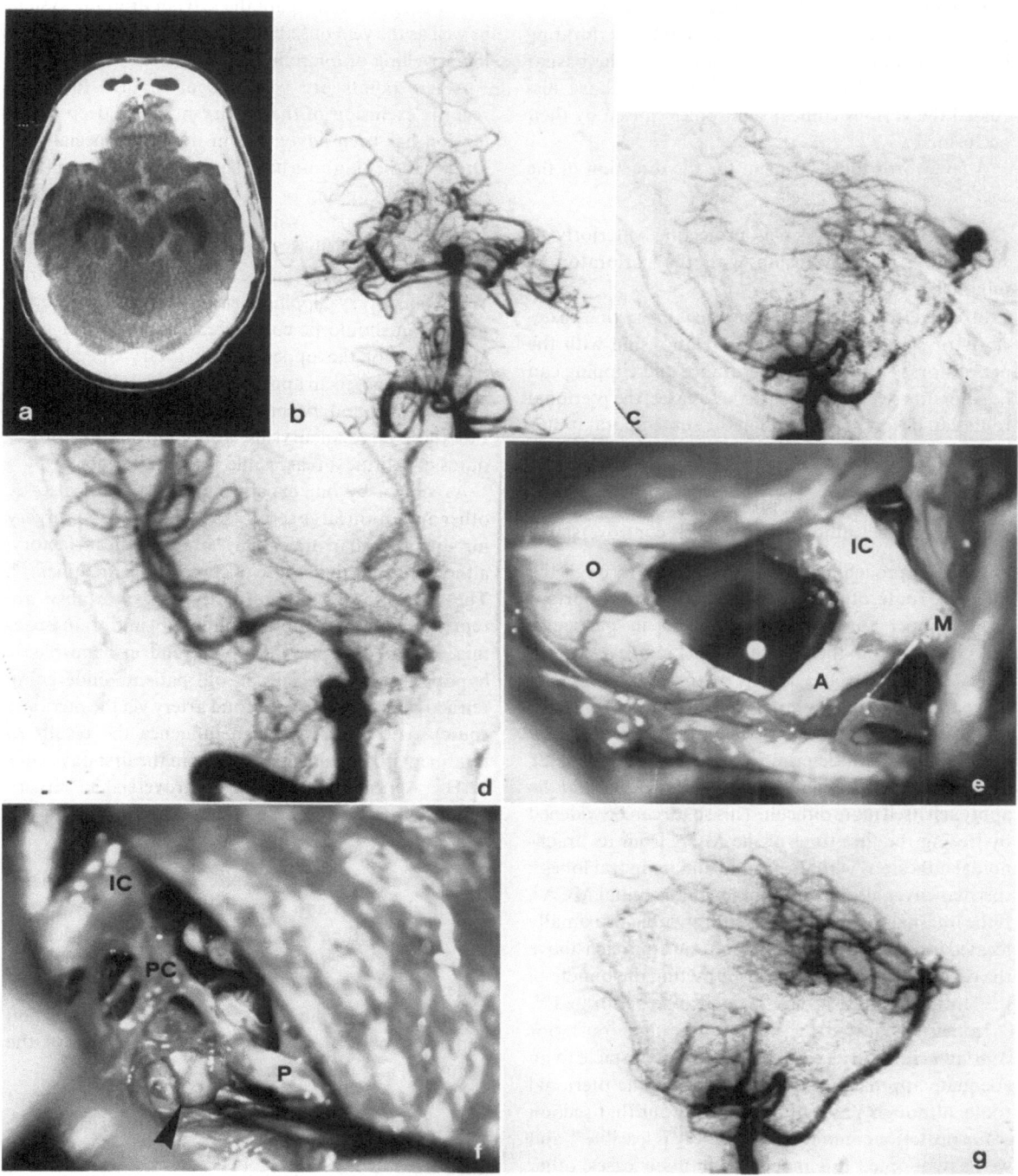

Fig. 2. (a) Thick subarachnoid hemorrhage in the basal cisterns, in a patient with (b) a basilar tip aneurysm with upward projection, diagnosed elsewhere; (c) preop. angiography 10 days after hemorrhage, showing moderate spasm of the basilar artery (note the height of the aneurysm over the posterior clinoid process); (d) rt carotid injection showing multisegmental spasm and a short internal carotid artery; (e) at surgery, short internal carotid artery and large space between optic and carotid; (f) aneurysm (arrow) eventually approached from anterior temporal route (variation of subtemporal approach); (g) postop. angiography, showing exclusion of the aneurysm; the patient presented a transient 3rd nerve palsy, and was neurologically intact 2 months after surgery. *O* optic nerve; *IC* internal carotid; *A* anterior cerebral; *M* middle cerebral; *PC* posterior communicating; *P* posterior cerebral

Previous studies on the microanatomy of the basilar apex have also described the pattern of the perforating branches coming from the last portion of the basilar artery and the P1 tracts[3,7,13,17,21,31] and have discussed the various clinical syndromes caused by their occlusion[17].

A few words must be spent for the direction of the sac:

a) when the aneurysm is projecting anteriorly or superiorly, its relationship with the perforators is minimal;

b) conversely, when the aneurysm is projecting posteriorly or supero-posteriorly, its relationship with the perforators is of outmost importance and clipping can be sometimes very difficult (in these cases, the pterional route can be less adequate than the subtemporal route);

c) when the sac projects laterally (as for superior cerebellar aneurysms), the approach – either pterional or subtemporal – should probably be from the non-dominant side[22], although this point is controversial[25].

When approaching basilar aneurysms through the pterional route, other anatomical details are important for a proper surgical exposure, and in particular the position and the length of the internal carotid artery. The approach is usually performed through the space between the internal carotid artery and the tentorium[27,30]; a laterally located and short internal carotid artery will determine a narrow space (Fig. 2), making the retraction of this artery dangerous and the approach itself more difficult. This space can be widened by freeing the first tract of the MCA from its arachnoidal adhesions with the frontal and temporal lobes[2]; this maneuver also avoids kinking of the initial MCA[2]. If the internal carotid artery is short (with a proximally located internal carotid bifurcation), an approach above the carotid bifurcation (gently retracting the bundle of the lenticulo-striate arteries) can also be performed[12].

In many istances, the presence of a large posterior communicating artery can constitute an obstacle to an adequate approach of the aneurysm by the pterional route; although Yaşargil has pointed out that section of the posterior communicating artery is feasible[30] and we have adopted this maneuver in a few cases, other authors have stressed the possibility of midbrain infarction following section of even a small p. comm.[20].

Finally, also the anatomy of the sylvian veins has its importance; it must be stressed that the temporal lobe – in this combined pterional/subtemporal approach – is alternatively retracted medially or laterally, and it is essential to spare the sylvian draining system as well as the vein of Labbe', in order to avoid temporal lobe swelling or infarction.

A few points are worth mention also for what regards exclusion of the aneurysm: while deep hypotension has been advocated in the past especially by Drake[5], other authors have suggested the convenience of transient clipping of the basilar artery (proximally to the aneurysm)[2,22]: with a tense sac, aneurysmal rupture can more easily occur and – due to the confined place – hemorrhage can be very difficult to control. When temporary clipping is employed, metabolic brain protection should be considered; moreover, for giant aneurysms of the upper basilar artery Spetzler has recently proposed an approach under circulatory arrest, hypothermia and barbiturate cerebral protection[26]. For these large aneurysms, also endovascular procedures constitute a reasonable way of treatment[1,9].

As shown by our experience and stressed also by other authors in large series[5,18,22] the results of surgery for upper basilar aneurysms are still unsatisfactory, although better than those of conservative treatment[28]. The main causes of morbidity and mortality are represented by: a) perforator injury, b) midbrain ischemia due to temporary clipping, and c) hemispheric hypoperfusion (especially in old patients undergoing retraction of the internal carotid artery via the pterional route). Also vasospasm can influence the results of treatment in patients operated on in the first days after SAH[2]. At this regard, it is controversial if surgery should be performed in the acute stage:

a) on one side, the surgical exposure in acute cases can be very limited, in spite of lumbar drainage, mannitol diuresis and hyperventilation;

b) on the other side, a disadvantage of a delayed operation is the presence of strong post-hemorrhagic adhesions in patients with a large-volume subarachnoid hemorrhage, compelling the surgeon to sharp dissection and to significant traction in the proximity of the aneurysm and perforators.

Injury to the 3rd nerve is generally transient: in most series, 3rd nerve palsy recovers in over 70% of cases[4,5,18], in agreement with our experience; for this reason, the third nerve should not influence the surgical plans, and it can be adequately retracted, provided that it is widely freed from its arachnoidal adhesions to the temporal lobe.

In conclusion, a combined pterional-subtemporal approach to upper basilar aneurysms allows a better exposure of most anatomical details required for a safe clipping. When compared to aneurysms in other location, morbidity and mortality for these aneurysms still remains high, especially if the patient has been damaged by the initial hemorrhage and the surgeon is faced with significant post-hemorrhagic adhesions during the operation.

References

1. Aymard A, Gobin P, Hodes JE, Bien S, Rufenacht D, Reizine D, George B, Merland JJ (1991) Endovascular occlusion of vertebral arteries in the treatment of unclippable vertebrobasilar aneurysms. J Neurosurg 74: 393–398
2. Batjer HH, Samson DS (1989) Causes of morbidity and mortality from surgery of aneurysms of the distal basilar artery. Neurosurgery 25: 904–916
3. Caruso G, Vincentelli F, Giudicelli G, Grisoli F, Xu T, Gouaze A (1990) Perforating branches of the basilar bifurcation. J Neurosurg 73: 259–265
4. Dolenc VV, Skrap M, Sustersic J, Skrbec M, Morina A (1987) A transcavernous-transsellar approach to the basilar tip aneurysms Br J Neurosurg 1: 251–259
5. Drake CG (1979) The treatment of aneurysms of the posterior circulations. Clin Neurosurg 26: 96–144
6. Fujitsu K, Kuwabara T (1985) Zygomatic approach for lesions in the interpeduncular cistern. J Neurosurg 62: 340–343
7. Grand W, Hopkins LN (1977) The microsurgical anatomy of the basilar artery bifurcation. Neurosurgery 1: 128–131
8. Hakuba A, Liu S, Nishimura (1986) The orbitozygomatic infratemporal approach. A new surgical technique. Surg Neurol 26: 271–276
9. Higashida RT, Halbach VV, Cahan LD, Hieshima GB, Konishi Y (1989) Detachable balloon embolization therapy of posterior circulation intracranial aneurysms. J Neurosurg 71: 512–519
10. Ikeda K, Yamashita J, Hashimoto M, Futami K (1991) Orbitozygomatic temporopolar approach for a high basilar tip aneurysm associated with a short intracranial internal carotid artery: a new surgical approach. Neurosurgery 28: 105–110
11. Jennett B, Bond M (1975) Assessment of outcome after severe brain damage: a practical scale. Lancet 1: 480–484
12. Kobayashi S, Sugita K, Nagawa G (1983) An approach to a basilar aneurysm above the bifurcation of the internal carotid artery. J Neurosurg 59: 1082–1084
13. Marinkovic S, Milisavljevic M, Kovacevic M (1986) Interpeduncular perforating branches of the posterior cerebral artery. Microsurgical anatomy of their extracerebral and intracerebral segments. Surg Neurol 26: 349–359
14. Muizelaar JP (1989) The use of electroencephalography and brain protection during operation for basilar aneurysms. Neurosurgery 25: 899–903
15. Neil – Dwyer G, Sharr M, Haskell R, Currie D, Hosseini M (1988) Zygomaticotemporal approach to the basis cranii and basilar artery. Neurosurgery 23: 20 – 22
16. Pasqualin A, Rosta L, Da Pian R, Cavazzani P, Scienza R (1984) The role of computed tomography in the management of vasospasm following subarachnoid hemorrhage. Neurosurgery 15: 344–353
17. Pedroza A, Dujovny M, Ausman JI, Diaz FG, Artero JC, Berman SK, Mirchandani HG, Umansky F (1986) Microvascular anatomy of the interpeduncular fossa. J Neurosurg 64: 484–493
18. Peerless SJ, Drake CG (1982) Management of aneurysms of posterior circulation. In: Youmans JR (ed) Neurological surgery, 2nd Ed, Vol 3. Saunders, Philadelphia, pp 1715–1763
19. Pitelli SD, Almeida GM, Nakagawa EJ, Marchese AT, Cabaral ND (1986) Basilar aneurysm surgery: the subtemporal approach with section of the zygomatic arch. Neurosurgery 18: 125–128
20. Regli L, de Tribolet N (1991) Tuberothalamic infarct after division of a hypoplastic posterior communicating artery for clipping of a basilar tip aneurysm: case report. Neurosurgery 28: 456–459
21. Saeki N, Rhoton AL Jr (1997) Microsurgical anatomy of the upper basilar artery and the posterior circle of Willis. J Neurosurg 46: 563–578
22. Samson DS, Hodosh RM, Clark WK (1978) Microsurgical evaluation of the pterional approach to aneurysms of the distal basilar circulation. Neurosurgery 3: 135–141
23. Sano K (1980) Temporopolar approach to aneurysms of the basilar artery at and around the distal bifurcation: technical note. Neurol Res 2: 361–367
24. Shiokawa Y, Saito I, Nobuhiko A, Mizutani H (1989) Zygomatic temporopolar approach for basilar artery aneurysms. Neurosurgery 25: 793–797
25. Solomon RA, Stein BM (1988) Surgical approaches to aneurysms of the vertebral and basilar arteries. Neurosurgery 23: 203–208
26. Spetzler RF, Hadley MN, Rigamonti D, Carter LP, Raudzens PA, Shedd SA, Wilkinson E (1988) Aneurysms of the basilar artery treated with circulatory arrest, hypothermia, and barbiturate cerebral protection. J Neurosurg 68: 868–879
27. Sugita K, Kobayashi S, Shinani A, Mutsuga N (1979) Microsurgery for aneurysms of the basilar artery. J Neurosurg 51: 615–620
28. Troupp H (1971) The natural history of aneurysms of the basilar bifurcation. Acta Neurol Scand 47: 350–356
29. Yaşargil MG (1984) Vertebrobasilar aneurysms. In: Microneurosurgery, Vol 2. Thieme, Stuttgart, pp 232–295
30. Yaşargil MG, Antic J, Laciga R, Jain KK, Hodosh RM, Smith RD (1976) Microsurgical pterional approach to aneurysms of the basilar bifurcation. Surg Neurol 6: 83–91
31. Zeal AA, Rhoton AL Jr (1978) Microsurgical anatomy of the posterior cerebral artery. J Neurosurg 48: 534–559

Correspondence: R. Da Pian, M.D., Department of Neurosurgery, City Hospital, I-37126 Verona, Italy.

Early Surgery for Ruptured Aneurysms of the Posterior Circulation – 60 Consecutive Cases

T. Moriyama, M. Kurosaki, and **T. Shiwaku**

Department of Neurosurgery, Hospital Moriyama, Tokyo, Japan

Summary

The authors have treated a total of 60 consecutive patients with ruptured aneurysms of the posterior circulation during the last ten years. Among them 54 patients were operated on by one of us (TM) within three days following the hemorrhage. These included 17 upper basilar aneurysms, 2 basilar trunk aneurysms, 31 VA-PICA complex aneurysms and 4 PCA aneurysms. Preoperatively 20 patients were in grade I–II (Hunt and Hess), 16 in grade III, and 18 in grade IV. The final outcome has been favorable in 38 patients (70%). Compared to our 200 consecutive cases with ruptured aneurysms of the anterior circulation operated on early, our experience suggests the following: 1) Early surgery for posterior circulation aneurysms may be more effective in improving the overall management outcome. This may be because posterior circulation aneurysms have a tendency to rebleed more frequently and the incidence of vasospasm is lower, especially in VA-PICA complex aneurysm. 2) Early operation can be carried out safely at any time after subarachnoid hemorrhage with the recent advances in neurosurgical techniques.

Keywords: Subarachnoid hemorrhage; early surgery; aneurysm of the posterior circulation; recurrent hemorrhage.

Introduction

Early surgery for anterior circulation aneurysms is now generally accepted except for giant aneurysms. However, the indication of early surgery for ruptured posterior circulation aneurysms is still controversial because of the technical difficulty at surgery. On the other hand, it has been pointed out that mortality and morbidity due to recurrent hemorrhage is very high[5,10,11,14,17]. Waiting for a few weeks before surgery makes the management of patients more complicated and will not help to prevent recurrent hemorrhage and vasospasm[1,3]. For the last ten years, we have experienced a number of early operations on patients with ruptured cerebral aneurysms. Based on our experience, we believe that early operation to prevent recurrent hemorrhage with aggressive treatment of postoperative spasm would be the best to improve the overall outcome. In this paper, we review 60 consecutive patients with ruptured posterior circulation aneurysms and discuss the validity of early surgery for posterior circulation aneurysms.

Clinical Material

In the period between June 1983 and May 1992, 60 patients suffering from subarachnoid hemorrhage due to ruptured posterior circulation aneurysms were treated in the acute stage. These cases included 12 basilar bifurcation (BA-BIF) aneurysms, 8 basilar-superior cerebellar (BA-SCA) aneurysms, 2 BA-trunk aneurysms, 17 vertebral-posterior inferior cerebellar (VA-PICA) aneurysms, 12 VA aneurysms, 5 distal PICA aneurysms and 4 posterior cerebral (PCA) aneurysms. Recurrent hemorrhage was confirmed in 22 patients (36.7%) with the interval between the episodes ranging from 2 hours to 15 days. Seven of 22 patients with basilar aneurysms, 14 of 31 patients with VA-PICA complex aneurysms and one patient with a P_1 aneurysm had a recurrent hemorrhage. Sixteen patients deteriorated suddenly by a recurrent hemorrhage and became comatose with severe respiratory disturbance. Two died before surgery, and 14 recovered in grade IV at surgery. The other six had a minor recurrent hemorrhage without any clinical deterioration. Early surgery was carried out on 54 patients. Two patients with large aneurysms were operated lately and 4 died before surgery. Clinical characteristics of the 54 patients are summarized in Table 1. Among the 54 patients, 25 were men and 29 were women, aged 26 to 82 with a mean age of 55 years. Preoperatively three patients were in grade I of the Hunt and Hess grading, 17 in grade II, 16 in grade III and 18 in grade IV.

All patients underwent computed tomography (CT) examinations prior to surgery and were classified by the amount and distribution of subarachnoid blood clots using Fisher's classification[6]. Twenty-one patients were in group 2, twenty-nine were in group 3, and four were in group 4. Nineteen patients in group 3, and four patients in group 4 had reflux of hematoma into the 4th and 3rd ventricle. This was an important CT finding to suspect the lesions of the posterior fossa, particularly of VA-PICA complex aneurysms. Acute hydrocephalus was observed in 16 patients mostly concomitant with thick and diffuse subarachnoid clots. Cerebral angiogram revealed 13 fusiform aneurysms (12 arising from the VA-PICA complex and one from PCA). The remainder had succular aneurysms. Fifty-one aneurysms were smaller than 12 mm in diameter.

Table 1. *Clinical Characteristics of 54 Surgical Cases*

		No. of cases			No. of cases	
1. Location of aneurysm			4. CT findings before surgery			
Basilar:	BA-BIF	10	a) SAH group	1		0
	BA-SCA	7	(Fisher)	2		21
	BA-trunk	2		3		29
				4		4
Vertebral:	VA-PICA	15				
	VA-dissecting	8	b) 3rd, 4th ventricle reflux of SAH			
	VA-fusiform	3				
	PICA-distal	5	Basilar, PCA aneurysm			8
			VA-PICA complex aneurysm			17
Posterior cerebral:	P$_1$	2	c) Acute hydrocephalus			16
	PCOM	2				
			5. Preoperative rebleeding			
2. Size of aneurysm						
Small (< 12 mm)		51	Basilar, PCA aneurysm			7
Large (12–25 mm)		3	VA-PICA complex aneurysm			13
Giant (> 25 mm)		0				
3. Preoperative grade						
(Hunt and Hess)	I	3				
	II	17				
	III	16				
	IV	18				
	V	0				

BA basilar artery; *BIF* bifurcation; *SCA* superior cerebellar artery; *VA* vertebral artery; *PICA* posterior inferior cerebellar artery; *PCOM* posterior communicating artery; *PCA* posterior cerebral artery; *SAH* subarachnoid hemorrhage.

Surgical Management and Results

Surgical management of the 54 patients is summarized in Table 2. We have undertaken early surgery on the patients with ruptured posterior circulation aneurysms under the same treatment regimen for anterior circulation aneurysms: immediate clipping of aneurysms on all grades I–IV patients and grade V patients with intracerebral hematoma, cisternal drainage for one to two weeks, postoperative administration of Ca^{++} antagonist, and intravascular volume expansion and induced hypertension if necessary. Technically, an appropriate approach, adequate brain relaxation, minimal brain retraction and minimal vessel manipulation are the fundamental surgical policy for safe handling of cerebral aneurysm in the acute stage. Furthermore, wider operating fields are required for better management of deeply located aneurysms of the posterior fossa.

Operations were carried out within 24 hours following the last hemorrhage in 36 patients, and between the second and third day in 18. Sixteen aneurysms arising from the upper basilar artery and 3 PCA aneurysms were approached by the transsylvian rout and occluded by neck clipping. One large posterior communica-

ting (PCOM) fusiform aneurysm was treated by PCOM clipping close to the internal carotid artery. Much wider working space was required than in a conventional transsylvian approach. Ordinarily a large frontotemporal craniotomy with partial zygomectomy and resection of the pterion to the anterior clinoid process was made. In certain cases with sclerotic internal carotid artery (ICA) or unusually short ICA, the resection of the anterior clinoid process and the opening of the cavernous sinus were necessary to mobilize the ICA-middle cerebral artery (MCA) arch. These procedures also provided a wider space around the ICA allowing the exposure of a highly situated BA-BIF aneurysm. The Sylvian fissure was dissected at least to the bifurcation of the MCA. Two fusiform basilar trunk aneurysms were wrapped with Biobond-cotton sheet through the right-sided subtemporal approach, but these two patients deteriorated and died from rebleeding of the aneurysms as a result of incomplete wrapping. One patient with very small BA-SCA aneurysm located low, was successfully clipped through the subtemporal approach. Thirty-one patients with VA-PICA complex aneurysms were operated on through the lateral suboccipital approach which was made as lateral as possible until exposing the sigmoid sinus.

Table 2. *Surgical Management for 54 Cases (Within 3 days)*

	No. of cases		No of cases
1. Time interval between surgery and final SAH		3. Aneurysm treatment	
		Clip occlusion of aneurysm	44
		Wrapping, coating	3
Within 24 hours	36	Proximal occlusion of parent artery (proximal VA occlusion 6)	7
(within 8 hours 17)			
Day 1–2	18		
		4. Temporary clip occlusion of parent artery	
2. Approach			
		Basilar (8–26 min.)	10
Pterional:		Vertebral (5–50 min.)	17
to upper basilar,	20	PCA (15 min.)	1
PCA aneurysm		5. Intraoperative aneurysm	
Subtemporal:	3[a]	rupture	9 (17%)
to BA-trunk aneurysm		Predissection	1
Lateral suboccipital:		Dissection	6
to VA-PICA complex aneurysm	31	Clip application	2
		6. Postoperative symptomatic	
		spasm	4[b] (7.5%)
		Transient ischemia	2
		Permanent disability or death	2

[a]One case with lowely situated BA-SCA aneurysm. [b]BA-BIF. BA-SCA aneurysm: 3, VA-PICA aneurysm: 1.

Twenty saccular aneurysms were clipped directly at the neck and one fusiform aneurysm was wrapped. Six patients with a dissecting VA aneurysm treated by a proximal clip occlusion, proximal to PICA[18] of the affected vertebral artery made full recoveries within several weeks. The affected vertebral arteries were nondominant in all six cases. Two patients with a dissecting aneurysm on the dominant vertebral artery and 2 with a fusiform aneurysm arising from the dominant vertebral artery (one aneurysm located at the low branching of PICA and the other located close to the VA junction from which three perforators were arising) were treated by a clip occlusion of the ruptured site of the aneurysm, followed by wrapping of the whole aneurysm. These procedures were successful through the extreme lateral suboccipital approach with partial condylectomy[2], which is very useful in handling deep-seated complicated VA-PICA complex aneurysms.

Temporary clip occlusion of the parent artery was an indispensable technique especially in early surgery to prevent a major intraoperative rupture during the critical stage of dissection and clipping[4]. We used this technique in 28 patients, ordinarily with an interval of five minutes. Temporary clip applications up to 26 minutes on the basilar artery and 50 minutes on the vertebral artery were used when an intraoperative rupture occurred without any apparent neurological

deficits. Postoperative angiogram in each case revealed no evidence of occlusion or injury of the artery.

Intraoperative rupture of the aneurysms occurred in nine patients (7.5%) mainly at final dissection of the aneurysm. The incidence of the intraoperative rupture was not significantly high compared to those of our 200 anterior aneurysms and of other reports[5,7]. Three had a major rupture with a difficult control even if a temporary clip was applied on the parent artery. Fortunately they recovered well. When the temporary clip applications are used at the critical stages of surgery, the intraoperative rupture is usually minor and easily controlled, thus avoiding disaster.

Four patients with diffuse and thick subarachnoid clots spreading into the supratentorial cisterns developed clinically delayed ischemic neurological deficits secondary to vasospasm. One became vegetative, one died of severe cerebral ischemia and the remaining two had transient ischemic symptoms with complete recovery. Excluding the cases dying immediately after surgery, postoperative symptomatic spasm was recognized in three out of 19 patients with upper basilar or PCA aneurysm (15.8%) and in one out of 25 with VA-PICA complex aneurysm (4.0%). Even though rather small number have been analized in the present study, the results suggest that the incidence of vasospasm in the upper basilar or PCA aneurysms is almost

Table 3. *Location of Aneurysm and Outcome*

Location		No. of cases	Outcome			
			Excellent	Good	Poor	Dead
Basilar	BA-BIF	10	5	2	2	1
	BA-SCA	7	4	0	1	2
	BA-trunk	2	0	0	0	2
Vertebral	VA-PICA	15	11	0	0	4
	VA-dissecting	8	5	1	0	2
	VA-fusiform	3	2	1	0	0
	PICA-distal	5	2	1	0	2
Post cerebral	P_1	2	2	0	0	0
	POM	2	2	0	0	0
Total		54	33	5	3	13

Table 4. *Preoperative Grade and Outcome (Posterior Circulation Aneurysm)*

Hunt and Hess	No. of cases	Outcome			
		Excellent	Good	Poor	Dead
I–II	20	17	2	0	1
III	16	11	0	2	3
IV	18	5	3	1	9
Total	54	33	5	3	13

Table 5. *Causes of Unfavorable Outcome*

		No. of cases
Primary brain damage due to SAH		6
Vasospasm		2
Medical complication		5
Hepatic coma	2	
Renal failure	1	
ARDS	1	
Tuberculosis (lung)	1	
Technical failure		3
Injury of thalamo-perforators	1	
Recurrent hemorrhage	2	
due to incomplete wrapping		

ARDS adult respiratory distress syndrome.

the same as in the anterior circulation aneurysms, but extremely low in VA-PICA complex aneurysms.

The overall results designated by the location of the aneurysm and by the preoperative neurological grade are summarized in Tables 3 and 4. At three months of surgery or later patients were evaluated and the results were as follows: excellent – able to work with no neurological handicaps; good – having a neurological deficit but able to care for self and to work independently; poor-suffering from severe disabling neurological deficits and depending on nursing or family help. Of the 54 patients with early surgical interventions, 38 (70%) were in favorable (excellent, good), and three in poor conditions, and 13 died.

The causes of poor and dead outcome are summarized in Table 5. Primary brain damage due to severe subarachnoid hemorrhage was the most common factor for patient deterioration in the postoperative course. Five patients died due to the effect of the hemorrhage without any improvement. Only one patient regained consciousness but remained severely disabled. One fatality was worthwhile to consider. A 62-year-old female in grade III with a small VA-PICA aneurysm underwent uneventful operation on the second day of hemorrhage, deteriorated soon after surgery and died. A postoperative CT scan revealed remarkable cerebellar swelling without hematoma or focal low density lesions. Probably the acute cerebellar swelling occurred as a result of the acute vasodilatation. Delayed cerebral ischemia secondary to vasospasm was noticed only in two patients, which indicated that vasospasm was less likely to be a main cause of poor outcome in patients with ruptured posterior circulation aneurysms. Of those three patients with a BA-BIF aneurysm whose postoperative CT Scan revealed the involvement of the thalamoperforating arteries, only one became persistently disabled.

Discussion

There have been several reports to suggest a high mortality (47–83%)[5,10,11,14,17] due to rebleeding from aneurysms of the posterior circulation and some difficulty in patient's management while waiting for a delayed surgery[1,3,9]. In our present study rebleeding was confirmed in 22 patients (36.7%) even if very early surgery was our general policy. For such dangerous and "nasty" lesions only a few neurosurgeons have carried out early surgery, and their surgical results have been poor especially in the case with BA-BIF aneurysm[8,13,16]. When these technical problems are solved, early surgery could be the best choice of treatment for preventing recurrent hemorrhage along with the aggressive treatment of postoperative vasospasm. Thus we have carried out early surgery under the treatment regimen mentioned above. Good recovery was made in 70% of the patients with posterior circulation aneurysms. On the other hand, out of 200 patients with early surgery for anterior circulation aneurysms 74% recovered in good condition (Table 7). When examining preoperatively good (grades I, II) and poor patients (grades III, IV), it is noticed that a favorable outcome was obtained in 90% and 55.9% respectively of the posterior circulation aneurysm patients, and in 91% and 60% of the patients with anterior circulation aneurysms. Our results indicate that the overall outcome of early surgery for ruptured posterior circulation aneurysms was almost similar to those of anterior circulation aneurysms. The outcome was not related to the location of the aneurysms, but significantly related to the neurological status prior to surgery. The same observations were made in the study of Peerless[14]. Of 86 patients with posterior circulation aneurysm operated on within 7 days following the last subarachnoid hemorrhage, 81% made good recoveries. This outcome was much better than in our study. In Peerless's study, 85% of the patients was preoperatively in good condition (grades I, II). In our study, on the other hand, 63% was in poor condition (grades III, IV).

Table 6. *Summary of 200 Consecutive Early Surgeries for Anterior Circulation Aneurysms (Within 3 days)*

	No. of cases		No. of cases
1. Location of aneurysm		4. Intraoperative aneurysm rupture	28 (14%)
ACOM	70	5. Postoperative symptomatic spasm	42 (21%)
A₂	12	Transient ischemia	17
ICA	61	Permanent disability or death	25
MCA	57		
2. Time interval between		6. Causes of unfavorable outcome	
surgery and SAH		Primary brain damage due to SAH	11
Within 24 hours	167	Vasospasm	25
(within 6 hours 63)		Medical complication	8
Day 1–2	33	Technical failure	8
3. Preoperative rebleeding	35/255 (14.7%)		

ACOM anterior communicating artery; *ICA* internal carotid artery; *MCA* middle cerebral artery.

Table 7. *Preoperative Grade and Outcome (Anterior Circulation Aneurysm)*

Hunt and Hess	No. of cases	Outcome				
		Excellent	Good	Fair	Poor	Dead
I–II	90	81	1	1	2	5
III	59	40	3	2	5	9
IV	51	19	4	3	10	15
Total	200	140	8	6	17	29

The differences in the overall outcome might be attributed to the differences in the clinical material. Concerning postoperative vasospasm, its incidence in posterior circulation aneurysms (7.4%) seemed much lower than in our series of anterior circulation aneurysms (21%) and in Peerless's study of posterior circulation aneurysms (16%). This result reflects the fact that the incidence of vasospasm was extremely low in VA-PICA complex aneurysms.

Recently it has been suggested that the cisternal irrigation with t-PA can remarkably reduce the postoperative vasospasm[12]. We now assume that early surgical obliteration of ruptured aneurysms and postoperative cisternal irrigation with t-PA for severe subarachnoid clots constitute the most effective therapy to obtain a favorable outcome.

References

1. Aritake K, Saito I, Segawa H, et al (1989) Overall management results in patients with ruptured aneurysms in the posterior fossa region. Surg Cereb Stroke 17: 1–5
2. Bertanffy, Seeger W (1991) The dorsolateral, suboccipital, transcondylar approach to the lower clivus and anterior portion of the craniocervical junction. Neurosurgery 29: 815–821
3. Chou SN, Ortiz-Suarez HJ (1974) Surgical treatment of arterial aneurysms of the vertebrobasilar circulation. J Neurosurg 41: 671–680
4. Drake CG, Perless SJ (1986) Posterior circulation aneurysms. In: Kikuchi H, et al (eds) Intracranial aneurysms – surgical timing and techniques. Proceedings of the First International Workshop on intracranial aneurysms. Nishimura, Niigata, pp 336–348
5. Duvoisin RC, Yahr MD (1965) Posterior fossa aneurysms. Neurology 15: 231–241
6. Fisher CM, Kistler JP, Davis JM (1980) Relation of cerebral vasospasm to subarachnoid hemorrhage visualized by computerized tomogrphic scanning. Neurosurgery 6: 1–9
7. Giannota SL, Oppenheimer JH, Levy ML, et al (1991) Management of intraoperative rupture of aneurysm without hypotension. Neurosurgery 28: 531–535
8. Gotoh T, Kikuchi K. Watanabe K (1990) Early surgical management of ruptured aneurysms of the vetebrobasilar arteries. In: Sugita K, et al (eds) Intracranial aneurysms and arteriovenous malformations. Proceedings of the 2nd International Workshop on Intracranial Aneurysms. Nagoya University Coop Press, Nagoya, pp 61–67
9. Hashimoto I, Sasaki T, Wada K, et al (1989) Early surgery for ruptured posterior circulation aneurysms. Surg Cereb Stroke (Tokyo) 17: 13–17
10. Hook O, Norien G, Guzman J (1963) Saccular aneurysms of the vertebrobasilar arterial system. A report of 28 cases. Acta Neurol Scand 39: 271–34
11. Locksley HS (1969) Natural history of subarachnoid hemorrhage. In: Sal AL, et al (eds) Intracranial aneurysms and subarachnoid hemorrhage. Lippincott, Philadelphia, pp 37–108
12. Mizoi K, Yoshimoto T, Sugawara T, et al (1990) Prevention of vasospasm by clot removal and intrathecal bolus injection of tissue-type plasminogen activator: preliminary report. In: Sano K, et al (eds) Cerebral vasospasm. Proceedings of the IVth International Conference on cerebral vasospasm. University of Tokyo Press, Tokyo, pp 317–320
13. Nukui H, Kaneko M. Mitsuka S, et al (1990) Early operation in cases with ruptured basilar aneurysms. In: Sugita K, et al (eds) Intracranial aneurysms and arteriovenous malformations. Proceedings of the 2nd International Workshop on intracranial aneurysms. Nagoya University Coop Press, Nagoya, pp 55–59
14. Peerless SJ, Nemoto S, Drake CG (1987) Acute surgery for ruptured posterior circulation aneurysms. In: Symon L, Brihaye J, Cohadon F, et al (eds) Advances and technical standards in neurosurgery, Vol 15. Springer, Wien New York, pp 115–129
15. Tanaka N, Fujitsu K, Fujii S, et al (1989) Consideration on early operation for ruptured basilar bifurcation aneurysms. Surg Cereb Stroke (Tokyo) 17: 60–65
16. Samson D. Batjer H (1986) Intraoperative aneurysmal rupture incidence, outcome and surgical management. In: Sano K, et al (eds) Intracranial aneurysms. Proceedings of the First International Workshop on intracranial aneurysms. Nishimura, Niigata, pp 123–131
17. Troupp H (1971) The natural history of aneurysms of the basilar bifurcation. Acta Neurol Scand 47: 350–356
18. Yamaura A (1988) Diagnosis and treatment of vertebral aneurysms. J Neurosurg 69: 345–349

Correspondence: T. Moriyama, M.D., Department of Neurosurgery, Moriyama Hospital, 6-15-24 Nishikasai Edogawaku, Tokyo 134, Japan.

Retrolabyrinthine Trans-Sigmoid (RLTS) Approach to Aneurysms of the Basilar Trunk and Vertebrobasilar Junction: an Update

S.L. Giannotta

Department of Neurosurgery, LAC-USC Medical Center, University of Southern California, School of Medicine, Los Angeles, California, U.S.A.

Summary

Traditionally, approaches for vertebral basilar junction and basilar trunk aneurysms have been complicated by excessive temporal lobe, brainstem, or cerebellar retraction, and by long reaches through narrow corridors bounded by interposed cranial nerves. The author has successfully developed and utilized an approach with a trajectory through the mastoid which reduces the working distance between the surface and the basilar artery and obviates the need for virtually any significant cerebellar retraction and no brainstem retraction. Mastoid air cells are removed anterior and posterior to the sigmoid sinus. The anterior extent of the removal is the posterior semicircular canal. The superior extent of removal is the superior petrosal sinus, and the inferior extent of removal is the jugular bulb. By including a small amount of bone removal posterior to the sigmoid sinus, the sigmoid sinus is then ligated at its junction with the jugular bulb and superior petrosal sinus and it and the dura are reflected anteriorly. With the patient in the supine position with the head turned 60 degrees away from the side of the approach, the pontine and medullary cisterns are easily accessible without cerebellar or brainstem retraction. Nine cases have been treated utilizing this approach. There was one death of a patient with a giant basilar trunk aneurysm which could not be successfully ligated and subsequently suffered a fatal recurrent subarachnoid hemorrhage four weeks post-operatively. The remaining eight patients made good recoveries. There were two lower cranial nerve deficits which resolved spontaneously. Hearing was preserved in all nine surviving cases. There have been no complications related to selective occlusion of the sigmoid sinus.

Keywords: Aneurysm; basilar trunk; mastoid; sigmoid sinus; vertebrobasilar junction.

Introduction

Aneurysms of the basilar trunk and vertebrobasilar junction are formidable challenges for the neurovascular surgeon from a number of standpoints. Their location under the brainstem, entangled in a web of cranial nerves, makes traditional approaches to this region much more hazardous. Approaches often proposed for these lesions require a retractor blade be placed on the brainstem or manipulation of the ninth and tenth cranial nerves, injury to which is probably tolerated least of all the cranial nerves[1-5,7,8,10-13,15,16]. The only approach devised to avoid these two complications, namely the trans clival approach, has its own set of drawbacks[14]. The retrolab-trans-sigmoid (RLTS) approach takes advantage of strategies developed from otological and cranial base procedures to affect a more basal-lateral trajectory in an effort to avoid any brainstem retraction and to minimize handling of the lower cranial nerves[6]. Since the original description of this technique, a larger experience has been gained allowing for further observations relative to the direction of approach, strategies for large and giant lesions, and alternatives to the approach.

Technique

The patient is positioned supine and the head is turned 45 degrees away from the side of the surgical procedure. The side of approach is predicated on the architecture of the aneurysm and the patency of and venous drainage pattern through the dural sinuses. The majority of vertebral basilar junction aneurysms and trunk aneurysms point either ventrally or dorsally and can be approached on the side of the smallest sigmoid sinus. Pin head rest fixation is optional since frequently no retractor system is necessary. This angle of the position of the head allows the cerebellum and brain stem to fall away from the clivus opening up the retroclival space and the pre-pontine cistern. A curvilinear incision approximately an inch and a half behind the ear crease is made and sel-retaining retractors are placed. A partial mastoidectomy is performed skeletonizing the posterior semicircular canal, the posterior fossa dura in front of the sigmoid sinus, the sigmoid sinus from its junction with the transverse sinus to its junction with the jugular bulb, and the posterior fossa dura for approximately 1 cm behind the sigmoid sinus. With relaxation afforded by intravenous mannitol, the posterior fossa dura both behind and in front of the sigmoid sinus at its junction with the transverse sinus and separately at its junction with the jugular bulb is opened and the sinus is ligated at both ends. The dura is opened using a flap based adjacent to the posterior semicircular canal. The cisterna magna is opened; and, with the dependent position of posterior fossa, spinal fluid egress is vigorous. This gives further relaxation to the cerebellar hemisphere. A #5 french suction tip resting on a cottonoid patty on the flocculus is all the retraction needed to begin dissection of the aneurysm. When the arachnoid of the pre-pontine and cerebellopontine angle cisterns is opened, the AICA and basilar arteries come into view. With further dissection, this vessel can be exposed from immediately adjacent to the vertebral artery junction up to a point where the superior cerebellar artery emerges. Depending on the size of intervening spaces, it may be expedient to work simultaneously on both sides of the auditory-facial nerve complex. This exposure allows adequate room for placement of temporary clips on the proximal vertebral vessels if necessary. Following satisfactory clip ligation of the aneurysm, a tight dural closure and placement of an autologous fat graft adjacent to all open air cells will obviate potential CSF otorhinorrhea.

Results

Nine cases of basilar trunk and vertebrobasilar junction aneurysms have been treated using this approach. Four patients harbored vertebrobasilar junction aneurysms, two had basilar trunk lesions, two had aneurysms of the vertebral artery above the takeoff of PICA, and one lesion was on AICA at the basilar artery junction (Table 1). Ages ranged from 26 to 63. Eight patients presented with subarachnoid hemorrhage, although the diagnosis was delayed more than several months in two; and one lesion was incidental to a previously ruptured one. At the time of surgery, 3 were grade 0, 4 were grade 1, one was grade 2, and one was grade 3. Two aneurysms were large, one was giant, and the remainder were small.

All patients had successful clip ligation of their aneurysms as demonstrated by post operative angiography except for the giant lesion. In that case, the large sac was approached on the side of a strongly lateralized fundus. Although proximal control of both vertebral arteries was easily accomplished, this did not slacken the sac enough to be able to negociate around the proximal dome to gain distal control. We were unable to secure the lesion, and while awaiting an endovascular procedure, the patient suffered a fatal rebleed (Table 2). Of the remaining 8 patients, 2 had temporary hoarseness with pneumonia. One case required a separate procedure for a CSF leak. Ultimately all made good recoveries, and have returned to the previous activities including employment (Table 3). No patient experienced

Table 1. *Location of Aneurysms Treated by RLTS Approach*

Location	n
Vertebrobasilar junction	4
Basilar trunk	2
Distal vertebral	2
AICA – basilar	1

Table 2. *Complications in 9 Cases Using RLTS Approach*

Complication	n
Lower cranial nerve paresis	2
CSF leak	2
Unable to clip	1

Table 3. *Outcome in 9 Cases Using RLTS Approach*

Outcome	n
Good recovery	8
Dead	1

hearing loss, and no patient suffered a complication secondary to occlusion of the sigmoid sinus.

Discussion

Among the benefits of the RTLS approach is the basolateral trajectory. By approaching the region of the clivus and the basilar artery trunk through the mastoid, the plane of the operative corridor is virtually parallel to the cranial base. This produces two dividends, namely the avoidance of any brainstem retraction, and the ability to work parallel to the lower cranial nerves instead of tangential to them. The removal of the retrolabyrinthine portion of the mastoid to access this region is analogous to utilizing the pterional approach for anterior circulation aneurysms, in which bone removal is accomplished in lieu of retraction of the frontal-temporal junction. Since the space between the labyrinthe and the anterior border of the sigmoid sinus is relatively restricted, in order to gain enough room to dissect and clip the aneurysm, the sigmoid sinus must be divided. In order to insure the safety of this manoeuvre, close scrutiny of the venous sinus collateral must be performed. In the case of a strongly dominant sigmoid or in a situation where a lateral sinus fails to connect with the torcular, either the approach should be made on the other side or an alternative strategy selected.

When the venous sinus anatomy does not dictate the side of the approach, the direction in which the aneurysm points does. In the case of small or large sacs, it is best to approach the lesion on the side to which it points. This avoids the need to work across the basilar artery and risk injuring unseen perforators to the brainstem. It also allows for the most advantageous visualization of the neck at the time of clip application. In the case of giant sacs where either the proximal or distal portion of the parent vessel is obscured making temporary occlusion difficult or impossible, the lesion may best be approached from the contralateral side. We failed to appreciate this in our case of a giant basilar trunk lesion. In retrospect, a contralateral approach should have been taken, or cardiopulmonary bypass with hypothermic arrest might have allowed collapse of the fundus such that clip application could have proceeded successfully.

When the sigmoid sinus cannot be sacrificed, two strategies are best considered. For those lesions located below the takeoff of the AICA, the so-called ELITE or extreme lateral inferior transcondylar exposure is advantageous[2,17]. This strategy embodies minor modifications of the so-called far lateral approach to the foramen magnum and lower posterior fossa as proposed by Heros and others[9]. The rim of the foramen magnum, posterior arch of C1, posterior tip of the mastoid and lateral half of the occipital condyle are all drilled away to affect an infero-to-superior, caudal-to-rostral trajectory along the vertebral artery, without significant lower brainstem retraction. Cranial nerves are still at risk, and the reach is long especially for lower trunk aneurysms.

For lesions of the basilar trunk at or above AICA, the retrolab-subtemporal combined approach can be an effective alternative[8]. By combining a retrolab mastoid approach with a temporal craniotomy, the superior petrosal sinus and tentorium can be divided, allowing retraction of the sigmoid sinus and a trajectory to the upper basilar trunk parallel to the 5th, 7th, and 9th cranial nerves.

As with most mastoid approaches where the dura is opened, CSF leak is a possible complication. To avoid this, we routinely place an autologous adipose graft in the mastoid defect. In the event of a leak, lumbar drainage for three days will invariably provide the solution.

The indications for the RLTS approach are relatively narrow. Obviously the decision to sacrifice a major venous sinus should not be taken lightly. Therefore we do not use the approach for lower vertebral aneurysms or PICA lesions. A lateralized retromastoid strategy is adequate in those situations. Lack of familiarization with the anatomy of the mastoid, can be remedied by practice in the skull-base lab, enrollment in one of a number of skullbase or temporal bone anatomy courses, or working in conjunction with an otologist.

Conclusion

The retrolabyrinthine trans-sigmoid approach for vertebrobasilar and basilar trunk aneuryms is a relatively simple technique which provides tangible benefits in terms of speed and acceptible morbidity at the expence of opening the mastoid and sacrificing the sigmoid sinus. It avoids time consuming and potentially complicated combined supratentorial-infratentorial approaches by allowing the most direct trajectory to lesions in this portion of the vascular tree.

References

1. Chou SN, Ortiz-Suarez HJ (1974) Surgical treatment of arterial aneurysms of the vertebrobasilar circulation. J Neurosurg 41: 671–680
2. Bertalanffy H, Seeger W (1991) The dorsolateral, suboccipital, transcondylar approach to the lower clivus and anterior portion of the craniocervical junction. Neurosurgery 29: 815–821
3. Drake CG (1969) The surgical treatment of vertebral-basilar aneurysms. Clin Neurosurg 16: 114–169
4. Drake CG (1979) The treatment of aneurysms of the posterior circulation. Clin Neurosurg 26: 96–144
5. Fox JL (1967) Obliteration of midline vertebral artery aneurysm via basilar craniectomy. J Neurosurg 26: 406–412
6. Giannotta SL, Maceri, DR (1988) Retrolabyrinthine transsigmoid approach to basilar trunk and vertebrobasilar junction aneurysms. J Neurosurg 69: 461–466
7. Hammon WM, Kempe LG (1972) The posterior fossa approach to aneurysms of the vertebral and basilar arteries. J Neurosurg 37: 339–347
8. Hashi K, Nin K, Shimotake K (1982) Transpetrosal combined supratentorial and infratentorial approach for midline vertebrobasilar aneurysms. In: Brock M (ed) Modern neurosurgery 1. Springer, Berlin Heidelburg New York, pp 442–448
9. Heros RC (1986) Lateral approach for vertebral and vertebrobasilar artery lesions. J Neurosurg 64: 559–562
10. Kasdon DL, Stein BM (1979) Combined supratentorial and infratentorial exposure for low-lying basilar aneurysms. Neurosurgery 4: 422–426
11. Kawase T, Toya S, Shiobara R, et al (1985) Transpetrosal approach for aneurysms of the lower basilar artery. J Neurosurg 63: 857–861
12. Ojemann RG, Crowell RM (1983) Surgical management of cerebrovascular disease. Williams and Wilkins, Baltimore, pp 223–232
13. Peerless SJ, Drake CG (1982) Management of aneurysms of the posterior circulation. In: Youmans JR (ed) Neurological surgery, 2nd Ed, Vol 3. Saunders, Philadelphia, pp 1715–1733
14. Sano K, Jinbo M, Saito I (1966) Vertebro-basilar aneurysms, with special reference to the transpharyngeal approach to basilar artery aneurysms. No To Shinkei 18: 1197–1203 (Jpn)
15. Sugita K, Koybayashi S, Shintani A, et al (1979) Microneurosurgery for aneurysms of the basilar artery. J Neurosurg 51: 615–620
16. Sugita K, Kobayashi S, Takemae T, et al (1987) Aneurysms of the basilar artery trunk. J Neurosurg 66: 500–505
17. Sen CN, Sekhar LN (1990) An extreme lateral approach to intradural lesions of the cervical spine and foramen magnum. Neurosurgery 27: 197–204

Correspondence: Steven L. Giannotta, M.D., Department of Neurosurgery, University of Southern California, School of Medicine, Box 239, 1200 State Street, Los Angeles, California 90033, U.S.A.

An Anterior Approach to Aneurysms of the Vertebro-Basilar Junction

W.A.S. Taylor[1], D. Uttley[1], and D.J. Archer[2]

[1]Department of Neurosurgery, Atkinson Morley's Hospital, Wimbledon, London, and [2]Department of Faciomaxillary Surgery, Royal Marsden Hospital, London, U.K.

Summary

The surgical treatment of anteriorly placed aneurysms of the posterior circulation crries a high morbidity which is mainly due to their inaccessibility. This is partly due to the need to retract the brainstem and cranial nerves. An anterior approach theoretically avoids this and we have used a Le Fort 1 maxillotomy to approach ten of these aneurysms.

Nine aneurysms were successfully clipped and one was wrapped. Morbidity was two cases of meningitis and one temporary sixth nerve palsy. There were no deaths and at six month follow up all patients had achieved a good outcome on the Glasgow Outcome Scale.

In conclusion this approach can be used with minimum morbidity and offers several advantages over posterior approaches.

Keywords: Dural repair; midline vertebrobasilar aneurysms; transclival approach.

Introduction

Vertebro-basilar aneurysms which lie anterior to the brainstem are relatively uncommon[1,3] and they carry a reputation of high surgical morbidity. This is due principally to their inaccessibility as conventional posterior or superior approaches may require significant retraction on the cranial nerves and brainstem. It would therefore seem that an anterior approach would have much to recommend it by avoiding these hazards but has failed to gain popularity for two main reasons. The first of these is that the exposure is said to be limited and thus compromises dissection of the aneurysm and the second is that a secure dural repair is difficult to achieve[2]. Despite these reservations in recent years we have used an anterior approach using a Le Fort I osteotomy[3] to treat a series of these aneurysms and the results are given in this report.

Patients and Methods

Clinical data was obtained retrospectively from the case records of a consecutive series of patients who had undergone surgery for aneurysms anterior to the brain stem following subarachnoid haemorrhage. The WFNS grade of the patients was recorded prior to surgery as was the timing of surgery in relation to the initial subarachnoid haemorrhage. Follow-up was obtained to at least six months in all patients and outcome was recorded according to the Glasgow Outcome Scale.

The surgical techniques employed were that all patients were operated on by a faciomaxillary surgeon and a neurosurgeon and the same technique was used each time. Under general anaesthesia a lumbar drain was sited and a Le Fort I maxillotomy performed and the posterior pharingeal wall divided in the midline and stripped from the clivus. An appropriate section of this was then removed to expose dura which was then opened away from the aneurysm to allow microsurgical dissection of the aneurysm. Mayfield–Kees aneurysm clips were used because of the small size of the spring which allowed it to be tucked inside the dura. The dural defect was then closed using a dural substitute and human fibrin glue, the maxillotomy repaired and a percutaneous pharingostomy performed for feeding post-operatively. Prophylactic antibiotics in the form of an intravenous cephalosporin were given at induction and continued for forty eight hours and lumbar drainage was continued for five days post-operatively and the patients subsequently mobilised.

Results

Between 1985 and 1992 ten patients underwent surgery for aneurysms anterior to the brainstem via an anterior approach and clinical details of these patients are given in Table 1. All patients were WFNS grades I and II at the time of surgery and the majority had delayed surgery. Five patients were delayed because of clinical vasospasm and one of these patients suffered a recurrent haemorrhage. There was no operative mortality and no significant extracranial morbidity in this series. Although there was no overt CSF leaks two patients suffered meningitis post-operatively which responded to appropriate antibiotics. One patient suffered a sixth nerve palsy post-operatively which ultimately resolved. The average duration in hospital post-operatively was sixteen days. At six months all patients had achieved a good outcome according to the Glasgow Outcome Scale and at final follow-up which ranged from six months

Table 1. *Patient Details*

Age	Sex	Site	Grade[a]	Timing[b]	Operation	Morbidity
46	F	PICA	I	2/12	clip	none
39	F	PICA	II	7/7	clip	meningitis
69	F	PICA	I	6/7	clip	meningitis
39	F	PICA	I	3/12	clip	VI palsy
45	F	PICA	II	1/12	clip	none
32	M	AICA	I	6/52	wrap	none
44	F	VA/BA	I	14/7	clip	none
27	F	PICA	I	12/7	clip	none
47	F	PICA	I	3/52	clip	none
30	F	VA/BA	I	5/7	clip	none

[a] WFNS grade.
[b] Interval between ictus and operation.

to two years all patients were functioning normally without neurological deficit.

Discussion

Aneurysms of the posterior circulation carry a higher morbidity than aneurysms at other sites and this is borne out by data from the recent co-operative study[1]. Fortunately they only account for between 5–7.6% of all aneurysms[1,3] and the majority of these are at either the basilar bifurcation or lateral to the medulla at the origin of the posterior inferior cerebellar artery. The aneurysms described in this study are in a minority in that all of these were anterior to the brainstem on the basilar trunk or on the distal vertebral vessels. These aneurysms provide the biggest surgical challenge in terms of access and there is debate as to which approach is most appropriate.

Approaches which have been suggested are either a supratentorial or a suboccipital approach or if either of these is inadequate a combined approach can be used[6]. It would seem logical that an anterior approach would have some advantages as it would avoid any retraction on the brain stem or proximal cranial nerves and would allow more direct access to the aneurysm. However this approach has not found favour because of the limited access provided and the risk of causing a CSF leak and meningitis[2]. We feel that the first of these arguments is not justified in light of our experience with this series. The Le Fort exposure allows the clivus to be exposed throughout its length and this can then be removed using a high speed drill and bone rongeurs. Once the dura is exposed the site of the aneurysm can be identified by yellowish purple staining allowing the dura to be opened away form the aneurysm. The whole length of the basilar trunk can be exposed via this approach and once the anatomy has been identified dissection and clipping of the aneurysm can be carried out.

The other main reservation about this technique has been that it leaves the patient at risk of CSF leak and meningitis because of the difficulty in obtaining a watertight dural repair. This occurred in two of our patients and remains a considerable cause for concern. However we feel that the use of dural substitutes, human fibrin glue and a protective lumbar drain keeps this complication at an acceptable level and should no longer be a limiting factor in using this approach.

One of the limitations of a study like this is that the number of patients is small and this reflects the rarity of the condition and is true of similar series employing different approaches. There is also selection in that only patients in good clinical grade were operated on and that the majority of cases were operated on late and these factors will influence the outcome of the surgically treated patients. Other surgical series are also affected by these limitations and the other reported series of similar groups of patients record an operative morbidity between 15–30%[2,6,7]. This series compares favourably to these results and we feel that the techniques used in this series do not carry an unacceptable morbidity and should have a increasing place in the management of these aneurysms.

References

1. Kassell NF, Torner JC, Haley EC, Jane JA, Adams HP, Kongable GL, and Participants (1990) The international co-operative study on the timing of aneurysm surgery: Part 1. Overall management results. J Neurosurg 73: 18–36
2. Peerless SJ, Drake CG (1985) Posterior circulation aneurysms. In: Wilkins RH, Rengachary SS (ed) Neurosurgery. Mc Graw Hill, New York, pp 1422–1437
3. Richardson AE (1969) Subarachnoid haemorrhage. BMJ 4: 89–92
4. Sasaki CT, Lowlicht RA, Astrachan DI, Friedman CD, Goodwin JW, Morales M (1990) Le Fort 1 osteotomy approach to the skull base. Laryngoscope 100: 1073–1076
5. Sekhar LN, Lanzino G (1990) Skull base surgery. Crit Rev Neurosurg 1: 211–216
6. Soloman RA, Stein BM (1988) Surgical approaches to aneurysms of the vertebral and basilar arteries. Neurosurgery 23: 203–207
7. Sugita K, Kobayashi S, Takemae T, Tada T, Tanaka Y (1987) Aneurysms of the basilar trunk. J Neurosurg 66: 500–505

Correspondence: W.A.S. Taylor, F.R.C.S., Department of Neurosurgery, Atkinson Morley's Hospital, Copsehill, Wimbledon, London SW20 One, U.K.

Anterior Transpetrosal Approach for Basilar Trunk Aneurysms – Further Experience

T. Kawase and **S. Toya**

Department of Neurosurgery, School of Medicine, Keio University, Tokyo, Japan

Summary

The anterior part of the petrous bone, not included the auditory structures, was resected epidurally through a subtemporal craniotomy to access the basilar trunk aneurysms. In 6 surgical cases, all the aneurysms were clipped even projecting posteriorly, without serious complications. The extradural access minimized the venous complication and retraction damage. Confining the resection of the petrous bone could preserve the auditory function. Possible other surgical complications such as CSF leakage, facial hypesthesia or lacrimation decrease were not seen in the recent cases. Technical points to prevent those complications are presented.

Keywords: Cerebral aneurysm; basilar artery; transpetrosal approach; surgical complication.

Introduction

In cases with basilar trunk aneurysms located lower than the Vth cranial nerve, exposure of the aneurysm is currently difficult either from the subtemporal or the suboccipital route, and extended retraction of the temporal lobe or lower cranial nerves is hazardous to the patient. The "transpetrosal approach" was originally developed in 1985[1] for such aneurysms to prevent these serious complications. The likely surgical complications of this method were: lacrimation decrease by sacrifice of the major petrosal nerve, abducens palsy or hearing loss by excessive petrous resection, and cerebrospinal fluid (CSF) rhinorrhea. This report presents the surgical points and refinements to avoid these possible complications, based on a nine year experience.

Operative Points

By the supine-lateral position, a scalp incision is made around the ear, and the anterior line is planned to spare the upper facial nerve and to create a craniotomy more anteriorly than that of the extended middle fossa approach used for acoustic tumor surgery[2] (Fig. 1). The temporal muscle is dissected long enough to cover the drilled petrous bone on closure. The craniotomy is centered above the mandibular joint. It is unnecessary to expose the sigmoid sinus, and if possible, mastoid air cells are not opened to avoid cerebrospinal fluid (CSF) leakage. The middle meningeal artery is coagulated and cut near the foramen spinosum.

It is easier to expose the anterior petrous bone, located beyond the eminentia arcuata, when the axis of the microscope is deviated anteriorly. The greater petrosal nerve, which is one of the important landmarks, must be spared and dissected from the dura, in order not to stretch the facial nerve; lacrimation decrease can be avoided when it is preserved. The eminentia arcuata, another important landmark, must not be opened. The area of drilling is surrounded by the tri-

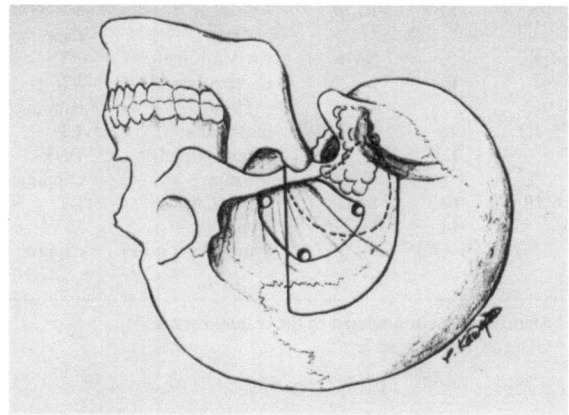

Fig. 1. Craniotomy site. Skin incision is planned to spare the upper facial nerve. The temporal muscle is preserved long enough to cover the drilled petrous bone: note the difference of craniotomy site from that of the extended middle fossa approach (posterior transpetrosal approach)

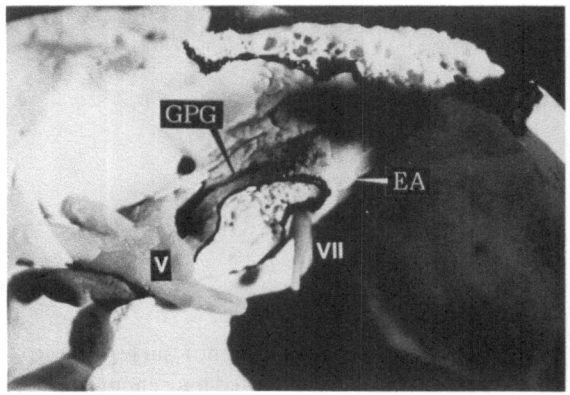

Fig. 2. Site of right petrous resection on a dried skull. *EA* eminentia arcuata, *GPG* greater petrosal groove

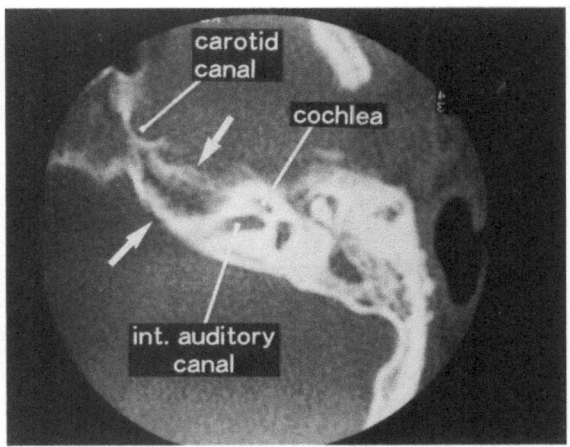

Fig. 3. Bone CT scan of right petrous bone. Note the difference of consistency between the petrous apex (arrows) and middle ear

Table 1. *Clinical Data of Patients*

Case	Age Sex	Onset Grade (Hunt and Hess)	Aneurysm location direction size	Surgery approach side level of CN[a] treatment of aneurysm	Surgical complications (temporary)	GOS[b] postoperative angiography
1. HK	49 F	SAH II	BA-VA junction posterior 6 mm	LT VI-VIII clipping	hearing disturbance incomplete VI, VIIth palsy (CSF rhinorrhea)	II completely clipped
2. TK	43 F	SAH III	BA-AICA posterior 10 mm	LT V-VI clipping	(bil. VIth palsy) (facial hypesthesia)	I completely clipped
3. IY	58 M	SAH I	mid-basilar posterior 4 mm	RT V clipping	(lacrimation decrease)	I completely clipped
4. KS	53 F	SAH I	BA-VA junction postero-lateral 10 mm	RT VI clipping	hearing disturbance (VIth palsy) (lacrimation decrease)	I completely clipped
5. KE	46 F	SAH I	mid-basilar antero-lateral 5 mm	LT IV-V clipping	None	I completely clipped
6. IR	64 M	SAH I	BA-AICA lateral 7 mm (broad neck)	RT V-VI clipping + wrapping	None	I clipped on the dome

[a] Aneurysm location related to the cranial nerves.
[b] Glasgow outcome scale.

geminal impression anteriorly, the eminentia arcuata posteriorly, the major petrosal groove laterally, and the carotid canal and internal auditory canal inferiorly (Fig. 2). The bone in this area does not contain organic structure, and is usually of softer consistency than the middle ear; this offers an important orientation during pyramid resection (Fig. 3). If the bone resection extends more laterally (Glasscock's triangle), the risk of injury to the carotid artery or the cochlea will be increased. Excessive bone resection toward the clivus increases the venous bleeding from the inferomedial triangle of the cavernous sinus, as well as injury of the VIth nerve.

After resection of the petrous bone, dural incisions are made above and below the superior petrosal sinus, which is incised using double Weck's clip. Care must be taken to the location of petrous vein behind the

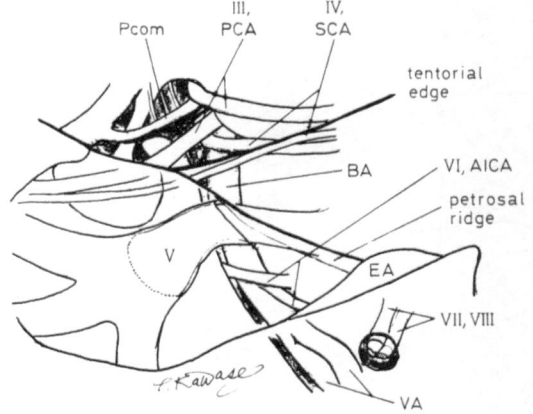

a

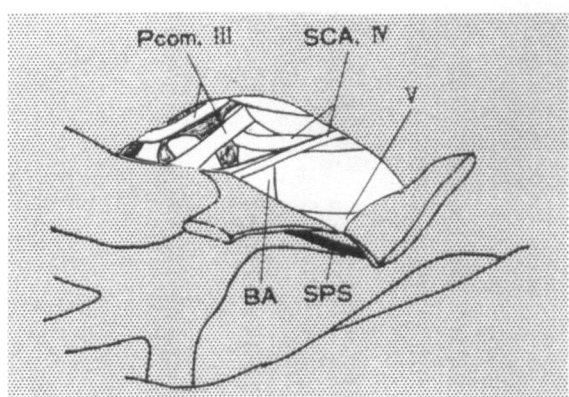

b

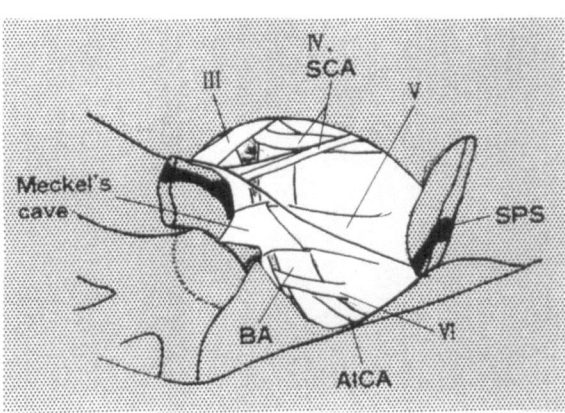

c

Fig. 4. (a) Lateral view of basilar artery, related with cranial nerves. Difference of surgical field between conventional subtemporal-transtentorial approach; (b) and anterior transpetrosal approach; (c) with opening of the Meckel's cave

tentorium. Complete incision and tacking of the tentorium offers an adequate view toward the basilar trunk. When the aneurysm locates behind the Vth nerve, the Meckel's cave can easily be opened to mobilize the nerve[3]. This procedure offers the advantage of enlarging the access route (Fig. 4).

The drilled petrous bone is covered with a temporal fascia strip, and coated with fibrin glue. In cases with large air cells, a muscle piece is packed into the cells. The margin of the dural defect is sutured to the inserted fascia.

Surgical Cases

Clinical data of 6 patients with a basilar trunk aneurysm are presented in Table 1. All had a ruptured saccular aneurysm, located on the mid-basilar artery (BA) (2 cases), on the bifurcation of anterior inferior cerebellar artery (BA-AICA) (2 cases) and on the basilar-vertebral (BA-VA) junction (2 cases). The aneurysm size ranged from 4 to 10 mms, and half of these projected toward the brainstem. The aneurysm was approached between the IVth and Vth nerves for mid-basilar aneurysms, between the Vth and VIIIth nerves for lower basilar aneurysm. The Meckel's cave was opened for aneurysms located behind the Vth nerve, or laterally projecting aneurysms in which a curved clip is applied (Fig. 5). A straight long clip was necessary for lower basilar aneurysms, because of a confined space (Fig. 6).

Surgical Complications and Technical Improvements

There was no complication caused by brain retraction. The surgical complications were focused on the cranial nerves from Vth to VIIIth.

– Facial hypesthesia: it occurred temporary in 1 case, when the retraction of the nerve was excessive.
– Abducens palsy: it occurred in 3 cases by manipulation near the aneurysm.
– Hearing disturbance: it occurred in 2 cases when the petrous resection was inadequately wide; the labyrinth was opened in case 1, and the cochlea in case 4.
– Lacrimation decrease; it occurred when the greater petrosal nerve was sacrificed.
– CSF leakage: it occurred only in the first case of this series, by careless opening of the middle year.

These surgical complications were less frequently observed in the recent cases due to the technical progress pointed out below.

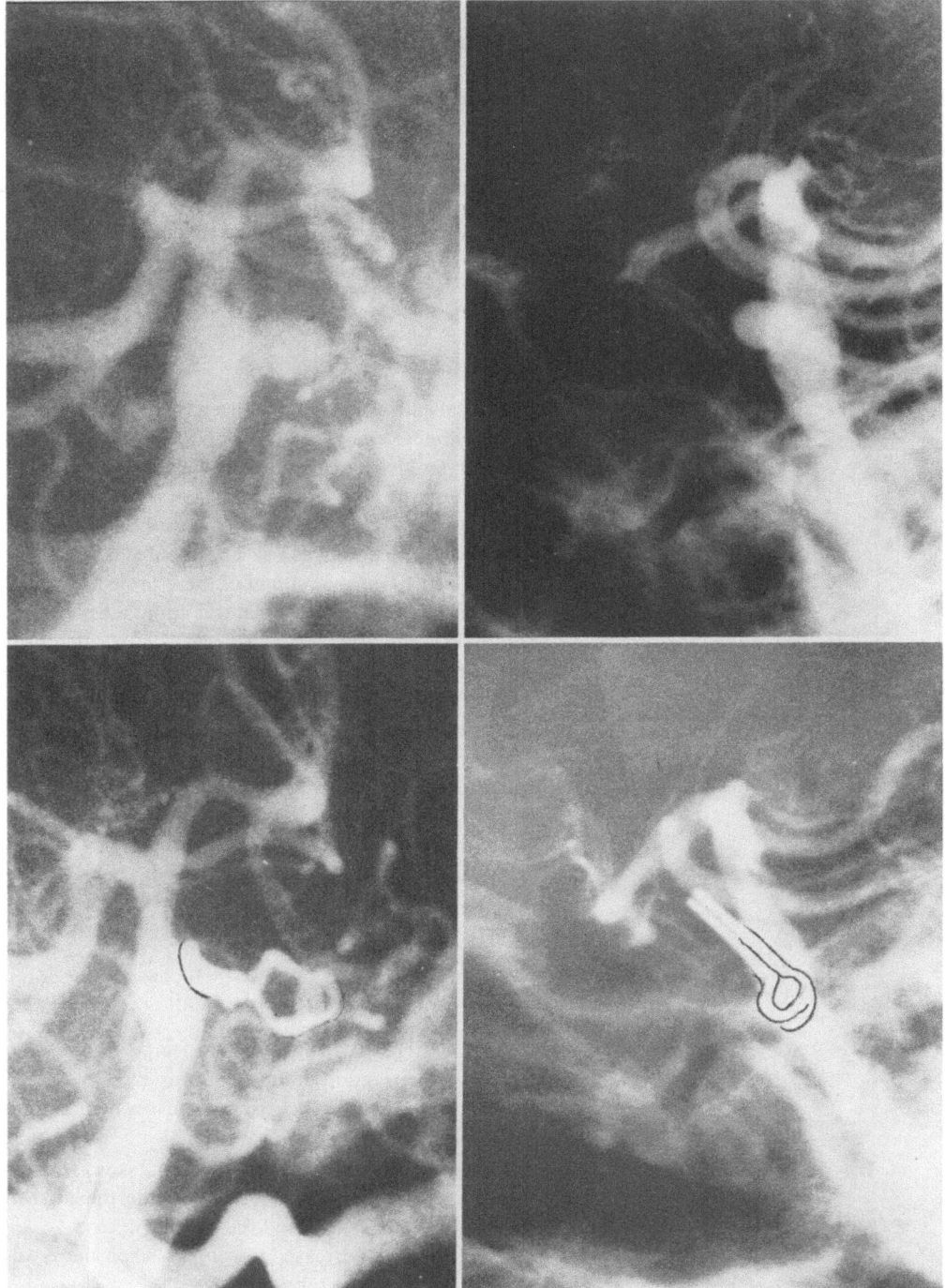

Fig. 5. Case 5, mid-basilar aneurysm projecting antero-laterally. The trigeminal nerve was mobilized by opening the Meckel's cave, for application of a curved clip

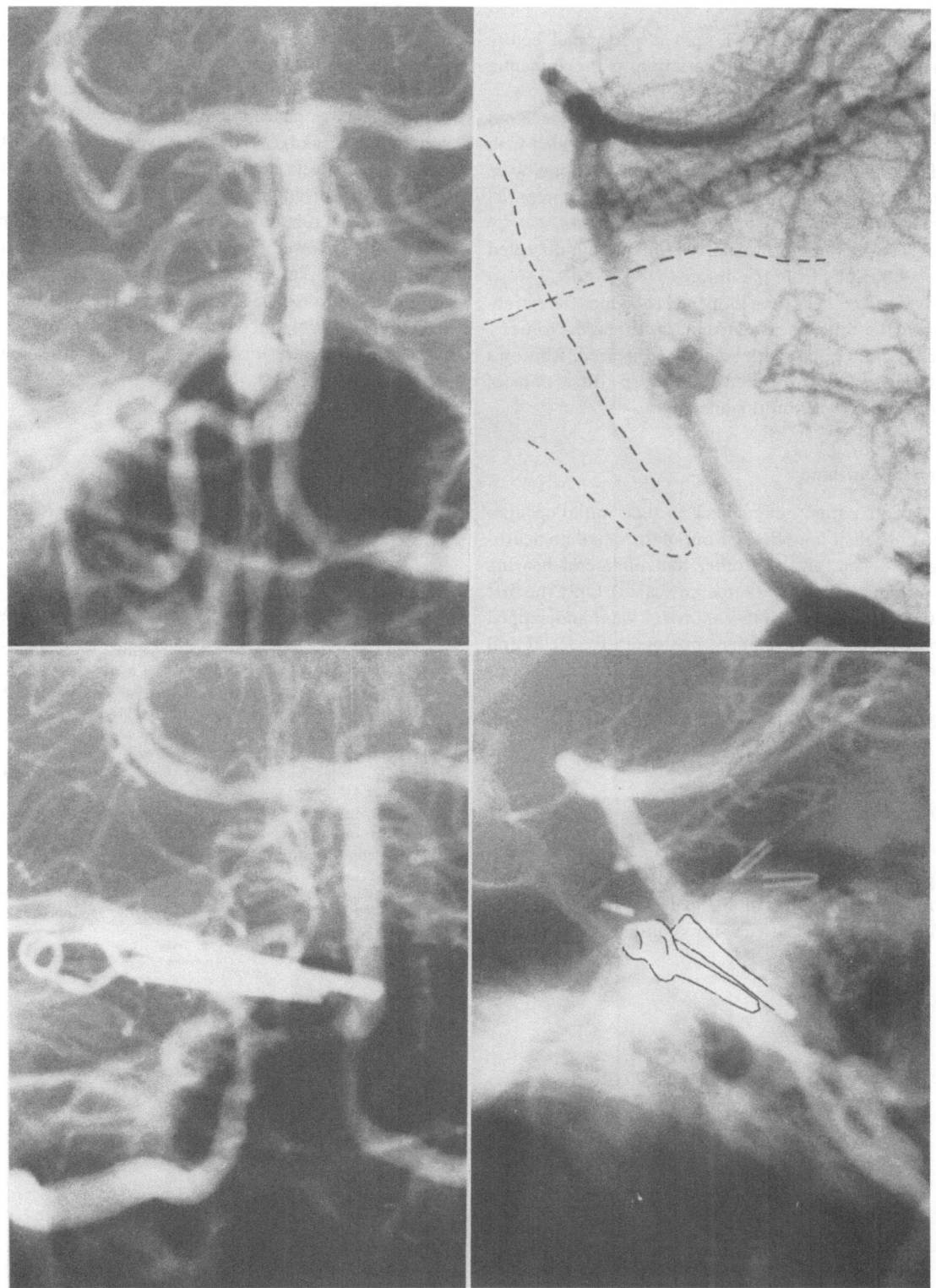

Fig. 6. Case 4, vertebro-basilar junction aneurysm projecting postero-laterally. Two straight long clips were applied

a) Thin sliced bone CT scan is performed before surgery in order to know the variations of the eminentia arcuata and the air cells in the petrous bone.

b) By an adequate and minimal craniotomy, mastoid air cells are not opened. If opened, they are sealed with a fascia flap and fibrin glue, not with bone wax. Enough length of the temporal muscle fascia is prepared for closure.

c) The greater petrosal nerve is not cut but dissected microsurgically from the dura.

d) The Meckel's cave is opened to reduce the retraction on the Vth nerve, and to enlarge the access route.

e) A clip applier with small head is used. Rhoton's microdissectors are used for sharp dissection of abducens nerve from the aneurysm.

Surgical Outcome

Five of six patients came back to their initial occupation or to their household. Four of them had no neurological deficit, and the other had unilateral hearing disturbance (Glasgow Outcome Scale I). Only the first patient operated on by this approach was handicapped (GOS II) by the permanent postoperative facial and abducens palsy. The aneurysm was completely clipped in all but one, which had a wide aneurysm neck. On the postoperative CT scan, no brain damage was found in the accessed side.

Discussion

In the recent years, various types of transpetrosal approaches have been developed for petroclival tumors[3-6], and extent of the petrous bone resection offers a wide surgical view for skull base surgery. For aneurysm surgery, however, a selective key hole resection of the petrous bone is important to shorten the time of operation and to minimize the surgical complications, such as hearing loss, facial palsy or cerebrospinal fluid leakage. The selective resection of the anterior petrous bone did not result in any functional or cosmetic disadvantage. This approach may be superior to the suboccipital approach, without a chance of hazardous lower cranial nerves injury, expecially when the aneurysm projected posteriorly. As the lower limit of the surgical view is the level of the VIIth nerve, the lateral suboccipital or the transcondylar route may be selected when the location of the aneurysm is lower than the internal auditory meatus.

References

1. Kawase T, Toya S, Shiobara R, Mine S (1985) Transpetrosal approach for aneurysms of the lower basilar artery. J Neurosurg 63: 857–861
2. Shiobara R, Ohira T, Kanzaki J, Toya S (1988) A modified extended middle cranial fossa approach for acoustic nerve tumors. J Neurosurg 68: 358–365
3. Kawase T, Shiobara R, Toya S (1991) Anterior transpetrosal-transtentorial approach for sphenopetroclival meningomas: surgical method and results in 10 patients. Neurosurgery 28: 869–876
4. Hakuba A, Nishimura S, Jang BJ (1988) A combined retroauricular and preauricular transpetrosal transtentorial approach to clivus meningiomas. Surg Neurol 30: 108–116
5. Samii M, Ammirati M (1988) The combined supra-infratentorial presigmoid sinus avenue to the petro-clival region. Surgical technique and clinical applications. Acta Neurochir (Wien) 95: 6–12
6. Sen CN, Sekhar LN (1990) The subtemporal and preauricular infratemporal approach to intradural structures ventral to the brain stem. J Neurosurg 73: 345–354

Correspondence: Takeshi Kawase, M.D., Department of Neurosurgery, School of Medicine, Keio University, 35 Shinanomachi, Shinjuku-ku, Tokyo 160, Japan.

Endovascular Treatment of Aneurysms

Standard and Giant Aneurysms: the Role of Endovascular Therapy

C.F. Dowd, R.T. Higashida, V.V. Halbach, T.P. Smith, K.W. Fraser, and G.B. Hieshima

Department of Neurological Surgery, University of California, San Francisco Medical Center, San Francisco, California, U.S.A.

Summary

Cerebral aneurysms are currently being treated by endovascular techniques when craniotomy and surgical clipping is not feasible. We have treated 301 aneurysms using interventional neurovascular methods since 1981. These aneurysms include 227 anterior circulation (140 extradural) and 74 posterior circulation aneurysms. Forty-two percent of the 161 intradural aneurysms in this series presented with subarachnoid hemorrhage. Embolic materials included detachable silicone balloons, fibered coils, and electrically detachable coils. Complications of endovascular therapy include stroke (5.9%) and mortality related to the aneurysm (7.6%). Fusiform, multilobular, giant, and previously treated aneurysms require special consideration because of the need for parent artery occlusion, combination of embolic material, and vigilance against recurrence of aneurysm neck or migration of embolic material into intra-aneurysmal thrombus. Endovascular therapy can provide effective therapy for cerebral aneurysms when surgical therapy is not feasible.

Keywords: Aneurysm; embolization; interventional neuroradiology; subarachnoid hemorrhage.

Introduction

Craniotomy, surgical exploration, and clipping remains the choice therapeutic option for patients with cerebral aneurysms. This is not feasible in certain clinical settings, as surgery may be precluded by inaccessible location of the aneurysm, excessive size of the aneurysm or its neck, or underlying medical condition precluding general anesthesia. Under such circumstances, aneurysm therapy using interventional neurovascular methods has become the standard alternative.

The first reports of endovascular aneurysmal therapy emerged in 1974, when Serbinenko[15] described his use of detachable balloons for intracranial aneurysms. Many technical advances have come forth in the intervening years, including improvement in imaging capabilities and development of new embolic materials. A number of centers now are able to provide endo-vascular therapy and nearly all types of intracranial aneurysms have been treated in this fashion.

Over the past 11 years, we have been involved in the treatment of 301 cerebral aneurysms using a variety of endovascular therapeutic techniques. This paper summarizes our experience.

Methods and Materials

Since 1981, we have treated a total of 301 patients with intracranial aneurysms using endovascular methods. All patients are initially considered for craniotomy and surgical clipping, which we consider to be the primary treatment method. Our indications for endovascular therapy include prior surgical exploration of the aneurysm with inability to properly place the clip, aneurysm in a surgically inaccessible anatomic region, aneurysm without a well-defined anatomic neck, and inability of the patient to tolerate general anesthesia because of an underlying medical condition. Therefore, our patient population represents a subset high-risk group. All patients were fully informed regarding the nature of the procedure and gave informed consent prior to treatment.

Our 301 aneurysms consisted on 227 anterior circulation (87 intradural) and 74 posterior circulation aneurysms (Table 1). Of 161 intradural aneurysms, 67 (42%) presented with subarachnoid hemorrhage (Table 2). Of the 87 intradural anterior circulation aneurysms, 58 (67%) presented with mass effect and 24 (28%) with subarachnoid hemorrhage. Of the 74 posterior circulation aneurysms, 43 (58%)

Table 1. *Aneurysm Locations*

Anterior circulation	227
Petrous ICA	7
Cavernous ICA	133
Supraclinoid ICA	73
Middle cerebral	6
Anterior cerebral	8
Posterior circulation	74
Vertebral	25
Basilar	43
Posterior cerebral	6

Table 2. *Intradural Aneurysms: Presenting Symptoms*

Anterior circulation	87	
Mass effect		58 (67%)
Subarachnoid hemorrhage		24 (28%)
Posterior circulation	74	
Mass effect		30 (41%)
Subarachnoid hemorrhage		43 (58%)

Table 3. *Embolic Materials*

Detachable silicone balloons	268 aneurysms
Fibered coils	8
Guglielmi detachable coils (GDC)	25

presented with subarachnoid hemorrhage and 30 (41%) with mass effect. The 301 aneurysms were treated with detachable balloons[10] (268 cases), fibered coils[2] (8), and the Guglielmi Detachable Coil (GDC)[5,6] (25).

All procedures were performed in the interventional neuroangiographic suite with direct fluoroscopic visualization. Unless contraindicated, the procedures are performed with local anesthesia to allow full neurological testing. Arterial access is gained via femoral artery puncture and a guiding catheter is navigated to the internal carotid or vertebral artery accessing the aneurysms. The embolization procedure is performed under full heparinization. In some instances, test occlusion of the affected artery is performed. In the internal carotid artery, a 7.0-French non-detachable fixed balloon catheter with a distal end port (Meditech, Inc., Watertown, Massachusetts) was used to test-occlude the internal carotid artery for 30 minutes under full heparinization and constant neurological monitoring. The end port allows arterial pressure measurements to be obtained before, during, and after balloon inflation.

Detachable silicone balloons (Interventional Therapeutics Corp., South San Francisco, California) were navigated to the aneurysm site or parent vessel occlusion site on a 2-French catheter. If placed directly within the aneurysm allowing parent vessel patency, a mixture of metrizamide and 2 hydroxyethyl methacrylate (HEMA)[4] was placed into the balloon to allow solidification and stabilization. Fibered coils ("Hilal" coils, Cook, Inc., Bloomington, Indiana) were placed into the aneurysm through a 2.2-French Tracker catheter (Target Therapeutics, Fremont, CA) with the use of a coil pusher. GDCs (Target Therapeutics) were placed into the aneurysm through a specially designed (0.010 or 0.018 inch) Tracker catheter, and a monopolar electric current was conducted along the coil to allow thrombus formation around the coil in the aneurysm and detachment of the coil at a predetermined location by electrolysis.

After the procedure, all patients were monitored in the hospital for at least 2 days. Skull radiographs or other imaging studies were used to insure that the embolic materials had not shifted or deflated and close neurological evaluation was carried out.

Post-embolization angiograms were obtained in all patients except for some who underwent parent artery occlusion. Follow-up angiography is performed at variable time intervals to assess degree of aneurysm occlusion.

Results

301 aneurysms were treated with either detachable silicone balloons, fibered coils, or electrically detachable coils (Table 3). In cases where the parent artery was preserved, embolic materials were placed into the aneurysm to either obliterate it completely, or as much as possible when placement of additional embolic material was precluded by the small residual aneurysm volume. Alternately, the parent artery was occluded either by placing detachable balloons proximal to the site of the aneurysm or via a "trapping procedure", with materials placed either across the aneurysm site or proximal and distal to the aneurysm.

Results and complications of endovascular therapy of posterior circulation aneurysms[8], cavernous carotid artery aneurysms[11], aneurysms with preserved parent arteries[9], and aneurysms in a large series of 215 patients[12] have been reported previously. Among the more difficult aneurysms to treat, 10 of 88 cases (11.4%) in which direct aneurysm embolization allowed parent artery preservation, a second endovascular procedure was required because of residual aneurysm filling on long-term control angiography[12].

In our current series of 301 patients, 18 (5.9%) suffered stroke as a result of the procedure with another 15 patients (4.9%) experiencing a reversible transient ischemic event. Twenty-three patients (7.6%) expired as a direct result of the aneurysm and its therapy, and another 6 patients (2.0%) as a result of other medical conditions (myocardial infarction, pulmonary embolus, etc.).

$\longrightarrow$

Fig. 1. 76 year old woman with orbital pain and a third cranial nerve palsy. (A) Transaxial contrast–enhanced computed tomography (*CT*) scan shows a giant, partially thrombosed right cavernous internal carotid artery (*ICA*) aneurysm, eroding the sella. Note aneurysm lumen (small closed arrows) and surrounding mural thrombus (large open arrows). (B) and (C) Right ICA arteriogram, frontal (B) and lateral (C) projections, shows the aneurysm lumen. Unusually small neck (C, arrow) is present for an aneurysm of the size, permitting direct embolization and preservation of the *ICA* in this elderly woman. (D) Superselective catheterization of the cavernous aneurysm, lateral projection, prior to detachable coil embolization. Note layering of contrast within aneurysm (arrows). (E) and (F) Right ICA arteriogram, frontal (E) and lateral (F) projections, after deposition of multiple Guglielmi Detachable Coils (GDCs). Small residual neck is identified (E, arrow). (G) Plain skull film, lateral projection, post-embolization, shows multiple redioopaque GDCs

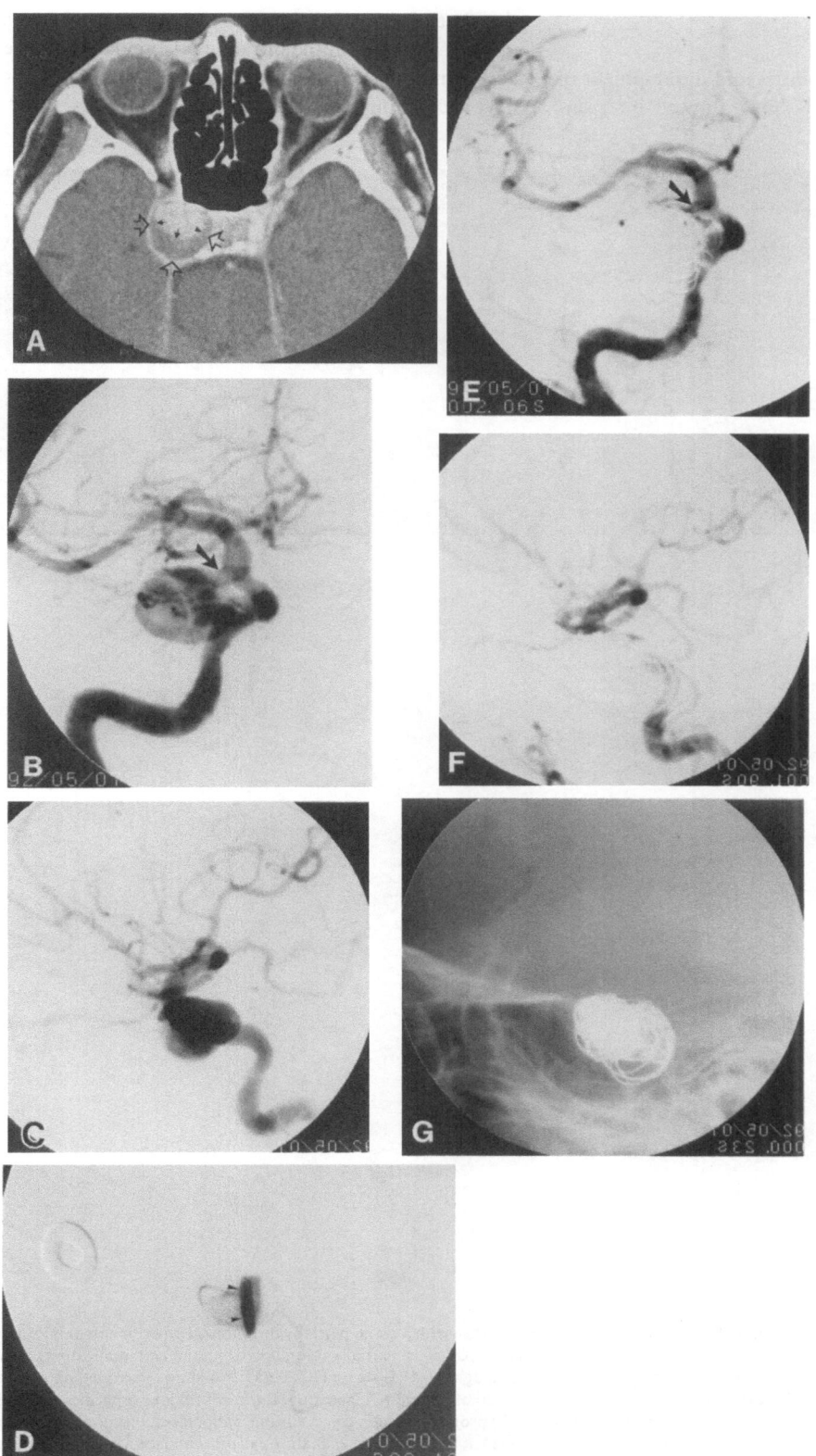

Discussion

Advances in imaging capabilities and development of improved embolic materials have allowed interven-

tional neuroradiologists to access and treat aneurysms in most locations in the intracranial circulation. Since Serbeninko's[15] seminal work in 1974, other groups have successfully used endovascular techniques[1,3,7,14].

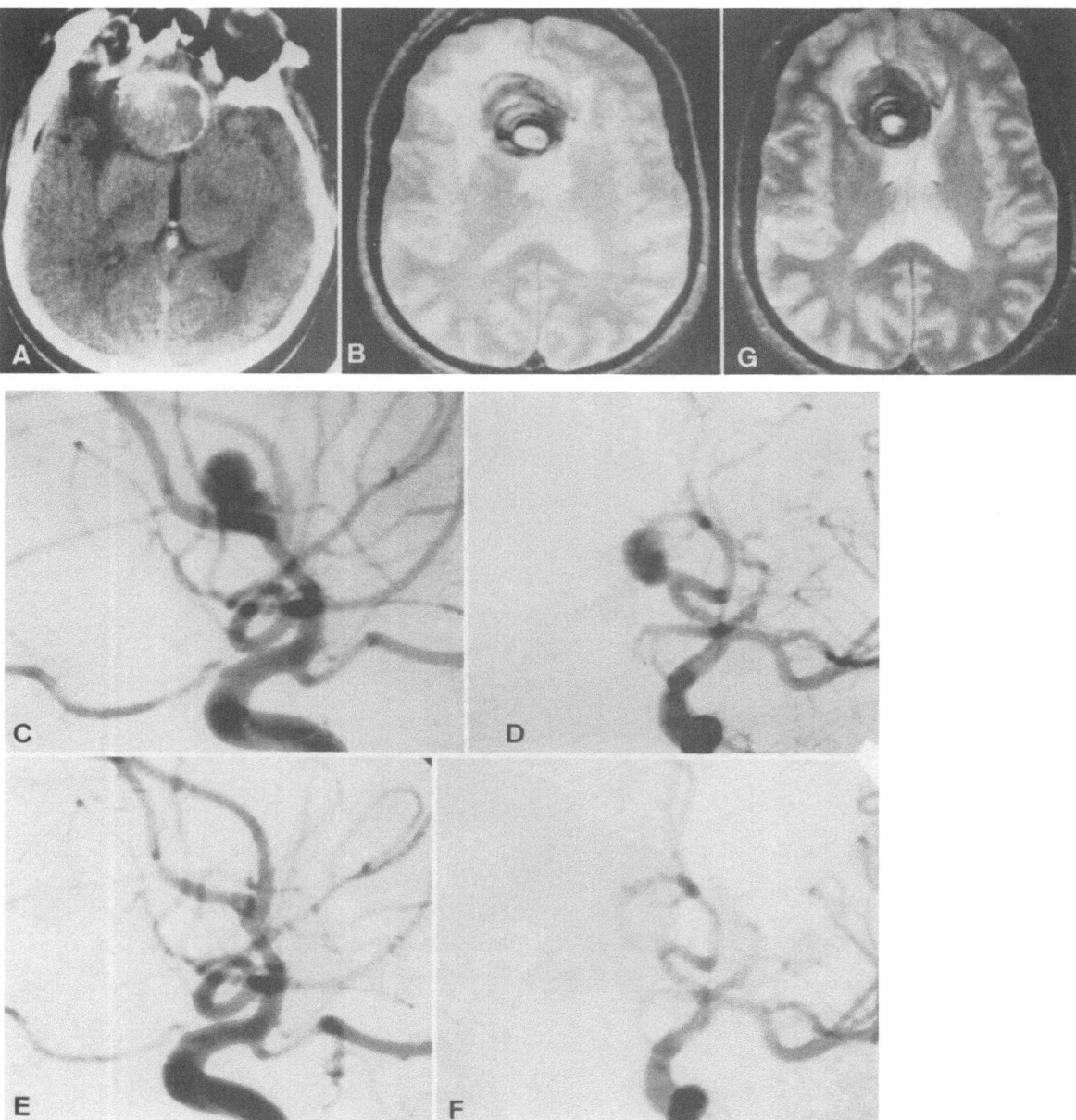

Fig. 2. Reduction in aneurysmal mass effect after embolization. 56 years old man with a giant, partially thrombosed anterior communicating artery aneurysm. (A) transaxial computed tomography (CT) scan shows a giant, calcified, partially thrombosed anterior communicating artery aneurysm, with surrounding edema. (B) Transaxial magnetic resonance imaging (MRI) scan (TR2800/TE 80) shows surrounding edema (high-signal) more clearly. (C) and (D) Left internal carotid (ICA) arteriogram, lateral (C), and frontal (D) projections, opacifies residual aneurysm lumen. (E) and (F) left ICA arteriogram, lateral (E), and fronal (F) projections, after direct silicone balloon embolization, shows no residual aneurysm filling. (G) transaxial MRI scan (TR 2800/TE 80) obtained at the same level as B, shows significant decrease in the amount of edema surrounding the aneurysm four months after embolization

The first large series was reported by Romodanov and Shcheglov[13] in 1982.

Our group has now achieved significant experience in endovascular therapy in higher risk aneurysms not amenable to standard neurosurgical therapy. Parent artery occlusion for the treatment of aneurysms for which parent artery patency can not be maintained has become an established endovascular procedure, especially with extradural internal carotid aneurysms, large or giant intradural carotid aneurysms, and fusiform vertebral aneurysms. The majority of our experience with parent vessel occlusion lies in the treatment of cavernous carotid aneurysms. Thrombosis of the aneurysm can be achieved in all cases by this technique and we have previously reported a 2.3% rate of delayed thromboembolic symptoms and a 4.6% stroke rate after therapy. In this patient population, no deaths occurred[11].

Direct aneurysm embolization, either with balloons or coils, is necessary in the majority of intradural aneurysms because of the risk of parent vessel occlusion. We do not consider an aneurysm fully treated if even a small neck remnant is present, and for this reason close angiographic follow-up is necessary. This higher risk group of aneurysms reflects the patient selection criteria at our institution, because we well accept for treatment only those patients who are not considered condidates for standard neurosurgical clipping. In particular, giant aneurysms provide special problems for the endovascular therapist (Fig. 1). Frequently, large or giant aneurysms exhibit a wide or absent (fusiform) aneurysm neck. This precludes preservation of the parent artery, because any embolic materials placed within the aneurysm will likely herniate into the parent vessel risking occlusion or thromboembolism. Many larger aneurysm demonstrate partial thrombosis prior to therapy. We have considerable experience in slicone balloon embolization of these partially-thrombosed large and giant aneurysms. Potential pitfalls include dislodging of thrombus to cause embolism in a normal distal vessel, and migration of the balloon into the thrombus allowing regrowth of the aneurysm neck. For this reason, close follow-up of these partially thrombosed aneurysms is necessary to exclude the development of this phenomenon and to allow early retreatment if necessary. This is true even a perfect angiographic result is achieved initially. Pre-therapy computed tomography (CT) or magnetic resonance imaging (MRI) scans will assist in determining whether partial thrombosis of an aneurysm has occurred and in predicting the potential for thromboembolism or

balloon migration into clot. We hope that the long-term data on therapeutic results of treatment with the GDC will demonstrate a smaller rate of migration of this embolic agent into the thrombus, but this information is not yet available. Large and giant aneurysms generally require more embolic material, thereby increasing the risk of this therapy to the patient with the addition of each balloon or coil. These aneurysms may also produce a significant amount of mass effect or edema within the brain which can be reduced by eliminating the residual aneurysm lumen (Fig. 2).

Long term data, as exist for standard neurosurgical treatment, regarding angiographic and clinical outcome and complications of endovascular therapy is not yet available in a very large number of these higher risk patients. As our experience accrues, the role of endovascular therapy in the treatment of cerebral aneurysms will be defined more clearly.

Acknowledgement

The authors would like to thank Joy Jacobson for her expert assistance in preparing this manuscript.

References

1. Debrun G, Fox A, Drake C, Peerless S, Girvin J, Ferguson G (1981) Giant unclippable aneurysms: treatment with detachable balloons. AJNR 2: 167–173
2. Dowd CF, Halbach VV, Higashida RT, Barnwell SL, Hieshima GB (1990) Endovascular coil embolization of unusual posterior inferior cerebellar artery aneurysms. Neurosurgery 27: 954–961
3. Fox AJ, Vinuela F, Pelz DM, et al (1987) Use of detachable balloons for proximal artery occlusion in the treatment of unclippable cerebral aneurysms. J Neurosurg 66: 40–46
4. Goto K, Halbach VV, Hardin CW, Highashida RT, Hieshima GB (1988) Permanent inflation of detachable balloons with a low viscosity, hydrophilic polymerizing system. Radiology 169: 787–790
5. Guglielmi G, Vinuela F, Sepetka I, Macellari V (1991) Electrothrombosis of saccular aneurysms via endovascular approach. Part 1: electrochemical basis, technique, and experimental results. J Neurosurg 75: 1–7
6. Guglielmi G, Vinuela F, Dion J, Duckwiler G (1991) Electrothrombosis of saccular aneurysms via endovascular approach. Part 2: preliminary clinical experience. J Neurosurgery 75: 8–14
7. Halbach VV, Higashida RT, Hieshima GB (1987) Treatment of intracranial aneurysms by balloon embolization. Semin Intervent Radiol 4: 261–268
8. Higashida RT, Halbach VV, Cahan LD, Hieshima GB, Konishi Y (1989) Detachable balloon embolization therapy of posterior circulation intracranial aneurysms. J Neurosurg 71: 512–519
9. Higashida RT, Halbach VV, Barnwell SL, Dowd C, Dormandy B, Bell J, Hieshima GB (1990) Treatment of intracranial aneurysms with preservation of the parent vessel: results of percutaneous balloon embolization in 84 patients. AJNR 11: 633–640
10. Higashida RT, Halbach VV, Dormandy B, Bell J, Hieshima GB (1990) Endovascular treatment of intracranial aneurysms with a

new silicone microballoon device: technical considerations and indications for therapy. Radiology 174: 687–691

11. Higashida RT, Halbach VV, Dowd C, Barnwell SL, Dormandy B, Bell J, Hieshima GB (1990) Endovascular detachable balloon embolization therapy of cavernous carotid artery aneurysms: results in 87 cases. J Neurosurg 72: 857–863

12. Higashida RT, Halbach VV, Dowd CF, Barnwell SL, Hieshima GB (1991) Intracranial aneurysms: interventional neurovascular treatment with detachable balloons. Results in 215 cases. Radiology 178: 663–670

13. Romodanov AP, Shcheglov VI (1982) Intravascular occlusion of saccular aneurysms of the cerebral arteries by means of a detachable balloon catheter. Adv Tech Stand Neurosurg 9: 25–48

14. Scialfa G, Vaghi A, Vaseccgu F, Bernardi L, Tonon C (1982) Neuroradiological treatment of carotid and vertebral fistulas and intracavernous aneurysms. Neuroradiology 24: 13–25

15. Serbinenko FA (1974) Balloon catherterization and occlusion of major cerebral vessels. J Neurosurg 41: 125–145

Correspondence: Christopher F. Dowd, M.D., Department of Neurological Surgery, University of California, San Francisco Medical Center, 505 Parnassus Ave., Room L-352, San Francisco, CA 94143-0628, U.S.A.

Endovascular Treatment of Intracranial Saccular Aneurysms with GDC Platinum Detachable Coils: Small-Necked Aneurysms

G. Guglielmi[1] and F. Vinuela[2]

[1] University of Rome Medical School, Rome, Italy, and [2] University of California, Los Angeles, California, U.S.A.

Summary

The rationale for treatment of small intracranial aneurysms is to avoid bleeding in unruptured ones or to prevent rebleeding in ruptured ones. In an effort to widen the therapeutic management of surgically difficult intracranial aneurysms, an endovascular approach utilizing platinum detachable coils and electrothrombosis has been developed[1,2].

To date about 250 patients have been treated with this technique, in a multicenter study involving several Institutions that have been approved by the Food and Drug Administration to determine the safety and efficacy of the method. The data included in this paper are results of a sub-group of 21 patients with 23 small-necked aneurysms out of 59 patients with 63 aneurysms treated at our Institution. The majority of cases had intracranial aneurysms considered to be technically difficult and to carry a high surgical risk; the remaining cases were either inoperable for medical reasons or had already undergone unsuccessful surgical exploration.

It was possible to enter all aneurysms with a microcatheter-microguidewire combination. It was always possible, before detachment, to retrieve the GDC coil from the aneurysm if inappropriate in size or position. Failure of electrolytic detachment did not occur.

An immediate, complete occlusion could be achieved in most (20) of these small-necked aneurysms. At follow-up angiograms, aneurysms that were completely occluded continued to be completely occluded. These results must be confirmed with longer-term angiographic follow-up.

Keywords: Aneurysms; endovascular treatment.

Introduction

In the neurosurgical literature aneurysms are classically subdivided in saccular and fusiform, depending on the presence or not of a definite neck. While a great deal of attention has been paid to the dimensions of the sac of saccular aneurysms (small, large, and giant), less informations are available on the size of the aneurysm neck. This is probably due to the fact that, in general, small aneurysms have a small neck whilst large and giant aneurysms have a wide neck. Therefore the concept "aneurysm neck size" is incorporated in the concept "aneurysm dimensions". From the neurosurgical perspective the factor that mostly affects the technical operative difficulties is the size of the sac, meant as an obstacle to expose the neck.

From the point of view of neuro-endovascular therapy with GDC coils, on the contrary, the diameter of the aneurysm neck, more than the dimensions of the sac, is the critical factor, particularly in foreseeing whether the treatment will be complete or not[3,5,6]. A small neck holds the GDC coils inside the aneurysm and allows dense coil packing without impingment on the parent vessel and with little risk of coil migration. Furthermore, the smaller the neck, the higher the probability that the mesh of coils bridges across the neck area, the neck being the location of the elastic lining defect initially responsible for aneurysm formation.

Materials and Methods

To date 59 patients with 63 intracranial saccular aneurysms have been treated with platinum electrically detachable coils and electro-thrombosis, via the endovascular approach. The technique and the patients selection criteria have already been reported[1-3].

Out of these 63 treated aneurysms, 23 had a small neck. The wide-neck versus small-neck border is arbitrarily considered to be 4 mm. The goal of this report is to present the results of treatment with the GDC coil technique in 21 patients harboring 23 small-necked intracranial aneurysms.

Fifteen patients presented with subarachnoid hemorrhage (SAH) (71.5%). Eight aneurysms were incidentally found (35%). Eight of the fifteen patients that presented with hemorrhage were in grade I or II, two were in grade III, and five were in grade IV or V. Treatment was performed in the acute phase after SAH (0 to 15 days post hemorrhage) in 12 cases. Eight aneurysms originated at the basilar artery bifurcation and four from the posterior inferior cerebellar artery. Internal carotid artery bifurcation (one case), internal carotid artery at the level of the ophthalmic artery (two cases) or of the posterior communicating artery (one case), intracavernous carotid (one case), middle cerebral artery (two cases), vertebro-basilar junction (two aneurysms), basilar artery trunk (one case), and P1 segment of the posterior cerebral artery (one aneurysm) represent the other locations. Twenty-one aneurysms were small (less than 12 mm), and two were large (12 to 25 mm).

The procedure technique has already been extensively reported[1-4]. However there are some details, particularly important in the treatment of small aneurysms, that is worthwhile to highlight.

1) Most procedures were performed using both local anesthesia at the groin and sedation with neuroleptic analgesia (16 out of 21 cases). Five patients in grades IV and V were already intubated before starting the procedure.

2) High quality (motionless) road mapping and subtraction fluoroscopy are mandatory for a safe catheterization of the aneurysm and for delivery, proper positioning, and detachment of the first coil. The microguidewire-microcatheter combination is less soft than the platinum portion of the GDC coils and should not touch the aneurysm wall (i.e. risk of aneurysm perforation). Without road mapping capability the risk of perforating the aneurysm with the delivery system is potentially high, particularly in small aneurysms. Road mapping also insures that, during the positioning of the first coil, none is deposited in the parent vessel. After first coil detachment, normal fluoroscopy may be used: the first coil constitutes a landmark that, indicating the position of the aneurysm neck, prevents any deposit of the second and subsequent coils in the parent vessel.

3) The combination Tracker 10 microcatheter-Seeker 10 (or Seeker 10 Lite) microguidewire is always used for small aneurysms. Consequently only GDC coils 0.010 in. in diameter are suitable for these aneurysms. The 0.015 in. GDC coils (that require the Tracker 18-Seeker 14 combination) are used for large unruptured and giant aneurysms.

4) The tip of the microcatheter must be steam shaped, if necessary, according to the geometric characteristics of the vascular complex parent vessel-aneurysm. The ideal position is when the microcatheter tip is floating in the middle of the aneurysm, without touching its inner walls. For internal carotid bifurcation aneurysms and for basilar bifurcation aneurysms it is usually not necessary to shape the microcatheter.

5) The importance of the proximal radiopaque markers as a safety feature has been already outlined in previous reports[3,5,6]. Their presence and usefulness is particularly relevant in small aneurysms, preventing aneurysm perforation with the stainless steel carrying portion of the GDC coils.

Results

An immediate and complete aneurysm occlusion was obtained in 20 aneurysms (87%) (Fig. 1). In two aneurysms a small triangular neck remnant was left patent. In one case a rectangular neck remnant was successfully clipped 3 months after endovascular treatment.

The angiographic follow-up, performed on 10 patients, ranged from 3 to 14 months (mean 5.3 months). The clinical follow-up period ranged from one month to 27 months (mean 14 months).

In this series of 21 cases there were two transient and two permanent neurologic deficit related to treatment. The transient neurologic deficit resolved within 48 hours after treatment. The permanent deficit were quadrantanopsia (one case) and memory deficit (one case).

One patient, harboring a recently ruptured posterior inferior cerebellar artery aneurysm, died in relation

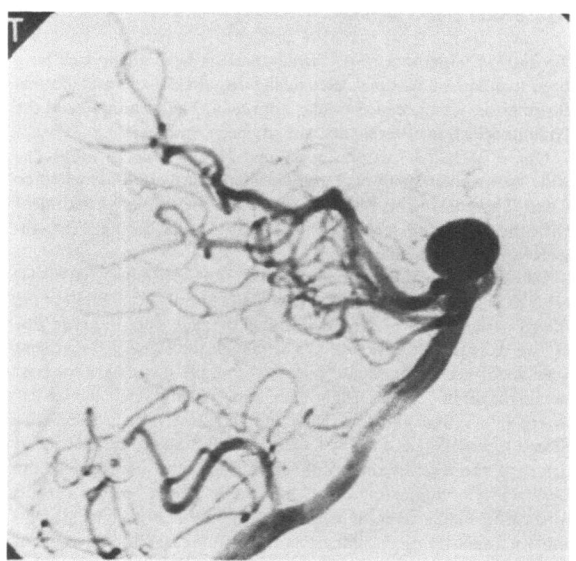 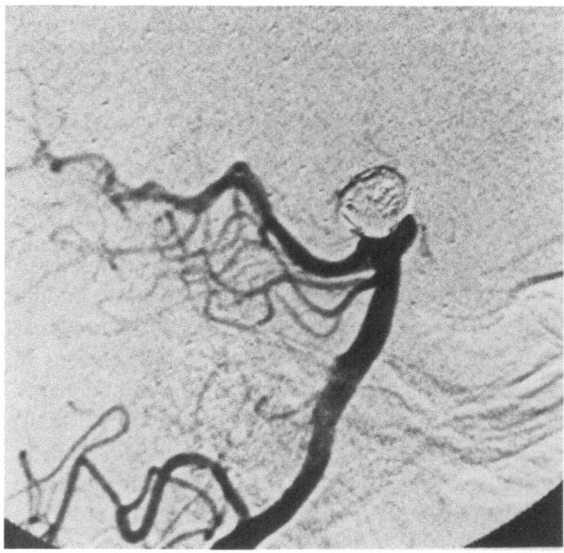

a   b

Fig. 1. (a) Left vertebral injection, lateral view, showing an unruptured basilar bifurcation aneurysm. (b) After detachment of four GDC coils for a total length of 85 cm, the aneurysm is completely occluded. A three months follow-up angiogram showed persistency of occlusion to the endovascular therapy. In this patient the aneurysm re-ruptured after detachment of a first coil, due to penetration of the fresh clot with the microcatheter. The patient, who was originally in grade V, died 5 days later. One patient, harboring a basilar bifurcation aneurysm, died one month after treatment because of an unrelated disease. The autopsy showed that marantic endocarditis had produced multiple organ infarctions. The patients treated while in grade IV (one case) or V (four cases) did not recover from the damage of the original bleeding and eventually died (four cases) or remained in a vegetative state (one case).

In grades 0, I, II and III patients, the morbidity/mortality rates related to technique are 12.5% and 0%, respectively.

Discussion

Currently, aneurysm treatment with preservation of the parent artery is performed by open surgical clipping. An alternative endovascular technique would be of benefit in patients that cannot undergo classic surgery. Selection of patients for this endovascular treatment is currently based on six criteria: 1) failure of surgical exploration; 2) poor surgical candidates secondary to hemorrhage (Hunt and Hess grade IV or V); 3) poor surgical candidates secondary to medical conditions; 4) inoperability secondary to anatomical considerations; 5) aneurysms considered to be difficult and to have too high a risk for surgery; 6) regrowth of the aneurysm after surgery. The advantages of the endovascular approach are that craniotomy and brain manipulation are unnecessary.

It is possible to achieve a dense aneurysm packing and complete occlusion in aneurysms with a small neck; a narrow aneurysm neck holds the coils inside the aneurysm allowing dense coil packing without impinging on the parent vessel. Small-necked aneurysms that were completely occluded remained occluded at follow-up angiograms. Longer-term follow-up angiographic studies are necessary, however, to assess the long term efficacy of this endovascular technique.

References

1. Guglielmi G, Vinuela F, Sepetka I, Macellari V (1991) Electrothrombosis of saccular aneurysms via endovascular approach. Part 1: electrochemical basis, technique and experimental results. J Neurosurg 75: 1–7
2. Guglielmi G, Vinuela F, Dion J, Duckwiler G (1991) Electrothrombosis of saccular aneurysms via endovascular approach. Part 2: preliminary clinical experience. J Neurosurg 75: 8–14
3. Guglielmi G, Vinuela F, Duckwiler G, Dion J, Lylyk P, Berenstein A, Strother C, Graves V, Halbach V, Nichols D, Hopkins N, Ferguson R, Sepetka I (1992) Endovascular treatment of posterior circulation aneurysm by electrothrombosis using electrically detachable coils. J Neurosurg 77: 515–524
4. Guglielmi G, Vinuela F, Briganti F, et al (1992) Carotid-cavernous fistula caused by a ruptured intracavernous aneurysm: endovascular treatment by electrothrombosis with detachable coils. Neurosurgery 31: 591–597
5. Guglielmi G (1992) Embolization of intracranial aneurysms with detachable coils and electrothrombosis. In: Vinuela F, et al (eds) Interventional neuroradiology: endovascular therapy of the central nervous system. Raven, New York, pp 63–75
6. Guglielmi G (1992) Endovascular treatment of intracranial aneurysms. In: Interventional neuroradiology. Neuroimaging Clinics of North America 2: 269–278

Correspondence: Guido Guglielmi, M.D., Servicio di Neuroradiologia II, Dip. di Scienze Neurologiche, Universita La Sapienza, Viale Dell' Universita 30, I–00185 Roma, Italy.

Internal Carotid Artery Balloon Test Occlusion Does Require Quantitative Assessment of CBF

J.-P. Witt[1], H. Yonas[1,2], and D.W. Johnson[2]

Departments of [1]Neurological Surgery and [2]Radiology, University of Pittsburgh Medical Center, Pittsburgh, Pennsylvania, U.S.A.

Summary

At our institution intra-arterial balloon test occlusions (BTOs) in combination with Stable Xenon enhanced CT (Xe/CT) cerebral blood flow (CBF) studies prior to radiological or surgical treatment have been performed in more than 400 patients since 1985 in order to evaluate the risk of temporary or permanent internal carotid artery (ICA) occlusion. We reviewed studies of 156 patients who passed the clinical BTO and underwent a Xe/CT CBF study in combination with a second BTO. The quantitative CBF data were analyzed for absolute changes as well as changes in symmetry. Fourteen patients showed CBF values between 20 and 30 cc/100g/min, an absolute CBF decrease, and a significant asymmetry in the middle cerebral artery (MCA) territory during BTO. These patients were considered at high risk for cerebral infarction following ICA occlusion. With one exception they belonged to a group of 61 patients at increased stroke risk who showed a bilateral or ipsilateral CBF decrease and a significant asymmetry with lower flow on the side of occlusion. The other 95 patients who showed a variety of CBF response patterns including ipsilateral or bilateral CBF increase, in our eyes, were at moderate or low stroke risk. In contrast to this, an exclusively qualitative CBF analysis lacks sensitivity and specificity to identify the patients at high risk. Thus, by an integration of a thorough analysis of quantitative CBF data before and during BTO we achieved a hemodynamic related overall stroke rate of 10% in 33 patients who underwent permanent clinical ICA occlusion.

Keywords: Balloon test occlusion; cerebral blood flow; cerebral infarction; internal carotid artery.

Introduction

Elective internal carotid artery (ICA) occlusion has remained the main stay of treatment for difficult intra-cavernous aneurysms[2,4,5,9,19]. For the treatment of many aneurysms ICA occlusion is sufficient to cause thrombosis, subsequently aneurysm shrinkage and the recovery of cranial nerve function. The major problem with this approach has been a relatively constant rate of subsequent stroke due presumably to both embolic and hemodynamic mechanisms[4,9,11,19].

In order to minimize hemodynamic compromise, some clinicians have elected to occlude only the common carotid artery allowing continued flow from the external to the internal carotid artery[21]. An alternative approach has been to assess the quality of collateral supply prior to ICA occlusion and therefore either taking measures to avoid occlusion or taking alternate approaches to ICA occlusion including vascular reconstruction or bypass procedures[19,5]. Strategies for collateral testing have evolved from temporary finger compression of the carotid to temporary endovascular balloon test occlusion (BTO) of the ICA[1,3,7,8,10,12,14,15,20,22]. In five to ten percent of patients balloon inflation is accompanied by the onset of neurological deficit which is rapidly reversible and clearly indicates a severe risk for elective permanent ICA occlusion[13,19]. While this approach has provided some valuable insights, patients that have passed this test have still had a roughly ten percent stroke rate with their strokes often being massive and life-threatening.

Methods

It has been our contention at the University of Pittsburgh that an additional group of patients could be identified that clinically pass BTO (therefore CBF > 15–20 ml/100 g/min) but still have compromised collaterals. Ipsilateral flow values in such patients might fall between 20–30 ml/100 g/min on the side of occlusion and therefore indicate a direct dependence on blood pressure for maintenance of adequate blood supply. A greater awareness of and particular attention to this group of patients at moderate stroke risk, we believe, allows us to further lessen what would likely be an increased stroke rate in this subgroup of about 10% of our patients.

We have utilized Stable Xe/CT CBF[6] studies performed during and immediately after temporary balloon test occlusion to identify the group presumably at moderate ischemic risk. The risk of this procedure has been acceptably low and with definition of patients where flow values fall to 20–30 ml/100g/min, alternate approaches to either early vascular reconstruction and or increased pharmacological protection during surgery have been implemented.

Results

A recent review of our series of 33 consecutive internal carotid artery occlusions performed both intraoperatively or with endovascular balloon placement in patients who passed clinical and CBF criteria also demonstrated 10 percent stroke rate[13]. These CT defined new lesions, however, were small borderzone lesions found in one still asymptomatic, one transiently symptomatic and one mildly symptomatic patient with no individual suffering a massive stroke as commonly reported with stroke following carotid occlusion.

Recently technically less demanding non-quantitative CBF methods had been proposed as substitutes for the type of quantitative flow assessment provided by Xe/CT CBF. While the benefits of quantitative CBF are still being defined, we have questioned whether the qualitative data obtained with SPECT utilizing tracers such as HMPAO or Iodamphetamine could yield equivalent results[16-18]. In order to examine this question we have examined our Xe/CT CBF data as if it were qualitative by subjecting it to an examination of asymmetry, i.e. $> 10\%$ lower on the side of occlusion. If asymmetry was found with a SPECT study, a repeat study (done on the next day) would be obtained to identify if symmetry had been present prior to BTO. In the article by Monsein et al.[16], in which a few patients also underwent a quantitative assessment of flow, it was noted that CBF response to BTO did include the possibility of an increase of CBF following BTO.

From an analysis of 156 pairs of CBF studies (Fig. 1) we conclude that the CBF response to brief ICA occlusion is highly variable with many territories developing symmetrical or asymmetrical elevations of CBF as developing symmetrical and asymmetrical decreases of CBF. Thus, of 58 individuals that are symmetrical with balloon test occlusion, only 29 were symmetrical during studies with the carotid artery being open (and none of these had flow values below 30 ml/100g/min). Asymmetrical flows were found on baseline studies in 29 individuals. In this group no patient, in fact, had flow below 30 ml/100g/min with balloon occlusion despite symmetry of flow. Conversely, of those individuals with lower flow values on the side of BTO (n = 81) 14 had ipsilateral flow reduction to less than 30 ml/100g/min (17%). 6 of the 42 individuals who had baseline symmetrical flows actually had flows

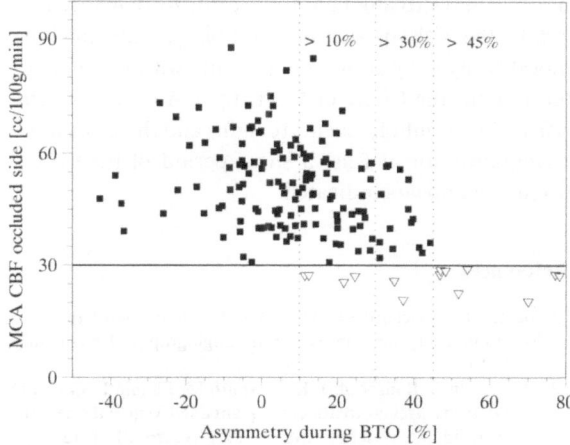

Fig. 1. CBF response pattern to BTO. Note number of CBF values <30cc/100g/min in each group referring to the BTO CBF study. Width of connecting line correlates with number of patients. Degree of asymmetry is symbolized by degree of line tilting

less than 30 ml/100g/min while 8 of 39 patients with baseline asymmetry and BTO asymmetry had flows less than 30 ml/100g/min. Asymmetrical CBF during BTO with lower flow on the contralateral side were found in 17 of 156 patients, of which only 1 patient developed CBF below 30 ml/100g/min.

Discussion

Therefore, the assumption that the only CBF response to balloon test occlusion are either a symmetrical fall of CBF or a reduction of flow only on the side of occlusion is false. As suggested by Monsein et al.[16], CBF response to BTO is complex and ranges from elevation to depression of CBF as well as symmetrical to asymmetrical responses depending on the quality of collateral blood supply about the Circle of Willis. Only with a quantitative assessment of absolute flow values can individuals who actually decrease flow to near ischemic levels with BTO be identified (about 10% of individuals who clinically pass BTO). Without such a quantitative database 5–10% of patients thought to be safe for permanent carotid occlusion will remain at risk and, conversely, 86% of individuals thought to be at risk would inappropriately not be offered carotid occlusion.

Balloon test occlusion with CBF assessment has helped guide towards safer ICA occlusion with the lessening of the severity of neurological sequelae of this procedure as well as guiding toward more selective use of procedures to augment CBF prior to ICA sacrifice. While the risk of delayed embolic events may be modified by subjecting only patients with good collateral about the Circle of Willis to ICA occlusion, the risk of distal embolic events remains and therefore anticoagulation for at least a short period of time postocclusion appears indicated.

References

1. Beatty RA, Richardson AE (1968) Predicting intolerance to common artery ligation by carotid angiography. J Neurosurg 28: 9–13
2. Berenstein A, Ransohoff J, Kupersmith M, Flamm E, Graeb D (1984) Transvascular treatment of giant aneurysm of the cavernous carotid and vertebral arteries. Surg Neurol 21: 3–12
3. Ehrenfeld WK, Stoney RJ, Wylie EJ (1983) Relation of carotid stump pressure to safety of carotid ligation. Surgery 93: 299–305
4. Fox AJ, Viñuela F, Pelz DM, Peerless SJ, Ferguson GG, Drake CG, Debrun G (1987) Use of detachable balloons for proximal artery occlusion in the treatment of unclippable cerebral aneurysms. J Neurosurg 66: 40–46
5. Gelber BR, Sundt TM Jr (1980) Treatment of intracavernous aneurysms by combined internal carotid ligation and extra- to intracranial bypass. J Neurosurg 52: 1–10
6. Gur D, Good WF, Wolfson SK Jr, Yonas H, Shabason L (1982) In vivo mapping of local cerebral blood flow by xenon-enhanced computed tomography. Science 215: 1267–1268
7. Gurdjian ES, Webster JE, Martin FA (1957) Carotid compression in the neck. Results and significance in carotid ligation. JAMA 163: 1030–1036
8. Hacke W, Zeumer H, Berg-Dammer E (1983) Monitoring of hemispheric or brainstem functions with neurophysiologic methods during interventional neuroradiology. AJNR 4: 382–384
9. Higashida RT, Halbach VV, Dowd C, Barnwell SL, Dormandy B, Bell J, Hieshima GB (1990) Endovascular detachable balloon embolization therapy of cavernous carotid artery aneurysms: result in 87 cases. J Neurosurg 72: 857–863
10. Kwaan JH, Peterson GJ, Connolly JE (1985) Stump pressure. An unreliable guide for shunting during carotid endarterectomy. Arch Surg 115: 1083–1085
11. Landoldt AM, Millikan CH (1970) Pathogenesis of cerebral infarction secondary to mechanical carotid artery occlusion. Stroke 1: 52–62
12. Leech PJ, Miller JD, Fitch W, Barker J (1974) Cerebral blood flow, internal carotid artery pressure, and the EEG as a guide to the safety of carotid ligation. J Neurol Neurosurg Psychiatry 37: 854–862
13. Linskey ME, Sekhar LN, Horton JA, Hirsch WL, Yonas H (1991) Aneurysms of the intracavernous carotid artery: a multidisciplinary approach to treatment. J Neurosurg 75: 525–534
14. Matas R (1914) Testing the efficiency of the collateral circulation as a preliminary to the occlusion of the great surgical arteries. JAMA 63: 1441–1447
15. Meinig G, Gunther P, Ulrich P (1982) Reduced risk of internal carotid artery ligation after balloon occlusion test. Neurosurg Rev 5: 95–98
16. Monsein LH, Jeffrey PJ, van Heerden BB, Szabo Z, Schwartz JR, Camargo EE, Chazaly J (1991) Assessing adequacy of collateral circulation during balloon test occlusion of the internal carotid artery with ^{99m}Tc-HMPAO SPECT. AJNR 12: 1045–1051
17. Moody EB, Dawson RC, Sandler MP (1991) ^{99m}Tc-HMPAO SPECT imaging in interventional neuroradiology: validation of balloon test occlusion. AJNR 12: 1043–1044
18. Peterman SB, Taylor A, Hoffman JC (1991) Improved detection of cerebral hypoperfusion with internal carotid balloon test occlusion and ^{99m}Tc-HMPAO cerebral perfusion SPECT imaging. AJNR 12: 1035–1041
19. Sen C, Sekhar LN (1992) Direct vein graft reconstruction of the cavernous, petrous and upper cervical internal carotid artery: lessons learned from 30 cases. Neurosurgery 30: 732–743
20. Sundt TM Jr, Sharbrough FW, Anderson RE, Michenfelder JD (1974) Cerebral blood flow measurements and electroencephalograms during carotidendarterectomy. J Neurosurg 41: 310–320
21. Swearingen B, Heros RC (1987) Common carotid artery occlusion for unclippable carotid aneurysms: an old but still effective operation. Neurosurgery 21: 288–295
22. Wilkinson HA, Wright RL, Sweet WH (1965) Correlation of reduction in pressure and angiographic cross-filling with tolerance of carotid artery occlusion. J Neurosurg 22: 241–245

Correspondence: Howard Yonas, M.D., Department of Neurological Surgery, B-400 Presbyterian University Hospital, 200 Lothrop Street, Pittsburgh, PA 15213, U.S.A.

Endovascular Treatment of Giant Intracranial Aneurysms by Balloon Occlusion of the Parent Vessel: Clinical and Diagnostic Follow-up

S. Perini, A. Pasqualin[1], P. Zampieri, M.G. Pecoraro, A. Talacchi[1], A. Maschio, L. Rosta, and A. Benati

Department of Neuroradiology and [1]Neurosurgery, City Hospital, Verona, Italy

Summary

From 1985 to 1991, 20 carotid artery aneurysms (12 intracavernous, 7 ophthalmic, 1 intra-petrous) and 2 vertebro-basilar aneurysms were treated in our Department by detachable balloon occlusion of the parent vessel. Presenting symptoms were the following: a) expanding lesion (15 cases); SAH (4 cases); c) severe epistaxis (1 case). In 3 patients ischemic brain lesions were observed. Occlusion of the parent vessel was performed using latex or silicone balloons which were detached by a coaxial micro-catheter system. Pre-treatment assessment included: 1) evaluation of the collateral blood supply (all cases); 2) analysis of CBF changes following carotid artery digital compression (Matas test) using the 133 Xe-inhalation technique (7 patients). Patient's neurological status was carefully monitored under complete heparinization, during a 30 min occlusion test. In one case only a neurological deficit occurred during the test (aphasia) and prevented definitive occlusion of the vessel.

No severe complication was observed during the procedure and in the follow-up period ranging from 1 to 6 years. Good clinical results were obtained in all cases mainly for the therapy of severe facial and orbital pain. No re-bleeding was seen in the follow-up of patients suffering from previous SAH. The outcome of the two giant fusiform vertebro-basilar aneurysms (causing in both cases a severe tetraparesis) was extremely satisfactory. Serial CT, MRI and angiographic controls performed in 9 cases during a follow-up period ranging from 1 to 6 years demonstrated the reduction of aneurysm size and the progressive decrease of the mass effect on the adjacent neural structures. This occurred even if a residual intra-aneurysmal lumen was patent in the first 6–12 months after the treatment.

Keywords: Cerebral aneurysms; embolization, interventional radiology; detachable balloon.

Introduction

Detachable balloon occlusion of the parent vessel was successfully utilized since 1974[3,17] for the treatment of intracranial aneurysms which were not amenable to a direct surgical approach, both in carotid and vertebral arteries. The procedure is simple and efficacious; low morbidity and mortality rates have been observed when a correct pre-treatment assessment of cerebral circulation was previously obtained[4,6,8]. Parent artery occlusion probably represents the method of choice for the therapy of giant fusiform aneurysms presenting with expanding mass symptoms; better than selective obliteration of the aneurysmal sac with permanently inflated balloons or platinum coils[10–13], this technique causes immediate decrease of arterial pulsations on adjacent neural structures and allows a progressive reduction of its mass effect[1,2,4,11,14,15]. After the procedure sequential studies well documented thrombus formation and organization inside the aneurysm and its reduction in size after complete thrombization[18]. On the other hand some authors have demonstrated the possibility of growth of a thrombosed giant aneurysm after parent artery occlusion, due to new hemorrhage within the arterial wall[9]; furthermore, a case of death due to massive, sudden endo-aneurysmal thrombosis has also been reported[7].

In order to assess the effect of the procedure on clinical symptoms and to evaluate the evolution of aneurysmal obliteration after treatment, we reviewed our series of patients treated from 1985 to 1991.

Materials and Methods

Table 1 summarizes the clinical presentation and the aneurysm location of the 22 patients of our series. All symptoms were severe and typical of the ICA and VA intracranial locations of the aneurysms. In all cases a fusiform shape or a large neck was present. Small calcifications were present in 6 cases. Intra-aneurysmal thrombi were present in 9/22 cases. Ischemic brain lesions were observed in 3 patients.

Our criteria to perform the procedure were the following: a) severity of the clinical symptoms due to mass effect; b) previous or present SAH.

Pre-treatment assessment was performed as follows: a) careful evaluation of collateral blood supply with cross-compression studies

Table 1. *Endovascular Treatment of Giant Intracranial Aneurysms by Occlusion of the Parent Vessel: 22 Cases (1985–1991)*

M: 8 – F: 14;	Age 13–64 (mean 51)	
Location		Clinical presentation
ICA intra-petrous	1	–severe visual loss	14
ICA intra-cavernous	12	–severe progressive ophthalmoplegia	12
		–severe facial and orbital pain	9
ICA ophthalmic	7	–previous SAH	4
		–ischemia	3
		–epistaxis	1
		–severe ponto-medullary	
VA intracranial	2	compression	2

(in all cases); b) 133 Xe-inhalation technique during Matas test (in 7 recent cases); c) 30 min. occlusion test under complete heparinization and accurate neurologic monitoring, before definitive ICA or VA balloon occlusion (in all cases).

CBF changes induced by carotid digital compression were assessed using Obrist[16] program and ISI parameter. After baseline flow measurements, two tests were carried out: one in the early and one in the late stage of ICA compression (1'–10' and 11'–22' respectively).

Although 3 cases showed an abnormal CBF pattern after the early stage and 4 after the late stage (in most cases global hypoperfusion), all patients were treated and all tolerated 30' occlusion test during the procedure. Only one patient (not submitted to rCBF Matas test) did not tolerate the occlusion test and suffered from transient dysphasia which disappeared immediately after balloon deflation.

The procedure of artery occlusion in all of the patients was performed by catheterization through femoral (18 cases), carotid (3 cases), and axillary (1 case) arteries. Latex or silicon balloons (volume 0,3–0,5 ml) were detached by means of a 3F/2F co-axial micro-catheter system. One or two "security" balloons below the first one were detached in each case following Debrun's technique. The ICA was always occluded close to the neck of the aneurysm, proximal to the ophthalmic artery origin; the vertebral artery was occluded in both cases at the C1 level, proximal to PICA origin.

Clinical results and complications were evaluated during a follow-up period ranging from 1 to 6 years (mean 2,2). Serial CT and MR images in association with traditional or MR angiograms were obtained in 9/22 patients, after artery occlusion; 5/9 patients were

examined by CT scan during the first 24–48 hours; all nine patients were examined 6, 12 or more months after the treatment. MRI angiograms were obtained in 5 cases.

Results

Table 2 summarizes the results of ICA and VA occlusion. The best results were observed in the treatment of severe facial and orbital pain (cured in all 9 cases), and in the treatment of severe ponto-medullary compression (2 cases: one cured and one improved); good results were obtained in ophthalmoplegia (12 cases), cured in 3/12, improved in 6/12 and stable in 3/12 cases. Less brilliant results were observed in patients suffering from severe visual loss (14 cases), cured in one case only, improved in 5/14, stable in 6 but worsened in 2 patients. No rebleeding was observed in the patients presenting with SAH.

All of the complications occurring during the procedure were transient: headache was the most frequent (16/22, 73%), ocular pain was observed in 8/22 cases (30%), paresthesias in 2/22 (9%), seventh nerve palsy and vertigo in 1/22 cases (4.5%). A complete recovery of these disturbances was observed in all cases, within 2–5 days from the procedure.

No permanent neurological deficit was observed.

No significant increase in the aneurysmal size was observed in the 5 patients who underwent CT scan during the first 48 hours after the treatment. A slight increase in CT density values was present in all cases, due to initial thrombization. Small new ischemic areas were present in 2 cases in late CT and MRI controls.

An important mass reduction was observed in all 9 patients after a period of 24 months or more. After this period signal intensity inside the aneurysm was uniform in MR T1WI and slightly disomogeneous in T2WI, attesting thrombus organization (Fig. 1). No refilling was observed from the collateral circulation. In 6 patients an important reduction of the aneurysmal

Table 2. *Results of ICA and VA Occlusion in 22 Patients with Giant Aneurysms*

Clinical signs	n	Cure	Improvement	Stable	Worsening	Follow-up
Severe visual loss	14	1	5	6	2	1–5y (mean 2.3)
Ophthalmoplegia	12	3	6	3	—	1–5y (mean 2.3)
Severe facial and orbital pain	9	9	—	—	—	1–5y (mean 2.3)
Severe ponto-medullary compression	2	1	1	—	—	1–5y (mean 1.5)
Hemorrhage	4	4	—	—	—	1–5y (mean 2.3)

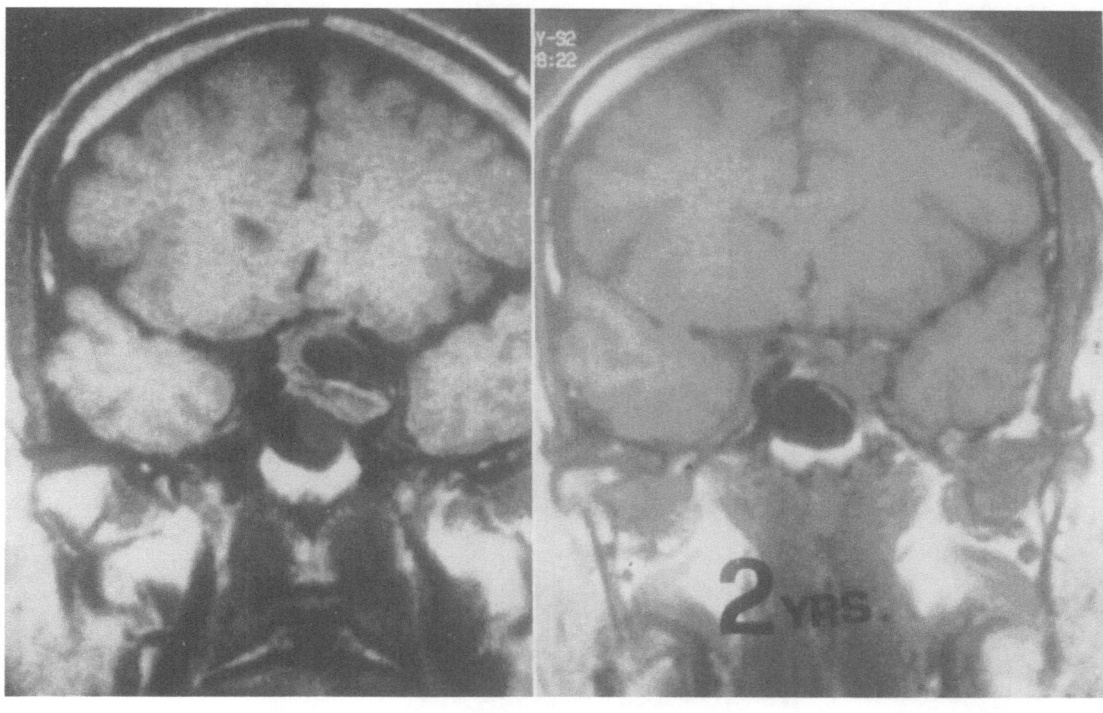

a   b

Fig. 1. Left intra-cavernous giant ICA aneurysm presenting with compression of the optic chiasm (MR T1WI). (a) Before treatment; (b) two years after ICA occlusion: complete obliteration of the aneurysmal sac with disappearance of mass effect

size was achieved already 6–12 months after the treatment. In 2 of them a complete thrombosis was demonstrated, while in the remaining 4 cases a residual lumen was still present: the aneurysmal sac re-filled from ECA (through the ophthalmic artery) or from the P.co.A (Fig. 2).

Both patients with giant vertebral aneurysms showed a remarkable improvement after VA occlusion. In both cases a hypo-plastic vertebral artery, ending at PICA, was present. A dramatic improvement was observed immediately after the treatment in the first patient (Fig. 3); although he presented severe respiratory failure (mechanical ventilation) and severe tetraparesis before the procedure he could walk at discharge, 2 weeks later. In the second patient a good recovery from a severe tetraparesis associated with cerebellar ataxia was observed 1–2 months after VA occlusion (Fig. 4).

Discussion

Complete obliteration of the aneurysmal sac due to organization of endosaccular thrombi and massive reduction of the size of the malformation represents the cure of giant fusiform and large neck aneurysms. This result is possible even if a residual intra-aneurysmal lumen remains patent with re-filling from collateral circulation in the first 6–12 months after parent artery occlusion. Therefore, in our opinion an incomplete thrombosis in the first period after the treatment does not represent a poor prognostic sign as regards decrease of mass effect and obliteration. This observation was previously reported[1] and is confirmed by our results (see Fig. 2); it seems important for the prognosis of some unclippable aneurysms which can cause SAH.

No complication was observed in our series as a consequence of sudden thrombization or of late aneurysmal hemorrhage. In our opinion a careful pretreatment MRI and CT evaluation must be performed to demonstrate any severe injuries or marked calcifications of the aneurysmal wall, and an accurate pretreatment angiography is required to show the origin of normal vessels from the aneurysmal sac.

Patients with vertebral artery aneurysms have a good recovery, if an adequate collateral circulation is present. An accurate neurological monitoring during a

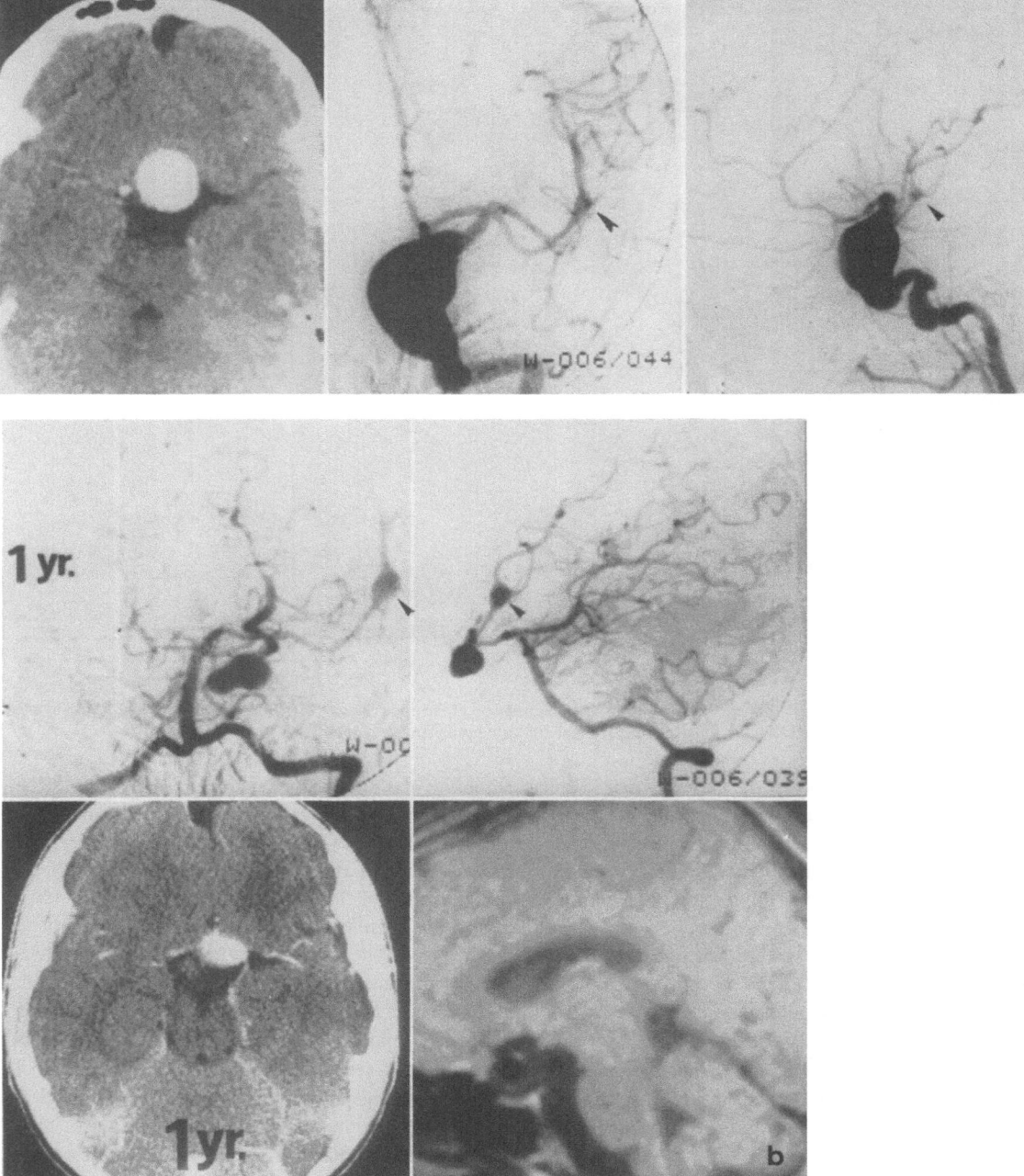

Fig. 2. Left giant fusiform ophthalmic aneurysm presenting with severe compression of the optic chiasm:(a) CT and angiographic pattern before treatment; an incidental sylvian aneurysm is evident at angiography (arrow). (b) One year after ICA occlusion a remarkable decrease of aneurysmal size is evident on the enhanced CT scan, or MR T1WI and on the control angiograms. The residual lumen is re-filled from left P.co.A.. The sylvian aneurysm is markedly enlarged (c) Four years after the treatment complete obliteration of both aneurysms is well demonstrated on MRI and MR angiograms on axial and coronal planes

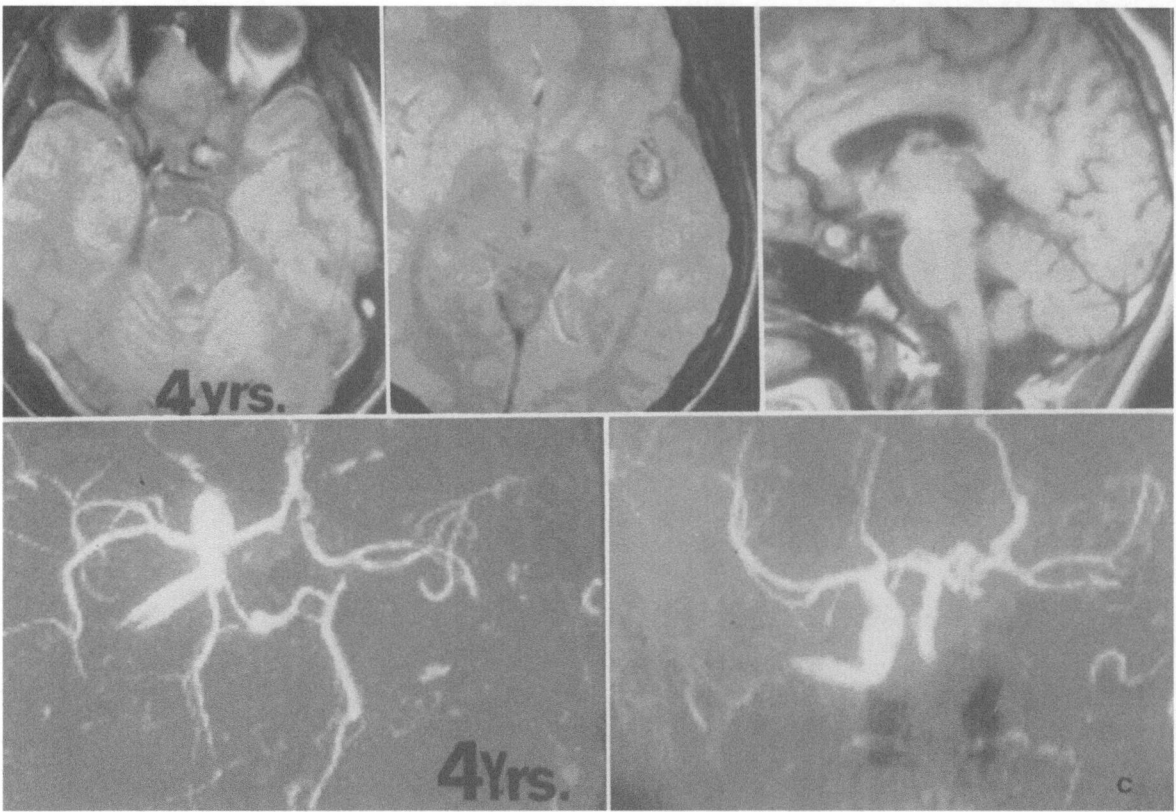

Fig. 2. (*continued*)

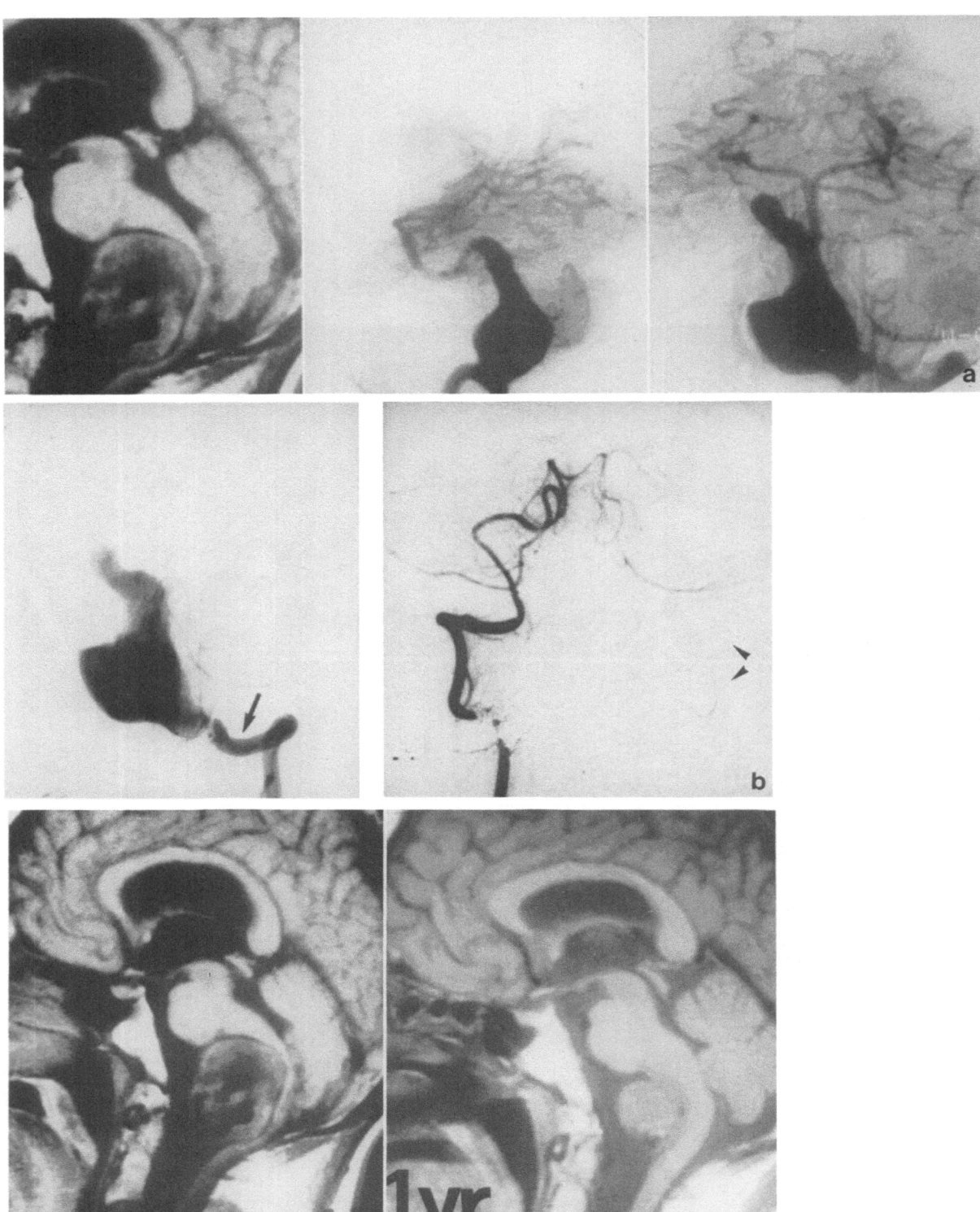

Fig. 3. (a) Left giant fusiform VA intra-cranial aneurysm presenting with severe bulbar compression. (b) VA occlusion was performed at C1 level, proximal to PICA origin (arrows). (c) One year after the treatment a remarkable reduction of aneurysmal size and mass effect with complete obliteration of aneurysmal sac is well demonstrated on sagittal MR T1WI

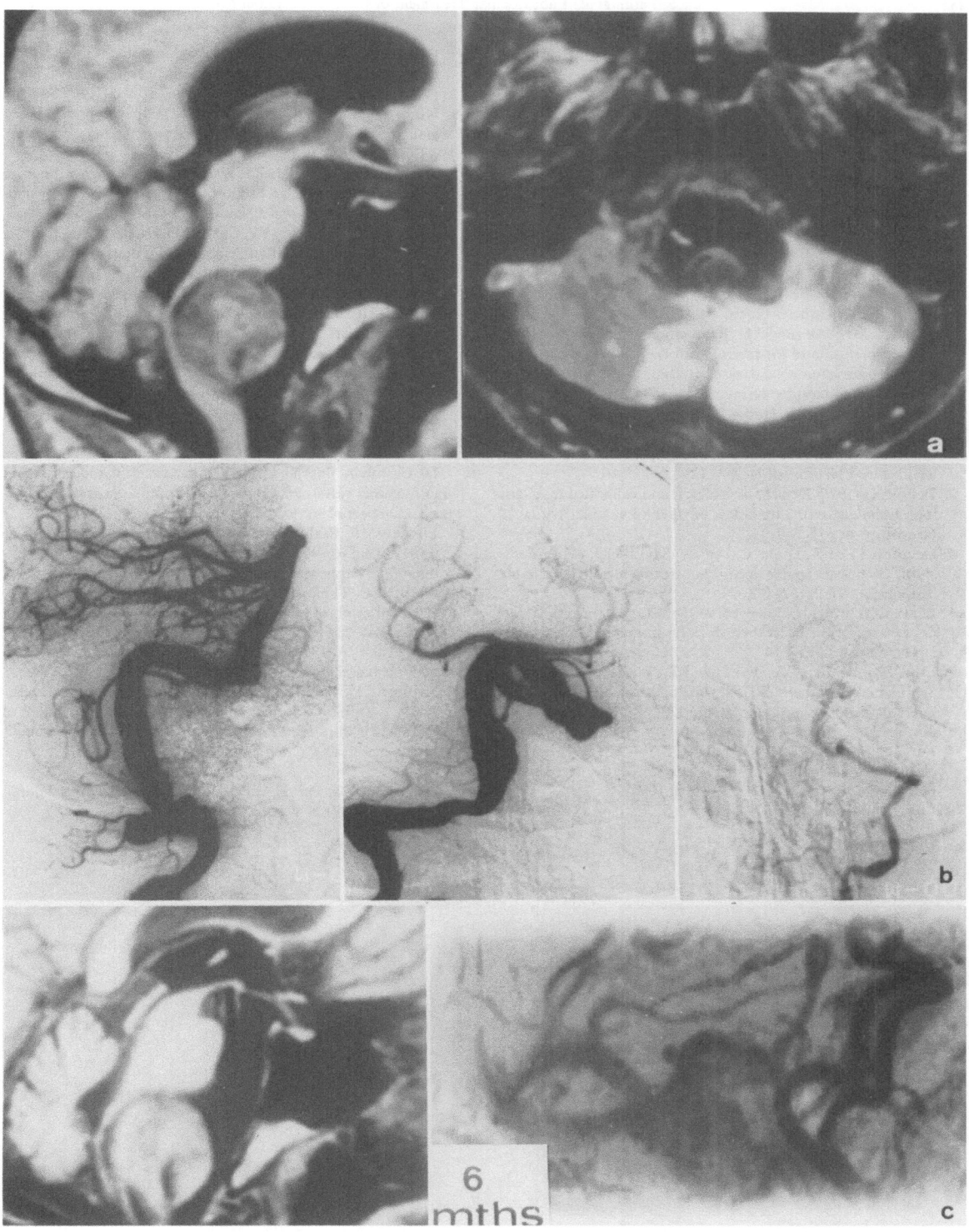

Fig. 4. Right giant fusiform aneurysm presenting with severe pontobulbar compression and cerebellar infarction: (a) MR T1WI on sagittal and axial planes; (b) angiographic pattern:left VA is hypoplastic and ends at PICA. (c) Six months after right vertebral occlusion signal intensity inside the aneurysmal sac is increased, aneurysmal size is not significantly reduced; MR control angiograms show a partial retrograde filling of the upper part of the aneurysmal sac from the basilar artery. A good clinical result was observed at 1 year follow-up

prolonged occlusion test is imperative. For giant aneurysms in this location, massive sudden thrombization may cause severe complications[5,7]. A partial re-filling of the aneurysmal sac (see Fig. 4) probabily allows a slower thrombization with consequent progressive aneurysmal obliteration. VA occlusion proximal to PICA origin seems to help in this process.

References

1. Añon VV, Aymard A, Gobin YP, Casasco A, Rüfenacht D, Khayata MH, Abizanda E, Redondo A, Merland JJ (1992) Balloon occlusion of the internal carotid artery in 40 cases of giant intracavernous aneurysm: technical aspects, cerebral monitoring, and results. Neuroradiology 34: 245–251
2. Aymard A, Gobin YP, Hodes JE, Bien S, Rüfenecht D, Reizine D, George B, Merland JJ (1991) Endovascular occlusion of vertebral arteries in the treatment of unclippable vertebrobasilar aneurysms. J Neurosurg 74: 393–398
3. Debrun G (1978) Detachable balloon and calibrated leak balloon technique in the treatment of cerebral vascular lesions. J Neurosurg 49: 635–649
4. Debrun G, Fox A, Drake C, Peerless S, Girvin J, Ferguson G (1981) Giant unclippable aneurysms: treatment with detachable balloons. AJNR 2: 167–173
5. Drake CG (1975) Ligation of the vertebral (unilateral or bilateral or basilar artery in the treatment of large intracranial aneurysms. J Neurosurg 43: 255–274
6. Erba SM, Horton JA, Latchaw RE, Yonas H, Sekhar L, Schramm V, Pentheny S (1988) Balloon test occlusion of the internal carotid artery with stable Xenon/CT cerebral blood flow imaging. AJNR 9: 533–538
7. Forsting M, Resch KM, Kummer R, Sartor K (1991) Balloon occlusion of a giant lower basilar aneurysm: death due to thrombosis of the aneurysm. AJNR 12: 1063–1066
8. Fox AJ, Vinuela F, Pelz DM, Peerless SJ, Ferguson GG, Drake CG, Debrun G (1987) Use of detachable balloons for proximal artery occlusion in the treatment of unclippable cerebral aneurysms. J Neurosurg 66: 40–46
9. Hecht ST, Horton JA, Howard Y (1991) Growth of thrombosed giant vertebral artery aneurysm after parent artery occlusion. AJNR 12: 449–451
10. Hieshima GB, Higashida RT, Wapenski J, Halbach VV, Bentson JR (1987) Intravascular balloon embolization of a large midbasilar artery aneurysm. J Neurosurg 66: 124–127
11. Higashida RT, Halbach VV, Cahan LD, Hieshima GB, Konishi Y (1989) Detachable balloon embolization therapy of posterior circulation intracranial aneurysms. J Neurosurg 71: 512–519
12. Higashida RT, Halbach VV, Dowd C, Barnwell SL, Dormandy B, Bell J, Hieshima GB (1990) Endovascular detachable balloon embolization therapy of cavernous carotid artery aneurysms: results in 87 cases. J Neurosurg 72: 857–863
13. Higashida RT, Halbach VV, Dowd CF, Barnwell SL, Hieshima GB (1991) Interventional neurovascular treatment of a giant intracranial aneurysm using platinum microcoils. Surg Neurol 35: 64–68
14. Hodes JE, Aymard A, Gobin YP, Rüfenacht D, Bien S, Reizine D, Gaston A, Merland JJ (1991) Endovascular occlusion of intracranial vessels for curative treatment of unclippable aneurysms: report of 16 cases. J Neurosurg 75: 694–701
15. Linskey ME, Sekhar LN, Horton JA, Hirsch WL, Yonas H (1991) Aneurysms of the intracavernous carotid artery: a multidisciplinary approach to treatment. J Neurosurg 75: 525–534
16. Obrist WD, Thompson HK, Wang HS, Wilkinson WE (1975) Regional cerebral blood-flow estimated by Xe-133 inhalation. Stroke: 245–256
17. Serbinenko JA (1974) Balloon catheterization and occlusion of major cerebral vessels. J Neurosurg 41: 125–145
18. Strother CM, Eldevik P, Kikuchiy Graves V, Curtis P, Merlis A (1989) Thrombus formation and structure and evaluation of mss effect in intra-cranial aneurysms treated by balloon embolization: emphasis on MR findings. AJNR 10: 787–796

Correspondence: S. Perini, M.D., Department of Neuroradiology, City Hospital, I-37126 Verona, Italy.

Severe Subarachnoid Hemorrhage, Unruptured and Intracavernous Aneurysms, Aneurysm Rests

Acute Medical and Surgical Management of Severely Ill Aneurysm Patients: a Review

J.M. Zabramski and **R.F. Spetzler**

Division of Neurosurgery, Barrow Neurological Institute, Phoenix, Arizona, U.S.A.

Summary

Perhaps no area of neurosurgery has undergone more rapid change than the management of patients with ruptured aneurysms. Only 10 years ago, early surgery was considered controversial; antifibrinolytic agents were used routinely at most major institutions; and the first publications emphasizing the importance of hypervolemic-hypertensive therapy were being published.

In 1992, early surgery for clipping of ruptured aneurysms is the norm; intracisternal fibrinolytic agents (e.g. rt-PA) are being studied for their ability to enhance the lysis of subarachnoid blood; and calcium antagonist and hypervolemic-hypertensive therapy are routine. In addition, new therapies (e.g. tirilazade) continue to be evaluated for the prevention and treatment of vasospasm.

The protocols followed at the authors institution, for the selection and treatment of patients with aneurysmal hemorrhage will be reviewed, including the results of ongoing trials.

Keywords: Aneurysmal subarachnoid hemorrhage; medical management; surgical management.

Introduction

Perhaps no area of neurosurgery has undergone more rapid change than the management of patients with ruptured aneurysms. Only 10 years ago, early surgery was considered controversial. Antifibrinolytic agents were used routinely at most major institutions, and the first articles emphasizing the importance of hyper-volemic-hypertensive therapy were being published.

In 1992, early surgery for clipping of ruptured aneurysms is the norm. Intracisternal fibrinolytic agents (e.g., rt-PA) are being studied for their ability to enhance the lysis of subarachnoid blood, and calcium antagonist and hypervolemic-hypertensive therapy are routine. In addition, new therapies (e.g., tirilizad) continue to be evaluated for the prevention and treatment of vasospasm.

The protocols followed at our institution for the selection and treatment of patients with aneurysmal hemorrhage are reviewed.

General Care

The preoperative care of the patient with aneurysmal subarachnoid hemorrhage is directed toward minimizing the risk of recurrent hemorrhage and toward accelerating the patient's clinical recovery.

Routine management should include admission to an intensive care unit, with cardiac monitoring and placement of an arterial line for the monitoring of blood pressure. Supportive care includes complete bed rest in a quiet room as well as sedation and pain medication as needed. For sedation and control of pain, we prefer small intravenous doses of morphine sulfate (1 to 4 mg/h), which has a short half-life and can be readily reversed if necessary to evaluate apparent changes in mental status.

Blood Pressure and Fluid Management

The decision of whether to treat hypertension, the choice of drugs, dosage schedules, and other elements of the management of blood pressure can be complex issues in the patient with aneurysmal subarachnoid hemorrhage. Hypertension may represent a response to increased intracranial pressure (ICP), pain, or anxiety. Blood pressure often returns to a normal range after the patient has been admitted to the hospital and these problems have been addressed.

In general, we do not recommend treatment of hypertension in patients with systolic blood pressures under 160 mm Hg. To control blood pressures above this level, we prefer one of the dihydropyridine class of calcium antagonists such as nimodipine or nicardipine. These agents have the advantage that while they lower systemic blood pressure, they tend to increase cerebral blood flow.

Nimodipine is the only agent presently approved by

the U.S. Food and Drug Administration for the prevention and treatment of delayed cerebral vasospasm and is thus started before other antihypertensives are instituted. Treatment with nimodipine (60 mg/4h, orally) for the first 21 days after hemorrhage has been shown to improve outcome significantly and to decrease the incidence of delayed ischemic deficits in patients with ruptured aneurysms[23]. We routinely treat all patients with aneurysmal subarachnoid hemorrhage with nimodipine, beginning therapy soon after they are admitted to the intensive care unit.

Occasionally patients are markedly sensitive to these agents, particularly the elderly and those taking multiple antihypertensive medications. Therefore, we begin therapy with 30 mg (orally or via nasogastric tube) every 4 hours and increase this dose to 60 mg every 4 hours if the patient remains clinically stable. If blood pressure remains consistently above 160 mm Hg before surgical clipping of the ruptured aneurysm, despite the initiation of therapy with nimodipine, small doses of labetolol or hydralazine-HCl can be given intravenously.

After the aneurysm is clipped, nimodipine is continued but other antihypertensive agents are withheld for the first 2 weeks after hemorrhage (when patients are at greatest risk of vasospasm) unless systolic blood pressure exceeds 200 mm Hg. Thereafter, medical management for hypertension is routine. Careful monitoring of neurologic function is essential during the administration of antihypertensive agents. If the patient's clinical status deteriorates after receiving antihypertensive medication, vasospasm should be suspected and the blood pressure should be briskly returned to a previously well-tolerated level.

A complete review of fluid and electrolyte management for the patient with aneurysmal subarachnoid hemorrhage is beyond the scope of this chapter. In general, however, we use prophylactic hypervolemic therapy (Table 1) for all patients during the initial 10 to 14 days after hemorrhage. Intravenous fluid therapy is gradually weaned in patients without clinical or transcranial Doppler evidence of vasospasm.

In patients who develop clinically symptomatic vasospasm, fluid therapy should be maximized and blood pressure should be elevated pharmacologically. Our protocol for the management of symptomatic spasm is outlined in Table 2. It is important to recognize early symptoms of clinically significant vasospasm before the onset of severe ischemic deficits. Worsening headache, hyponatremia, and increasing

Table 1. *Prophylactic Hypervolemic Fluid Therapy*

Low risk vasospasm protocol
(CT scan – little or no SAH[a])
  Normal saline – 150 ml/h
  Serum sodium level daily
    If serum sodium < 132 meq/l
    switch to high risk protocol

High risk vasospasm protocol
(CT scan – moderate or large SAH)
  Swan Ganz catheter
  Normal saline – 150 ml/h
  Plasminate – 100 ml/h PRN
    PAD[b] < 10 mm.hg

Serum sodium level twice daily
3% Sodium chloride sol'n – 30 to
  50 ml/h PRN serum sodium
  Less than 132 meq/l
  (hold for pad < 16 moh g)

[a] Subarachnoid hemorrhage.
[b] Pulmonary artery diastolic pressure.

Table 2. *Hypervolemic-Hypertensive Protocol for Treatment of Symptomatic Vasospasm*

Swan Ganz catheter
Normal saline – 150 ml/h
Plasminate 100 ml/h PRN
    PAD[a] > 12 mm.bg

DDAVP 1 to 2 ml intravenously
  prn urine output > 200 ml/h
  (hold for PAD < 16 mm.hg, or
  serum sodium < 132 meq/l

Neosynephrine infusion (50 mg in 250 ml
  normal saline) – titrate to maintain
  systolic blood pressure 180 to 220 mm/hg
  and reversal of ischemic deficits
  (hold for SVR[b] > 1500 dynes-s/m^2)

Dopamine infusion PRN cardiac output
  less than 5 liters/min, or maximum
  SVR on neosynephrine and persistent
  ischemic deficits

Serum sodium level every 8-hours
3% sodium chloride sol'n 30 to 50 ml/h
  PRN serum sodium < 134 meq/l

[a] Pulmonary artery diastolic pressure.
[b] Systemic vascular resistance.

lethargy 5 to 10 days after hemorrhage are the most frequent harbingers of vasospasm.

Ventricular Drainage

Hydrocephalus is a constant threat in the patient with subarachnoid hemorrhage. When computed tomography (CT) reveals evidence of hydrocephalus or

Table 3. *Hunt and Hess Scale for Classification of Patients with Intracranial Aneurysms*

Grade 0	unruptured aneurysms
Grade I	asymptomatic, or minimal headache and slight nuchal rigidity
Grade II	moderate to severe headache, nuchal rigidity, no neurological deficit other than cranial nerve palsy
Grade III	drowsiness, confusion, mild focal deficit
Grade IV	stupor, moderate to severe hemiparesis, possibly early decerebrate rigidity and vegetative disturbances
Grade V	deep coma, decerebrate rigidity, moribund appearance

intraventricular hemorrhage or when the patient has a depressed level of consciousness (i.e., Hunt and Hess Grade III–V, Table 3), an external ventriculostomy should be placed. If ICP is above 15 mm Hg, the ventriculostomy is opened intermittently to drain at a level of 10 cm above the external auditory meatus. Cerebrospinal fluid (CSF) drainage at these levels maximizes cerebral perfusion and often improves clinical status by one to two grades on the Hunt and Hess Scale.

Monitoring ICP is also useful in deciding whether to proceed with surgery in poor grade patients (Hunt and Hess Grades IV and V; see section on Timing of Surgery). Postoperatively, the drain is left open to constant drainage at 10 to 15 cm H_2O until CSF output falls below 30 to 40 ml per shift, or until the 14th day after hemorrhage when the drain is progressively elevated in an attempt to wean the patient from the ventriculostomy. In our experience, about 30% of patients will require a CSF shunt.

Risk of infection from external ventriculostomy can be minimized by observing meticulous sterile technique, including a full surgical preparation during placement of the catheter, prophylactic antibiotics (we prefer cefuroxime 1.5 g/8h started immediately before placement of the catheter and continued until its removal), and tunneling the ventriculostomy catheter a minimum of 4 cm subcutaneously from the insertion site. Finally, it is important that the catheter be connected to a closed drainage system that does not require opening the system directly to air for zeroing or obtaining CSF samples (Becker External Drainage System, PS Medical, Goleta, CA, 93117). CSF samples are obtained twice weekly on a routine basis for cell counts, gram stain, and culture.

Using this protocol, we have not found it necessary to change the ventriculostomy site every 2 to 3 days as some authors have recommended[18,32]. We routinely leave ventricular drainage catheters in place for as long as 2 to 3 weeks and have only a 3% to 5% incidence of infection.

Antifibrinolytic Therapy

Amicar and other antifibrinolytic agents that were once widely used to reduce the incidence of early rebleeding while patients awaited surgery (usually a period of 10 to 14 days) have fallen into disfavor. One reason for this change is that aneurysms can be clipped early with modern microsurgical techniques without increasing the operative morbidity and mortality. More importantly, however, evidence from a number of studies has demonstrated that while therapy with antifibrinolytic agents significantly reduced the risk of early rebleeding by as much as 50%, their use was associated with an equally significant increase in the risk of ischemic complications[7,12,29,30]. In addition, the use of antifibrinolytic agents has been linked to an increased risk of hydrocephalus[8,12,21,24]. Overall, these studies fail to demonstrate any clear benefit associated with antifibrinolytic therapy, and this treatment can no longer be recommended.

Timing of Surgery for Ruptured Aneurysms

The timing of surgery for the patient presenting with aneurysmal subarachnoid hemorrhage remains controversial. Much of the debate arises from the failure of earlier authors to consider the historical developments in this field. Before the general introduction of the operating microscope in the early 1970s, the risks of early surgery for the clipping of ruptured aneurysms clearly outweighed any potential benefit secondary to reduction in rebleeding. In the late 1970s and early 1980s, a small number of authors reported good outcomes in patients undergoing early surgery for ruptured aneurysms[10,15,26,31]. Simultaneously, the emphasis on the management of these patients shifted from operative morbidity and mortality rates to overall management outcome.

In a 1981 report, the Cooperative Aneurysm Study Group[1] analyzed the overall results of early medical management and delayed surgery for clipping of the ruptured aneurysm in 249 patients. The authors reported a favorable outcome in only 46% of patients with a mortality rate of 36.2%. Of patients admitted in good condition with a potential for complete recovery, only 55.7% had a favorable outcome and 28.7% died.

Other authors have reported similar results with an overall management mortality for delayed surgery between 40% and 60%[6,11,19,25]. As a result, early surgery was proposed by an increasing number of authors in an attempt to improve upon these disappointing figures.

This issue was addressed by the recently published International Cooperative Study on the Timing of Aneurysm Surgery[13,14]. Between January 1981 and June 1983, 3521 patients who were hospitalized within 3 days of subarachnoid hemorrhage were enrolled in the cooperative multi-institutional protocol. This was an intention-to-treat study: When the patient was admitted, the surgeon stated the time of scheduled surgery. Results were analyzed on the basis of outcome assessed 6 months after hemorrhage.

Intracranial operations were performed in 92% of patients who had surgery planned for Days 0–3. However, 24% of the patients originally scheduled for surgery for 11–14 days after hemorrhage and 38% of those with surgery scheduled at 15+ days did not undergo clipping of their aneurysm. These patients died or had complications related to rebleeding and/or vasospasm that contraindicated surgery. Among alert patients, those operated within 48 hours of rupture did as well as those undergoing surgery 2 weeks after hemorrhage. Early operation was not accompanied by a significantly higher rate of surgical complications than those associated with delayed operation. The overall results of management were almost identical in patients with surgery planned within 3 days of hemorrhage and in those with surgery scheduled for 11 to 14 days. The mortality was 20%, and 60% had good outcomes. Vasospasm was the major cause of death and poor outcome.

Early surgery eliminates the morbidity and mortality associated with rebleeding. In addition, with the aneurysm clipped, delayed ischemic deficits secondary to vasospasm can be treated more effectively and safely. In good grade patients (Hunt and Hess Grades I–III), multiple groups have reported that early surgery, the use of calcium antagonists, and hypervolemic-hypertensive therapy can reduce overall management mortality to 10% or less, with good outcomes in 75% or more of those who survive[2–4,16,17,20,27,28].

Methods

We reviewed our experience at the Barrow Neurological Institute from 1988 to 1990. During these 2 years, we operated early on all patients with documented aneurysmal subarachnoid hemorrhage regardless of their clinical grade (excluding only patients without evidence of brain stem function). Early surgery (within 72 hours of hemorrhage) was performed in 90 patients. All patients were treated with aggressive fluid management, including hypervolemic-hypertensive therapy in those that developed evidence of cerebral vasospasm.

Results

At 3-month follow-up, 81% of patients had good outcomes, 8% had poor outcomes, and 11% had died. In good grade patients (Hunt and Hess Grades I–III), 88% had a good outcome, and only 7% died. In 23 poor grade patients (Hunt and Hess Grades IV and V), 54% had good outcomes and 26% died. Three patients had severe deficits, and one was vegetative.

Discussion

Our experience parallels that reported in other recent series. Early surgery, combined with calcium antagonists and aggressive fluid management, improves survival and outcome. We now operate on all good grade patients (Hunt and Hess Grades I-III) regardless of the timing of presentation. When patients are referred on a delayed basis (4 or more days after hemorrhage) and are neurologically stable, we routinely maximize fluid-volume status and proceed with surgery; however, many surgeons will repeat angiography and delay operative clipping of the aneurysm if angiographic evidence of vasospasm is present.

Although angiographic vasospasm may affect surgical outcome, its effect on overall management outcome is an issue that has not been addressed in clinical trials. When surgery is delayed because of angiographic evidence of vasospasm, patients are exposed to the risks of rebleeding. Furthermore, if the arterial spasm becomes clinically symptomatic, it cannot be treated safely in an aggressive fashion. Until this issue is more thoroughly studied, we think that angiographic evidence of vasospasm should not be considered an absolute contraindication to surgery. Special care should be taken in these patients to limit the risks of ischemic injury by preventing even mild intraoperative hypotension. Reductions of systemic arterial pressure of more than 10% to 15% below preoperative levels should be avoided.

The decision of when and whether to operate on poor grade patients (Hunt and Hess Grades IV and V) after aneurysmal hemorrhage is much more contro-

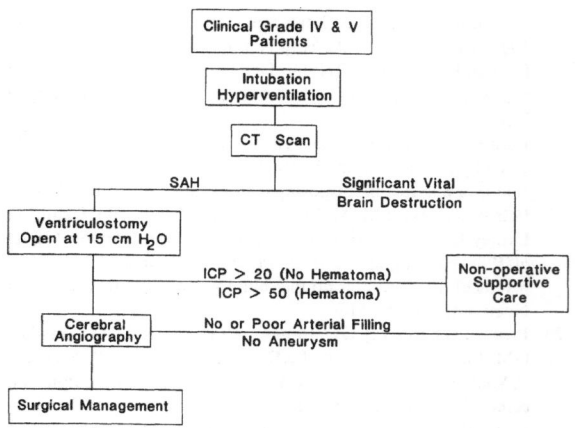

Fig. 1

versial. Nevertheless, it is clear that occasional patients admitted in poor condition soon after hemorrhage will have a good outcome. Based on our experience with this population, we have developed a protocol for the selection of operative candidates based on data from CT, ICP measurements, and angiographic findings (Fig. 1)[5]. Briefly, all patients presenting with subarachnoid hemorrhage in Grades IV and V have a ventriculostomy placed except those who show radiographic evidence of irreversible brain destruction. For example, a large hematoma in the dominant basal ganglia would preclude active treatment. In addition, operative intervention is withheld for three reasons after ventriculostomy: (1) if ICP cannot be controlled below 20 cm H_2O in the patient without hematoma, (2) if ICP is greater than 50 cm H_2O in the patient with hematoma, or (3) if intracranial filling is poor or absent on angiography. Once medically stable, all other patients have early surgery for aneurysm clipping and evacuation of any intracranial hematomas, irrespective of their neurological examination. Postoperatively, patients are treated with calcium antagonists and aggressive hypervolemic-hypertensive therapy.

Certainly, patients in worse neurological condition are expected to have a poorer outcome; however, clinical examination alone soon after aneurysmal hemorrhage is not a good criterion for predicting outcome[5,9,22]. In a prospective study that evaluated our protocol in 54 poor grade patients, 35 patients (20 Grade IV and 15 Grade V) were selected for active treatment. Nineteen (54%) had good outcomes at 3 months and were independent for all activities of daily living; 4 (11%) were dependent for some activities but were not housebound; 4 patients were institutionalized with poor

outcomes; and 8 (23%) patients died[5]. There were no survivors in the nonoperative group. Clearly, an aggressive surgical approach based on appropriate selection criteria is warranted in Grade IV and V patients.

While the decision tree outlined in Fig. 1 is helpful in selecting patients for surgery, the decision of whether to operate in the poor grade patient often rests on associated clinical variables. For example, while most surgeons would operate to clip a posterior communicating artery aneurysm in a young, Hunt and Hess Grade IV patient, few would attempt intervention in an elderly, Grade 4 patient with a large basilar tip aneurysm.

Conclusion

Changes in the management of patients with aneurysmal subarachnoid hemorrhage over the last 10 years have significantly improved the outcome. Routine management at most major institutions now includes early surgery for clipping of the ruptured aneurysm, combined with the use of calcium antagonists and hypervolemic-hypertensive therapy for the treatment of vasospasm. Morbidity and mortality in those patients admitted in good condition (Hunt and Hess Grades I–III) have been reduced to 10% to 15%.

Morbidity and mortality in patients admitted in poor clinical condition after aneurysmal rupture (Hunt and Hess Grades IV-V) remains high; however, it is clear that with aggressive management a small percentage of these patients will have a good outcome. The use of appropriate selection criteria (Fig. 1) can help identify the subgroup of these poor grade patients in whom surgical intervention is indicated.

References

1. Adams HP, Kassel NF, Torner JC, Nibbelink DW, Sahs AL (1981) Early management of aneurysmal subarachnoid hemorrhage: a report of the Cooperative Aneurysm Study. J Neurosurg 54: 141–145
2. Auer LM (1984) Acute operation and preventive nimodipine improve outcome in patients with ruptured cerebral aneurysms. Neurosurgery 15: 57–66
3. Auer LM, Brandt L, Ebeling U, Gilsbach J, Groeger U, Harders A, Liunggren B, Oppel F, Reulen HJ, Saeveland H (1986) Nimodipine and early aneurysm operation in good condition SAH patients. Acta Neurochir (Wien) 82: 7–13
4. Auer LM, Schneider GH, Auer I (1986) Computerized tomography and prognosis in early aneurysm surgery. J Neurosurg 65: 217–221
5. Bailes JE, Spetzler RF, Hadley MN, Baldwin HZ (1990) Management morbidity and mortality of poor-grade aneurysm patients. J Neurosurg 72: 559–566

6. Drake CG (1981) Management of cerebral aneurysm. Stroke 12: 273–283

7. Fodstad H (1982) Antifibrinolytic treatment in subarachnoid haemorrhage: present state. Acta Neurochir (Wien) 63: 233–244

8. Graff-Radford NR, Torner JC, Adams HP Jr, Kassell NF (1989) Factors associated with hydrocephalus after subarachnoid hemorrhage. A report of the Cooperative Aneurysm Study. Arch Neurol 46: 744–752

9. Hochman MS (1986) Reversal of fixed pupils after spontaneous intraventricular hemorrhage with secondary acute hydrocephalus: report of two cases treated with early ventriculostomy. Neurosurgery 18: 777–780

10. Hugenholtz H, Elgie RG (1982) Considerations in early surgery on good-risk patients with ruptured intracranial aneurysms. J Neurosurg 56: 180–185

11. Kassell NF, Drake CG (1982) Timing of aneurysm surgery. Neurosurgery 10: 514–519

12. Kassell NF, Torner JC, Adams HP Jr (1984) Antifibrinolytic therapy in the acute period following aneurysmal subarachnoid hemorrhage. Preliminary observations from the Cooperative Aneurysm Study. J Neurosurg 61: 225–230

13. Kassell NF, Torner JC, Haley EC Jr, Jane JA, Adams HP, Kongable GL, and participants (1990) The International Cooperative Study on the timing of aneurysm surgery. Part 1: overall management results. J Neurosurg 73: 18–36

14. Kassell NF, Torner JC, Jane JA, Haley EC Jr, Adams HP, and participants (1990) The International Cooperative Study on the timing of aneurysm surgery. Part 2: surgical results. J Neurosurg 73: 37–47

15. Ljunggren B, Brandt L, Kagstrom E, Sundbarg G (1981) Results of early operations for ruptured aneurysms. J Neurosurg 54: 473–479

16. Ljunggren B, Brandt L, Saveland H, Nilsson PE, Cronqvist S, Anderson KE, Vinge E (1984) Outcome in 60 consecutive patients treated with early aneurysm operation and intravenous nimodipine. J Neurosurg 61: 864–873

17. Ljunggren B, Saveland H, Brandt L, Zygomunt S (1985) Early operation and overall outcome in aneurysmal subarachnoid hemorrhage. J Neurosurg 62: 547–551

18. Mayhall CG, Archer NH, Lamb VA, Spadora AC, Baggett JW, Ward JD, Narayan RK (1984) Ventriculostomy-related infections. A prospective epidemiologic study. N Engl J Med 310: 553–559

19. Milhorat TH, Krautheim M (1986) Results of early and delayed operations for ruptured intracranial aneurysms in two series of 100 consecutive patients. Surg Neurol 26: 123–128

20. Ohman J, Heiskanen O (1989) Timing of operation for ruptured supratentorial aneurysms: a prospective randomized study. J Neurosurg 70: 55–60

21. Park BE (1979) Spontaneous subarachnoid hemorrhage complicated by communicating hydrocephalus: epsilon amino caproic acid as a possible predisposing factor. Surg Neurol 11: 73–80

22. Petruk KC, West M, Mohr G, Weir BK, Benoit BG, Gentili F, Disney LB, Khan MI, Grace M, Holness RO, Karwon MS, et al (1988) Nimodipine treatment in poor-grade aneurysm patients: results of a multicenter double-blind placebo-controlled trial. J Neurosurg 68: 505–517

23. Pickard JD, Murray GD, Illingworth R, Shaw MDM, Teasdale GM, Foy PM, Humphrey PRD, Lang DA, Nelson R, Richards P, Sinar J, Bailey S, Skene A (1989) Effect of oral nimodipine on cerebral infarction and outcome after subarachnoid haemorrhage: British aneurysm nimodipine trial. BMJ 298: 636–642

24. Pinna G, Pasqualin A, Vivenza C, DaPian R (1988) Rebleeding, ischaemia and hydrocephalus following anti-fibrinolytic treatment for ruptured cerebral aneurysms. A retrospective clinical study. Acta Neurochir (Wien) 93: 77–87

25. Ropper AH, Zervas NT (1984) Outcome 1 year after SAH from cerebral aneurysm: management morbidity, mortality and functional status in 112 consecutive good-risk patients. J Neurosurg 60: 909–915

26. Samson DS, Hodosh RM, Reid WR, Beyer CW, Clark WK (1979) Risk of intracranial aneurysm surgery in the good grade patient: early versus late operation. Neurosurgery 5: 422–426

27. Saveland H, Ljunggren B, Brandt L, Messeter K (1986) Delayed ischemic deterioration in patients with early aneurysm operation and intravenous nimodipine. Neurosurgery 18: 146–150

28. Vapalahti M, Ljunggren B, Saveland H, Hernesniemi J, Brandt L, Tapaninaho A (1984) Early aneurysm operation and outcome in two remote Scandinavian populations. J Neurosurg 60: 1160–1162

29. Vermeulen M, Lindsay KW, Murray GD, Chea F, Hijora A, Muizellar JP, Schannong M, Teasdale GM, van Crevel H, van Gign J (1984) Antifibrinolytic treatment in subarachnoid hemorrhage. N Engl J Med

Correspondence: c/o Editorial Office, Joseph M. Zabramski, M.D., Barrow Neurological Institute, 350 West Thomas Road, Phoenix, AZ 85013-4496, U.S.A.

Strategy of Surgical Treatment in Severely Ill Patients After Aneurysmal Subarachnoid Hemorrhage

V. Seifert, H.A. Trost, D. Stolke, and **H. Dietz**

Neurosurgical Clinic, University of Essen and Neurosurgical Clinic, Medical School Hannover, Federal Republic of Germany

Summary

In order to clarify whether the surgical timing in severely ill patients after aneurysmal subarachnoid hemorrhage is an important factor in regard to the management morbidity and mortality of these patients, the clinical data of 131 patients admitted to the Neurosurgical Clinics of the University of Essen and the Medical School of Hannover being in Grades IV and V after aneurysm rupture were analyzed. 91 patients (69.4%) were in Grades IV and 40 patients (30.6%) were in Grade V. The aneurysmall location of the 131 patients was as follows: ICA: 22 patients (16.8%), MCA. 39 patients (29.8%), ACA: 54 patients (41.2%), VBA: 16 patients (12.2%). Surgery was performed in 77 patients, 62 in Grades IV and 15 in Grade V. In Grade IV patients with surgical intervention, combined severe morbidity and mortality was 62%, while a satisfactory outcome was achieved in 34%. Of the Grade V patients, combined surgical morbidity and mortality was 93%, with only 7% of good results. In 54 patients no surgical treatment was performed (29 Grade IV, 25 Grade V). In 35 patients no surgery was undertaken, because the disastrous effect of the initial hemorrhage was judged to be too severe to attempt any surgical intervention. Of these patients 34 died and one survived in a vegetative state. 19 patients died before the scheduled delayed surgery could be performed. 8 patients died from lethal rebleeding, and 11 patients died from the sequelae of the initial hemorrhage, cerebral ischemia and/or severe medical complications. Thus mortality in Grades IV and V patients in the nonsurgical group was 98%.

Keywords: Aneurysm rupture; subarachnoid hemorrhage; early aneurysm surgery; Grades IV and V patients.

Introduction

Early surgery in low risk aneurysm patients (Hunt and Hess I–III) has led to a considerable improvement of the perioperative management morbidity and mortality and is now an almost generally accepted regimen of treatment. Except for those patients with a space occupying intracerebral hematoma, patients in Grades IV and V Hunt and Hess are often not considered to be surgical candidates. Thus surgery is delayed, hoping that with improvement of the clinical condition the patient will be later amenable to aneurysm clipping.

However with this form of treatment many of these patients will finally die from recurrent haemorrhage or from the effect of delayed ischemic deficits. The following study was performed in order to examine the clinical management of a population of Grades IV and V patients with the aim to clarify, whether certain variables of treatment, including early surgery, could be defined, that might help to improve the so far almost hopeless outlook for the stuporous or comatose patient after aneurysm rupture.

Material and Methods

755 patients who had been admitted to the Neurosurgical Clinics of the University of Essen and the Medical School Hannover within a period of 8 years suffering from acute subarachnoid hemorrhage form the clinical background of our study (Fig. 1). After neurological examination and grading of the patients according to the Hunt and Hess scale[2], diagnosis of SAH was confirmed in all patients by computerized tomography. 191 (25,3%) of the SAH patients were poor risk patients, 114 (15,1%) Grades IV and 77 (10,2%) Grade V respectively. In case of acute hydroephalus an immediate ventriculostomy and continuous external CSF drainage was performed. Four-vessel angiography was undertaken in 137 of these 191 patients (71,7%), who were considered to be potential surgical candidates. The strategy of surgical or nonsurgical treatment in each patient was left to the decision of the surgeon being responsible for the individual patient. Surgery was performed under neurolept anesthesia using standard microsurgical techniques including washout of the basals cisterns from subarachnoid blood collections. Postoperatively induced hypertension and hypervolemia was installed. All surviving patients were reexaminded 6–12 months post surgery and graded according the criteria of the Glasgow Outcome Scale[3].

Results

131 of the 191 poor risk patients (68,6%) suffered from aneurysmal SAH. 14 patients (7,3%) had bled from an arteriovenous malformation, 23 patients (12,0%) had SAH of unknown origin assumed by "negative angio-

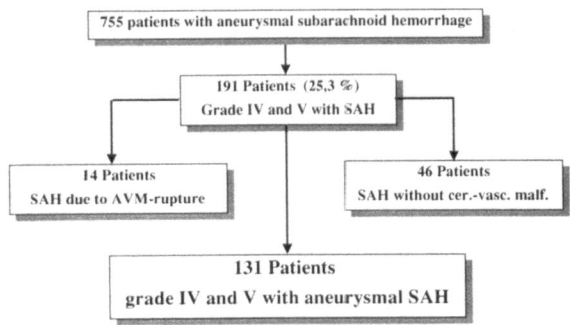

Fig. 1. Flow diagram demonstrating the clinical distribution of 755 patients with aneurysmal subarachnoid hemorrhage

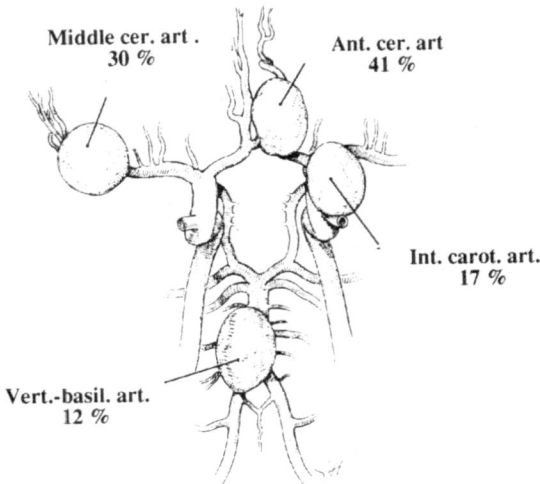

Fig. 2. Localization of intracranial aneurysms in 131 patients, Grades IV and V, n = 131

graphy" or proved by autopsy, and in further 23 patients (12,0%) the origin of SAH remained unclear, because neither angiography nor autopsy was undertaken. 58% of our patients were admitted within 24 hours after SAH, 87% were admitted within the first 72 hours after SAH. No difference could be found between the surgery and the nonsurgical group concerning age, sex and admission pattern. The ruptured aneurysm was located at the anterior communicating artery complex in 54 patients (41,2%), in 39 patients (29,8%) at the middle cerebral artery, at the internal carotid artery in 22 patients (16,8%) and at the vertebrobasilar artery

complex in 16 patients (12,2%) (Fig. 2). 14 patients had multiple aneurysms (11 times 2 aneurysms, 3 times 3 aneurysms). 77 patients (58,8%) were operated on: 52 patients (39,7%) were operated on early, 25 patients (19,1%) had delayed surgery. 13 patients (10,0%) died within few hours after admission, not allowing enough time for diagnostic procedures and operation. 4 patients

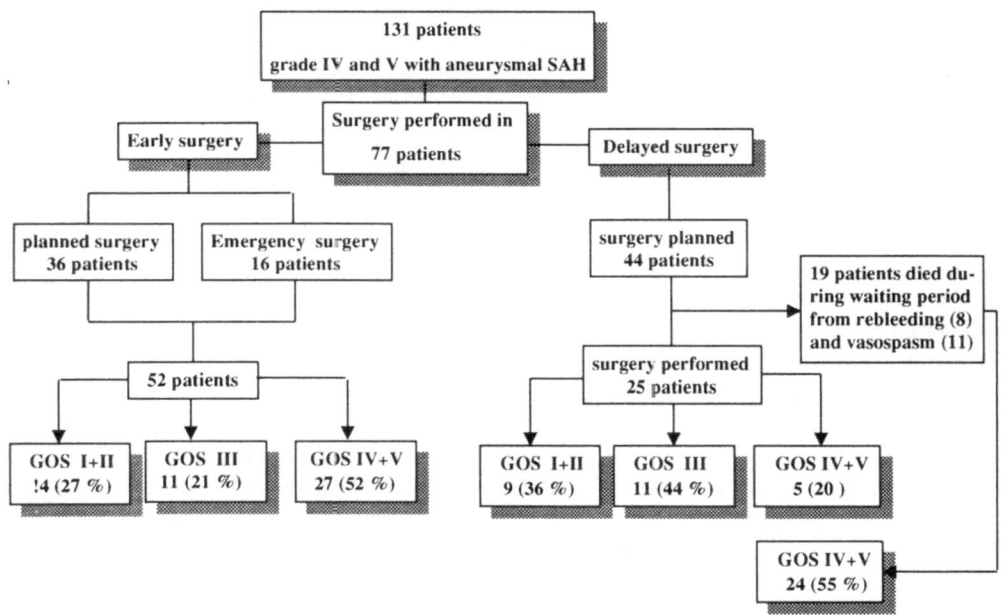

Fig. 3. Flow diagram of clinical outcome in 131 patients, Grades IV and V

(3,1%) had false negative angiography. 18 (13,7%) patients were not considered to be surgical candidates because of age, poor clinical condition or otherwise poor prognosis. 36 (27,5%) of the 52 early operated patients had been operated on schedule. The remaining 16 (12,2%) patients had emergency operation for space occupying hemorrhage (12 patients) or rebleeding (4 patients) respectively. 44 (33,6%) patients were scheduled for delayed surgery; 19 (14,5%) of them died while waiting for the operation, 8 (6,1%) patients as a result of fatal rebleeding, 11 (8,4%) from sequelae of the initial hemorrhage, of vasospasm or medical complications. 25 patients (19,1%) managed to live long enough for delayed surgery.

In Grade V patients mortality was 54%. In the non-surgical group only 1 out of 26 patients survived severely disabled (4%). In the surgery group we had excellent outcome in one patient (7%), who recovered well after drainage of acute hydrocephalus and had delayed surgery. Another 7 patients (47%) survived severely disabled. The 69 grade IV patients did somewhat better. Mortality in the early surgery group was 48%, 50% in emergency operations and 47% in operation on schedule respectively. An excellent or good outcome were reached in 32% of the early surgery group. Decision for delayed surgery in 25 patients led to 40% mortality, 7 patients (28%) dying while waiting for operation. 18 patients finally operated on late had a 17% mortality and a 44% rate of excellent or good outcome (Fig. 3).

Discussion

Despite the fact that poor risk patients after aneurysmal SAH represent between 15 and 30% of all aneurysm patients reported in large series, detailed analysis of the management morbidity and mortality are surprisingly scarce and recomendations for treatment are vague, based mostly on personal experience and intuition[1,4,5]. Our data demonstrate that patients subjected to aneurysm clipping had a far better outcome (mortality 42%) as compared to those who were treated non-operatively (mortality 98%). Timing of poor risk aneurysm surgery is still under discussion. In 1990 we recommended early diagnosis and operation in Grade IV patients and a wait and see policy in Grade V patients based on our results during 1983 to 1987[7]. The

more aggressive treatment in grade IV patients in 1988 to 1990 led to a rise in operative mortality (34% versus 39%) and a fall in good surgical outcome (GOS 1 + 2) (49% versus 35%). This changed the relation between severely disabled (10% versus 18%) and good outcome (31% versus 24%); the overall mortality in these patients however remained stable (58%). In Grade V patients we had another 3 severely disabled and 11 fatal outcomes, and the overall mortality remained at about 80%, the rest being severely disabled (15% versus 18%) with one lucky excellent outcome. Treatment of grade V patients remains disappointing. Mortality in non-surgical treatment is almost 100%, decision for early surgery leads to 75% mortality as well as a decision for delayed surgery. A wait and see policy in these patients seems to be justified, since the only excellent outcome was achieved after secondary improvement after ventriculostomy followed by delayed surgery. In Grade IV patients we still advocate early diagnosis and operative treatment, since aneurysm clipping facilitates treatment of delayed ischemic deficits by administration of hypervolemic hypertension, tissue plasminogen activator or nimodipine[6], and prevents rebleeding.

References

1. Bailes JE, Spetzler RF, Hadley MN, Baldwin HZ (1990) Management morbidity and mortality of poor-grade aneurysm patients. J Neurosurg 72: 559–566
2. Hunt WE, Hess RM (1968) Surgical risk as related to time of intervention in repair of intracranial aneurysm. J Neurosurg 28: 14–19
3. Jennet B, Bond M (1975) Assessment of outcome after severe brain damage. Lancet i: 480–484
4. Kassell NF, Torner JC, Haley EC, et al (1990) The International Cooperative Study on the Timing of Aneurysm Surgery. Part 1: overall management results. Part 2: surgical results. J Neurosurg 73: 18–36, 37–47
5. Petruk KC, West M, Mohr G, et al (1988) Nimodipine in poor grade aneurysm patients. Results of a multicenter double-blind placebo-controlled trial. J Neurosurg 505–517
6. Seifert V, Eisert WG, Stolke D, Goetz C (1989) Efficacy of single intracisternal injection of recombinant tissue plasminogen activator to prevent delayed cerebral vasospasm after experimental subarachnoid hemorrhage. Neurosurgery 25: 590–598
7. Seifert V, Trost HA, Stolke D (1990) Management morbidity and mortality in Grades IV and V patients with aneurysmal subarachnoid haemorrhage. Acta Neurochir (Wien) 103: 5–10

Correspondence: V. Seifert, M.D., Neurochirurgische Klinik, Universität GH5 Essen, Hufelandstrasse 55, D-45147 Essen, Federal Republic of Germany.

Unruptured Intracranial Aneurysms – Current Concepts and Future Directions*

D.O. Wiebers

Mayo Foundation, Rochester, Minnesota, U.S.A.

Unruptured intracranial aneurysms constitute a significant public health problem which is growing in magnitude. This is due in part to the increasing age of the population. In addition, the widespread use of CT and MR scanning, and the improving quality of these techniques have increased the numbers of aneurysms discovered incidentally.

In formulating an approach to the management of patients with unruptured intracranial aneurysms, it is important to recognize potential differences in behavior between these lesions and previously ruptured intracranial aneurysms. Among patients with unruptured intracranial aneurysms, there should be a distinction between patients without a history of subarachnoid hemorrhage and patients with an unruptured aneurysm who have a prior history of subarachnoid hemorrhage from a different aneurysm which has been successfully repaired.

Among patients with unruptured intracranial aneurysms (UIA) and no history of prior subarachnoid hemorrhage from a different source, the size of the aneurysm at the time of discovery appears to be the greatest determinant of future rupture. In prior natural history studies[1], size was the only individual variable of unquestionable significance for predicting aneurysmal rupture ($p < .0001$). However, when combinations of variables were analyzed, the interaction term of aneurysm size and patient age was even more significant than aneurysm size alone ($p < .00001$)[1].

In 23 patients, the product of aneurysm size (in mm) times the patient's age (in years) exceeded 1,000. Of these, 11 patients had subsequent ruptures (all of whom died), and 7 patients died from other causes during the followup period. Conversely, only 4 of 100 patients had rupture when their size times age values were < 1000.

Patients with unruptured intracranial aneurysms without prior SAH from a different source, with aneurysms 10 mm in angiographic diameter or larger have a fairly high probability of experiencing subsequent rupture and many of these ruptures occur within a few months of identification of the aneurysm.

For unruptured aneurysms less than 10 mm in diameter in patients without prior subarachnoid hemorrhage, the risk of subsequent rupture appears to be very low but not zero.

It is certainly possible that patients with an unruptured aneurysm who have a history of subarachnoid hemorrhage from a different source have a different prognosis than patients who have never had subarachnoid hemorrhage. In other words, whatever caused the initial rupture may make it more likely for such patients to have rupture of a second or third aneurysm and the risk associated with size may be different or conceivably irrelevant in these patients.

The management of patients with unruptured intracranial aneurysms remains controversial and widely varied throughout the world for a variety of reasons. Available data regarding natural history and operative morbidity and mortality remain sparse. There is a need to better understand the unruptured intracranial aneurysm as a risk factor for subarachnoid hemorrhage (SAH), to define other SAH risk factors, and to optimize the management of patients with these conditions.

The International Study of Unruptured intracranial Aneurysms (ISUIA) has been organized to address these issues.

This group has undertaken an initial epidemiological study to address what we believe to be the most cri-

*Keywords: Intracranical aneurysm; subarachnoid hemorrhage.

tical clinical issues in regard to unruptured intracranial aneurysms.

The project involves 44 centers including 16 in the United States, 6 in Canada, and 22 in Europe. Altogether, this study involves 3500 patients including 1500 retrospective and 2000 prospective, all with unruptured intracranial aneurysms. The project will run from 1991 to 1996.

The three primary hypotheses to be addressed by this study are as follows:

1) Among patients without a history of subarachnoid hemorrhage with unruptured intracranial aneurysms, there is a critical size above which there is a significant risk of aneurysmal rupture, neurological morbidity, and mortality. This hypothesis relates to one of the major controversies about management. Although most neurologists and neurosurgeons seem to agree that among patients with unruptured aneurysms without a history of subarachnoid hemorrhage, larger aneurysms are more likely to rupture than smaller ones, there is little or no agreement on what if any size range has a low enough future rupture rate to warrant conservative management.

2) Among patients with unruptured intracranial aneurysm and a history of subarachnoid hemorrhage from another source, the risk of future rupture of UIA, disability, and death is greater than patients without a history of SAH and varies directly with aneurysmal size. Clearly, even more confusion exists about this group of patients. The natural history data available at this time do not allow determination about whether or not future rupture is in any way dependent on aneurysmal size.

3) The risk of death and significant disability from surgery to isolate unruptured intracranial aneurysms from the intracranial circulation varies according to the size of the aneurysm, the location of the aneurysm, history of subarachnoid hemorrhage from another source, and confounding variables such as age and associated medical conditions.

Another major difficulty in making management decisions concerning patients with UIA relates to relatively scant and conflicting data about operative morbidity and mortality. The largest series to date by Nishimoto et al.[2] reports an operative mortality of 7 percent which is considerably higher than other recent series[3,4].

A variety of *secondary hypotheses* will also be addressed involving 17 other variables which may be associated with an increased risk of subsequent rupture of UIA.

References

1. Wiebers DO, Whisnant JP, Sundt TM Jr, O'fallon WM (1987) The significance of unruptured intracranial saccular aneurysms. J Neurosurg 66: 23–29
2. Nishimoto A, Ueta K, Onbe H, Kitamura K, Omae T, Goto F, Ohneda G, Chigasaki H, Tsuru M, Suzuki J, Wada T, Sano K, Mannen T, Yoshioka M, Nakai O, Kageyama N, Nomura T, Handa H, Tanaka K (1985) Nationwide co-operative study of intracranial aneurysm surgery in Japan. Stroke 16: 48–52
3. Wirth FP, Laws ER Jr, Piepgras D, Scott RM (1983) Surgical treatment of incidental intracranial aneurysms. Neurosurgery 12: 507–511
4. Rice BJ, Peerless SJ, Drake CG (1990) Surgical treatment of unruptured aneurysms of the posterior circulation. J Neurosurg 73: 165–173

Correspondence: D.O. Wiebers, M.D., Mayo Foundation, Department of Neurology, 200 First St.sw, Harrich Room 672, Rochester, Minnesota 55905, U.S.A.

Validity of Surgical Treatment of Unruptured Aneurysms

N. Yasui, A. Suzuki, and **H. Hadeishi**

Department of Surgical Neurology, Research Institute for Brain and Blood Vessels-Akita, Akita, Japan

Summary

The results of surgically treated cases of unruptured aneurysm, in which mean hemispheric cerebral blood flow (CBF) values were above the critical flow level, are reported. The operations were performed in the chronic stage of cerebral ischemia when the patient had a cerebral infarction as the basic pathology. Analysis of these patients suggest the option of operating on cases of unruptured aneurysms. Permanent neurological deficits (PND) were not observed when pre-operative CBF was maintained above the critical flow level. Most PND occurred after the surgical treatment of large or giant aneurysms. Low cerebral flow values alone did not cause PND, although they could be the basic causative factor of transient neurological deficits (TND).

Keywords: Unruptured aneurysm; surgical treatment; critical cerebral blood flow; surgical procedure.

Introduction

From the results of our previous analysis (1976–1985) of 121 cases of unruptured aneurysms, surgical treatment was indicated in cases where the mean hemispheric cerebral blood flow (mCBF) values were above the critical level; moreover surgery was indicated only in the chronic stage of cerebral ischemia, when the patient had a cerebral infarction as the basic pathology[16]. In this paper, the results of surgically treated cases of unruptured aneurysms are reported according to our previously mentioned criteria.

Method and Material

Surgery was performed in 108 cases of unruptured aneurysms from 1986 to 1990. Sixty-six cases were female and 42 cases were male. Their ages ranged from 30 to 74, and the mean age was 57.9 years. The location of the aneurysms were as follows: 33 of internal carotid artery, 33 of middle cerebral artery, 22 of anterior cerebral artery including anterior communicating artery, 10 of vertebro-basilar artery and 10 of multiple. Forty five were small aneurysms (less than 5 mm), 49 were moderate size aneurysms (between 6 and 14 mm), 12 were large aneurysms (between 15 and 24 mm) and 2 were giant aneurysms (larger than 25 mm in maximum diameter). The basic pathology in 38 cases was cerebral infarction (INF). Also 14 cases with intracerebral hemorrhage (ICH), 34 cases with subarachnoid hemorrhage (SAH) and 22 cases with the other condition (Alia) – such as headache or head injury – were noted.

Mean hemispheric cerebral blood flow (mCBF) values were measured using the 10 mci of ^{133}Xe intravenous injection method with a CBF BI-1400 analyzer (Valmet Oy Instrument, Finland). The mCBF was calculated by mean values of initial slope index in the brain. Pre-operative resting mCBF was measured in 66 cases to evaluate the relationship between pre-operative CBF and the surgical results.

Comparisons of the surgical results and other factors – such as the basic pathology, aneurysm location and size, operative procedures and pre-operative CBF – were made. In cases with multiple aneurysms, the largest aneurysm was considered for the surgical outcome. Surgical results were evaluated in comparison with pre-operative condition. "Without deficit" was a case who had no post-operative additional neurological deficit. When the additional post-operative neurological deficit disappeared at the time of discharge, the patient was considered as presenting a transient neurological deficit (TND). If the additional post-operative symptom continued, the patient was considered as presenting a permanent neurological deficit (PND).

For statistic analysis, Fisher's test, chi-square test in a contingency table or Wilcoxon ranked sign test were used. A p-value < 0.05 was considered significant.

Results

1) Basic Pathology and Surgical Results

Surgical results of the whole region are summarized in Table 1. There was no mortality. 81 cases (75%) had no additional deficits after the aneurysm surgery. There was no significant difference in the incidence of the different pathologies in cases with PND, but the incidence of INF was significantly higher in cases with TND. The mean age of the group without deficits was lower than in both groups with neurological deficit. There was no age difference between the PND and the TND groups.

Permanent neurological deficits (PND) were noted in 8 cases (7.5%), secondary to the following causes, ischemic disturbances caused by clipping procedures for giant and large aneurysms (5 cases), perforator

Table 1. *Basic Pathology and Surgical Results*

	Without deficit	Neurological deficit	
		Permanent	Transient
INF	24	1	13
ICH	12	2	0
SAH	30	1	3
Alia	15	4	3
Total	81	8	19
Mean age	55.6	62.3	62.8

INF cerebral infarction, *ICH* intracerebral hemorrhage, *SAH* subarachnoid hemorrhage, *Alia* other condition.

injury (1 case), hemorrhage caused by tear of frontal bridging vein (1 case), and cerebral infarction caused by brain retraction (1 case). Observed clinical findings were hemiparesis (4 cases), psychiatric dysfunction (2 cases), aphasia (1 case) and vegetative state (1 case).

Transient neurological deficits (TND) such as psychiatric dysfunction (8 cases), epileptic seizures (6 cases), hemiparesis (5 cases) and dysphasia (2 cases) occurred in 19 cases (17.8%). The causes of TND were excessive brain retraction (9 cases), perforator injury (2 cases), brain contusion (1 case), temporary clipping (1 case) and unknown (6 cases). Three of these cases revealed areas of small infarction on CT scan.

2) Location and Size of the Aneurysms and Surgical Results

Surgical results in relation to aneurysmal location and size are presented in Tables 2 and 3.

The location of the aneurysm did not affect the

Table 2. *Aneurysm Location and Surgical Results*

	Without deficit	Neurological deficit	
Location		Permanent	Transient
IC	27	1	5
MC	26	3	4
ACA	13	2	7
VB	7	2	1
Mult.	8	0	2
Total	81	8	19

IC internal carotid artery aneurysm, *MC* middle cerebral artery aneurysm, *ACA* anterior cerebral artery aneurysm, *VB* vertebrobasilar artery aneurysm, *Mult.* multiple aneurysms.

Table 3. *Aneurysm Size and Surgical Results*

	Without deficit	Neurological deficit	
Size		Permanent	Transient
≦ 5 mm	41	0	4
6–14 mm	34	3	12
15–24 mm	6	3	3
25 mm ≦	0	2	0
Total	81	8	19

Table 4. *Pre-Operative Mean Hemispheric Blood Flow and Surgical Results*

	CBF (ml/100g/min)	
	Mean	< 35
Without deficit	46.0	3/45
Transient deficit	38.2	7/14
Permanent deficit	41.1	1/ 7

incidence of PND, but a TND was a frequent occurrence for anterior communicating artery aneurysms (ACoA An): five out of 7 cases of TND occurred in patients with ACoA aneurysms larger than 8 mm. There was no TND and no PND in 6 cases of small ACoA An. Three out of 4 cases with TND – whose aneurysm size was small – had epileptic seizures after surgery. There were no cases of PND after surgery in small aneurysms; most of the PND occurred in large or gian aneurysms.

3) Pre-Operative Cerebral Blood Flow and Surgical Results

In patients with PND, mCBF values were above 35 ml/100g/min in all cases except in one and average CBF was 41.7 ml/100g/min. In patient with TND, 7 of 14 cases showed mCBF values below 35 ml/100g/min and average CBF was 38.1 ml/100g/min. CBF reduction in the TND group was significant, when compared to the group with no deficits (Table 4). This finding indicates that low cerebral perfusion values could be the main causative factor for TND.

Discussion

There have been many recent advances in neurological diagnosis, such as CT scan, digital subtraction angiography and magnetic resonance imaging; these advances have made a reliable diagnosis of cerebral aneurysms possible before rupture. Inspite of this, surgical treatment of an unruptured aneurysm is still controversial.

The incidence of intracranial aneurysms was reported as less than 1% to 8% by autopsy studies[3,8,9,11] but the premorbid incidence is not known. The probability of rupture is about 1% or less per year according to several reports[4,6,10], but Atkinson *et al.*[2] reported in 1989 that unruptured aneurysms have a higher probability of rupture than was previously thought. This conclusion was based on the comparison of current statistics concerning patients with subarachnoid hemorrhage exhibiting a low frequency of asymptomatic aneurysm at the time of the angiographic study. Stehbens[14] reviewed the etiology of intracranial aneurysms, and felt that the most plausible explanation was that aneurysms were an acquired degenerative lesion. He felt that the effect of hemodynamic stress would affect the aneurysm formation, growth and rupture.

From this, we have considered a plan for preventing the rupture of unruptured aneurysms. The most certain means of preventing aneurysmal rupture remains surgical treatment. In recent years, also intravascular methods have been introduced, allowing direct obliteration of cerebral aneurysms[7,13]. These methods are not widely accepted, due to the difficulty of the technique and complications of the procedures.

There are several problems in the surgical treatment of unruptured aneurysms. Most surgical risks have been reported in cases that were complicated by ischemic cerebro-vascular disease[12,15]. The risk of surgery was especially related to the pre-operative CBF level. Abumiya *et al.*[1] reported the regional effect of craniotomy performed in cases of unruptured aneurysms on cerebral circulation and oxygen metabolism using positron emission tomography. He concluded that the regional effect of craniotomy was acceptable when refined microneurosurgical procedures were used. Hadeishi *et al.*[5] compared preoperative CBF and surgical results, and concluded that lower pre-operative CBF values may indicate a risk of brain damage; all cases reviewed, except one, showed transient deficits which resolved within 2 weeks following surgery.

Several activation CBF studies such as CO_2 inhalation, autoregulation and intravenous injection of acetazolamide, have been reported for evaluating the viable brain function in patients with cerebral ischemia. Although the activation CBF measurement was not done in this study, this would be able to become a method for evaluating the operative indication of an unruptured aneurysm, especially in the cases of INF. Cerebral vascular reactivity was disturbed in most cases in the acute stage of cerebral ischemia, so that the operative procedure (including anesthesia) may constitute a risk for brain damage in these cases even though the patient's CBF value was above the critical flow leve. Disturbance of the cerebral vascular reserve capacity may also be one of the causative factor of postoperative TND in patients with unruptured aneurysm.

From our previous analysis of unruptured aneurysms[16], we have been performing surgical treatment for these cases since 1986–90. The cause of post-operative complications in regards to permanent neurological deficits were the same as for ruptured aneurysms. Predisposing factors – such as CBF values – had an influence on neurological deficits, but most were only transient effects.

Microneurosurgical procedures are continually being refined and there is knowledge that minimal brain retraction improves the surgical outcome of aneurysms with cerebral ischemia. Therefore, the surgical treatment of unruptured aneurysms is acceptable when the pre-operative CBF is maintained above the critical flow level. Improvement in the surgical treatment of large or giant unruptured aneurysms remains an area for future investigation.

References

1. Abumiya T, Sayama I, Asakura K, Hadeishi H, Mizuno M, Suzuki A, Yasui N, Shishido F, Uc..ura K (1990) Regional effects of craniotomy on cerebral circulation and metabolism: PET study on the unruptured aneurysmal surgery. Neurol Surg 18: 837–844
2. Atkinson JLD, Sundt TM Jr, Houser OW, Whisnant JP (1989) Angiographic frequency of anterior circulation intracranial aneurysms. J Neurosurg 70: 551–555
3. Chason JL, Hindman WM (1958) Berry aneurysms of the circle of Willis. Results of a planned autopsy study. Neurology 8: 41–44
4. Dell S (1982) Asymptomatic cerebral aneurysm: assessment of its risk of rupture. Neurosurgery 10: 162–166
5. Hadeishi H, Yasui N, Suzuki A (1991) Risks of surgical treatment for unruptured intracranial aneurysms. Neurol Surg 19: 945–949
6. Heiskanen O (1981) Risk of bleeding from unruptured aneurysms in cases with multiple intracranial aneurysms. J Neurosurg 55: 524–526
7. Higashida RT, Hablach VV, Dowd C, Barwell SL, Dormandy B, Bell J, Hieshima GB (1990) Endovascular detachable balloon embolization therapy of cavernous carotid artery aneurysms; results in 87 cases. J Neurosurg 72: 857–863
8. Housepian EM, Pool JL (1958) A systematic analysis of intracranial aneurysms from the autopsy file of the Presbyterian Hospital. J Neuropathol Exp Neurol 17: 409–423

9. Inagawa T, Hirano A (1990) Ruptured intracranial aneurysms: an autopsy study of 133 patients. Surg Neurol 33: 117–123
10. Jane JA, Kassell NF, Torner JC, Winn HR (1985) The natural history of aneurysms and arteriovenous malformations. J Neurosurg 62: 321–323
11. McCormic WF, Nofzinger JD (1065) Saccular intracranial aneurysms. An autopsy study. J Neurosurg 22: 155–159
12. Nagashima M, Nemoto M, Hadeishi H, Sayama I, Suzuki A, Yasui N (1988) Surgical treatment of unruptured aneurysms associated with ischemic cerebrovascular diseases. Surg Cereb Stroke 16: 219–223 (Japanese)
13. Romodanov AP, Shcheglov VI (1982) Intravascular occlusion of saccular aneurysms of the cerebral arteries by means of a detachable balloon catheter. In: Krayenbuhl H (ed) Advances and technical standards in neurosurgery, Vol 9. Springer Wien, New York, pp 25–48
14. Stehbens WE (1989) Etiology of intracranial berry aneurysms. J Neurosurg 70: 823–831
15. Wirth FP, Laws ER Jr, Piepgras D, Scotto RM (1983) Surgical treatment of incidental intracranial aneurysms. Neurosurgery 12: 507–511
16. Yasui N, Nemoto M, Nagashima M, Asakura K, Sayama I, Suzuki A, Mizuno M (1987) Surgical problems of the treatment for nonruptured aneurysm. Abstracts of the 46th Congress of the Japan Neurosurgical Society. Neurol Med Chir (Tokyo): 31 (Japanese)

Correspondence: Nobuyuki Yasui, M.D., Department of Surgical Neurology, Research Institute for Brain and Blood Vessels-Akita, 6–10, Senshu-Kubota machi, Akita 010, Japan.

The Fate of Patients with Incidental Intracavernous Carotid Artery Aneurysms (ICCAA)

J. Hernesniemi[1], J. Rinne[1], M. Puranen[2], and T. Saari[2]

Departments of [1]Neurosurgery and [2]Radiology (Neuroradiology), University Hospital of Kuopio, Kuopio, Finland

Summary

Of 1150 patients with cerebral aneurysms, 35 had a total of 37 intracavernous carotid artery aneurysms (ICCAA); 27 were incidental findings. These aneurysms are associated with female sex, advanced age, hypertension and multiplicity – and their presence should prompt four vessel angiography. The mean aneurysm size of the 27 incidental aneurysms was 5.2 mm. In no case had clinical symptoms developed or was any growth of ICCAAs observed in angiographic controls during a mean follow-up time of 5.4 years (range 1–11 years). These asymptomatic aneurysms should be left alone, even with a very low risk therapeutic regimen.

Keywords: Cerebral aneurysm; cavernous sinus; internal carotid artery; outcome.

Introduction

In the presence of large size or fistula, patients with intracavernous carotid artery aneurysms (ICCAAs) are often referred to specialized neurosurgical centers. This selection gives a heavily skewed picture of giant size aneurysms in published cases[1-25]. In a general sample ICCAAs compromise 3–5% of all aneurysms; however, in many studies concerning subarachnoid hemorrhage they are neglected and not included in the series[1-25]. These aneurysms are mainly saccular or arteriosclerotic, seldom traumatic or mycotic. As ICCAAs very seldom rupture into the subarachnoid space, a conservative attitude in treating these cases has been the usual and accepted policy. Recent developments in endovascular surgery and direct intracavernous sinus surgery have made a study on the natural course of these aneurysms necessary. This is an analysis of all ICCAAs diagnosed at one institution over a defined period with a defined catchment area with a stable population and careful follow-up.

Patients and Methods

Of 1444 patients with cerebrovascular malformations (spontaneous intracerebral hemorrhage ICH excluded) treated in the only neurosurgical unit in eastern Finland (total population of 870,000 in the catchment area) from 1977 to 1990, 1150 had a diagnosed cerebral aneurysm with or without SAH. In these 1150 cases, 1001 right-sided and 957 left-sided carotid angiograms were performed. Bilateral carotid angiography was done in 868 patients (75.5%). Aneurysm size was measured in angiograms or CT scans: the largest diameter of the aneurysm in any direction was selected as the aneurysm size and the largest diameter of the neck was selected as the neck size. No corrections for magnification were made. In 24 of the 1150 cases, angiograms were not available and the aneurysms were classified according to radiological, clinical and operative notes as small (0–6 mm), medium (7–14 mm), large (15–24 mm) and giant (25 mm or more).

The aneurysm was considered to be within the cavernous sinus if it arose proximal to the ophthalmic artery. One case with spontaneous carotid cavernous fistula was included, as in this case the aneurysm was visualized and measured easily.

Presentation of ICCAA

The results can be seen in Tables 1–5. There were 35 patients with 37 ICCAA. Twenty-five were females. The aneurysm size in the 10 symptomatic aneurysms ranged from 2 mm (fistula) to 55 mm, with a mean of 19.7 mm. Mean aneurysm size in 24 of the 27 incidental aneurysms was 5.2 mm (range 1–12 mm). In three cases x rays were not available: in two cases the aneurysm was small and in one case medium-sized according to the records. The presenting signs and symptoms can be seen in Table 2. Thirty-three cases were saccular aneurysms, two cases were considered arteriosclerotic fusiform and two cases congenital fusiform. All except one (congenital fusiform) of the asymptomatic aneurysms were saccular.

Distribution according to age, size and sex can be seen in Table 3. Twenty-five patients (71%) had multiple

Table 1a. *Age and Sex Distribution in 35 Cases with ICCAA*

Age years	Female	Male	Total
<19	0	0	0
20–29	0	1	1
30–39	1	2	3
40–49	2	2	4
50–59	9	4	13
60–69	8	1	9
>70	5	0	5
Total	25	10	35

Table 1b. *Age and Sex as Related to Symptoms in 35 Cases with ICCAA*

Presentation	Mean age		
	Females	Males	Total
Symptomatic	60.3	46.0	57.4
Asymptomatic	57.5	47.4	54.2
Total	58.4	47.1	55.1

Table 2. *Presenting Signs and Symptoms of 37 Aneurysms of ICCA*

	Patients	Per cent
Asymptomatic	27	73
SAH	4	11
Mass lesion	5	14
Fistula	1	3

Table 3. *Aneurysm Size by Sex in 35 Cases with ICCAA*

Size	Female	Male	Total
Small	15	8	23
Medium	7	2	9
Large	2	0	2
Giant	2	1	3
Total	26	11	37

Table 4. *Distribution of 92 Aneurysms Seen in 35 Cases with ICCAA*

	Exact site of aneurysm	No. of patients
Internal carotid artery 51	unilateral ICCAA	33
	bilateral ICCAA	2
	ophthalmic	5
	medial wall distal	1
	posterior communicating	8
	anterior choroidal	2
Middle cerebral artery 19	proximal	4
	bifurcation	14
	distal	1
Anterior cerebral artery 16	A1	1
	CoA forward	5
	CoA forward-upward	1
	CoA upward	2
	CoA backward	1
	CoA down	1
	pericallosal (genu)	5
Vertebrobasilar 4	basilar SCA	2
	basilar bifurcation	1
	P1	1
Total		92

Table 5. *Follow-up in 25 Patients with Incidental ICCAAs*

4 early deaths due to SAH

⇓

21 survivors:
one death due to recurrent SAH (Middle cerebral artery aneurysm)
three deaths due to unrelated causes

⇓

17 long term survivors:
– No aneurysm became symptomatic (cranial nerve compression, headache, fistula or SAH) during the follow-up time which ranged from 1 to 11 years (mean 5.3 years).
– No aneurysmal growth in angiographic controls (10 cases)

aneurysms, a total of 92 aneurysms were seen in these 35 cases (Table 4). One occipital AVM was seen, and two patients had contralateral carotid occlusion.

Outcome in Symptomatic Aneurysms

Ten symptomatic cases had the following treatment: no operation (2), shunt operation for relief of hydrocephalus (1), unsuccessful ligation of a large aneurysm by direct surgery (1), trapping (1), carotid ligation in neck (3) and intracranially (2). One patient died after carotid ligation and one patient remained severely disabled, both after a severe SAH and in Grade III preoperatively. The patient with severe disability died later on from rebleeding. Six patients were in excellent condition and two moderately disabled after a mean follow-up of 5.8 years (range 1 to 11 years).

Follow-up of Incidental ICCAA

Twenty-seven ICCAAs were incidental findings associated with symptomatic aneurysms in other locations,

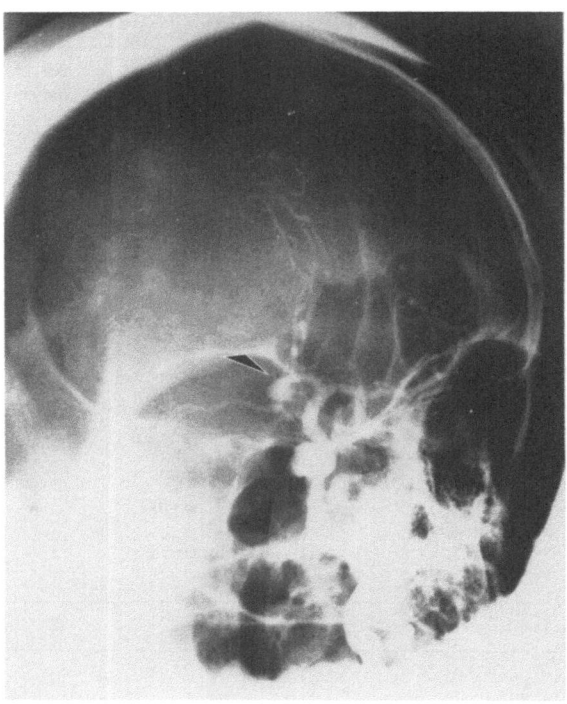

Fig. 1. A medium-sized (8 mm, large arrow head) incidental intracavernous internal carotid artery aneurysm seen in an oblique view
of left carotid angiography of a 56-years-old male patient in 1983.
The small arrow head points to the symptomatic anterior communicating aneurysm. No change in size was observed in a control study
nine years later

usually presenting with SAH. The fates of these 25
patients can be seen in Table 5. No aneurysm became
symptomatic (cranial nerve compression, headache,
fistula or SAH) during the follow-up time, which
ranged from 1 to 11 years (mean 5.4 years in the 20
patients surviving more than one year). One patient
had a fatal rebleed of her symptomatic middle cerebral
artery aneurysm five years after her first SAH and
conservative treatment. Three patients died during the
follow-up from unrelated causes.

Ten of the 17 survivors had angiographic controls
without any anatomical changes in the ICCAA size
or shape (Fig. 1).

Discussion

These aneurysms are associated with female sex, advanced age, hypertension and multiplicity. The strong
female preponderance is in contrast to common findings in Finnish aneurysm series[7,17]. Male patients

seem to have smaller aneurysms at a younger age.
Sizes of ICCAA seem generally to be rather small and
this series differs – in any case as one of the largest
series – from others by being a uniform series from a
catchment area without any special admission policies
such as those associated with most metropolitan neurosurgical units[1–6,8,9,12,18–25]. No other associated vascular anomalies were seen in our patients except
two carotid occlusions – maybe related to aneurysm
formation – and one rather low flow AVM.

Multiple aneurysms were seen in 71% of the cases.
The presence of ICCAA should prompt four vessel
angiography, which was not always done in this series
so some aneurysms may have been missed. Two cases
had bilateral ICCAAs, which are rather seldomly
described[13]. Eighteen associated carotid aneurysms in
other sites were seen in these 35 cases (Table 3).

This is the series with the highest incidence of
asymptomatic ICCAA (73%). We believe this represents
the true situation, as: 1) all patients come from a
defined catchment area with a defined population. No
patients outside of this area were accepted in treatment
here, and no patients were treated elsewhere; 2) the
number of all cases with aneurysms is given. The eleven
per cent incidence of SAH is in good agreement with
earlier series[1–25].

These aneurysms are harmless if found incidentally,
and we doubt at the moment that there is any therapeutic regimen to concur with the good natural course
of these aneurysms. Why some of these aneurysms
become symptomatic is a mystery to us – we could
find no differences in patients characteristics between
the symptomatic and asymptomatic groups. Maybe
our follow-up time is too short. As these aneurysms
are usually found at an older age, the life span of these
patients is reduced, and so is the risk of the aneurysm
becoming symptomatic.

References

1. Barr HWK, Blackwood W, Meadows SP (1971) Intracavernous
   carotid aneurysm: a clinical pathological report. Brain 94:
   607–622
2. Berenstein A, Ransohoff J, Kupersmith M, Flamm E, Graeb D
   (1984) Transvascular treatment of giant aneurysms of the cavernous carotid and vertebral arteries. Surg Neurol 21: 3–12
3. Brihaye J (1979) Intracavernous carotid artery aneurysms. In:
   Pia HW, Langmaid C, Zierski J (eds) Cerebral aneurysm:
   advances in diagnosis and therapy. Springer, Berlin Heidelberg
   New York, pp 67–78
4. Diaz FG, Ohaegbulam S, Dujovny M, Ausman JI (1988)
   Surgical management of aneurysms in the cavernous sinus. Acta
   Neurochir (Wien) 91: 25–28

5. Dolenc V, Cerk M, Sustersic J, Pregel R, Skrap M (1986) Treatment of the intracavernous aneurysms of the internal carotid artery and carotid cavernous fistulas by direct approach. In: Proceedings of the International Symposium of the cavernous sinus. Ljubljana, Yugoslavia, June–July, pp 190–200

6. Drake CG (1979) Giant intracranial aneurysms, experience with surgical treatment in 174 patients. Clin Neurosurg 26: 12–95

7. Fogelholm R (1981) Subarachnoid hemorrhage in Middle-Finland: incidence, early prognosis, and indications for neurosurgical treatment. Stroke 12: 296–301

8. Fox AJ, Vinuela F, Pelz DM, Peerless SJ, Ferguson GG, Drake CG, Debrun G (1987) Use of detachable balloon for proximal artery occlusion in the treatment of unclippable cerebral aneurysms. J Neurosurg 66: 40–46

9. Gelber BR, Sundt TM (1980) Treatment of intracavernous and giant carotid artery aneurysms by combined internal carotid ligation and extra- to intracranial bypass. J Neurosurg 51: 1–10

10. Jefferson G (1938) On the saccular aneurysms of the internal carotid artery in the cavernous sinus. Br J Surg 26: 267–301

11. Jha AN, Lye RH (1986) Aneurysms of the intracavernous internal carotid artery, outcome following carotid ligation or conservative treatment. In: Proceedings of the International Symposium of the cavernous sinus. Ljubljana, Yugoslavia, June–July, p 413

12. Keraver Y, Sindou M, Gaston A (1986) Surgical occlusions of the carotid artery for treatment of giant aneurysms in the cavernous sinus. In: Proceedings of the International Symposium of the cavernous sinus. Ljubljana, Yogoslavia, June–July, pp 235–253

13. Linskey ME, Sekhar LN, Hirsch W Jr, Yonas H, Horton JA (1990) Aneurysms of the intracavernous carotid artery: clinical presentation, radiographic features, and pathogenesis. Neurosurgery 26: 71–79

14. Lombardi G, Passerini A, Migliavacca F (1963) Intracavernous aneurysms of the internal carotid artery. AJR 89: 361–371

15. Meadows SP (1959) Intracavernous aneurysms of the internal carotid artery, their clinical features and natural history. Arch Opthalmol 62: 566–574

16. Ohmoto T, Nagao S, Mino S, Ito T, Honma Y, Fujiwara T (1991) Exposure of the intracavernous carotid artery in aneurysm surgery. Neurosurgery 28: 317–324

17. Pakarinen S (1967) Incidence, aetiology, and prognosis of primary subarachnoid haemorrhage. A study based on 589 cases diagnosed in a defined urban population during a defined period. Acta Neurol Scand 43 [Suppl] 29: 1–128

18. Parkinson D (1979) Surgical approach to cavernous sinus aneurysms. In: Pia HW, Langmaid C, Zierski J (eds) Cerebral aneurysm: advances in diagnosis and therapy. Springer, Berlin Heidelberg, New York, pp 224–228

19. Parkinson D (1965) Surgical approach to cavernous portion of the carotid artery: anatomical studies and case report. J Neurosurg 23: 474–483

20. Pendl G, Vorkapic P, Richlin B, Koos WT (1986) Strategies in intracavernous saccular aneurysms. In: Proceedings of the International Symposium of the cavernous sinus. Ljubljana, Yugoslavia, June–July, pp 211–215

21. Perneczky A, Knosp E (1986) Para- and infraclinoid aneurysms: direct microsurgical repair. In: Proceedings of the International Symposium of the cavernous sinus. Ljubljana, Yugoslavia, June–July, pp 202–210

22. Sahs AL, Perret GE, Locksey HB, Nishioka H (eds) (1969) Intracranial aneurysms and subarachnoid hemorrhage: a Co-operative Study. Lippincott, Philadelphia

23. Sano H, Jain VK, Kato Y, Kamei Y, Asai T, Katada K, Kanno T (1988) Bilateral giant intracavernous aneurysms. Technique of unilateral operation. Surg Neurol 29: 35–38

24. Sekhar LN, Burgess J, Atkin O (1987) Anatomical study of the cavernous sinus emphasizing operative approaches and related vascular and neural reconstruction. Neurosurgery 21: 806–816

25. Weil SM, VanLoveren HR, Tomsick TA, Quallen BL, Tew JM (1987) Management of inoperable cerebral aneurysms by the navigational balloon technique. Neurosurgery 21: 296–302

Correspondence: Juha Hernesniemi, M.D., Ph.D. Department of Neurosurgery, University Hospital of Kuopio, SF-70210 Kuopio, Finland.

Surgical and Endovascular Approaches to Intracavernous Aneurysms

T. Ohmoto, K. Kinugasa, S. Asari, and **M. Sakurai**

Department of Neurological Surgery, Okayama University Medical School, Okayama, Japan

Summary

Five patients with transitional internal carotid aneurysms and 5 patients with large paraclinoid aneurysms underwent direct surgery through an ipsilateral pterional intradural approach. The anterior part of the cavernous sinus anterior to the third nerve was opened to expose the intracavernous portion of the internal carotid artery proximal to the aneurysm. Successful clipping without permanent deficits was accomplished in all cases.

Four aneurysms were treated by injecting a liquid material (cellulose acetate polymer; CAP) into the dome of the aneurysms through an endovascular approach. Three aneurysms arose from the intracavernous portion of the internal carotid artery, one from the transitional area of the internal carotid artery. The transitional aneurysm with poor clinical grade in the acute stage of subarachnoid hemorrhage was successfully treated with CAP at the time of initial angiography. In one patient with a large intracavernous aneurysm, the parent artery was occluded after successful thrombosis of the entire dome of the aneurysm with CAP. These patients are under follow-up with a good clinical condition.

For transitional internal carotid aneurysms, we consider that CAP can be applied to occlude the part of the aneurysm dome to prevent early rupture at the time of initial angiography and that the complete obliteration of the aneurysm neck should be reserved for direct surgical approach.

Keywords: Intracavernous aneurysm; direct intradural approach; intravascular approach; cellulose acetate polymer.

Introduction

Aneurysms arising from the dural transitional area of the internal carotid artery may lead to subarachnoid hemorrhage (SAH)[2,9,15]. Such transitional aneurysms include intracavernous aneurysms bulging into the carotid cistern and paraclinoid aneurysms extending into the cavernous sinus. These transitional aneurysms are generally difficult to approach directly, because the dural transitional area exhibits a complex arrangement of osseous and dural structures and cranial nerves around the internal carotid artery[7,12].

Currently in our department, poor grade patients in the acute stage of SAH have been treated by injecting a liquid material (cellulose acetate polymer; CAP) into the dome of an aneurysm through an endovascular approach at the time of initial angiography. The surgical and endovascular approaches are described including the indication for the combined treatment and the timing of surgery.

Procedures and Results

Surgical Approach

Five patients with transitional internal carotid aneurysms (Table 1, Fig. 1) and 5 patients with large paraclinoid aneurysms underwent direct surgery through an ipsilateral approach[14]. After reaching the carotid cistern, the anterior clinoid process, optic canal roof and optic strut were removed intradurally, facilitating wide exposure of the intradural portion of the aneurysm and its extension through the dura of the cavernous sinus. The anterior siphon knee and the horizontal portion of the intracavernous carotid artery were exposed by cutting the lateral wall of the cavernous sinus along the antero-superior margin of the third nerve. The intracavernous aneurysm was isolated after the cavernous roof was incised along the dome. A fenestrated angled clip was used in most of the cases (Figs. 2–4). No postoperative complications were noted in this series of transitional aneurysms, except for mild oculomotor paresis occurred in one case for a few days. Two patients (cases 3 and 4) were operated upon in the acute stage of SAH, though the ruptured aneurysm was only one (20%) out of 5 transitional aneurysms.

Endovascular Approach

We developed a liquid material, CAP, for direct thrombosis of intracranial aneurysms via an endovascular approach[10,11]. CAP is superior to conventional balloon embolization, since it can conform to the contours of even irregularly-shaped aneurysms without raising the risk of rupture.

Three patients with large intracavernous aneurysms and one patient with a ruptured transitional aneurysm were treated by injecting CAP into the dome of aneurysms. One case out of three intracavernous aneurysms (case 6) had mild hemiparesis due to occlusion of the parent artery.

Case 6: A 58-year-old woman suffered from gradually increasing opthalmoplegia. Cerebral angiogram showed an aneurysm measuring 16×20 mm in the intracavernous internal carotid artery. Direct thrombosis of the aneurysm with CAP was attempted, but the parent artery was occluded at the origin of the aneurysm.

Table 1. *Clinical Summary of Patients with Transitional Internal Carotid Aneurysms*

Case	Age, Sex	Initial symptoms	Site of aneurysm	Preoperative grade	Associated lesions
1	23, F	seizure	Rt transitional IC	0	Rt parietal AVM
2	62, F	headache	Lt transitional IC	0	Rt IC aneurysm
3	60, F	SAH	Lt transitional IC	I	none
4	52, F	SAH	Rt transitional IC	II	Rt MC aneurysm
5	43, F	SAH	Rt transitional IC	0	Lt MC aneurysm

Case 7: A 61-year-old man suddenly lost consciousness because of SAH and was semicomatose at the time of admission. Cerebral angiography demonstrated an aneurysm (8 × 11 mm) arising from the dorsal wall of the proximal internal carotid artery (Fig. 5). Direct thrombosis with CAP was attempted at the time of the initial angiography. A tracker-18 catheter was carefully introduced into the sac of the aneurysm, 0.47 ml of CAP was slowly injected under carotid compression to prevent the migration of CAP. Consecutive angiograms revealed that the aneurysm was almost totally obliterated and the parent vessel preserved (Fig. 6). Five months after the procedure, the patient is neurologically intact except for unsteadiness of his gait.

Discussion

Aneurysms arising anywhere from the anterior siphon knee to the origin of the posterior communicating artery on the internal carotid artery are named intracavernous aneurysm, carotid-ophthalmic aneurysm, infraclinoidal aneurysm[15], paraclinoid aneurysm[5], superior hypophyseal artery aneurysm[1], or carotid cave aneurysm[8], according to the location. Many authors have reported on the approaches to these proximal intradural carotid aneurysms. Regarding the intracavernous aneurysm, Dolenc[3] described an approach through an extradural route, whereas Diaz[2] and Hakuba[4] preferred an intradural approach through the roof of the cavernous sinus.

Of these, the ipsilateral pterional intradural approach is useful to access both intradural and extradural aneurysms, considering that it is easy to proceed with the operation while confirming the anatomical orientation in the operative field. It is necessary first to remove the anterior clinoid process and then to drill off the roof of the optic canal to retract the optic nerve medially. This procedure facilitates an easy exposure of the cavernous roof and isolation of an intradural aneurysm.

When one attempts to reach the horizontal portion of the intracavernous ICA, the drilling should be carried further anterolaterally along the lesser sphenoid wing to the superior orbital fissure and deeper into the optic strut that obscures the view of the carotid siphon knee. Most of the optic strut can be removed by proceeding with drilling deep along the lateral and ventral borders of the optic nerve sheath. By opening the lateral wall of the cavernous sinus anterior to the third nerve, the siphon knee can be exposed, but the

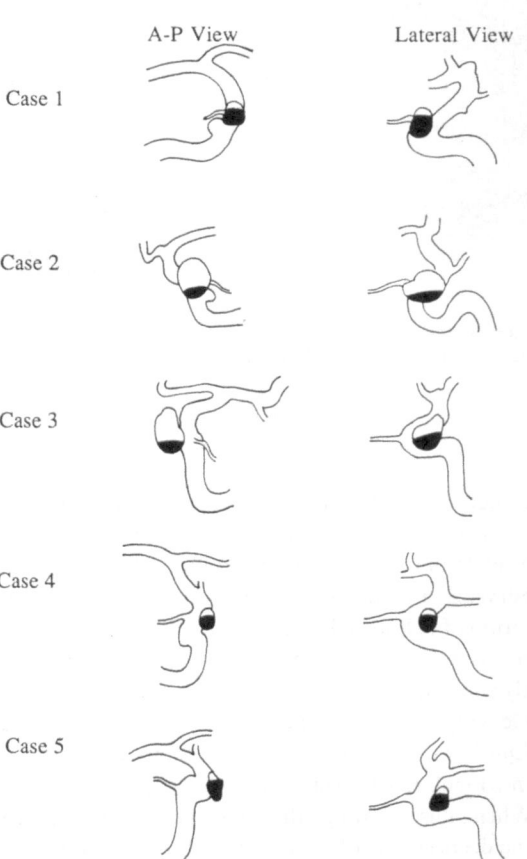

A-P View   Lateral View

Case 1

Case 2

Case 3

Case 4

Case 5

Fig. 1. Angiographic features of transitional internal carotid aneurysms. Tracings of carotid angiograms illustrate the size and location of transitional aneurysms in A–P view (left) and lateral view (right). The shadow part of aneurysm indicates the intracavernous portion of an aneurysm in each case confirmed by surgery

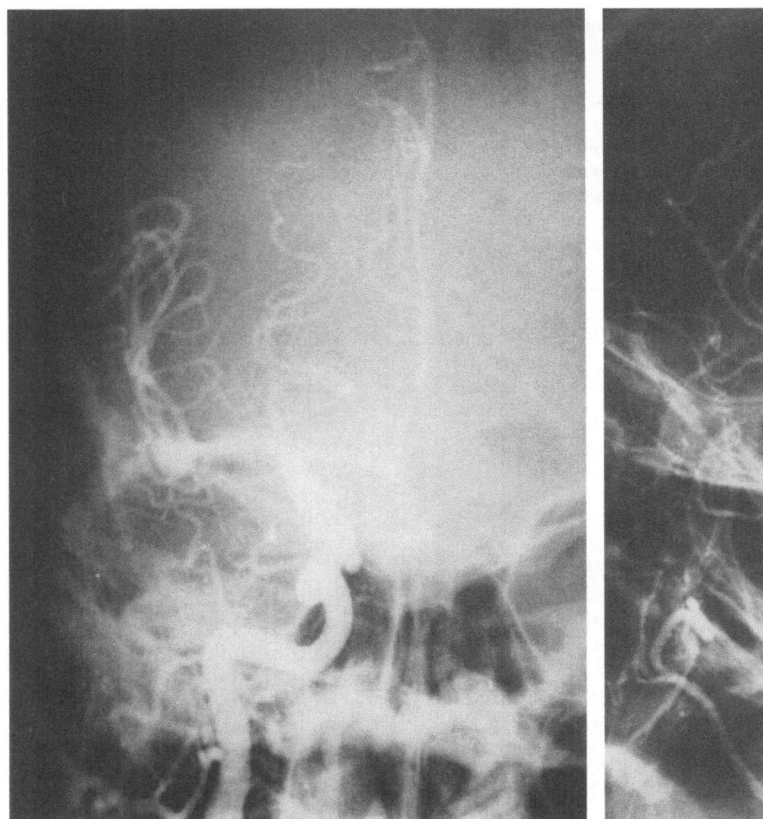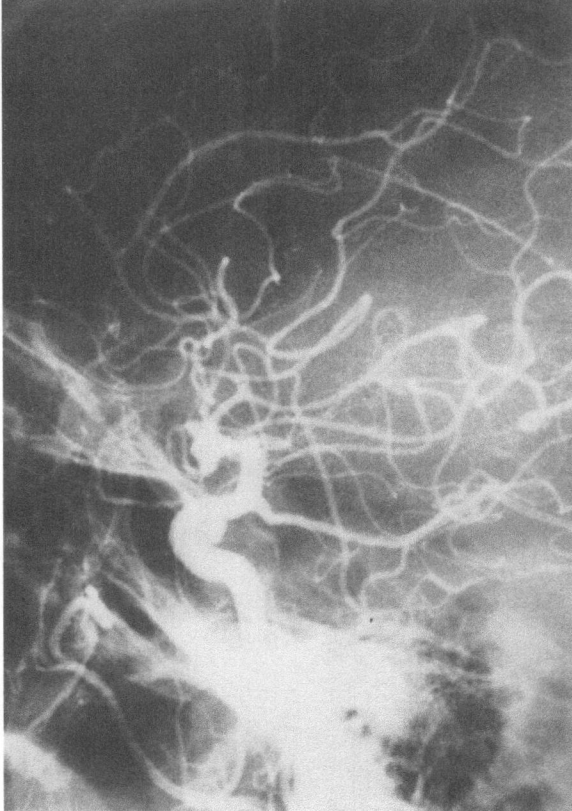

Fig. 2. Preoperative right carotid angiograms (case 4). A–P view (left) and lateral view (right) demonstrate aneurysms arising from the right middle cerebral artery and from the medial aspect of the anterior siphon knee projecting medially and posteriorly

horizontal portion cannot. By opening the roof of the cavernous sinus around the dome, most of the horizontal portion of the internal carotid artery can be approached[14].

During the direct approach to an intracavernous aneurysm, temporary occlusion of the internal carotid artery proximal to the neck is usually repeated to prevent intraoperative rupture. The direct approach is therefore recommended in good grade patients or in the chronic stage of SAH, even through a careful monitoring of cerebral blood flow is carried out during surgery[13].

In many aneurysms treated with intravascular balloon embolization, parts of the neck may not be filled completely. When this happens, circulatory flow and turbulence often cause the aneurysm to grow and form a thrombus around the balloon. There are several re-

ports concerning the growth and rupture of an aneurysm after incomplete obliteration with balloons[6,16]. These complications arise from difficulties of obliterating aneurysms completely with any one balloon or combination of balloons. It is unlikely, at the present time, that any balloon, regardless of its size or shape, perfectly conforms to the shape of an aneurysmal sac without leaving a remnant of neck. Therefore, we developed a liquid material which gives the same contours to even irregularly-shaped aneurysms.

When infused through the tip of a catheter positioned in the deepest part of the aneurysmal sac, CAP begins to solidify upon contact with the inner surface of the sac. It can be infused until the aneurysm neck is occupied keeping the lumen of the parent vessel open. CAP hardens within 5 minutes after the infusion[10,11]. The complete obliteration of the neck, however, may

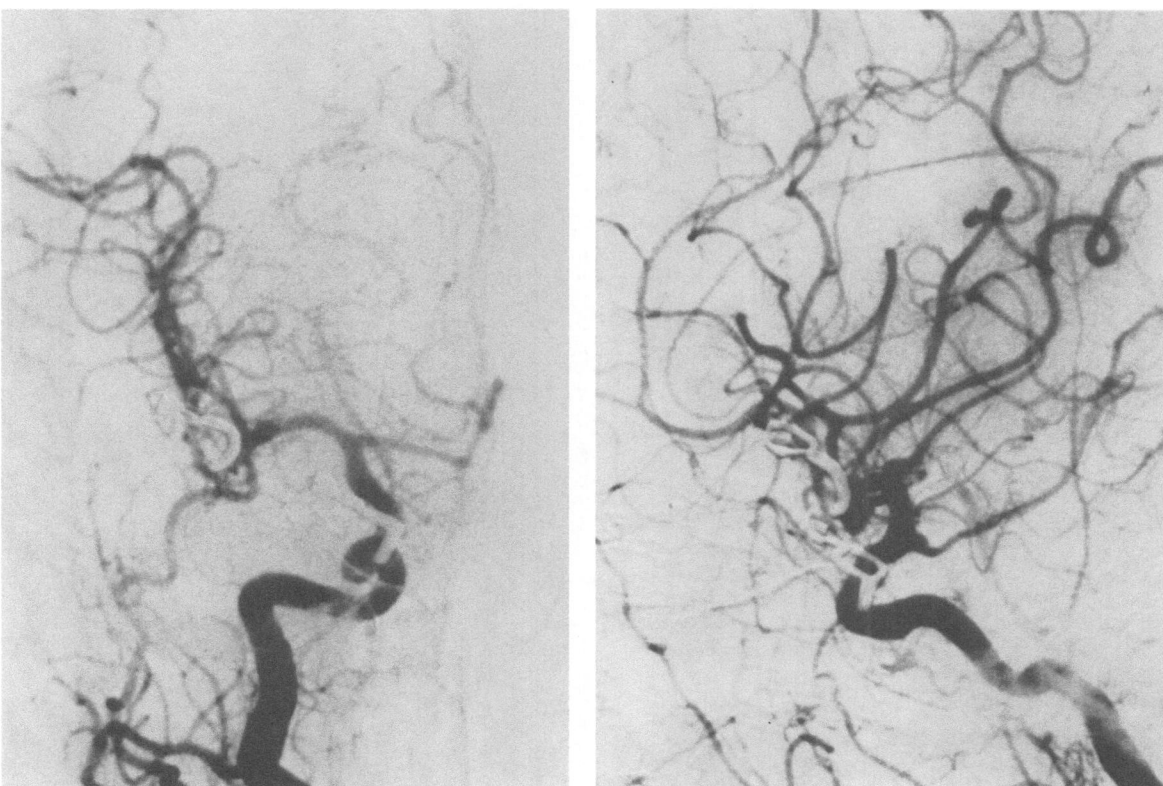

Fig. 3. Postoperative right carotid angiograms (case 4). A–P view (left) and lateral view (right) show complete clipping of both aneurysms

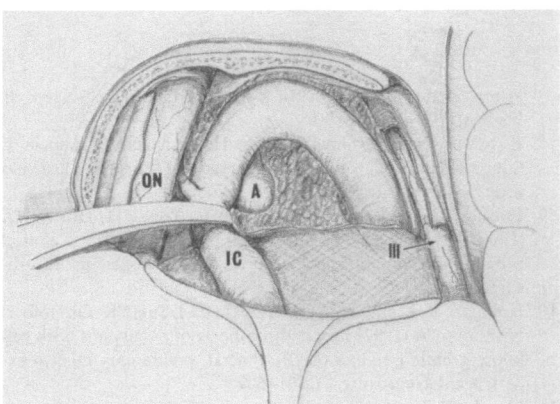

Fig. 4. Final exposure of the intracavernous aneurysm (case 4). The aneurysm and the horizontal portion of the intracavernous carotid artery are exposed between the optic nerve and the thrid nerve. The venous plexus has been coagulated and covered with oxidized cellulose. The lateral wall of the cavernous sinus was opened after removal of the anterior clinoid process and optic canal roof and optic strut through a pterional intradural approch. *A* aneurysm; *ON* optic nerve; *IC* internal carotid artery; *III* third nerve

have a risk of occlusion of the parent artery during solidification, as shown in the patient with a large intracavernous aneurysm (case 6). A fragment of solidified CAP cannot migrate into the distal vessel because blood flow is controlled through carotid compression or microballoon inflation during the procedure.

Since the time we have developed CAP for direct thrombosis of intracranial aneurysms, poor grade patients in the acute stage of SAH are the candidates for this treatment at the time of initial angiography. Our current policy to apply this procedure to ruptured aneurysms is to reduce the risk of rebleeding in the acute stage and to surgically treat the aneurysm after waiting until the patients show uphill course in their neurological status.

Further experience in combined surgical therapy with endovascular thrombosis with CAP will give us advantages to treat the transitional internal carotid aneurysm, which is always in danger of uncontrollable bleeding.

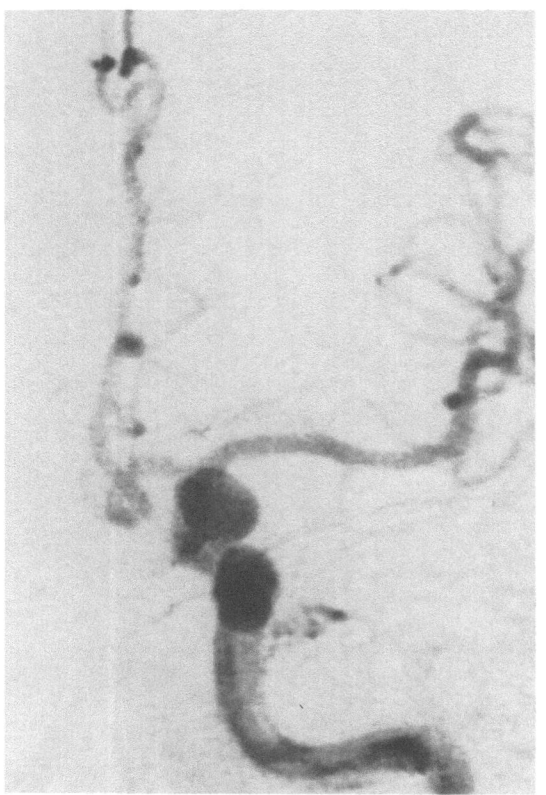

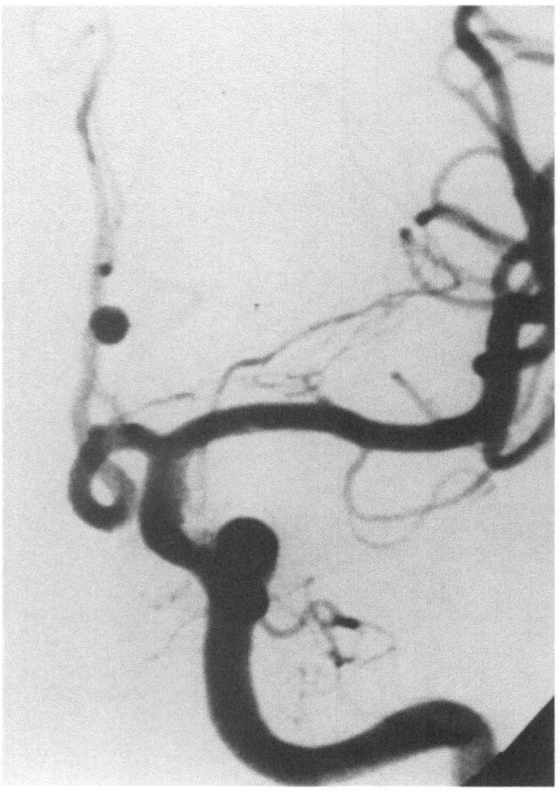

Fig. 5. Left carotid angiogram (A–P view). An initial left carotid angiogram on day 0 showing an aneurysm arising from the dorsal wall of the internal carotid artery and projecting dorsally

Fig. 6. Left carotid angiogram (A–P view). A left carotid angiogram after intraluminal thrombosis with CAP showing a nearly complete obliteration of the aneurysm

References

1. Day AL (1990) Clinicoanatomic features of supraclinoid aneurysms. Clin Neurosurg 36: 256–274
2. Diaz FG, Ohaegbulam S, Dujovny M, Ausman JI (1989) Surgical alternatives in the treatment of cavernous sinus aneurysms. J Neurosurg 71: 846–853
3. Dolenc VV (1990) Surgery of vascular lesions of the cavernous sinus. Clin Neurosurg 36: 240–255
4. Hakuba A, Matsuoka V, Suzuki T, Komiyama M, Jin TB, Inoue V (1987) Direct approaches to vascular lesions in the cavernous sinus via the medial triangle. In: Dolenc VV (ed) The cavernous sinus. A multidisciplinary approach to vascular and tumorous lesions. Springer, Berlin Heidelberg New York Tokyo, pp 272–284
5. Heros RC, Nelson PB, Ojemann RG, Crowell RM, Debrun G (1983) Large and giant paraclinoid aneurysms: surgical techniques, complications, and results. Neurosurgery 12: 153–163
6. Hodes JE, Fox AJ, Pelz DM, Peerless SJ (1990) Rupture of aneurysms following balloon embolization. J Neurosurg 72: 567–571
7. Knosp E, Müller G, Perneczky A (1988) The paraclinoid carotid artery: anatomical aspects of a microneurosurgical approach. Neurosurgery 22: 896–901
8. Kobayashi S, Kyoshima K, Gibo H, Hedge SA, Takemae T, Sugita K (1989) Carotid cave aneurysms of the internal carotid artery. J Neurosurg 70: 216–221
9. Linskey ME, Sekhar LN, Hirsch WJr, Yonas H, Horton JA (1990) Aneurysms of the intracavernous carotid artery: clinical presentation, radiographic features, and pathogenesis. Neurosurgery 26: 71–79
10. Kinugasa K, Mandai S, Terai Y, Kamata I, Sugiu K, Ohmoto T, Nishimoto A (1992) Direct thrombosis of aneurysms with cellulose acetate polymer (CAP): Part II, preliminary clinical experience. J Neurosurg 77: 501–507
11. Mandai S, Kinugasa K, Ohmoto T (1992) Direct thrombosis of aneurysms with cellulose acetete polymer (CAP): Part I, the nature of CAP and the results of thrombosis in experimental aneurysms. J Neurosurg 77: 497–500
12. Nutik SL (1988) Removal of the anterior clinoid process for exposure of the proximal intracranial carotid artery. J Neurosurg 69: 529–534
13. Ohmoto T, Nagao S, Mino S, Fujiwara T, Honma Y, Ito T, Ohkawa M (1991) Monitoring of cortical blood flow during

temporary arterial occlusion in aneurysm surgery by the thermal diffusion method. Neurosurgery 28:49–55

14. Ohmoto T, Nagao S, Mino S, Ito T, Honma Y, Fujiwara T (1991) Exposure of the intracavernous carotid artery in aneurysm surgery. Neurosurgery 28:317–324

15. Perneczky A, Knosp E, Vorkapic P, Czech T (1985) Direct surgical approach to infraclinoidal aneurysms. Acta Neurochir (Wien) 76:36–44

16. Strother CM, Lunde S, Graves V, Toutant S, Hieshima GB (1989) Late paraophthalmic aneurysm rupture following endovascular treatment. Case report. J Neurosurg 71:777–780

Correspondence: Takashi Ohmoto, M.D., Department of Neurological Surgery, Okayama University Medical School, 2-5-1 Shikatacho, Okayama, 700, Japan.

Aneurysm Rests in a Surgical Series of 275 Patients (Five Years): Incidence, Prognostic and Therapeutic Implications

P. Mennonna, F. Ammannati, L. Bordi, G. Cagnoni, R. Gagliardi, G.C Guizzardi, F. Mariotti, and **R. Morichi**

U.O. di Neurochirurgia, U.S.L. 10/D, Firenze, Italy

Summary

The authors present a surgical series of 275 consecutive cases operated in a five years period between 1986 and 1991. This group represents about 26% of the total number of 1033 aneurysms operated on in the Neurosurgical Department of Florence City Hospital since its establishment in 1966. The majority of these patients underwent early surgery and, as a rule, they had calciumantagonist therapy and post-operative (control) angiography.

The incidence of aneurysm rests is evaluated together with its prognostic significance and possible therapeutic approach.

Keywords: Aneurysm rest; post-operative angiography; cerebral aneurysm regrowth.

Introduction

The continuous improvment of microsurgical and anaesthesiological techniques, combined with the always increasing availability of high standard neuroradiological facilities (in particular angiography), has dramatically reduced the risk of direct surgical treatment of cerebral aneurysms. Direct surgical treatment still represents the "golden standard" for the management of endocranial aneurysms, even taking into account the preliminary, although spectacular, results of endovascular procedures[7,8,12].

The incidence, the prognostic significance and the management of post-operative aneurysm rests are still poorly investigated in the literature, despite the large and exaustive surgical series reported; their assessment and possible treatment remains controversial[7,19,20].

According to Drake et al.[7,8] post-operative aneurysm rest should possibly be treated surgically with a second operation; in their experience the aneurysm rest represents anyway a starting point for the regrowth of a new aneurysm, with the associated risk of rupture and subsequent rebleeding. On the other hand, other authors[11] report that the chance of spontaneous obliteration of post-operative aneurysm rest is good and the risk of rebleeding is negligible. These two positions are opposite and very well show how the issue remains debatable.

Clinical Material and Methods

Between January 1986 and December 1990, 275 consecutive patients were operated on in the Department of Neurosurgery of Florence City Hospital for intracranial bleeding aneurysms. This group constitutes about 26% of the 1033 patients operated on for intracranial aneurysms since the establishment of the Neurosurgical Unit in Florence in 1966.

Age ranged between 18 and 72 years (mean 45). According to the Hunt and Hess grading system, 124 (45%) patients were in the first grade at the time of admission to our hospital; 86 (31.2%) in grade two; 55 (20%) in grade three and the remaining 10 patients (7.2%) were in grade four. 81 (29.4%) of the 275 patients were admitted to the hospital within 24 hours from haemorrhage; 104 (37.8%) between 24 and 72 hours from haemorrhage; 63 (33.9%) were admitted between the 4th and the 7th day post-SAH; 18 (6.5%) between the 8th and the 14th day and the remaining 9 (3.2%) arrived after the 14th day from bleeding. 178 patients (65.1%) underwent "early surgery" (within 72 hours), while the remaining 97 (35.3%) were treated with "late surgery" (after 7 days). There were 244 (88.7%) aneurysms in the supratentorial compartment and 31 (11.3%) arising from the vertebro-basilar circulation. 37 patients (13.5%) had multiple aneurysms. 24 (8.7%) aneurysms were "small", ranging from 1 to 6 mm; 143 (52%) were of "medium" size, between 7 and 10 mm of diameter; 85 (30.9%) were considered "large", with a diameter of 11 to 25 mm and 23 (8.4%) were "giant" aneurysms being 25 mm or more in diameter.

In 242 patients of this series (88.6%), it was possible to perform post-operative (control) angiography and, according to neuroradiological evaluation, there were 9 (3.7%) aneurysm rests.

Results

According to the literature[7,8,20] the aneurysm rest is defined as "a small segment at the base of the aneurysm, proximal to the clip, which still fills with contrast on the post-operative control angiogram". Its size is measured between the clip and the parent artery on the best picture of the angiographic series and adjusted according to the radiographic enlargment factor. Follow-up in our series ranged between 2 and 6 years.

There were 6 aneurysm rests (2.8%) in the 215 supratentorial aneurysms and 3 rests (11.1%) in the 27 aneurysms arising in the infratentorial compartment (Table 1 and 2). The 9 patients harbouring aneurysm rests were followed up clinically at 3–6 months intervals. One of the nine patients rebled and required a second operation; the other eight patients remained free of complications (Table 3).

Among the other clinical, epidemiological and surgical variables submitted to analysis in our series, it was clear that age, sex and clinical grade of the patient were not statistically significant to the incidence of aneurysm rests.

Table 1. *Aneurysm Rests*

Incidence (on 242 cases)	9	(3,7%)
Supratentorial (on 215 cases)	6	(2,8%)
Infratentorial (on 27 cases)	3	(11,1%)

Table 2. *Aneurysm Rests*

Timing		
Early surgery	178	(64,7%)
Late surgery	97	(35,3%)
Site		
Supratentorial aneurysms	244	(88,7%)
Infratentorial aneurysms	31	(11,3%)
Multiple aneurysms	37	(13,5%)
Size		
Small (1–6 mm)	24	(8,7%)
Middle 7–10 mm)	143	(52%)
Large (11–25% mm)	85	(30,9%)
Giant (over 25 mm)	23	(8,4%)

Table 3. *Aneurysm Rests-Follow-up*

Case	Site	Follow-up	Outcome
1	basilar tip	6 years	excellent (no rebleeding)
2	basilar tip (+MCA)	6 "	excellent (no rebleeding)
3	ACoA	6 "	good (no rebleeding)
4	carotid siphon	6 "	excellent (no rebleeding)
5	carotid-ophthalmic (giant)	5 "	good (no rebleeding)
6	basilar tip	3 "	excellent (no rebleeding)
7	ACoA (+ pericallosal A)	3 "	excellent (no rebleeding)
8	ACoA	3 "	excellent (no rebleeding)
9	ACoA	2 "	good (rebleeding after 2 months and re-operation)

Two illustrative cases are given below:

Case 1: This 47 year old man was admitted to our hospital after a SAH due to the rupture of a "bulbous" aneurysm arising from the basilar tip. The operation took place on the 12th day post-haemorrhage through a trans-sylvian approach; apparently the aneurysm was clearly exposed and a Sugita clip was placed across its neck to exclude it from the circulation. The aneurysm sac was subsequently pierced and the surgeon was absolutely convinced of the complete exclusion of the aneurysm. Control angiography showed the persistence of a considerable aneurysm rest proximal to the clip. The clinical post-angiographic course was uneventful, but the patient refused consent to a second operation. One year later the patient was found in excellent clinical condition at routine follow-up.

Case 2: This 65 year old man was operated on acutely for an anterior communicating artery aneurysm which had bled. The post-operative course was uneventful and 15 days post-operation a control angiogram was done. This showed a marked vasospasm of the ACA A CoA system and an apparently complete exclusion of the original aneurysm from the circulation. The patient was discharged with no neurological signs. Two months post-operatively a new SAH occurred and angiography at that time disclosed a quite large aneurysm rest which was clearly detected in absence of vasospasm. A second operation was done. At surgery the clip was repositioned across the aneurysm neck. A further (control) angiogram showed a complete and definitive occlusion of the aneurysm without vasospasm. The clinical condition of the patient at follow up was excellent.

Discussion

The incidence of aneurysm rests varies among different reports between 1% and 5%[6,7,9,11,12,15,19,20,22]. We report an incidence of 3.7%, which obviously cannot be considered negligible and represents a potentially serious problem despite the general agreement of various Authors on a basically benign prognosis of the aneurysm rests, if their size is less than 2 mm.

In our cases, "early surgery" (64.7%) prevails on "late surgery" (35.3%). We failed to observe any significant difference of incidence of aneurysm rests between the two groups of treatment. We emphasize the marked difference in localization of the aneurysm rests in our 9 cases: only 2.8% in the supratentorial compartment,

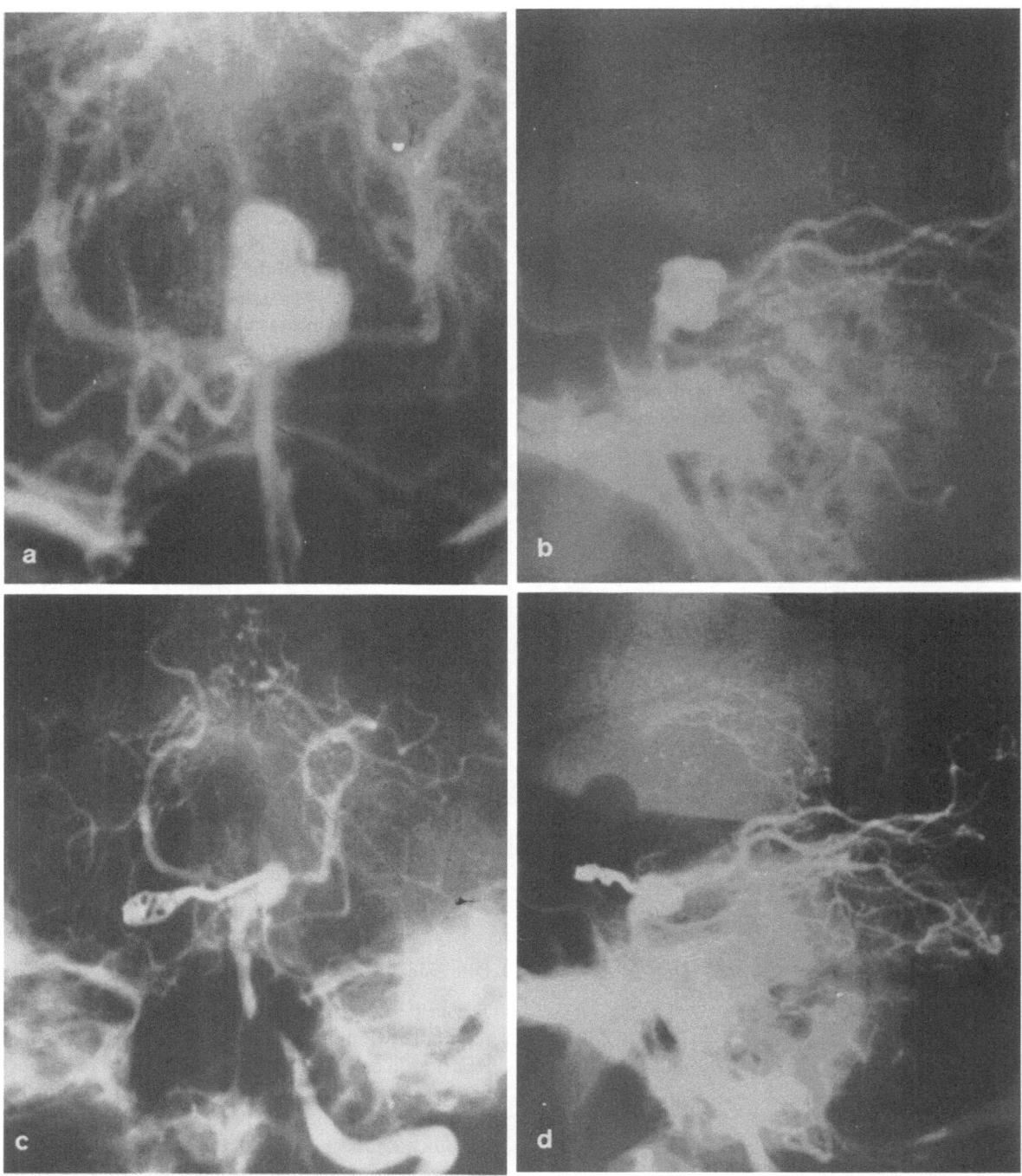

Fig. 1. Case 1. (a, b) "Bulbous" aneurysm of the basilar tip. (c, d) Post-operative control: presence of aneurysm rest

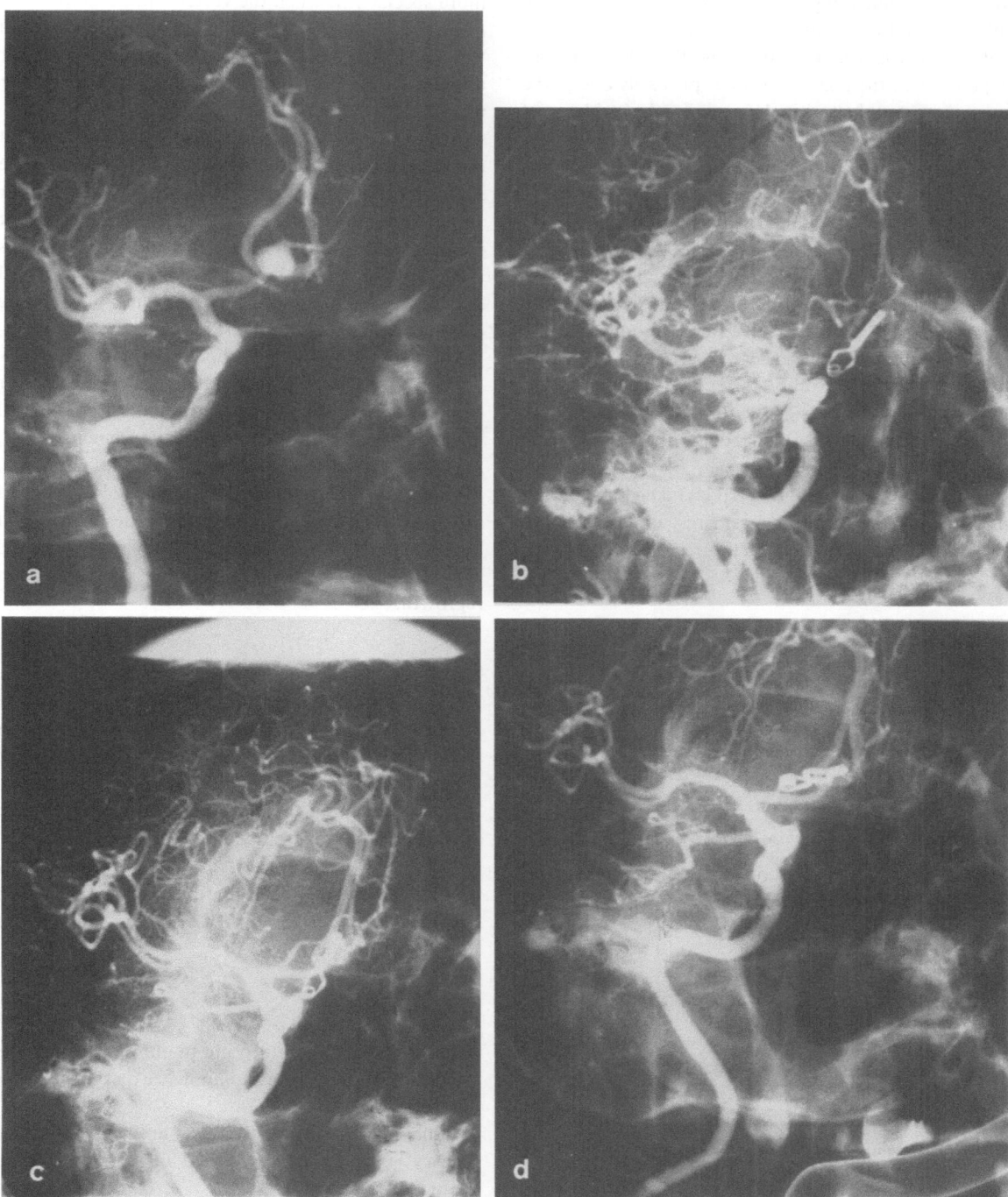

Fig. 2. Case 2. (a) ACoA aneurysm. (b) Post-operative angiogram: presence of vasospasm; the aneurysm is apparently excluded. (c) Control angiogram after two months: an aneurysm rest is clearly seen. (d) Second post-operative angiogram: complete obliteration of the aneurysm

versus the much higher percentage of 11.1 in the infratentorial one. This acquisition has little statistic value, but it is useful to underline that the surgeon's experience at the aneurysm site is probably one of the most important factors in determining the incidence of aneurysm rests.

Generally speaking, it is obvious that the aneurysms arising deeply from the posterior circulation are operated on with much more difficulty and their dissection requires great effort and is a more time-consuming process compared with the supratentorial localization. As underlined by other Authors[2,6,15,20], it is mandatory to evaluate the post-operative (control) angiography very carefully in the presence of focal vasospasm of the arteries next to the clip: this could easily lead to misdiagnosis. Even a significant aneurysm rest could be completely missed, being cut off by the spastic segment of the proximal artery.

We reviewed the possible variables taken into account in the evolution of an aneuysm rest on the basis of the data reported in the literature and of our own experience.

1. Age

The phenomenon of aneurysm rest is more frequent in young people where[3,5,10,21] the growth of intracranial aneurysms is more rapid than in older individuals.

The mean age of our group of patients is 56 years.

2. Sex

Statistically the incidence of aneurysm rests seems to be slightly higher in female patients[3,5,16,18].

3. Size

The so called "minimal rests", which have a diameter of less than 2 mm, do not have evolutive capacities and they are generally considered to have a benign prognosis[6]. However, the possibility of the rest's enlargement has to be taken into account and, if this is proved with control angiography, the possibility of rebleeding immediately rises[6,7].

4. Morphology

The incidence of aneurysm rests is higher with "bulbous" aneurysms with a wide base or when functionally important vessels are close to the aneurysm sac or, even more specifically, when the vessel originates from the aneurysm wall, which could also be very sclerotic. In this case it is difficult to reconstruct the local vascular anatomy, even with the use of fenestrated clips or microsutures.

According to the literature, it has also to be said that the aneurysm regrowth bears no relationship with the size or morphology of the original aneurysm itself, nor with time elapsed[6,7]; therefore, not taking into account the morphology and the size of the aneurysm rest, this is always to be regarded very carefully, from a theoretical and practical point of view, particularly in young people. For this reason the rest has to be checked angiographically not only post-operatively, as routinely done (on the 8th-15th day), but also regularly at 3 or 6 months intervals. Non-invasive neuroradiological techniques (CT with contrast enhancement, MRI, angio-MRI) are to be used for late investigation. Moreover there are pathological (congenital or acquired artery disease, e.g. the collagenopathies or arterial hypertension) or physiological (pregnancy) factors which may contribute to a surprisingly rapid aneurysm regrowth.

5. Site

The aneurysms arising from the posterior circulation are more commonly sites of rests. This is evident in our series and it is certainly due to the depth of these aneurysms and to the difficulty of a complete dissection. In this localization the difference is made, more than anywhere else, by the surgeon's experience.

The theory that aneurysm rests enlarge more rapidly if arising from sites of haemodinamic stress (carotid bifurcation, bifurcation of MCA, basilar apex) is not statistically proved.

6. Surgical Timing

According to the literature and to our own experience, the timing of surgery has no influence on the incidence of aneurysm rests[5,7,14,19,20,21].

It has to be noticed that in our institution "late surgery" is routinely performed on vertebro-basilar aneurysms.

There are other elements which should be studied and statistically assessed in large series, concerning the rests' incidence:

– the type and shape of clip used;
– the possible use of fenestrated clips;

– the reshaping of the aneurysm neck with bipolar coagulation before clipping and subsequent opening and shrinking of the sac;

– the use of controlled hypotension or temporary clipping to allow better dissection of the neck;

– wrapping and coating of the remnants not included in the clip.

We underline the necessity of routine post-operative control angiography (there are no angiographic complications in our series), particularly when during the operation there has been the doubt of "dog ear" persistence or when the surgeon has voluntarily left behind an "unavoidable" rest, as when a functionally important vessel originates from the aneurysm wall.

If vasospasm is found on pre or post-operative angiography, it becomes mandatory to repeat a late control: we know from our experience that vasospasm may easily mask an aneurysm rest which may dangerously evolve in time. Pre-operative angiography cannot be sufficient to solve this problem.

In conclusion, it is possible to say that an aneurysm rest smaller than 2 mm statistically bears a benign prognosis; however it remains an element of doubt, to be followed carefully both after microsurgical and endovascular treatment[6,7,12,14,20]. Larger aneurysm rests should require reoperation, particularly in young people.

References

1. Allcock JM, Canham PB (1976) Angiographic study of the growth of incranial aneurysm. J Neurosurg 45: 617–621
2. Allcock JM, Drake CG (1963) Postoperative angiography in case of ruptured intracranial aneurysm. J Neurosurg 20: 752–759
3. Andrews RJ, Spiegel PK (1979) Intracranial aneurism. Age, sex, blood pressure and multiplicity in an unselected series of patients. J Neurosurg 51: 27–32
4. Bonnal J, Stevenaert A (1969) Thrombosis of intracranial aneurysm of the circle of Willis after incomplete obliteration by clip or ligature across the neck. J Neurosurg 30: 158–164
5. Crompton MR (1959) Mechanism of growt and rupture in cerebral berry aneurysm. J Neurol Neurosurg Psychiatry 22: 259–266
6. Drake CG, Allock JM (1973) Postoperative angiography and the "slipped" clip. J Neurosurg 39: 683–689
7. Drake CG, Friedmann AH, Peerless SJ (1984) Failed aneurysm surgery. Reoperation in 115 cases. J Neurosurg 61: 848–856
8. Drake CG, Vanderbinden RG (1967) The late consequences of incomplete surgical treatment of cerebral aneurysms. J Neurosurg 27: 226–238
9. Ebina K, Suzuki M, Andoh A, et al (1982) Recurrence of cerebral aneurysm after initial neck clipping. Neurosurgery 11: 764–768
10. Ferguson GG (1972) Physical factors in the initiation, growth and rupture of human intracranial saccular aneurysms. J Neurosurg 37: 666–677
11. Feuerberg I, Lindquist C, Lindqvist M, et al (1987) Natural history of postoperative aneurysm rests. J Neurosurg 66: 30–34
12. Fox AJ, Drake CG (1987) Aneurysm neck remnant following baloon embolization. J Neurosurg 67: 321–323
13. Fried LC, Ybolle A (1972) Rapid formation of giant aneurysm: a case report. J Neurol Neurosurg Psychiatry 35: 527–530
14. Kwan ES et al (1991) Enlargement of basilar artery aneurysm following balloon occlusion. Report of two cases. J Neurosurg 75: 963–968
15. Lin T, Fox AJ, Drake CG (1989) Regrowth of aneurysm residual neck following aneurysm clipping. J Neurosurg 70: 556–560
16. McCormick WF, Acosta-Rua GJ (1970) The size of intracranial saccular aneurysms. An outopsy study. J Neurosurg 33: 422–427
17. McKissok W (1965) Recurrence of an intracranial aneurysm after excision. Report of a case. J Neurosurg 23: 547–548
18. Ostergaard JR, Hog E (1985) Incidence of multiple intracranial aneurysms. Influence of arterial hypertension and gender. J Neurosurg 63: 49–55
19. Sato S, Suzuki J (1971) Prognosis in cases of intracranial aneurysm after incomplete dire ct operations. Acta Neurochir (Wien) 24: 245–252
20. Suzuki J, Kwak R, Katakura R (1979) Angiographical consideration of residual aneurysms following direct operations on intracranial aneurysms. In Suzuki J (ed) Cerebral aneurysms; experience with 1000 directly operated cases. Neuron, Tokyo, pp 619–630
21. Suzuki J, Ohara H (1978) Clinicopathological study of cerebral aneurysms. Origin, rupture, repair and growth. J Neurosurg 48: 505–514
22. Wein B, Drake CG (1991) Rapid growth of residual aneurysmal neck during pregnancy. Case report. J Neurosurg 75: 780–782

Correspondence: Pasquale Mennonna, M.D. U.O. di Neurochirurgia U.S.L. 10/D, Policlinico di Careggi, Viale Morgagni, 85, I-50134 Florence, Italy.

Recurrent Subarachnoid Hemorrhage After Aneurysm Surgery

M. Takeda, Y. Yonekawa, H. Miyake, T. Tsukahara, and **A. Kobayashi**

Department of Neurosurgery, National Cardiovascular Center, Fujishirodai, Suita, Osaka, Japan

Summary

We investigated the pathogenesis and risk factors for recurrent subarachnoid hemorrhage (SAH) in 590 patients with aneurysmal SAH. Out of these, 12 suffered a recurrent SAH after surgery. The main causes of recurrence were aneurysm rest in the early rebleeding group, and de novo aneurysm in the late rebleeding group. All patients with recurrence except one had hypertension, and none of the 5 normotensive patients with an aneurysm rest suffered recurrence. Hypertension and history of SAH itself are considered to be the risk factors for recurrent SAH. We emphasize the importance of medication for hypertension after surgery in patients with a history of SAH with or without an aneurysm rest.

Keywords: Subarachnoid hemorrhage; recurrence; hypertension; de novo aneurysm.

Introduction

Neck clipping is thought to be the most curative treatment for intracranial aneurysms. Surgery, however, does not always result in permanent cure. We investigated the pathogenesis and risk factors for recurrent SAH in 590 patients with aneurysmal SAH who had undergone direct surgery.

Clinical Material and Methods

Out of 857 patients with ruptured intracranial aneurysm seen at the National Cardiovascular Center between 1978 and 1990, 590 had undergone direct surgery (Table 1). The patient group included 252 males and 338 females ranging in age from 2 to 88 years, with a mean age of 54.0 years (Fig. 1). The mean follow-up period was 57.0 months and follow-up periods ranged from 2 days to 7 years. Surgical treatment employed in each patient is shown in Table 2. Surgery was performed with Yasargil's clip or Sugita's clip, except for some patients in early years. Aneurysm rests were wrapped with muscle or fascia, or coated with Biobond.

Results

The clinical features of the 12 patients who suffered a recurrent SAH are summarized in Table 3. There were 4 males and 8 females, with a mean age of 53.2 years.

Recurrent SAH occurred within 2 months in 5 patients (early rebleeding group), and later than 4 years in 7 (late rebleeding group). Four out of 5 patients in the early rebleeding group suffered a recurrent SAH from aneurysm rests, and 6 out of 7 patients in the late rebleeding group from de novo aneurysms which had not been visualized on the initial angiograms. The ruptured aneurysm was located on the anterior communicating artery (Acom) in 3, internal carotid artery (ICA) in 3, basilar artery (BA) in 3, middle cerebral artery (MCA) in 2, and distal anterior cerebral artery (ACA) in 1. In no patients had multiple aneurysms been detected on the initial angiograms. Azygous ACA was found in 1 patient (Case 6), and no patient had cerebrovascular occlusive disease. All patients except 1 (Case 3) had hypertension.

Three patients in addition to those described above suffered a recurrent SAH after the proxymal ligation of the parent artery with EC/IC bypass.

Case Report

Case 3

This 36-year-old man suffered a severe headache of sudden onset and vomiting. Angiograms revealed a Acom aneurysm, which was clipped on day 1. The postoperative course had been favorable until day 13, when he suddenly became semicomatose. Repeated angiograms revealed an aneurysm adjacent to the clip, which was larger than the one visualized on the initial angiograms (Fig. 2). At the second operation, a pulsating aneurysm with an extremely thin wall was found adjacent to the edge of the clip.

Case 7

This 31-year-old woman suffered a headache of sudden onset. Initial angiograms revealed an Acom aneurysm

Table 1. *Location of Aneurysms*

Internal carotid artery	190
IC top	16
IC-posterior communicating artery	129
IC-anterior choroidal artery	24
IC-ophthalmic artery	22
etc.	14
Middle cerebral artery	199
M1–M2	193
etc.	14
Anterior cerebral artery	249
anterior communicating artery	211
distal anterior cerebral artery	34
etc.	9
Posterior circulation	60
basilar artery	30
vertebral artery	23
etc.	9

IC internal carotid artery.

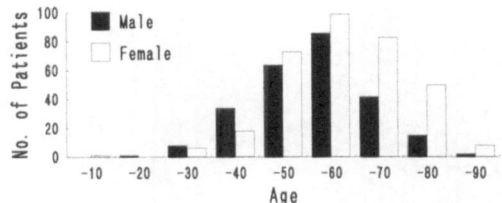

Fig. 1. Age and sex distribution in 590 patients with aneurysmal SAH treated surgically at NCVC between 1978 and 1990

Table 2. *Surgical Treatment*

Clipping	568
complete	550
incomplete	18
Coating/wrapping	9
Trapping	7
Proximal ligation	3
etc.	3

Table 3. *Patients with Recurrent SAH After Clipping Aneurysms*

Case	Age	Sex	Location 1st	2nd	Pathogenesis	Interval
1	75	M	Acom	rerupture	aneurysm rest	4 days
2	65	F	Lt IC-PC	rerupture	slipped-out clip	4 days
3	36	M	Acom	rerupture	aneurysm rest	12 days
4	73	M	BA top	rerupture	aneurysm rest	14 days
5	41	M	Acom	rerupture	aneurysm rest	52 days
6	49	F	DACA	DACA	de novo	4 years
7	31	F	Acom	Rt MCA	de novo	4 years
8	52	F	BA top	rerupture	slipped-out clip	6 years
9	71	F	Lt IC-PC	Rt IC-PC	de novo	6 years
10	40	M	Lt MCA	Rt MCA	de novo	7 years
11	41	F	Acom	BA top	de novo	7 years
12	65	F	Lt IC-PC	Rt IC	de novo	10 years

Acom anterior communicating artery; *DACA* distal anterior cerebral artery; *IC-PC* internal carotid artery-posterior communicating artery; *MCA* middle cerebral artery; de novo: de novo aneurysm; *BA* basilar artery.

and a small projection at the left MCA bifurcation but no abnormality of the right MCA. Surgery was performed on day 3, and she was discharged without any neurological deficit. Four years after surgery, she suffered a recurrent SAH. Repeated angiograms revealed a de novo aneurysm at the right MCA (Fig. 3).

Discussion

Since McKissock[14] described a case of recurrent aneurysm and reported that excision of the aneurysm after occlusion of the neck does not necessarily result in permanent cure, various mechanisms of recurrent

SAH have been reported[1,3,8,13,19] (Fig. 4). Drake and Vanderlinden[8] reported the late consequences of incomplete surgical treatment of cerebral aneurysms; 11 of 25 patients in whom the obliteration was incomplete rebled, and 9 of them died from the rebleeding. On the other hand, in patients in whom the obliteration was complete, there has been no known rebleeding. They emphasized the importance of the complete treatment of the aneurysm. Recurrent SAH, however, sometimes occurs after complete clipping. Injury of the arterial wall due to surgical maneuver or the edge of the clip[1,9,19], postoperative change in hemodynamic flow pattern[3,13], and microscopic aneurysm rest[9] have all

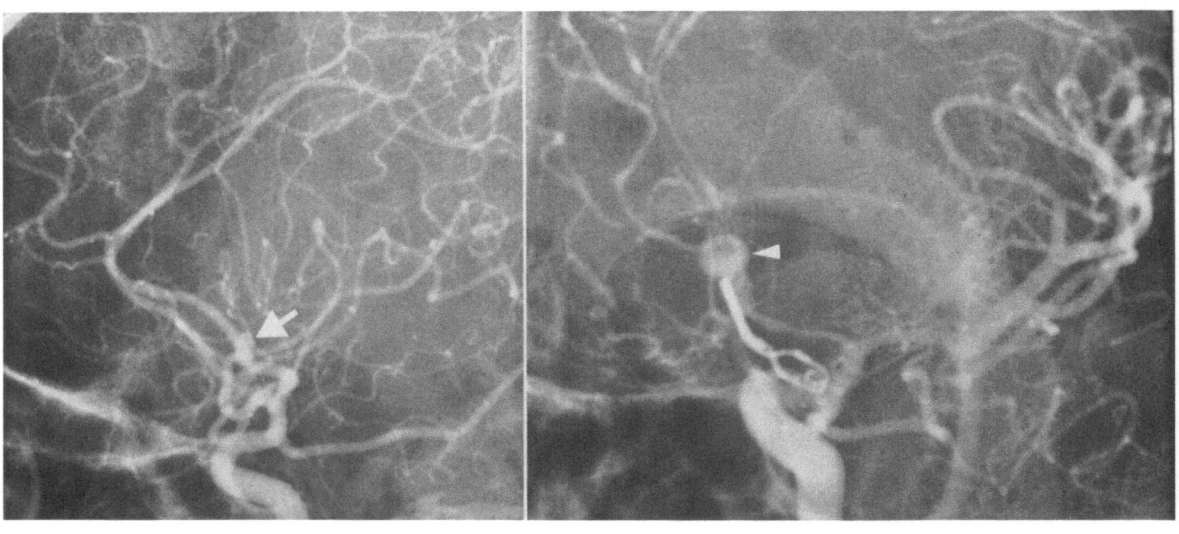

Pre-op   Post-op

Fig. 2. Case 3: left carotid angiogram. Small aneurysm (arrow) at anterior communicating artery on the initial angiogram (left), and larger aneurysm (arrow head) on the postoperative angiogram (right)

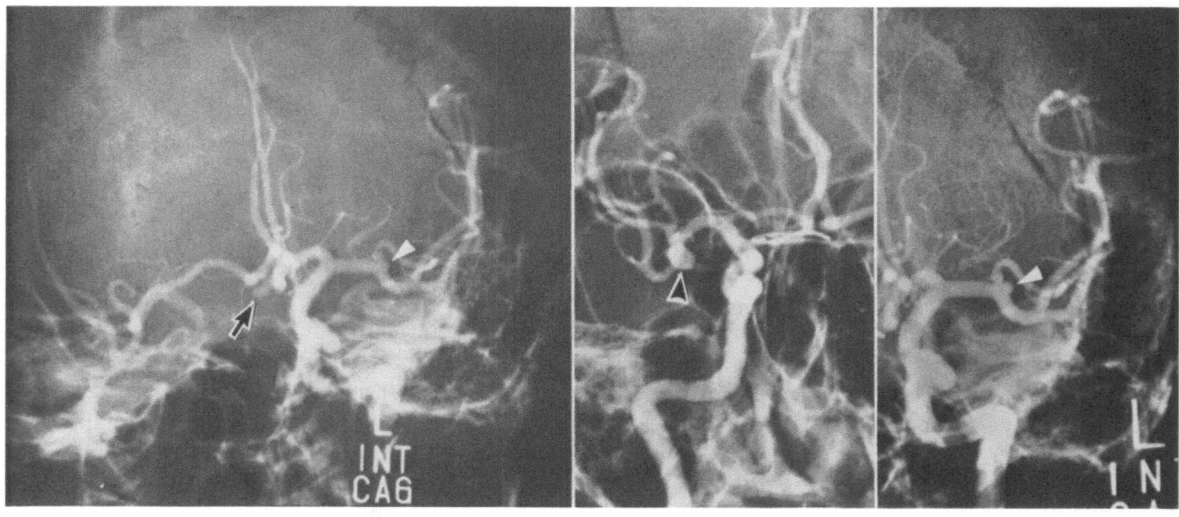

Pre-op   Post-op

Fig. 3. Case 7: bilateral carotid angiogram. Acom aneurysm (arrow) and a small projection (white arrow head) at left MCA on the initial angiogram (on the left); de novo aneurysm (black arrow head) at right MCA (in the middle); slightly grown-up aneurysm (white arrow head) at left MCA (on the right); on the postoperative angiograms

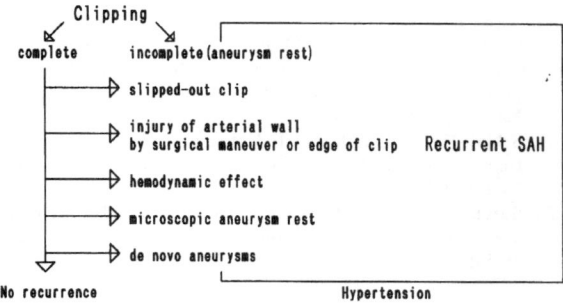

Fig. 4. Pathogenesis of recurrent SAH

been considered to be involved in the pathogenesis of recurrent SAH.

In our series, 4 out of 5 patients in early rebleeding group rebled from an aneurysm rest. However, no patients have had recurrent SAH from aneurysm rests in the chronic stage, which is reported to be a rare event in the literature[2,7]. Suzuki[20] reported that in some aneurysms the wall is thinner at the neck than at the dome. The outcome in patients in whom the obliteration of the aneurysm has been incomplete seems to depend upon the fragility of the aneurysm rest.

It is noteworthy that 6 of our 7 patients in the late rebleeding group suffered a recurrent SAH from de novo aneurysms. The study of the formation of "de novo" aneurysm, a term introduced by Graf and Hamby[10], can illuminate the etiology of intracranial aneurysms. Miller et al.[15] reported that de novo aneurysms were observed in 7 of 620 consecutive patients with intracranial aneurysms. This incidence is almost the same as that in the present study. De novo aneurysms play an important part in the pathogenesis of recurrent SAH.

Intracranial aneurysms are considered to result from a combination of congenital and/or acquired vascular vulnerability and hemodynamic effects (Fig. 5). Analysis

of the clinical features of the patients with a history of SAH can be expected to provide some information regarding risk factors for recurrent SAH. The reported incidence of aneurysmal SAH ranged from about 3 to 10 per 100,000 per year[5,16,17]. In our group of 590 patients with a history of SAH with a mean follow-up period of 57.0 months, 6 suffered a recurrent SAH from de novo aneurysms. This would give a rate of about 214 per 100,000 per year. A history of SAH itself can be a risk factor for SAH. Hypertension is one of the risk factors which influences the hemodynamic environment of the aneurysm[6,18]. All of our patients with recurrent SAH except 1 (Case 3) had hypertension. Furthermore, repeated angiograms performed in 5 normotensive patients with aneurysm rest revealed no significant change in the size of the aneurysm.

Conclusions

Even if surgical treatment is complete, some patients suffer a recurrent SAH. Hypertension and history of SAH itself are considered to be the risk factors for recurrent SAH. We enphasize the importance of medication for hypertension in patients with history of SAH with or without an aneurysm rest.

References

1. Alexander E, Adams JE, Davis CH (1963) Complication in the use of temporary intracranial arterial clip. J Neurosurg 20: 810–811
2. Allcock JM, Drake CG (1963) Postoperative angiography in cases of ruptured intracranial aneurysm. J Neurosurg 20: 752–759
3. Asari S, Kunishiro K, Sunami N, Yamamoto Y (1968) Rapid growth and rupture of newly originated aneurysm near the clipped middle cerebral artery aneurysm. Neurol Surg 14: 587–591
4. Bjorkesten G, Troupp H (1962) Changes in the size of intracranial arterial aneurysms. J Neurosurg 19: 583–588
5. Crawford MD, Sarner M (1965) Ruptured intracranial aneurysms. Community study. Lancet ii: 1254–1257
6. Crompton MR (1966) Recurrent hemorrhage from cerebral aneurysm and its prevention by surgery. J Neurol Neurosurg Psychiatry 29: 164–170
7. Drake CG, Allcock JM (1973) Postoperative angiography and the "slipped" clip. J Neurosurg 39: 683–689
8. Drake CG, Vanderlinden RG (1967) The late consequences of incomplete surgical treatment of cerebral aneurysms. J Neurosurg 27: 226–238
9. Ebina K, Suzuki M, Andoh A, Saitoh K, Iwabuchi T (1982) Recurrence of cerebral aneurysm after initial neck clipping. Neurosurgery 6: 764–768
10. Graf CJ, Hamby WB (1964) Report of a case of cerebral aneurysm in an adult developing apparently de novo. J Neurol Neurosurg Psychiatry 27: 153–156
11. Hashimoto N, Handa H, Hazama F (1979) Experimentally induced cerebral aneurysms in rats: Part III. Pathology. Surg Neurol 11: 299–304

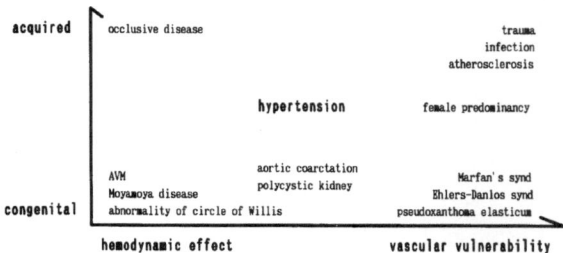

Fig. 5. Pathogenesis of intracranial aneurysms

12. Hashimoto N, Kim C, Kikuchi H, *et al* (1987) Experimental induction of cerebral aneurysms in monkeys. J Neurosurg 67: 903–905

13. Maeda Y, Fujita T, Yamamoto S, Karino M (1989) Recurrent cerebral aneurysm suggestive of misplaced clipping. Neurol Med Chir (Tokyo) 29: 319–323

14. McKissock W (1965) Recurrence of an intracranial aneurysm after excision. J Neurosurg 23: 547–548

15. Miller CA, Hill SA, Hunt WE (1985) "De novo" aneurysms, a clinical review. Surg Neurol 24: 173–180

16. Parkinen S (1967) Incidence, etiology, and prognosis of primary subarachnoid hemorrhage. A study based on 589 cases diagnosed in a defined urban population during a defined period. Acta Neurol Scand 43 [Suppl] 29: 1–28

17. Ramussen P, Busch H, Haase J, Hansen J, Harmsen A, Knudsen V, Marcussen E, Midholm ST, Olsen RB, Rosenorn J, Schmidt K, Voldby B, Hansen L (1980) Intracranial aneurysms. Results of treatment in 851 patients. Acta Neurochir (Wien) 53: 1–17

18. Sacco RL, Wolf PA, Bharucha NB, Meeks SL, Kannel WB, Charette LJ, Mcnamara PM, Palmer EP, D'Agostino R (1984) Subarachnoid and intracerebral hemorrhage. Natural history, prognosis, and precursive factors in the Framingham study. Neurology 34: 847–854

19. Sekino H, Kitoh Y, Kanki T, Nakamura N (1985) Iatrogenic traumatic intracranial aneurysm. Neurol Med Chir (Tokyo) 25: 945–951

20. Suzuki J, Ohara H (1978) Clinicopathological study of cerebral aneurysms: origin, rupture, repair, and growth. J Neurosurg 48: 505–514

Correspondence: Makoto Takeda, M.D., Department of Neurosurgery, National Cardiovascular Center, 5–125 Fujishirodai, Suita, Osaka, Japan.

Intracranial Arteriovenous Malformations

Classification of Cerebral AVMs

Classification of Arteriovenous Malformations

K.A. Smith and **R.F. Spetzler**

Division of Neurological Surgery, Barrow Neurological Institute, Phoenix, Arizona, U.S.A.

Summary

Cerebral arteriovenous malformations (AVMs) are complex lesions with variable resectability. Multiple grading systems have been proposed that aim to predict the risk of surgical treatment in individual patients based on several radiographical and clinical characteristics of AVMs. A grading system is only useful if it can accurately predict the surgical risks prospectively. Furthermore, it must be simple enough to be applied reliably by general neurosurgeons with minimal interpretational error and without additional testing requirements. The application of a standardized grading scheme enables accurate comparisons between different treatment paradigms and assists in the process of choosing the appropriate management for individual cases. The grading system proposed by Spetzler and Martin divides cerebral AVMs into five clinical grades based on AVM size, proximity to eloquent tissue, and the presence or absence of deep venous drainage. This system has been applied retrospectively and prospectively and has been found to predict surgical morbidity accurately. This system also has the advantage of being simple and reliable, and it requires no additional testing other than a conventional angiogram. It compares favorably with other proposed grading systems in terms of simplicity, accuracy, and reliability.

Keywords: Cerebral AVM; grading system; surgical morbidity.

Introduction

Cerebral arteriovenous malformations (AVMs) are a complex group of lesions that have a propensity to hemorrhage. They often cause devastating neurological deficits if untreated. Other common nonhemorrhagic symptoms include headaches, seizures, and various neurological symptoms caused by vascular steal[14,21]. Treatment of AVMs is intended to prevent intracerebral hemorrhage and to preserve neurologic function. A patient only clearly benefits from treatment if the risk of hemorrhage is completely eliminated without undue cost in neurological function[13,14,19]. AVMs vary greatly in complexity and therefore in resectability. Some lesions are small and superficial and can be removed safely. Other lesions are massive, involve eloquent areas of the brain, and drain into the deep venous structures. Such lesions are almost impossible to resect without causing a neurological deficit. Most cerebral AVMs fall somewhere between these two extremes. Current treatment modalities for cerebral AVMs include surgical excision, embolization[10], radiation therapy[7,20], and combinations of all three. The "gold standard" of AVM treatment remains complete surgical resection since only the complete removal of the AVM can prevent an intracranial hemorrhage.

Rational decision making regarding the treatment of AVMs requires a grading system that accurately predicts risks of treatment of individual patients in a prospective fashion. Stratification of lesions into groups in a reproducible fashion permits accurate and meaningful comparisons between different treatment modalities. A useful grading system must also be simple enough to be applied by general neurosurgeons in a consistent fashion without the need for additional testing or data available only at specialized centers.

An ideal grading system would define the degree of difficulty of resecting individual AVMs with respect to operative morbidity and mortality. A grading system must also be comprehensive enough to include all variations of AVMs but yet allow assimilation into large enough groups to make comparisons between groups statistically meaningful. Previously proposed grading systems have failed, either because they were too simple or too complex and awkward[6,9,12]. A system based on size of AVMs alone does not incorporate other characteristics that are relevant to the feasibility of resection. For example, a 5-cm right frontopolar AVM carries less surgical risk than a 2-cm deep thalamic AVM with deep venous drainage. Other classification systems are too complex. For example, the scheme proposed by Pasqualin et al.[12] uses 11 anatomical locations, calculated volumes, four variations in venous drainage, and scaled flow velocity as measured on Doppler ultrasonography. Although such information can be useful in individual cases, the system is cumbersome. It produces such a large number of subdivisions that comparisons between treatment groups has little meaning due to the small number of patients in each group.

Ultimately, a grading system is useful only if it consistently correlates with operative morbidity when tested clinically. Hollerhage et al.[6] retrospectively reviewed 93 surgically treated cerebral AVM patients and assigned the patients into groups according to the classification systems proposed by Leussenhop and Genarelli[9], Shi[15], and Spetzler and Martin[16]. The Spetzler and Martin[16] scheme was the best predictor of clinical outcome in this comparison. In fact, the other two classifications systems only correlated weakly with clinical outcome. Originally Spetzler and Martin[16] applied their grading system retrospectively to 100 consecutively treated cerebral AVM patients and found an excellent correlation with predicted clinical outcome based on preoperative grade. We are using the Spetzler-Martin grading scheme prospectively and continue to be able to predict the safety of resection based on the preoperative grade of an AVM[18]. With rare exceptions, different physicians consistently assign the same grade to an AVM. When differences of opinion do exist, it is always by only one grade and usually attributable to the assigned eloquence of the location of the AVM.

Description of Grading System

Graded Variables

The most important factors relating to the difficulty and safety of surgical resection of cerebral AVMs are size, location, surgical accessibility, proximity to adjacent eloquent brain areas and vascular structures, flow velocity, degree of steal, the number of feeding vessels, and patterns of venous drainage. As stated, a grading system that would incorporate all of these variables would be too cumbersome. However, many of these factors are so interrelated that one of the variables can account for several others. In most cases, three graded variables – size of the AVM, pattern of venous drainage, and eloquence of the brain adjacent to the AVM – include features of the other variables. With only three variables, the system is simple and applied easily with much less chance for interpretational error.

Size of the AVM

The size of the AVM is responsible for much of the technical difficulty of resection. Larger AVMs take longer to dissect from adjacent brain and, by mere chance, a larger AVM has a greater likelihood of proximity to vital regions of the brain and to be fed by multiple vessels. The longer operating times required and the risk for anesthetic-related complications are naturally increased for larger AVMs. The degree of vascular steal and rate of flow are also largely a function of size. Consequently, size is the predominant factor of the AVM grade.

The size of the AVM is determined by the largest diameter of the AVM nidus on conventional angiography. When magnification is used, the measurement must account for the degree of magnification. We do not calculate volume, as suggested by other grading systems, to maintain simplicity and to avoid further error from inherent problems with volume calculations based on routine angiographic data. A small AVM, less than 3 cm in greatest dimension, is assigned 1 point. Medium-sized AVMs, larger than 3 cm but less than 6 cm, are assigned 2 points. Large AVMs, which are greater than 6 cm, are assigned 3 points.

Pattern of Venous Drainage

The pattern of venous drainage is clearly associated with resectability of the AVMs. Deep venous drainage complicates AVM excision. Small arterialized subependymal veins of the deep venous component are typically friable, difficult to cauterize, and tend to retract and bleed into the ventricle or brain parenchyma when disrupted. Coagulation or disruption of major draining veins of the deep system is associated with venous hypertension and postoperative hemorrhage following AVM resection[2]. Superficial cortical draining veins are usually much less problematic. The collateral venous outflow is greater, and the veins are accessible and typically easy to cauterize and divide[17]. Therefore, AVMs with deep venous drainage are assigned higher grades than those with superficial venous drainage.

The pattern of venous drainage is determined by careful inspection of the angiogram. If all the draining veins from the AVM are of the cortical venous system, the AVM is assigned 0 points for venous drainage on the grading scale. If there are any draining veins into the deep system, the AVM is assigned one point for venous drainage. Superficial vessels in posterior fossa

AVMs are considered to be only those that drain directly into the transverse or straight sinuses.

Eloquence of Adjacent Brain

The safety of an AVM resection depends on its proximity to vital anatomical structures. The degree of importance of different brain locations becomes difficult to define. Certainly, assignment of eloquence to one area of the brain and not to another is arbitrary. For the purpose of the grading scheme, however, eloquent brain regions are those that, if injured, result in a readily identifiable neurologic deficit. Noneloquent areas are those associated with more subtle neurologic function in which injury does not produce a permanent disabling deficit. For clarity and to avoid interpretational error, eloquent areas are defined as the following: the sensorimotor, language, and visual cortex; the

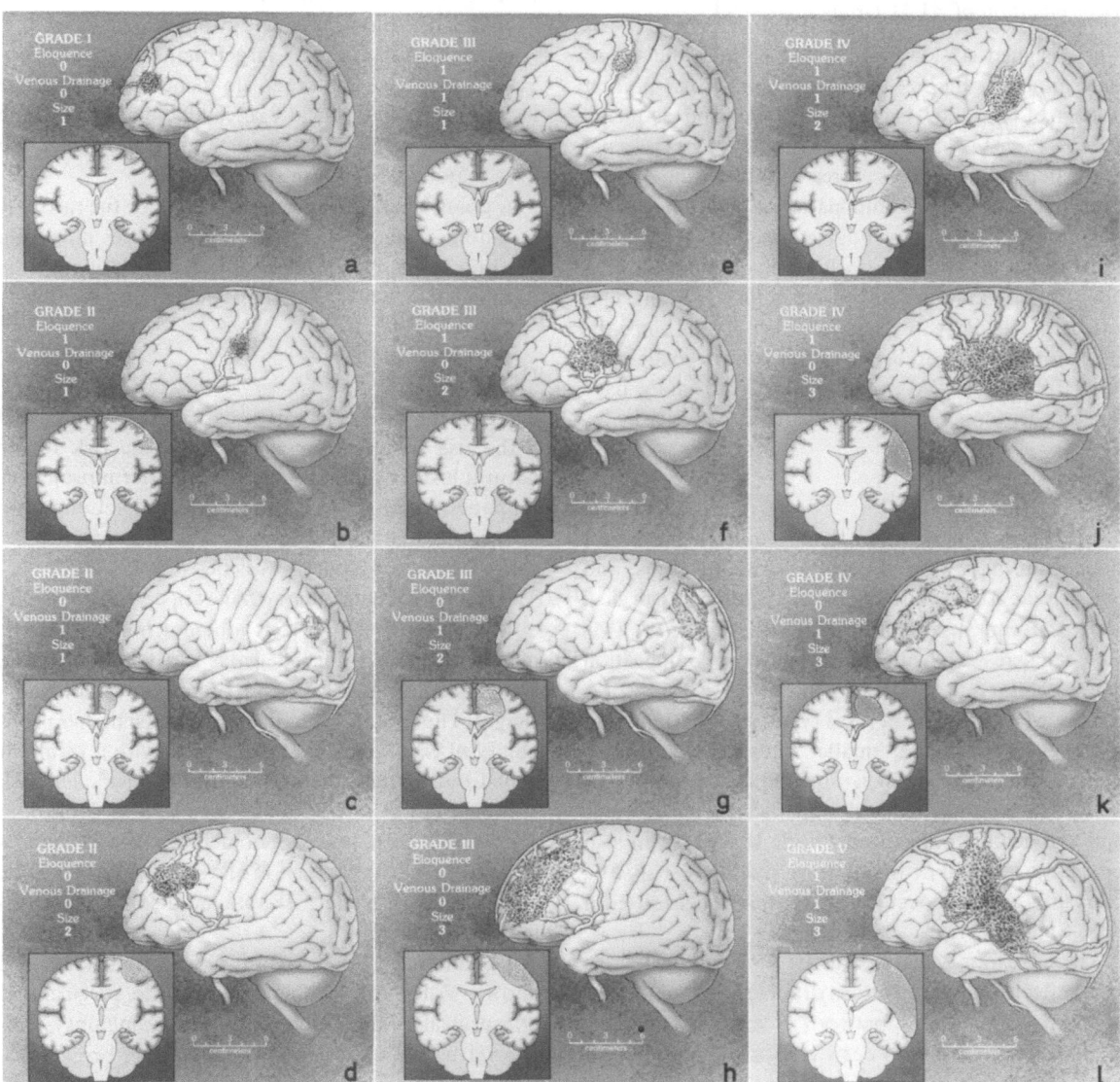

Fig. 1. (a–l) Diagrammatic representation of the combinations of graded variables (size, eloquence, and venous drainage) that are possible for each grade of arteriovenous malformation. There is one combination each for Grades I (a) and V (l) three combinations each for Grades II (b–d) and IV (i–k), and four possible combinations for Grade III (e–h)

thalamus and hypothalamus; the internal capsule; the brain stem; cerebellar peduncles; and the deep cerebellar nuclei. An AVM in any of these locations is assigned an additional point for eloquence. Noneloquent areas are defined as the anterior portion of the frontal and temporal lobes and the cerebellar hemispheres. Normal anatomical location for function is assumed, and there is no requirement for electrophysiological mapping or WADA testing in this scheme.

Determination of AVM Grade

The assigned AVM grade is the sum of the points determined by the size of the AVM (1, 2, or 3 points), pattern of venous drainage (0 or 1 point), and eloquence (0 or 1 point). Thus all AVMs are graded between 1 and 5 depending on these three variables. Angiograms are inspected for size and patterns of drainage. We have found magnetic resonance imaging (MRI) to be most useful in correlation with the angiograms, especially in determining eloquence of adjacent brain. This is true particularly in posterior fossa AVMs since the proximity to the cerebellar nuclei is most evident on MRI imaging. AVMs of the same grade may have variable features but share similar operative risks.

Examples of AVM Grades

Grade I lesions are smaller than 3 cm in their greatest dimension, have only superficial draining veins, and are distant from eloquent brain regions. In surgical series that have used this grading scale, grade I AVMs were safely resected with a minimal risk of complication (0% morbidity and mortality in our series).

Grade II AVMs are of three types: smaller than 3 cm in an eloquent region, smaller than 3 cm with deep venous drainage but in a noneloquent location, or between 3 and 6 cm with only superficial draining veins and a noneloquent location. Grade II AVMs can also be safely resected with minimal operative risk (0% mortality and 5% occurrence of minor neurological deficit in our series).

There are four types of grade III AVMs: large lesions (>6 cm) without deep venous drainage and in noneloquent regions, lesions between 3 and 6 cm in their greatest dimension with deep venous drainage but in noneloquent areas, AVMs between 3 and 6 cm with only superficial draining veins and in eloquent areas, or small lesions (<3 cm) with both deep venous drainage and an eloquent location. Grade III AVMs can

typically be resected but carry a higher surgical risk than grade I and II AVMs (0% mortality, 12% minor morbidity, and 4% major morbidity in our series).

Grade IV AVMs are of three different types: medium-sized lesions (>3 cm <6 cm) with both deep venous drainage and in eloquent areas, large AVMs (>6 cm) in noneloquent areas with deep venous drainage, and large AVMs (>6 cm) in eloquent brain areas but with superficial drainage. Grade IV AVMs can be safely resected but carry significant surgical risk (20% occurrence of minor neurological deficit and 7% occurrence of major neurological deficit in our series).

Grade V AVMs are all larger than 6 cm, have deep venous drainage, and are in eloquent locations. These lesions are also technically resectable but carry a high risk of postoperative deficit (19% minor morbidity and 12% major morbidity in our series).

A grade VI classification is reserved for the rare case of a diffuse, very large AVM that occupies most of a cerebral hemisphere and deep brain nuclei with deep drainage. These AVMs are considered nonresectable.

Discussion

The decision to resect a cerebral AVM is only indicated if the risk of operation is less than the risk of the natural history of the AVM. The long-term prognosis for patients with AVMs appears to be grim. Long-term data reveal that the annual risk of intracranial hemorrhage from a cerebral AVM is between 2% to 3%[3,4,5]. The risk for a second hemorrhage appears to be higher, at least in the first year after a hemorrhage[5]. The risk of permanent neurologic deficit is 50% with each event, and the risk of death is about 10% with each hemorrhage[4]. Thus young patients have a much higher probability of experiencing a hemorrhage with a resultant deficit during their lifetime than otherwise[8]. The risk approaches 100% at 30 to 40 years. Indeed, some data suggest that there is an age of increased risk of hemorrhage from AVMs between 15 and 40 years[11]. Therefore, children have a higher risk than adults of hemorrhaging in their lifetime[1].

The alternative risk of surgical resection is less well known. Without a reliable grading scale, surgical and nonsurgical series, until recently, had been nonsystematic retrospective reviews. The results of prospective analyses of the Spetzler-Martin grading system, however, suggest that most low-grade AVMs can be resected with good result and less risk than associated with the natural history. Certainly, Grades 1, 2, and

3 AVMs should be considered surgically curable. Grade 4 and 5 AVMs are more formidable and require individual consideration. These lesions often require preoperative and intraoperative embolization as well as multiple stage resections. In young patients, however, especially in the presence of neurologic symptoms, attempts of surgical removal are justifiable since the surgical risk, although high, is still less than that of the natural history[18]. In middle-aged and older adults with minimal symptoms, a conservative approach seems more reasonable since the surgical risk may not be less than that of the natural history.

Conclusion

The Spetzler-Martin grading scheme for cerebral AVMs is a simple yet useful system for classifying AVMs into categories of variable resectability reflecting the safety of resection. This system benefits from being easily applied, both retrospectively and prospectively based on universally available imaging studies. This grading scheme is also comprehensive enough to group all conceivable AVMs according to size, pattern of venous drainage, and eloquence of adjacent brain. The grade of AVM assigned by incorporating these three variables has been proven to be better than other classification schemes for predictably grouping patients according to surgical risk[6]. Consequently, the clinician can more accurately predict operative morbidity in individual cases. This grading system makes the process of treatment decision more objective. Furthermore, alternative treatment strategies and alternative therapies can be compared meaningfully in a prospective fashion with utilization of this system.

References

1. Celli P, Ferrante L, Palma L, Cavedon G (1984) Cerebral arteriovenous malformations in children. Clinical features and outcome of treatment in children and in adults. Surg Neurol 22: 43–49
2. Drake CG (1979) Cerebral arteriovenous malformations: considerations for and experience with surgical treatment in 166 cases. Clin Neurosurg 26: 145–208
3. Forster DMC, Steiner L, Hakanson S (1972) Arteriovenous malformations of the brain. A long-term clinical study. J Neurosurg 37: 562–570
4. Fults D, Kelly DL Jr (1984) Natural history of arteriovenous malformations of the brain: a clinical study. Neurosurgery 15: 658–662
5. Graf CJ, Perret CE, Torner JC (1983) Bleeding from cerebral arteriovenous malformations as part of their natural history. J Neurosurg 58: 331–337
6. Hollerhage HG, Zumkeller M, Dewenter KM (1990) Pronostic value of grading systems in cerebral arteriovenous malformations. Neurochirurgia 33 (3): 59–64
7. Kjellberg RN, Hanamura T, Davis KR, Lyons SL, Adams RD (1983) Bragg-peak proton-beam therapy for arteriovenous malformations of the brain. N Engl J Med 309: 269–274
8. Luessenhop AJ (1984) Natural history of cerebral arteriovenous malformations. In: Wilson CB, Stein BM (eds) Intracranial arteriovenous malformations. Williams and Willkins, Baltimore, pp 12–23
9. Luessenhop AJ, Gennarelli TA (1977) Anatomical grading of supratentorial arteriovenous malformations for determining operability. Neurosurgery 1: 30–35
10. Luessenhop AJ, Presper JH (1975) Surgical embolization of cerebral arteriovenous malformations through internal carotid and vertebral arteries. Long-term results. J Neurosurg 42: 443–451
11. Parkinson D, Bachers G (1980) Arteriovenous malformations. Summary of 100 consecutive supratentorial cases. J Neurosurg 53: 285–299
12. Pasqualin A, Barone G, Cioffi F, Rosta L, Scienza, Da Pian R (1991) The relevance of anatomic and hemodynamic factors to a classification of cerebral arteriovenous malformations. Neurosurgery 28 (3): 370–379
13. Pellettieri L, Carlsson CA, Grevsten S, Norlen G, Uhlemann C (1980) Surgical versus conservative treatment of intracranial arteriovenous malformations. A study in surgical decision-making. Acta Neurochir (Wien) [Suppl] 29: 1–86
14. Perret G, Nishioka H (1966) Report on the Cooperative Study of Intracranial Aneurysms and Subarachnoid Hemorrhage. Section VI. Arteriovenous malformations. An analysis of 545 cases of craniocerebral arteriovenous malformations and fistulae reported to the Cooperative Study. J Neurosurg 25: 467–490
15. Shi YQ (1984) A proposed scheme for grading of intracranial arteriovenous malformations. Chung Hua Shen Ching Ching Shen Ko Tsa Chih 17 (2): 65–68
16. Spetzler RF, Martin NA (1986) A proposed grading system for arteriovenous malformations. J Neurosurg 65: 576–583
17. Spetzler RF, Wilson CB, Weinstein P, Medhorn M, Townsend J, Telles D (1978) Normal perfusion pressure breakthrough theory. Clin Neurosurg 25: 651–672
18. Spetzler RF, Zabramski JM (1990) Grading and staged resection of cerebral arteriovenous malformations. Clin Neurosurg 36: 318–337
19. Stein BM, Wolpert SM (1980) Arteriovenous malformations of the brain. I. Current concepts and treatment. Arch Neurol 37: 1–5
20. Steiner L (1984) Treatment of arteriovenous malformations by radiosurgery. In: Wilson CB, Stein BM (eds) Intracranial arteriovenous malformations. Williams and Wilkins, Baltimore, pp 295–314
21. Wilkins RH (1985) Natural history of intracranial vascular malformations: a review. Neurosurgery 16: 421–430

Correspondence: Robert F. Spetzler, M.D., c/o Editorial Office, Barrow Neurological Institute, 350 West Thomas Road, Phoenix, AZ 85015, U.S.A.

A New Grading System for Cerebral Arteriovenous Malformations

G.M. Malik[1], A. Pasqualin[2], and J.I. Ausman[3]

[1]Department of Neurological Surgery, Henry Ford Hospital, Detroit, Michigan, U.S.A., [2]Department of Neurological Surgery, Verona City Hospital, Verona, Italy, and [3]Department of Neurosurgery, University of Illinois, Chicago, Illinois, U.S.A.

Summary

The basic aim of the proposed grading system is to provide for a simple, easily adoptable scheme to categorize the AVMs and assess the outcome of different treatments. It is well recognized that the AVMs present in wide variety of shapes, sizes and locations and each case is almost unique in its characteristics. After evaluating the necessary parameters and previously proposed classifications, it became obvious that three variables turned out to be the most important, namely location, size and arterial feeders. Measurement of size in terms of volume reduces the variability and the formula used for calculating the volume is simple and easily adoptable. The proposed system incorporates location both in terms of function and depth, size in the form of volume and arterial supply in the presence or absence of deep feeders. The Karnofsky rate is recommended to be used for functional assessment of patients pre and postoperatively.

Keywords: Cerebral arteriovenous malformations (AVMs); AVM grading system; AVM volume; AVM location.

Introduction

Arteriovenous malformations (AVMs) by nature present with variety of sizes, shapes and locations within the brain. Their treatment, or lack thereof, carry definite risks. With variability of treatments considered as well as experience of particular surgeon in the management of AVMs make it difficult to compare the outcome of patients. Despite thoughtful attempts by many in the past[2,3,6,7,8], there is no universally agreed upon system. The World Federation of Neurosurgical Societies appointed a committee some years ago to develop such a system. It became obvious after the first meeting and a draft proposal that additional background and statistical information was needed to accomplish this task. Pasqualin *et al.*[5] undertook the responsibility of looking at their cases. They assessed the relevance of anatomical and hemodynamic factors affecting the AVMs and influencing the outcome.

Analysis of Previous Classifications

Among the classification systems previously proposed, the ones by Drake[2] and Spetzler and Martin[7] are used more frequently. Drake proposed dividing the malformations into small, moderate, and large. This is based on the maximum linear dimension, thus small being 2.5 cm, moderate 2.5–5.0 cm, and the large > 5.0 cm. This is the most simple and practical method. However, there is significant variability of size within each category if volume is taken into consideration. If we assume an AVM to be a sphere, its volume V is defined as $4/3\pi r^3$ or $4.2\,r^3$: with 4.2 a constant and r its radius. In Drake's classification, AVMs with dimensions of 2.8 cm and 4.8 cm would be of moderate size. The volume of an AVM 2.8 cm would be (4.2×1.4^3) 11.55^3 cm while that of 4.8 cm (4.2×2.4^3) dimension 58^3 cm, thus at least a five fold difference. Wilson[8] suggested similar system but AVMs less than 2.0 cm were considered small, 2.0–4.0 cm moderate and more than 4.0 cm as large.

The grading system proposed by Spetzler and Martin is similarly simple to use. It again utilizes largest dimension as the basis of size. One grade point is assigned to AVMs less than 3.0 cm, two points to AVMs 3.0–6.0 cm and three points to AVMs with largest dimension more than 6.0 cm. In this particular proposal variability of size becomes even more significant. For example AVMs 3.2 cm and 5.8 cm will be given same grade as far as the size is concerned but according to the above formula the volume would be 17.22^3 cm and 102.48^3 cm, a six fold difference. The second component of the grading system is deep venous drainage which is assigned a grade point. Generally deep drainage points to deep location, however, it has become quite obvious recently, while analyzing venous drainage that a significant number of superficial malformations can have deep drainage depending on variability of venous system. Therefore, a malformation located in the thalamus or periventricular region having deep venous drainage is assigned an extra grade and this rightfully reflects its complexity. But an AVM located in the sylvian fissure with drainage mainly through basal vein of Rosenthal, because of lack of available superficial drainage gets an extra grade, even though it does not reflect upon its complexity. The third part of this system is location in "eloquent areas of the brain" and this also gets an additional grade. Eloquent areas are "those that speak to readily identifiable neurological function, and, if injured, result in a disabling neurological deficit". Sensorimotor, language and visual cortex, hypothalamus and thalamus, internal capsule, brain stem, cerebral peduncles and deep cerebellar nuclei are considered as eloquent areas. The major difficulty with this grading system is lack of inclusion of the location of the AVM[4]. Obviously as noted before, the size grade is not necessarily reflective of all of the AVMs in that category also. A malformation in the sylvian fissure with largest dimension of 4.0 cm and deep venous drainage would be considered grade III and similarly a 3.0 cm malformation in the brain stem would be grade III. It is quite obvious that these two are not the same malformations from the standpoint of complexity or morbidity associated with treatment. Similarly an AVM of 6.5 cm in the anterior frontal region without deep venous drainage would be grade III, and again compared to a grade III AVM in the brain stem, thalamus or basal ganglia, would carry less morbidity in its resection.

Pasqualin et al.[5] evaluated different parameters that affect the outcome and need to be considered in any classification system in their 248 cases. Size was evaluated as volume rather than single largest dimension. The formula utilized to calculate the volume used multiplication of 3 dimension of the AVM from standard lateral and anteroposterior angiogram films corrected for magnification and divided by two. This provides closest approximation of volume as shown by Brock[1] and is simplest to use. It was noted that malformations with volume > 20.0 cm[3] carried higher morbidity and risk of hyperemic complications. Location was similarly analyzed. The malformations were divided into frontal, rolandic, posterior parietal, occipital, temporal, callosal/cingular, inferior limbic, insular, nuclear, cerebellar and brain stem. For the sake of comparison, they considered eloquence as defined by Spetzler and Martin. It was concluded that precise anatomic location was

necessary and when this was available the term eloquent provided only limited definition.

In assessing the arterial supply and venous drainage, it was noted that deep venous drainage did not influence the outcome unless the malformations were large. Presence of arterial feeders, including lenticulostriate, anterior and posterior choroidals, thalamoperforators, and anterior inferior cerebellar, definitely increased the occurrence of complications. They also looked at mean flow velocities in the main feeding vessels using transcranial doppler and noted that mean flow velocities more than 120 cm/s were associated with significant increase in postoperative complications.

Shi and Chen[6] proposed a grading system based on size, location and depth, arterial supply and venous drainage. Each of these variables was then divided into four grades. Size is again assessed as the largest dimension. Location and depth help divide malformations into definable categories. Basically it represents the division into superficial and deep and then into relatively critical functional areas and less functional ones. The arterial feeding vessels and venous drainage were also categorized into four groups each which actually makes the final use of classification more complex.

Proposed Classification

Based upon the above facts and after having input from colleagues around the world including neurosurgeons and neuroradiologists, the following grading system is being recommended. The intent is to have a system which can be easily adopted around the world. This has to be simple but at the same time reflective of the complexity of malformations and should allow for meaningful comparison between different series as well as different treatments. We, therefore, propose evaluating arteriovenous malformations using a scheme based on its A) anatomic location, B) size as determined by volume, and C) the presence or absence of deep arterial feeders (Tables 1 and 2).

A. Location

This is divided into four categories and generally follows the concept of Shi and Chen[6].

I. Cortical (simple): This includes malformations located superficially in the non-critical and easily accessible areas of frontal lobe, most of temporal lobe

Table 1. *Location/Size (Volume)/Arterial Feeders*

---

1. 3 cm × 2 cm × 2.5 cm right frontal AVM supplied by MCA and ACA branches

   $$\text{Volume} = \frac{3 \times 2 \times 2.5}{2} = 7.5 \, \text{cm}^3$$

   Cortical (simple) grade I

2. 2.5 cm × 2.0 cm × 2.5 cm right parietal AVM supplied by MCA, ACA

   $$\text{Volume} = \frac{2.5 \times 2.0 \times 2.5}{2} = 6.25 \, \text{cm}^3$$

   Cortical (functional) grade I

3. 4.0 cm × 3.5 cm × 3.0 cm left parietal AVM supplied by superficial branches of MCA and PCA

   $$\text{Volume} = \frac{4.0 \times 3.0 \times 3.0}{2} = 18.0 \, \text{cm}^3$$

   Cortical (functional) grade II

4. 3.5 cm × 3.0 cm × 2.5 cm right mesial temporal AVM supplied by ant. chor., MCA (cortical and lenticulostriate) and PCA

   $$\text{Volume} = \frac{3.5 \times 3.0 \times 2.5}{2} = 13.0 \, \text{cm}^3$$

   Deep (non-vital) grade II-A

5. 2 cm × 1.5 cm × 1.5 cm corpus callosum AVM supplied by both ACAs

   $$\text{Volume} = \frac{2.0 \times 1.5 \times 1.5}{2} = 2.25 \, \text{cm}^3$$

   Deep (non-vital) grade I

6. 5 cm × 4.5 cm × 4.0 cm left frontoparietal AVM supplied by ACA, MCA (cortical and lenticulo-striate), PCA and meningeal vessels

   $$\text{Volume} = \frac{5.0 \times 4.5 \times 4.0}{2} = 45 \, \text{cm}^3$$

   Cortical (functional) grade V-A

7. 6 cm × 4.5 cm × 4.0 cm right frontal AVM supplied by MCA and ACA branches including lenticulostriates

   $$\text{Volume} = \frac{6.0 \times 4.5 \times 4.0}{2} = 54.0 \, \text{cm}^3$$

   Cortical (simple) grade VI-A

8. 4.0 cm × 3.5 cm × 3 cm cerebellar AVM supplied by SCA, PICA, and AICA

   $$\text{Volume} = \frac{4.0 \times 3.5 \times 3.0}{2} = 21.0 \, \text{cm}^3$$

   Deep (non-vital) grade III-A

9. 2.5 cm × 2.0 cm × 2.0 cm brain stem AVM supplied by AICA and brain stem perforators

   $$\text{Volume} = \frac{2.5 \times 2.0 \times 2.0}{2} = 5 \, \text{cm}^3$$

   Deep (vital) grade I-A

ACA anterior cerebral artery; *MCA* middle cerebral artery; *PCA* posterior cerebral artery; *ant chor* anterior choroidal; *SCA* superior cerebellar artery; *AICA* anterior inferior cerebellar artery; *PICA* posterior inferior cerebellar artery.

except speech areas, cerebellar hemispheres without involvement of deep cerebellar nuclei and occipital lobe. The latter assumes that visual field defect is not judged as a significant neurological deficit.

II. Cortical (functional): Sensory motor cortex, speech areas.

III. Deep (non-vital): Insula, basal ganglia, anterior limb of internal capsule, corpus callosum, deep medial temporal lobe, intra and periventricular and cerebellar nuclei.

IV. Deep (vital): Genu and posterior limb of internal capsule, thalamus, hypothalamus, brain stem and large lesions extending into them.

B. Size

Size is calculated as volume and based on the formula, length × width × height divided by two. These measurements are taken in late arterial/early venous phase on AP and lateral angiogram films corrected for magnification. Volume gives less variability between different malformations. Radiosurgery is also based upon the volume. With increasing availability of magnetic resonance imaging and newer software, it would be possible to get even more accurate volume measurements and therefore MRI in the future may be substituted for angiography in assessing the volume of AVMs. To minimize the variability, the AVMs are divided into the following grades based upon volume.

Grade I < 10 cm³   Grade IV 30–40 cm³
Grade II 10–20 cm³   Grade V 40–50 cm³
Grade III 20–30 cm³   Grade VI > 50 cm³

C. Arterial Supply

Deep arterial feeders, particularly lenticulostriate, Huebner's, thalamo-perforators, anterior and posterior choroidals and perforating vessels of the brain stem including anterior inferior cerebellar carry significant importance from surgical standpoint. These are most difficult to secure during resection of an AVM and add to surgical morbidity. The deep venous drainage on the other hand merely points to deeper location or is reflective of an anomalous venous drainage. As pointed out by Pasqualin[5], deep venous drainage did not appreciably influence the outcome while deep arterial supply definitely contributed to morbidity. Counting different feeders and adding to the grading system will again make it more complex. Therefore, it would be sufficient to indicate the presence or absence of deep feeding vessels (Table 2). If these are present, add letter A to the size grade. If the total supply is from superficial vessels, then nothing is added to the size grade (see Table 1 for examples).

Table 2

Cortical Simple	Functional	Location nonvital	Deep vital
Frontal	sensory motor	insula	internal capsule
Temporal[a]	speech	medial temporal	genu and posterior limb
Occipital[b]		internal capsule	thalamus
Cerebellar hemispheres		anterior limb	hypothalamus
		corpus callosum	brain stem
		ventricles	
		cerebellar nuclei	
		basal ganglia	

Volume	Arterial supply	
	Superficial	Deep
Grade 1 = < 10 cm³		lenticulostriate
Grade 2 = 10–20 cm³		thalamoperforators
Grade 3 = 20–30 cm³		choroidals
Grade 4 = 30–40 cm³		brain stem perforators
Grade 5 = 40–50 cm³		(including AICA)
Grade 6 = > 50 cm³		

[a] Except speech areas.
[b] Assuming visual field deficit not considered major complication.

Table 3. *Karnofsky Rating*

100	Normal: no complaints; no evidence of disease
90	Able to carry on normal activity: minor symptoms
80	Normal activity with effort: some symptoms
70	Cares for self: unable to carry on normal activity
60	Requires occasional assistance: care for most needs
50	Requires considerable assistance and frequent care
40	Disabled: requires special care and assistance
30	Severely disabled: hospitalized, death not imminent
20	Very sick: active supportive treatment needed
10	Moribund: fatal processes are rapidly progressing

Clinical Status

There are multiple variables to be considered in assessing the clinical status. Since many factors like age, medical condition, neurological function have significant influence on mortality and morbidity from AVMs, both considering natural history and different therapies, any grading system incorporating all these factors becomes extremely complex. In the majority of cases, the AVM is treated on an elective basis and therefore change in the clinical status is of more significance than initial status. It is the Committee's feeling that Karnofsky's rating (Table 3) offers the most suitable system. It addresses both the asymptomatic patients and allows for assessment of degree of disability in those who are impaired both pre and postoperatively.

References

1. Brock M (1964) Indikation zur total Extirpation von arteriovenosen Angiomen als funktionell hochwertig angesehenen Hirngebieten. Doctoral thesis. University of Köln, Köln, Federal Republic of Germany
2. Drake CG (1979) Cerebral arteriovenous malformations: considerations for and experience with surgical treatment in 166 cases. Clin Neurosurg 26: 145–208
3. Leussenhop A, Gennarelli T (1977) Anatomical grading of supratentorial arteriovenous malformation for determining operability. Neurosurgery 1: 30–35
4. Malik GM, Ausman JI, Mann R (1987) Grading systems for AVMs. Letter to the editor. J Neurosurg 67: 473
5. Pasqualin A, Barone G, Cioffi F, Rosta L, Scienza R, Da Pian R (1991) The relevance of anatomical and hemodynamic factors to a classification of cerebral arteriovenous malformations. Neurosurgery 28: 370–379
6. Shi YQ, Chen XC (1986) A proposed scheme for grading intracranial arteriovenous malformations. J Neurosurg 65: 484–489
7. Spetzler RF, Martin NA (1986) A proposed grading system for arteriovenous malformations. J Neurosurg 65: 476–483
8. Wilson CB, U HS, Domingue J (1979) Microsurgical treatment of intracranial vascular malformations. J Neurosurg 51: 446–454

Correspondence: Ghaus M. Malik, M.D., Henry Ford Hospital, 2799 West Grand Boulevard, Detroit, MI 48202, U.S.A.

Use of the Callosal Grid System for Cortical Localization

R. Lehman[1] and **A. Olivier**[2]

[1]UMDNJ-Robert-Wood-Johnson-Medical-School, Division of Neurosurgery, New Brunswick, New Jersey, U.S.A. and [2]Department of Neurosurgery, Montreal Neurological Institute and Hospital, Montreal, Quebec, Canada

Summary

The callosal grid system based on stereoscopic arteriovenous DSA and MRI imaging facilitates the identification of the central sulcus by its relationship to the midcallosal plane. Imaging in either modality allows superimposition of identical landmarks. Adjacent neurovascular structures can be compartmentalized within subdivisions of the grid system. This permits pre-operative planning and intraoperative recognition of the central artery and sulcus to coordinate resection within the central area.

Keywords: Callosal grid; central sulcus; stereoscopic arteriovenous DSA; MRI.

Introduction

Anatomical mapping and cortical localization begin in the pre-operative period[24]. The central sulcus is a pivotal landmark whose identification remains, at times, difficult. The angiographic localization of the central sulcus has been described by Ring and Waddington[14], Szikla et al.[18]. Stereoscopic arteriovenous digital subtraction angiography (DSA) enhances the visual recognition of the location and variable branching patterns of the arteries and veins. By using the corpus callosum, seen indirectly on DSA and directly on Magnetic Resonances Imaging (MRI), the two image modalities can be superimposed to clarify the central sulcus[10,12]. The authors have previously described a proportional grid system based on the corpus callosum to further study localization of the central sulcus and adjacent neurovascular structures[6]. A similar methodology using the Talairach proportional grid system for anatomical localization of the central area in the surgery of arteriovenous malformations has been described by Kunc[3,4]. With modern imaging a more comprehensive and accurate methodology has been achieved with the callosal grid system.

Materials and Methods

To summarize briefly our previously described methodology, the corpus callosum can be identified indirectly on the lateral arteriovenous DSA by the pericallosal (A 2, 3) portions of the anterior cerebral artery and posteriorly by the vein of Galen, and directly on the midsagittal MRI (Fig. 1)[7]. A horizontal plane (HP) is constructed through the inferior border of the genu and the splenium of the corpus callosum. Three vertical planes perpendicular to HP are created: anterior callosal plane (AC) tangential to the anterior border of the genu, a posterior callosal plane (PC) tangential to the posterior border of the splenium, and a midcallosal plane (MC) that is midpoint between AC and PC (Fig. 2)[8].

Initially, using this callosal grid system the DSA and MRI images of 100 consecutive patients without mass lesions or arteriovenous malformations (AVM) were analyzed by film and 3-D computer terminal display[9,13]. Forty cases were studied in detail as to the relationship within the callosal grid of not only the central artery, but the entire central sulcus, the amygdala, insula, and temporal plane. The length of corpus callosum, entire brain length, and anterior and posterior pole lengths created by the vertical planes were recorded (Figs. 3–5). Additionally, 24 patients with focal epilepsy arising in the central area with or without focal lesion, including cortical dysplasia, glioma, or AVM were studied in a similar manner[5]. The stereoscopic computer terminal (tetronix) permitted the 3-D visualization of the DSA and in a small 2-D frame the MRI images in any plane of choice. The cursor was interactive in identical neighborhoods in either image modality. Further updating of this computer terminal allows rapid construction of the callosal grid system in either image which allows cross-correlation of any anatomic point within the grid system (Figs. 9 and 10). Recently, after co-registration computer 3-D reconstruction MRI images can be interactive, intraoperatively, with the computer stereoscopic DSA images.

Dissection and analysis of 20 cadaver brain hemispheres after the cerebral vasculature was perfused with latex was performed. Using a plastic template, probes were passed through this template in the planes of the callosal grid system aligned to the corpus callosum and the relationship of the grid system to the central artery and sulcus could be noted as the probes pierced the cortex of the lateral hemisphere (Figs. 6–8). Adjacent sulci and arteries in relationship to the grid system were demonstrated. By sectioning the brain in these callosal planes, cortical and subcortical structures could be compartmentalized, using this proportional grid system, based on their location within the vertical and horizontal grid planes.

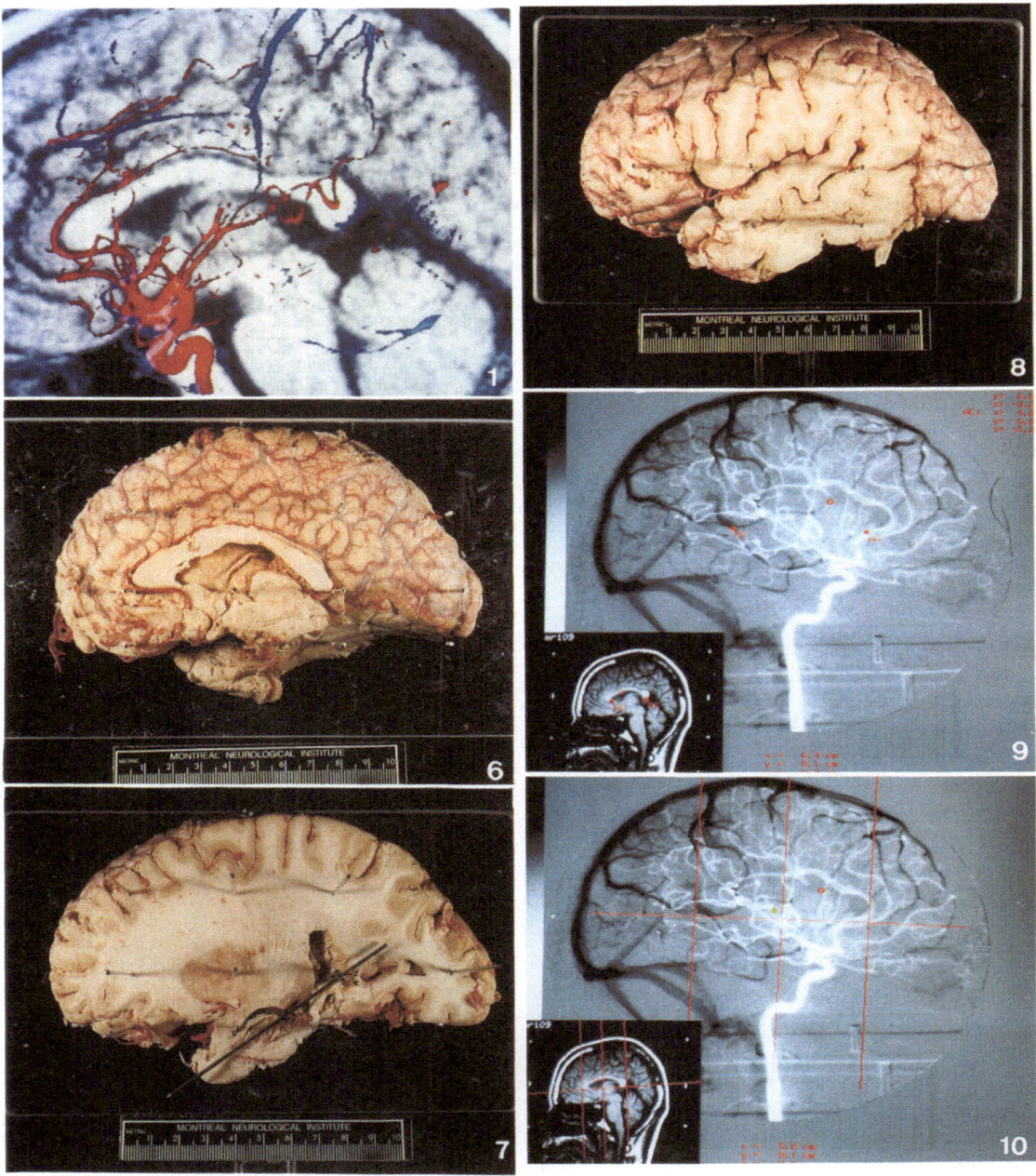

Figs. 1, 6, 7, 8–10. Fig. 1. Identification of corpus callosum superimposed DSA and MRI. Fig. 6. Callosal grid template. Fig. 7. Callosal grid template. "Limbic" parasagittal. Fig. 8. Callosal grid template cortical parasagittal. Note: MC in relation to inf. central sulcus. Fig. 9. 3-D computer combines DSA and MRI. to HP. Identification of horizontal plane (HP). Fig. 10. Construction of vertical planes to HP. Note: Relationship of MC to central artery

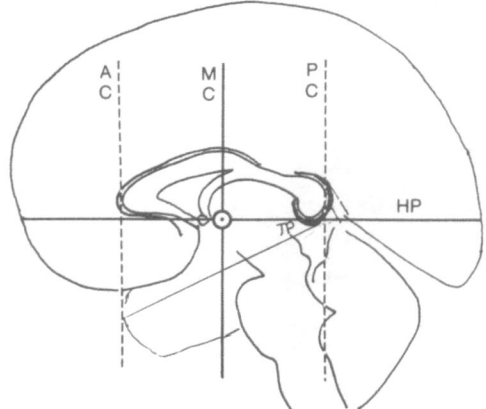

Fig. 2. Callosal grid System

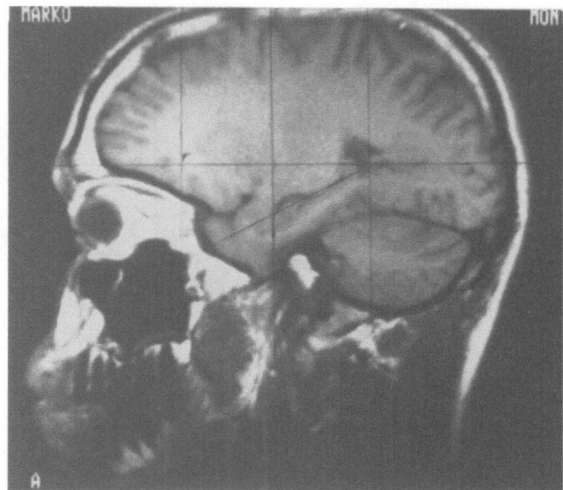

Fig. 4. "Limbic" parasagittal MRI

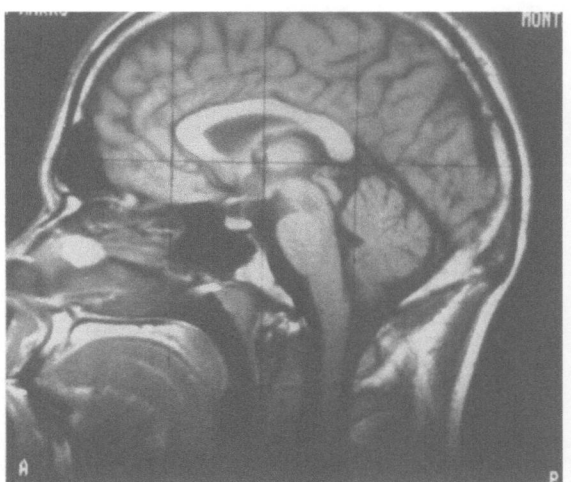

Fig. 3. Midsagittal MRI

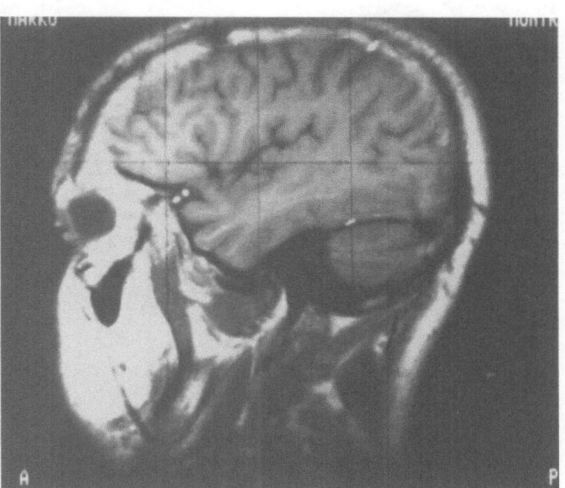

Fig. 5. "Cortical" parasagittal MRI. Note: MC in relation to inf. central sulcus

Results

Our studies have shown that the midcallosal plane intersects the central sulcus inferiorly at a point where the central artery enters the central sulcus. The mean deviation was $0.3 +/- 1.2$ mm posterior to MC. The superior extent of the central sulcus at the midline was a mean of 4 mm anterior to PC. The ascending limb of the callosal marginal sulcus was a mean of 6.2 mm posterior to PC[6]. Cadaver brain dissections revealed similar findings. At the computer work station the stereotactic coordinates of a DSA locus would be visualized with the identical coordinates and location in the MRI image. Further, by following stereoscopically

the loops and bends of any particular branch of the anterior, middle, or posterior cerebral artery on the DSA, one could map the sulci and gyri by the arterial course, and confirm it with the MRI image.

In all of the central area cases even with a mass or vascular malformation the recognition of the individual vessels, whether, facilitated by the callosal grid system, would predict the location of the sulci and gyri on the MRI and at the time of intraoperative electrophysiological mapping (Figs. 11 and 12)[5]. Post operative MRI

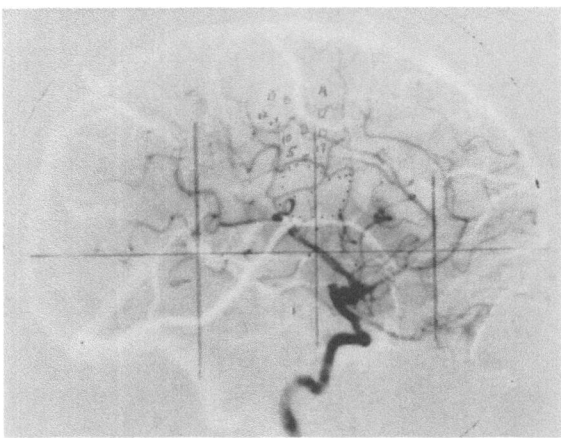

Fig. 11. DSA with superimposed stimulation ticket loci and resection area in relation to callosal grid

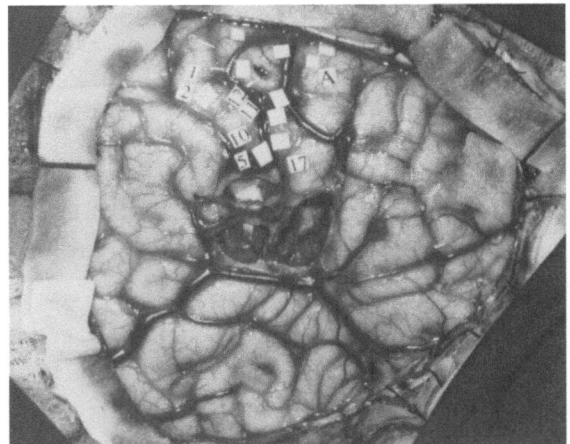

Fig. 12. Post resection inferior central area

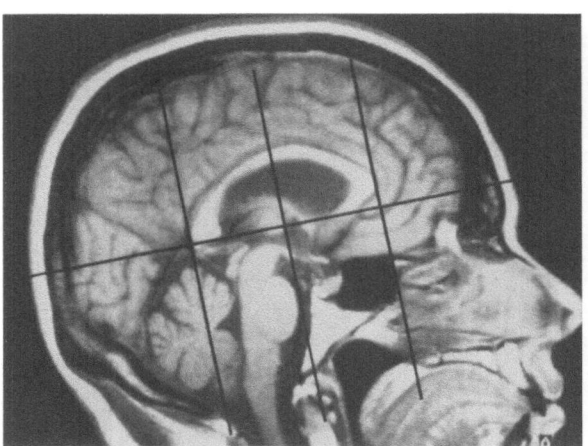

Fig. 13. Post-operative MRI to confirm location of resection with superimposed callosal grid. Midsagittal MRI.

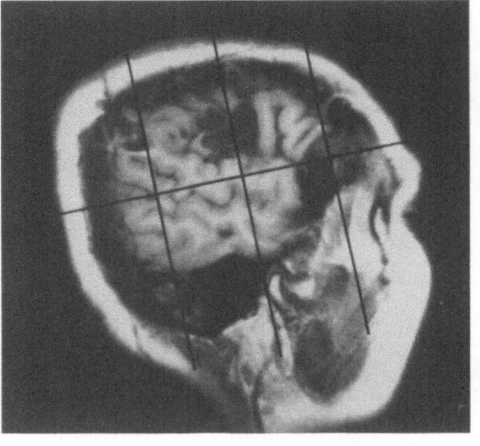

Fig. 14. Lateral cortical MRI

imaging confirmed the predicted resection in relation to the callosal grid (Figs. 13 and 14). Additional computer analysis to confirm the identical loci by superimposition of DSA and MRI is ongoing. Use of the callosal planes and imaging in the horizontal plane of the corpus callosum for combined positron-emission tomography (PET) – MRI is being studied to determine whether it would afford a more anatomically relevant image.

Discussion

Orthogonal tele-angiography with stereoscopic visualization for the localization of cortical structures was developed by Szikla and Talairach[20,21]. Their laboratory anatomical work was based in part on Duret's study which revealed the course of the cortical arteries was determined by the growth and formation of the gyri[2]. The foldings of the brain cause the arteries to enter and leave the sulci in order to pass from one gyrus to the next. Stereoscopic viewing of the angiogram allows the recognition of these bends and loops of the arteries as they delineate the gyri and sulci. By combining ventriculography with the outlining of the diencephalic anterior and posterior commissures a proportional grid system was established that allowed the integration of angiography and ventriculography for the stereotactic localization of any intracerebral structure. The intercommissural line was the horizontal plane and two vertical planes perpendicular to the horizontal plane were created through the anterior and posterior commissure. This formed the basic unit of measurement for their grid system[22]. The inferior central sulcus and artery fell between these 2 vertical planes. Electrophysiologic data supported this[19]. Kunc has reported using the Talairach proportional grid system for anatomical mapping and intraoperative recognition of normal and abnormal vessels in the surgical management of 24 patients with arteriovenous malformations in the speech and sensorimotor regions[3]. However, Steinmetz, using real time cinematographic display of MRI images of 40 cerebral hemispheres to evaluate the anatomic variability of the inferior central, precentral and postcentral sulci, found 1.5 to 2 cm variation zone of the precentral, central and postcentral sulci in relation to the Talairch proportional grid system based on the anterior-posterior commissure[19]. Similarly, the use of the anterior-posterior commissure line for localization of thalamic nuclear groups has been found unreliable by Brierly and Beck[16].

MRI imaging provides a bold landmark of the corpus callosum. This structure provides a more suitable basis for a grid system based on a series of horizontal and vertical planes. Further, this structure allows superimposition of the DSA and MRI, and reformatting parasagittally, one can see the central artery, inferiorly, enter the central sulcus. It is at this point that the midcallosal plane passes through laterally in a constant and reliable manner[6]. The remainder of the central sulcus can be identified and compartmentalized between the vertical planes MC and PC[6]. Pandya, using radioactive amino acids in monkeys, has shown a relationship of the crossing cortical sensorimotor fibers to the mid-point of the corpus callosum[11]. By using stereoscopic arteriovenous DSA with the callosal grid system, the gyri and sulci can be more easily identified and compartmentalized based on the recognition of the parent arteries and their branches within the callosal planes. Of equal importance, is the recognition and location of the veins and their relationship to the arteries and sulci.

Stein has reported using a template of the arterial and venous phases of the arteriogram with stereoscopic views to afford better anatomical detail in the surgical management of supratentorial arteriovenous malformation[15]. End and passing vessels that feed an arteriovenous malformations can be localized, facilitating their operative recognition and dissection as described

by Yamada[23]. Mass effect or a large AVM still allows recognition of the central sulcus by stereoscopic visualization of the DSA aided by the callosal grid system and identification of adjacent structures, or the more proximal or distal portion of the central artery or sulcus. Similarly, using the grid system with MRI images, a distal or proximal portion of the central sulcus or adjacent structure within MC-PC planes will allow recognition of the displaced central sulcus. Event related PET scanning has confirmed the relationship of the central sulcus within MC-PC portion of the callosal grid system. PET imaging in the horizontal plane of the corpus callosum will allow superimposition of this data with DSA and MRI. Intraoperatively, with or without a mass lesion, electrophysiologic mapping has consistently confirmed our preoperative anatomically mapping. Recently Suzuki and Yasui have described difficulty relying only on cortical somato-sensory evoked potentials for intraoperative localization of the central sulcus in brain tumors[17]. This data, including electrocorticography, stereoencephalography, evoked potential, and cortical stimulation can be coordinated within the callosal grid system on the MNI brain map, anatomical text, or integrated with DSA or MRI.

Acknowledgement

Grateful appreciation is given to Ms. Rosanna Gnudi for assistance with the manuscript.

References

1. Brierly JB, Beck E (1959) The significance in human stereotactic brain surgery of individual variation in the diencephalon and globus palidus. J Neurol Neurosurg Psychiatry 22: 287–298
2. Duret H (1974) Recherches anatomiques sur la circulation de l'Encephale. Archives de Psychologie Normal et Pathologique 2: 60–91, 316–353, 646–693, 919–957
3. Kunc Z (1974) Surgery of arteriovenous malformations in the speech and motorsensory regions. J Neurosurg 40: 293–303
4. Kunc Z (1965) The possibility of surgical treatment of arteriovenous malformations in anatomically important cortical regions. Acta Neurochir (Wien) 13: 361–249
5. Lehman RM, Olivier A (1992) Use of the callosal grid system for the pre- and post-operative assessment of resection in the central area. J Neurosurg 76: 387A
6. Lehman RM, Olivier A, Moreau J-J, Tampieri D, Henri C (1992) Use of the callosal grid system for the preoperative identification of the central sulcus. Stereotact Funct Neurosurgery 58: 179–188
7. Olivier A (1991) Extratemporal resections in the surgical treatment of epilepsy. In: Spencer S, Spencer D (eds) Surgery for epilepsy. Blackwell, pp 150–167
8. Olivier A, Marchand E, Peters T, Tyler J (1987) In: Engel J (ed) Surgical treatment of the epilepsies. Depth electrode implanta-

tion at the Montreal neurological institute and hospital. Raven, New York, pp 595–601

9. Olivier A, Peters T, Bertrand G (1985) Stereotaxic system and apparatus for use with MRI, CT and DSA. Proceedings of the International Society Stereotactic and Functional Neurosurgery, Toronto Appl Neurophysiol 48: 94–96

10. Olivier A, Peters T, Clark J, Marchand G, Mawko G, Bertrand G, Vanier M, Ethier R, Tyler J, De Lotbiniere A (1987) Integration de l'angiographie numerique dela resonance magnetique, de la tomodensitometrie et de la tomographie par emission de positrons en stereotaxie. EEG Neurophysiol Clin 25–43

11. Pandya D, Rosene D (1985) Some observations on trajectories and topography of commissural fibers. In: Reeves (eds) Epilepsy of the corpus callosum. Plenum, New York, pp 21–29

12. Peters T, Clark J, Olivier A, et al (1986) Integrated stereotaxic imaging with CT, MRI and digital subtraction angiography. Radiology 161: 821–826

13. Peters T, Henri C, Pike B, Clark J, Collins L, Olivier A (1990) Integration of stereotactic DSA with three-dimensional image reconstruction for stereotactic scanning. Proceedings of the Tenth Meeting of the World Society for Stereotactic and Functional Neurosurgery, Maebashi, Japan, October 1989. Stereotact Funct Neurosurg 55: 471–476

14. Ring BA, Waddinton MM (1967) Angiographic identification of the motor strip. J Neurosurg 26: 249–254

15. Stein BM (1985) Supratentorial arteriovenous malformations in cerebrovascular surgery. In: Fein JM Flamm ES (eds) Vol IV. Springer, Wien New York, pp 1097–1115

16. Steinmetz H, Furst G, Freund JJ (1990) Variation of perisylvian and calcarine anatomic landmarks within stereotaxic proportional coordinates. AJNR 11: 1123–1130

17. Suzuki A, Yasui N (1992) Intraoperative localization of the central sulcus by cortical somatosensory evoked potentials in brain tumor. J Neurosurg 76: 867–870

18. Szikla G, Bouvier G, Hori T, Petrov V (1977) Angiography of the human brain cortex. Atlas of vascular patterns and stereotactic cortical localization. Springer, Berlin Heidelberg New York

19. Szikla G, Talairach J (1965) Coordinates of the rolandic sulcus and topography of cortical and subcortical motor responses to low frequency stimulation in a proportional stereotaxic system. Confin Neurol 26: 471–475

20. Talairach J, David M, Tournoux P, Corredor H, Kvasina T (1957) Atlas d'anatomie stereotaxique des noyaux gris centrau. Masson and Ce, Paris

21. Talairach J, Szikla G (1967) Atlas of Stereotaxic Anatomy of the Telencephalon. Anatomo-radiological studies. Masson and Ce, Paris

22. Talairach J, Tournoux P (1988) Co-planar stereotaxic atlas of the human brain. Thieme, New York

23. Yamada S, Brauer FS, Knierim (1990) Direct approach to arteriovenous malformations in functional areas of the cerebral hemisphere. J Neurosurg 72: 418–425

24. Yasargil MG (1988) AVM of the brain, clinical considerations, general and special operative techniques, surgical results, non-operated cases, canvernous and venous angiomas, neuroanesthesia. In: (eds) Microneurosurgery, Vol III B. Thieme, Stuttgart

Correspondence: Richard M. Lehman, M.D., UMDNJ-Robert Wood Johnson Medical School, Division of Neurosurgery, One Robert Wood Johnson Place, CN-19, New Brunswick, New Jersey 08903–0019, U.S.A.

Hemodynamics of Cerebral AVMs and Perioperative Management

Hemodynamics of Cerebral Angiomas: Perioperative Angiography, Transcranial and Intraoperative Doppler Studies

W. Hassler[1] and R. Burger[2]

[1]Department of Neurosurgery, Municipal Clinic of Duisburg, Duisburg and [2]Department of Neurosurgery, University of Würzburg, Würzburg, Federal Republic of Germany

Summary

Documentation of characteristic hemodynamic changes in angiomas as high flow velocities, decreased intraluminal pressure in the arterial supplying feeders and increased flow and pressure on the venous side with dilatation of vessels, decrease of intraluminal pressure in the angioma nidus and diminished vasomotor reaction is possible by combining descriptive methods as perioperative angiography, monitoring of flow velocity in basal cerebral arteries by transcranial doppler and of the angioma nidus and directly supplying vessels on the brain surface by intraoperative doppler. Angiography shows topography of angioma in detail, dilated vessels, steal effects and postoperative early angiography stagnating arteries as sign of higher intravascular stream resistance; intraoperative doppler shows the flow velocities and changes of intravascular resistance directly in the nidus or feeders; and transcranial doppler shows preoperative steal effects and influences to basal cerebral arteries as postoperative changes after angioma removal. So the hemodynamic influences of AVM's to the surrounding brain regions and the Circle of Willis are detectable. A pressure breakthrough phenomenon could not be observed in our 125 patients after operation or combined treatment with embolization.

Keywords: Arteriovenous malformations; transcranial Doppler; intraoperative Doppler; normal pressure breakthrough theory.

Introduction

Doppler sonography permits continuous, noninvasive monitoring of flow velocities in the basal cerebral arteries, in the feeding arteries and in the angioma nidus[1,2,8]. This makes it possible to monitor the influence of the flow velocities in arteriovenous malformations, or angiomas, on the surrounding brain region by measuring the changes of flow spectra in the circle of Willis or nidus. Hence the hemodynamic features of angiomas can be demonstrated by doppler, angiography, CBF and laser-Doppler using miniprobes[1,3,6-8,14-16]. The typical changes in angiomas are high flow velocities in supplying arteries and draining veins, diminished intravascular pressure in arteries, and increased pressure in veins[7,13,18,19]. The diameters of arteries and veins are enlarged and CO_2 reactivity is diminished or abolished[2,8,11]. Intraluminal pressure decreases in the angioma nidus. In contrast to the hemodynamic situation of the angioma, the perfusion pressure in neighbouring vessels supplying normal brain is decreased. Intraluminal pressure in draining veins is increased and steal effects occur in basal cerebral arteries, particularly in precommunicating arteries of the anterior and posterior cerebral arteries. In large angiomas, a breakthrough phenomenon has been proposed[17] to be the cause of postoperative complications, which include swelling and rebleeding. Our investigations as early postoperative angiography, intra- and transcranial doppler studies have revealed that flow velocities in the former arteries are diminished and demonstrate higher resistance profiles, which is a sign of restored auroregulation[7,9,10].

Method

Pre- and postoperative transcranial Doppler investigations in 125 patients were performed by using a pulsed wave, range-gated 2 MHz doppler and the intraoperative measurements in 42 of 125 patients by a 20 MHz Doppler. The following parameters were observed: first the timed mean flow velocity (FVmean) of the Doppler spectrum and second, the pulsatility-index (PI), a ratio between systolic, diastolic and mean flow velocity. (Systolic minus diastolic flow velocity, divided by the mean flow velocity) as parameter for estimating stream resistance in arterioles[5]. TCD normal values for timed mean flow velocitiy in basal cerebral arteries have been reported by several authors[1,4,7,9]. For the PI, Lindegaard et al.[11,12] described a mean value of $0.71 + 0.10$ in the middle cerebral artery. (mean value + standard deviation). Low peripheral stream resistance leads to a decreasing pulsatility-index between $0,4 - 0,2$. Normal values for intraoperative measurements do not exist.

Small Changes of TCD Flow Velocity are Seen in Cases with

- Long-distances between proximal basal cerebral artery and angioma nidus;
- small angiomas (< 2 cm);
- Increasing number of supplying feeders;
- small shunt volume;
- small cross-sectional plane of feeders.

Severe Flow Accelerations in TCD are Seen in Cases with

- Short distances between suppling feeders and the circle of Willis;
- large angiomas;
- decreasing number of angioma feeders;
- high shunt volume;
- large cross-sectional plane of feeders; in this cases steal effects appear quite often.

A grading system for arteries supplying the angioma, depending on flow velocities and pulsatility, is described in Fig. 1 as exclusively, mainly and partially supplying. Normal flow velocites and pulsatility in feeding arteries are detectable in arteriovenous malformations which are very small or distally located and which functional supplying arteries are mainly supplying normal brain. These arteries can only be indentified by an interhemispheric difference in corresponding vessels of 20 cm/s and a disturbed vasomotor reactivity.

Altered CO_2 Reactivity and Steal Effects Monitored by TCD in AVM's

With the CO_2-reactivity test, the vasomotor response of the distal vascular bed can be investigated. During hyperventilation distal arterioles get constricted in presence of unchanged diameter of the basal cerebral arteries. The stream resistance increases with consequent diminishing of flow velocities. High levels of CO_2 (Hypoventilation) lead to a dilatation of the distal arterial bed with decrease of the stream resistance, thus resulting in higher flow velocities.

Since angiomas have non reactive vessel walls, flow velocities do not change with altering the CO_2 concentration. The CO_2-reactivity test is helpful to detect small angiomas with quite normal flow velocities in their feeders.

Figure 2 shows changes of intracerebral CO_2-reactivity in angioma feeders and brain supplying portions, in left PCA and the right-sided brain supplying vessels in the case of a left-sided angioma under the following 3 conditions: Normocapnia, hypercapnia and hypocapnia.

At normocapnia, the proximal angioma feeders show high flow velocities due to low resistance in the distal arterioles. High flow rates in the main feeding arteries cause diminished blood flow in the surrounding brain areas with compensatory vasodilation and reduced flow velocities. Flow velocity and diameter of arterioles on the contralateral side are not influenced.

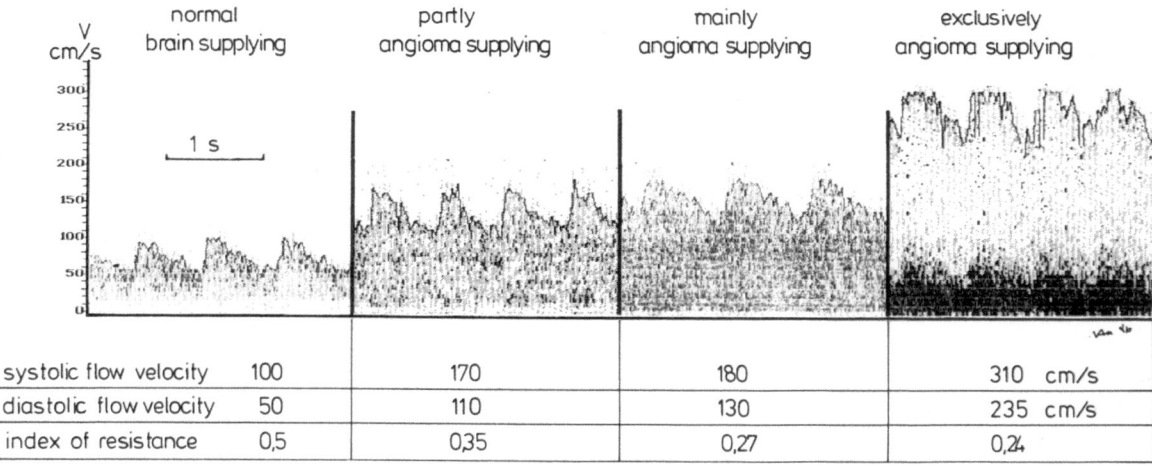

	normal brain supplying	partly angioma supplying	mainly angioma supplying	exclusively angioma supplying
systolic flow velocity	100	170	180	310 cm/s
diastolic flow velocity	50	110	130	235 cm/s
index of resistance	0,5	0,35	0,27	0,24

Fig. 1. Flow characteristics of angioma feeders in relation to the degree of contribution to the arterial supply

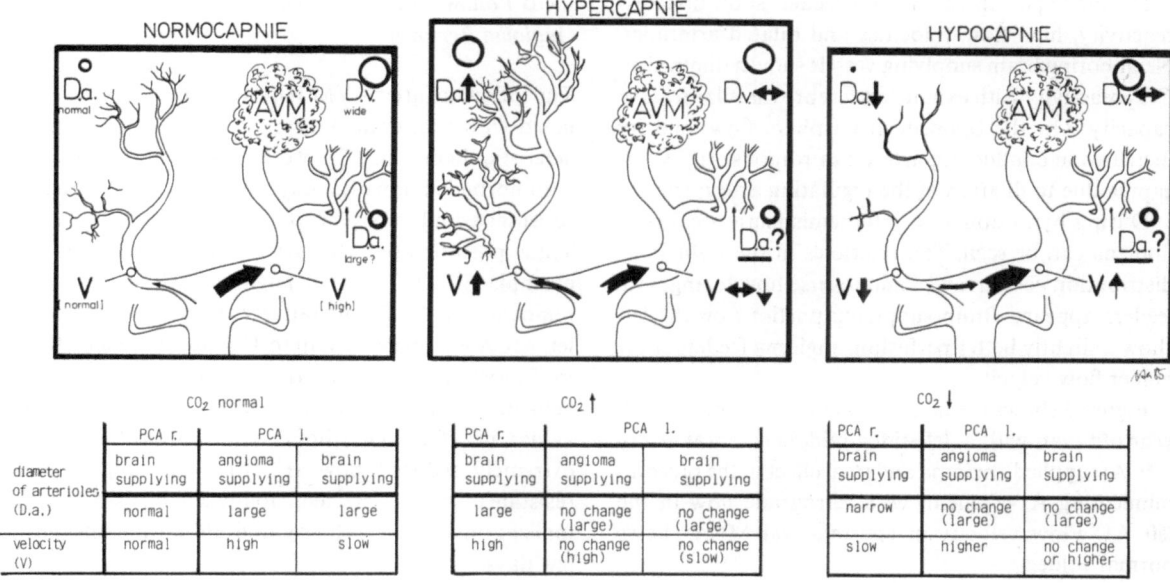

Fig. 2. Illustration of CO_2 reactivity and interhemispheric cerebral steal under normocapnia, hypercapnia and hypocapnia

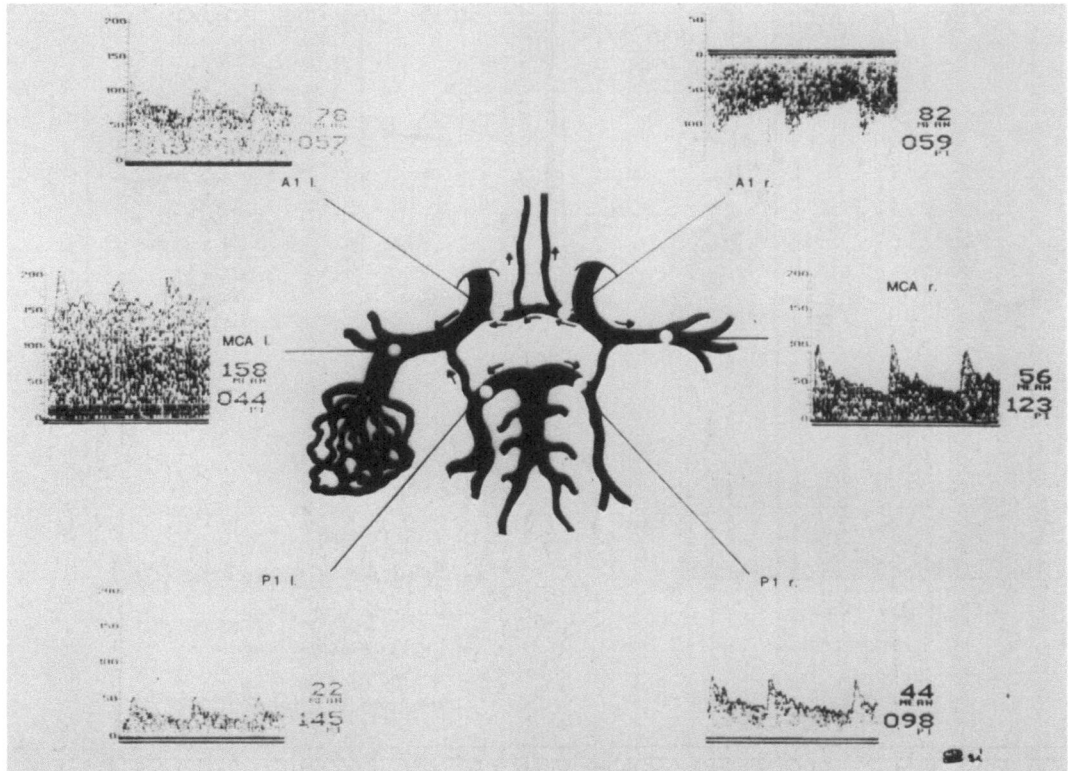

Fig. 3. Illustration of flow velocity changes and anterior precommunicating steal effect in the circle of Willis in left middle cerebral artery supplied large arteriovenous malformation

During hypercapnia angioma feeders show no CO_2-reactivity, high flow velocities and dilated arterioles. Neighboring brain supplying vessels show a diminished CO_2 reactivity with exhausted cerebrovascular reserve capacity. On the opposite hemisphere flow velocity increases in conducting arteries in response to hypercapnia due to dilation of the regulating arterioles.

During hypocapnia an interhemispheric steal phenomena can be seen. The arterioles in the right PCA distribution get narrowed and reverse flow to angioma feeders appears. Brain supplying portions on the left show a slightly better perfusion, angioma feeders show higher flow velocities.

Figure 3 shows the hemodynamic conditions of a 20 year old man with a, left-sided middle cerebral artery (MCA) supplied angioma and steal effect in the precommunicating A1-segment, with retrograde flow in the left A1. Flow velocity in contralateral MCA shows normal values.

TCD Follow-up Investigations After Angioma Removal

The follow-up after AVM removal can also be investigated with transcranial doppler. After removal characteristic changes in TCD were seen: low flow velocities with normalization after days or weeks, a high stream resistance and recovery of CO_2 reactivity (Fig. 4). These postoperative changes are demonstrated in an example of a left sylvian angioma before and after removal (Fig. 5). Preoperatively the mean velocity in left MCA was increased up to 170 cm/s with a distinct low resistance flow pattern and high diastolic flow velocities. The contralateral MCA showed normal values in TCD. Two hours after surgical excision, extremely reduced flow velocities with high distal resistance were detected, followed by slow normalization of flow velocity and PI during the next few days.

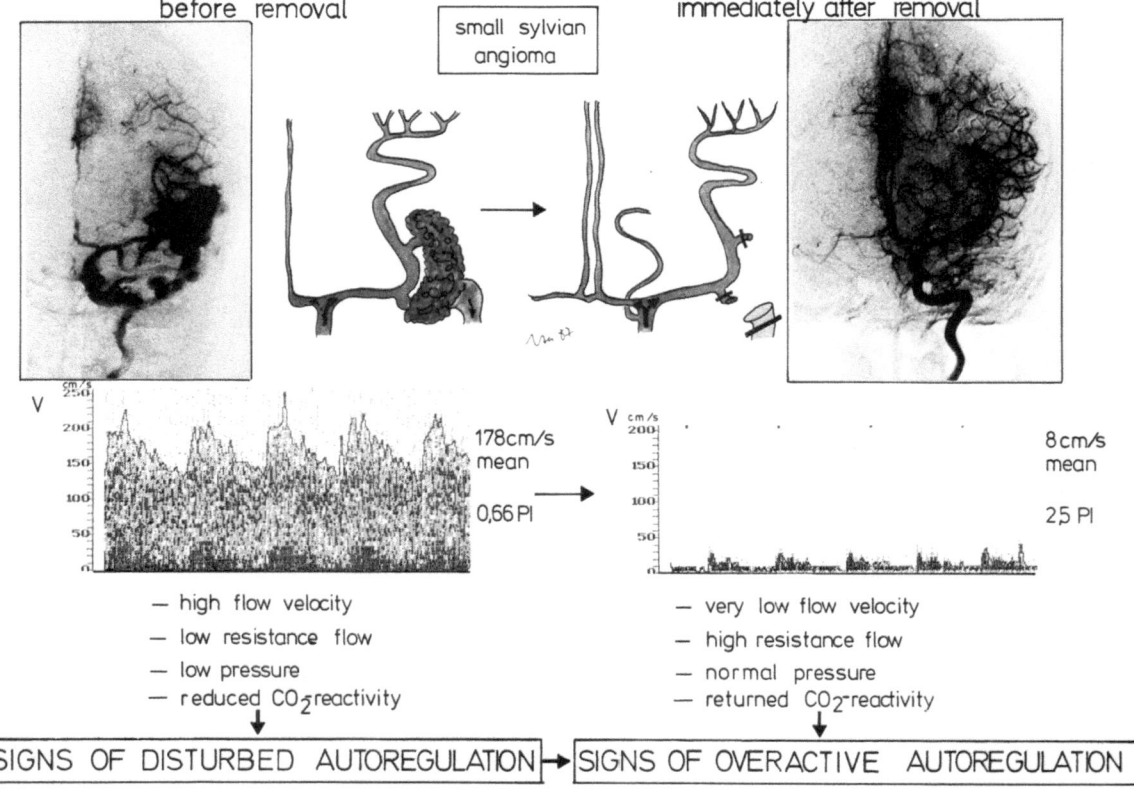

Fig. 4. Hemodynamic flow characteristics of angioma feeder demonstrated in a small sylvian AVM before and after removal of angioma

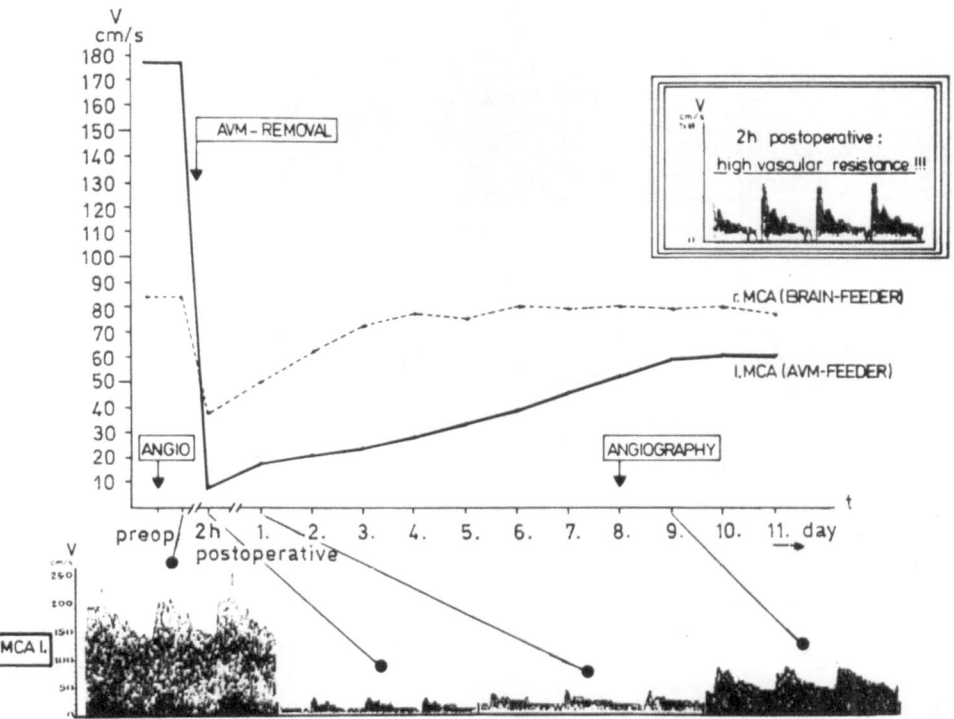

Fig. 5. Time course of flow velocity on TCD before and after removal of a middle cerebral artery supplied left sylvian angioma

Results

I. Preoperative Angiography in AVMs

The preoperative angiography shows the topography in detail, size, dilated supplying feeding arteries, a disturbed blood distribution and steal effects. This angiography is important for planning of operation strategy and shows signs of angioma specific angiographic changes. After removal, blood distribution normalizes, previously not – specified vessels are again visible and the angioma supplying vessels in the early postoperative angiography are perfused very slowly, as sign of a higher stream resistance in these vessels. These vessels are called stagnating arteries and can be occluded by thrombosis in the next days. Sometimes this causes ischemic complications when the thrombosed feeders have supplied also normal brain regions.

II. Transcranial Doppler in AVMs

TCD measurements in 125 angioma patients showed in angioma supplying feeding arteries characteristic pathological hemodynamic changes as high flow velocities, low pulsatility – indices and a disturbed vasomotor reactivity. These changes depend on the following angioma specific factors: size, location, number and length of main feeders, as well as shunt volume and cross sectional area of feeder arteries.

Interpretation of Increased Flow Velocities in Special Cases with Arteriovenous Malformations

A) Cerebral Vasospasm

It's important to mention that bleeding from angiomas often is associated with subarachnoid blood. Vasospasm after subarachnoid hemorrhage (SAH) produces, as in angioma feeders, increases in flow velocity and a quite identical flow spectrum on TCD. In contrast to angioma feeders with hyperperfusion, flow acceleration after SAH is due to spasm of the basal arteries and is usually limited to a period between 5 and 20 days after bleeding. Diastolic flow velocities are lower and pulsatility – Index higher than in patterns seen in patients with AVM. Since moderate and severe vasospasm

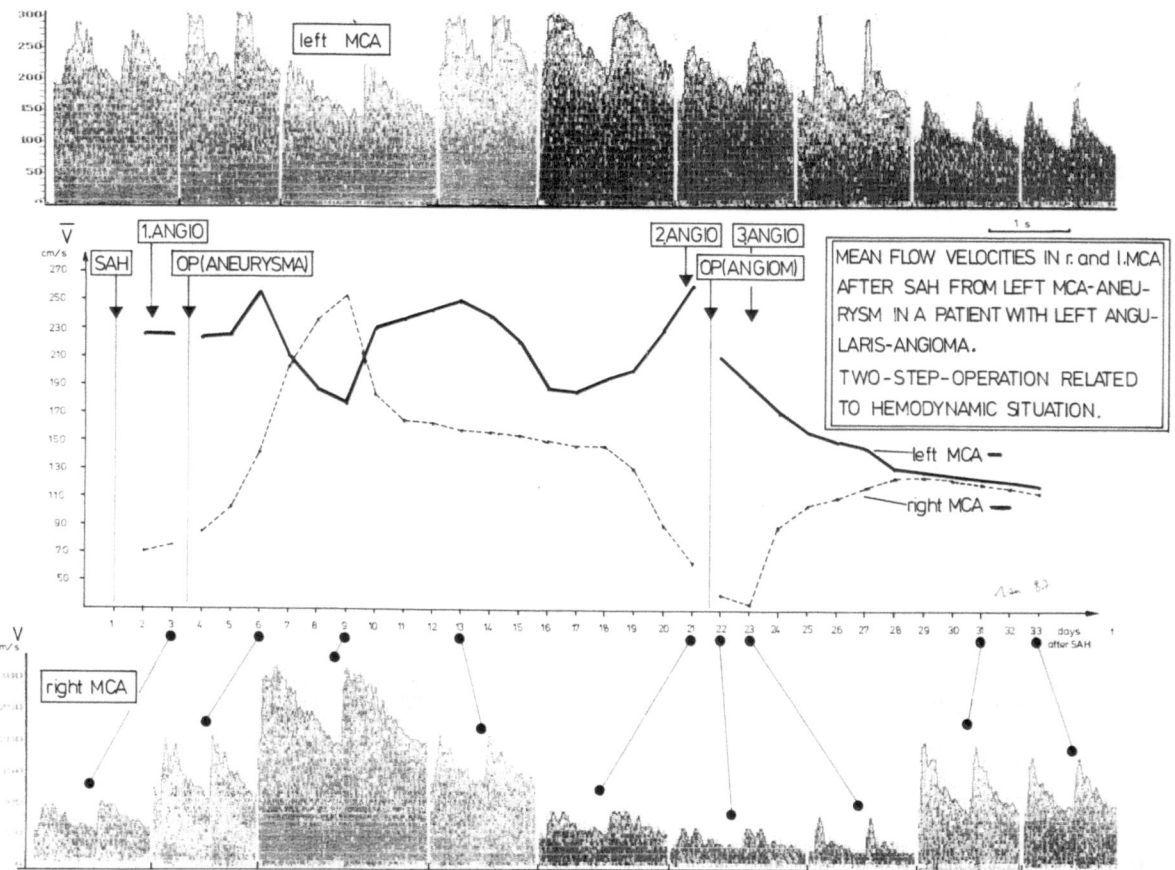

Fig. 6. Time course of flow velocity on TCD after rupture and clipping of a left middle cerebral artery aneurysm and a second operation to excise an angioma in a left angular region

also causes a reduction of the cerebrovascular reserve capacity (CVRC) with diminished CO_2 reactivity, the grade of reactivity is not a reliable parameter to differentiate between these two conditions causing flow acceleration. Figure 6 shows a 30 year old woman after SAH (Grade II Hunt and Hess) with angiographic indentification of a left-sided MCA-aneurysm and an angioma supplied by the MCA in the angular region. After the first step of a staged operation, following clipping of aneurysm, she developed severe spasm in both MCAs between the 6th and 19th day after bleeding. When the spasm declined, flow velocities remained high in the left MCA, the main feeder of the angioma. The second operation was performed on the 22nd day after bleeding. Postoperative angiography showed a complete elimination of the angioma; the Doppler spectrum returned to normal values in both sides.

B) Interaction of Intracranial Pressure Due to Acute Hydrocephalus and Hemodynamics of AVM

After rebleeding of a left anterior cerebral artery (ACA) malformation with intracerebral and biventricular bleeding, the patient developed obstructive hydrocephalus. Figure 7 shows Doppler monitoring of the contralateral MCA and the ACA feeding the angioma, before and after ventricular puncture.

High flow velocities, up to 144 cm/s in the angioma feeder, and normal values in the contralateral MCA were measured after the initial bleeding. Rebleeding occured with subsequent hydrocephalus, which produced increased intracranial pressure (ICP). This produced increased resistance in the right MCA and decreased flow velocities in the ACA feeding the angioma.

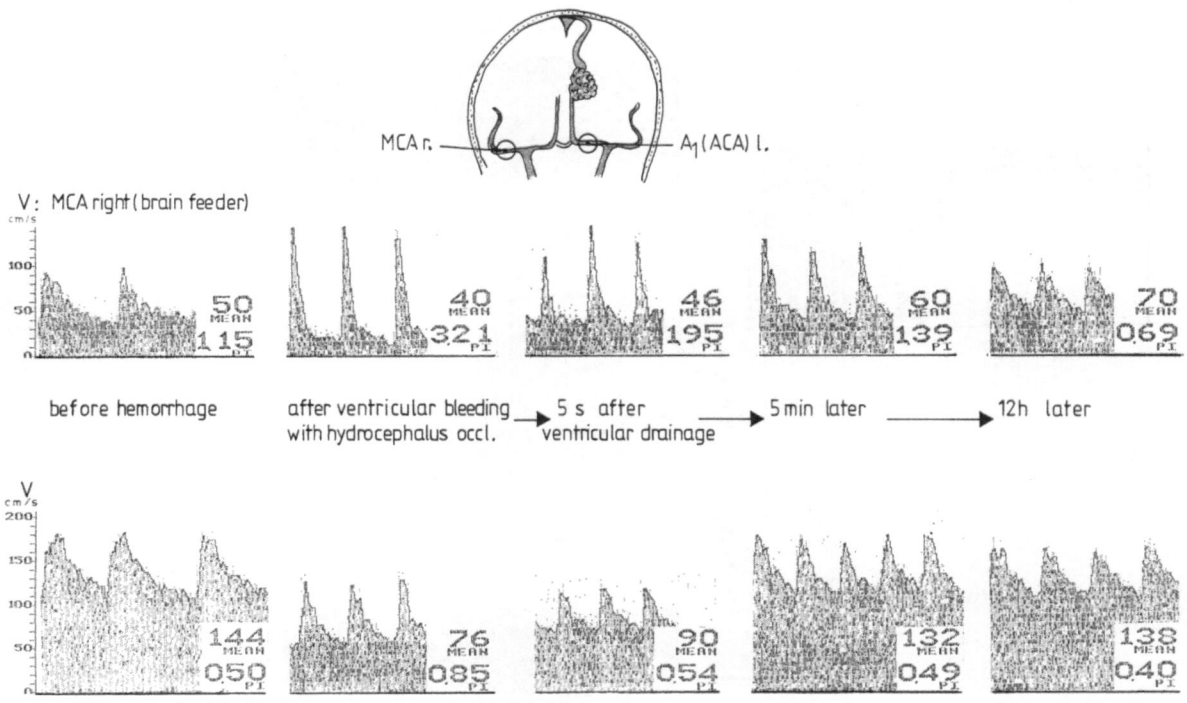

Fig. 7. Time course of flow velocities in brain and angioma feeders after rebleeding of an anterior cerebral artery supplied angioma in presence of hemorrhagic obstructive hydrocephalus before and after ventricular puncture

In contrast to the opposite side, with high PI (up to 3, 21), the PI in the feeding artery increased only slightly. Five seconds after ventricular drainage, the flow velocities began to increase bilaterally toward their initial values.

III. Intraoperative Doppler in AVMs

Intraoperative measurements were performed in 42 of 125 patients during operative angioma removal. Thereby selective monitoring of flow velocities and intravascular pressure changes in feeding arteries, the angioma nidus and normal brain supplying branches are possible. In the beginning the feeders and the angioma nidus show high flow velocities and a decreased intravascular pressure, the draining veins increased flow velocities and a high intravascular pressure. Before occlusion of the main feeding arteries and draining veins the nidus will be skeletonized. When the feeding arteries are occluded, flow velocities and intravascular pressure in the nidus and veins decrease, the intravascular pressure increases tremendously in the proximal part of the former feeding artery, whereas the flow

velocity is reduced. Flow velocity decreases and intravascular pressure increases in brain supplying vessels as sign of restored cerebral autoregulation with higher distal stream resistance (Fig. 8 demonstrates a typical example).

Discussion

Transcranial and intraoperative Doppler sonography are simple, noninvasive methods for pre-, intra- and postoperative monitoring of altered hemodynamic conditions in cerebral AVM's. Together with preoperative angiography it might be possible, if the angioma is large and has very high flow velocities and an abolished CO_2 reactivity, to assess the risk of postoperative complications[17]. In our intraoperative doppler and postoperative TCD measurements after removal of angiomas in 125 patients we could not find hemodynamic signs of a normal pressure breakthrough phenomenon (NPBP) as described by Spetzler[17]. He postulated that bleeding, swelling and ischemia after removal of an angioma is caused by a suddenly increased cerebral perfusion with defective cerebral autoregulation.

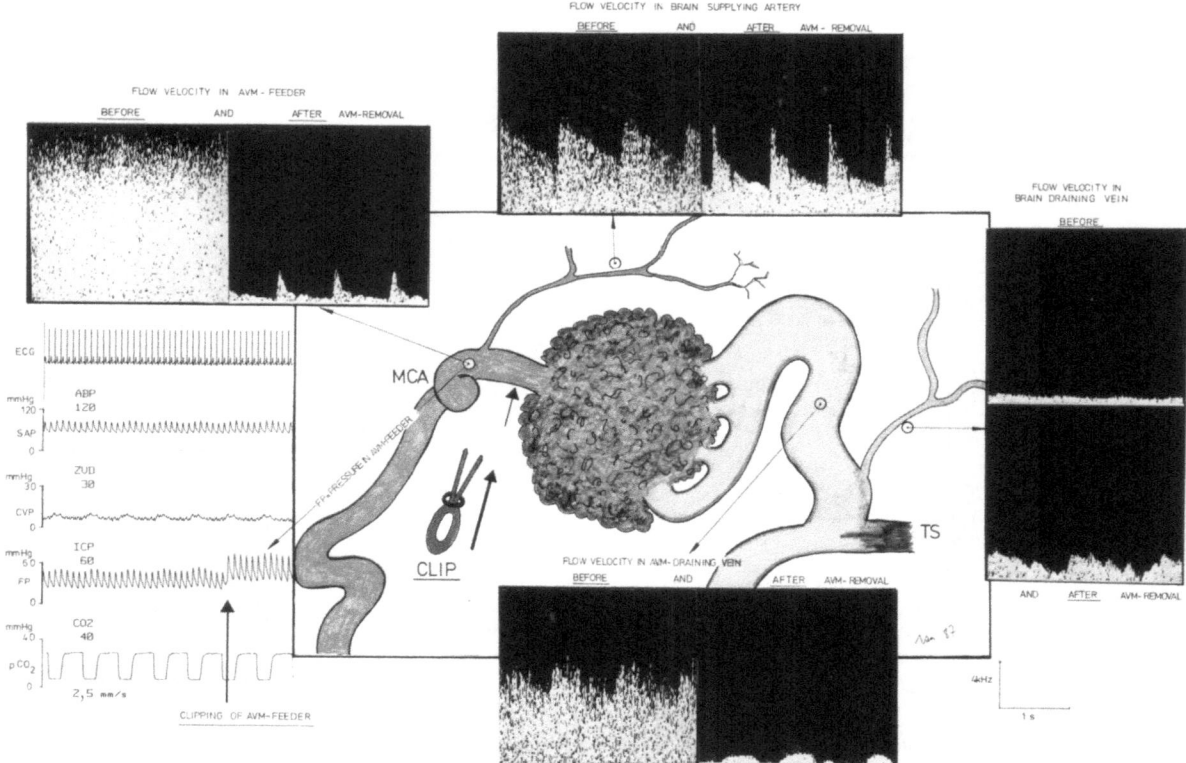

Fig. 8. Illustration of the typical intraoperative doppler flow velo-cities in the feeder and draining vein before and after AVM removal and of intravascular pressure changes before and after clipping of the feeding artery

Our results showed that the autoregulation is established immediately after removal. In our opinion the NPBP is caused by a wrong operative strategy, incomplete angioma removal with pressure dependent rupture of angioma vessels, postoperative thrombosis of veins and arteries and *iatrogenic* vessel occlusion by the surgeon.

Some critical remarks to the value of transcranial and intraoperative doppler in angioma patients have to be mentioned. With TCD the identification of a feeder for angiomas with basal location is difficult and often it is only possible to detect the angioma itself. The identification of distal lying, small angiomas below a diameter of 2 cm is quite uncertain. High flow velocities do not only occur in angioma feeders, but also in case of vasospasm or hyperemia. Grading of the operative risk is not possible with TCD. Also the topographic localization of angioma is not possible; only the main vessel trunks supplying the angioma can be identified. The identification of brain supplying arteries adjacent

to the angioma is very difficult and often impossible. The first intraoperative doppler presents only a spectral analysis without quantitative measurements of flow velocity and pulsatility. To date, by judging only the wave and proportion between diastolic and systolic flow velocity, it was impossible to present quantitatively reliable data. In the future perhaps transcranial-color-coded real time sonography, with a better topographic orientation, will give more information than transcranial doppler sonography.

References

1. Aaslid R, Markwalder T-M, Nornes H (1982) Noninvasive transcranial Doppler ultrasound recording of flow velocities in basal cerebral arteries. J Neurosurg 57: 769–774
2. Aaslid R (1986) Transcranial Doppler sonography. Springer, Wien New York
3. Aaslid R, Huber P, Nornes H (1984) Evaluation of cerebrovascular spasm with transcranial Doppler ultrasound. J Neurosurg 60: 37–41

4. Arnolds JA, von Reutern G (1986) Transcranial Doppler sono-graphy. Examination technique and normal reference values. Ultrasound Med Biol 12: 115–123

5. Gosling RG, King DH (1974) Arterial assessment of Doppler shift ultrasound. Proc R Soc Med 67: 447–449

6. Harders A (1986) Neurological applications of transcranial Doppler sonography. Springer, Wien New York, pp 94–107

7. Hassler W (1986) Hemodynamic aspects of cerebral angiomas. Acta Neurochir (Wien) [Suppl] 37

8. Hassler W, Steinmetz H (1987) Cerebral hemodynamics in angioma patients: an intraoperative study. J Neurosurg 67: 822–831

9. Hassler W, Burger R (1992) Arteriovenous malformation. In: Newell DW, Aaslid R (eds) Transcranial Doppler. Raven, New York, pp 123–135

10. Hassler W, Burger R (1992) Transcranial doppler sonography in cerebral arteriovenous malformations. In: Limoni P, Cerisoli M, Masson SpA (eds) Ultrasound in neuroscience. Parigi, Barcelona, pp 67–73

11. Lindegaard KF, Grolimund P, Aaslid R, Nornes H (1986) Evaluation of cerebral AVM's using transcranial Doppler ultra-sound. J Neurosurg 65: 335–344

12. Lindegaard KF, Bakke SJ, Grolimund P, et al (1985) Carotid artery disease: assessment of intracranial hemodynamic pat-tern by noninvasive transcranial Doppler ultrasound. J Neuro-surg 63: 890–898

13. Luessenhop AJ, Gennarelli ThA (1977) Anatomical grading of supratentorial arteriovenous malformations for determining op-erability. Neurosurgery 1: 30–35

14. Nornes H, Grip A, Wikeby P (1979) Intraoperative evaluation of cerebral hemodynamics using directional doppler technique. Part 1: arteriovenous malformations. J Neurosurg 50: 145–151

15. Okabe T, Mayer JS, et al (1983) Xenon-enhanced CT CBF measurements in cerebral AVM's before and after excision. Contribution to pathogenesis and treatment. J Neurosurg 59: 21–31

16. Rosenblum BR, Bonner RF, Oldfield FH (1987) Intraoperative measurement of cortical blood flow adjacent to cerebral AVM using Laser doppler velocimetry. J Neurosurg 66: 396–399

17. Spetzler RF, Wilson CB, Weinstein P, et al (1978) Normal perfusion pressure break-through theory. Clin Neurosurg 25: 651–672

18. Spetzler RF, Martin NA (1986) A proposed grading system for arteriovenous malformations. J Neurosurg 65: 476–483

19. Wilkins RH (1985) Natural history of intracranial vascular malformations: a review. Neurosurgery 16: 421–450

Correspondence: W. Hassler, M.D., Department of Neurosurgery, Municipal Clinic, Duisburg, Zu den Rehwiesen 9, Im Kalkweg, D-47055 Duisburg, Federal Republic of Germany.

Cerebrovascular Reserve Capacity in AVM Patients

A. Piepgras, G. Leinsinger, and **P. Schmiedek**

Department of Neurosurgery, University of Munich, Federal Republic of Germany

Summary

Cerebrovascular reserve capacity (CVRC) was tested in 18 patients with arteriovenous malformations by means of 133-Xe inhalation technique and stimulation of cerebral blood flow (CBF) with 1 g acetazolamide i.v. Mean hemispheric cerebral blood flow at rest and after stimulation did not differ significantly from 35 healthy controls. Focal high flow areas exceeding 120% of intraindividual mean resting CBF were found in 11 patients ipsilaterally, a focally decreased CVRC adjacent to a high flow area was present in 6 of these. In 7 patients with small AVMs high flow areas were missed. In 5 cases there were contralateral findings at rest as well, in 4 of them with an equally depressed CVRC.

The 133-Xe inhalation technique presents several methodological problems in assessment of hemodynamic changes in AVMs that are further discussed.

Keywords: Arteriovenous malformation; 133-Xe regional cerebral blood flow; cerebrovascular reserve capacity; acetazolamide (Diamox).

Introduction

Arteriovenous malformations are commonly understood as high flow areas with low resistance. Intraoperative measurements in feeding vessels have proven flow up to 550 ml/min in single feeding vessels. To investigate whether these findings are reproducible with a Xe-Inhalation technique we performed measurements of cerebral blood flow in patients with AVMs. To prove the hypothesis that the large, non-nutritional shunt volume causes dysautoregulation in the surrounding tissue we additionally tested the cerebrovascular reserve capacity in these patients.

Material and Methods

In a retrospective study over the past 4 years, 18 patients, 9 female, 9 male were included. Mean age was 33 ± 13 years. Leading clinical symptoms were seizure disorders in 10 patients, headaches in 3 and transient ischemic attacks in 2 patients. 3 patients had suffered an intracranial bleeding several weeks prior to the blood flow study. Angiographically determined volume of the malformation ranged from 1 to 137 cm³ with a mean volume of 32 cm³. 8 AMSs were smaller than 20 cm³. Broken down according to the Spetzler-classification the majority of patients was classified as of grade 3.

Quantitative measurements of cerebral blood flow were obtained by means of the 133-Xe Inhalation D-SPECT technique in two slices above the canthomeatal line. Each slice is of 2 cm thickness and there is a gap of 2 cm between both slices. The slices were divided in 12 regions of interest of equal size. After an initial determination of CBF at rest 1 g Diamox i.v. was administered and the cerebrovascular reserve capacity calculated as the net increase in CBF in each ROI 15 minutes after this stimulus. Diamox causes an increase in normal brain tissue blood flow by dilatation of small resistance vessels.

The results were compared to 35 healthy controls.

Focal hyperperfusion was defined as an area of flow exceeding 20% of the individual mean global cerebral blood flow. Reduced cerebrovascular reserve capacity was defined as an area with a lower 10% increase in CBF after stimulation with Diamox.

Results

Mean hemispheric CBF (ml/100 g/min) ipsilateral to the AVM was not significantly different from the contralateral hemisphere and not significantly different from 35 normal controls in both slices (Table 1). After stimulation, mean hemispheric CBF increased normally, again with no differences between ipsilateral and contralateral hemisphere.

All 288 regions of interest relative to the respective mean global CBF are plotted in Fig. 1. High flow areas exceeding 120% were measured in 11 patients ipsilaterally. 5 high flow areas of the same magnitude were detected contralaterally – in 2 cases there were ipsi- and contralateral findings, in 3 patients we found

Table 1. *Mean Hemispheric CBF (ml/100 g/min)*

Slice	Ipsilateral	Contralateral	Controls
II	60.1 ± 10.5	58.7 ± 8.9	61.1 ± 6.5
III	54.1 ± 10.1	52.4 ± 10.9	56.3 ± 7.1

Mean stimulated hemispheric CBF (ml/100 g/min) after 1 g Diamox®

Slice	Ipsilateral	Contralateral	Controls
II	$83.8 - 15.2$	$84.3 - 13.9$	$84.9 - 7.4$
III	82.2 ± 15.5	81.0 ± 17.3	86.2 ± 7.4

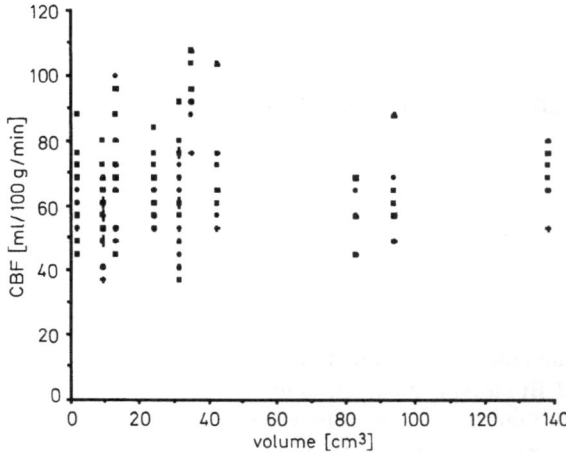

Fig. 1. CBF rest vs. volume; n = 18

contralateral high flow areas only. Mean volume of the AVM's in the 7 patients that had no high flow areas at rest was 9.6 cm^3 (1–31 cm^3, range).

A focally decreased cerebrovascular reserve capacity (CVRC) was noted ipsilaterally to the malformation in 8 patients, in 6 cases there were contralateral findings of the same magnitude as well. A decrease CVRC could be attributed to an adjacent high flow area ipsilaterally in 6 patients, additionally contralateral in 4 of them.

Discussion

Since the first description of the "cerebral steal syndrome" by Feindel et al.[1] being understood as an interference of the surrounding microcirculation with an arteriovenous malformation, several reports focused on non-invasive measurements of cerebral blood flow in these patients. Various means of measurement have been utilized with differing results regarding the issue, whether or not there is an ischemic and dysregulated adjacent borderzone[2–8].

Problems in the accuracy of the 133-Xe inhalation technique include Compton scatter, an arbitrarily set partition coefficient that might be insufficient for angiomatous tissue, tracer recirculation, prolonged initial input of the tracer and potential pathophysiological reasons as arterial thrombosis, cerebral edema, neuronal depression etc. A major drawback of the method used in this study is the rather large thickness of slices and especially the 2 cm gap between, that leads to inaccurate results in small AVM's.

Therefore, we do not believe in reliable measurements being possible with this technique within the nidus.

A depressed CBF in the contralateral hemisphere has been described before[7,9], however, a depressed CVRC adjacent to contralateral high-flow areas, most often mirror-like, is a new finding and lets us speculate about interhemispheric neuronal activation/depression.

In conclusion, the 133-Xe inhalation method appears to be unsuitable for the reliable quantification of very high flow within an AVM nidus due to various methodological considerations, a depressed CVRC adjacent to an AVM is indicative for vascular dysregulation that might even affect the contralateral hemisphere, as contralateral high flow areas in combination with a decreased CVRC are present in some patients.

References

1. Feindel W, Yamamoto YL, Hodge CP (1971) Red cerebral veins and the cerebral steal syndrome. Evidence from fluorescein angiography and microregional blood flow by radioisotopes during excision of an angioma. J Neurosurg 35: 167–180
2. Shenkin HA, Spitz EB, Grant FC, Kety SS (1948) Physiological studies of arteriovenous anomalies of the brain. J Neurosurg 5: 165–172
3. Lassen NA, Munck O (1956) Cerebral blood flow in arteriovenous anomalies of the brain determined by the use of radioactive krypton 85. Acta Psychiatr 31: 71–80
4. Spetzler RF, Selman WR (1984) Pathophysiology of cerebral ischemia accompanying arteriovenous malformations. In: Wilson CB, Stein BM (eds) Intracranial arteriovenous malformations. Williams and Wilkins, Baltimore, pp 24–31
5. Homan RW, Devous MD, Stokely EM, Bonte FJ (1986) Quantification of intracerebral steal in patients with arteriovenous malformation. Arch Neurol 43: 779–785
6. Menon D, Weir B (1979) Evaluation of cerebral blood flow in arteriovenous malformations by the xenon-133 inhalation method. Can J Neurol Sci 6: 411–416
7. Takeuchi S, Kikuchi H, Karasawa J, Naruo Y, Hashimoto K, Nishimura T, Kozuka T, Hayashi M (1987) Cerebral hemodynamics in arteriovenous malformations. Evaluation by single-photon emission CT. AJNR 8: 193–197
8. Batjer HH (1992) Role of cerebral blood flow imaging in the evaluation of subarachnoid hemorrhage and intracranial arteriovenous malformations. In: Schmiedek P, Einhäupl K, Kirsch CM (eds) Stimulated cerebral blood flow. Springer, Berlin Heidelberg New York Tokyo, pp 84–93
9. Okabe T, Meyer JS, Okayasu H, Harper R, Rose J, Grossman RG, Centeno R, Tachibana H, Lee YY (1983) Xenon-enhanced CT CBF measurements in cerebral AVMs before and after excision. J Neurosurg 59: 21–31

Correspondence: P. Schmiedek, M.D., Klinikum der Stadt Mannheim, Theodor-Kutzer-Ufer, D-68167 Mannheim, Federal Republic of Germany.

Vasodilatory Challenge with rCBF Measurement in Patients with Cerebral AVMs: a Preliminary Report

A. Talacchi, F. Sala, A. Pasqualin, and **A. Bricolo**

Department of Neurosurgery, City Hospital, Verona, Italy

Summary

In an attempt to evaluate the pathophysiology of arteriovenous malformations (AVMs) and the prognostic factors in patients undergoing surgery, pre-operative cerebral blood flow (CBF) measurements were performed in 14 patients: the examinations were repeated after acetazolamide infusion (1g i.v.) in order to investigate residual vascular reserve and vasoreactivity for regional and hemispheric assessment. The 133-Xe inhalation technique was used and the data processed through the M2 model elaborated by Prohovnik. Fourteen patients were studied; the mean volume was 26 cm3; 4 patients experienced post-operative hyperemic complications. Mean resting CBF values (54 ml/100 g/min) showed a variable increase after acetazolamide (average 35%, ranging from 5 to 52%), higher in the patients affected by hyperemic complications (41 vs. 26%). Moreover: a) regional activated-CBF showed a correlation with the baseline values, with higher response in patients with lower values; b) hemispheric activated-CBF was influenced by AVM volume, showing lower increase in larger AVMs. A common mechanism has been suggested to explain these unexpected features.

Keywords: Cerebral arteriovenous malformations; cerebral blood flow; acetazolamide test; hyperemic complications.

Introduction

In patients harbouring arteriovenous malformations (AVMs), the common condition leading to clinical impairment and post-operative clinical deterioration is the reduced perfusion in the brain around the AVM, due to the presence of the shunt flow[1,14,19]. In an attempt to avoid ischemia, cerebral autoregulation can lead to vasodilation and increased oxygen extraction: once this mechanism cannot meet further reduction of the perfusion pressure, ischemia occurs[7].

In order to evaluate vasoactive changes – avoiding hypotensive tests that may be uncomfortable for the patient – in many clinical trials acetazolamide has substituted hypercarbia in testing vasodilatory challenge, because of easy administration and scant side effects: the drug is an inhibitor of erytrocyte carbonic anhydrase and induces a rapid and marked increase in CBF, leaving metabolism unchanged[4,6,18].

Our purpose was to evaluate cerebral perfusion reserve in relation to the residual vasodilation capacity, as well as to assess the regional vasoreactivity. Both these aspects were related to the baseline CBF values and to the clinical and radiological factors influencing hemodynamics in patients with cerebral AVMs.

Material and Methods

In an attempt to evaluate surgical risks and indications to surgery, 14 patients were studied by means of CBF measurements in the Department of Neurosurgery of Verona from September 1989 to February 1992. There were 8 males and 6 females, ranging in age between 19 and 66 years (average 36 yrs). On clinical examination, neurological impairment unrelated to hemorrhage was disclosed in 3 patients: 1 presented hemiparesis, 1 presented organic brain syndrome and one suffered from intracranial hypertension. Angiography and CT scan were performed in all cases; 11 cases were also evaluated with magnetic resonance imaging (MRI). On angiography, AVM size was determined through its volume, obtained by the multiplication of the three diameters by 0.52[11]. In the present series the mean volume was 25 cm³. As regards AVM location, 3 AVMs were frontal, 3 temporal, 5 parietal, 2 occipital, 1 callosal. Eight AVMs were located in the right hemisphere, 5 in the left, 1 in the midline (callosal). Eleven patients were submitted to surgical resection of the AVM: in 4 of them hyperemic complications occurred. Hyperemic complications were defined as intra-operative blood loss over 2000 ml, post-operative hemorrhage (not due to residual AVM), and post-operative cerebral edema on CT scan, associated with either impairment in the level of consciousness or focal neurological signs[11].

CBF studies were performed pre-operatively in resting and activated states. The test consists in CBF measurement before and 20 minutes after acetazolamide infusion (1 g i.v.)[18]. It is difficult to obtain normative data for statistical comparison in activated CBF because of a certain variability in the test response. In our laboratory a 30% increase with respect to the baseline values has been considered the mean for control patients.

The method used for CBF measurements was the 133-Xe inhalation with the Novo Cerebrograph (the instrument is equipped with 32 epicranial detectors); the clearance curves were analyzed in a mono-compartimental fashion by the ISI parameter and processed through the M2 model elaborated by Prohovnik[10,12,13]. For statistically significant comparison, an age-matched control population (n = 85 cases) was adopted, divided agewise into two groups (under and over 45 yrs.), with mean values of 57 and 47 ml/100 g/min respectively. Hemispheric hypoperfusion and hemispheric asymmetry were considered for both resting and activated CBF. Statistical significance of observed differences (> 2 SD) was assessed by the Z test[5]. Baseline CBF data were expressed in terms of absolute values (ml/100 g/min) and inter-exams differences (resting vs. activated) in terms of percent both for hemispheric and regional values.

Results

Mean hemispheric CBF in the 14 patients was 50 ml/100 g/min; only in 1 case global CBF was significantly decreased. In 2 patients it was asymmetric (p < 0.05), with lower values in the hemisphere ipsilateral to the

AVM: both underwent hyperemic complications after surgical resection of the malformation. At baseline CBF, the 3 patients with neurological impairment at admission showed: hemispheric asymmetry in the patient presenting with hemiparesis; global hypoperfusion (not reaching the level of significance) in the patient with organic brain syndrome, and normal CBF values in the patient with intracranial hypertension.

After acetazolamide test the average augmentation of hemispheric CBF was 35% (ranging from 5% to 52%). One of the 2 patients showing hemispheric asymmetry at resting CBF, presented normal CBF values at the activated examination; the other patient showed a more marked asymmetry (from p < 0.05 to p < 0.001) when compared with the controls. Among

Table 1. *Acetazolamide Test (11 Operated Cases)*

	Baseline CBF (ml/100 g/min)	Increase
No hyperemic complications (7 c.)	45	26%
Hyperemic complications (4 c.)	55	41%

Table 2. *Acetazolamide Test. CBF Augmentation Related to AVM Volume*

AVM < 20 cm³	(6 cases)	38%
AVM 20–30 cm³	(4 cases)	37%
AVM > 30 cm³	(4 cases)	24%

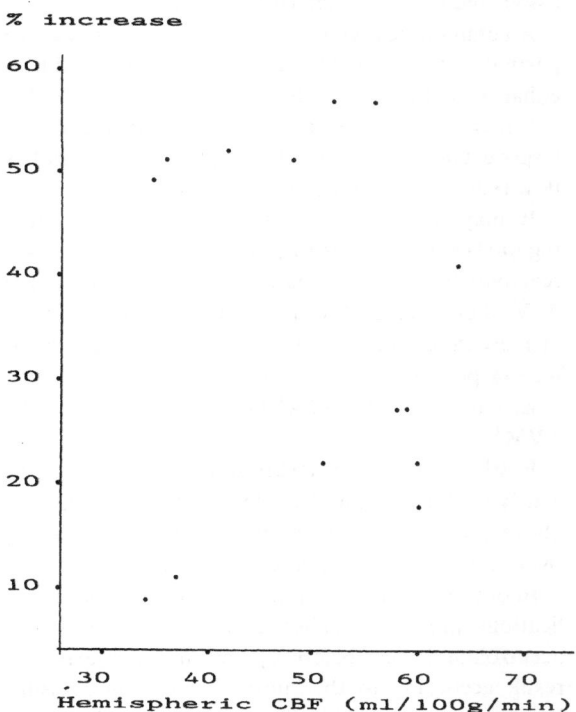

Fig. 1. The relation between resting hemispheric CBF and percentage increase after activation shows two different groups regardless of resting values (see the text for further explanation)

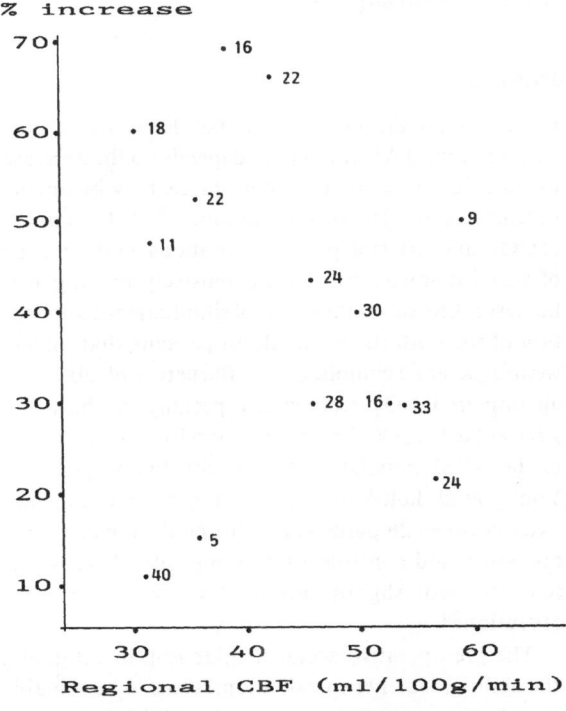

Fig. 2. The relation between lowest regional resting values adjacent to the AVM and percentage increase after activation shows a trend towards a direct relationship between lower baseline values and higher increase after the test. The numbers inside the graphic are the volume of each case: lower enhancement is detected in large AVM

the activated CBF, 4 new patients disclosed hemispheric asymmetry: 2 of them were operated on and 1 suffered from a hyperemic complication. Considering the patients (4 cases) undergoing hyperemic complications as a group, mean CBF at rest and percentage increase after acetazolamide test were compared in Table 1 to the results obtained from patients that fared well.

In Fig. 1 baseline hemispheric CBF was correlated with the percentage increase after acetazolamide test. Two distinct groups were recognized: patients with increase under 30%, and patients with increase over 50% in activated CBF. The mean volume for each group was 29 and 17 cm^3 respectively. Furthermore no difference was found in the degree of increase in relation to baseline values and in relation to post-operative course. There was a lower increase in larger AVMs (Table 2).

For each patient the lowest regional resting values adjacent to the AVM were plotted against the percentage increase after the test in the same areas (Fig. 2): a trend towards a linear relation was observed between lower baseline values and higher increase after activation (and viceversa). Furthermore lower enhancement was detected in larger AVMs.

Discussion

Even though the mechanism that leads to chronic vasodilation, in AVM patients, depends on the decrease of perfusion pressure, the same vessels may be unable to react to several physiological stimuli[9,14]. The impact of CO_2 and perfusion pressure variations on the change of vessel diameter has been extensively investigated, but less is knwon on the result of simultaneous application of the both these stimuli. In patients that underwent hyperemic complications, Barnett et al. observed an impaired CO_2 reactivity, especially in the areas adjacent to the AVM, as it was found by Takeuchi et al. in the AVM population tested with hypocapnia[1,16]. Young et al. failed to note differences in CO_2 reactivity between 26 patients monitored during and after operation and controls; on the opposite, there was a trend towards slightly increased vasoreactivity after operation[20].

The pre-operative acetazolamide test, investigating the ability to further vasodilation, seems to be valuable in selecting a population at risk of hemodynamic complications, because cerebral vessels in these patients may be maximally vasodilated, and presumably unable to constrict[14]. Furthermore acetazolamide infusion

allows an evaluation of cerebral perfusion reserve in relation to the residual vasodilation capacity[15]. Tyler et al. in 1990 using PET scan investigated metabolic and hemodynamic parameters in AVM patients. Cerebral blood volume was often and widely increased, but oxygen extraction remained in the normal limit, with a trend to increase in larger AVM[17].

Our results are consistent with those illustrated by Morgan et al. on experimental ground and by Batjer et al. on clinical grounds, respectively induced by CO_2 changes and by acetazolamide test. Both authors found a higher response of baseline CBF to CO_2 variations, suggesting implications on the peri-operative respiratory management or proposing prognostic indications according to the CBF response to acetazolamide test[2,8].

In our experience, as concerns hemispheric CBF, the degree of percent increase after acetazolamide infusion was irrespective of resting values, but was influenced by the volume, with a lower increase in larger AVMs. Regions surrounding the AVMs were most prone to hypoperfusion and showed a higher response after activation. As the AVM volume increased, after activation the increase in hemispheric CBF was lower and associated to a lower inter-regional difference.

A common behavior is thought to exist, influenced partially by the size of the lesion: higher regional flow enhancement in hypoperfused areas of smaller AVMs is somewhat lost in larger AVMs, possibly due to a larger extension of the steal phenomenon that renders flow redistribution unrelevant.

It may be speculated that the abnormally high regional response is due to: a) an exaggerated local vasoreactivity (or only vasodilation)[3]; b) a reduction of the A–V shunt via a flow redistribution owing to an increase in cerebral volemia; c) an inverse steal phenomenon possibly due to a pressure gradient between vessels remote from the AVM and those around the AVM[1].

Further studies and larger series are necessary to clarify the basic pathophysiology of these lesions and above all the relation between these abnormalities and the occurrence of hyperemic complications.

In our series, patients undergoing hyperemic complications presented higher hemispheric response to acetazolamide test before operation, an unexpected result according to the "normal perfusion pressure breakthrough theory"[14]. The possible explanations are still speculative: Batjer et al. – who presented in 1988 two pilot studies about activated states in AVM

patients – postulated that vasoconstrictive and vasodilatory capacities could be dissociated in these patients[3]. The same authors, in a recent study (in a series
of 35 patients) confirmed these data and suggested that
the sudden redistribution of blood after AVM removal
can lead to inappropriate vasodilation and finally to
edema or hemorrhage[2].

These preliminary data provide promising perspective either in regard to AVM pathophysiology
either in the assessment of peri-operative hyperemic
complications.

References

1. Barnett GH, Little JR, Ebrahim ZY, Jones CS, Friel HT (1987)
   Cerebral circulation during arteriovenous malformation operation. Neurosurgery 20: 836–842
2. Batjer HH, Devous MD (1992) The use of acetazolamide-
   enhanced regional cerebral blood flow measurement to predict
   risk to arteriovenous malformation patients. Neurosurgery 31:
   213–218
3. Batjer HH, Devous MD, Meyer YJ, Purdy PD, Samson DS
   (1988) Cerebrovascular hemodynamics in arteriovenous malformation complicated by normal perfusion pressure breakthrough.
   Neurosurgery 22: 503–509
4. Cotev S, Lee J, Severinghaus JW (1968) The effects of acetazolamide on cerebral blood flow and cerebral tissue pO_2.
   Anesthesiology 29: 471–477
5. Downie NM, Heath RW (1974) Basic statistical methods.
   Harper Row, New York
6. Ehrenreich DL, Burns RA, Alman RW, Fazekas JF (1961)
   Influence of acetazolamide on cerebral blood flow. Arch Neurol
   15: 125–130
7. Gibbs JM, Wise RJS, Leenders KL, Jones T (1984) Evaluation
   of cerebral perfusion reserve in patients with carotid-artery
   occlusion. Lancet ii: 310–314
8. Morgan MK, Anderson RE, Sundt TM (1989) The effects of
   hyperventilation on cerebral flow in the rat with an open and
   closed carotid-jugular fistula. Neurosurgery 25: 606–612
9. Nornes H, Grip A (1980) Hemodynamic aspects of cerebral
   arteriovenous malformations. J Neurosurg 53: 456–464
10. Obrist WD, Thompson HK, King CH, Shon Wang H (1967)
    Determination of regional cerebral blood flow by inhalation of
    133-Xenon. Circ Res 20: 124–135
11. Pasqualin A, Barone G, Cioffi F, Rosta L, Scienza R, Da Pian
    R (1991) The relevance of anatomic and hemodynamic factors
    to a classification of cerebral arteriovenous malformations.
    Neurosurgery 28: 370–379
12. Prohovnik I, Knudsen E, Risberg J (1983) Accuracy of models
    and algorithms for determination of fast-compartment flow by
    noninvasive Xe-133 clearance. In: Magistretti PL (ed) Functional
    radionuclide imaging of the brain. Raven, New York, pp 87–115
13. Risberg J, Ali Z, Wilson EM, Wills EL, Halsey J (1975) Regional
    cerebral blood flow by Xenon-133 inhalation. Stroke 6: 142–148
14. Spetzler RF, Wilson CB, Weinstein P, Mehdorn M, Townsend J,
    Telles D (1978) Normal perfusion pressure breakthrough theory.
    Clin Neurosurg 25: 651–672
15. Sullivan HG, Kingsbury TB, Morgan ME, Jeffcoat RD, Allison
    JD, Goode JJ, McDonnel DE (1987) The rCBF response to
    diamox in normal subjects and cerebrovascular disease patients.
    J Neurosurg 67: 525–534
16. Takeuchi S, Kikuchi H, Karasawa J, Naruo Y, Hashimoto K,
    Nishimura T, Kozuka T, Hayashi M (1987) Cerebral hemo-
    dynamics in arteriovenous malformations: evaluation by single-
    photon emission CT. AJNR 8: 193–197
17. Tyler JL, Leblanc R, Meyer E, Dagher A, Yamamoto LY, Diksic
    M, Hakim A (1989) Hemodynamic and metabolic effects of
    cerebral arteriovenous malformations studied by position emis-
    sion tomography. Stroke 20: 890–898
18. Vorstrup S, Henriksen L, Paulson OB (1984) Effect of acet-
    azolamide on cerebral blood flow and cerebral metabolic rate for
    oxygen. J Clin Invest 74: 1634–1639
19. Wade JPH, Hachinski VC (1987) Cerebral steal: robbery or
    maldistribution. In: Wood JH (ed) Cerebral blood flow. Mc
    Graw Hill, New York, pp 467–480
20. Young WL, Prohovnik I, Ornstein E, Ostapkovich N, Sisti MB,
    Solomon RA, Stein MB (1990) The effect of arteriovenous
    malformation resection on cerebrovascular reactivity to carbon
    dioxide. Neurosurgery 27: 257–267

Correspondence: A. Talacchi, M.D., Department of Neurosurgery,
City Hospital, I-37126 Verona, Italy.

Clinical Evaluation of Cerebral Perfusion in AVM Patients

H.H. Batjer, D.S. Samson, and **P.D. Purdy**

Department of Neurological Surgery, University of Texas Southwestern Medical Center, Dallas, Texas, U.S.A

Summary

The presence of an arteriovenous malformation (AVM) exerts a significant and occasionally profound effect on overall cerebral hemodynamic patterns. It is likely that the high-flow low-resistance nature of the shunt occasionally results in ischemic sequelae in surrounding brain tissue and may in some way relate to perioperative hyperemic consequences. In order to better understand the global and regional impact of these hemodynamic disturbances, 62 AVM patients referred to our Center who underwent microsurgical resection were subjected to preoperative single photon emission computed tomography (SPECT) regional cerebral blood flow (rCBF) quantitative measurements using xenon-133 inhalation. Attempts were made to correlate specific clinical, radiographic, and hemodynamic patterns with end points including the occurrence of perioperative hyperemia and outcome. In addition, 35 patients were studied preoperatively with and without acetazolamide activation in an attempt to identify patterns which might predict hemodynamic disturbances.

The occurrence of hyperemic complications was associated with: a) recruitment of perforating vessels, b) angiographic steal, c) large size, d) large sum of diameter of feeding vessels, e) intermediate contralateral steal severity, f) dramatic increase in hemispheric rCBF after embolization, g) enhanced vasodilation to acetazolamide stimulation. Unfavorable outcome appeared to be associated with: a) older patients, b) recruitment of perforating vessels, c) right hemispheric AVMs, d) large size, e) decreased total brain flow, f) mild ipsilateral steal severity, g) mild contralateral steal severity, h) hyperemic complications, i) enhanced vasodilation to acetazolamide stimulation.

Keywords: Arteriovenous malformation; cerebral hemodynamics.

Introduction

Intracranial AVMs at least in part are composed of high-flow and low-resistance arteriovenous shunts. It is well known that these low-resistance arteriovenous connections can selectively capture a large portion of intracranial flow. This phenomenon has historically been used to assist in flow directed embolization of AVMs. Occasionally, however, the presence of rapid shunting can lead to hypoperfusion of surrounding brain tissue[33]. Consistent with this observation, Nornes

and Gripp have described decreased metabolite delivery to this involved tissue perhaps due in part to excessive venous pressures[23]. In clinical practice, it is not uncommon to see patients presenting with clinical syndromes suggesting transient or progressive ischemic deficits who are found to have appropriately situated AVMs[20,27]. The term "steal" was coined by Feindel and Perot to describe the poor and delayed angiographic opacification of adjacent cerebral arteries[13]. Reversal of this angiographic phenomenon following treatment for the AVM was noted by Norlen in 1949[22]. Perhaps the most substantial evidence in support of the existence of steal phenomena may be found in pathological observations in which remote neuronal dropout was noted in an AVM patients[11].

An occasional patient during surgery for an intracranial AVM or in the immediate post-operative period will develop a clinical syndrome in which brain edema and punctuate as well as confluent hemorrhage are consistent manifestations[5,12,21]. When severe and fulminant, these hemodynamic events can be disabling or fatal. Successful therapy has been described using induced hypotension and barbiturate coma[2,12]. Not infrequently, late in dissection of a large AVM, brain distension is noted which progressively obscures the deeper aspects of the dissection planes. This brain fullness may be accompanied by the eruption of bleeding sites in previously hemostatic regions. On most occasions, these events are reversible using standard neuro-anesthetic maneuvers, it is our hypothesis that similar pathophysiologic mechanisms explain these relatively minor events as well as more fulminant events. Several clinical and radiographic findings have been associated with the development of these hyperemic disturbances including ischemic clinical symptoms, hypoperfusion adjacent to the AVM, large size, high flow, and long tortuous feeding arteries[23,33,34]. In an interesting clinical experiment, Pertuiset *et al.* attempted to prevent this complication in patients at high risk by partially occluding the cervical carotid artery at the time of excision[28].

A number of clinical methods have been developed in an attempt to further delineate the actual hemodynamic physiology existing due to the presence of an AVM and to observe alterations occurring at different points in the execution of therapy. Using intraoperative Doppler studies, Nornes *et al.* observed flow in feeding vessels up to 500 ml/min and found that total AVM flow could reach 900 ml/min[23,24]. Also using an open technique, Barnett *et al.* measured local cortical blood flow in cerebral tissue adjacent to AVM margins and at remote sites[3]. These investigators noted that prior to excision, cortical flow was significantly depressed and CO_2 reactivity impaired at sites remote from the AVM. Following excision, significantly increased flow was noted in this tissue. Similar events have been observed intraoperatively by Young and co-workers[39,40]. Transcranial doppler techniques have also proven particularly useful for the measurement of flow patterns in feeding and unrelated arteries[1,14,18,31]. The availability of cerebral blood flow measurement performed both invasively[3,16,23,30] and non-invasively[10,17-19, 25,31,37] has produced substantial new insights into the underlying pathophysiology of this condition. In particular the three dimensional non-invasive studies using emission tomography and stable-xenon enhanced computed tomography have clearly demonstrated evidence of hypoperfusion in certain regions and definite flow asymmetry. In addition, striking physiologic evidence of substantial flow redistribution into surrounding brain tissue at the time of AVM resection has been well documented by the above-mentioned intra- and post-operative measurements[3,5,10,17,25,39,40].

Due to the availability of single photon (SPECT) techniques at our Institution as well as the presence of a large AVM referral practice, we felt that it might be possible to identify parameters associated with untoward hemodynamic and clinical sequelae. Patients were selected for study largely by the clinical and angiographic nature of their presentation in which we felt there to be a high likelihood of some circulatory disturbance.

Methods

Over a 4-year period, 77 patients with radiographically proven intracranial AVMs were evaluated with SPECT at our Institution.

Sixty-two of these patients underwent treatment and as such form the subjects of this report. The pre- and post-operative clinical and radiographic data from these treated patients have been collected and analyzed. In addition to sex, age, and handedness, the presenting symptoms were noted including intracranial hemorrhage (ICH), seizures, headaches, and progressive neurological deficit. CT and angiographic studies were carefully studied to note characteristics that might be expected to impact on cerebral blood flow patterns and surgical results. These data included location, angiographic AVM diameter (< 3 cm, 3–6 cm, > 6 cm)[32], the presence of an intracerebral hematoma > 2 cm, the number of major feeding vessels, recruitment of perforating arteries, the pattern of venous drainage (superficial, deep, or both), and the sum of diameters of all angiographically visible feeding arteries (determined by direct measurement). Angiographic evidence of steal was defined by a paucity of normal vessels opacifying in the mid-arterial phase adjacent to the nidus. Redistribution phenomena were not considered evidence of steal, i.e. capture of both anterior cerebral artery distributions by a single carotid injection related to frontal AVM which reverts to normal patterns after resection. Peri-operative hyperemic complications were liberally defined as the occurrence of unexpected or abnormal degrees of intraoperative brain swelling or hemorrhage unrelated to technical error or concealed intraventricular hemorrhage. This designation also included post-operative CT evidence of edema not related to inadvertent proximal vascular occlusion or hemorrhage after *angiographically proven* complete AVM resection. Outcome was determined at the six-month followup examination and was scored as good (capable of independent life), poor (not capable of independent life), of dead.

Dynamic SPECT

Regional CBF was determined by monitoring the cerebral transit of xenon-133 using the Tomomatic 64 SPECT (Medimatic A/S, Copenhagen, Denmark) designed by Stokely *et al.*[35]. This instrument consists of four detector arrays each containing 16 NaI (T1) scintillation crystals. The arrays are mounted in a hollow-square configuration that rotates around the subjects at 6 rpm. Special focus collimators define three transverse tomographic cross sections with centers 4 cm apart. Xenon-133 is administered in an air/oxygen mixture (10 mCi/l) during one minute of a four-minute wash-in/wash-out procedure. During the four-minute measurement period, activity in the lung is monitored by a scintillation probe placed on the chest, and this activity is assumed to correspond to the arterial blood concentration of xenon-133 in the brain. Regional CBF is calculated in ml/100 g/min according to the double-integral method. Voxel flow values are displayed in a 64 × 64 matrix using a 16-shade scale that can be normalized to the highest flow value. Cerebral blood flow was also numerically recorded with values characterizing the whole hemisphere. *Total brain flow* was calculated by averaging right and left hemispheric flow values. Because each patient had some region of hypoperfused brain tissue and these regions were of varying size, shape, and degree of rCBF depression, some method of incorporating these factors and quantifying the severity of "steal" was needed. A *steal index* was therefore calculated to allow quantitation of the volume of tissue involved and the severity of rCBF depression, as well as provide a means to analyze the relationship between steal severity and the clinical and radiographical parameters. The rCBF in a hand-drawn region of hypoperfusion in the ipsilateral hemisphere in each patient was divided by the total brain flow to yield an ipsilateral steal index as a measure of steal severity:

$$\text{Steal Index (ipsilateral, contralateral)} = \frac{\text{rCBF (steal area)}}{\text{total brain flow}}.$$

System resolution (full width at half maximum) measured with a xenon-133 line source in water varies from 1.7 cm at the center of each slice to 1.0 cm at the edge transversely. Subjects were positioned in the tomograph so that the 3 transverse cross sections were located 2, 6, 10 cm above and parallel to the canthomeathal line. These rCBF studies were obtained after informed consent was given by the patients in accordance with a policies of the Institutional Review Board of the University of Texas Southwestern Medical Center at Dallas. No rCBF studies were obtained before a 3-week waiting period in patients who had suffered intracranial hemorrhage.

Acetazolamide Studies

Vasoreactivity was also assessed pre-operatively in 35 patients by the administration of acetazolamide, a cerebral vasodilator that acts via carbonic anhydrase inhibition in the red cell and which impairs the removal of CO_2 from brain tissue[15,36,38]. For this study, the subject received a baseline rCBF study and 30 minutes later acetazolamide (1 g) was injected rapidly intravenously. Twenty minutes after this injection, a vasodilator-stimulated rCBF SPECT measurement was obtained. In normal subjects, acetazolamide leads to a $35 \pm 3\%$ increase in rCBF throughout the entire brain.

Each patient studied with acetazolamide had at least one area ipsilateral and contralateral to the AVM that was hypoperfused as determined on the resting rCBF study by visual inspection by an observer blinded to all clinical and radiographic data. Because these areas varied in size, shape, and depth of rCBF depression, some means of quantifying the severity of "steal" was needed. An ipsilateral and contralateral "steal index" was calculated by dividing the actual flow value averaged over the hand-drawn steal region by the flow value in a normal area of cerebellum. Thus an ipsilateral and contralateral steal index was determined on each resting study. In addition, a maximum steal index was calculated by determining the region with the most severe rCBF depression and dividing the flow measured in this region by the normal cerebral flow value. After acetazolamide was administered, the flow values in each of the regions of interest were again determined. A series of "Delta" values were then calculated by subtracting the resting steal index from the acetazolamide index. Therefore the vasoreactive properties of each of these regions could be quantitated relative to the behavior of normal brain tissue. Within these guidelines, three separate patterns of vasoactive behavior would be possible:

a) If "Delta" = 0, the CBF in the steal region behaves identically to normal brain tissue following acetazolamide (Group A).

b) If "Delta" > 0, the steal region vasodilates more than normal brain tissue following acetazolamide (Group B).

c) If "Delta" < 0, the steal region fails to vasodilate as much as normal brain tissue (Group C).

Comparisons were made in this group between clinical and radiographic parameters and vasoreactivity as calculated by the various "Delta" values. Statistical significance was determined by the Chi-square test. For this purpose "Delta" values were categorized into three groups based on the median value and standard deviation for the total population. In the case of small observed numbers in any classification in any category, significance was based on Fisher's exact test.

Embolization

A number of patients studied in this protocol underwent flow directed or superselective embolization using particles of polyvinyl alcohol sponge with or without reinforcement with platinum micro-coils[29]. Occasionally, superselective Wada testing was used to determine the eloquence of certain feeding arteries.

Results

Clinical Relationships

This patients series proved to be relatively representative of most large series of patients: nearly 50% presented with intracranial hemorrhage, 34% presented with progressing neurological deficits, 44% had a history of seizures, and 18% had a serious headache history. Intracranial hematomas were detected in 13%, angiographic steal phenomena were documented in 37%, and perforating arteries were recruited into the feeding system in 31% of patients. As defined, hyperemic complications occurred in 21% of cases. Analysis of the purely clinical and radiographic data demonstrated a number of interesting relationships[7]. Older patients were found to more frequently present with progressing deficits; 44% of those patients greater than 50 years of age had ischemic symptoms while only 16% of those patients younger than 30% had similar complaints (p < 0.05). The presence of perforator recruitment into the feeding system was associated with progressing neurological deficits; 53% of patients *with* perforator recruitment had ischemic deficits while only 26% of those *without* perforator recruitment had similar findings (p < 0.05). Interestingly, the presence or absence of angiographically documented steal phenomena was not predictive of patients found to have progressive neurological deficits. Clinical and radiographic factors were analyzed to determine which of these characteristics were associated with the development of hyperemic complications. We found that the presence of angiographic steal was associated with hyperemic events: 35% of those *with* angiographic steal ultimately developed hyperemia while only 13% of those *without* angiography steal developed similar complications (p < 0.05). A striking relationship was noted in patients with perforator recruitment: while only 7% *without* perforators recruited into their feeding systems developed hyperemia, 53% of those *with* perforator recruitment developed those complications (p < 0.001). Clinical outcome was surprisingly independent of most clinical and radiographic findings except the recruitment of perforating vessels and age of the patient. Eighty-eight percent of patients without perforators recruited ultimately had a good outcome while only 68% of those with perforator recruitment had a good outcome (p = 0.07). Of patients less than 30 years of age 92% had a good outcome, whereas only 86% of the 30–50 years group and 44% of the patients over 50 years had a favorable recovery. This impact of age is statistically significant (p < 0.05). Hyperemic complications had a profound influence on outcome such that 92% of the patients who did not develop hyperemic complications ultimately recovered well while less than half of those patients developing hyperemic complications had similar favorable recoveries (p < 0.001).

Baseline rCBF Relationships

While all patients were found to have some visually identifiable brain region which was hypoperfused on rCBF imaging, these areas of steal were categorized as severe, moderate, or mild. These categories were defined such that approximately one-third of patients fell in each group[6,8,9]. Interestingly, the severity of steal thus measured was clearly associated with progressing neurological deficits whereas angiographic steal phenomena had not been. Ninety percent of patients presenting with progressing deficits had steal indices of severe or moderate degree while 41% of patients without progressing deficits were found to have steal indices in the mild categories (p < 0.05). A converse relationship was noted in patients who had presented with intracranial hemorrhage. Forty-three percent of those patients who had initially bled had a steal index in the mild category, while of the patients who had not suffered hemorrhage, 47% were found to have severe steal, 34% had intermediate steal severity, and only 19% were noted to have a steal index in the mild range (p = 0.08). A substantially larger patient series and perhaps prospective study would be required to determine if two independent subgroups of patients exists: a) those with depressed CBF around their malformatoin who may be at low risk of subsequent hemorrhage but at high risk of ischemic sequelae, and b) a group with higher flow around the AVM (less severe steal) who may be at higher risk of hemorrhage due to increased stress on the fragile vasculature. No relationship was noted between the severity of ipsilateral steal (as calculated by steal index) and the size of the malformation, the number of feeding vessels involved, the presence of a hematoma, perforator involvement, angiographic steal, or the pattern of venous drainage. An interesting paradoxical relationship was frequently observed between angiographic criteria of hypoperfusion and rCBF evidence of steal. A number of pa-

tients with apparent angiographic steal phenomena were found to have surprisingly normal rCBF images while some patients with very early angiographic opacification of adjacent brain parenchyma were found to have severely depressed adjacent rCBF.

Acetazolamide Studies

Early in our experience, we were performing acetazolamide-activated rCBF studies in patients with occlusive cerebrovascular disease in hopes of identifying patients with threatened perfusion reserve. The same provocative maneuver appeared to be an ideal mechanism to identify patients potentially at risk of hyperemic therapeutic complications. Our initial thoughts about relating potential patterns of vasoreactivity to Spetzler's model of "normal perfusion pressure breakthrough"[34] seemed to suggest that acetazolamide might be an ideal provocative indicator. If the adjacent brain parenchyma of AVM patients behaved as tissue rendered chronically ischemic from occlusive cerebrovascular disease, one would predict two possible responses to the administration of acetazolamide. In the circumstance of intact vasoreactivity, one would expect to see flow augmentation in normal brain regions as well as in ischemic "steal" regions surrounding the AVM. In cases with failed vasoreactivity, one would expect to see normal flow augmentation in normal brain tissue but to see no further dilation in the maximally dilated steal region. This maximally vasodilated tissue would logically be presumed to be at acute risk at the time of sudden flow redistribution during shunt obliteration. Evidence quickly accumulated that our original hypothesis was likely incorrect. A patient reported previously[5] was studied both with and without acetazolamide activation preoperatively. This man ultimately developed fatal intraoperative and postoperative hyperemic complications resulting in severe hemorrhage and brain edema. He harbored a large and high flow frontal AVM and the results of his pre- and post-embolization rCBF studies were compared with four other patients with similar supratentorial malformations treated in similar fashion with aggressive preoperative embolization in whom baseline and acetazolamide studies were performed preoperatively and after embolization. These four control patients had uneventful perioperative courses and made normal recoveries. Several interesting features were noted from analysis of these rCBF studies.

a) The patient with fatal outcome had significantly depressed rCBF before treatment in both ipsilateral and contralateral hemispheres compared to the control group.

b) Therapeutic embolization resulted in a dramatic increase in rCBF in both hemispheres in this patient while changes in the control group were slight.

c) Acetazolamide augmented rCBF in the patient with fatal outcome both before and after embolization significantly more than in the control patients in the ipsilateral hemisphere.

This pathological and paradoxical augmentation of flow to acetazolamide was a significant surprise. One would expect vessels in the surrounding brain regions to have been maximally dilated and totally unable to further respond to a vasodilator. This finding led us to postulate that there might be a dissociation in vasoreactive properties in vessels surrounding an AVM such that pharmacologic or metabolic stimuli (or a sudden volume challenge) might induce further vasodilation, but that in certain patients protective vasoconstriction might not be prompted by acute hemodynamic redistribution during treatment. These surprising results led us to pursue provocative acetazolamide studies in additional patients[4].

A total of 35 patients were studied with preoperative baseline and acetazolamide-activated studies. Twenty (57%) of the patients were male. Eighteen (51%) were less than 31 years of age, 13 (37%) were between 30–50 years, and 4 (11%) were over 50 years of age. Clinical presentation included intracranial hemorrhage in 19 (54%), progressive neurological deficit in 12 (34%), seizure disorder in 14 (40%), and headaches in 5 (14%). Radiographic categorization according to size demonstrated 10 (29%) less than 3 cm in diameter, 15 (43%) between 3 and 6 cm, and 10 (29%) measuring greater than 6 cm. Intracerebral hematomas > 2 cm in diameter on CT scanning were present in 6 (17%). Angiographic steal or hypoperfusion involving surrounding parenchyma was noted in 13 (37%). Lenticulostriate and/or thalamoperforating vessels were found to supply the AVM in 12 cases (34%). Seven patients (20%) developed some evidence of a peri-operative or postoperative hyperemic disturbance using criteria for definition as previously noted.

A number of interesting relationships between clinical and CBF characteristics were noted using vasodilatory quantitation in hypoperfused brain regions following acetazolamide administration. Increased or pathological vasodilation (greater than normal brain tissue; high "Delta" values) was noted in patients with perforator recruitment. In contralateral steal regions identified in resting rCBF studies, 58% were found to have strongly positive "Delta" values (> 0.083) when perforator recruitment was present while similar high values were noted in only 22% of cases without perforator involvement (p < 0.05). A similar trend was noted in ipsilateral steal regions (p = 0.16). A strong association was seen in patients with angiographic steal phenomena when the rCBF region of maximal flow depression was evaluated. These critical brain regions were found to be hyper-responsive to acetazolamide stimulation and have high "Delta" values (p < 0.01). A trend toward pathologically high vasoreactivity was noted in ipsilateral rCBF steal regions in patients noted to have evidence of angiographic steal (p = 0.09). Patients developing hyperemic complications were found to have surprising hyper-responsiveness to acetazolamide in certain brain regions. In ipsilateral steal regions, significantly increased vasodilation was noted (higher "Delta" values) in patients becoming hyperemic (p < 0.05). Trends were noted toward similarly increased vasodilation in contralateral steal regions (p = 0.069) and regions of maximal flow depression (p = 0.059) in these same patients. A trend was also noted towards elevated vasodilatory capacity in ipsilateral steal regions in patients with poor neurological outcome in (p = 0.12). No apparent relationship was noted between these parameters of vasoreactivity and the sex or age of the patient, the mode of clinical presentation, the size of the AVM, or the presence of intracerebral hematoma.

Discussion

Intracranial AVMs remain a problem for clinicians in several respects. The best natural history data available stems from the experience of Troupp in Finland in which an annual bleeding risk of 4% was documented regardless of whether prior hemorrhage had occurred[26]. Most clinicians suspect that subgroups exist within this overall AVM population. We have all seen patients whose AVMs repetitively bled or in whom neurological deficits relentless progressed to death or disability. There are currently few means of prospectively identifying these subgroups. We are increasingly being asked to evaluated patients whose AVMs were diagnosed either incidentally after routine screening examinations or after minimal or trivial neurological complaints. Due to the availability of multiple therapeutic modalities including primary embolization, stereotactic radiation therapy, and traditional microsurgery, or combinations of these modalities, it is becoming increasingly important to tailor therapy to the individual patient particularly the elderly or infirm. For these reasons an accurate determination of the specific etiology of the patient's symptoms becomes important. Whether or not current medical and surgical therapy offer a legitimate option to the patient critically hinges on our ability to adequately predict the risk of such therapy and compare that risk to his expected natural history. Current attempts at identifying risk factors for various therapeutic options are quite crude and concern the size and eloquence of the malformation, the patients general medical condition, and an awareness of the surgeon's own unique skill and experience. Attempts at classification of AVMs have proven quite helpful but to date concern only radiographic criteria[32]. The risk of embolization therapy as a primary mode of treatment is difficult to predict but in our experience involves approximately 5% risk of hemorrhage for each endovascular procedure performed. The risk of stereotactic radiation therapy will become increasingly obvious as this modality is offered to wider populations but clearly brain necrosis, cranial neuropathy, and cerebral ischemia are well known sequelae. Due to the potentially severe morbidity and mortality associated with perioperative hemodynamic disturbances, means of prospectively identifying predictive characteristics offer not only the advantage of detecting those patients at high risk but also of selecting patients in whom alternate strategies or innovative therapies may be considered.

Much of our current concept of hyperemic surgical complications stems from the innovative laboratory investigations of Spetzler and colleagues more than a decade ago[34]. In response to a number of disastrous clinical events, these investigators performed a series of feline experiments. Thirty cats underwent the creation of an arteriovenous fistula between the rostral cervical carotid and the caudal internal or external jugular vein after division of both vessels. Resultant afferent fistula flow was obtained by retrograde flow down the ipsilateral carotid artery "stealing" blood from the contralateral carotid and basilar arteries via the circle of Willis. Over a six-week followup interval, the fistula size remained constant or diminished in size in 25 cats, but markedly dilated in five cats. All animals with patent fistulae demonstrated loss of autoregulatory and PCO_2 control. With temporary fistula occlusion, autoregu-

latory and PCO_2 control was immediately re-established in all but the five cats with enlarged shunts. Two of these five cats demonstrated hemiparesis following shunt occlusion. These experimental data and clinical experience led the authors to postulate that small hemispheric vessels maximally vasodilate to divert flow from an AVM and lose autoregulatory capacity. In rare cases, this derangement could lead to an inability to vasoconstrict to protect the brain from the redistribution of flow at the time of AVM resection. This attractive theory termed "normal perfusion pressure breakthrough" explains clinical phenomena occurring in AVM cases and suggests that hypoperfused vasculature in AVM patients may behave in a similar manner to that in patients suffering chronic ischemia from occlusive cerebrovascular disease.

The investigations reported in this presentation particularly regarding the acetazolamide-activated studies[4] are at substantial variance with the traditional "normal perfusion pressure breakthrough" theory. Despite the fact that the statistical methods employed in this analysis did not precisely categorize vasoreactive characteristics into the theoretical groups A, B, and C, mentioned above (i.e. "Delta" $> 0, 0, < 0$), patterns of vasoreactive behavior can be reasonably deduced from the acquired data. By applying the "normal perfusion pressure breakthrough" theory to the current study, one would predict that patients with no peri- or postoperative hyperemic complications would be those with preserved autoregulatory and PCO_2 control in hypoperfused brain regions. They would have been expected to have similar vasodilation capabilities in tissue surrounding the AVM to that of normal brain tissue. By our methodology, this group would have had "Delta" values of *zero* (Group A). The normal perfusion breakthrough theory would predict that these patients are not maximally vasodilated at rest and therefore should have the capacity to tolerate acute flow redistribution without decompensation. Those patients who should be at highest risk of hyperemia according to the perfusion breakthrough theory would be those with maximal vasodilation at rest who are vasoparalyzed and unable to protectively vasoconstrict once confronted with an acute flow challenge. This physiologic state should be represented by the hypothetical Group C in the present schema as those patients whose surrounding brain regions do not vasodilate as much as normal brain tissue to acetazolamide challenge. The "Delta" values in this group of patients whould be *negative*. Surprisingly, only one of twelve (8%) in our group with the lowest ipsilateral Delta values had evidence of hyperemia. The "normal perfusion pressure breakthrough" theory would not have predicted the existence of Group B in our schema with vasodilation in the surrounding brain regions that is more pronounced than in normal brain. One might anticipate that, if at all present, this physiologic response would represent preserved autoregulation and hemodynamic reserve. In fact, this is the group which we found to have the highest risk of hyperemia.

This aspect of our studies suggests that *enhanced vasodilation* to acetazolamide challenge in brain tissue around AVMs may indicate the highest risk of intraoperative and postoperative hyperemic disturbance by failure to effectively confront an increased tissue perfusion by protective vasoconstriction. Why this category of vasoreactivity is potentially harmful (or even exists) is a matter of speculation. It is possible that physiologically deranged vasculature may be present in the AVM patient either as a response to chronic hemodynamic stress or as a congenital epiphenomenon occurring with another congenital cerebrovascular anomaly (the AVM itself). It is tempting to speculate that in these particular patients, the sudden redistribution of large quantities of previously shunted blood does not provoke vasoconstriction or result in simple dysautoregulated vasoparalysis, but rather leads to bizarre vasodilatory states dramatically increasing the blood volume in the involved hemisphere. This engorgement might initially be primarily intravascular but subsequent events could lead to passive transudation, increasing extracellular fluid and the development of clinically significant edema. The commonly observed hemorrhagic mottling or frank intracerebral hematomas could feasibly result from simple reactive overdistension of the fragile microvasculature at the arteriolar level. It is hoped that if these vasoreactive data prove valid in larger populations, the use of provoked preoperative non-invasive rCBF imaging might then become a clinically useful predictor of therapeutic risk. It is clear from our earlier studies that the presence of peri-operative hyperemia (as previously defined) carries a much higher risk of neurological morbidity after treatment. It is possible that these bizarre vasodilatory states may be responsive to vasoactive agents. Investigation of this potential could lead to useful interventional and/or prophyllactic pharmacological therapy. It is also possible that the use of provoked rCBF studies might provide very helpful clinical information to help determine the

optimal extent of preoperative embolization, the optimal intervals between embolization attempts, and between the final embolization procedure and subsequent surgical resection.

In summary, analysis of clincal, radiographical, and rCBF data in our series has lead to the conclusion that certain characteristics may be associated with hyperemic complications and unfavorable outcome. The occurrence of hyperemic complications was associated with the following variables: a) recruitment of perforating vessels, b) angiographic steal, c) large AVM size, d) larger sum of diameter of feeding vessels, e) intermediate contralateral steal severity, f) dramatic increase in hemispheric rCBF after embolization, g) enhanced vasodilation to acetazolamide. Unfavorable outcome appeared to be associated with: a) older patients, b) recruitment of perforating arteries, c) right hemispheric AVMs, d) large AVM size, e) depressed total brain blood flow, f) mild ipsilateral steal severity, g) mild contralateral steal severity, h) enhanced vasodilation to acetazolamide, i) hyperemic complications. It is of note that f) and g) above imply relatively higher flow in the areas around the AVM.

References

1. Aaslid R, Markwalder TM, Nornes H (1982) Non-invasive transcranial doppler ultrasound recording of flow velocity in basal cerebral arteries. J Neurosurg 57: 769–774
2. Aoki N, Mizutani H (1985) Arteriovenous malformation in the territoy of the occluded middle cerebral artery with massive intraoperative brain swelling, case report. Neurosurgery 16: 660–662
3. Barnett GH, Little JR, Ebrahim ZY, Jones SC, Friel HT (1987) Cerebral circulation during arteriovenous malformation resection. Neurosurgery 20: 836–842
4. Batjer HH, Devous MD (1992) The use of acetazolamide-enhanced rCBF measurement to predict risk to AVM patients. Neurosurgery 31: 213–218
5. Batjer HH, Devous MD Sr, Meyer YJ, Purdy PD, Samson DS (1988) Cerebrovascular hemodynamics in arteriovenous malformation complicated by normal perfusion pressure breakthrough. Neurosurgery 22: 503–509
6. Batjer HH, Devous MD Sr, Seibert GB, Purdy PD, Ajmani AK, Delarosa M, Bonte FJ (1988) Intracranial arteriovenous malformation: relationships between clinical and radiographic factors and ipsilateral steal severity. Neurosurgery 23: 322–328
7. Batjer HH, Devous MD Sr, Seibert GB, Purdy PD, Bonte FJ (1989) Intracranial arteriovenous malformation: relationship between clinical factors and surgical complications. Neurosurgery 24: 75–79
8. Batjer HH, Devous MD Sr, Seibert GB, Purdy PD, Ajmani AK, Delarosa M, Bonte FJ (1989) Intracranial arteriovenous malformation: relationships between clinical and radiographic factors and cerebral blood flow. Neuro Med Chir (Tokyo) 29: 395–400

9. Batjer HH, Devous MD Sr, Seibert GB, Purdy PD, Ajmani AK, Delarosa M, Bonte FJ (1989) Intracranial arteriovenous malformation: contralateral steal phenomena. Neurol Med Chir (Tokyo) 29: 401–406

10. Batjer HH, Purdy PD, Giller CA, Samson DS (1989) Evidence of redistribution of cerebral blood flow during treatment for an intracranial arteriovenous malformation. Neurosurgery 25: 599–605

11. Constantino A, Vintners HV (1986) A pathogenic correlate of the "steal" phenomena in a patient with cerebral arteriovenous malformation. Stroke 17: 103–106

12. Day A, Friedman W, Sypert G, Mickle P (1982) Successful treatment of the normal perfusion breakthrough syndrome. Neurosurgery 11: 625–630

13. Feindel W, Perot P (1965) Red cerebral veins: a report on arteriovenous shunts in tumors and verebral scars. J Neurosurg 22: 315–325

14. Giller CA, Hodges K, Batjer HH (1990) Transcranial Doppler pulsatility in vasodilation and stenosis. J Neurosurg 72: 901–906

15. Hauge A, Nicolaysen G, Thoresen M (1983) Acute effects of acetazolamide on cerebral blood flow in man. Acta Physiol Scand 117: 223–229

16. Hassler W, Steinmetz H (1987) Cerebral hemodynamics in angioma patients: an intraoperative study. J Neurosurg 67: 822–831

17. Leblanc R, Little JR (1989) Hemodynamics of arteriovenous malformations. Clin Neurosurg 36: 299–317

18. Lindegaard KF, Grolimund P, Aaslid R, Nornes H (1986) Evaluation of cerebral AVMs using transcranial Doppler ultrasound. J Neurosurg 65: 335–344

19. Menon D, Weir B (1979) Evaluation of cerebral blood flow in arteriovenous malformation by Xenon-133 inhalation method. Can J Neurol Sci 6: 411–416

20. Mohr JP (1984) Neurological manifestations and factors related to therapeutic decision. In: Wilson CB, Stein BM (eds) Intracranial arteriovenous malformations. Williams and Wilkins, Baltimore, pp 1–11

21. Mullan S, Brown F, Patronas N (1979) Hyperemic and ischemic problems of surgical treatment of arteriovenous malformations. J Neurosurg 51: 757–764

22. Norlen G (1949) Arteriovenous aneurysms of the brain: report of 10 cases of total removal of lesion. J Neurosurg 6: 475–494

23. Nornes H, Grip A (1980) Hemodynamic aspects of cerebral arteriovenous malformations. J Neurosurg 53: 456–464

24. Nornes H, Grip A, Wikeby P (1979) Intraoperative evaluation of cerebral hemodynamics using directional doppler technique: Part I. Arteriovenous malformations. J Neurosurg 50: 145–151

25. Okabe I, Meyer JS, Okayasu H, Harper R, Rose J, Grossman RG, Centeno R, Tachibana H, Lee YY (1983) Xenon-enhanced CT CBF measurements in cerebral AVMs before and after excision. J Neurosurg 59: 21–31

26. Ondra SL, Troupp H, George ED, Schwab K (1990) The natural history of symptomatic arteriovenous malformation of the brain: a 24-year follow-up assessment. J Neurosurg 73: 387–391

27. Paterson JH, Mckissock W (1956) A clinical survey of intracranial arteriovenous aneurysms with special reference to their mode of progression and surgical treatment. A report of 110 cases. Brain 233–266

28. Pertuiset B, Ancri D, Arthuis F, Basset JY, Fusciardi J, Nakano H (1985) Shunt induced hemodynamic disturbance in supratentorial arteriovenous malformations. J Neuroradiol 12: 165–178

29. Purdy PD, Samson D, Batjer HH, Risser RC (1990) Preoperative embolization of cerebral arteriovenous malformation with poly-vinyl alcohol particles: experience in 51 adults. AJNR 11: 501–510

30. Rosenbloom BR, Bonner RF, Oldfield EH (1987) Intraoperative measuremrnts of cortical blood flow adjacent to cerebral AVM using Laser Doppler velocimetry. J Neurosurg 66: 396–399

31. Schwartz A, Hennerici M (1986) Non-invasive transcranial doppler ultrasound in intracranial angiomas. Neurology 36: 626–635

32. Spetzler R, Martin N (1986) A proposed grading system for arteriovenous malformations. J Neurosurg 65: 476–483

33. Spetzler RF, Selman WR (1984) Pathophysiology of cerebral ischemia accompanying arteriovenous malformation. In: Wilson CB, Stein BM (eds) Intracranial arteriovenous malformations. Williams and Wilkins, Baltimore, pp 24–31

34. Spetzler RF, Wilson CB, Weinstein P, Mehdorn M, Townsend J, Telles D (1978) Normal perfusion pressure breakthrough theory. Clin Neurosurg 25: 651–672

35. Stokely E, Sveinsdotter E, Lassen N, Rommer P (1980) A single photon dynamic computer assisted tomograph (DCAT) for imaging brain function in multiple cross sections. J Comput Assist Tomogr 4: 230–240

36. Sullivan HG, Kingsbury TB, Morgan ME, Jeffcoat RD, Allison JD, Goode JJ, McDonnell DE (1987) The rCBF response to acetazolamide in normal subjects and cerebrovascular disease patients. J Neurosurg 67: 525–534

37. Takeuchi S, Kikuchi H, Karasawa J, Naruo Y, Hashimoto K, Nishimura T, Kozuka T, Hayashi M (1987) Cerebral hemodynamics in arteriovenous malformations: evaluation by single photon emission CT. AJNR 8: 193–197

38. Vorstrup S, Hendriksen L, Paulsen OB (1984) Effect of acetazolamide on cerebral metabolic rate for oxygen. J Clin Invest 74: 1634–1639

39. Young WL, Prohovnik I, Ornstein E, Sisti MB, Solomon RA, Stein BM, Ostapkovich N (1988) Monitoring of intraoperative cerebral hemodynamics before and after arteriovenous malformation resection. Anesth Analg 67: 1011–1014

40. Young WL, Solomon RA, Prohovnik I, Ornstein E, Weinstein J, Stein BM (1988) Xe-133 blood flow monitoring during arteriovenous malformation resection. A case of intraoperative hyperperfusion with subsequent brain swelling. Neurosurgery 22: 765–769

Correspondence: H. Hunt Batjer, M.D., Department of Neurological Surgery, 5323 Harry Hines Blvd., Dallas, Texas 75235-8896, U.S.A.

The Role of Hemodynamic Assessment in Patients with Cerebral AVMs

A. Talacchi, A. Pasqualin, F. Sala, and **A. Bricolo**

Department of Neurosurgery, City Hospital, Verona, Italy

Summary

In order to investigate cerebral hemodynamics in arteriovenous malformations (AVM), 27 patients – after a complete angiographic study – undertook cerebral blood flow (CBF) measurements and 17 of them also transcranial Doppler (TCD) sonography. On admission, 12 patients presented neurological impairment unrelated to previous hemorrhage. The mean AVM volume was 27 cm^3. In 17 patients the lesion was surgically removed; in 12 of them embolization was performed pre-operatively. Five patients underwent moderate to severe hyperemic complications. Clinical aspects (neurological presentation and post-operative deterioration due to hyperemic complications) were related to the following radiological and instrumental factors: AVM volume, AVM location, angiographic steal (adjacent and/or remote), hemispheric hypoperfusion, regional hypoperfusion (adjacent and/or remote), and mean flow velocity on AVM feeders. As compared to patients without deficits, patients with neurological deficits unrelated to previous hemorrhage presented higher AVM volume (31 cm^3 vs. 26 cm^3), lower hemispheric CBF (45 vs. 50 ml/100g/min) and higher flow velocity on TCD (133 vs. 122 cm/s); no relation was found with respect to angiographic steal (type and incidence), AVM location and regional hypoperfusion. As compared to patients without hyperemic complications, patients with post-operative hyperemic complications presented a higher incidence of angiographic steal, adjacent and remote (3/5 vs. 1/12), a higher AVM volume (29 vs. 21 cm^3 as mean), a higher hemispheric CBF (61 vs. 46 ml/100g/min; p < 0.05) and a higher flow velocity on TCD (137 vs. 111 cm/s). Hyperemic complications were less frequent in patients with frontal AVMs, who also presented the lowest CBF values. Regional steal detected on angiography and regional hypoperfusion were not associated, neither flow velocity was significantly increased in patients presenting any of these two features; nevertheless all of these aspects were influenced by volume and location of the AVM. In conclusion, angiographic steal, regional hypoperfusion and increased TCD velocity presented a correlation with AVM volume and location; moreover clinical deficits (on admission) and hyperemic complications were both related with higher AVM volume and TCD velocity, but were associated with different CBF patterns.

Keywords: Cerebral arteriovenous malformation; cerebral blood flow; transcranial Doppler sonography; hyperemic complications.

Introduction

It is now well accepted that blood diversion from nutritional vessels through an A–V shunt exerts a deep influence on cerebral hemodynamics. It has been demonstrated by presenting symptoms, angiographic steal and operative observations that areas adjacent to the AVM are primarily affected, even if degree and extension of the cerebro-vascular derangement has not yet been assessed [4,5,8,14,26–28].

The size of an AVM is considered to be an important factor influencing either the operative difficulty and the occurrence of post-operative hyperemic complications [18,23,25]. Nevertheless little is known to which extent cerebral perfusion is altered in patients with AVMs of different size. Since embolization can reduce the shunt flow in large AVMs, indications to surgery have been broadened by the use of pre-operative embolization, and increasing attention has been paid to the precise evaluation of flow derangement [4,6].

The aim of this study is to investigate the relation between angiographic/clinical data and cerebral hemodynamics, evaluated by combined cerebral blood flow (CBF) and transcranial Doppler (TCD) measurements.

Clinical Material

Between September 1989 and January 1992, 27 patients with cerebral AVMs were evaluated in the Department of Neurosurgery of Verona. Seventeen patients were male, 10 female; average age was 37 years (ranging from 18 to 65 years). Mean duration of symptoms was 8 years (ranging from 4 days to 31 years.) The initial and following clinical events are reported in Table 1. On admission, neurological examination disclosed clinical signs in 11 cases: memory impairment (4 cases), paresis (3), hemianopia (3), cerebellar deficits (1), papilledema (1); the remaining 16 patients were intact.

All patients undertook angiography, CT scan and MRI. AVM feeders were classified as a) superficial, b) deep, c) originating from the external carotid artery; they were also related to the location and the volume of the AVM (Table 2). AVM volume was determined through multiplication of the 3 AVM diameters by 0.52, according to the volume calculation proposed by our group in a recent paper [18]. The mean AVM volume was 27 cm^3. Three volume subgroups were considered: under 20 cm^3, between 20 and 30 cm^3 and over 30 cm^3 (the so-called "large AVMs"). AVM location was as follows: frontal (6 cases), parietal (9), temporal (6), occipital (4). The corresponding

Table 1. *Clinical Course in 27 Patients: Initial and Following Events*

Initial event		Following events	
		i.h.	n.d.
Intracerebral hemorrhage (i.h.)	(1 case)	–	–
Seizures (s.e.)	(15 cases)	3	3
Neurological deficit (n.d.)	(5 cases)	–	–
Headache (head.)	(6 cases)	–	4
Total	(27 cases)	3	7

Table 2. *Relation Between AVM Location and Number and Type of Feeders*

AVM location		AVM mean volume (cm³)	Number of feeders			
			Tot.	Superf.	Deep.	ECA
Frontal	(6 c.)	22	12	11	1	–
Temporal	(4 c.)	20	10	7	1	2
Parietal	(9 c.)	39	23	19	4	–
Occipital	(6 c.)	23	13	10	2	1

ECA external carotid artery. One cerebellar and 1 callosal AVM excluded. c. cases.

mean AVM volumes for each location were: 22 cm³, 39 cm³, 20 cm³, 23 cm³. Fourteen AVMs were located in the right hemisphere, 11 in the left, 1 in the cerebellum (48 cm³) and 1 in the corpus callosum (24 cm³).

All patients were submitted to baseline CBF test and 17 undertook baseline TCD flow velocity measurements. Among the 17 embolized patients, 10 were examined with CBF measurements, for a total of 14 studies, and 13 with TCD examination, for a total of 24 studies.

Seventeen out of the 27 patients were operated on (12 after embolization); the remaining 10 patients received embolization only (5 cases) or no treatment. Hyperemic complications were defined as: a) intraoperative blood loss over 2000 ml, b) post-operative hemorrhage not due to a residual AVM, and c) post-operative edema, associated to neurological impairment. The first evenience (a) occurred in 3 cases, the second (b) in 2 cases (one of them belonging also to the group "a"), the third (c) occurred in 1 case, so that the overall incidence of hyperemic complications was 29% (5 out of the 17 patients operated on).

Methods

Angiographic steal was defined as the reduction of vascular filling in the area adjacent to the AVM, observed in the midarterial phase (Fig. 1); even a remote steal was observed in the distal branches of arteries that did not supply the AVM (Fig. 2). The evaluation of "steal" was done considering the complete angiographical study; in fact in some cases, particularly for temporal and parietal AVMs, the ipsilateral anterior cerebral artery, not visualized from the injection of the ipsilateral carotid artery, was normally opacified from the controlateral carotid artery through the anterior communicating artery (this angiographic effect was considered a "redistribution phenomenon")[4,6,12,27] (Fig. 3).

rCBF was measured by the 133-Xe inhalation method, using a Novo Cerebrograph 32C. The instrument was equipped with 16 collimated scintillation head detectors containing NaI crystals for each side of the head. The M2 model was used: it consisted of the Prohovnik version of the Obrist original model, which includes additional coefficients for the upper air passages artifact and for the arterial artifact (in this way contamination of the surrounding areas from hyperemia of the AVM is avoided or at least reduced)[16,20]. The ISI parameter, a non-compartmental index, was chosen[21]. The location of each detector is shown in Fig. 4 together with the map obtained by a computerized planar reconstruction of cortical areas corresponding to the detectors[22]. The hemispheric results were expressed in terms of absolute values (ml/100g/min) and asymmetry, the regional results in terms of absolute values, asymmetry and percent of the hemispheric mean. In order to evaluate the statistical significance, the overall data were compared with two population: the first consisted of subjects under 45 years (60 cases, with a mean CBF value of 57 ml/100g/min), the second of subjects over 45 years (23 cases, with mean CBF value of 47 ml/100g/min). Both groups were used for the evaluation of the individual cases (adopting the Z test)[7] and the lower-age group also for the comparison with the AVM population and its sub-groups (adopting the Student t test).

For a better comprehension of the regional redistribution of blood flow induced by AVM location, a suitable program was made to move on the right side the AVM located in the left hemisphere in order to obtain homogeneous maps for each location (thus keeping the AVMs always on the right side).

Transcranial Doppler (TCD) EME TC 64 was used[1,6,9,11]. Flow velocities measured on anterior cerebral artery (ACA), middle cerebral artery (MCA) and posterior cerebral artery (PCA) were considered pathological when higher than 120 cm/s for the anterior and middle cerebral, and higher than 90 cm/s, for the posterior cerebral. The examinations performed immediately before operation were related to the occurrence of hyperemic complications.

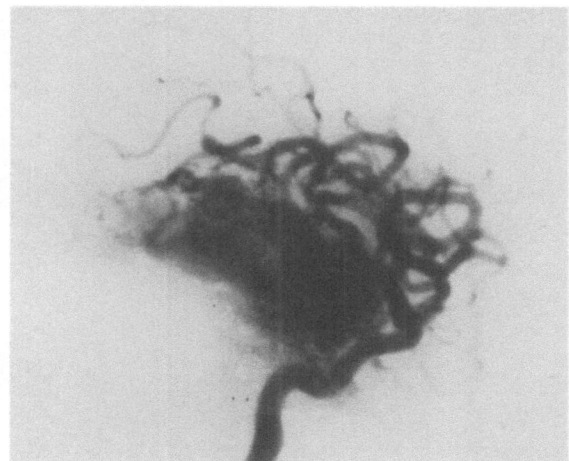

Fig. 1. Demonstration of adjacent angiographic steal: a patient with a large right temporal AVM, with poorly visualized distal branches of MCA

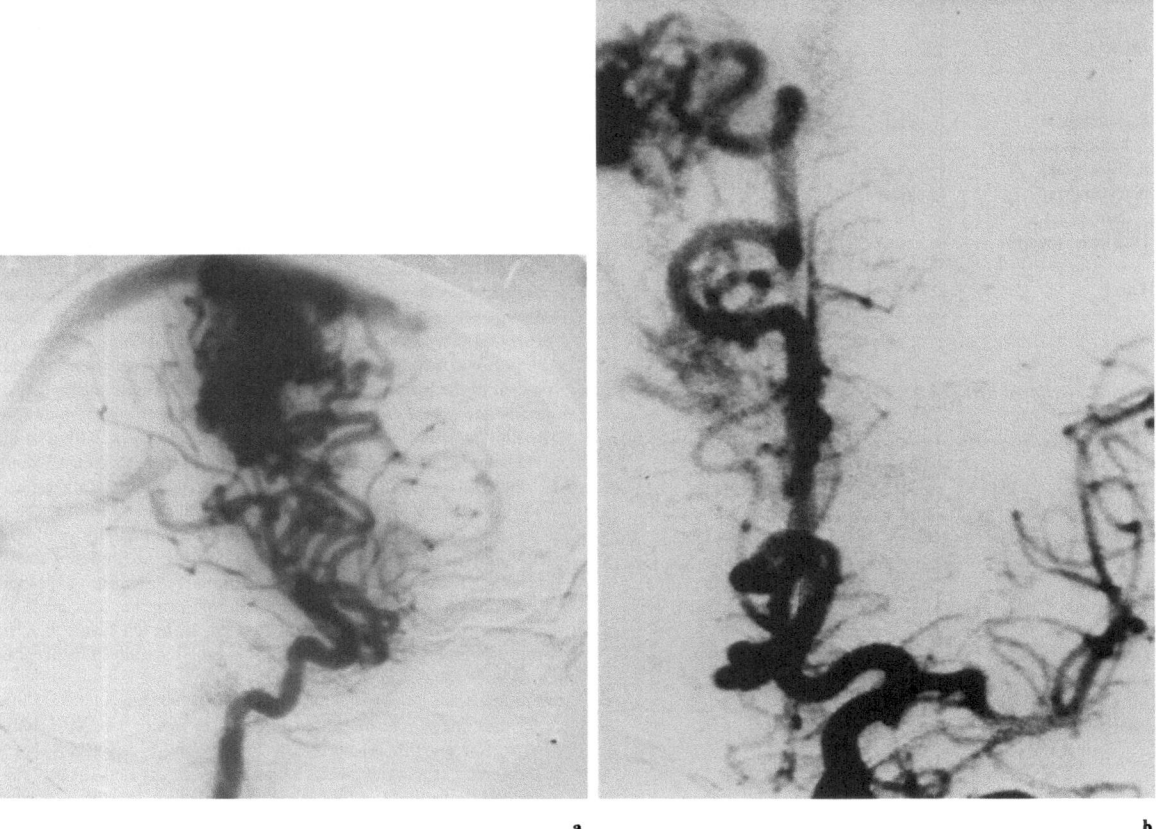

a   b

Fig. 2. Demonstration of remote steal: (a) a patient with a large right rolandic AVM and right ACA scantly visualized; (b) the right ACA is properly filled from controlateral angiography, but the distal branches of the left ACA are poorly opacified

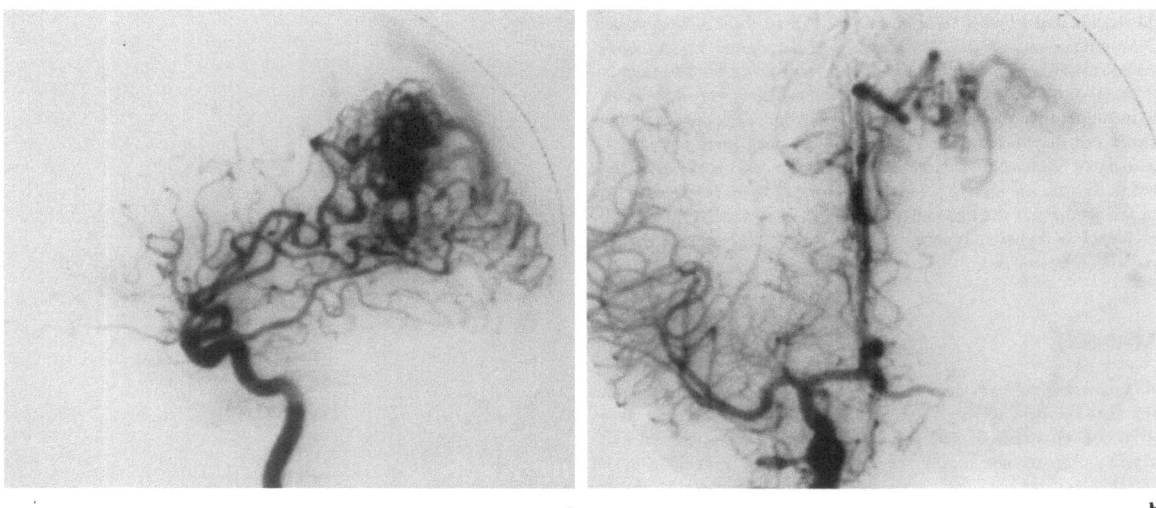

a   b

Fig. 3. Demonstration of "redistribution phenomenon": (a) a patient with a left posterior parietal AVM; (b) the ipsilateral ACA is visualized only from controlateral angiography

Results

Angiographic Features

Angiographic steal in areas adjacent to the AVM occurred in 13 cases, in remote areas in 10 cases (both patterns being detected in 8 cases). There was a relation between increasing AVM volume and angiographic steal: in particular adjacent and remote steal together were significantly more frequent ($p < 0.01$) in patients with AVMs larger than 20 cm^3 (Table 3).

Steal (adjacent or remote) and redistribution were also related to AVM location, as shown in Table 4. A close relationship was found between parietal or temporal AVMs and adjacent steal in the MCA territory, remote steal in the controlateral ACA territory and redistribution phenomena in the ipsilateral ACA territory.

Angiographic features as AVM location and steal in patients with neurological impairment were not different from those of the remaining patients, while AVM volume was slightly higher in patients with neurological impairment (31 vs. 26 cm^3).

Those patients undergoing hyperemic complications (5 cases) had a mean AVM volume of 29 cm^3: 3 of them disclosed steal (adjacent and remote) on angiography. The patients that fared well (12 cases) showed a lower mean volume (21 cm^3), and angiographic steal (adjacent and remote) in only 1 case. The incidence of hyperemic complications was lower in frontal AVMs than in other locations (1/5 vs. 4/7).

CBF Evaluation

As regards CBF studies, global hypoperfusion was demonstrated in 4 cases, hemispheric asymmetry in 2, adjacent hypoperfusion in 3, remote hypoperfusion in 7, both adjacent and remote hypoperfusion in 6 cases.

Mean global CBF was significantly reduced when compared with the control population (48 ml/100g/min; $p < 0.001$); regional aspects – when examined as percent of the hemispheric mean – disclosed a pattern similar to the controls, with significant hypoperfusion in the border-zone areas (Fig. 5).

The volume sub-groups had different mean hemispheric CBF, with significantly lower values under 20 cm^3 and over 30 cm^3 (Table 5). As regards location,

Table 3. *Relation Between AVM Volume and Angiographic Steal Patterns*

Volume (cm^3)	Angiographic steal			
	Adjacent only	Remote only	Adjacent + remote	None
<20 (6 cases)	1	1	–	4
20–30 (7 cases)	2	1	4	–
>30 (7 cases)	2	–	4	1
Signif. (<20 vs. >20; Fisher's test)	NS	NS	$p < 0.01$	$p < 0.05$

Seven cases excluded because of incomplete angiography.

Table 5. *Relation Between AVM Volume and Mean Hemispheric CBF*

AVM volume (cm^3)	Mean hemispheric CBF (ml/100g/min)	Signif. (Student t test)[a]
<20	46.6	$p < 0.001$
20–30	52.6	NS
>30	45.5	$p < 0.001$

[a]Compared to control population.

Table 4. *Relation Between AVM Location and Angiographic Abnormalities*

AVM Location	Angiogr. steal territory		Redistribution territory
	Adjacent	Remote	
Frontal (4 cases)	ACA (n = 2)	ACAc (n = 2)-MCAi (n = 1)	–
Parietal (7 cases)	MCA (n = 5)	ACAc (n = 3)	ACAi (n = 4)
Temporal (6 cases)	MCA (n = 5)	ACAc (n = 3)	ACAi (n = 5)-PCAc (n = 1)
Occipital (3 cases)	PCA (n = 3)	PCAc (n = 1)-MCAi (n = 1)	ACAi (n = 1)-PCAc (n = 1)

Seven cases excluded because of incomplete angiography.

Ac controlateral artery; *Ai* ipsilateral artery.

Table 6. *Relation Between Angiographic Steal and Patterns of Regional Hypoperfusion*

	Regional		Hypoperfusion	
	Adjacent	Remote	Adjacent + remote	None
Adjacent steal (5 cases)	1	2	1	1
Remote steal (2 cases)	–	–	–	2
Adj. + rem. steal (8 cases)	–	2	4	2 .
No steal (5 cases)	1	2	–	2
Total	2	6	5	7

Seven cases excluded because of incomplete angiography.

Table 7. *Relation Between AVM Volume and Patterns of Regional Hypoperfusion*

	Regional hypoperfusion			
Volume (cm^3)	Adjacent only	Remote only	Adjacent + remote	None
<20 (10 cases)	–	4	2	4
20–30 (7 cases)	–	1	1	5
>30 (9 cases)	3	2	3	1
Signif. (<30 vs. >30; Fisher's test)	$p < 0.05$	NS	NS	$p < 0.05$

One patient with cerebellar AVM excluded.

Table 8. *Relation Between AVM Location and Vessels with Pathological Flow Velocity*

AVM Location	Vessels with pathological flow velocity	
	Ipsilateral	Controlateral
Frontal (3 cases)	MCAi (n = 3)	MCAc (n = 1)
Temporal (4 cases)	MCAi-PCAi (n = 4) (n = 3)	ACAc (n = 2)
Parietal (6 cases)	MCAi-PCAi; (n = 6) (n = 3)	ACAc-PCAc (n = 5) (n = 1)
Occipital (4 cases)	MCAi-PCAi (n = 2) (n = 2)	ACAc-PCAc (n = 1) (n = 1)

Ai ipsilateral artery; *Ac* controlateral artery.

a significant hypoperfusion was observed in frontal and parietal AVMs (parietal AVM having a higher mean volume than all other locations) (Fig. 6). Hemispheric CBF was not significantly different in patients with neurological signs as compared to the remaining patients (45 vs. 50 ml/100g/min). Surprisingly, hemispheric CBF in patients with uneventful post-operative course was significantly lower (46 ml/100g/min) than in controls ($p < 0.01$), while patients that underwent hyperemic complications showed flow values in the normal range (61 ml/100g/min), with a significant difference ($p < 0.05$) between these two groups.

As regards regional CBF, the relation between regional hypoperfusion and angiographic steal is reported in Table 6: no correlation between angiographic steal and hypoperfusion emerged from these data. Analyzing the influence of AVM volume on regional hypoperfusion, adjacent hypoperfusion was the pattern most commonly associated with larger AVMs (> 30 cm^3) (Table 7), as well as with temporal and occipital AVMs (exhibiting hemispheric CBF in the normal range). Differently from the angiographical pattern on the controlateral ACA territory, in parietal and temporal AVMs CBF examination showed that frontal hypoperfusion (when examined in asymmetry) was more marked on the ipsilateral side. Patients with preoperative neurological signs and patients developing hyperemic complications did not present significant differences in the regional CBF adjacent to the AVM when compared either to the remaining patients or to the control population.

TCD Evaluation

The volume of the AVM influenced the mean flow velocity on the main feeder, since the mean velocity was 12% higher than the upper limit considered (120 cm/s for ACA and MCA, 90 cm/s for PCA) for AVMs under 20 cm^3, 26% higher for AVMs between 20 and 30 cm^3 and 36% higher for AVMs larger than 30 cm^3.

As regards angiographic steal, the mean velocity value on the main feeder was 145 cm/s when angiographic steal was present; in cases without angiographic steal the mean velocity on the main feeder was 138 cm/s, suggesting a poor correlation between angiographic steal and increased flow velocity.

Evaluating TCD velocity in 2 groups of patients chosen by absence or presence of adjacent regional hypoperfusion, the obtained mean flow velocity were 158 and 137 cm/s respectively.

Evaluating the abnormal patterns recorded by TCD for AVMs in certain locations, parietal and – to a lesser extent – occipital and temporal malformations presented flow velocity increased on the controlateral

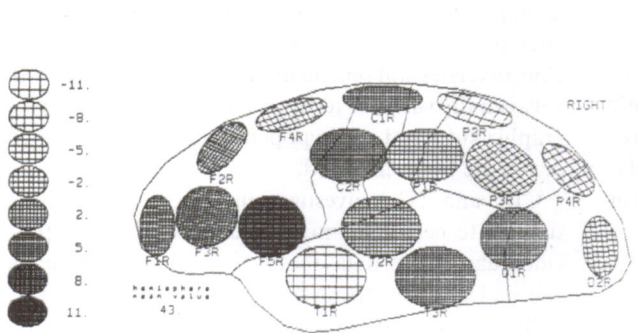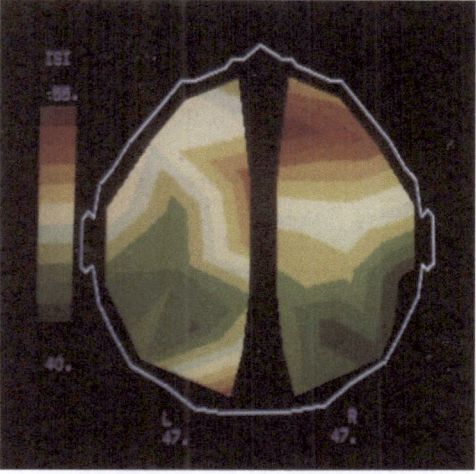

a

b

Fig. 4. (a) Representation of cortical areas assessed by 16 head detectors in each hemisphere (*F* frontal; *C* central; *P* partietal; *T* temporal; *O* occipital); (b) the map produced by computer elaboration, with planar reconstruction of cortical areas, is expressed by a color scale reflecting absolute flow values (ml/100g/min)

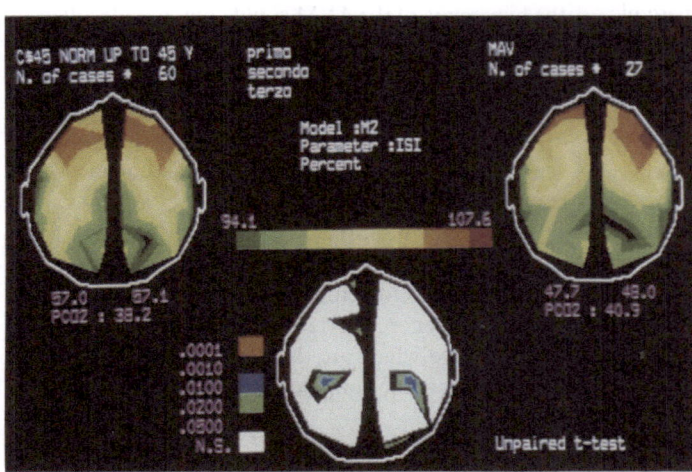

Fig. 5. A computerized elaboration demonstrating regional hypoperfusion. The upper left map shows the cerebral perfusion of the control population; the upper right map represent the AVM population (mean hemispheric values are 47 ml/100g/min); color variations represent different grades of perfusion (expressed in percent values of the hemispheric mean) as indicated in the color scale in the center; the lower map represents areas that differ significantly from the control group (the adjacent color scale represents the levels of significance versus control values)

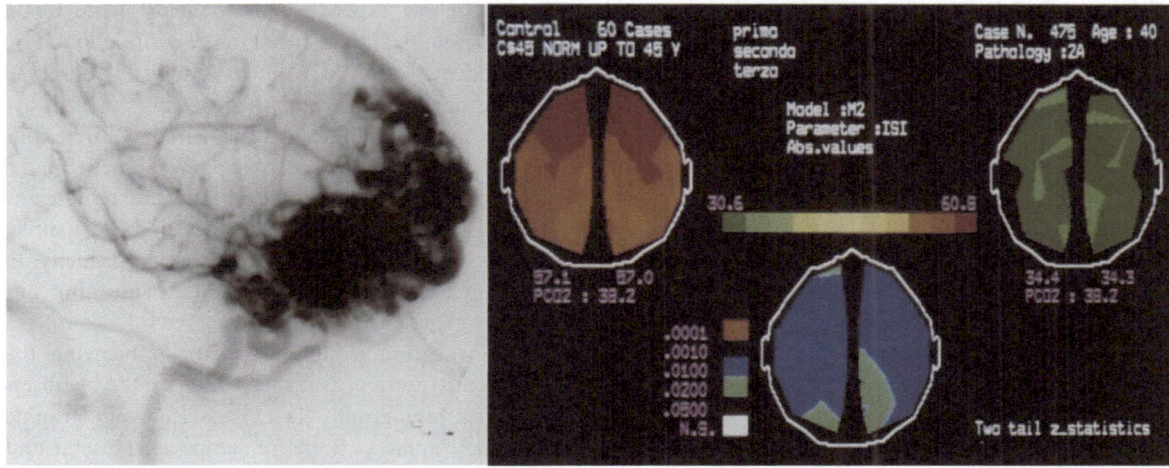

a

b

Fig. 6. Demonstration of global hypoperfusion in frontal AVMs: (a) angiography shows a large right frontal AVM (40 cm^3); (b) the rCBF map shows global hypoperfusion (on the upper right), with the level of significance in the lower map. In this patient, the post-operative course was uncomplicated

ACA, coupled with pathological velocities on the ipsilateral MCA, similarly to what mentioned regarding the angiographical "redistribution phenomenon" (Table 8).

In neurologically impaired vs intact patients, mean flow velocity was 133 vs. 122 cm/s respectively. Four out of the 5 patients that suffered from hyperemic complications were submitted to TCD before operation; all of them showed pathological flow velocity, with a mean of 137 cm/s (against 111 cm/s recorded in patients not developing hyperemic complications).

Discussion

The presence of a cerebral AVM is frequently associated with a less or more severe derangement in cerebral hemodynamics; an assessment of the hemodynamic impairment may have a practical importance, since it is very likely responsible for the hyperemic complications (mainly hemorrhage or edema) occurring either during and after surgery, and bearing a negative influence on the clinical outcome[3,4,5,24,26]. The impairment of autoregulation or vasoreactivity observed in patients with AVMs can cause hypoperfusion around the AVM pre-operatively and hyperemia after operation, and these aspects seem to be linked to each other, as stated by Spetzler *et al.*[26].

Some factors involved in the basal vascular disorder as well as in the pathogenesis of hyperemic complications are: a) regional hypoperfusion in the areas adjacent to the AVM; b) impairment of vasoreactivity and/or autoregulation; c) low perfusion pressure in the cerebral vessels around the AVM. Other hemodynamic factors occurring in the post-operative course are: d) restoration of the normal perfusion pressure in the areas that were previously hypoperfused, and e) increase of cerebral blood flow[2,3,13,24,26,27].

Although in AVM patients the individual variability is high, in this study we attempted to combine the data pertinent to the hemodynamic assessment of an AVM, in order to: a) evaluate the prognostic value of clinical and instrumental data (clinical presentation, angiographic features, rCBF and TCD values), and b) verify, in the clinical practice, which are the mechanisms that concur to the development of perfusion breakthrough and hyperemic complications.

As regards angiographic features, in the prognostic classifications appeared in the literature size and number of feeders are the factors influencing surgical results as well as flow abnormalities and hyperemic complica-

tions[18,23,25]. However AVM size should be considered the main risk factor, being the number of feeders closely related to AVM size[18,19]. It is questionable whether angiographic data still offer a reliable interpretation of altered cerebral hemodynamics in AVM patients[4]. Controversies still remain about a possible correlation between the vascular territories involved in the angiographic steal and the hypoperfused areas adjacent to or remote from the AVM.

CBF and TCD investigations are obviously more suitable to hemodynamic studies, since they can provide quantitative data about regional cerebral perfusion and flow velocity on the feeding vessels. As regards CBF, several studies have appeared in the literature, even if different methods of measurement were used[2,4,8,10,12,13,17,27,29]. In most studies, hypoperfused areas adjacent or remote to the AVM were described[4,8,10,12,17,27]. In the former evenience, it was pointed out that the hyperemia of the AVM could contaminate adjacent areas[17]; as concerns remote areas, a correlation between hypoperfusion and angiographic steal was suggested. A relation was found by Marks *et al.* between these two aspects (perfusional and angiographic); on the contrary, Batjer *et al.* did not find any correlation in a wider clinical series[4,12].

The studies performed during and after operation demonstrated how precocious is the flow redistribution after AVM removal and what is the impact of this phenomenon. Nevertheless, until now it has not been clarified which are the baseline features that can predict hyperemic complications[2,5,6,9,15,29].

Radiological/Instrumental Data

Assessing the influence of AVM volume on hemodynamics, in our experience mean hemispheric blood flow was significantly reduced in the entire population independently of AVM volume. Among the observed patterns of regional hypoperfusion, only adjacent hypoperfusion was significantly more frequent in lesions larger than 30 cm^3. As regards angiographic steal, the more frequent pattern was the adjacent and remote one in AVMs larger than 20 cm^3. As regards TCD, a direct relation was observed between increasing velocity on the main feeder and larger AVMs, confirming our previous experience[6].

AVM location is another factor influencing the blood redistribution, as it was demonstrated by observations on angiography, TCD and CBF. Angiographic and sonographic patterns of temporal, parietal and occipital AVM showed common characteristics, i.e. flow diversion from the controlateral A1 to the ipsilateral A2 thorough the anterior communicating artery; in these cases blood flow measurements, if evaluated in asymmetry, did not disclose significant impairment in the side controlateral to the AVM, as opposed to the vascular paucity observed on angiography in the distal branches of the controlateral anterior cerebral artery ("remote steal"). As concerns CBF measurements: a) frontal AVMs showed significant reduction of the hemispheric values when compared with the controls; b) temporal and occipital AVM presented adjacent areas significantly hypoperfused, ipsilaterally for the former, bilaterally for the latter.

Angiographic steal was not associated with regional hypoperfusion in the corresponding areas. Furthermore there was no relation between pathological flow velocities and incidence of either regional hypoperfusion or angiographic steal.

Influence on Clinical Aspects

In patients who underwent hyperemic complications, mean hemispheric blood flow and the mean volume were both higher than in the remaining patients; mean flow velocity on the main AVM feeder and the incidence of adjacent and remote angiographic steal were also higher in these patients. These features, i.e. high blood flow (either in the nutritional vessels or through the A–V shunt, especially if of large size) can lead to drammatic consequences, if aggressive treatment is performed. Batjer *et al.* noted a decreased incidence of regional hypoperfusion (expressed by the "steal index") in the patients who died[4]. On the other side – in our series – frontal AVMs, which presented the lowest CBF values, also showed the lowest incidence of hyperemic complications.

Similarly to what observed for hyperemic complications, patients that presented – at admission – neurological impairment not related to previous hemorrhage exhibited a higher AVM volume and mean flow velocity; on the contrary hemispheric CBF in these patients was either slightly lower than in the others (45 vs. 50 ml/100g/min) or significantly lower than in the patients undergoing hyperemic complications (45 vs. 61 ml/100g/min).

In conclusion, these results confirm that – among the radiological data – AVM volume and location are those exhibiting a closer relation with hemodynamic derangement, since angiographic steal seems to have a marginal importance. Moreover CBF and TCD add very important informations, which higher CBF values and TCD velocities in patients developing hyperemic complications.

References

1. Aaslid R, Markwalder TM, Nornes H (1982) Noninvasive transcranial Doppler ultrasound recording of flow velocity in basal cerebral arteries. J Neurosurg 57: 769–774
2. Barnett GH, Little JR, Ebrahim ZY, Jones CS, Friel HT (1987) Cerebral circulation during arteriovenous malformation operation. Neurosurgery 20: 836–842
3. Batjer HH, Devous MD, Meyer YJ, Purdy PD, Samson DS (1988) Cerebrovascular hemodynamics in arteriovenous malformation complicated by normal perfusion pressure breakthrough. Neurosurgery 22: 503–509
4. Batjer HH, Devous MD, Seibert GB, Purdy PD, Ajmani AK, Delarosa M, Bonte FJ (1988) Intracranial arteriovenous malformation: relationships between clinical and radiographic factors and ipsilateral steal severity. Neurosurgery 23: 322–328
5. Batjer HH, Purdy PD, Giller CA, Samson DS (1989) Evidence of redistribution of cerebral blood flow during treatment for an intracranial arteriovenous malformation. Neurosurgery 25: 599–605
6. Chioffi F, Pasqualin A, Beltramello A, Da Pian R (1992) Hemodynamic effects of preoperative embolization in cerebral arteriovenous malformation: evaluation with transcranial Doppler sonography. Neurosurgery 31: 877–885
7. Downie NM, Heath RW (1974) Basic statistical methods. Harper Row, New York
8. Hachinski V, Norris JW, Cooper PW, Marshall J (1977) Symptomatic intracranial steal. Arch Neurol 34: 149–153
9. Hassler W, Steinmetz H (1987) Cerebral hemodynamics in angioma patients: an intraoperative study. J Neurosurg 67: 822–831
10. Homan RW, Devous MD, Stokely EM, Bonte FJ (1986) Quantification of intracerebral steal in patients with arteriovenous malformation. Arch Neurol 43: 779–785
11. Lindegaard KF, Grolimund P, Aaslid R, Nornes H (1986) Evaluation of cerebral AVM's using transcranial Doppler ultrasound. J Neurosurg 65: 335–344
12. Marks MP, O'Donahue J, Fabricant JI, Frankel KA, Phillips MH, DeLaPaz RL, Enzmann DR (1988) Cerebral blood flow evaluation of arteriovenous malformations with stable xenon CT. AJNR 9: 1169–1175
13. Morgan MK, Johnston I, Besser M, Baines D (1987) Cerebral arteriovenous malformations, steal, and the hypertensive breakthrough threshold. J Neurosurg 66: 563–567
14. Nornes H, Grip A (1980) Hemodynamic aspects of cerebral arteriovenous malformations. J Neurosurg 53: 456–464
15. Nornes H, Grip A, Wikeby P (1979) Intraoperative evaluation of cerebral hemodynamics using directional Doppler technique. J Neurosurg 50: 145–151
16. Obrist WD, Thompson HK, King CH, Shon Wang H (1967) Determination of regional cerebral blood flow by inhalation of 133-Xenon. Circ 20: 124–135
17. Okabe T, Meyer JS, Okayasu H, Harper R, Rose J, Grossman RG, Centano R, Tachibana H, Ya Yen Lee (1983) Xenon-enhanced CT CBF measurements in cerebral AVM's before and after excision. J Neurosurg 59: 21–31
18. Pasqualin A, Barone G, Cioffi F, Rosta L, Scienza R, Da Pian

    R (1991) The relevance of anatomic and hemodynamic factors to a classification of cerebral arteriovenous malformations. Neurosurgery 28: 370–379

19. Pellettieri L, Carlsson CA, Grevsten S, Norlen G, Uhlemann C (1980) Surgical versus conservative treatment of intracranial arteriovenous malformations. A study in surgical decision making. Acta Neurochir (Wien) [Suppl] 29: 1–86

20. Prohovnik I, Knudsen E, Risberg J (1983) Accuracy of models and algorithms for determination of fast-compartment flow by noninvasive Xe-133 clearance. In: Magistretti PL (ed) Functional radionuclide imaging of the brain. Raven, New York, pp 87–115

21. Risberg J, Ali Z, Wilson EM, Wills EL, Halsey J (1975) Regional cerebral blood flow by Xenon-133 inhalation. Stroke 6: 142–148

22. Rosadini G, Cossu M, De Carli F, Marenco S, Nobili F, Rodriguez G (1989) Evaluation of cerebral blood flow data in stroke patients using a mapping system. Stroke 20: 1182–1189

23. Shi Y, Chen X (1986) A proposed scheme for grading intracranial arteriovenous malformations. J Neurosurg 65: 484–489

24. Solomon RA, Michelsen WJ (1984) Defective cerebrovascular autoregulation in regions proximal to arteriovenous malformations of the brain: a case report and topic review. Neurosurgery 14: 78–82

25. Spetlzer RF, Martin NA (1986) A proposed grading system for arteriovenous malformations. J Neurosurg 65: 476–483

26. Spetlzer RF, Wilson CB, Weinstein P, Mehdorn M, Townsend J, Telles D (1978) Normal perfusion pressure breakthrough theory. Clin Neurosurg 25: 651–672

27. Takeuchi S, Kikuchi H, Karasawa J, Naruo Y, Hashimoto K, Nishimura T, Kozuka T, Hayashi M (1987) Cerebral hemodynamics in arteriovenous malformations: evaluation by single-photon emission CT. AJNR 8: 193–197

28. Wade JPH, Hachinski VC (1987) Cerebral steal: robbery or maldistribution. In: Wood JH (ed) Cerebral blood flow. Mc Graw Hill, New York, pp 467–480

29. Young WL, Solomon RA, Prohovnik I, Ornstein E, Weinstein J, Stein MB (1988) Xenon-133 blood flow monitoring during arteriovenous malformation resection: a case of intraoperative hyperperfusion with subsequent brain swelling. Neurosurgery 22: 765–770

Correspondence: A. Talacchi, M.D., Department of Neurosurgery, City Hospital, I-37126 Verona, Italy.

Selective Flow Modulation of Proximal Feeding Arteries in Surgery of High-Flow Cerebral Arteriovenous Malformations

N. Tamaki, K. Ehara, T. Shirakuni, T. Nagashima, M. Asada, K. Korosue, and K. Fujita

Department of Neurosurgery, Kobe University School of Medicine, Kobe, Japan

Summary

Cerebral hemodynamics were evaluated in 7 patients with large high-flow arteriovenous malformations (AVMs) using an intra-operative thermo-gradient flowmeter. The maximum post-excision/pre-excision blood flow ratio was determined. Special clamps made from silicone tubes with absorbable threads were applied on the proximal feeding arteries.

Two patients with 7 large AVMs (> 4 cm) developed postoperative hematoma. Their flow ratio were larger than 1.9. In 4 patients, blood flow was reduced from an initial ratio > 2.0 to < 1.5. These patients did not develop hemorrhagic complications. Postoperative complications due to the hyperperfusion after excision of high-flow AVMs would be eliminated by this flow modulation technique.

Keywords: High-flow AVM; flow modulation; normal perfusion pressure breakthrough; intraoperative monitoring.

Introduction

The aim of this study was to investigate cerebral hemodynamics in arteriovenous malformations (AVMs) in relation to two important prognostic factors; the size of the AVM, and the hemodynamic changes immediately after AVM excision. On the basis of the results obtained from intraoperative measurement of cortical blood flow, the degree of postexcision hyperperfusion was evaluated. According to these data, special clamps made from silicone tubes with absorbable threads were applied on the proximal feeding arteries in several cases of high-flow AVMs to modulate the excessive increase in blood flow after excision. Surgical results and intra-operative hemodynamic changes were also analyzed after flow modulation.

Material and Methods

Cortical blood flow was measured in 7 patients with large AVMs (> 4 cm) before and after excision. A thermal blood flow monitor (Biomedical Science Inc., Tokyo, Japan) was used. A clinical summary of the patients is shown in Table 1. The blood flow was measured on several parts of the surrounding cortex about 2 cm away from the AVM in each patient. The ratio of postexcision/preexcision cortical blood flow was determined, and the maximum value of the ratio (P–P ratio) was compared to the size of the AVMs. The P–P ratio was also compared to the surgical outcome. Total excision was confirmed by intraoperative or postoperative angiography.

Intraoperative cortical blood flow is measured before and after excision in the same portion as described above. If the P–P ratio is greater than 2.0 in some regions, special clamps made from silicone tubes (Silascon, medical grade silicon tubes, Dow Corning Japan Co. Ltd., Tokyo, Japan) with absorbable threads (#8 – 0 Coated Vicryl, Ethicon Inc. Somerville, NJ, U.S.A.) are applied around the most proximal portion of the main feeding arteries, as it is shown in Fig. 1. The feeding arteries are then constricted by tightening the threads until the P–P ratio is reduced below 1.5. Thus, the sudden increase in blood volume after AVM excision is redirected to the contralateral carotid and posterior circulation or to the ipsilateral intact cerebral arterial systems. These silicone clamps can safely be left in the subarachnoid space.

Results

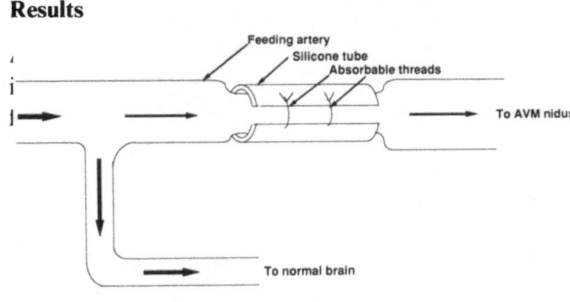

Fig. 1. Diagram of blood flow modulation; the proximal segments of the main feeding arteries are constricted using silicone clamps with absorbable threads. This technique allows to redirect the excessive blood from the dysautoregulated vessels to the intact vascular system after excision of a large AVM

Table 1. *Clinical Summary of Intra-Operative Blood Flow Monitoring in Patients with Large AVMs*

	Case	Age	Sex	Size (cm)	Location	Flow modulation	Postoperative complication	Outcome
Group 1								
	1	46	male	4.0 × 3.5 × 3.0	Lt. parietal	no	ICH	fair
	2	14	male	4.0 × 3.5 × 2.5	Rt. frontal	no	ICH	fair
	3	42	male	4.0 × 3.0 × 3.0	Lt. temporal	no	none	good
Group 2								
	4	62	male	8.0 × 5.5 × 4.5	Rt. temporal	yes*	none	good
	5	29	male	4.0 × 2.5 × 2.5	Rt. parietal	yes**	none	excellent
	6	25	male	4.0 × 2.0 × 1.5	Lt. parietal	yes**	none	excellent
	7	61	male	5.0 × 4.0 × 3.0	Rt. sylvian	yes**	INF	fair

* Blood flow modulation with constriction of the common carotid artery.
** Selective blood flow modulation with constriction of feeding arteries. *ICH* postoperative intracerebral hematoma; *INF* cerebral infarction due to intraoperative deep hypotention.

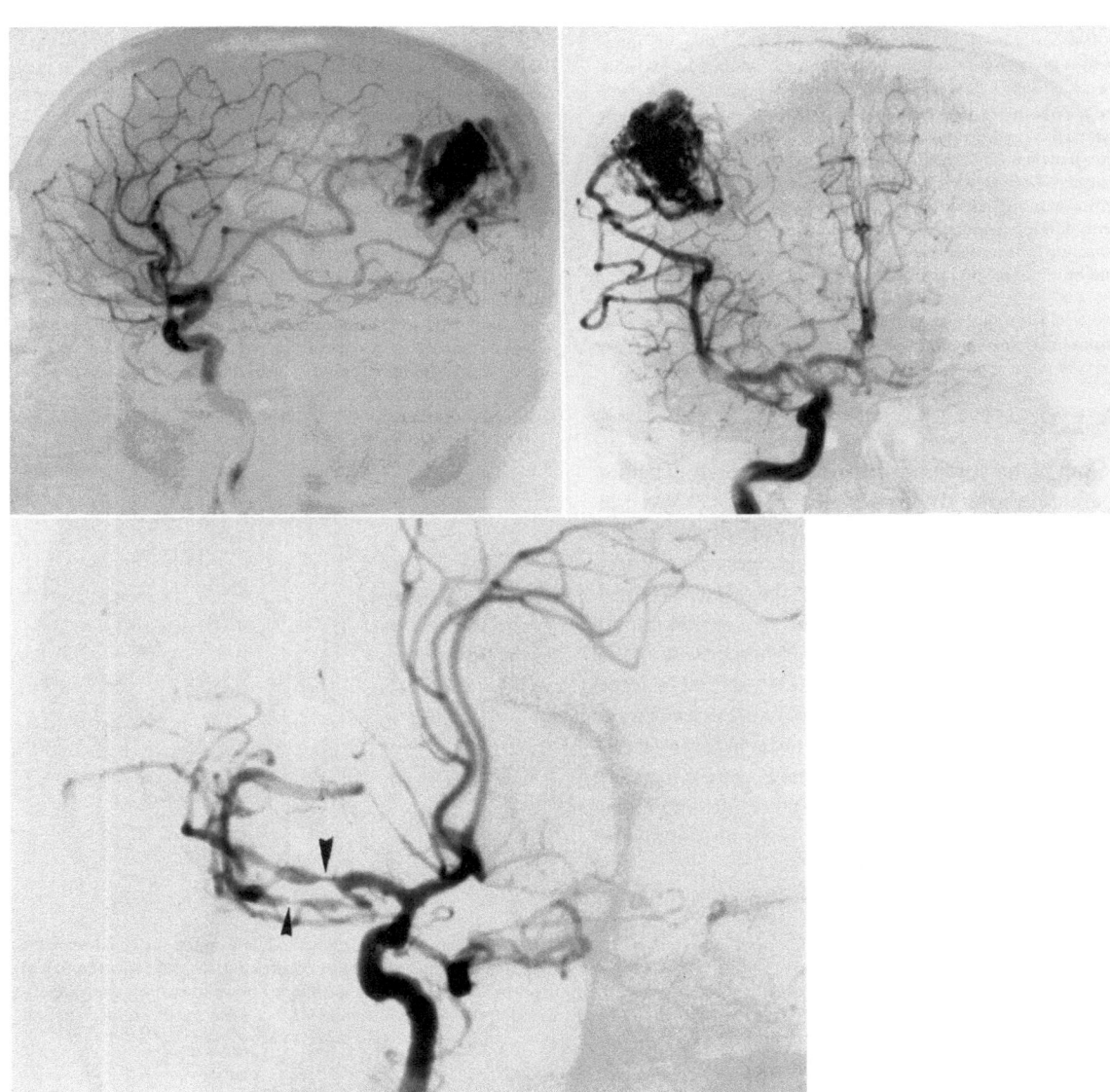

AVMs of 4 cm in diameter, where no special procedure to reduce an increase in cortical blood flow after excision was undertaken. Group 2 consisted of 4 patients, with AVMs ranging in diameter from 4 to 8 cm (mean; 5.0 cm); in this group the sudden increase in blood flow in the surrounding cortex was modulated by constricting either the dilated carotid artery (Case 4) or the proximal segment of the dilated feeding arteries (Case 5, 6 and 7) until the ratio decreased to below 1.5.

There were two patients in the group 1 who developed postoperative hemorrhagic complications (Case 1 and 2) despite the complete removal was confirmed by an intraoperative or postoperative angiography. The remaining 14 patients had no hemorrhagic complications.

The P–P ratio increased as the AVM enlarged, and exceeded > 2.0 as most of AVMs approached 4 cm in diameter (group 1 and 2). Two out of three in group 1 patients developed postoperative intracerebral hematoma. The flow ratio of these two patients was larger than 1.9.

In the group 2 patients with large AVMs, blood flow was reduced from an initial ratio > 2.0 to 1.5 using these special clamps (Case 5, 6 and 7) or extracranial carotid Selverstone clamps (Case 4). These patients did not develop any hemorrhagic complications.

Figure 2 demonstrate the preoperative and postoperative angiogram of a 29-year-old man (Case 5). Preoperative right carotid angiograms showed AVM fed by the parietal and angular arteries, as well as by the parietooccipital artey. The postoperative carotid angiogram demonstrated total excision of the AVM. The proximal segments of the major feeding arteries remained constricted by silicone clamps (arrow heads). The patient was discharged without neurological deficits.

Discussion

Hyperemic complications, defined as unusual hemorrhage or edema immediately after excision of high-flow AVMs, were described as the normal perfusion pressure breakthrough syndrome[10]. Intraoperative cortical blood flow measurement in this study demonstrated the blood flow at post-excision increased more than twice as that of pre-excision in most cases of large AVMs over 4 cm in size. These results suggested that the rate of increase in blood flow after excision correlated closely with the size of the AVM, and with a greater risk of developing postoperative hemorrhagic complications.

For prevention of these hyperemic complications, the following strategies have been tried: 1) multiple-staged operations, 2) preoperative embolization of the feeding arteries followed by surgical excision, 3) intraoperative embolization combined with feeding artery ligation followed by surgical excision, and 4) ligation of several feeding arteries followed by later excision[1,6,7,9].

Gradual stepwise reperfusion of the surrounding ischemic hemisphere after a staged reduction of shunt flow seems a reasonable approach to reestablishing autoregulation. In contrast, the hemodynamic change induced by preoperative embolization may cause an additional risk of ischemic or hemorrhagic complications[2]. Some surgeons also question the benefits of staged surgical excision of an AVM, since this may induce acute intraoperative hypoperfusion superimposed on chronic preoperative hypoperfusion[4,5]. Partial occlusion of the carotid artery has previously been used to prevent or to treat NPPB in the one-stage excision of high-flow AVMs[3,8,11-13]. Selective flow modulation by constricting the proximal segments of main feeding arteries would be indicated if the size of AVMs is from 4 to 6 cm and if the cortical blood flow after excision is more than twice as much as preexcision value according to the intraoperative blood flow monitoring.

In patients with these large high-flow AVMs, an excessively large volume of blood flows into the brain, and then flows out the intracranial cavity through the AVM. Following excision of an AVM, this flow modulation technique allows re-distribution of the sudden increase in blood flow from the dysautoregulated vessels to the intact arterial system. Postoperative complications due to hyperperfusion after excision of high-flow AVMs would be eliminated by this flow modulation technique.

References

1. Andrews BT, Wilson CB (1987) Staged treatment of arteriovenous malformations of the brain. Neurosurgery 21: 314–323

Fig. 2. Upper right and left: preoperative right carotid angiograms of Case 5. The AVM is fed by the large, tortuous parietal and angular arteries, as well as by the parietooccipital artery. Lower: Oblique view of the postoperative carotid angiogram of Case 5. The AVM was totally excised and proximal segments of the major feeding arteries remained constricted with silicone clamps (arrow heads)

2. Batjer HH, Devous MD, Meyer YJ, Purdy PD, Samson DS (1988) Cerebrovascular hemodynamics in arteriovenous malformation complicated by normal perfusion pressure breakthrough. Neurosurgery 22: 503–509

3. Bonnal J, Born JD, Hans P (1989) One-stage excision of high-flow arteriovenous malformations. J Neurosurg 762: 128–131

4. Morgan MK, Sundt Jr TM (1989) The case against staged operative resection of cerebral arteriovenous malformations. Neurosurgery 25: 429–436

5. Mullan S, Brown FD, Patronas NJ (1979) Hyperemic and ischemic problems of surgical treatment of arteriovenous malformations. J Neurosurg 51: 757–764

6. Pelz DM, Fox AJ, Vinuela F, Drake CC, Ferguson GG (1988) Preoperative embolization of brain AVMs with isobutyl-2-cyanoacrylate. AJNR 1988: 9 :757–764

7. Pertuiset B, Ancri D, Clergue F (1982) Preoperative evaluation of hemodynamic factors in cerebral arteriovenous malformations for selection of a radical surgery tactic with special reference to vascular autoregulation disorders. Neurol Res 4: 209–233

8. Pertuiset B, Ancri D, Sichez JP, Chauvdn M, Gunax E, Metzger J, Gardeur D, Basset Y (1983) Radical surgery in cerebral AVM-tactical procedures based upon hemodynamic factors. Adv Tech Stand Neurosurg 10: 83–143

9. Spetzler RF, Martin NA, Carter LP, Flom RA, Raudzens PA, Wilkinson (1978) Surgical management of large AVMs by staged embolization and operative excision. J Neurosurg 67: 17–28

10. Spetzler RF, Wilson CB, Weinstein P, Mechdoron M, Townsend J, Telles D (1978) Normal perfusion pressure breakthrough theory. Clin Neurosurg 25: 651–672

11. Tamaki N, Lin T, Asada M, Fujita K, Tominaga S, Kimura M, Ehara K, Matsumoto S (1990) Modulation of blood flow following excision of a high-flow cerebral arteriovenous malformation. Case report. J Neurosurg 72: 509–512

12. Tamaki N, Ehara K, Lin T, Kuwamura K, Obora Y, Kanazawa Y, Yamashita H, Matsumoto S (1992) Cerebral arteriovenous malformations: factors influencing the surgical difficulty and outcome. Neurosurgery 29: 856–863

13. Tamaki N, Ehara K (1992) Arteriovenous malformations–indications and strategies for surgery. In: Raimondi A *et al* (eds) Cerebrovascular disease in children. Principle in pediatric neurosurgery. Springer, Berlin Heidelberg New York Tokyo, pp 59–74

Correspondence: N. Tamaki, M.D., Department of Neurosurgery, Kobe University School of Medicine, 7-5-1 Kusunoki-cho, Chuoko, Kobe 650, Japan.

The Importance of Transcranial Doppler Sonography in the Management of Cerebral AVMs: Pre-Treatment Evaluation and Post-Embolization Changes

F. Chioffi, A. Pasqualin, G. Acerbi[1], and G. Pavesi

Department of Neurosurgery, Verona City Hospital and [1]Division of Neurosurgery, Pescara City Hospital, Italy

Summary

94 patients with cerebral arteriovenous malformations were evaluated with transcranial Doppler sonography. Ultrasonographic and neuro-radiological characteristics of severely altered cerebral hemodynamics were associated with the presence of intravascular mean flow velocity > 120 cm/s, pulsatility index < 0.5 and AVM volume > 30 cm^3. Cerebrovascular reactivity was evaluated in 9 patients by means of autoregulation to hypotension (sodium nitroprusside) and in 25 patients by means of vasomotor response to hypocapnia: it was defective proportionally to the volume of the AVMs. In 43 patients serial TCD investigation were performed during the stages of embolizations: significant mean flow velocity reduction ($> 60\%$) occurred in 72% of cases after the first embolization, in 45% of cases after the second embolization and in no case after the third embolization. A flow velocity redistribution on basal vessels (defined as an increase in flow velocity of at least 30% of the initial value) occurred only after the first endovascular treatment (62% of the cases). It is concluded that TCD sonography is a valuable method for noninvasive hemodynamic assessment of shunt flow in arteriovenous malformations and permits a physiological monitoring of hemodynamic changes after embolization.

Keywords: Arteriovenous malformations; cerebro-vascular reactivity; embolization; transcranial Doppler sonography.

Introduction

The neuroradiological imaging by means of angiography, CT scan and MRI provide invaluable informations in patients with cerebral AVMs, such as anatomical location, size, arterial supply and venous drainage of the lesion[6]; combined computed tomographic (CT) scan and regional cerebral blood flow (rCBF) methods, and in particular the single photon emission computed tomography (SPECT) add useful informations on cerebral perfusion, although not always reliable in detecting hypoperfused areas around the AVM[9,11,18].

In the last years, a new hemodynamic measurement has been introduced in the management of these patients, by means of transcranial Doppler sonography[1,10]. This method determines the degree of hemodynamic involvement of the single basal arteries, in multi-supplied AVMs, through atraumatic measurements of intravascular flow velocities (systolic, diastolic and mean) and the calculation of the pulsatility index (PI). Besides it permits a physiological monitoring of cerebro-vascular reactivity to different tests (autoregulation to hypotension, vasomotor response to hypocapnia) and assessment of hemodynamic changes occurring during multi-staged treatment of AVMs.

The aim of this study was to draw some general rules regarding the hemodynamic behaviour of cerebral AVMs, in order to plan the best treatment for each patient.

Material and Methods

From October 1986 to February 1992, 94 patients with cerebral AVMs were evaluated by TCD sonography. TCD investigations were carried out with a 2-MHz pulsed frequency transcranial Doppler device with a built-in 64-point Fast Fourier Transformation spectrum analyzer (EME, Ueberlingen, Germany). Systolic, mean, and diastolic flow velocities were measured in centimeters/second and displayed on the screen. The pulsatility index (PI) was defined according to Gosling and King[7] as: $PI = (Vs\text{-}Vd)/Vm$. The proximal intracranial segments (M1, A1, P1) of middle cerebral artery (MCA), anterior cerebral artery (ACA) and posterior cerebral artery (PCA) were insonated from the temporal window; the vertebral artery from the mastoid region; and the basilar artery from the foramen magnum window.

Patients were divided into five subgroups according to AVM volume: 0 to 10 cm^3, 11 to 20 cm^3, 21 to 30 cm^3, 31 to 50 cm^3, and > 50 cm^3. The calculation of AVM volume was made in the mid-to late arterial phase of the angiogram by multiplying the product of the three main diameters (horizontal and vertical diameters in the anteroposterior projection, and longitudinal diameter in the lateral projection) by 0.52, as proposed by our group in a recent paper[12].

Table 1. *Therapeutic Procedures in 94 Patients Evaluated with TCD*

Volume (cm³)	Direct surgery	Emboliz-ation and surgery	Emboliz-ation	Other treatments
0–11 (n = 11)	6(54%)	5(45%)	–	–
11–20 (n = 21)	3(14%)	12(57%)	5(24%)	1(5%)
21–30 (n = 22)	1(5%)	11(50%)	8(36%)	2(9%)
31–50 (n = 28)	1(4%)	12(43%)	15(53%)	–
> 50 (n = 12)	–	3(25%)	8(67%)	1(8%)
Total	11(12%)	43(46%)	36(38%)	4(4%)

Table 2. *Basal TCD Values According to AVM Volume (94 Patients)*

| Volume (cm³) | Velocity (cm/s ± SEM) | | | |
	Systolic	Diastolic	Mean	PI
0–10 (n = 11)	119 ± 9	64 ± 7	76 ± 6	0.8 ± 0.02
11–20 (n = 21)	150 ± 7	86 ± 9	97 ± 10	0.63 ± 0.04
21–30 (n = 22)	162 ± 7	94 ± 8	118 ± 13	0.52 ± 0.04
31–50 (n = 28)	186 ± 10	124 ± 12	140 ± 10	0.41 ± 0.01
> 50 (n = 12)	182 ± 15	127 ± 11	142 ± 12	0.37 ± 0.01
	<0.001*	<0.001*	<0.001*	<0.001*

* Significance [except (31–50) vs. (> 50)].

The therapeutic procedures adopted in these patients are shown in Table 1.

Pre-Treatment Evaluation

Basal measurements were considered TCD investigations before any kind of interventional therapeutical procedures. In some cases – during basal measurements – we studied cerebrovascular reactivity. Autoregulation to hypotension was studied in 9 cases of supratentorial AVMs (1 small, 4 medium, 4 large) and in 3 voulonteers. The procedure consisted in a slow infusion of sodium nitroprusside (SNP) through a cubital vein omolateral to the radial artery incannulated for mean arterial pressure (MAP) monitoring. The drip of SNP was set up in order to get a MAP reduction of 20% for 30 minutes and then stopped. In all cases the test was well tolerated. Transcranial Doppler measurements were performed at short intervals (5 minutes) both in feeder arteries and in non-feeder arteries.

Cerebrovascular reactivity was studied by a 30 seconds test of maximal hyperventilation with continuous transcranial Doppler measurements of systolic, mean, diastolic flow velocities. 25 patients with cerebral AVMs of different volumes (8 small, 9 medium, 8 large) were compared to a control group (n = 47).

Post-Embolization Changes

49 patients were submitted to preoperative embolization. Selective embolization was performed – in all of the patients – with surgical sutures (polyene threads) by means of a microcatheter system; flow-directed embolization with Silastic sponge was associated with selective embolization in 2 patients (a total of 4 procedures). All procedures were done through the transfemoral route. The data were evaluated using one-way analysis of variance to test whether the means of the five samples (categories of volume: 0–10, 11–20, 21–30, 31–50, and > 50 cm³) were different. If so, we used Sheffe's method to determine which samples were different from the others.

Results

Pre-Treatment Evaluation

Basal Measurements

Considering mean flow velocity and pulsatility index the most meaningful ultrasonographic parameters of endocranial arteries[1,8], we recorded mean flow velocity

over 120 cm/s in many cases of AVMs sized over 20 cm³ and in all cases of AVMs sized over 30 cm³. The arterial pulsatility index, whose value normally ranges between 0.65 and 0.8, has been close to normal in cases of small AVMs and pathologically low in cases of large AVMs (Table 2).

When intravascular mean velocity was over 120 cm/s and PI lower than 0.5 – at least in one cerebral artery – we have frequently seen pathologically low values of mean flow velocity in the precommunicating segment of the anterior and posterior cerebral artery ipsilateral to the AVM and in some cases even reversal of flow direction with high flow velocity in the controlateral A1 (or P1). We have defined this situation as "altered blood flow distribution", in agreement with the corresponding angiographical patterns. Figure 1 is an example: the left parietal AVM makes a sort of "sucking" effect on basal vessels determining a blood supply from ipsilateral MCA and controlateral ACA; the ipsilateral ACA is not visualized on angiography and its intravascular flow velocity is lower than the controlateral.

Cerebro-Vascular Reactivity

As regard *autoregulation to hypotension*, intravascular flow velocities did not change – in the control group – during the test. In the patient with a small AVM (< 10 cm³) hypotension produced a reduction of mean flow velocity of 10% on the arterial feeder (ACA) of the AVM and no modifications on non-feeders arteries. In the patients with medium-sized AVM (11–20 cm³) hypotension produced a reduction of mean flow velocity of 25% on the arterial feeders of the AVMs and no modifications on non-feeder arteries. In patients with large AVMs (> 20 cm³) hypotension produced a reduction of mean flow velocity ranging from 30 to 60% on the arterial feeders; similar modifications were

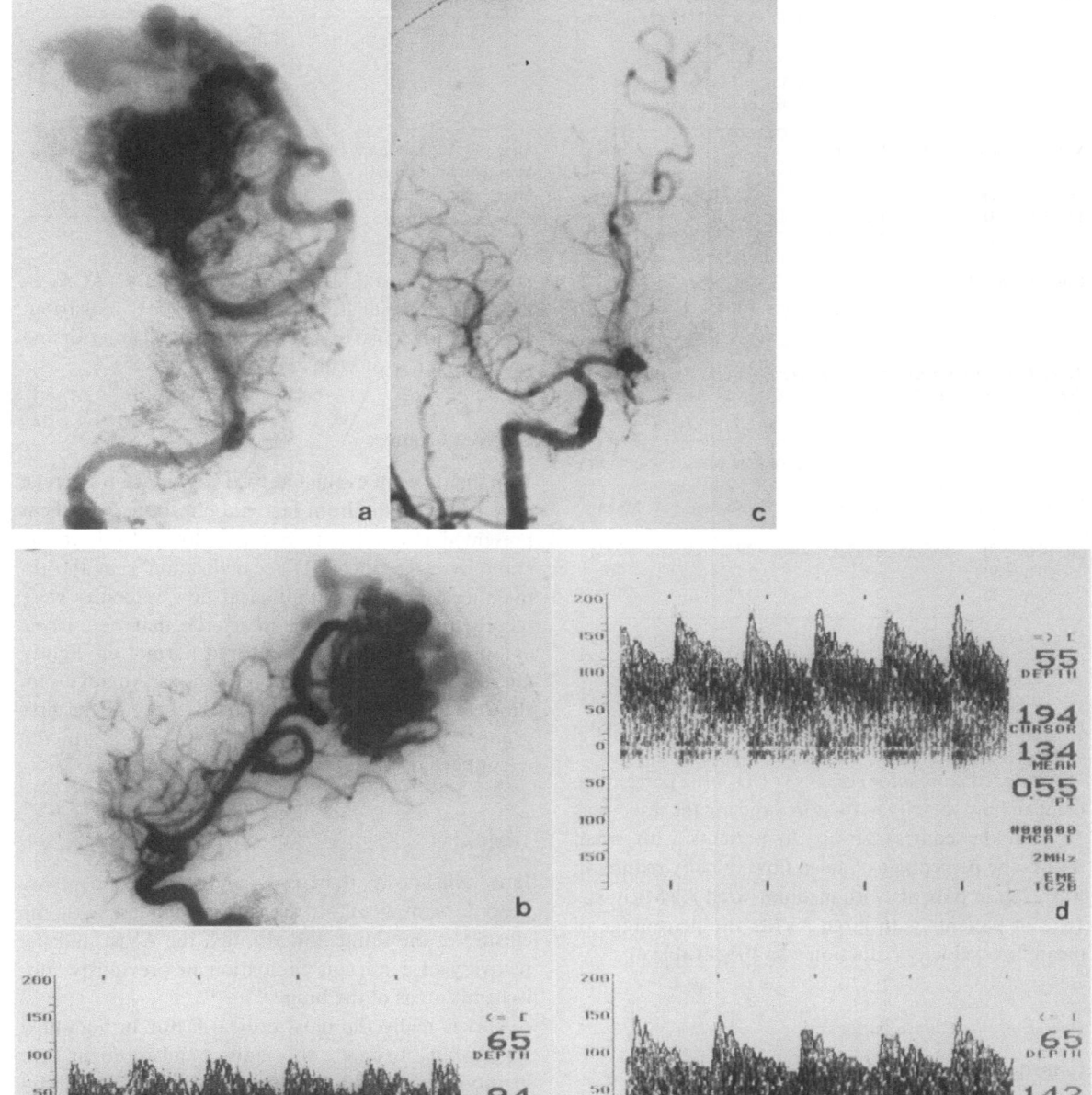

Fig. 1. (a, b) Left posterior parietal AVM (24 cm³) with ectatic feeders from middle cerebral artery (MCA) and no injection of ipsilateral anterior cerebral artery (ACA); (c) the left ACA – also feeding the AVM – also feeding the AVM – is injected from the right side; (d) on TCD, high time-mean velocity (134 cm/s) and low PI (0.55) on left MCA; (e) normal velocity on left ACA; (f) high timemean velocity on right ACA (104 cm/s)

Table 3. *TCD Evaluation of Autoregulation to Hypotension (with Sodium Nitroprusside) in 9 Patients with Cerebral AVMs and in 3 Controls*

| Volume (cm^3) | Mean flow velocities changes (>30% of initial value) | |
	Feeder artery	Normal artery
0–10 (n = 1)	–	–
11–20 (n = 4)	1(25%)	–
> 20 (n = 4)	4(100%)	2(50%)
Controls (n = 3)		–

Table 4. *Vasomotor Response to Hypocapnia (by Hyperventilation for 30 Seconds), in 25 Patients with Cerebral AVMs and in 47 Controls*

| Volume (cm^3) | Percentage of flow velocity reduction | | |
	Systolic	Diastolic	Mean
0–10 (n = 8)	−13%	−29%	−22%
11–20 (n = 9)	−7%	−17%	−10%
> 20 (n = 8)	−8%	−14%	−10%
Controls (n = 47)	−22%	−48%	−40%

recorded on non-feeder arteries in 2 out of 4 patients (Table 3).

As regard *vasomotor response (CO_2)* the percentage of mean flow velocity reduction – during the test – was 40%, in the control group. In patients with small AVMs the percentage of mean flow velocity reduction was 22%; in patients with medium-sized AVMs it was 16%; in patients with large AVMs the percentage of mean flow velocity reduction was 10% (Table 4).

Post-Embolization Changes

Immediate Changes

Considering hemodynamically significant a mean flow velocity reduction >60%[10], we obtained this result in 72% of patients after the first embolization, in 45% of patients after the second embolization and in none of the patients submitted to three or more embolizations (Table 5).

After the first embolization we frequently saw a flow velocity redistribution among basal arteries, that is an increase of mean flow velocity (at least 30% of the basal value) in arteries not embolized Table 5. The most frequent redistribution occurred between ipsi-

Table 5. *TCD Evaluation 1 Day After Embolization (43 Patients)*

	Flow velocity reduction >60%	Flow velocity reduction <20%	Flow redistribution
After 1 embolization (n = 43)	31(72%)	3(7%)	29(67%)
After 2 embolization (n = 12)	6(50%	3(25%)	–
After 3 embolization (n = 9)	–	6(66%)	–

lateral MCA and ipsilateral/controlateral ACA, in large, paramedian supratentorial AVMs; redistributions occurred also between the ipsilateral anterior and posterior circle of Willis.

Delayed Changes

13 patients were evaluated by TCD after an average time of 6 months from last embolization; 7 of them presented a complete recovery of flow velocity in the embolized artery ("TCD recanalization"); in the remaining 6 patients pathological flow velocities were recorded for the first time in arteries that were never embolized and that had appeared normal or slightly altered on previous TCD examinations. Angiography showed the recanalization of the vessel – in the first group – and the recruitment of new feeders – in the second group.

Discussion

It is well known that intra- and post-operative hyperemic complications are strictly related with the closure of the shunt flow through the AVM and the recovery of a normal circulation in previously sub-ischemic areas of the brain[3,8,14-16].

This is really the most critical factor in high-flow AVMs, but – to date – only indirect and approximative methods were available for a preoperative hemodynamic evaluation of cerebral AVMs.

Our experience, by means of transcranial Doppler sonography, demonstrates a clear correlation between intravascular flow velocity on feeder arteries and AVM volume; in particular the "altered blood flow distribution" – demonstrated both on TCD and on angiography – appears as an effect of well identified ultrasonographic and neuroradiological characteristics: mean flow velocity >120 cm/s, PI <0.5 and volume >20 cm^3. Under these conditions we believe reasonable to use the term "high-flow AVMs".

Furthermore the same hemodynamic and volumetric patterns have been associated, in our study, with severe functional alterations of cerebral circulation. The autoregulative capacities – apt to maintain a constant cerebral blood flow under hypotension – are defective in patients with medium/large AVMs; the vasoconstrictive response to hypocapnia – in the same kind of patients – is so altered that no significant variations of mean flow velocity occur.

From these premises (large, high-flow and vasoparalyzed AVM), it is reasonable to consider a staged preoperative treatment of shunt flow reduction, by means of superselective embolization.

We have obtained good results with serial embolizations at short intervals (1–2 weeks); experiences of other authors[2,4,5,13,17] confirm this point as a general rule. The 60% of mean flow velocity reduction – after embolization – seems to be, in our experience, indicative of a successful shunt flow reduction. After this hemodynamic change, we have seen that the vessel filling slows down and that the nidus becomes clearer on angiography. It is of interest that flow velocity reduction was most likely to occur after the first embolization attempt and that multiple procedures were often futile. In our opinion the reasons are: 1) AVMs submitted to multiple embolizations are usually large, high-flow, multi-supplied malformations, so that any attempt of shunt flow reduction can be unsuccessful; 2) when the time interval between sequential embolizations is too long, the embolized vessel may recanalize its lumen – as occurred in 54% of our patients controlled by TCD after 6 months from last embolization–; or 3) the collateral circulation – based on pial anastomoses usually pre-existing but not functioning, or consisting of a newly formed network of medullary vessels – may activate itself, neutralizing to a great extent the attempt to reduce AVM shunt flow.

A point for the future is to check if an hemodynamically significant shunt flow reduction – after embolization – determines a parallel improvement of cerebrovascular reactivity.

In conclusion we believe that this easily mastered atraumatic methodology, applied to the hemodynamic characteristics of cerebral arteriovenous malformations, may have important therapeutic implications in the management of these patients, especially if associated with more refined reactivity tests and possibly if combined with more reliable rCBF methods.

References

1. Aaslid R, Markwalder TM, Nornes H (1984) Noninvasive transcranial Doppler ultrasound recording of flow velocity in basal cerebral arteries. J Neurosurg 57: 769–774
2. Andrews BT, Wilson CB (1987) Staged treatment of arteriovenous malformations of the brain. Neurosurgery 21: 314–323
3. Batjer HH, Devous MD, Meyer YJ, Purdy PD, Samson DS (1988) Cerebrovascular hemodynamics in arteriovenous malformation complicated by normal perfusion pressure breakthrough. Neurosurgery 22: 503–509
4. Batjer HH, Purdy PD, Giller CA, Samson DS (1989) Evidence of redistribution of cerebral blood flow during treatment for an intracranial arteriovenous malformation. Neurosurgery 25: 599–605
5. Benati A, Beltramello A, Colombari R, Maschio A, Perini S, Da Pian R, Pasqualin A, Scienza R, Rosta L, Piovan E, Scarpa A, Zamboni G (1989) Preoperative embolization of arteriovenous malformations with polylene threads: techniques with wing microcatheter and pathologic results. AJNR 10: 579–586
6. Drake CG (1983) Arteriovenous malformations of the brain. The options for management. N Engl J Med 309–310
7. Gosling RG, King DH (1974) Continuous wave ultrasound as an alternative and complement to X-rays in vascular examinations. In: Reneman RE (ed) Cardiovascular applications of ultrasound. North-Holland, Amsterdam, pp 266–282
8. Hassler W (1986) Hemodynamic aspects of cerebral angiomas. Acta Neurochir (Wien) [Suppl] 37: 77–79
9. Marks MP, O'Donahue J, Fabricant JI, Frankel KA, Phillips MH, DeLaPaz RL, Enzmann DR (1988) Cerebral blood flow evaluation of arteriovenous malformations with stable Xenon CT. AJNR 9: 1169–1175
10. Mohr JP, Petty GW, Massaro AR (1990) Transcranial Doppler studies in arteriovenous malformations. AJNR 11: 223
11. Okabe T, Meyer JS, Okajasu H, Harper R, Rose J, Grossman RG, Centeno R, Tachibana H, Lee YY (1983) Xenon enhanced CT CBF measurements in cerebral AVMs before and after excision. Contribution to pathogenesis and treatment. J Neurosurg 59: 21–31
12. Pasqualin A, Barone G, Cioffi F, Rosta L, Scienza R, Da Pian R (1991) The relevance of anatomic and hemodynamic factors to a classification of cerebral arteriovenous malformations. Neurosurgery 28: 370–379
13. Pasqualin A, Scienza R, Cioffi F, Barone G, Benati A, Beltramello A, Da Pian R (1991) Treatment of cerebral arteriovenous malformations with a combination of preoperative embolization and surgery. Neurosurgery 29: 358–368
14. Spetzler RF, Wilson CB, Weinstein P, Mehdorn J, Townsend J, Telles D (1978) Normal perfusion pressure breakthrough theory. Clin Neurosurg 25: 651–672
15. Spetzler RF, Martin NA, Carter LP, Flam RA, Raudzens PA, Wilkinson E (1987) Surgical management of large AVMs by staged embolization and operative excision. J Neurosurg 67: 17–28
16. Stein BM, Wolpert SM (1977) Surgical and embolic treatment of cerebral arteriovenous malformations. Surg Neurol 7: 359–369
17. Vinuela F, Fox AJ (1983) Interventional neuroradiology and the management of arteriovenous malformations and fistulas. Neurol Clin 1: 131–154
18. Yaşargil MG (1987) Hemodynamics. In: Yaşargil MG (ed) Microneurosurgery, Vol IIIA. Thieme, Stuttgart, pp 213–239

Correspondence: F. Chioffi, M.D., Department of Neurosurgery, Verona City Hospital, I-37126 Verona, Italy.

Perioperative Management of High-Flow Arteriovenous Malformations: Hemodynamic Monitoring and Anesthetic Considerations

W.L. Young[1,2] and **E. Ornstein**[1]

Departments of [1]Anesthesiology and [2]Neurological Surgery, Columbia University College of Physicians and Surgeons, New York, New York, U.S.A.

Summary

High-flow AVMs represent formidable management challenges. Since AVM resection is almost never emergent, a thoughtful management plan can be formulated with attention to goals for blood pressure management. In addition to routine monitoring, pulmonary artery catheters, or at least central venous lines, are recommended. Monitoring cerebral hemodynamics can assist in 1) titration of drug effects for cerebral protection (e.g. barbiturates) or brain relaxation (e.g. hypocapnia), 2) monitoring for the occurrence of cerebral hyperperfusion, 3) monitoring for the occurrence of regional cerebral ischemia during vascular manipulation, 4) monitoring for the occurrence of global cerebral ischemia during induced hypotension, 5) differentiating arterial and venous structures, 6) identifying patients at high risk for post-operative hyperfusion complications. Methods currently available include transcranial Doppler ultrasound, microvascular Doppler, thermal clearance CBF, laser Doppler CBF, 133-Xe CBF, EEG and direct intravascular pressure measurement.

Choice of anesthesia is primarily directed at optimizing brain relaxation and cerebral protection, which is achievable with a large number of anesthetic techniques. Potent agents have the advantage of superior systemic blood pressure control. Barbiturate loading during critical periods may offer additional cerebral protection at the expense of delayed emergence. The anesthesia team must be prepared to induce hypotension, especially during deeper dissection. The possibility of rapid and massive blood loss must be anticipated and adequate replacement and venous access should be available. Alpha- and beta-adrenergic antagonists such as labetolol and esmolol are ideal hypotensive agents, with a minimal effect on the cerebral circulation. Fluid replacement should be aimed at maintaining normovolemia and isotonicity with avoidance of hyperglycemia. Because of recent evidence for a strong cerebroprotective effect of very modest hypothermia, the normal temperature decrease seen with induction of anesthesia should be allowed to persist (34–35 °C) throughout most of the procedure. When closure is imminent, rewarming towards 37 °C should be started.

A primary goal for immediate post-operative management is to minimize complications of brain swelling and hemorrhage. Immediate post-operative angiography is an attractive strategy to minimize risk of hemorrhage due to occult residual AVM. Patients who exhibit large increases in cerebral blood flow or have abnormal autoregulation to changes in arterial pressure after resection may be at higher risk for the development of hyperperfusion or circulatory breakthrough. The AVM patient tends to exhibit a hyperdynamic systemic circulation post-operatively, and adrenergic antagonists can be used to aggressively prevent systemic hypertension. Poorly controlled systemic blood pressure in the immediate post-operative period is felt to increase the risk of cerebral hyperperfusion complications. Patients thought to be at especially high risk should have blood pressure maintained in the low normal range, provided that no evidence of cerebral ischemia is present.

Keywords: Cerebral arteriovenous malformation; anesthetic management; cerebral blood flow monitoring; induced hypotension.

Introduction

High-flow AVMs represent formidable management challenges. Since the general anesthetic care of the neurosurgical patient can be found in many other excellent sources, this review will focus on particular points germane to the AVM patient.

Preoperative

Since AVM resection is almost never emergent, a careful review of the patient's perioperative status and assessment of the likelihood of encountering intraoperative difficulties is possible. Preexisting medical conditions should be optimized and neurologic dysfunction, either as a result of presenting hemorrhage, presumed effect of the AVM or pre-operative embolization (infarction or edema), should be factored into the intraoperative management plan regarding choice of monitoring, vascular access, anesthetic agents, vasoactive drugs and muscle relaxants. A critical consideration that looms large throughout the operative period is the potential for massive and rapid blood loss. Choice of intraoperative monitoring is tempered by this eventuality and adequate blood, and access for its administration, must be at hand.

Intraoperative

Hemodynamic Monitoring

Systemic Monitoring

In addition to routine monitors such as EKG, pulse oximeter, end-tidal CO_2 and direct arterial pressure transduction, central access is recommended. A central venous line is probably adequate in most uncomplicated cases. Unfortunately, it is not always possible to predict pre-operatively which patient is going to become a "complicated" case during resection, subsequently requiring extraordinary levels of induced hypotension or aggressive volume therapy. Happily, such cases are a minority, but pulmonary artery catheters are indispensable for management of such complicated patients.

Route of access for central cannulation deserves mention. In most intraoperative settings, the preferred site of cannulation is the internal jugular vein. Because the AVM patient may have abnormalities of venous drainage that have as yet an undetermined influence on perioperative complications, any temptation to cannulate the internal jugular should cause one to at least pause for reflection. If inspection of the angiogram suggests that one of the jugular veins seems to dominate cerebral venous drainage, it may be of value to cannulate the non-dominant side.

We routinely place a pulmonary artery catheter through the antecubital approach*. The only disadvantage to this approach is that it is less well suited for post-operative monitoring, because the catheter tip position may migrate with movement of the arm in the awake patient. In practice, however, those patients who need the catheter for the initial post-operative period tend to be either comatose or sedated.

Knowledge of cardiac filling pressures and cardiac output allows the clinician to maintain optimal volume status, which is critical for smooth conduct of induced hypotension, volume replacement and rational use of systemic vasodilators and adrenergic blocking agents. Although pediatric patients may develop heart failure because of a cerebral shunt, the AVM fistula does not usually affect cardiac output in adults[71]. In the future, non-invasive monitoring of cardiac output may supplant the thermodilution method via a pulmonary artery catheter[69].

Cerebral Monitoring

Monitoring cerebral hemodynamics during AVM resection is desirable for several reasons. The ideal goals for hemodynamic monitoring are shown in Table 1. Unfortunately, our ability to monitor the central nervous system lags far behind our ability to monitor other systems and the development of suitable technologies is still in its infancy. There is no consensus about optimum monitoring techniques, primarily because there is a dearth of commercially available technologies.

Along with absolute CBF measures, a promising avenue for future development is the use of deliberate physiologic perturbations to unmask underlying autoregulatory defects. Examples would be small changes in $PaCO_2$ or systemic blood pressure, but newer methods need to be developed. In the extraoperative setting, visually evoked autoregulatory challenge[1] and assessment of the "transient hyperemic response" to carotid compression have been proposed[22].

Following is a brief description of the currently available modalities.

Ultrasound Methods

Transcranial Doppler (TCD) may be applied in the intraoperative and postoperative settings, and the subject is reviewed elsewhere[35,37,48]. TCD is undergoing an enormous amount of development. Currently available probes can be affixed over the contralateral, if not the ipsilateral, temporal bone window. Although the MCA is the easiest vessel to image, it is possible to position the probe to view the ACA and PCA as well.

---

*We prefer to use a 8.5 F rapid-infuser catheter instead of the customary long introducer sheath employed for internal jugular cannulation. As a result, there appear to be fewer problems with local post-operative phlebitis.

Table 1. *Goals for Cerebral Hemodynamic Monitoring*

---

1. To have the ability to titrate drug effects for cerebral protection (barbiturate) or brain relaxation (hypocapnia)
2. To monitor for the occurrence of cerebral hyperperfusion
3. To monitor for the occurrence of regional cerebral ischemia during vascular manipulation
4. To monitor for the occurrence of global cerebral ischemia during induced hypotension
5. To assist the surgeon in differentiating arterial and venous structures
6. To identify patients at high risk for post-operative complications (no good guidelines exist at present)

TCD information is limited, for the present, to continuous assessment of the systolic, diastolic and mean flow velocities in the target vessel and calculation of the resistive or pulsatility indices. TCD's greatest advantages are that it is relatively inexpensive, non-invasive, non-radioactive and furnishes beat-to-beat (i.e., continuous) information about the cerebral circulation.

Direct Doppler ultrasound interrogation of surface vessels exposed during neurosurgical procedures is possible using a higher frequency (e.g., 20 MHz) probe[23,24]. Although primarily a research tool at present, this has potential application during AVM resection to gauge local hemodynamic effects as well as to aid in differentiating between venous and arterial structures.

A significant advance presently just over the horizon is the use of albumin "microspheres"[55] to increase the sensitivity of existing ultrasound techniques, and this would open up the possibility of making quantitative measurements of intravascular transit time. Furthermore, it may be possible to simulate "autoradiography" of the exposed brain by interrogating a field of view during passage of the tracer[50].

Thermal Clearance

Carter has recently reviewed the use of thermal diffusion CBF monitoring[9]. The thermal diffusion CBF technique has been used to describe autoregulatory dysfunction in a number of operative settings, including cerebral aneurysm[11,31,32,46,64] and AVM surgery[4,43]. The greatest strength of thermal diffusion is the ability to have continuous, on-line and at least semi-quantitative assessment of cortical perfusion. The time resolution is 1–2 seconds. The probe measures perfusion in a relatively small (and indeterminate) area of cortex in the vicinity of the temperature sensors. If CBF changes take place in an entire vascular supply territory (e.g., MCA), the focal flow changes in the probe's vicinity should reflect the regional changes.

Extraneous thermal influences, such as operating room lights, electrocautery interference and irrigation of the surgical field, may result in erroneous CBF changes. A further nettlesome problem is frequent separation of the probe from the cortical surface. Any detected CBF change must therefore be carefully related to activity in the operative field.

Since the methodology does not require sophisticated equipment, does not use ionizing radiation and is theoretically easy to use, it deserves further development for use during neurosurgery[46]. In our view, the biggest obstacle with current technology is the probe design. They do not give stable and reliable measurements. Reliability could be enhanced with probes that have multiple sensing ports, in conjuction with a true multichannel device or a single channel multiplexed configuration. Hopefully, newer instruments will offer such improvements.

Laser Doppler

Laser Doppler is similar in application to thermal diffusion as a direct cortical method. It measures a very limited area of tissue perfusion. It has been used in the setting of AVMs to describe changes in regional blood flow[53]. The CBF information is highly focal in nature, since the probe reflects perfusion in an area of cortex of only several cubic millimeters. Similar to thermal diffusion, it is relatively inexpensive, does not involve ionizing radiation and furnishes continuous information. Additionally, it is possible to adjust the time resolution to look at events with a very short time constant, such as the effects of pulsatile pressure on local flow phenomena[38]. It is non-invasive in the sense that it may be used with an open skull at operation with no additional preparation. It is well suited to animal studies[12] and, with improved probe design, may be adaptable for routine human use[38,60].

The same problems of probe design mentioned for thermal clearance apply to laser Doppler.

133-Xe CBF

We utilize 133-Xe CBF measurements to monitor for hemispheric flow changes during the course of resection[72]. One detector is placed ipsilateral to the AVM, 5–6 cm from the nidus margin but within the same major arterial supply territory. Another detector is placed contralaterally in homologous position. An i.v. bolus of 10–20 mCi of 133-Xe in saline is injected for each CBF measurement and the tracer washout is recorded for 11 minutes. We have found the technique useful in monitoring for large increases in hemispheric CBF, which appear to be related to the development of post-operative hyperperfusion problems[29]. We are currently assessing the use of pressure challenges to further unmask autoregulatory dysfunction which may portend post-operative calamity[29]. Inadequate probe design rears its head here as well. Current probes are difficult to place in the operative field where perhaps the highest likelihood of detecting changes exists.

Electrophysiologic

Intraoperative EEG monitoring achieves several of the stated goals of hemodynamic monitoring. Titration of barbiturates to burst-suppression can be done with simple hemispheric leads and a one- or two-channel system. A bihemispheric system can be of aid in ruling out global ischemia during the conduct of induced hypotension.

Although we routinely use hypocapnia as an adjunct to brain relaxation, even during induced hypotension, it has been suggested that this may be associated with post-operative complications[42]. Notwithstanding, we have had no instances of hemispheric cerebral ischemia during combined hypocapnia and induced hypotension.

Monitoring for regional or local ischemia may be accomplished using electrode strips placed directly on the cortical surface[72a]. Such highly localized recording may be of use in assessing interruption of vessels, possibly supplying normal tissue in addition to verifying that functional areas around the nidus are not adversely affected by induced hypotension.

Pressure Measurements

Technically, direct puncture of feeding arteries and draining veins is a relatively simple procedure with little if any associated morbidity.

We have transduced pressures using both 26-g and 30-g short needles. Although 30-g needles significantly dampen the arterial waveform, the fidelity of the tracings with 26-g needles is remarkably good, even with long extension tubing interposed between measuring site and transducer. Increasing needle size larger than 26-g does not seem to *visually* improve the waveform. Vascular pressures have been reported by several groups[5,25,45,57]. The patients with the lowest arterial and highest draining venous pressure (hence the largest pressure gradient) may be those patients at greatest risk for post-operative hemodynamic complications[45]. Pressure measurements may also have some use in differentiating arterial and venous structures in certain cases. Unfortunately, the surgical anatomy does not allow measurement in all cases. Development of reliable microtonometers would be useful in this setting.

In a related application, pressure measurements may be of value during the course of cerebral embolization procedures. Pressure measurements in this setting have been reported[15,17,28]. We find such measurements useful for gauging the effect of shunt obliteration. Furthermore, intermittent pressure transduction of the intracranial vascular catheters can also indicate damage to the lumen or wall of the catheter.

Anesthetic Technique

ICP control, so often discussed regarding anesthetic care of neurosurgical patients, is rarely a problem with the AVM patient coming for elective resection[10]. Notwithstanding, these patients may have decreased intracranial compliance, so the usual caveats about avoiding cerebral vasodilators are reasonable. More importantly, excellent brain relaxation is required for optimal access to the operative site with a minimum of retraction and manipulation. Rational vasopressor and anesthetic choice are equally as important as spinal drainage, mannitol, good head positioning and modest hypocapnia.

Excepting cerebral vasodilators, the specific choice of anesthesia should be guided primarily by other cardio- and cerebro-vascular considerations.

We employ an isoflurane/N_2O technique, because it offers superior systemic blood pressure control over most techniques. Total intravenous anesthetic techniques, or combinations of inhalational and intravenous methods can be effectively used as well[51]. Some centers use additional barbiturate loading during the resection to afford additional protection against cerebral ischemia, resulting in perhaps a greater degree of brain relaxation and protection against acute hyperemia[58]. Barbiturates can be titrated to an EEG response of burst-suppression as an endpoint. The main price to be paid for barbiturate use is delayed emergence and the foregoing of early post-operative neurologic exams. Cardiac depression is not a problem in the patient without concomitant heart disease[61,62]. There is no compelling evidence that any anesthetic agent-other than barbiturates[56] – is superior in terms of cerebral protection[39,44]. Etomidate[68] and, more recently, propofol[30,52] are attractive alternatives, but the evidence for cerebral protection is not as compelling as for the barbiturates. If found to be protective, propofol-induced burst-suppression would offer the prospect of a more rapid recovery than with barbiturates.

Nimodipine has now found a place in the treatment and prevention of ischemic complications in the patient with aneurysmal subarachnoid hemorrhage. Should nimodipine be used routinely in all high-risk neuro-surgical patients? It is an intuitively appealing propo-sition, but there are no studies to base this on. As far as intraoperative management is concerned, there appears to be no argument against its use as hemody-namic stability is maintained and it has a tendency to lower systemic arterial pressure[63]. Available evi-dence suggests that excessive cerebral vasodilation from nimodipine should not be a problem[18,19].

Induced Hypotension

Profound levels of induced hypotension may occasi-onally be necessary during AVM resection and know-ledge of cardiac filling pressures is a tremendous aid. The subject of induced hypotension is discussed exten-sively in the neuroanesthesia literature. There is little to add here regarding the choice of agents except our bias that cerebral vasodilators are best avoided in the AVM patient. Vasoactive agents may affect different aspects of autoregulatory behavior, as illustrated by recent evidence that nitroprusside impairs the ability of the circulation to maintain CBF when CPP is lowered but not when CPP is increased[59]. In the setting of the AVM patient post-treatment, this may have the theoretical disadvantage of exacerbating cere-bral hyperemia. The prevalence, extent and clinical significance of such effects are far from clear at present. But, in the already murky waters that surround the cerebral hemodynamic changes in the perioperative period, one less unknown variable is preferable.

For intraoperative induced hypotension, we prefer to use alpha- and beta-adrenergic antagonists such as labetolol and esmolol, often in conjunction with in-creasing the inspired concentration of isoflurane.

The interaction of induced hypotension and hypo-capnia remains an ill-defined area. During *global* ischemia, the lower limit of autoregulation does not seem to be effected by hypocapnia[2]. And during *regional* ischemia, hypocapnia may improve CBF to critical areas[3,47]. Although we routinely maintain modest hypocapnia during hypotension, some authors recommend normocapnia[14].

An important interface between "anesthesia" and "blood pressure control" is likely to develop with the advent of newer alpha-2 adrenergic agonists. Clonidine is the prototype of this class of agents. Not only does it appear to smooth out the course of intraoperative blood pressure changes[21,36] but it has additional anesthetic properties[16]. Experience with neurosurgical

patients is still limited[20]. Dexmedetomidine is under investigation as a more specific alpha-2 agonist[13].

Fluid Replacement

Fluid restriction is a time-honored means of guarding against brain swelling in the neurosurgical patient. Adequate volume status to maintain stable systemic hemodynamics, especially with the application of in-duced hypotension, may require liberal fluid adminis-tration. Recent evidence reconciles these two apparently divergent goals. There is an emerging body of evidence that it is tonicity of replacement therapy, not oncotic pressure, that determines water movement into both normal and damaged brain[26,65,66,73]. Even mildly hypotonic fluids such as lactated Ringers solution, if given in sufficient quantity, may aggravate brain swell-ing more than do isotonic crystalloid or colloids. *Isotonic* fluid replacement with either blood, saline or hetastarch after forebrain ischemia in the rat appears to yield similar results in terms of cerebral edema formation[67]. The most important point is that fluid should never be withheld at the expense of a stable cardiovascular status. Serum tonicity can be easily monitored if large volumes of crystalloid are needed.

There is considerable evidence that glucose aggra-vates cerebral injury (see the lucid review by Lanier[33]). Routine perioperative steroid use invariably causes hyperglycemia.

In 40 non-diabetic AVM patients undergoing iso-flurane anesthesia the mean ($\pm$ SE) preoperative glu-cose was 98 ± 5 mg/dl, increasing to 129 ± 6 mg/dl at 2.8 ± 0.1 hours from induction, and to 140 ± 7 mg/dl at 66 ± 0.4 hours from induction (all significantly dif-ferent, $p < .0001$). These are levels of hyperglycemia that may place the brain at risk for worsened outcome as demonstrated in a primate model[34]. Studies are in progress to determine at what point therapy is indicated to lower plasma glucose levels (David S. Warner, Personal Communication).

Glucose-containing fluids have no place in the intraoperative management of the high-risk neuro-surgical patient, except possibly in the management of the neonate or diabetic patient with recent or current insulin therapy.

Temperature

A fall in body temperature during general anesthesia and surgery is common for many reasons, including exposure of skin and body cavities, administration of i.v. fluids, irrigation, anesthetic effects on temperature regulation and mechanical ventilation with dry gases. Decreases in temperature below 34 °C are associated with many well-known adverse effects, including increased risk of infection, peripheral vasoconstriction (with post-rewarming vasodilation), increased blood viscosity, decreased respiratory drive to hypercapnia or hypoxia, post-operative shivering (and increased whole body oxygen consumption) and cardiac arrhythmias. In the otherwise uncomplicated neurosurgical patient, two important concerns are the interaction between mild hypothermia and (a) the reversal of neuromuscular blockade[41] and (b) the residual anesthetic effects and neurologic sequelae of the procedure, which may cause delayed emergence.

There is, however, accelerating interest in using small reductions in body temperature to either treat or prevent cerebral ischemic injury. Although profound hypothermia is routinely used for protection of the central nervous system, anesthesiologists and surgeons have traditionally struggled to prevent even modest drops in body temperature during surgery. However, it is becoming increasingly apparent that even decreases in body temperature to 33–34 °C can have a dramatic effect on neurological damage[6-8]. In fact, modest temperature reduction appears to be much more powerful than choice of anesthesia as a determinate of outcome from cerebral ischemia[54].

A fall in body temperature of 1 or 2 °C is commonly observed during surgery. This may be partially prevented or reversed by use of heating blankets and humidification of inspired gases. Modest falls in temperature are probably not associated with adverse systemic complications, although the issue has not yet been studied prospectively. We have retrospectively examined a recent series of 59 elderly carotid endarterectomy patients at our institution with a mean ($\pm$ SD) age of 68 ± 8 yrs. Esophageal temperature at 3.1 ± 0.5 h after induction (20 minutes prior to emergence) was 35.62 °C. None of these patients had clinically significant episodes of shivering or myocardial ischemia in the immediate post-operative period.

In another series of AVM patients, temperature at dural closure was $35.5 \pm .1$ (n = 84, range: 32.7 to 37.7) at 7.6 ± 0.2 hours after induction (range 4 to 13.2 hours) without obvious clinical complications attributable to this temperature reduction.

We currently believe the normal temperature decrease seen with induction of anesthesia (34–35 °C)

should be allowed to persist until closure is imminent and only then should the heating blankets and humidifiers be called into active play and warming towards 37 °C started. However, before firm recommendations for deliberate mild hypothermia can be made, additional studies of safety need to be performed. Rebound hyperthermia is a concern[5].

Emergence and Initial Recovery: Blood Pressure Control

A particularly challenging aspect of perioperative care is emergence and initial recovery. It is our impression that the AVM patient tends to be systemically (and in the worst case, cerebrally) hyperdynamic, and evidence for this has been recently presented[49].

After phenylephrine-induced blood pressure augmentation during drying of the operative bed and discontinuation of isoflurane, we routinely use large doses of labetolol (300 to 1000 mg) and, after a 0.5 to 1 mg/kg loading dose, a variable esmolol infusion to maintain the patient's blood pressure within 10% below the usual ward values.

Postoperative

Blood Pressure Control

The points related to intraoperative blood pressure management apply here; we find esmolol to be an effective agent to smoothly cap the blood pressure swings common in the initial ICU period. There are seemingly refractory cases of post-operative hypertension, however, and the clinician must be prepared to draw upon all the agents in the available armamentarium[40]. A possible advantage of barbiturate loading may be a smoother emergence from anesthesia, although emergence may be more protracted and without the benefit of neurologic exams.

The sword of aggressive blood pressure control can cut both ways. There are rare cases of ischemic deficits due to intraoperative sacrifice of, for example, an *en passage* feeding vessel, which may result in a deficit ascribed to brain retraction or the resection itself. Marginally perfused areas may be critically dependent on collateral perfusion pressure. Maintenance of low or even normal blood pressure may be inadequate and result in infarction if unrecognized. Unfortunately, the only reliable means of verifying this at the present time in most centers is immediate post-operative angiography or, more rarely, intraoperative angiography.

Temperature

Whether post-ischemic hypothermia of any degree improves[27] or does not improve[70] the outcome from a cerebral ischemic event is not clear at present. But it certainly seems prudent to aggressively treat fever and strictly maintain normothermia.

Acknowledgements

The authors wish to thank Joyce Ouchi for assistance in preparation of the manuscript.

References

1. Aaslid R (1987) Visually evoked dynamic blood flow response of the human cerebral circulation. Stroke 18: 771–775

2. Artru AA, Katz RA, Colley PS (1989) Autoregulation of cerebral blood flow during normocapnia and hypocapnia in dogs. Anesthesiology 70: 288–292

3. Artru AA, Merriman HG (1989) Hypocapnia added to hypertension to reverse EEG changes during carotid endarterectomy. Case report. Anesthesiology 70: 1016–1018

4. Barnett GH, Little JR, Ebrahim ZY, Jones SC, Friel HT (1987) Cerebral circulation during arteriovenous malformation operation. Neurosurgery 20: 836–842

5. Baker KZ, Young WL, Stone JG, Kader A, Baker CJ, Solomon RA (1993) Deliberate mild intraoperative hypothermia for craniotomy (abstract). Anesthesiology 79: A225

6. Busto R, Dietrich WD, Globus MY-T, Ginsberg MD (1989) The importance of brain temperature in cerebral ischemic injury. Stroke 20: 1113–1114

7. Busto R, Dietrich WD, Globus MY-T, Valdes I, Scheinberg P, Ginsberg MD (1987) Small differences in intraischemic brain temperature critically determine the extent of ischemic neuronal injury. J Cereb Blood Flow Metab 7: 729–738

8. Busto R, Globus MY-T, Dietrich WD, Martinez E, Valdes I, Ginsberg MD (1989) Effect of mild hypothermia on ischemia-induced release of neurotransmitters and free fatty acids in rat brain. Stroke 20: 904–910

9. Carter LP (1991) Surface monitoring of cerebral cortical blood flow. Cerebrovasc Brain Metab Rev 3: 246–261

10. Chimowitz MI, Little JR, Awad IA, Sila CA, Kosmorsky G, Furlan AJ (1990) Intracranial hypertension associated with unruptured cerebral arteriovenous malformations. Ann Neurol 27: 474–479

11. Dernbach PD, Little JR, Jones SC, Ebrahim ZY (1988) Altered cerebral autoregulation and CO_2 reactivity after aneurysmal subarachnoid hemorrhage. Neurosurgery 22: 822–826

12. Dirnagl U, Pulsinelli W (1990) Autoregulation of cerebral blood flow in experimental focal brain ischemia. J Cereb Blood Flow Metab 10: 327–336

13. Doze VA, Chen B-X, Maze M (1989) Dexmedetomidine produces a hypnotic-anesthetic action in rats via activation of central alpha-2 adrenoceptors. Anesthesiology 71: 75–79

14. Drummond JC, Shapiro HM (1990) Cerebral physiology. In: Miller RD (ed) Anesthesia, 3rd Ed, Vol 1. Churchill Livingstone, New York, pp 621–649

15. Duckwiler G, Dion J, Vinuela F, Jabour B, Martin N, Bentson J (1990) Intravascular microcatheter pressure monitoring: experimental results and early clinical evaluation. AJNR 11: 169–175

16. Flacke JW, Bloor BC, Flacke WE, et al (1987) Reduced narcotic requirements by clonodine with improved hemodynamic and adrenergic stability in patients undergoing coronary bypass surgery. Anesthesiology 67: 11–19

17. Fleischer LH, Young WL, Pile-Spellman J, terPenning B, Kader A, Mohr JP, Stein BM (1993) The relationship of transcranial Doppler flow velocities and arteriovenous malformation feeding artery pressures. Stroke 24: in press

18. Gaab MR, Haubitz I, Brawanski A, Korn A, Czech T (1985) Acute effects of nimodipine on the cerebral blood flow and intracranial pressure. Neurochirurgia (Stuttg) 28: 93–99

19. Gaab MR, Rode CP, Schakel EH, Haubitz I, Bockhorn J, Brawanski A (1985) The influence of the Ca-antagonist nimodipine on regional and global cerebral blood flow. Klin Wochenschr 63: 8–15

20. Gaumann D, Tassonyi E, Rivest R, Fathi M, Reverdin A (1990) Effects of clonidine premedication in neurosurgical patients. Anesthesiology 73: A1211

21. Ghignone M, Calvillo O, Quintin L (1987) Anesthesia and hypertension: the effect of clonidine on perioperative hemodynamics and isoflurane requirements. Anesthesiology 67: 3–10

22. Giller CA (1991) A bedside test for cerebral autoregulation using transcranial Doppler ultrasound. Acta Neurochir (Wien) 108: 7–14

23. Gilsbach J, Hassler W (1984) Intraoperative Doppler and real time sonography in neurosurgery. Neurosurg Rev 7: 199–208

24. Hassler W (1986) Hemodynamic aspects of cerebral angiomas. Acta Neurochir (Wien) [Suppl]37: 1–36

25. Hassler W, Steinmetz H (1987) Cerebral hemodynamics in angioma patients: an intraoperative study. J Neurosurg 67: 822–831

26. Hindman BJ, Funatsu N, Cheng DCH, Bolles R, Todd MM, Tinker JH (1990) Differential effect of oncotic pressure on cerebral and extracerebral water content during cardiopulmonary bypass in rabbits. Anesthesiology 73: 951–957

27. Hoffman WE, Werner C, Baughman VL, Thomas C, Miletich DJ, Albrecht RF (1991) Postischemic treatment with hypothermia improves outcome from incomplete cerebral ischemia in rats. J Neurosurg Anesth 3: 34–38

28. Jungreis CA, Horton JA, Hecht JA, Hecht ST (1989) Blood pressure changes in feeders to cerebral arteriovenous malformations during therapeutic embolization. AJNR 10: 575–578

29. Young WL, Kader A, Prohovnik I, Ornstein E, Fleischer LH, Ostapkovich N, Jackson LD, Stein BM (1993) Pressure autoregulation is intact after arteriovenous malformation resection. Neurosurgery 32: 491–497

30. Kochs E, Hoffman WE, Werner C, Thomas C, Albrecht RF, Esch JSa (1992) The effects of propofol on brain electrical activity, neurologic outcome, and neuronal damage following incomplete ischemia in rats. Anesthesiology 76: 245–252

31. Koshu k, Hirota S, Sonobe M, et al (1987) Continuous recording of cerebral blood flow by means of a thermal diffusion method using a Peltier stack. Neurosurgery 21: 693–698

32. Kuwayama N, Takaku A, Harada J, Fukuda O, Endo S, Saito T (1991) Modified thermal diffusion flow probe for the continuous monitoring of cortical blood flow. Neurosurgery 29: 583–589

33. Lanier WL (1991) Glucose management during cardiopulmonary bypass: cardiovascular and neurologic implications. Editorial. Anesth Analg 72: 423–427

34. Lanier WL, Stangland KJ, Scheithauer BW, Milde JH, Michenfelder JD (1987) The effects of dextrose infusion and head position on neurologic outcome after complete cerebral ischemia in primates: examination of a model. Anesthesiology 66: 39–48

35. Lindegaard K-F, Grolimund P, Aaslid R, Nornes H (1986) Evaluation of cerebral AVM's using transcranial Doppler ultrasound. J Neurosurg 65: 335–344

36. Longnecker DE (1987) Alpine anesthesia: can pretreatment with clonidine decrease the peaks and valleys? Editorial. Anesthesiology 67: 1–2

37. Massaro AR, Young WL, Kader A, Ostapkovich N, Tatemichi TK, Stein BM, Mohr JP (1994) Characterization of arteriovenous malformation feeding vessels by CO_2 reactivity AJNR Jan/Feb: in press
38. Meyerson BA, Gunasekera L, Linderoth B, Gazelius B (1991) Bedside monitoring of regional cortical blood flow in comatose patients using laser Doppler flowmetry. Neurosurgery 29: 750–755
39. Michenfelder JD, Sundt TM, Fode N, Sharbrough FW (1987) Isoflurane when compared to enflurane and halothane decreases the frequency of cerebral ischemia during carotid endarterectomy. Anesthesiology 67: 336–340
40. Miller LR, Drummond JC, Lamond RG (1991) Refractory arterical and intracranial hypertension in the intensive care unit: successful treatment with isoflurane. Anesthesiology 74: 946–949
41. Miller RD (1981) Anesthesia, 1st Ed, Vol 1. Churchill Livingstone, New York, p 762
42. Morgan MK, Johnston IH, Sundt TM Jr (1989) Normal perfusion pressure breakthrough complicating surgery for the vein of Galen malformation: report of three cases. Neurosurgery 24: 406–409
43. Nagao S, Ueta K, Mino S, et al (1989) Monitoring of cortical blood flow during excision of arteriovenous malformations by thermal diffusion method. Surg Neurol 32: 137–143
44. Nehls DG, Todd MM, Spetzler RF, Drummond JC, Thompson RA, Jonshon PC (1987) A comparison of the cerebral protective effects of isoflurane and barbiturates during temporary focal ischemia in primates. Anesthesiology 66: 453–464
45. Nornes H, Grip A (1980) Hemodynamic aspects of cerebral arteriovenous malformations. J Neurosurg 53: 456–464
46. Ohmoto T, Nagao S, Mino S, Fujiwara T, Honma Y (1991) Monitoring of cortical blood flow during temporary arterial occlusion in aneurysm surgery by the thermal diffusion method. Neurosurgery 28: 49–55
47. Paulson OB, Strandgaard S, Edvinsson L (1990) Cerebral autoregulation. Cerebrovasc Brain Metab Rev 2: 161–192
48. Petty GW, Massaro AR, Tatemichi TK, et al (1990) Transcranial Doppler ultrasonographic changes after treatment for arteriovenous malformations. Stroke 21: 260–266
49. Porembka D, Ebrahim Z, Bloomfield E, Stuebing R (1991) The postoperative hyperdynamic cardiovascular response following intracranial excision of arterial venous malformation (AVM). Abstract. Anesthesiology 75: A215
50. Rampil IJ (1991) Cerebral perfusion mapping with ultrasound contrast. Anesthesiology 75: A1006
51. Ravussin P, Tempelhoff R, Modica PA, Bayer-Berger M-M (1991) Propofol vs. thiopental-isoflurane for neurosurgical anesthesia: comparison of hemodynamics, CSF pressure, and recovery. J Neurosurg Anesth 3: 85–95
52. Ridenour TR, Warner DS, Todd MM, Gionet TX (1992) Comparative effects of propofol and halothane on outcome from temporary middle cerebral artery occlusion in the rat. Anesthesiology 76: 807–812
53. Rosenblum BR, Bonner RF, Oldfield EH (1987) Intraoperative measurement of cortical blood flow adjacent to cerebral AVM using laser Doppler velocimetry. J Neurosurg 66: 396–399
54. Sano T, Drummond JC, Patel PM, Grafe MR, Watson JC, Cole DJ (1992) A comparison of the cerebral protective effects of isoflurane and mild hypothermia in a model of incomplete forebrain ischemia in the rat. Anesthesiology 76: 221–228
55. Schlief R (1991) Ultrasound contrast agents. Curr Opin Radiol 3: 198–207
56. Shapiro HM (1985) Barbiturates in brain ischaemia. Br J Anaesth 57: 82–95
57. Spetzler RF, Martin NA, Carter LP, Flom RA, Raudzens PA, Wilkinson E (1987) Surgical management of large AVM's by staged embolization and operative excision. J Neurosurg 67: 17–28
58. Spetzler RF, Martin NA, Carter LP, Flom RA, Raudzens PA, Wilkinson E (1987) Surgical management of large AVM's by staged embolization and operative excision. J Neurosurg 67: 17–28
59. Stange K, Lagerkranser M, Sollevi A (1991) Nitroprusside-induced hypotension and cerebrovascular autoregulation in the anesthetized pig. Anesth Analg 73: 745–752
60. Steinmeier R, Fahlbusch R, Powers AD, Dotterl A, Buchfelder M (1991) Pituitary microcirculation: Physiological aspects and clinical implications. A laser-Doppler flow study during transsphenoidal adenomectomy. Neurosurgery 29: 47–54
61. Stone JG, Young WL, Khambatta HJ, et al (1991) Effect of massive intraoperative thiopental loading on cardiovascular hemodynamics and myocardial performance. Case report. J Neurosurg Anesth 3: 132–135
62. Stone JG, Young WL, Marans ZS, Khambatta HJ, Solomon RA, Smith CR, Ostapkovich N, Jamdar SC, Diaz J (1993) Cardiac performance preserved despite thiopental loading. Anesthesiology 79: 36–41
63. Stullken EH, Johnston WE, Prough DS, Balestrieri EF, McWhorter JM (1985) Implications of nimodipine prophylaxis of cerebral vasospasm on anesthetic management during intracranial aneurysm clipping. J Neurosurg 62: 200–205
64. Tenjin H, Hirakawa K, Mizukawa N, et al (1988) Dysautoregulation in patients with ruptured aneurysms: Cerebral blood flow measurements obtained during surgery by a temperature-controlled thermoelectrical method. Neurosurgery 23: 705–709
65. Todd MM, Tommasino C, Moore S (1985) Cerebral effects of isovolemic hemodilution with a hypertonic saline solution. J Neurosurg 63: 944–948
66. Tommasino C, Moore S, Todd MM (1988) Cerebral effects of isovolemic hemodilution with crystalloid or colloid solutions. Crit Care Med 16: 862–868
67. Warner DS, Boehland LA (1988) The effects of iso-osmolal hemodilution on post-ischemic brain water content in the rat. Anesthesiology 68: 86–91
68. Watson JC, Drummond JC, Patel PM, Sano T, Akrawi W, U HS (1992) An assessment of the cerebral protective effects of etomidate in a model of incomplete forebrain ischemia in the rat. Neurosurgery 30: 540–544
69. Weissman C, Ornstein E, Young WL (1991) Arterial pulse contour analysis tending of cardiac output: hemodynamic manipulations during neurosurgery. Abstract. Anesthesiology 75: A469
70. Welsh FA, Harris VA (1991) Postischemic hypothermia fails to reduce ischemic injury in gerbil hippocampus. J Cereb Blood Flow Metab 11: 617–620
71. Young WL, Ornstein E, Prohovnik I, Ostapkovich N, Solomon RA, Stein BM (1991) Cardiac output does not influence cerebral hyperemia after arteriovenous malformation shunt ablation. Abstract. J Cereb Blood Flow Metab 11 [Suppl 2]: S48
72. Young WL, Prohovink I, Ornstein E, et al (1990) The effect of arteriovenous malformation resection on cerebrovascular reactivity to carbon dioxide. Neurosurgery 27: 257–267
72. a. Young WL, Solomon RA, Pedley TA, Ross L, Schwartz AE, Ornstein E, Matteo RS, Ostaprovich N (1989) Direct cortical EEG monitoring during temporary vascular occlusion for cerebral aneurysm surgery. Anesthesiology 71: 794–799
73. Zornow MH, Todd MM, Moore SS (1987) The acute cerebral effects of changes in plasma osmolality and oncotic pressure. Anesthesiology 67: 936–941

Correspondence: William L. Young, M.D., Neuroanesthesia, Room 901, 161 Ft. Washington Ave., New York, NY, 10032 U.S.A.

Deep Barbiturate Anesthesia in the Multi-Staged Treatment of Large Deep AVMs

H.S. U[1], **J.C. Drummond**[2], and **M.M. Todd**[3]

[1]Division of Neurosurgery, [2]Department of Anesthesia, University of California San Diego, San Diego, California, U.S.A., and [3]Department of Anesthesia, University of Iowa College of Medicine, Iowa City, Iowa, U.S.A.

Summary

Surgical treatment of large AVMs (greater than 4 cm in diameter) of the cerebral hemisphere which are associated with significant arteriovenous shunting can lead to the occurrence of sudden catastrophic cerebral swelling and/or hemorrhage with resultant morbidity and mortality. In order to reduce the incidence of this unfavorable outcome, multi-stage excision of large AVMs has evolved. Even though the incidence of malignant swelling and/or hemorrhage has been reduced and the outcome of treatment has improved, sudden swelling and/or hemorrhage nevertheless does occasionally occur. In these situations, the emergent administration of high doses of barbiturates has been most effective in reducing increased intracranial pressure. Even then, severe impairment of the extruded cerebrum can ensue leading to marked disability. In order to prevent and protect the brain from these insults, we developed and instituted the use of an anesthetic technique consisting of the elective administration of high dose barbiturate combined with moderate hypothermia. The intent was to achieve the lowest possible cerebral blood flow and cerebral blood volume at the time of AVM resection so as to minimize vascular engorgement and the magnitude of any sudden hemodynamic changes in the AVM and the surrounding tissues. With the institution of this anesthetic regimen, the incidence of sudden cerebral swelling/hemorrhage has been reduced. The attendant treatment results have also improved suggesting that the use of elective, high dose barbiturate anesthesia may have a role in the surgical treatment of large high flow AVMs.

Keywords: Barbiturate anesthesia; large AVM; staged therapy.

Introduction

Arteriovenous malformations (AVMs) divert blood from the surrounding brain. When this vascular shunting or 'steal' becomes significant, hypoperfusion of surrounding tissues may result leading to vascular dysautoregulation and ischemia[3,12,14]. During progressive elimination of an AVM with significant flow through the AV shunts, a catastrophic condition may develop where the brain suddenly and rapidly becomes very swollen and hemorrhages occur at sites distant from the AVM bed[1,2,4,9,10,13,17-19]. The involved cerebrum often extrudes through the craniotomy. Left untreated, this condition is frequently fatal. Standard maneuvers designed to relax the brain such as hypotension, hyperventilation, head elevation, and the administration of mannitol are often not successful. The infusion of high doses of barbiturates is commonly necessary to salvage an otherwise hopeless situation[8]. Even then, marked disability from damage to the extruded brain can result.

We reasoned that, while the emergent administration of barbiturates is often adequate as a salvage maneuver, the elective use of a high dose barbiturate anesthetic in the surgical treatment of these high flow AVMs might further facilitate our multi-stage elimination of these lesions[5,6,15,16]. When barbiturate anesthesia is induced prior to AVM resection, global cerebral blood flow and blood volume is likely to be markedly reduced. This might be expected to minimize vascular engorgement and thus the effects of any sudden changes of hemodynamics around the AVM. In addition, the brain would be much relaxed and this would also minimize the need for extensive brain retraction and facilitate exposure of deep brain structures[17,18].

Material and Methods

Patient Population

Elective deep barbiturate anesthesia was evaluated in a population of 17 patients having deep periventricular AVMs. This included 12 women and 5 men with an average age of 32 years (range 12–60 years). There were two small (< 2 cm in diameter), five moderate (2–4 cm in diameter), and 10 large (> 4 cm in diameter) lesions.

Operative Regimen

All patients were treated with staged excision of their lesions after preoperative embolization. The operative approach taken were either through initial exposure of the feeding arteries in the sylvian fissure prior to AVM dissection (the first four patients) or through a transfrontal, transventricular approach with exposure of the AVM through the ependymal surface and isolation of the lesion from the rest of the ventricular system (the subsequent 13 patients).

Anesthetic Regimen

The first four patients received routine fentanyl/N_2O/relaxant anesthetics for a total of 11 operations. In view of the occurrence of three episodes of malignant brain swelling/hemorrhage which had to be treated with the emergent administration of high doses of barbiturates, the anesthetic regimen for the subsequent operations was modified to involve an elective, high dose barbiturate anesthetic.

In all patients who received a deep barbiturate anesthetic, systemic and pulmonary arterial pressures, EEG, EKG, oxygen saturation, expired gases and temperature were monitored. Anesthesia was induced with thiopental (3–6 mg/kg) followed by fentanyl (8–15 µg/kg) and a non-depolarizing relaxant. Anesthesia was initially maintained with N_2O and isoflurane, while $PaCO_2$ was adjusted to 25–30 mm Hg. Cooling blankets were used to maintain a temperature of 30–32 °C by the time of dural opening. During opening of the skull, an infusion of pentobarbital (loading dose: 10–15 mg/kg given over 30–60 min) was begun. The rate of infusion was titrated to achieve and maintain deep burst-suppression of the EEG. Isoflurane was then discontinued. These patients were usually moderately hypotensive (systolic BP 90–100 mm Hg). At the completion of an uneventful operation, pentobarbital administration was discontinued and rewarming was begun at a rate of 1 °C per hour. An ICP monitor was placed and the $PaCO_2$ was elevated to normal as long as the ICP was acceptable. Paralysis and sedation were maintained for 24 hours during which time arterial pressures were strictly controlled.

Results

During the 11 staged operations for the first four patients, three episodes of sudden brain swelling/hemorrhage occurred (Table 1). In each case, swelling became fully manifest within one minute. The protruding cerebral cortex was hyperemic. All standard methods to relax the brain were unsuccessful. The emergent administration of high doses of barbiturates was invariably necessary. Even when the patient survived, significant impairment referable to the herniated region of the cerebral cortex was invariably evident. In patient 3, intraventricular hemorrhage also occurred. The resultant brain compression was ultimately fatal.

The subsequent 13 patients received a total of 27 operations for excision of their AVMs. All operative

Table 1

Total number of operations (stages)	38
Number of operations without barbiturate anesthesia	11
Incidence of malignant brain swelling/hemorrhage	3
Number of operations with deep barbiturate anesthesia	27
Incidence of malignant brain swelling/hemorrhage	1

stages were performed under elective deep barbiturate anesthesia. The brain was much more relaxed, and this facilitated the transfrontal exposure of the ventricular system and the feeding vessels to the AVMs. As a result of the delayed initiation of barbiturate administration, the use of intraoperative cooling and the early termination of barbiturate administration, emergence from the drug-induced coma was complete within 36 to 48 hours. Blood pressure fluctuations were minimal and generally easily controlled. Only one episode of malignant cerebral swelling/hemorrhage occurred leading to extensive intracerebral and intraventricular hematomas. The patient was markedly impaired but recovered sufficiently to be a functional member of her family. This same patient also developed significant cerebral pulsation in a previous operation. That operation was immediately terminated uneventfully.

Discussion

Neurologic dysfunction referable to cerebral regions surrounding large AVMs is presumed to result from ischemia due to the shunting of blood from these regions through the AV shunts. Impairment of autoregulatory mechanisms in these areas has also been demonstrated[3,12,14]. When these AVMs are located in the central gray, involvement of vasoactive centers may theoretically occur[7,11]. Surgical treatment of large and centrally situated AVMs may occasionally be complicated by the sudden onset of massive and rapid cerebral swelling/hemorrhage in the peri-AVM tissues[1,2,4,9,10,13,17–19]. Since these occurrences are ill understood and unpredictable, their treatment must, of necessity, occur under emergency circumstances and high doses of barbiturates are frequently required[8]. The outcome is far from satisfactory.

In order to reduce the incidence of malignant cerebral swelling/hemorrhage, we instituted an elective high dose barbiturate anesthesia in combination with moderate hypothermia in the surgical treatment of large, deep AVMs[5,6,8,15,16,18]. The rationale is that by the marked suppression of metabolic demand, any ischemia as a result of increased intracranial pressure from swelling and/or hemorrhage would be better tolerated. In addition, severe metabolic suppression should reduce cerebral blood flow and volume to very low levels. This may in turn enable the surrounding, dysregulated vascular bed to better accommodate the blood redistributed to it from the AVM as a result of progressive AVM elimination. Alternatively, this would reduce the volume of blood available to fill a paralyzed vascular system arising from damage to deep vasomotor centers. Our experience suggests that the institution of elective high dose barbiturate anesthesia combined with moderate hypothermia may have contributed to the reduced incidence of malignant brain swelling/ hemorrhage since our basic microsurgical technique in the staging of the operations and in AVM dissection was not altered. It is unlikely that the change from the sylvian to the transventricular approach contributed substantially to the reduced incidence of malignant swelling as this was directed to the prevention of unnoticed intraventricular hemorrhages and direct AVM exposure. In addition to the reduced incidence of brain swelling/hemorrhage, the degree of hemodynamic fluctuation (hypertension in particular) attendant upon emergence from anesthesia also appears to have been reduced. Thus a more controlled post-operative course has resulted.

In summary, the employment of an elective deep barbiturate anesthesia in combination with moderate hypothermia in the surgical treatment of large deep AVMs appears to have reduced the incidence of malignant brain swelling/hemorrhage with an overall improved outcome. The mechanisms involved remain unknown, however, and need to be investigated.

Acknowledgement

The authors would like to thank the UCSD Operating Room and Intensive Care Unit personnel as well as Neurosurgical and Anesthesia house-staff and faculty for unfailing and dedicated support; and R. Morgan for excellent editorial assistance.

References

 1. Batjer HH, Devous MD Sr, Meyer YJ, Purdy PD, Samson DS (1988) Cerebrovascular hemodynamics in arteriovenous malformation complicated by normal perfusion pressure breakthrough. Neurosurgery 22: 503–509
 2. Batjer HH, Purdy PD, Giller CA, Samson DS (1989) Evidence of redistribution of cerebral blood flow during treatment for an intracranial arteriovenous malformation. Neurosurgery 25: 599–605
 3. Batjer H, Samson D (1992) Clinical evaluation of cerebral perfusion in AVM patients. New trends in management of cerebro-vascular malformations: abstracts. Verona, pp 111–112
 4. Day AL, Friedman WA, Sypert GW, Mickle JP (1982) Successful treatment of the normal perfusion pressure breakthrough syndrome. Neurosurgery 11: 625–630
 5. Drummond JC, Todd MM, U HS (1985) The effect of high dose sodium thiopental on brain stem auditory and median nerve somatosensory evoked responses in humans. Anesthesiology 63: 249–254
 6. Drummond JC, Tood MM, Schubert A, U HS (1987) Effect of the acute administration of high dose pentobarbital on human brain stem auditory and median nerve somatosensory evoked responses. Neurosurgery 20: 830–835
 7. Iadecola C, Mraovitch S, Meeley MP, Reis DJ (1983) Do cholinergic neurons of the basal forebrain cholinergic system mediate the cortical vasodilation elicited by fastigial nucleus stimulation in rats? J Cereb Blood Flow Metab 3: S178–S179
 8. Marshall LF, U HS (1983) Treatment of massive intraoperative brain swelling. Neurosurgery 13: 412–414
 9. Morgan MK, Johnston I, Besser M, Baines D (1987) Cerebral arteriovenous malformations, steal, and the hypertensive breakthrough threshold. J Neurosurg 66: 563–567
10. Mullan S, Brown FD, Patronas NJ (1979) Hyperemic and ischemic problems of surgical treatment of arteriovenous malformations. J Neurosurg 51: 757–764
11. Nakai M, Iadecola C, Reis DJ (1982) Global cerebral vasodilation by stimulation of rat fastigial cerebellar nucleus. Am J Physiol 243: H226–H235
12. Piepgras A, Leinsinger G, and Schmiedek P (1992) Cerebrovascular reserve capacity in AVM patients. New trends in management of cerebro-vascular malformations: abstracts. Verona, p 109
13. Spetzler RF, Wilson CB, Weinstein P, Mehdorn M, Townsend J, Telles D (1978) Normal perfusion pressure breakthrough theory. Clin Neurosurg 25: 651–672
14. Talacchi A, Pasqualin A, Chioffi F (1992) The role of hemodynamic assessment in the management of cerebral AVMs. New trends in management of cerebro-vascular malformations: abstracts. Verona, p 113
15. Todd MM, Drummond JC, U HS (1985) The hemodynamic consequences of high-dose thiopental anesthesia. Anesth Analg 64: 681–687
16. Todd MM, Drummond JC, U HS (1987) Hemodynamic effects of high dose pentobarbital: studies in elective neurosurgical patients. Neurosurgery 20: 559–563
17. U HS (1985) Microsurgical excision of paraventricular arteriovenous malformations. Neurosurgery 16: 293–303
18. U HS, Kerber CW, Todd MM (1992) Multi-modality treatment of deep basal cerebral arteriovenous malformations. Surg Neurol 38: 192–203
19. Young WL, Solomon RA, Prohovnik I, Ornstein E, Weinstein J, Stein BM (1988) ^{133}Xe blood flow monitoring during arteriovenous malformation resection: a case of intraoperative hyperperfusion with subsequent brain swelling. Neurosurgery 22: 765–769

Correspondence: Hoi Sang U, M.D., Division of Neurosurgery, University of California, San Diego, CA 92103-8893, U.S.A.

Surgery of Deep-Seated and Posterior Fossa AVMs

Medial Hemisphere and Tentorial Ring AVMs

B.M. Stein, R.A. Solomon, and **A. Kader**

Neurological Institute of the Columbia-Presbyterian Medical Center, New York, New York, U.S.A.

Summary

Our experience with deep and obscure AVMs located along the medial hemisphere and those related to the tentorial ring numbers approximately 30.

Because most of these areas are obscure and the AVMs cannot be approached in a perpendicular fashion, surgical techniques have to be modified in dealing with these lesions. Brain retraction may become a problem in terms of effecting an appropriate exposure and therefore the various roots and challenges related to the exposure will be detailed in this discussion.

The group of malformations in these regions often involve portions of the limbic system and significant effects may be noticed on the memory systems. It would appear that the most significant effect on memory is related to cerebral dominance and this raises some interesting implications in terms of the processing of memory.

The postoperative results have been excellent in this group of difficult cases and justifies surgical intervention toward complete obliteration of these lesions.

Keywords: Microsurgery; AVMs; vascular malformations of the brain.

Introduction

This group of arteriovenous malformations (AVMs) which generally follow the limbic system deserves special mention because of: (1) their location in relatively obscure areas of the brain, (2) their relative inaccessibility, suggesting inoperability, and (3) their moderate proportion of all AVMs, approximately 15%.

While convexity AVMs whether on the surface or subsurface are straightforward in terms of surgical approach[3] (perpendicular to the lesion), this group of AVMs by their obscure location requires specialized surgical approaches which are often tangential to the lesion[1,2,4,6-13]. Brain retraction is a problem, therefore measures for brain relaxation are essential in the surgical management of these lesions. Furthermore, the arterial supply is often deep to the malformation and approached during the latter stages of the operation.

Materials and Methods

We have divided the regions of the medial hemisphere according to the diagram of Fig. 1[11]. As noted, these lesions tend to follow the limbic system and the more anteriorly placed ones are approached either when superior by an interhemispheric anterior transcallosal approach, or when inferior by a sylvian splitting or parahippocampal approach[4]. Those located in the area of the trigone as represented by C in Fig. 1, are in a "no man's land" and are approached with difficulty by the various routes so indicated. In these cases, it may be necessary to approach transcortically even though the lesion is deep, especially when located on the nondominant hemisphere.

To those lesions that are situated close to the tentorial ring[5], there are basically three exposures as shown in Fig. 2A illustrates an interhemispheric posterior approach to the vein of Galen and midbrain region, the parahippocampal gyrus and the trigonal region of the lateral ventricle. The approach represented in Fig. 2B is particularly useful for those lesions located around the midbrain or pineal region and is over the cerebellum via the posterior fossa. The approach represented in 2C is subtentorial with retraction of the temporal lobe or on occasion with resection of a small portion of the inferior

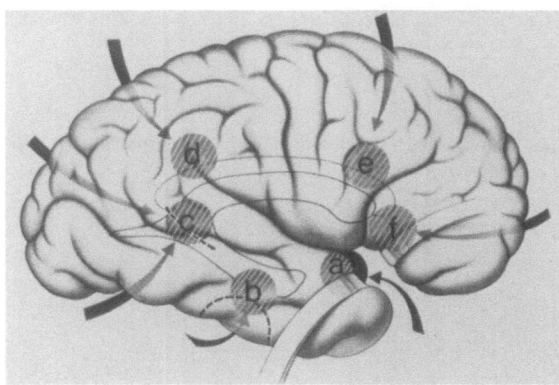

Fig. 1. Drawing of location of medial hemisphere lesions. As noted in the text, various exposures as illustrated by the arrows in the drawing can be utilized to remove the lesions. Most difficult are those located at site c, and these can be approached from three directions: (1) infratemporal, (2) interhemispheric paraparietal and in rare cases via the dotted line approach which is transcortical utilizing the posterior middle temporal gyrus

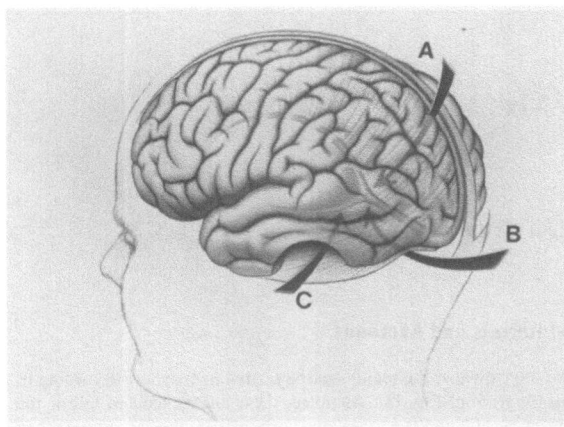

Fig. 2. Drawing of the three (*A, B, C*) basic routes to the tentorial incisura (explanation in text)

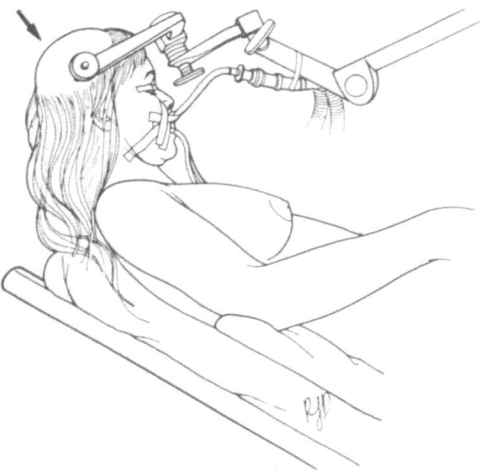

Fig. 3. Sitting-slouch position used for interhemispheric approach to more posterior lesions

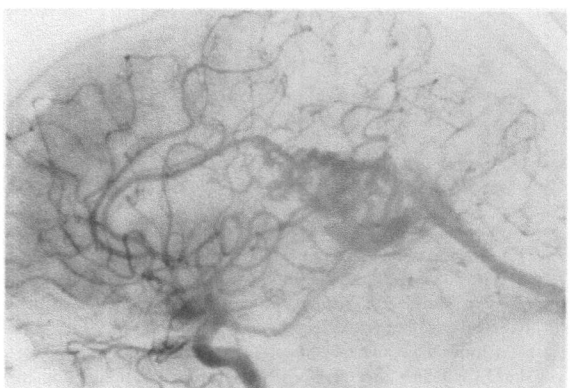

Fig. 4. Lateral right carotid arteriogram showing arteriovenous malformation of the posterior corpus callosum, cingulate gyrus, parahippocampal area, approached by an interhemispheric paraparietal route

temporal gyrus, care being taken that there is no injury or occlusion of the vein of Labbé.

For the interhemispheric transcallosal approach, a semisitting-slouch position is utilized for the more posteriorly palced lesions (Fig. 3) and a supine position with the head flexed for the more anteriorly placed lesions.

A number of cases are illustrated in the following Figs. 4–7 and 8. These represent the different regions and the various approaches used for them (please note in particular the legends with these figures). In some of the lesions, especially those located in the diencephalic region, the lesion has been associated with a small aneurysm on one of the penetrating arteries (Fig. 6). These aneurysms have been controlled at the time of the AVM obliteration by microsurgical techniques.

Most of these lesions are modest in size and fed by relatively small but high flow, perforating arteries. They do not lend themselves well to preoperative embolization unless there is major feeding from one of the three primary circulations: anterior, middle or posterior.

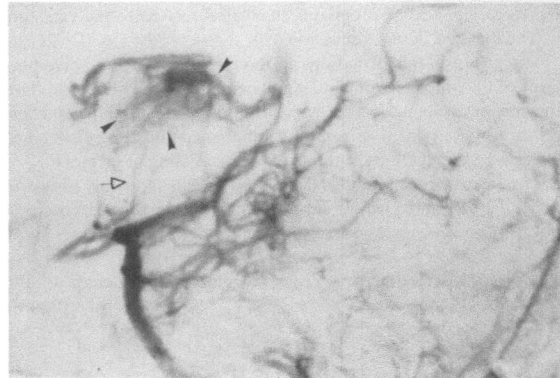

Fig. 5. Right lateral vertebral arteriogram showing thalamic AVM (arrowheads) fed by thalamoperforate arteries (open arrow). This lesion was successfully obliterated by a posterior interhemispheric transcallosal exposure

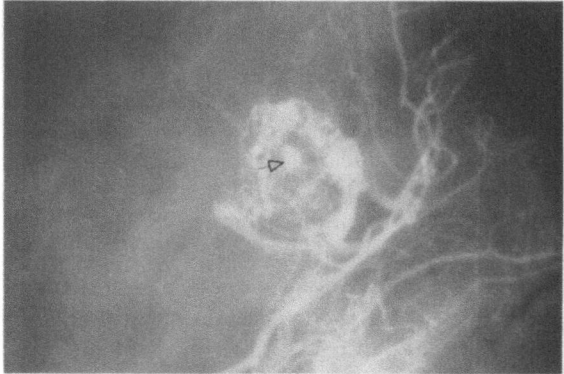

Fig. 6. Lateral vertebral arteriogram showing a complex but small AVM of the trigone region and an associated choroidal artery aneurysm (open arrow). Both lesions were successfully removed by a posterior interhemispheric exposure

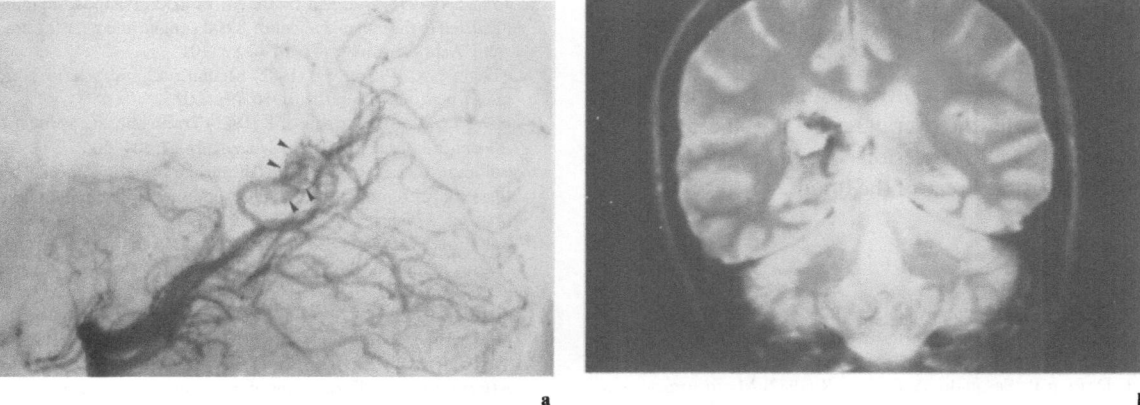

Fig. 7. (a) Lateral vertebral arteriogram showing small AVM of the trigone (arrowheads). (b) Coronal MRI scan emphasizing the anatomy and relationships gleaned from the MRI, so important to the posterior interhemispheric exposure of these AVMs.

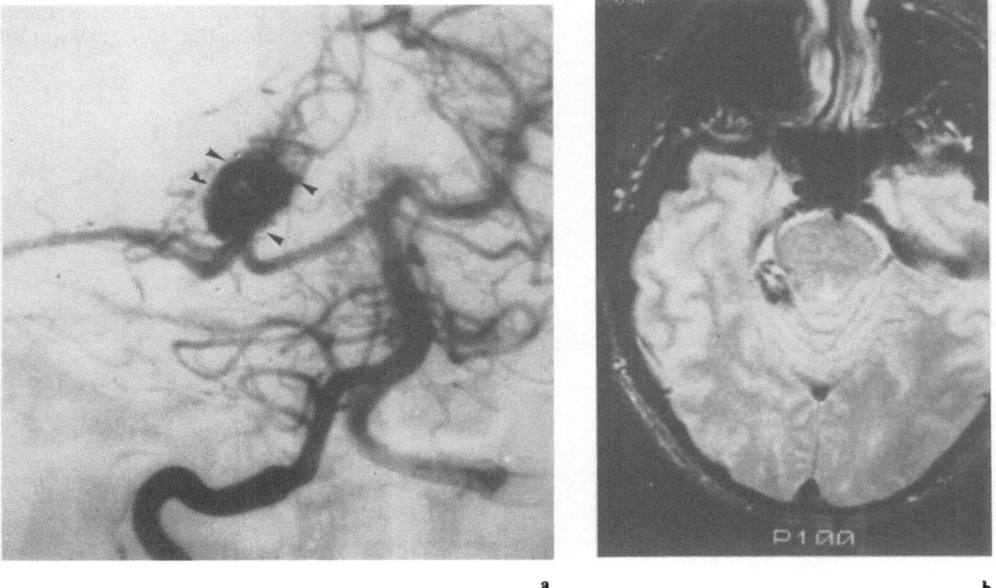

Fig. 8. (a) AP vertebral arteriogram showing subtentorial AVM fed by the superior cerebellar artery (arrowheads). This lesion was successfully removed by a subtemporal transtentorial exposure. (b) Axial MRI showing relation of AVM to brain stem, cerebellum and temporal lobe

Conclusions

These medial hemisphere and tentorial ring AVMs represent a unique group of cases. They represent a surgical challenge in terms of exposure and in terms of removal, all related to the anatomy of the lesion. Specialized surgical approaches must be used to deal with such lesions[2,5,7,11,12]. The physiological out-

comes of the surgery depend on the location being intimate to the limbic system. Accordingly, those lesions which are associated with thalamocaudate anatomy, especially on the dominant side, have been associated with memory problems. These problems can occur from hemorrhage or surgical resection. They are mainly related to the acquisition of memory and interference with that function. Fortunately these problems are temporary and in all but the rare case, the patient will return to normal memory control after a period of time.

In spite of the difficulty encountered in the surgery of these lesions, the overall results have been excellent and equate well with lesions of similar size located in more accessible areas of the brain.

References

1. DaPian R, Pasqualin A, Scienza R, Vivenza C (1980) Microsurgical treatment of ten arteriovenous malformations in critical areas of the cerebrum. Microsurgery 1: 305–320
2. DaPian R, Pasqualin A, Scienza R (1982) Microsurgical treatment of juxtapeduncular angiomas. Surg Neurol 17: 16–29
3. Drake CG (1983) Arteriovenous malformations of the brain. The options for management. Engl J Med 309: 308–310
4. Garrido E, Stein BM (1978) Removal of an arteriovenous malformations from the basal ganglion. J Neurosurg Psychiatr 41: 992–995
5. Heros RC (1982) Arteriovenous malformations of the medial temporal lobe. Surgical approach and neuroradiological characterization. J Neurosurg 56: 44–52
6. Juhasz J (1978) Surgical treatment of arteriovenous angiomas localized in the corpus callosum, basal ganglia and near the brain stem. Acta Neurochir (Wien) 40: 83–101
7. Martin NA, Wilson CB (1982) Medial occipital arteriovenous malformations. J Neurosurg 56: 798–802
8. Nehls D, Marano S, Spetzler R (1985) Transcallosal approach to the contralateral ventricle. J Neurosurg 62: 304–306
9. Solomon RA, Stein BM (1987) Interhemispheric approach for the surgical removal of thalamocaudate arteriovenous malformations. J Neurosurg 66: 345–351
10. Solomon RA, Stein BM (1986) Surgical treatment of arteriovenous malformations that follow the tentorial ring. Neurosurgery 6: 708–715
11. Stein BM (1984) Arteriovenous malformations of the medial cerebral hemisphere and the limbic system. J Neurosurg 60: 23–31
12. Yaşargil MG, Jain KK, Antic J, Laciga R, Kletter G (1976) Arteriovenous malformations of the anterior and middle portion of the corpus callosum: microsurgical treatment. Surg Neurol 5: 67–80
13. Yaşargil MG, Jain KK, Antic J, Laciga R (1976) Arteriovenous malformations of the splenum of the corpus callosum: microsurgical treatment. Surg Neurol 5: 5–14

Correspondence: Bennett Stein, M.D., Neurological Surgery, College of Physicians and Surgeons of Columbia University, 710 West 168th Street, New York, NY 10032, U.S.A.

Surgical Experience with Callosal-Cingular and Inferior Limbic AVMs

R. Da Pian, A. Pasqualin, R. Scienza, B. Cappelletto, and **C. Licata**

Department of Neurosurgery, City Hospital, Verona, Italy

Summary

From 1970 to 1992, 51 patients with limbic AVMs were operated on in our department with a direct microsurgical approach. 31 malformations were located in the corpus callosum and/or gyrus cinguli, 20 in the uncal, juxtapeduncular or parasplenial area (= inferior limbic AVMs). On angiography, deep feeders were present in 26% of callosal-cingular and 45% of inferior limbic AVMs; a deep drainage was observed in 65% of callosal-cingular and in 85% of inferior limbic AVMs. Preoperative embolization was undertaken in 4 callosal-cingular and in 4 inferior limbic AVMs. Adopted surgical approaches were: ipsilateral interhemispheric for callosal-cingular AVMs, combined pterional-subtemporal for uncal AVMs, subtemporal for juxtapeduncular AVMs, and posterior interhemispheric for parasplenial AVMs. During surgery paraventricular bleeding was very rare for AVM volumes within 10 cm³; over this size, it was observed in about half of cases. Postoperative hematomas were observed rarely for both locations, and only for AVMs over 10 cm³. Transient postoperative deficits were observed in about one third of cases, regardless of AVM location. Permanent postoperative deficits were never observed for callosal-cingular AVMs, while they were not infrequent for inferior limbic AVMs. Two patients died: one was operated on in deep coma, and the other developed acute postoperative renal failure. It is concluded that for these patients: a) results of surgery are mainly dependent upon AVM volume; b) preoperative embolization can be useful for lesions over 10 cm³; c) there is a substantial risk of ischemic complications for uncal AVMs.

Keywords: Cerebral AVMs; AVM volume; corpus callosum; limbic system.

Introduction

Supratentorial deep-seated arteriovenous malformations remain a challenge for the neurosurgeon. Their removal requires a thorough understanding of the midline and deep anatomical structures and an adequate experience of the various surgical approaches, always with the aim to avoid injury to the functional parenchyma adjacent to the AVM.

The aim of this paper is to present our experience in the operative treatment of 51 patients with callosal-cingular and mesial temporal (or inferior limbic) AVMs and to discuss the problems presented by these lesions.

Clinical Material and Methods

From 1970 to 1992, 54 patients with deep-seated AVM were submitted to microsurgical removal in our Department, out of a total of 308 patients with cerebral AVMs operated on in the same period: except 3 AVMs located in the basal ganglia, 31 were located in the corpus callosum and/or gyrus cinguli and 20 in the inferior limbic region.

The mean age of the 51 patients was 29.3 years (ranging from 5 to 69 years); there were 26 female and 25 male patients. For callosal-cingular AVMs, the mean age was 29.2 years and 42% of patients were male; for inferior limbic AVMs, the mean age was 29.7 years and 60% of patients were male.

As for clinical history, intracranial hemorrhage only was observed in 77% of patients with callosal/cingular and in 50% of patients with inferior limbic AVMs, epilepsy only in 13% of patients with callosal/cingular and in 15% of patients with inferior limbic AVMs, epilepsy and hemorrhage in 6% of patients with callosal/cingular and in 20% of patients with inferior limbic AVMs, and other disturbances (mainly headache) in 3% of patients with callosal/cingular and in 15% of patients with inferior limbic AVMs.

The callosal-cingular AVMs were located in the genu in 13 cases, in the pars media in 11 cases and in the splenium in 7 cases (Fig. 1); the inferior limbic AVMs were located in the uncal area in 2 cases (Fig. 2), in the juxtapeduncular area in 12 cases (Figs. 3 and 4) and in the parasplenial area in 6 cases (Fig. 5). Important angiographical features are presented in Table 1; the volume calculation and the classification of the draining system appearing here have been proposed in a recent paper by our group[20].

The majority of patients were submitted to direct microsurgical removal without preoperative embolization; 4 patients with callosal/cingular AVMs (2 with volume within 10 cm³ and 2 over 10 cm³) and 4 patients with inferior limbic AVMs (1 with volume within 10 cm³ and 3 over 10 cm³) were also submitted to preoperative embolization, mostly performed with superselective catheterization of feeders and embolization with threads, as recently reported by our group[3,21].

Preoperative examination was negative in 68% of patients with callosal/cingular and in 75% of patients with inferior/limbic AVMs; mild deficits were observed in 10% of patients with callosal/cingular and in 25% of patients with inferior limbic AVMs; severe motor deficits were observed in 16% of patients with callosal/cingular AVMs; 1 patient with a callosal/cingular AVM was operated on in coma for the presence of a life-threatening hematoma.

All patients with callosal/cingular AVMs were operated on through an ipsilateral interhemispheric approach. A combined pterional/subtemporal approach was used for patients with uncal AVMs, a subtemporal approach for patients with juxtapeduncular

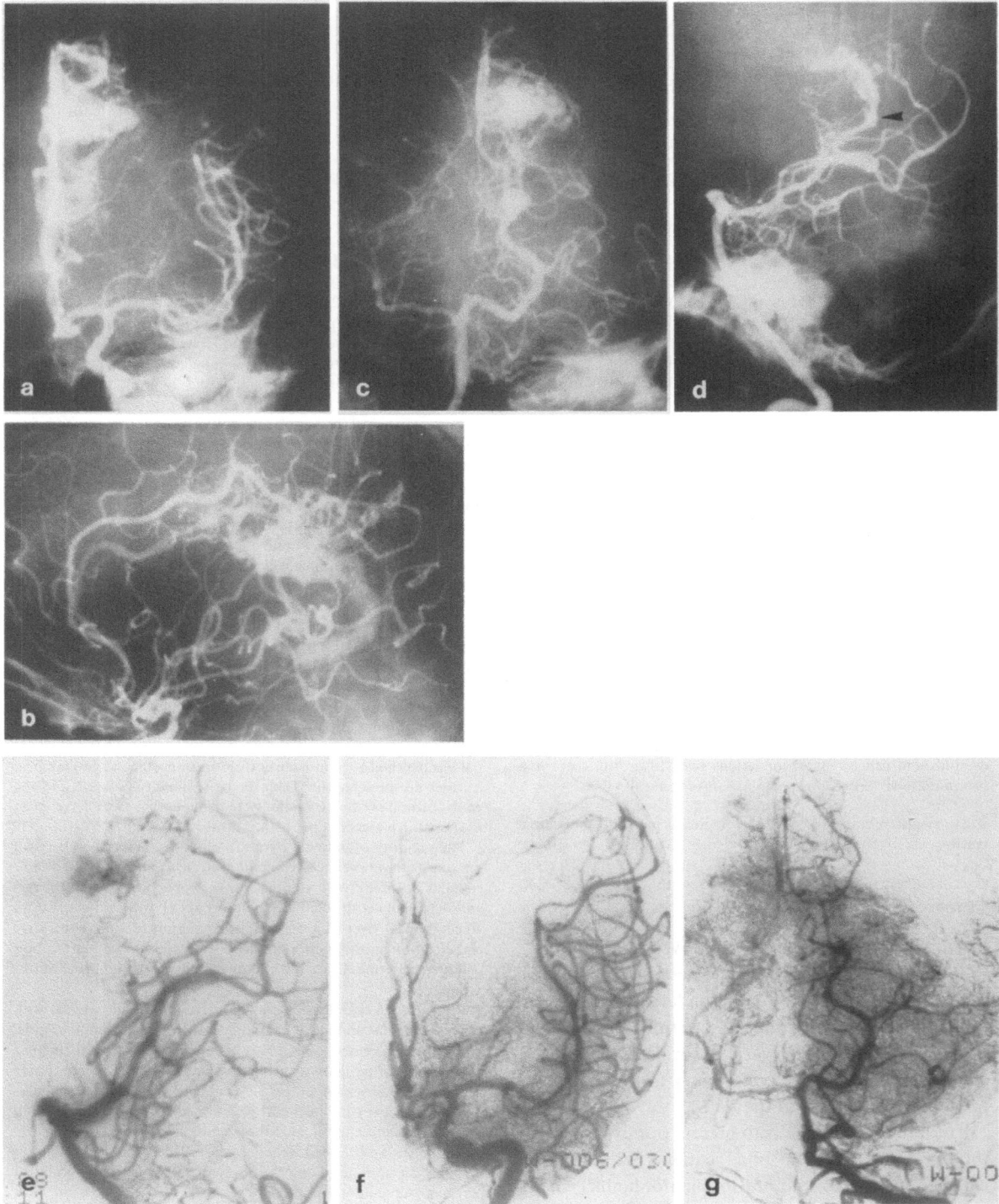

Fig. 1. (a, b) 48 year-old woman with a left splenial AVM (9 cm³), supplied by ectatic left ant. pericallosal artery and by left calloso-marginal artery; (c, d) vascular supply also from the posterior cerebral artery (*PCA*), with large post. pericallosal artery (arrow); (e) result after embolization of PCA; (f, g) postoperative lt. carotid and lt. vertebral angiography. The patient had an uneventful postop. course and was neurologically intact at discharge

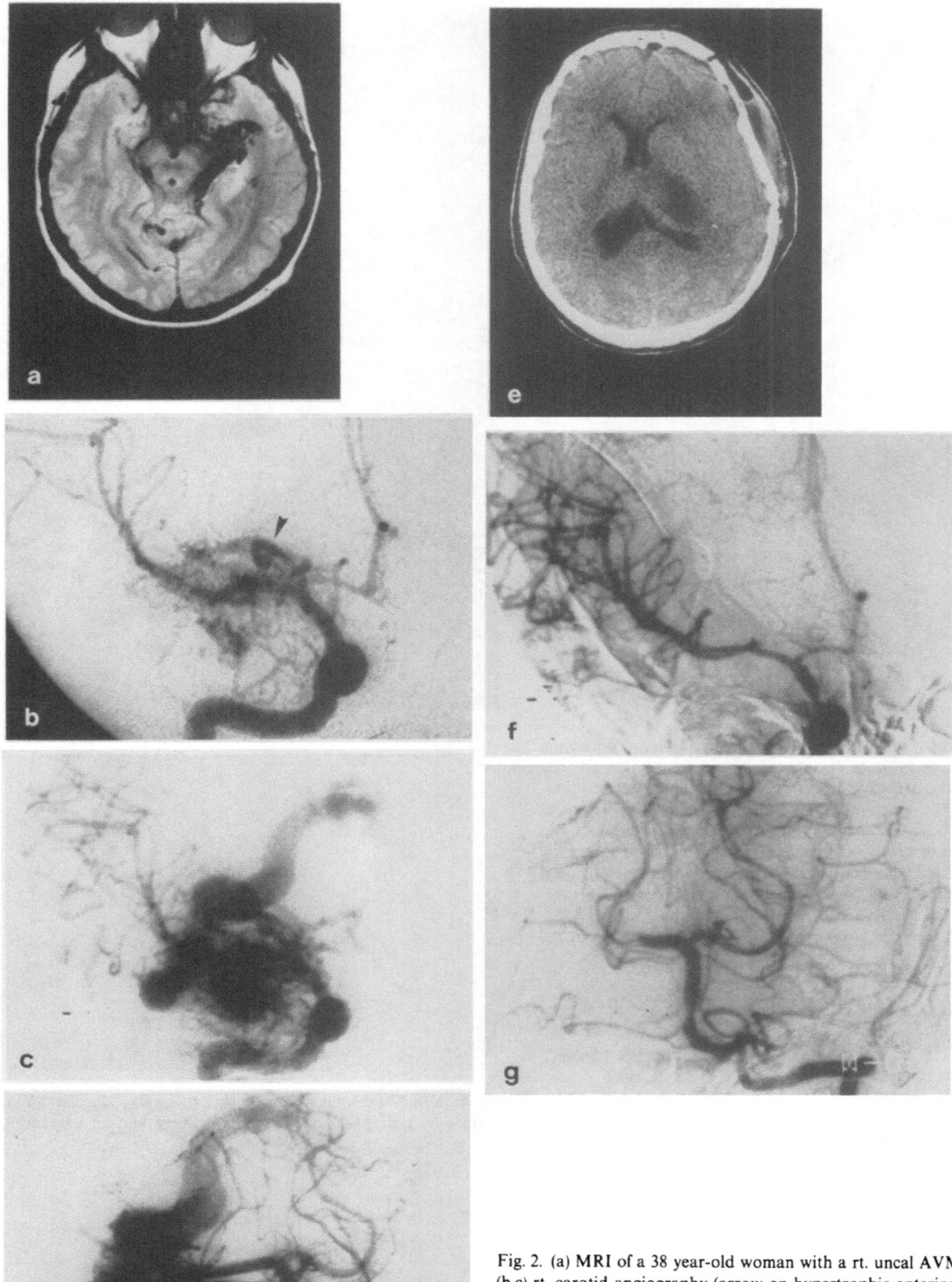

Fig. 2. (a) MRI of a 38 year-old woman with a rt. uncal AVM (14 cm³); (b,c) rt. carotid angiography (arrow on hypertrophic anterior choroidal artery); (d) lt. vertebral angiography, with large PCA also supplying the AVM; (e) postop. CT scan, showing rt. capsulo-thalamic infarction; (f,g) postop. rt. carotid and lt. vertebral angiography. After surgery, the patient developed a severe left hemiparesis and a transient rt. 3rd nerve palsy; 1 year after surgery, the patient can walk independently, but is unable to move her left hand

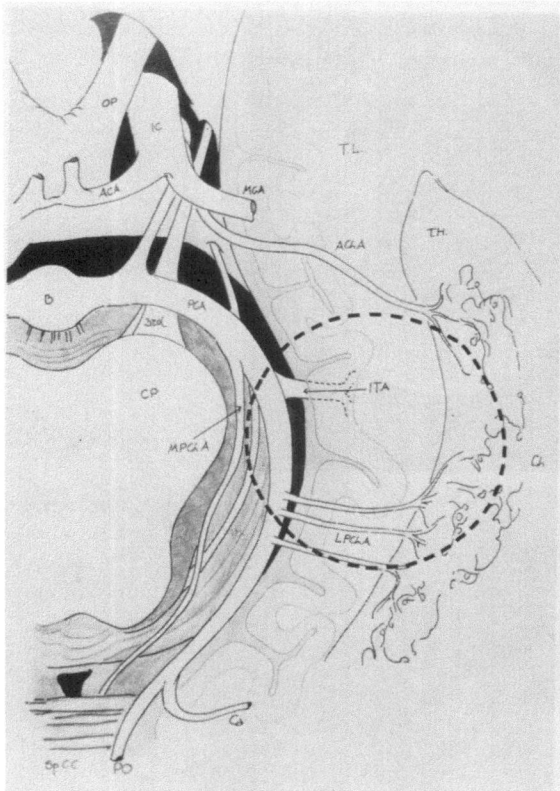

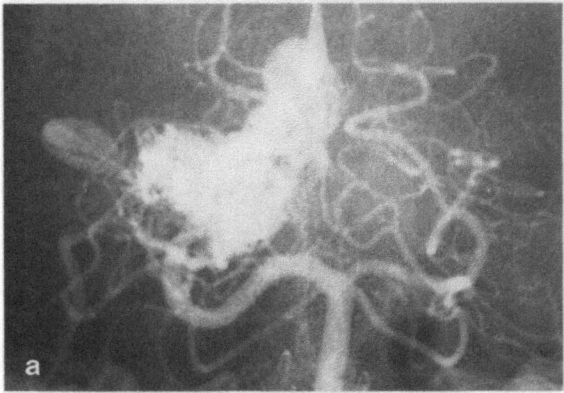

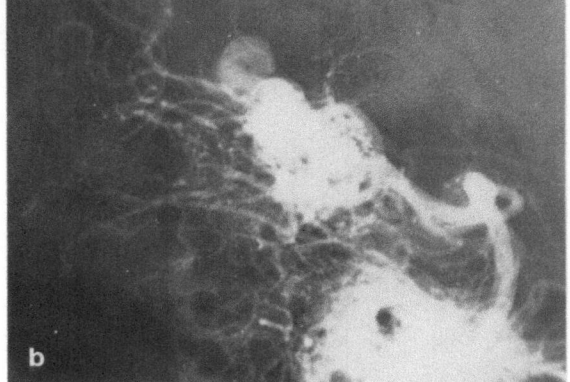

Fig. 3. Vascular supply to juxtapeduncular AVMs, in horizontal section. *OP* optic chiasm; *IC* internal carotid artery; *ACA* anterior cerebral artery; *MCA* middle cerebral artery; *AChA* anterior choroidal artery; *TL* temporal lobe; *TH* temporal horn of the lateral ventricle; *Ch* choroid plexus of the temporal horn; *B* basilar fundus; *3rd* oculomotor nerve; *PCA* posterior cerebral artery; *CP* cerebral peduncle; *ITA* inferior temporal artery (ies); *MPChA* posteromedial choroidal artery; *LPChA* posterolateral choroidal arteries; *4th* trochlear nerve; *Ca* calcarine artery; *PO* parietooccipital artery; *SpCC* splenium of corpus callosum. The area of AVM is indicated by the dashed circle

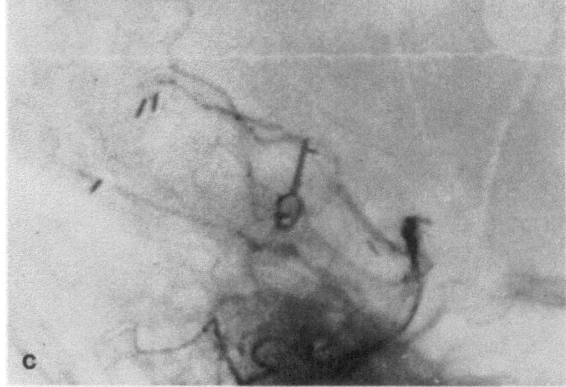

Table 1. *Angiographical Features (51 Patients)*

	Callosal/Cingular (31 cases)		Inferior Limbic (20 cases)	
Large size (volume > 20 cm³)	2	(6%)	5	(25%)
Deep feeders	8	(26%)	9	(45%)
Deep drainage	20	(65%)	17	(85%)
Extensive draining system (grade 3–4)*	5	(16%)	7	(35%)

*See Ref.[20]

Fig. 4. (a, b) 27 year-old woman with a rt. juxtapeduncular AVM (8 cm³); (c) postop. angiography. The patient had an uneventful postop. course and was neurologically intact at discharge

Fig. 5. (a, b) 49 year-old man with a rt. parasplenial AVM (8 cm³) fed by a large rt. PCA; (c) MRI in the same patient; (d) decrease in nidus opacification after embolization; (e, f) postop. angiography. After surgery, the patient developed a complete left hemianopia, slightly improved at follow-up, 1 year later

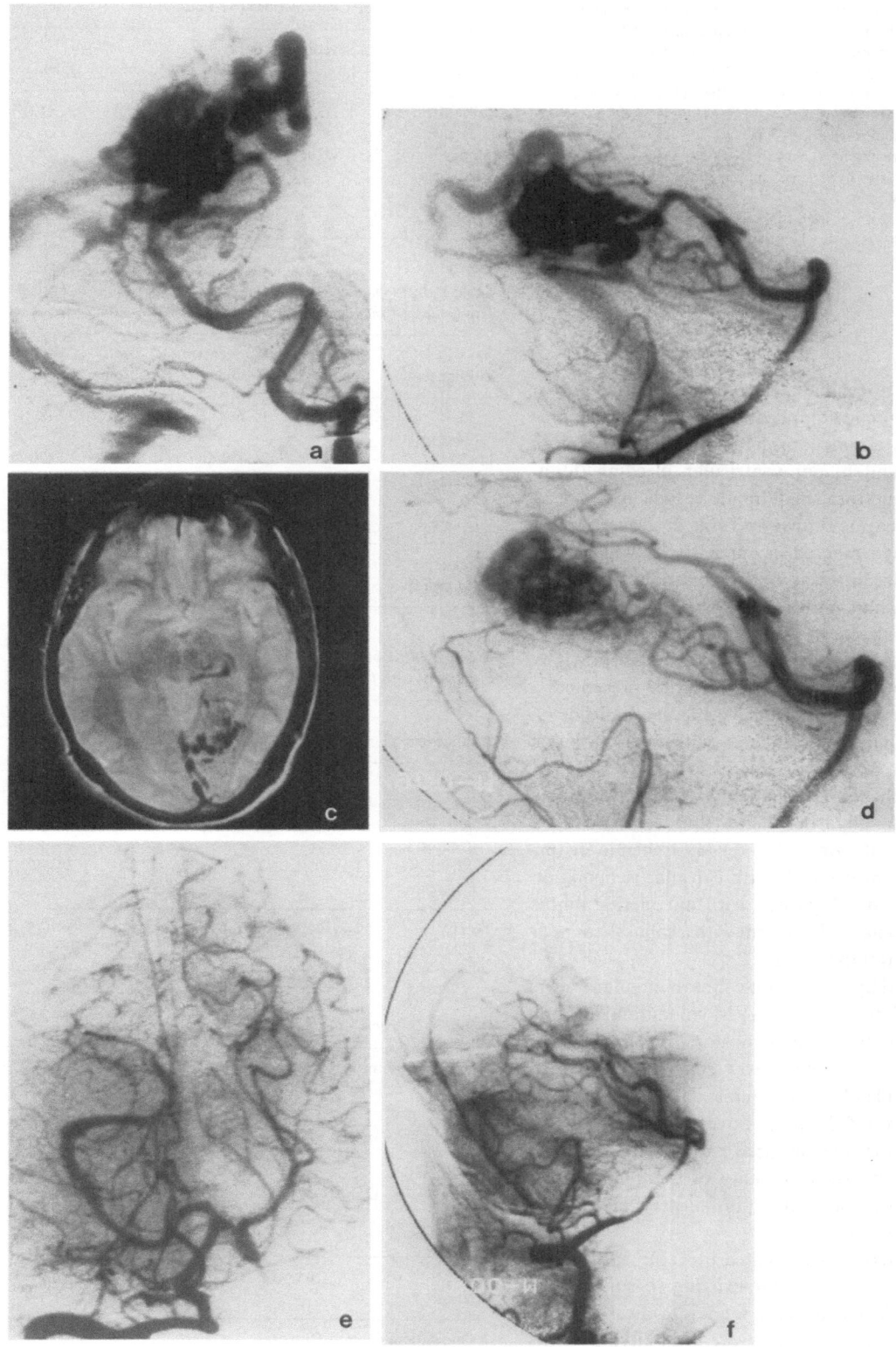

AVMs, and a posterior interhemispheric approach for patients with parasplenial AVMs. During surgery, deep controlled hypotension (induced by sodium nitroprusside at approximately 60 mm/Hg of systolic blood pressure) was used in 15 patients. In all patients, postoperative angiography documented the radical removal of the AVM (one patient with a splenial AVM underwent a second operation for a small rest).

The results of treatment were evaluated by the rate of intraoperative and postoperative hyperemic complications and by the morbidity and mortality rates.

The chi-square test was used to determine statistical significance. Fisher's exact test was used when the sample size was too small for the chi-square test.

Results

As reported in previous papers by our group[20,21] we have separately evaluated intraoperative and postoperative hyperemic complications. For intraop. complicacations, we have considered: a) severe blood loss (>2000 ml), and b) paraventricular bleeding (long-lasting bleeding from small fragile vessels in the paraependymal area); as shown by Table 2, a severe blood loss was rarely observed in our patients, while paraventricular bleeding was not uncommon in patients with inferior limbic AVMs. For postop. complications, we have considered: a) hematoma with midline shift, and b) cerebral edema with midline shift. As shown by Table 2, only 2 patients in our series presented a significant postop. hematoma, while cerebral edema was not uncommon in patients with inferior limbic AVMs. In the postoperative course – apart from hyperemic complications – 3 patients with inferior limbic AVMs presented hydrocephalus (shunted in 1 case), 2 patients with inferior limbic AVMs ischemic disturbances (both uncal AVMs with capsular ischemia on postop. CT scan), 1 patient with an inferior limbic AVM pneumonia, and 1 patient with a callosal/cingular AVM a subdural hygroma.

As presented by Table 3, for callosal-cingular AVMs there was a relation between AVM volume and intraop. hyperemic complications or postop. hematoma, with worse results for volumes over 20 cm³. For inferior limbic AVMs (Table 4), hyperemic complications were already observed for volumes over 10 cm³. Owing to the small number of embolized patients, there was no clear relation between modality of treatment (direct surgery versus embolization plus surgery) and hyperemic complications.

Clinical outcome is presented in Table 5 (for "old" we have meant a deficit pre-existing to surgery; for "minor" a deficit causing a moderate disability; for "major" a deficit causing a severe disability). Patients

Table 2. *Hyperemic Complications (51 Patients)*

Location	Severe blood loss		Paraventr. bleeding		Hematoma		Edema	
Callosal/cingular (31 cases)	1	(3%)	4	(13%)	1	(3%)	3	(10%)
Inferior limbic (20 cases)	2	(10%)	6	(30%)	1	(5%)	5	(25%)
Significance	n.s.		n.s.		n.s.		n.s.	

Table 3. *Intraop. and Postop. Hyperemic Complications in Patients with Callosal-Cingular AVMs, According to AVM Volume*

Volume (cm³)	Severe blood loss		Paraventr. bleeding		Hematoma		Edema	
0–10 (24 cases)	–		1	(4%)	–		2	(8%)
11–20 (5 cases)	–		2	(40%)	–		1	(20%)
>20 (2 cases)	1	(50%)	1	(50%)	1	(50%)	–	
Total (31 cases)	1	(3%)	4	(13%)	1	(3%)	3	(10%)

Table 4. *Intraoperative and Postoperative Hyperemic Complications in Patients with Inferior Limbic AVMs, According to AVM Volume*

Volume (cm³)	Severe blood loss		Paraventr. bleeding		Hematoma		Edema	
0–10 (9 cases)	–		1	(11%)	–		2	(22%)
11–20 (6 cases)	1	(17%)	3	(50%)	1	(17%)	1	(17%)
>20 (5 cases)	1	(20%)	2	(40%)	–		2	(40%)
Total (20 cases)	2	(10%)	6	(30%)	1	(5%)	5	(25%)

Table 5. *Outcome After Surgery (51 Patients)*

Location	Transient deficit		Old perm. deficit		New perm. deficit: minor		major		death	
Callosal/ cingular (31 cases)	9	(29%)	6	(19%)	–		–		2	(6%)*
Inferior/ limbic (20 cases)	5	(25%)	3	(15%)	6	(30%)	2	(10%)	–	
Significance	n.s.		n.s.		p = 0.0002				n.s.	

* One patient comatose preop.

Table 6. *Outcome in Patients with Callosal/Cingular AVMs, According to AVM Volume*

Volume (cm^3)	Transient deficit	Old permanent deficit	New permanent deficit: minor	major	death
0–10 (24 cases)	5 (21%)	6 (25%)	–	–	1 (4%)*
11–20 (5 cases)	3 (60%)	–	–	–	–
>20 (2 cases)	1 (50%)	–	–	–	1 (50%)
Total (31 cases)	9 (29%)	6 (19%)	–	–	2 (6%)*

* One patient comatose preop.

Table 7. *Outcome in Patients with Inferior Limbic AVMs, According to AVM Volume*

Volume (cm^3)	Transient deficit	Old permanent deficit	New permanent deficit: minor	major	death
0–10 (9 cases)	3 (33%)	–	2 (22%)	1 (11%)	–
11–20 (6 cases)	1 (16%)	1 (16%)	2 (33%)	1 (16%)	–
>20 (5 cases)	1 (20%)	2 (40%)	2 (40%)	–	–
Total (20 cases)	5 (25%)	3 (15%)	6 (30%)	2 (10%)	–

with inferior limbic AVMs showed a lower recovery rate and a significantly higher permanent morbidity than patients with callosal/cingular AVMs; in particular new permanent deficits were observed only for inferior limbic AVMs. One death occurred in a patient operated on in coma, with a large hematoma; the other death was in a patient with a large callosal-cingular AVM (>20 cm^3) developing acute renal failure in the postop. period.

A possible relation between AVM volume and clinical outcome is considered in Tables 6 and 7. For callosal/cingular AVMs, volume did not seem to influence clinical outcome (except for a fatality in a patient with a large callosal/cingular AVM). For inferior limbic AVMs, the rate of old and new minor deficits increased with larger volumes; however, major deficits (both due to ischemia) were not influenced by AVM volume.

Discussion

As already proposed by Yaşargil[33] and Stein[28], we have grouped together callosal AVMs and AVMs located in the medial portion of the temporal lobe, under the term "limbic AVMs", i.e. AVMs located along the limbic system. Moreover, we have adopted the term "inferior limbic AVMs" for lesions of the medial temporal lobe, which have been further divided into uncal-juxtapeduncular AVMs (amygdalo-hippocampal AVMs, according to Yaşargil) and parasplenial AVMs (same as Yaşargil[33]; we have also enlarged the group of callosal AVMs to those located in the cingulate gyrus, that give similar problems in the surgical approach[33,34,35]. Limbic AVMs present the common feature of a deep location, forcing the surgeon to approach these lesions through preferential routes, in order to respect the functional parenchyma adjacent to the AVM and yet to gain the best possible exposure of the AVM.

Callosal-Cingular AVMs

As proposed by Yaşargil[33,34,35] these AVMs can be conveniently divided into anterior and middle callosal – which are both approached through a frontal interemispheric route – and posterior callosal (or splenial)

(Fig. 1) – which are approached through a parieto-occipital interhemispheric route. Another feature that separates these 2 groups is constituted by the feeding pattern: while anterior and middle callosal AVMs are fed almost exclusively by the anterior cerebral artery, splenial AVMs are also fed by the posterior cerebral artery, through the posterior pericallosal (or splenial) artery (Fig. 1) and sometimes through the postero-medial choroidal arteries[4,15,32–34,35]. Apart from these differences, callosal/cingular AVMs exhibit common features:

a) when the AVM involves the corpus callosum, the pericallosal artery (or arteries) cover(s) the AVM; conversely the pericallosal artery(ies) is (are) covered by the AVM when the lesion extends to the cingulate gyrus (in this second case, also the calloso-marginal artery can feed the AVM);

b) callosal AVMs often extend to one side and are rarely on the midline; when the lateral extension is marked, the AVM can reach the lateral ventricle and can even receive one or more lentriculostriate or choroidal arteries; generally only one pericallosal artery feeds the angioma directly, while the other sends small branches or is independent of the AVM system;

c) the main feeding artery is often ectatic, and sends many small comb-like branches to the AVM nidus[7,16,33–35]; after the angioma, the pericallosal artery is frequently atresic[32]; in large cingular AVMs, one or more calloso-marginal branches can terminate into the AVM itself;

d) for callosal AVMs, the draining system is often deep, generally towards the internal cerebral vein[33–35], and in this way the draining vein will be approached at the end of the procedure; for cingular AVMs, the draining system is more often towards the superior longitudinal sinus, and – when it is widely represented – it can cause problems in the surgical approach; conversely when the cingular AVM is small, the draining vein can be easily traced backward, in order to better localize the AVM[7,23,33].

From a surgical point of view, the anterior inter-hemispheric approach is always employed in the supine position; for the posterior interhemispheric approach, it is controversial if the patients should stay in the semi-sitting position as suggested by most authors[1,8,28,32,33], in the prone position as suggested by Batjer[2], or in the park-bench position as in some of our cases. Generally the approach is from the non-dominant side if the AVM is on the midline, and from the ipsilateral side if the AVM extends laterally[33–35], although in this latter case some authors have proposed a controlateral interhemispheric approach[1,18]. It is convenient that the flap is wide along the longitudinal sinus, in order to choose – in the individual case – the best route between the veins draining to the longitudinal sinus; it should be added that some of these veins can be carefully dissected for a certain length before entering the sinus, thus enlarging the surgical route. In the callosal AVMs, it is often necessary to open the lateral ventricle in order to close the draining vein; in this area – especially when choroidal and/or lenticulo-striate arteries feed the AVM – the surgeon can face a tedious bleeding[32,33], probably due to the presence of extensive anastomoses among the small fragile subependymal vessels[10,24,25,37].

Inferior Limbic AVMs

As proposed by Yaşargil[33], we have divided inferior limbic AVMs into 2 different groups: the anterior ones, or uncal-juxtapeduncular (amygdalo-hyppocampal, for Yaşargil) and the posterior ones, or parasplenial.

Uncal-juxtapeduncular AVMs are all located in the medial and inferior portion of the temporal lobe, involving the amygdala, the hippocampus, the para-hippocampal and sometimes the fusiform gyrus, and not infrequently the temporal horn of the lateral ventricle; they sit above the tentorium and may extend into the cisterna ambiens through the tentorial notch, in close relationship with the upper brainstem and with the cerebral peduncle (Fig. 3)[6,8,9,13,14,22,28,33]. Uncal AVMs are fed mainly by the anterior choroidal artery and secondarily by the middle cerebral artery and the posterior cerebral artery. Besides to its main branches to the choroid plexus of the lateral ventricle, the anterior choroidal artery (A. Cho. A.) feeds a critical vascular territory: part of the optic tract, the lateral part of the geniculate body, part of the posterior limb of the internal capsule, the globus pallidus, and part of the cerebral peduncle[12,24]. Although its closure is not always followed by neurological deficits[11,24] – probably for the terminal anastomoses with the posterior communicating and posterior cerebral artery[24] – we have observed the development of severe motor deficits in 2 patients with uncal AVMs fed by branches of the anterior choroidal artery (Fig. 2). In both cases we have preserved the main trunk of the artery (i.e. the "cisternal" segment)[12,24] and we have interrupted the continuation of the artery in the ventricle (i.e. the "plexal" segment)[12,24]; in retrospective: a) a few secondary branches may have left the anterior choroidal artery in the ventricle, with a recurrent direction to the cerebral peduncle or to the internal capsule, or b) the upper part of the malformation may have involved the inferior border of the basal ganglia and internal capsule, as illustrated by Heros for similar cases[13]. Based on our experience, we recommend that the A.Cho.A. is carefully followed and preserved along its course in every case, closing only the branches directed to the nidus.

For juxtapeduncular AVMs, the A.Cho.A. is not a constant feeder; on the opposite, the posterior cerebral artery is the main feeder through: a) the inferior temporal arteries, arising as a single trunk or as separate branches (hippocampal, anterior, middle and posterior temporal arteries), and b) the lateral posterior choroidal artery (as a single trunk or as separate branches), feeding the region surrounding the temporal horn and the choroid plexus of the lateral ventricle (Fig. 3)[19]. Anomalies of the posterior cerebral artery (PCA) are relatively common in juxtapeduncular AVMs: in particular, the presence of a "fetal" type of PCA originating directly from the carotid artery, with an absent or poorly developed precommunicating segment (this anomaly has caused some difficulties in the recognition of deep anatomical structures in one of our early cases, owing to the abnormal course of the artery)[6,19,25,37].

From a surgical point of view, uncal AVMs are approached through a pterional route or through a combined pterional – subtemporal route in order to adequately expose the A.Cho.A., the posterior communicating and – when needed – the posterior cerebral artery[28,33,36]. Juxtapeduncular AVMs are approached through a subtemporal route, possibly removing – by suction – part of the parahippocampal gyrus overlying the angioma[6,9]; alternatively, Heros has suggested a transcortical approach to the temporal horn and to the AVM through the inferior temporal gyrus (or through the fusiform gyrus for smaller AVMs)[13].

Parasplenial AVMs are located medially to the trigone of the lateral ventricle, in the region of the isthmus cinguli, posterior parahippocampal gyrus, lingular gyrus and inferior part of the precuneus, lying anterior to the calcarine sulcus (Fig. 5)[33]; they have been differently defined as subtrigonal, juxtathalamic, incisural or occipito-cerebellar-mesencephalic by other authors[26,28,30,33]. These AVMs are lateral, posterior and inferior to true splenial AVMs. They often extend to the trigone of the lateral ventricle and should be differentiated from true trigonal AVMs[2,31]; they can also extend to the quadrigeminal cistern, gaining strict relations with the vein of Galen. The feeders to parasplenial AVMs come prevalently from the PCA, through the transverse and calcarine fissures, although in some cases also the anterior pericallosal artery can feed a portion of the AVM. To this regard it is important to identify the bifurcation of the PCA on preop angiography and surgery. The bifurcation point may vary considerably in different patients, and even in the hemispheres of the same patient[19,37]: the identification of this point facilitates anatomical orientation and should prevent inadvertent closure of the calcarine artery or its branches.

From a surgical point of view, parasplenial AVMs are approached through a large parieto-occipital craniotomy, with exposure of the superior longitudinal and transverse sinuses[17]; as mentioned above in regard to splenial AVMs[2,26,28,33] there is some controversy on the patient's positioning. Moreover, when a parasplenial AVM extends far laterally, reaching the trigone, some authors have suggested a posterior subtemporal or a transcortical approach through the middle temporal gyrus[2,8,9,28], although this approach is very risky in the dominant hemisphere; for large AVMs Stein has even suggested a two-stage approach[28]. It should be added that for the more common approaches the occipital lobe must be moved laterally and also superiorly, in order to expose the falcotentorial junction, where the feeders from the PCA can be identified and followed towards the AVM[17].

As for callosal AVMs, also for parasplenial and uncal/juxtapeduncular AVMs extension to the lateral ventricle can determine a tedious paraventricular bleeding during surgery, which generally ends when all the choroidal feeders are coagulated in the ventricle.

Other Observations

The importance of AVM volume should be emphasized for these deep-seated AVMs, where the risk of injury to the adjacent neural parenchyma is possible even for small lesions; with a volume over 20 cm^3, removal of an AVM from the medial hemisphere is coupled with high risks, as illustrated by our cases. To this regard, the introduction of preoperative embolization may decrease the operative risk[21].

A deep venous drainage has been regarded by some authors as a clue to inoperability[14,22] or as a substantial risk factor[27]; based on our experience, we cannot agree on this point, while we consider the presence of deep feeders as a more significant risk factor[20]. It should be added that the majority of our patients with callosal/cingular or inferior limbic AVMs have presented a medially directed venous drainage (65% of patients with callosal/cingular and 85% of patients with inferior limbic AVMs); this anatomical feature has not prevented – nor made more difficult – the radical removal of the AVM.

As an adjunct to surgery, lumbar drainage has shown a particular usefulness for these deep-seated AVMs, where space is of crucial importance[28,33]. Intraoperative deep hypotension (used in the early cases) has been abandoned in the recent years, for a possible responsability in postoperative hyperemia.

The introduction of radiosurgery[5,29] has probably limited surgical indications for deep-seated AVMs; however, while direct surgery of basal ganglia AVMs remains a matter of controversy, especially for large lesions, operative removal of AVMs in the corpus callosum and in the infero-medial temporal lobe seems preferable to radiosurgical treatment, considering the long period between radiosurgery and cure and the 80% obliteration rate reported by the most experienced authors[5,29] with radiosurgery.

In conclusion, callosal/cingular and inferior limbic AVMs can be adequately treated with a direct microsurgical approach, although results of surgery are dependent upon AVM volume, with high risks for AVMs over 20 cm^3; there is a substantial risk of ischemic complications for inferior limbic AVMs fed by the anterior choroidal artery, regardless of AVM volume.

References

1. Almeida GM, Shibata MK, Nakagawa EJ (1984) Contralateral parafalcine approach for parasagittal and callosal arteriovenous malformations. Neurosurgery 14: 744–746
2. Batjer H, Samson D (1987) Surgical approaches to trigonal arteriovenous malformations. J Neurosurg 67: 511–517
3. Benati A, Beltramello A, Colombari R, Maschio A, Perini S, Da Pian R, Pasqualin A, Scienza R, Rosta L, Piovan E, Scarpa A, Zamboni G (1989) Preoperative embolization of arteriovenous malformations with polylene threads: techniques with wing microcatheter and pathological results. AJNR 10: 579–586
4. Bonnal J, Petrov V, Gillet J (1978) Aneurysmes arterio-veineux interessant la toile choroidienne du III ventricule. Neurochirurgie 24: 15–21
5. Colombo F, Benedetti A, Pozza F, Marchetti C, Chierego G (1989) Linear accelerator radiosurgery of cerebral arteriovenous malformations. Neurosurgery 24: 833–840
6. Da Pian R, Pasqualin A, Scienza R (1982) Microsurgical treatment of juxtapeduncular angiomas. Surg Neurol 17: 16–29
7. Da Pian R, Pasqualin A, Scienza R, Vivenza C (1980) Microsurgical treatment of ten arteriovenous malformations in critical areas of the cerebrum. J Microsurg 1: 305–320
8. Drake CG (1979) Cerebral arteriovenous malformations: considerations for and experience with surgical treatment in 166 cases. Clin Neurosurg 26: 145–208
9. Drake CG, Amacher AL (1969) Aneurysms of the posterior cerebral artery. J Neurosurg 30: 468–474
10. Fujii K, Lenkey C, Rhoton AL Jr (1980) Microsurgical anatomy of the choroidal arteries: lateral and third ventricles. J Neurosurg 52: 165–188
11. Fujita K, Matsumoto S (1984) Anterior choroidal artery arteriovenous malformation. Its clinical manifestations and surgical treatment. Surg Neurol 21: 347–352
12. Goldberg HI (1974) The anterior choroidal artery. In: Newton TH, Potts DG (eds) Radiology of the skull and brain, Vol II, Book 2. Mosby St. Louis, pp 1628–1658
13. Heros RC (1982) Arteriovenous malformations of the medial temporal lobe. Surgical approach and neuroradiological characterization. J Neurosurg 56: 44–52
14. Juhasz J (1978) Surgical treatment of arteriovenous angiomas localized in the corpus callosum, basal ganglia and near the brain stem. Acta Neurochir (Wien) 40: 83–101
15. Kosary IZ, Braham J, Shacked I, Kronenberg Y (1978) Vascular malformation of the posterior corpus callosum: surgical treatment. Surg Neurol 10: 345–347
16. Laine E, Jomin M, Clarisse J, Combelles G (1981) Les malformations arterio-veineuses cerebrales profondes. Classification topographique. Possibilities et resultats therapeutiques a propos de 46 observations. Neurochirurgie 27: 147–160
17. Martin NA, Wilson CB (1982) Medial occipital arteriovenous malformations. Surgical treatment. J Neurosurg 56: 798–802
18. Nehls DG, Marano SR, Spetzler RF (1985) Transcallosal approach to the contralateral ventricle. Technical note. J Neurosurg 62: 304–306
19. Newton TH, Hoyt WF, Margolis MT (1974) The posterior cerebral artery. Sections I, II and III. In: Newton TH, Potts DG (eds) Radiology of the skull and brain: angiography, Vol I, Book 2. Mosby, St. Louis, pp 1540–1627
20. Pasqualin A, Barone G, Cioffi F, Rosta L, Scienza R, Da Pian R (1991) The relevance of anatomic and hemodynamic factors to a classification of cerebral arteriovenous malformations. Neurosurgery 28: 370–379
21. Pasqualin A, Scienza R, Cioffi F, Barone G, Benati A, Beltramello A, Da Pian R (1991) Treatment of cerebral arteriovenous malformations with a combination of preoperative embolization and surgery. Neurosurgery 29: 358–368
22. Pertuiset B, Sachs M, Guyot JF (1963) Les aneurysmes arterioveineux des parois juxta-pedonculaires de la fente de Bichat. Presse med 71: 2341–2342
23. Pertuiset B, Sichez JP (1978) The backward technique in the total excision of cerebral arteriovenous malformations: experience with 86 cases. In: Wullenweber R *et al* (eds) Advances in neurosurgery, Vol 6. Springer, Berlin Heidelberg New York, pp 148–153
24. Rhoton AL Jr, Fujii K, Fradd B (1979) Microsurgical anatomy of the anterior choroidal artery. Surg Neurol 12: 171–187
25. Saeki N, Rhoton AL Jr (1977) Microsurgical anatomy of the upper basilar artery and the posterior circle of Willis. J Neurosurg 46: 563–578
26. Solomon RA, Stein BM (1986) Surgical management of arteriovenous malformations that follow the tentorial ring. Neurosurgery 18: 708–715
27. Spetzler RF, Martin NA (1986) A proposed grading system for arteriovenous malformations. J Neurosurg 65: 476–483

28. Stein BM (1984) Arteriovenous malformations of the medial cerebral hemisphere and the limbic system. J Neurosurg 60: 23–31

29. Steiner L (1984) Treatment of arteriovenous malformations by radiosurgery. In: Wilson CH, Stein B (eds) Intracranial arteriovenous malformations. Williams and Wilkins, Baltimore, pp 295–313

30. Vigouroux RP, Baurand C, Reynier Y (1978) A propos des malformations arterio-veineuses du diedre occipito-cerebello-mesencephalique. Neurochirurgie 24: 363–373

31. Waga S, Shimosaka S, Kojima T (1985) Arteriovenous malformations of the lateral ventricle. J Neurosurg 63: 185–192

32. Wilson CB, Martin NA (1984) Deep supratentorial arteriovenous malformations. In: Wilson CB, Stein BM (eds) Intracranial arteriovenous malformations. Williams and Wilkins, Baltimore, pp 184–208

33. Yaşargil MG (1988) Supratentorial (Central) AVMs. In: Yaşargil MG (ed) Microneurosurgery, Vol IIIb. Thieme, Stuttgart, pp. 211–293

34. Yaşargil MG, Jain KK, Antic J, Laciga R (1976) Arteriovenous malformations of the splenium of the corpus callosum: microsurgical treatment. Surg Neurol 5: 5–14

35. Yaşargil MG, Jain KK, Antic J, Laciga R, Kletter G (1976) Arteriovenous malformations of the anterior and the middle portions of the corpus callosum: microsurgical treatment. Surg Neurol 5: 67–81

36. Yaşargil MG, Teddy PJ, Roth P (1985) Selective amygdalo-hippocampectomy. Operative anatomy and surgical technique. In: Advances and technical standards in neurosurgery, Vol 12. Springer, Wien New York, pp 93–123

37. Zeal AA, Rhoton AL (1978) Microsurgical anatomy of the posterior cerebral artery. J Neurosurg 48: 534–559

Correspondence: R. Da Pian, M.D., Department of Neurosurgery, City Hospital, I-37126 Verona, Italy.

Stereotactic Uses in the Treatment of Deep "Inaccessible" AVMs and a Comparison with Radiosurgery

B.M. Stein, M.B. Sisti, and **A. Kader**

Neurological Institute of the Columbia-Presbyterian Medical Center, New York, New York, U.S.A.

Summary

We have had significant but limited experience in the use of stereo-tactic-guided craniotomy for AVMs that are sub-surface and otherwise difficult to locate. Our experience and technique utilizing arteriographic and CT data is these cases is reviewed. In addition a comparison of the results of stereotactic radiosurgery which we perform with a linear accelerator and microsurgery for these deep otherwise approachable AVMs that are under 3 cms is reviewed.

Keywords: Arteriovenous malformations; cerebrovascular; micro-neurosurgery; radiosurgery; stereotactic surgery.

Introduction

Stereotactic techniques have been used both for therapy and localization in the treatment of small, deeply placed and sometimes considered inaccessible AVM. We have reported on the use of stereotactic localization techniques, assisting craniotomy for the approach to these malformations[7]. Localization techniques include the use of CT scan, angiogram, and MRI. In addition, stereotactic techniques have been utilized in focusing radiation treatment to obliterate small AVMs[12]. The results of the surgical series numbering 67 patients and those of major radiosurgery centers will be discussed.

Materials and Methods

The stereotactic-guided craniotomy has been used in the localization and microsurgical obliteration of AVMs in 14 patients[7]. Examples include lesions that are located deep in eloquent areas such as the frontal operculum (Fig. 1).

In addition many of the smaller AVMs which are located close to known landmarks such as the ventricular regions or the surface of the brain stem have been approached directly without the need of stereotactic guidance[3,8,9] (Fig. 2a–c). Because of the specificity and reproducibility of the landmarks, these lesions have been approached by various techniques including interhemispheric, trans-callosal, and posterior fossa approaches to the brain stem.

Many of these small deep lesions are associated with "bizarre" aneurysms which are probably related to the hemorrhage occurring with these malformations (Fig. 2c). These aneurysms would not respond to radiation therapy or the response would be delayed and not preclude recidivous hemorrhage. An example of such a case is

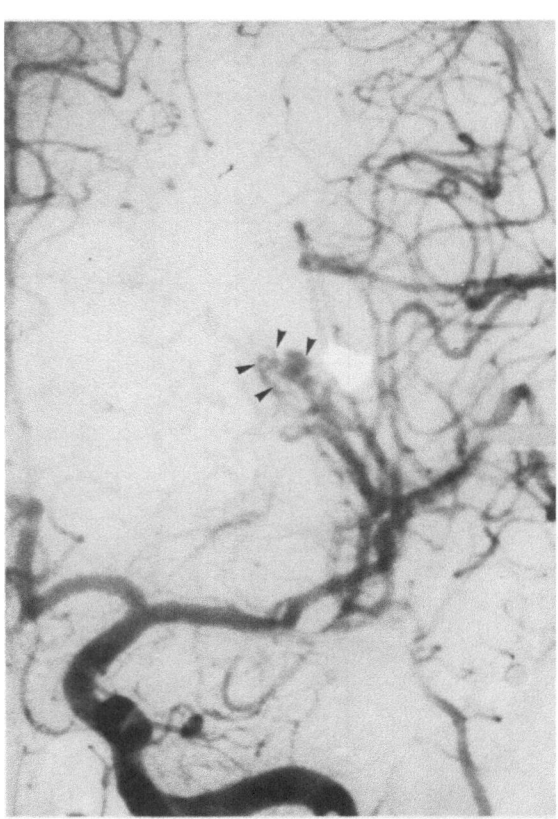

Fig. 1. AP carotid arteriogram showing AVM deep to the dominant frontal operculum (arrowheads). This lesion which hemorrhaged was successfully removed by microsurgical stereotactic guided craniotomy

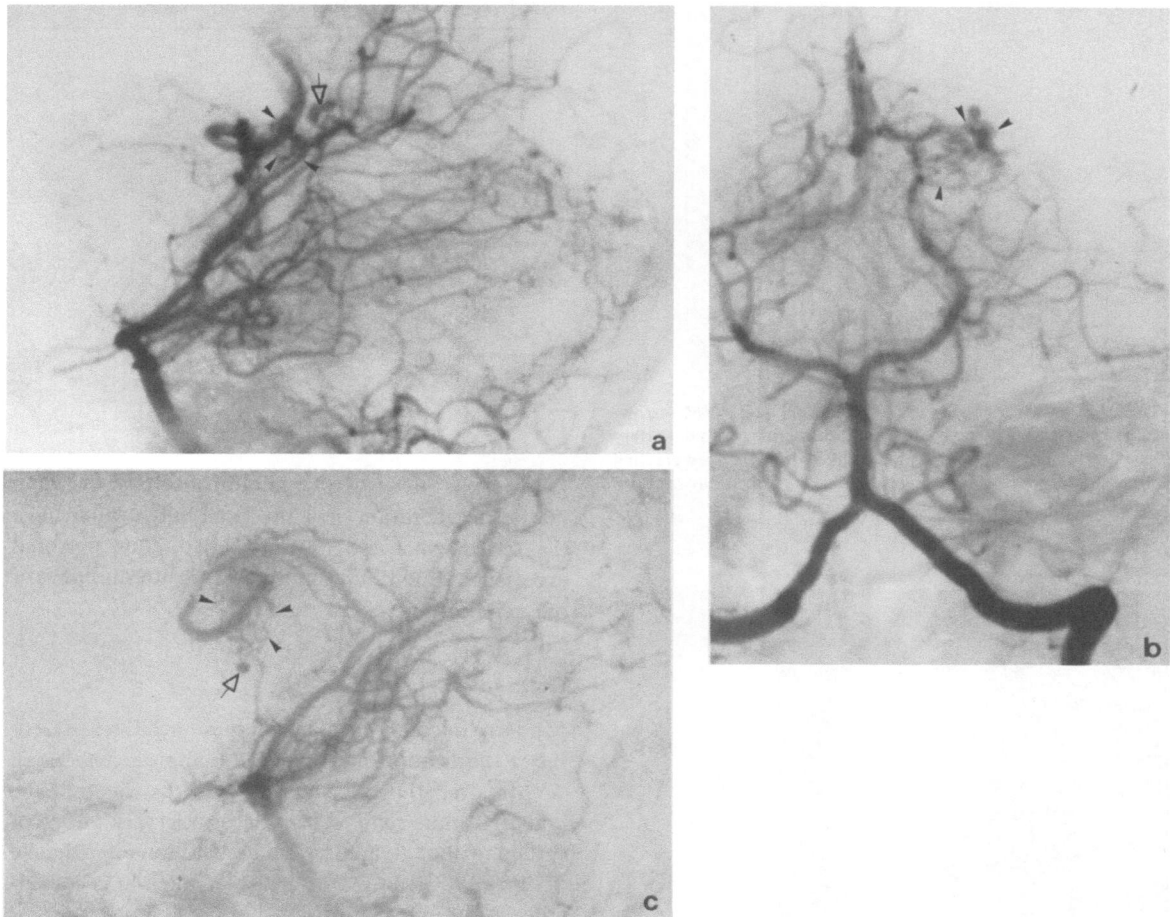

Fig. 2. (a) Lateral vertebral arteriogram, left side, showing small medial trigonal AVM (arrowheads) with small arterial aneurysms from the choroidal artery (open arrow). This lesion was successfully removed without neurological deficit via a transcallosal interhemispheric approach. (b) Same patient as in Fig. 2a. AP vertebral arteriogram showing the AVM (arrowheads) located in the left trigone. (c) Lateral right vertebral arteriogram showing thalamic AVM (arrowheads) with associated aneurysm (open arrow) arising from thalamoperforate arteries. Both lesions were successfully obliterated by a microsurgical approach, interhemispheric transcallosal

illustrated in Fig. 3 where an AVM located in the pulvinar was associated with a pulvinar hemorrhage, probably due to the associated aneurysm. These lesions were approached directly by microsurgical techniques and the aneurysm and AVM obliterated at the same operation.

There were 67 patients with AVMs under 3 cm which were subjected to microsurgical removal. Forty-five percent of these were located in deep diencephalic or brain stem regions. Total removal was accomplished in all of the hemispheric lesions and in 94% of all of the lesions considered under 3 cm in maximal diameter. Stereotactic craniotomy was useful to precisely locate AVMs that were sub-surface and might otherwise be considered inaccessible. There was no incomplete removal in 14 cases of stereotactic-guided craniotomies.

In comparison to the surgical series, we reviewed the radiosurgical treatment of AVMs under 3 cm from 5 major centers[1,2,5,11,12]. We have had limited experience in the follow-up of patients treated by radiosurgery. However, our experience would indicate that the treatment is not without long-term side effects such as radionecrosis or white matter degeneration at some distance from the treated AVM (Fig. 4). In our overall series of AVMs we would consider no more than 3% of those under 3 cm as being in inoperable locations.

Results

The surgical series of 67 AVMs located in various regions of the brain (45% being in deep otherwise inaccessible locations) had a favorable outcome. There was a 94% cure rate, 1.5% modest neurological deficit, no rebleeds, and no mortality. In comparison the statistics from radiosurgery centers would indicate

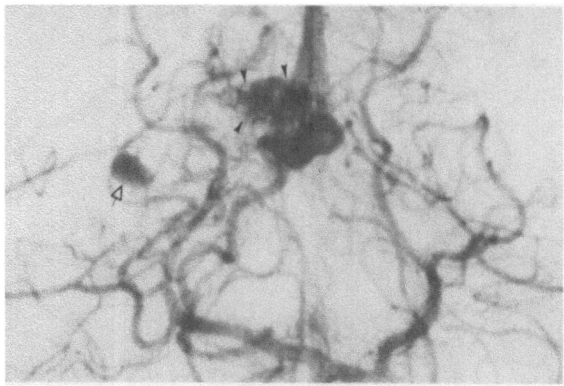

Fig. 3. AP vertebral arteriogram showing pulvinar AVM (arrowheads) and associated aneurysm from the anterior choroidal artery (open arrow). The aneurysm had most likely hemorrhaged creating a hematoma between the two lesions. Both were successfully removed by an interhemispheric, transcallosal approach

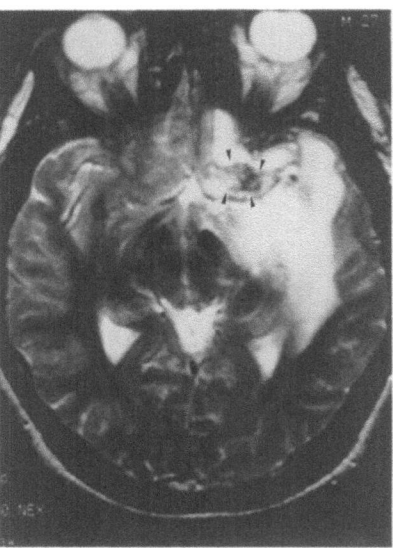

Fig. 4. MRI (T-2) with extensive white matter changes three years after Gamma Knife radiosurgery which successfully obliterated an AVM associated with the middle cerebral artery (arrowheads). The white matter changes extended far up into the hemisphere of the dominant side and created a progressive neurological syndrome

approximately an 80% cure rate (in some instances lower), after the 2-year waiting period when radiosurgery is expected to maximize obliteration[4,6]. In addition, during this period there was an average of 6% bleeding rate and serious neurological deficits in the range of 5%. There was a very small mortality.

Table 1. *Treatment of AVMs Under 3 cm*

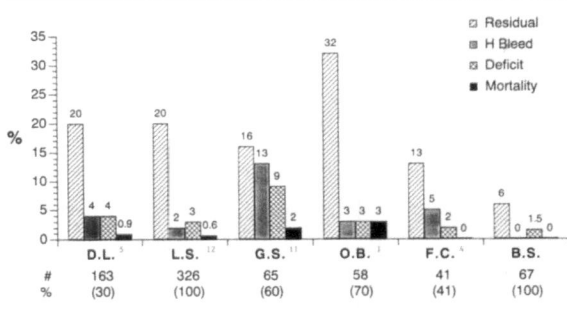

#	163	326	65	58	41	67
%	(30)	(100)	(60)	(70)	(41)	(100)
	D.L.[5]	L.S.[12]	G.S.[11]	O.B.[1]	F.C.[4]	B.S.

\# Total number Rx
% Percent followed 2 or more years;
D.L.[5]; L.S.[12]; G.S.[11]; O.B.[1]; F.C.[4] = see references.

Late results in terms of radiation necrosis or white matter degeneration have not been fully evaluated in the series which we have reviewed. Our personal experience would indicate that this is not an unheard of complication.

Conclusion

Modern microsurgical techniques including stereotactic localization have made the approach to small AVMs, even those located deep in the diencephalic and the brain stem, safe. Microsurgery is the most certain method to accomplish obliteration immediately of an AVM. Even when the 2-year interval is considered, radiosurgery falls far short of the cure rate of microsurgery in the treatment of these lesions[10,13] (Table 1). In addition radiosurgery may have unrealized long-term complications of radiation-induced injury. The immediate complication rate of neurological deficit, and rebleeding during the treatment interval is much higher than microsurgery.

All of these factors must be considered in selecting patients for the most appropriate and safest form of treatment of small AVMs, especially those located in abscure locations.

References

1. Betti OO, Munari C, Rosler R (1989) Stereotactic radiosurgery with the linear accelerator: treatment of arteriovenous malformations. Neurosurgery 24: 311–321
2. Colombo F, Benedetti A, Pozza F, Marchetti C, Chierego G (1989) Linear accelerator radiosurgery of cerebral arteriovenous malformations. Neurosurgery 24: 833–840
3. Garrido D, Stein BM (1978) Removal of an arteriovenous malformation from the basal ganglion. J Neurosurg Psychiatry 41: 992–995

4. Heros RC, Korosue K (1990) Radiation treatment of cerebral arteriovenous malformations. N Engl J Med 323: 127–129

5. Lunsford LD, Kondziolka D, Flickinger JC, Bissonette DJ, Jungreis CA, Maitz AH, Horton JA, Coffey RJ (1991) Stereotactic radiosurgery for arteriovenous malformations of the brain. J Neurosurg 75: 512–524

6. Ogilvy CS (1990) Radiation therapy for arteriovenous malformations: a review. Neurosurgery 26: 725–735

7. Sisti MB, Solomon RA, Stein BM (1991) Stereotactic craniotomy in the resection of small arteriovenous malformations. J Neurosurg 75: 40–44

8. Solomon RA, Stein BM (1987) Interhemispheric approach for the surgical removal of thalamocaudate arteriovenous malformations. J Neurosurg 66: 345–351

9. Solomon RA, Stein BM (1986) Management of arteriovenous malformations of the brain stem. J Neurosurg 64: 857–864

10. Stein BM, Mohr JP, Sisti MB (1991) is radiosurgery all that it appears to be? Letters to the editor. Arch Neurol 48: 19–20

11. Steinberg GK, Fabrikant JI, Marks MP, Levy RP, Frankel KA, Phillips HK, Shver LM, Silverberg GD (1990) Stereotactic heavy-charged particle Bragg-peak radiation for intracranial arteriovenous malformations. N Engl J Med 323: 96–101

12. Steiner L, Lindquist CH (1987) Radiosurgery in cerebral arteriovenous malformation. In Tasker RR (ed) Neurosurgery: state of the art reviews, stereotactic surgery, Vol 2. Hanley and Belfus, Philadelphia, pp 329–336

13. Wascher TM, Spetzler RF (1992) Radiosurgery of arteriovenous malformations. Letter to the editor. J Neurosurg 76: 1045–1046

Correspondence: Bennett Stein, M.D., Neurological Surgery, College of Physicians and Surgeons of Columbia University, 710 West 168th Street, New York, NY 10032, U.S.A.

Surgical Removal of Thalamic Arteriovenous Malformation – Transventricular Approach, Sitting Position, Intraoperative Angiography

Y. Yonekawa, Y. Kaku, K. Yamashita, S. Yoshida, K. Niijima, T. Kawano, and **W. Taki**

Department of Neurosurgery, National Cardiovascular Center, Japan

Summary

Management of deep-seated arteriovenous malformations AVMs remains a problem, although alternative methods of surgical excision such as stereotactic radiosurgery and superselective embolization have recently been developed. We report the methods and results of the surgical excision of thalamic AVM up to 4 cm in size, mainly via the parieto-occipital transventricular approach in the sitting position using intraoperative angiography. Complete removal was possible in some cases with a low morbidity.

Keywords: Thalamic arteriovenous malformation; transventricular approach; sitting position; intraoperative angiography.

Introduction

Arteriovenous malformations (AVMs) of the basal ganglia and the thalamus are reported to comprise 20% of all brain AVMs[1,6,11]. Around 50% of them have been reported to bleed producing intracerebral and/or intraventricular hematomas, with a resultant poor prognosis[6]. The surgical management of such AVMs has been reported sporadically[1,2,4,5,6,7,11,13], but the management of those confined to the thalamus has not been reported, except by Yaşargil[12], to our knowledge. This article covers the surgical management of thalamic AVMs with emphasis on the importance of selection of the transventricular approach in conjunction with the sitting position and the concurrent use of intraoperative angiography.

Patients and Methods

Ten patients with AVMs located in the thalamus proper were admitted to the Department of Neurosurgery at the National Cardiovascular Center (NCVC) in Japan during the last five years (1987–1991) out of a total of 85 cases of cerebral AVM. The clinical features of these ten patients are summarized in Table 1. There were six males and four females with ages ranging from 8 to 38 years. The left and right sides were almost equally involved. Intraventricular hemorrhage (IVH) with or without intracerebral hematoma (ICH) was the mode of presentation in all except one case, in which the AVM was detected incidentally (Case 6). Hemorrhage occurred once in six cases and more than once in 3 cases (Case 3, Case 7, Case 9). The main feeding artery was the anterior choroidal artery, followed by the lateral posterior choroidal artery, the thalamoperforating arteries, the thalamogeniculate artery, and the lateral lenticulostriate arteries. The main draining vein was always the same, the internal cerebral vein (ICV). Seven out of the ten patients

Table 1. *Arteriovenous Malformations of the Thalamus (1987–1991 NCVC)*

	Case	Onset	Location	Feeder	Drainer	Removal	Stage	Result
1.	F 18	IVH	lt thalamus	ACHO	ICV	total	1	excellent
2.	M 30	IVH	rt thalamus	LLST	ICV	total	1	excellent
3.	F 29	IVH, ICH	lt thalamus	LPCHO	ICV	total	2	good
4.	M 38	IVH	rt thalamus	ACHO	ICV	total	2	good
5.	M 11	IVH, ICH	lt thalamus	ACHO	ICV	s-total	2	excellent
6.	F 8	incid	lt thalamus	ACHO	ICV	none		unchanged
7.	M 19	IVH	rt thalamus	TP, TG	ICV	part	emb	unchanged
8.	M 29	IVH	rt thalamus	ACHO	ICV	part	1	excellent
9.	M 19	IVH, ICH	rt thalamus	LPCHO	ICV	s-total	2	good
10.	F 17	IVH, ICH	lt thalamus	TP	ICV	none		unchanged

IVH intraventricular hemorrhage; *ICH* intracerebral hemorrhage; *ACHO* anterior choroidal artery; *LLST* lateral lenticulostriate arteries; *LPCHO* lateral posterior choroidal artery; *TP* thalamoperforating arteries; *TG* thalamogeniculate artery; *ICV* internal cerebral vein.

underwent surgery for four total removals and three subtotal removals. We used the following approaches: the parieto-occipital transventricular approach in the sitting position in five cases (Cases 1, 3, 5, 8, and 9), the anterior transcallosal approach in Cases 2 and 3, the posterior transcallosal approach in Case 5, and the trans Sylvian approach in Case 4. A staged operation was performed in four cases because of residual AVM. Two of them had still residual AVM. One of them was sent to Gamma-knife therapy, resulting in its complete nonvisualization in 1.5 year (Case 5). The other residual AVM (Case 9) bled into subcortex, compelling to evacuation of the hematoma and to partial removal of the residual AVM. The patient then underwent Gamma-knife therapy. A large AVM occupying the whole thalamus (Case 7) was partially embolized, and the incidentally discovered AVM (Case 6) is still under observation, disclosing a marked regression angiographically in 5 years. A small AVM (Case 10) fed by the thalamoperforating arteries (which bled into the third ventricle) was sent primarily to the stereotactic Gamma-knife therapy.

The results of surgery were excellent (without any sequelae) in four patients and good in three other patients, who had residual minor neurological deficits such as homonymous hemianopia (Cases 3, 4 and 9), slight motor dysphasia (Case 3), and slight hemiparesis (Case 4). Cases with subtotal removals revealed regrowth of the AVM rest (Case 5 and Case 9) within 2 years; the former case was submitted to Gamma-knife therapy and the latter bled severely and was submitted to removal of a big intracerebral hematoma (5 cm in diameter) as mentioned above.

Representative Cases

Case 3

This 29-year-old female suffered from a sudden onset of disturbance of consciousness on January 21, 1988.

On admission to our department on the next day, she was drowsy but had no focal neurological deficits. CT scan and MRI displayed a left thalamic hematoma with ventricular hemorrhage (Fig. 1). Angiography revealed a left thalamic AVM with various feeding arteries: the medial lenticulostriate arteries, posterior thalamoperforating arteries, and medial and lateral posterior choroidal arteries. The nidus was located in the dorsomedial to ventrolateral part of the thalamus

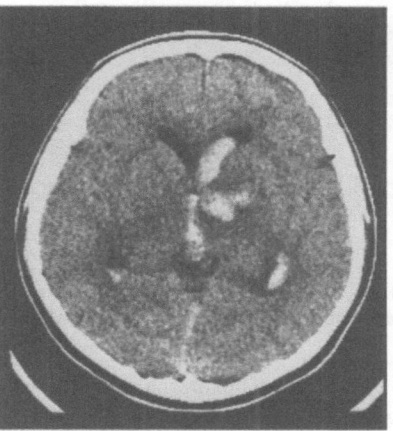

Fig. 1. CT scan of Case 3 displaying a hematoma in the left thalamus that has extended into the ventricular system

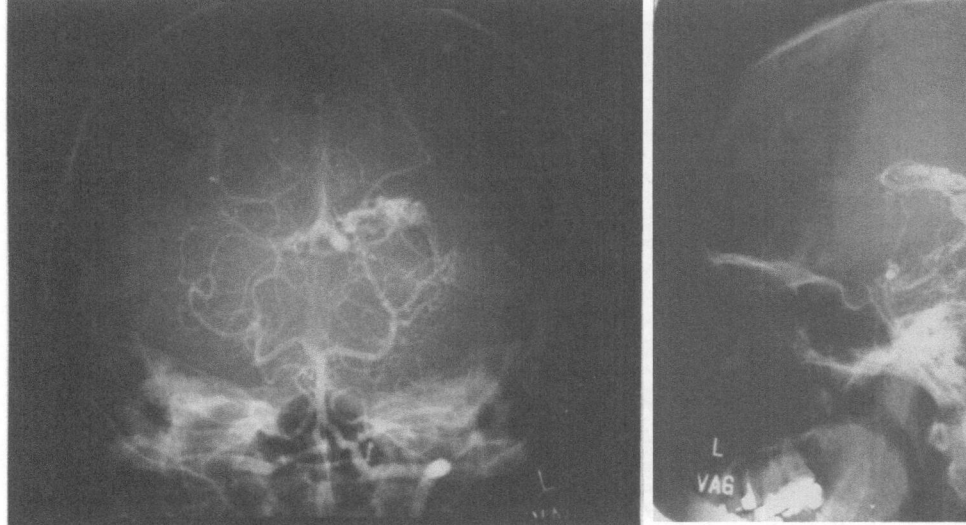
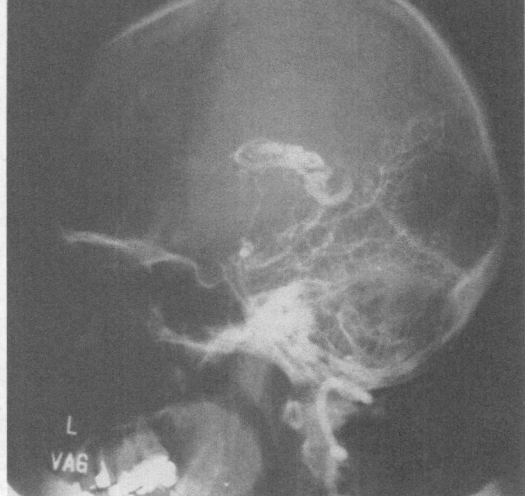

a   b

Fig. 2. Vertebral angiogram of Case 3. (a) A–P view, revealing a nidus fed mainly by the posterior lateral choroidal artery and drained by the internal cerebral vein. (b) Lateral view, displaying the nidus fed also by the posterior thalamoperforating arteries

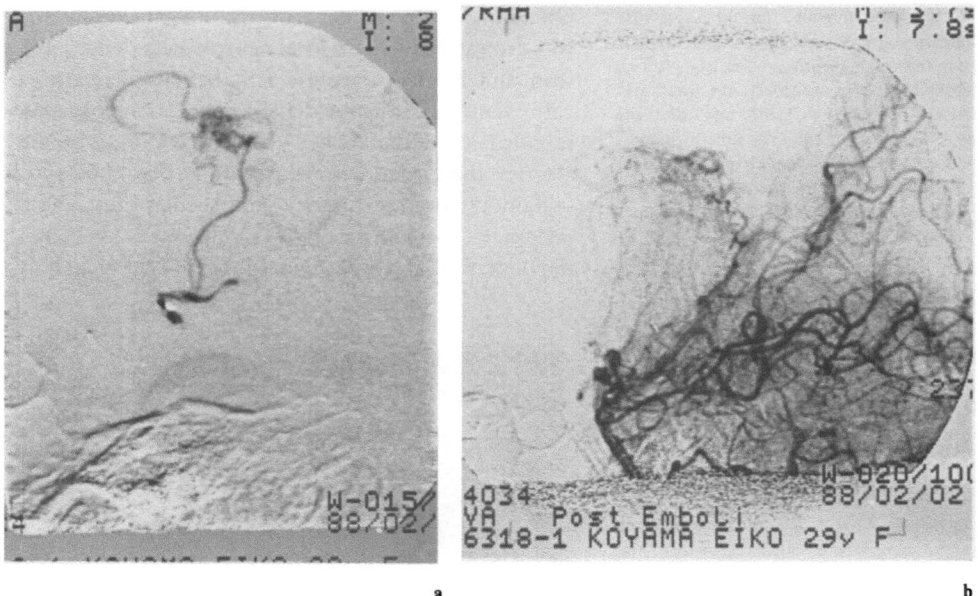

a   b

Fig. 3. Selective embolization with EVAL. (a) Selective angiography of the lateral posterior choroidal artery was performed with a micro-balloon catheter, and 0.5 ml of EVAL was injected. (b) The AVM was partially embolized

and was $3 \times 2 \times 2$ cm in size. The internal cerebral vein was the draining vein (Fig. 2).

Neuroradiological intervention was performed on February 1 via the main feeder, the lateral posterior choroidal artery, using 0.5 ml of ethylvinylalcohol

(EVAL) as the embolic agent, subsequent to a thiopental test which revealed no abnormality. The AVM could be effectively embolized, (Fig. 3) but a right homonymous hemianopia, motor weakness of the right lower extremity, and mild aphasia developed.

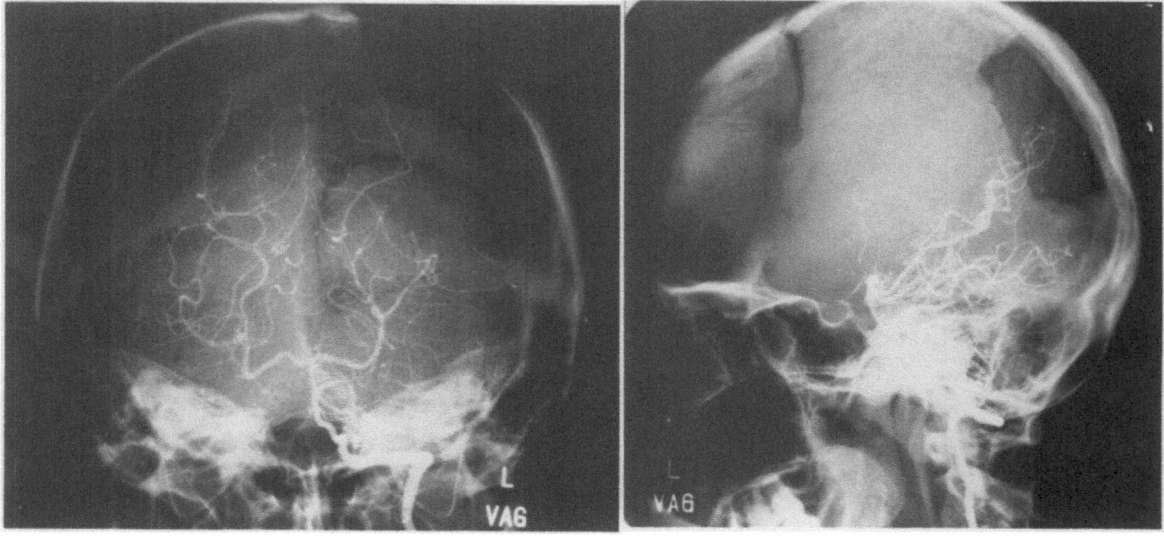

a   b

Fig. 4. Follow-up vertebral angiography showed no residual AVM (a), although the posterior thalamoperforating artery was still dilated (b)

Left parieto-occipital craniotomy was performed in the sitting position on February 9, which enabled removal of half of the nidus via a transventricular approach. The procedure was interrupted by some episodes of air embolism.

The residual nidus located anteriorly was extirpated using the anterior transcallosal approach on March 2, 1988. Follow-up angiography revealed total removal of the AVM, although some of the thalamoperforating arteries still remained dilated (Fig. 4). The patient was discharged on April 28, 1988, with mild dysphasia and a complete homonymous hemianopia.

Comment: This patient underwent preoperative super-selective embolization via the lateral posterior choroidal artery using the new embolic material EVAL[10], which resulted in the complication of homonymous hemianopia. Although the AVM was reduced in size, this procedure might have not been necessary retrospectively. Also, the second operation could have been obviated if episodes of air embolism had not interrupted the first procedure, as one would have been able to reach the lesion just posterior to the foramen of Monroe. Intraoperative angiography might have been very useful to demonstrate the residual AVM.

Case 5

This 11-year-old male suffered from a severe headache of sudden onset on April 4, 1989. An emergency CT scan revealed a thalamic hemorrhage with ventricular bleeding. Cerebral angiography at that time showed a thalamic AVM ($4 \times 2 \times 2$ cm) fed mainly by the anterior choroidal artery and drained by the internal cerebral vein (Fig. 5). The patient was admitted to our department on May 29, 1989. Neurological findings were completely normal at that time. On June 1, selective embolization of the anterior choroidal artery was performed at its plexal segment using 0.45 ml of EVAL. The procedure was complicated by a right homonymous hemianopia which improved gradually. About two thirds of the AVM were occluded and one third was still fed by the lateral and medial posterior choroidal arteries as well as the posterior thalamo-perforating and thalamogeniculate arteries (Fig. 6). On June 8, 1989, removal of the remaining nidus was performed via the posterior transcallosal approach in the sitting position. Follow-up angiography revealed subtotal removal, with a small nidus remaining in the vicinity of the medial posterior choroidal artery. The patient was discharged on July 10, 1989, with only an upper quadrant hemianopia.

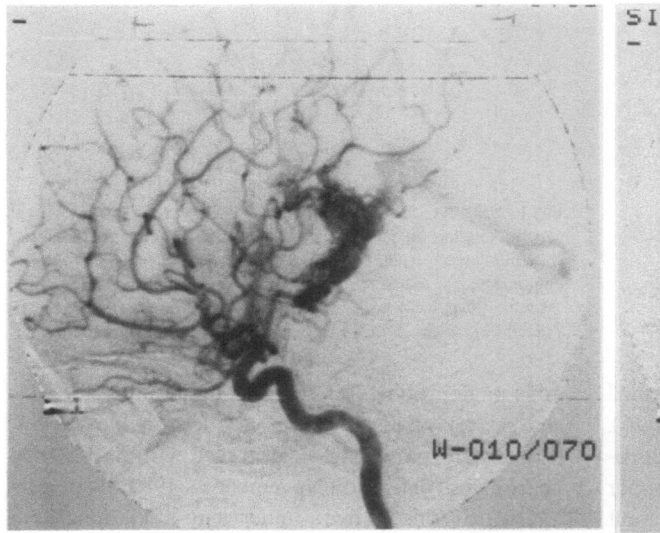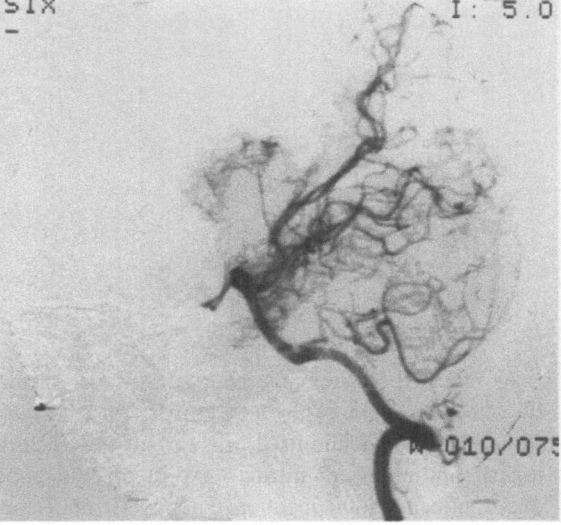

a   b

Fig. 5. Angiogram of Case 5. (a) Carotid angiogram shows an AVM fed mainly by the anterior choroidal artery and drained by the internal cerebral vein. (b) Vertebral angiogram shows that the AVM is also fed by the lateral and medial posterior choroidal arteries and the anterior thalamoperforating arteries

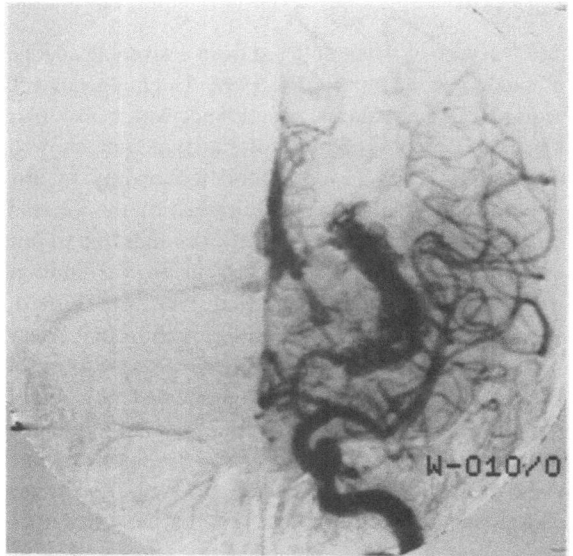

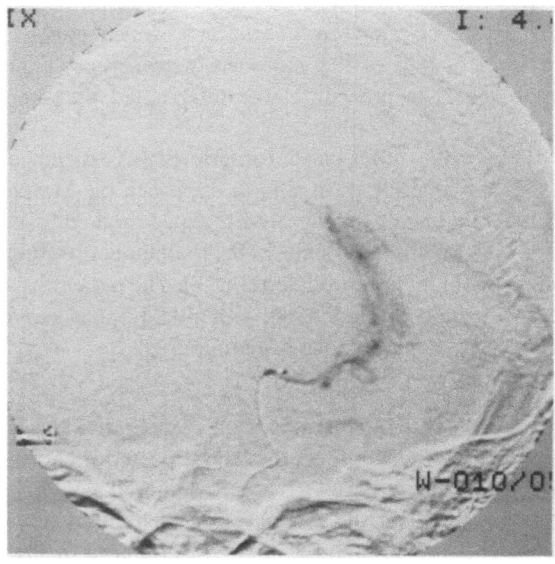

a   b

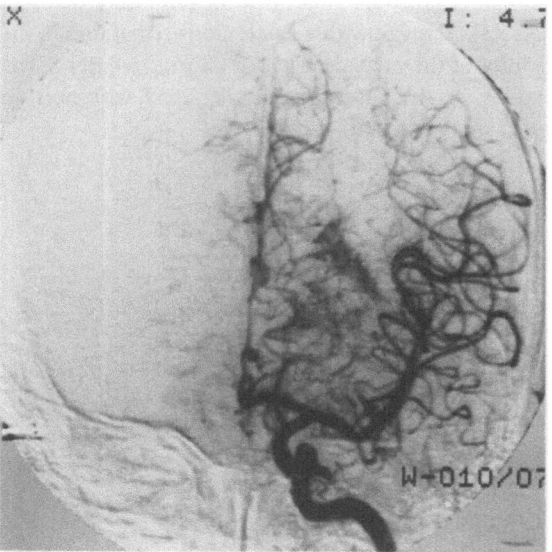

c

Fig. 6. Selective embolization with EVAL. (a) A–P view of the carotid angiogram shows the AVM fed by the dilated anterior choroidal artery draining into the internal cerebral vein. (b) Selective angiography of the anterior choroidal artery with a microballoon catheter. The AVM was subsequently embolized with EVAL. (c) Postembolization carotid angiogram indicates a residual nidus

As regrowth of the remaining nidus was confirmed by follow-up angiography on October 2, 1989 (Fig. 7), the patient was readmitted on November 6. Neurological findings were normal, except for the upper quadrant hemianopia mentioned above. He underwent a repeated parieto-occipital craniotomy on November 8, 1989, and the residual AVM was removed via the transcortical transventricular approach in the sitting position. Total removal was confirmed by intraoper-

ative angiography; follow-up angiography before discharge revealed, however, a questionable residue (Fig. 8). The patient was discharged without any new neurological deficits on November 28, 1989. Six months afterwards this patient underwent a Gamma-knife therapy as the regrowth of the AVM was observed.

Comment: A thalamic AVM on the dominant side fed mainly by the anterior choroidal artery was success-

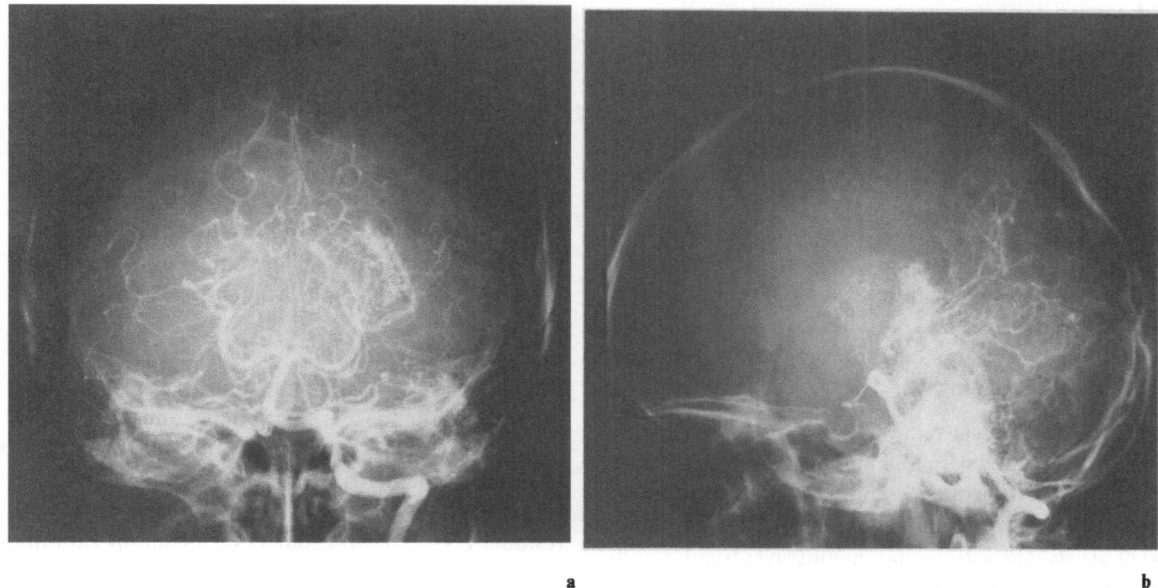

Fig. 7. Follow-up angiogram prior to the second operation demonstrates the residual nidus. (a) A–P view, (b) lateral view

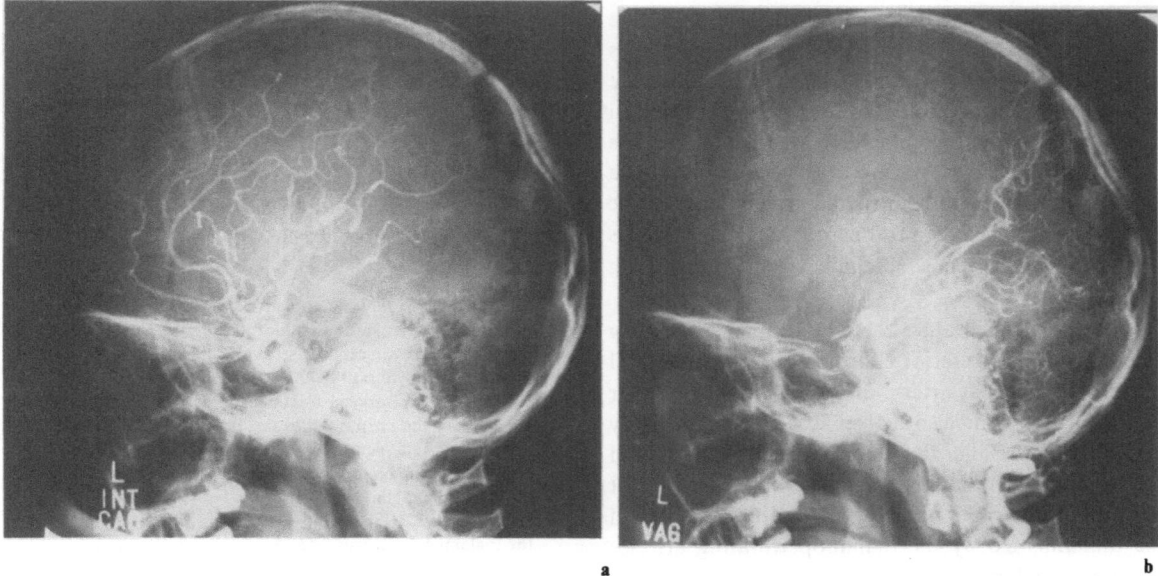

Fig. 8. Postoperative angiogram shows no evidence of an AVM. The anterior choroidal artery, anterior thalamoperforating arteries, and lateral and medial posterior choroidal arteries are well outlined. (a) Carotid angiogram. (b) Vertebral angiogram

fully subtotally embolized without any serious complications. The residual AVM was extirpated via the posterior transcallosal approach. A small AVM detected by follow-up angiography that was fed by the thalamoperforating arteries enlarged over the course of three months. The AVM could be removed almost totally via the transcortical transventricular approach, in the sitting position with the use of intraoperative angiography. Because of regrowth of the residual AVM, however, the patient underwent radiosurgery later on.

Discussion

Pure thalamic AVMs are considered to comprise half of the AVMs located in the basal ganglia-thalamic region from our experience. AVMs in this region, as compared to those in the cerebral hemispheres, have been reported to have the following characteristics[6]:

1. The risk of rebleeding of deep-seated AVMs is three times higher than that of superficial lesions.

2. Rebleeding tends to take place within 2–3 years from the initial bleed.

3. Long-term follow-up for more than 10 years has disclosed a rebleeding rate of 90%.

Thus, the surgical removal of such AVMs appears to be justified, and a limited number of patients having the following features have undergone microsurgical extirpation with reasonable results[1,5,7,11]. The AVMs were associated with hematoma (intraventricular and/or parenchymal hematoma), were small to moderate in size (up to 3–4 cm in diameter), and were located paraventricularly, subependymally, anteriorly, or posterosuperiorly.

We emphasize here that thalamic AVMs should be separated from those of the anterior basal ganglia, as the feeding arteries differ and, therefore, so does the surgical approach. Although the posterior transcallosal approach has been recommended for thalamic AVMs by some surgeons[2,12], we are of the opinion that the parieto-occipital transventricular approach in the sitting position using intraoperative angiography is the surgical treatment of choice for the following reasons.

This approach enables the management of feeding arteries from the anterior choroidal artery, the lateral posterior choroidal artery, and the medial posterior choroidal artery and also enables access to an anteriorly located AVM as far as the foramen of Monro. It should be, however, emphasized that this approach is not appropriate in cases with the nidus in the center of the thalamus fed by the thalamoperforating arteries or by the thalamogeniculate arteries, as observed in our Case 10.

The approach itself does not induce major neurological deficits of the dominant hemisphere, except for lower quadrant hemianopia in some cases.

In addition, the sitting position enables microsurgical extirpation in a clean operative field and also allows easy neuroanatomical orientation, despite the inherent risk of complications such as air embolism.

Finally, intraoperative angiography might minimize the risk of a residual AVM, which tends to regrow rapidly as observed in Case 5 and Case 10. A stereotactic radiosurgery should be seriously considered in cases with residual AVM difficult to manage surgically.

Although selective embolization prior to microsurgical removal (especially with EVAL) has been revealed to be useful[9], this procedure might induce complications like homonymous hemianopia (as observed in Case 5).

Stereotactic irradiation[3,8] is considered to be promising but to have limited indications. The AVM should be smaller than $3\,cm^3$ in volume and the risk of rebleeding remains considerable until the final disappearance of the AVM years later. A stereotactic radiosurgery should be seriously considered in cases with residual AVM or with feeders of thalamoperforating arteries and thalamogeniculate arteries as well. These cases are difficult to manage surgically.

It is concluded that some thalamic AVMs can be extirpated safely via the parieto-occipital transventricular approach in the sitting position using intraoperative angiography.

References

1. Drake CG (1979) Cerebral arteriovenous malformations: considerations for and experience with surgical treatment in 166 cases. Clin Neurosurg 26: 145–208
2. Garrido E, Stein B (1978) Removal of an arteriovenous malformation from the basal ganglia. J Neurol Neurosurg Psychiatry 41: 992–995
3. Hosobuchi Y (1988) Stereotactic heavy-particle irradiation of intracranial arteriovenous malformations. In: Suzuki·J (ed) Advances in surgery in cerebral stroke. Springer, Berlin Heidelberg New York Tokyo, pp 190–201
4. Juhasz J (1978) Surgical treatment of arteriovenous angiomas localized in the corpus callosum, basal ganglia, and near the brain stem. Acta Neurochir (Wien) 40: 83–101
5. Kikuchi H, Yamagata S, Karasawa J (1987) Treatment of AVMs in the basal ganglia. Neurosurgeons 6: 246–250 (in Japanese)
6. Ochiai C (1987) Treatment of AVMs in the basal ganglia and the thalamus. Neurosurgeons 6: 258–259 (in Japanese)
7. Saito I (1983) Treatment of AVMs in the basal ganglia. Mt Fuji Workshop on CVD 2: 67–74 (in Japanese)
8. Steiner L (1984) Treatment of arteriovenous malformations by radiosurgery. In: Wilson CB, Stein BM (eds) Intracranial arteriovenous malformations. Williams and Wilkins, Baltimore, pp 295–313
9. Taki W, Yonekawa Y, Handa H (1987) Embolization of AVMs in thalamus and basal ganglia. Neurosurgeons 6: 251–253 (in Japanese)
10. Taki W, Yonekawa Y, Iwata H, Uno A, Yamashita K, Amemiya H (1990) New liquid material for embolization of arteriovenous malformations. AJNR 11: 163–168

11. Wilson CB, Martin NA (1984) Deep supratentorial arteriovenous malformations. In: Wilson CB, Stein BM (eds) Intracranial arteriovenous malformations. Williams and Wilkins, Baltimore, pp 184–208
12. Yaşargil MG (1988) Thalamic AVMs. In: Yaşargil MG (ed) Microneurosurgery, Vol 3B. Thieme, Stuttgart, pp 301–317
13. Yonekawa Y, Handa H, Taki W (1983) Total removal of a brain stem arteriovenous malformation. Neurosurgery 13: 443–446

Correspondence: Yasuhiro Yonekawa, M.D., Neurochirurgische Klinik, Universitätspital Zürich, Raemistrasse 100, CH-8091 Zürich, Switzerland.

Treatment of Deep Basal Cerebral Arteriovenous Malformations

H.S. U

Division of Neurosurgery, University of California San Diego, San Diego, California, U.S.A.

Summary

The surgical treatment of arteriovenous malformations located in deep periventricular regions poses significant technical challenges since approaches through functional regions limit adequate exposure of the lesions, while surgical dissection is sometimes complicated by acute severe brain swelling/hemorrhage in the surrounding tissues. In our approach to deep AVMs, our regimen has evolved from direct staged microsurgical excision under routine fentanyl/N$_2$O/relaxant anesthesia (first four patients) to the use of elective high dose barbiturate anesthesia (subsequent 13 patients). In the first group, 11 operations were performed. Two patients improved with one returning to normal neurologically. There were three episodes of acute brain swelling/hemorrhage resulting in mild deterioration in one patient and death in the other. In the second group, all but two lesions were eliminated completely. Among the 11 patients in whom the AVM was completely obliterated, seven improved, six of whom achieved a good to excellent outcome. Three patients regained full neurological function. Three patients worsened (one as a result of acute brain swelling/hemorrhage). There was no death in this group. Only one incidence of acute brain swelling/hemorrhage occurred out of 27 operations. Our intraoperative observations and postoperative results would suggest that our evolved multi-modality regimen, such as staged excision and the use of deep barbiturate anesthesia, was likely to have contributed to the improved treatment results of these formidable lesions.

Keywords: Treatment of deep AVM.

Introduction

Treatment of deep seated lesions in periventricular regions continues to present significant technical challenges despite advances in microsurgery and neuroradiology since exposure of deep lesions are limited by the need to circumvent functionally critical areas and yet to minimize brain retraction[11,17,18,23]. Secondly, elimination of large AV shunts has been complicated by the occurrence of sudden severe brain swelling/hemorrhage from the peri-AVM brain tissues[2-4,13,14,19,23,25]. In an effort to facilitate our treatment of these deep lesions, a therapeutic regimen has evolved which now includes preoperative embolization followed by the

Table 1. *Presentation of Deep Seated Arteriovenous Malformations*

Intracranial hemorrhage	9
Progressive neurologic deficits	4
Headaches → progressive neural deficits	3
Seizures → progressive neural deficits	1

transventricular, multi-staged microsurgical excision of the lesion using a high dose barbiturate anesthetic[5-7,9,10,16,20-23]. This report details the evolution of our experience in treating 17 patients between 1979 and 1991[24].

Methods and Material

Patient Population

This report involves 17 patients treated between 1979 and 1991 who harbored AVMs situated in the basal ganglia, thalamus, hypothalamus, internal capsule or deep (at least 1 cm below the cerebral cortex) in the periventricular regions.

Pre-operative Evaluation and Embolization

Preoperative angiography was performed to assess the AVM vascular anatomy as well as to identify any associated aneurysm. CT or MRI scanning was performed to delineate the relationship between the malformation and the ventricular and basal nuclei systems. Intravascular embolization was performed before each operative intervention to reduce vascular engorgement and the number of stages necessary for total AVM excision. Agents used were polyvinyl alcohol foam particles, silk or Dacron suture strands, or cyanoacrylates. Superselective Amytal injection (25–45 mg) was used for reversible functioning testing.

Operative Approach

Large peri-ventricular lesions draining through cortical veins were approached by following these venous anomalies to the AVM located in the deep white matter. Lesions located in the basal regions were approached through the sylvian fissure to occlude lenticular feeding vessels early in the operation (Patients 1 to 3). The ventricular system was not entered. Due to the occurrence of unanticipated and fatal intraventricular and peri-AVM hemorrhage in patient 3, this approach was abandoned in favor of a mid-frontal gyrus approach to the ventricular system[23,24]. The entire ventricular system was then isolated from the AVM which presented through the ependyma. Dissection was undertaken as that for cortical AVMs.

Anesthetic Technique

The first four patients received routine fentanyl/N_2O/relaxant anesthetics for a total of 11 operations. In view of the poor outcome associated with the occurrence of sudden malignant cerebral swelling and hemorrhage which had to be treated with the emergent institution of barbiturate therapy, we subsequently employed an elective, high dose barbiturate anesthetic in the surgeries for the next 13 patients[5,6,21-24]. Hypothermia was used to reduce the anesthetic dose.

Intraoperative Angiography

In order to assess the adequacy of operative excision, all patients were examined with digital intraoperative angiography since November 1988.

Results

Patient Population

Seventeen patients (12 women and 5 men, ages 12–60 years) harboring deep AVMs were treated. Seven lesions were located in the dominant left hemisphere while the remaining 10 AVMs resided in the right hemisphere. There were two small (<2 cm in diameter), five moderate (2–4 cm in diameter), and 10 larger (>4 cm in diameter) lesions.

Nine patients presented with intracranial hemorrhage while four manifested progressive neurologic deficits. Three patients presented with headache while one had a seizure initially but all developed progressive deficits before treatment. Most lesions were intimately associated with the internal capsule; thus, hemiplegia was the most common presenting finding (12 patients). In three patients, additional deficits included rapidly deteriorating sensorium, decreased intellectual function, and memory loss. The remaining patients presented with expressive dysphasia (two), hemianopsia (one), and loss of urinary control (one). All treatments were elective except for two patients who were operated on acutely for massive hemorrhages.

Staged Treated of AVMs (Table 2)

Preoperative embolization significantly reduced the volume of the AVM in six patients. In the first three patients treated through the sylvian approach using

Table 2. *Outcome of Treatment – Deep Seated Arteriovenous Malformations*

	Without barbiturate anesthesia	With barbiturate anesthesia
Neurologically intact	1	3
Improved	1	5
Unchanged	–	2
Deteriorated	1	3*
Death	1	–

* One patient had a postoperative hemorrhage due to hypertension (methohexital used as anesthetic).
One patient deteriorated from malignant brain swelling and hemorrhage. One patient developed a mild hemiparesis during intraoperative angiography.

standard fentanyl/N_2O/relaxant techniques, patient 1 recovered completely from hemiplegia and returned to full employment. Patient 2 remained hemianopic but is fully functional and gainfully employed. Patient 3 developed massive brain swelling and intraventricular hemorrhage. The outcome was fatal. As a result, part of the treatment in the fourth patient and treatment of all subsequent 13 patients was modified to involve a midfrontal gyrus approach to the ventricular system prior to AVM dissection to prevent inadvert intraventricular hemorrhage. In addition, an elective deep barbiturate anesthetic was employed to reduce cerebral metabolism, blood demand, flow, and volume. The resultant brain relaxation facilitated AVM dissection with minimal brain retraction. This enabled us to remove the AVM completely in 11 patients. Three regained full neurologic function while five improved. Three patients worsened – one from acute intraoperative brain swelling/hemorrhage, one from hypertensive hemorrhage from unexpected awakening when a short acting barbiturate agent was evaluated, and one from cerebral swelling during intraoperative angiography. There was no mortality in this group. The AVM was not totally removed in three patients. One patient with a small multi-compartmental caudate AVM and another with a moderate basal ganglia lesion both refused further surgeries. One improved while the other remained unchanged. In the third patients, acute hemorrhage and swelling occurred at the time of wound closure after an uneventful operative stage for a large basal ganglia AVM. She eventually awoke from prolonged coma and is leading a meaningful life as an active member of her family despite severe intellectual and motor impairment. Her AVM was finally obliterated with proton beam irradiation.

Discussion

Our approach to deep periventricular AVMs has evolved to one involving preoperative embolization followed by staged microsurgical excision under deep barbiturate anesthesia. With this therapeutic regime, the treatment results show improved morbidity and no mortality. One of the most davastating outcome of treatment of large deep AVMs is the occurrence of sudden massive cerebral swelling/hemorrhage[2-4, 13,14,19,23,25]. Hemorrhage from residual AVM clusters is usually focal. Hemorrhage and swelling involving the entire hemisphere or at sites distant from the AVM bed are more difficult to explain. This may be due to insult to vasomotor centers in the deep gray matter[8,15]. Alternatively, swelling/hemorrhage may result from the over-redistribution of blood to the surrounding brain regions rendered incapable of adequate autoregulation as the result of prolonged hypoperfusion[20]. In order to prevent these catastrophic occurrences, staged elimination of the AVM shunts has been employed to assist the surrounding vasculature to accommodate this acutely changing hemodynamic state[1,20,23,24]. Despite this, catastrophic swelling nevertheless still occurred in the first four patients in this series. The administration of high doses of barbiturates was invariably necessary for brain relaxation[12]. Even then, impairment of the extruded cortex had ensued. With the use of elective deep barbiturate anesthetic, however, we have been able to further reduce the occurrence of acute brain swelling/hemorrhage to a minimum (twice in the last ten years). The resultant brain relaxation also faciliated AVM dissection with significantly improved results.

In the treatment of these deep seated lesions, the introduction of intraoperative angiography has ensured that each lesions is completely eliminated. Had this been available to us, we would have detected and removed the residual AVM components in the two patients with incompletely treated lesions. Incompletely treated AVMs are just as lethal as untreated ones especially since smaller clusters are more prone to hemorrhage. Every attempt must be made to obliterate the AVM completely.

In conclusion, the treatment of large deep basal AVMs has evolved with improved neuroradiological, microsurgical, and anesthetic techniques. Our experience demonstrates that even though these lesions remain a formidable challenge, their treatment should improve in the future.

Acknowledgement

The author wishes to thank C. Kerber, J. Drummond, and M. Todd for their invaluable assistance in the treatment of these difficult lesions; and R. Morgan for unfailing editorial assistance.

References

1. Andrews BT, Wilson CB (1987) Staged treatment of arteriovenous malformations of the brain. Neurosurgery 21: 314–323
2. Batjer HH, Devous MD Sr, Meyer YJ, Purdy PD, Samson DS (1988) Cerebrovascular hemodynamics in arteriovenous malformation complicated by normal perfusion pressure breakthrough. Neurosurgery 22: 503–509
3. Batjer HH, Purdy PD, Giller CA, Samson DS (1989) Evidence of redistribution of cerebral blood flow during treatment for an intracranial arteriovenous malformation. Neurosurgery 25: 599–605
4. Day AL, Friedman WA, Sypert GW, Mickle JP (1982) Successful treatment of the normal perfusion pressure breakthrough syndrome. Neurosurgery 11: 625–630
5. Drummond JC, Todd MM, U HS (1985) The effect of high dose sodium thiopental on brain stem auditory and median nerve somatosensory evoked responses in humans. Anesthesiology 63: 249–254
6. Drummond JC, Todd MM, Schubert A, U HS (1987) Effect of the acute administration of high dose pentobarbital on human brain stem auditory and median nerve somatosensory evoked responses. Neurosurgery 20: 830–835
7. Eskridge JM, Hartling RP (1989) Preoperative embolization of brain AVMs using surgical silk and polyvinyl alcohol. AJNR 10: 882
8. Iadecola, C, Mraovitch S, Meeley MP, Reis DJ (1983) Do cholinergic neurons of the basal forebrain cholinergic system mediate the cortical vasodilation elicited by fastigial nucleus stimulation in rats? J Cereb Blood Flow Metab 3: 178–179
9. Kerber C (1976) Balloon catheter with a calibrated leak. Radiology 120: 547–550
10. Kricheff II, Madayag M, Braunstein P (1972) Transfemoral catheter embolization of cerebral and posterior fossa arteriovenous malformations. Radiology 103: 107–111
11. Malik GM, Umansky F, Patel S, Ausman JI (1988) Microsurgical removal of arteriovenous malformations of the basal ganglia. Neurosurgery 23: 209–217
12. Marshall LF, U HS (1983) Treatment of massive intraoperative brain swelling. Neurosurgery 13: 412–414
13. Morgan MK, Johnston I, Besser M, Baines D (1987) Cerebral arteriovenous malformations, steal, and the hypertensive breakthrough threshold. J Neurosurg 66: 563–567
14. Mullan S, Brown FD, Patronas NJ (1979) Hyperemic and ischemic problems of surgical treatment of arteriovenous malformations. J Neurosurg 51: 757–764
15. Nakai M, Iadecola C, Reis DJ (1982) Global cerebral vasodilation by stimulation of rat fastigial cerebellar nucleus. Am J Physiol 243: H226–H235
16. Pelz DM, Fox AJ, Vinuela F, Drake CC, Ferguson GG (1988) Preoperative embolization of brain AVMs with isobutyl-2 cyanoacrylate. AJNR 9: 757–764
17. Shi YQ, Chen XC (1987) Surgical treatment of arteriovenous malformations of the striatothalamocapsular region. J Neurosurg 66: 352–356
18. Solomon RA, Stein BM (1987) Interhemispheric approach for the surgical removal of thalamocaudate arteriovenous malformations. J Neurosurg 66: 345–351

19. Spetzler RF, Wilson CB, Weinstein P, Mehdorn M, Townsend J, Telles D (1978) Normal perfusion pressure breakthrough theory. Clin Neurosurg 25: 651–672
20. Spetzler RF, Martin NA, Carter LP, Flom RA, Raudzens PA, Wilkinson E (1987) Surgical management of large AVMs by staged embolization and operative excision. J Neurosurg 67: 17–28
21. Todd MM, Drummond JC, U HS (1985) The hemodynamic consequences of high-dose thiopental anesthesia. Anesth Analg 64: 681–687
22. Todd MM, Drummond JC, U HS (1987) Hemodynamic effects of high dose pentobarbital: studies in elective neurosurgical patients. Neurosurgery 20: 559–563

23. Hoi Sang U (1985) Microsurgical excision of paraventricular arteriovenous malformations. Neurosurgery 16: 293–303
24. Hoi Sang U, Kerber CW, Todd MM (1992) Multi-modality treatment of deep basal cerebral arteriovenous malformations. Surg Neurol 38: 192–203
25. Young WL, Solomon RA, Prohovnik I, Ornstein E, Weinstein J, Stein BM (1988): [133]Xe blood flow monitoring during arteriovenous malformation resection: a case of intraoperative hyperperfusion with subsequent brain swelling. Neurosurgery 22: 765–769

Correspondence: Hoi Sang U, M.D., Division of Neurosurgery, University of California, San Diego, CA 92103-8893, U.S.A.

The Surgery of Posterior Fossa Arteriovenous Malformations

D. Samson, H. Batjer, and **P. Purdy**

Department of Neurological Surgery, Division of Neuroradiology, University of Texas Southwestern Medical Center, Dallas, Texas, U.S.A.

Summary

Arteriovenous malformations of the posterior fossa are relatively rare yet form a surprisingly heterogeneous array of clinical problems. The shared vascular supply with critical brain stem centers and the intimate proximity of these lesions to eloquent neural tissue and cranial nerves mandate a somewhat different philosophical and technical approach than with the more common supratentorial malformations. Superselective embolization procedures have proven to be extremely helpful surgical adjuncts and have been employed in nearly half of our cases.

From 1977 through 1991, 75 cases of posterior fossa arteriovenous malformations have been treated at our Center. Seventy-four of these lesions have been completely removed microsurgically. Management morbidity has been 8% (seven patients) and mortality has been 6.6% (six patients). Careful anatomically-based pre-operative planning and the liberal use of interventional radiology allows the successful management of the majority of such lesions whose nidus is outside the brain stem.

Keywords: Cerebellar arteriovenous malformation; brain stem arteriovenous malformation.

Introduction

Arteriovenous malformations of the vertebral-basilar system are relatively uncommon, representing only some 7% of intracranial, intradural arteriovenous malformations[2,3,5,6]. Most malformations of the posterior circulation present with intraparenchymal hemorrhage (greater than 60%)[2-6], and in such cases the initial surgical focus should be the treatment of any mass effect and/or hydrocephalus which are frequently associated with such posterior fossa hemorrhage. When possible, such patients should be managed without initial surgical intervention, being treated medically for a period of some four to six weeks from the time of the last hemorrhage prior to definitive removal of the malformation. In the small group of patients whose initial mass effect is life threatening, an optimal surgical approach is subtotal removal of the clot and adjacent edematous brain without attempting to deal with the arteriovenous malformation at the initial surgical sitting. Postoperatively, these patients may be managed medically until their clinical condition has stabilized and there is CT/MRI evidence of resolution of any residual mass effect. At that point definitive resection of the malformation can be undertaken. An occasional patient undergoing early hematoma evacuation will require, because of intraoperative hemorrhage, complete resection of the arteriovenous malformation. In this situation, every attempt should be made to spare all viable cerebellar tissue, and to minimize the extent of sacrifice of both arteries and veins in the immediate region of the malformation. The following discussion will describe our philosophy regarding the case of patients with posterior fossa malformations and techniques which have proven helpful in our Center.

Methods

Interventional Neuroradiology

Surgery of almost all arteriovenous malformations has been made simpler and more straightforward in the past decade by the advent and increasing use of preoperative embolization procedures[7]. The overwhelming majority of malformations located in the posterior fossa are amenable to at least partial devascularization by these techniques, and it is strongly recommended that preliminary embolization of malformations, coupled with obliteration of their major feeding arteries, be undertaken at a period of some five to seven days prior to definitive resection of the malformation. Embolization is not a treatment in and of itself, but an adjunct to the surgical management of these lesions. If protracted time is allowed to lapse between embolization and definitive resection, the surgeon will discover that in the interval, the malformation has come to be supplied by a large number of difficult-to-access nutrient arteries, whose copious flow effectively negates any beneficial effect of the previous embolization procedures.

Surgical Management of Specific Malformations

Malformations of the cerebellum may be anatomically separated into those of the vermis, the cerebellar hemisphere, and the cerebellar tonsils. AVMs located primarily in the cerebellar vermis occur with relative equal frequency to those of the cerebellar hemisphere. Vermian malformations receive their arterial input from superior cerebellar arteries and posterior/inferior cerebellar arteries and not infrequently have bilateral arterial supply. Venous drainage of these lesions is initially via the vermian venous system, but ultimately drain laterally across the cerebellar hemisphere into the petrosal sinuses, or more commonly directly superiorly into the galenic system. Almost invariably, AVMs of the vermis have some degree of ventricular representation but almost never extend ventrally into the middle cerebellar peduncle and brain stem.

The "concorde position"[1] coupled with an extensive midline bony exposure, offers an ideal approach to vermian arteriovenous malformations. Following dural opening, the surgeon should initially sever any arachnoid adhesions between cerebellum and tentorium to permit the cerebellum to "settle" into the posteior fossa and maximize exposure of the superior vermis. Superior cerebellar artery feeders should be identified and tracked into the vermis itself prior to sacrifice; proximal occlusion of these vessels on the superior surface of the cerebellum is unnecessary, and will produce ischemia and infarction of the cerebellar nuclei with severe postoperative appendicular ataxia, etc. Posterior inferior cerebellar artery branches can be accessed at the medial margins of the cerebellar tonsils near the midline.

The folia of the cerebellar vermis should be opened in the sagittal plane, respecting all arterialized veins, and the malformation's periphery encountered and dissected in a circumferential fashion. Retraction is often not necessary if an ample vermian incision is employed, and the malformation, rather than normal brain, can be compressed and displaced as dissection deepens into the vermis. Despite methodical circumferential dissection of these malformations with sequential sacrifice of all visible feeding arteries, vermian lesions many times remain impressively distended with arterial blood well into the later stages of dissection. Close inspection of the vermian venous peduncles in such instances will identify large arterial branches, usually stemming from the superior cerebellar arteries, incased in arachnoid and tightly bound to the enlarged and distended draining veins. Sequential identification and sacrifice of these vessels will permit further mobilization and ultimate resection of the entire arteriovenous malformation following transection of the draining veins.

Because of the frequency of ventricular wall involvement in malformations of the vermis, the roof of the fourth ventricle will be opened in the resection of almost every vermian lesion. Once the ventricular limit is entered, it should be carefully marked with a cottonoid patty and the ventricular wall closely inspected both prior to and following removal of the lesion to ensure that residual malformation is not overlooked. At the time of closure, ventricular hemostasis should be immaculate and the ventricle should be lavaged clean of any accumulated hematoma.

Malformations of the cerebellar hemisphere vary in size from extremely small lesions with trivial arterial input to holohemispheric malformations of impressive extent in enormous flow. The arterial supply to hemispherical lesions is almost always unilateral and may include branches of both superior cerebellar artery and posterior inferior cerebellar arteries; these branches are frequently the sight of associated and sometimes symptomatic arterial aneurysms. Involvement of the anterior inferior cerebellar artery in the supply of the malformation often suggest that the AVM itself involves not only the cerebellar hemisphere, but also the lateral aspect of the roof of the fourth ventricle and the adjacent middle cerebellar peduncle.

Venous drainage of these malformations is often via both the lateral hemispherical veins and the midline vermian venous plexus.

For malformations involving the rostral portions of the hemisphere above the horizontal fissure, the concorde position and a large superiorly located bony exposure provide an optimal operative approach. When dealing with more laterally- or inferiorly-placed lesions, the lateral position in a large laterally-situated bone flap should be employed. Arterial input from the superior cerebellar arteries and posterior inferior cerebellar arteries should be accessed as outlined for vermian lesions; feeding vessels originating from the anterior inferior cerebellar artery can be identified at or near the foramina of Luschka and should be followed into the brain parenchyma prior to cautery and sacrifice.

The medial margins of the AVM initially should be exposed by incising the cerebellar folia, and then the malformation dissected from medial to lateral, lifting the lesion out of the hemisphere and avoiding excessive retraction on the cerebellum itself. Such malformations can often be hinged on their lateral venous peduncle and their anterior pia margins exposed through the brain by elevation and dissection of the deeper part of the malformation, thus approaching its anterior and lateral pia margins beneath the AVM itself. Malformations of the hemisphere rarely have any ventricular representation, and thus routinely the fourth ventricle does not need to be opened in almost all circumstances.

Tonsil arteriovenous malformations are, as a rule, limited in size and produce problems in exposure only if their very caudal location is not appreciated. These lesions may be best approached with the patient lateral, and the neck fully flexed. Low midline or paramedian excision which permits wide opening of the foramen magnum (and removal of the arch of C1) from the midline to the sigmoid sinus is preferred, and the dura mater should be opened below the inferior margin of the involved tonsil.

After the cisterna magna has been opened and evacuated of spinal fluid, a cotton strip is placed in the vallecula, and the cerebellar tonsil elevated to identify the lateral and posterior medullary segments of the enlarged posterior cerebellar artery. This vessel can then be followed in the subarachnoid space until its major branches to the AVM enter the tonsil itself where they should be cauterized and cut at the margin of the malformation. A limited opening of the inferior aspect of the inferior vermis will provide additional exposure of the rostral aspect of the tonsil if needed; once arterial input has been secured and the medial aspect of the tonsil dissected free, the tonsil itself should be resected on block from medial to lateral, cauterizing and cutting the inferior vermian veins which represent the malformation's sole venous drainage.

Brain stem arteriovenous malformations located on the lateral aspect of the pons and presenting in the cerebellar pontine angle may be either entirely epipial or have a varying degree of parenchymal involvement. As a rule, arterial supply to these lesions is derived from enlarged branches of the anterior inferior cerebellar artery and enters the malformation directly from the subarachnoid space rostral to the foramina of Luschka. Venous drainage via enlarged lateral pontine veins also occupies the subarachnoid space of the cerebellar pontine angle, and ultimately reaches the petrosal and or galenic systems. Enlarged afferent and efferent vasculature, the pia presentation of the AVM itself, and the surrounding lower cranial nerves serve to produce a complex and potentially confusing anatomical puzzle within the crowded confines of the cerebellar pontine angle.

Such malformations should be approached with the patient in the true lateral position, with care being taken to avoid rotation of the head toward the floor. The paramedian excision followed by an extensive, far lateral craniotomy exposing the entire length of the sigmoid sinus should be employed to both maximize exposure of the complete cerebellar pontine angle and to minimize cerebellar and brain stem retraction. The arachnoid cistern of the cerebellar pontine angle should be widely opened from the level of the dural entry of the vertebral artery to the root entry zone of the fifth cranial nerve prior to beginning dissection of the malformation.

As is routinely true, dissection of the malformation should begin with the identification and occlusion of all feeding vessels. Unfortunately, such indentification may be difficult if not impossible in its anatomical situation, and the inadvertent occlusion of normal arterial channels within the cerebellar pontine angle may result in catastrophic brain stem ischemia. A reasonable approach, predicated on the very superficial extent of almost all these lesions, entails the preliminary identification of the posterior pia margin of the malformation, an extension of this pia dissection to both rostral and caudal poles of the AVM with subsequent subpial elevation of the lesion from its bed in the lateral aspect of the pons. This approach will undercut the malformation and displace it into the angle as it is gradually dissected free from the intertwined cranial nerves and normal vasculature, and will permit progressive identification and obliteration of the abnormal arterial supply to the malformation and yet allow for preservation of the multiple draining veins until the malformation is completely liberated from the pons itself. This dissection is tedious and often made more difficult by the inability to reliably and safely eliminate arterial supply to the lesion prior to beginning resection of the malformation itself, but is much safer and more effective than a more aggressive approach to these somewhat difficult malformations.

Malformations of the anterior basis pontis, medullary and pontine floor of the fourth ventricle and cerebellar peduncles are distinctly unusual and fortunately quite rare. These lesions uncommonly present with subarachnoid hemorrhage, more frequently coming to clinical attention because of unusual and often progressive neurologic syndromes more commonly seen with demyelinating disorders or occasional intrinsic glioma of the brain stem[9]. Such malformations receive their arterial input directly from perforating vessels of the vertebral and basilar systems, vessels which enter the malformation in its ventral aspect and frequently pass through normal brain tissue to access the AVM. The principal venous drainage of these lesions is most commonly via intraventricular ependymal veins into the galenic system.

The unique and forbidding aspect of these malformations is their intimate association with clinical brain stem parenchyma and their arterial supply which both transgresses and provides arterial input to normal surrounding brain stem structures. The latter of these facts makes preoperative embolization of these lesions difficult if not impossible, and their association with a normal brain stem parenchyma makes their surgical removal fraught with risks to injury of critical pontine medullary and mid brain structures. Occasionally, a small superficial lesion of this type, especially when associated with a prior intraparenchymal hemorrhage, may be amenable to complete surgical resection with minimal neurological consequence, but much more commonly the degree of surgical trauma and vascular occlusion required to completely resect such a lesion is attendent with overwhelming neurological morbidity. In the absence of documented intraparenchymal hemorrhage and progressive neurologic dysfunction, these patients are poor candidates for microsurgical resection and should instead be considered for alternative modes of therapy, more specifically focused radiotherapy.

Postoperative Angiography

Immediate postoperative angiography is recommended in all patients having undergone arteriovenous malformation resection. The goal of the operative procedure is complete elimination of the malformation, and the risk of hemorrhage subsequent to the surgical procedure is not eliminated unless complete malformation removal is verified by angiographic study. Furthermore, the appropriate diagnosis and treatment of the most common postoperative complications necessitate definitive knowledge that residual malformation does not exist. For these reasons an immediate intraoperative or postoperative arteriogram is recommended to document that malformation resection has been complete. In this operative series, five patients (6.6%) demonstrated residual AVM on their immediate postoperative angiogram.

Results

During the period from 1977 through 1991, the authors have managed 75 malformations located in the cerebellum or brain stem. Pre-operative selective embolization has been done in almost 50% of cases and has become the rule in the last five years of our experience. Embolization has been followed by resection in all cases and 74 out of 75 malformations have been completely removed, with this removal documented by postoperative angiography. Management mortality has been 6.6% (six patients) and management morbidity has been 8% (seven patients).

Discussion

In light of this experience, it is our belief that arteriovenous malformations located in the cerebellum (vermis, hemispheres, tonsils) and some lesions of the superficial aspect of the brain stem, especially those presenting in the cerebellar pontine angle, are routinely amenable to microsurgical resection with relatively low morbidity and mortality. Intrinsic malformations of the anterior basis pontis and cerebral peduncles which receive their principle arterial supply from perforating vessels of the vertebral or basilar arteries may occasionally be completely removed with good surgical results; however, in general the morbidity and mortality attendant to complete surgical extirpation of these brain stem lesions is forbiddingly high.

References

1. Bloomfield SM, Sonnatag VKH, Spetzler RF (1985) Pineal region lesions. BNI Quarterly 1(3): 10–24
2. Ciminello VJ, Sach E (1975) Arteriovenous malformations of the posterior fossa. J Neurosurg 41: 23–31
3. Drake CG (1979) Cerebral arteriovenous malformations: considerations for and experience with surgical treatment in 166 cases. Clin Neurosurg 26: 145–208
4. Drake CG, Friedman AH, Peerless SJ (1986) Posterior fossa arteriovenous malformations. J Neurosurg 64: 1–10
5. Lapras C (1975) Angiomas of the cerebellum and brain stem. In: Pia HW, Gleave JRW, Grote E, *et al* (eds) Cerebral angiomas:

advances in diagnosis and therapy. Springer, Berlin Heidelberg New York, pp 136–144

6. Martin NA, Stein BM, Wilson CB (1984) Arteriovenous malformations of the posterior fossa. In: Wilson CB, Stein BM (eds) Intracranial arteriovenous malformations. Williams and Wilkins, Baltimore, pp 209–221

7. Purdy PD, Samson D, Batjer HH, Risser RC (1990) Preoperative embolization of arteriovenous malformations with polyvinyl alcohol particles. AJNR 11: 501–510

8. Stahl SM, Johnson KP, Malamud N (1980) The clinical and pathological spectrum of brain-stem vascular malformation: longterm course simulates multiple sclerosis. Arch Neurol 37: 25–29

Correspondence: Duke Samson, M.D., Department of Neurological Surgery, University of Texas Southwestern Medical Center, 5323 Harry Hines Blvd., Dallas, Texas 75 235–9155, U.S.A.

Surgical Experience with Cerebellar AVMs

R. Da Pian, A. Pasqualin, R. Scienza, B. Cappelletto, and **G. Barone**

Department of Neurosurgery, City Hospital, Verona, Italy

Summary

From 1970 to 1992, 22 patients with cerebellar AVMs were surgically treated in our Department. Nineteen patients presented with an intracranial hemorrhage, two patients with increased intracranial pressure; in the remaining patient the AVM was an incidental discovery. According to angiography, we classified cerebellar AVMs into four groups: 1) superior (12 cases); 2) inferior (6 cases); 3) cerebello-pontine angle (3 cases); holohemispheric (1 case). In 19 patients, the AVM volume was within 20 cm³, in 3 over this size. In the last years, preoperative embolization was undertaken in 4 of these patients, harbouring large AVMs. Preoperative examination was negative in 7 patient; 13 patients presented a variable degree of neurological impairment and 2 patients were comatose. The AVM was totally resected in all patients, as documented by postoperative angiography. During the postoperative course 2 patients presented an acute ventricular dilatation, treated with a shunt; 1 patient developed a cerebellar hematoma (evacuated in a second operation) and 1 patient presented thrombosis of the venous sinuses (treated with anticoagulants). At follow-up, 12 patients were neurologically intact, 3 had minimal disturbances and 7 exhibited mild ataxia and/or dysmetria; there was no severe disability and no mortality. In conclusion, direct microsurgical excision is advised for all cerebellar AVMs, especially considering the high frequency of hemorrhage in the clinical history and the low surgical morbidity; for the largest lesions, preoperative embolization can be a reasonable adjunct.

Keywords: Cerebellar AVMs; embolization; microsurgery; AVM volume.

Introduction

Infratentorial arteriovenous malformations (AVMs) are rare, representing from 5 to 20% of all cerebral AVMs[9,14,15,17,23]. Recent reports on the natural history of infratentorial AVMs[10,24] have pointed out that these lesions are linked with a worse prognosis than supratentorial AVMs; on the other hand – owing to recent diagnostic, operative and anesthesiological advances – radical resection of an infratentorial AVM has become less hazardous, with favourable results in over 70% of cases[9].

The aim of this study is to present our experience in the surgical treatment of 22 patients with cerebellar AVMs and to discuss the proper approach for the various types of cerebellar AVMs.

Clinical Material and Method

From 1970 to 1992, 22 patients with cerebellar AVMs were operated on in the Neurosurgical Department of Verona, out of a total of 308 patients operated on for cerebral AVMs. 12 patients were male, 10 female. Age ranged between 5 and 63 years, with 3 patients younger than 20 years (mean age 34 years).

19 patients presented with an intracranial hemorrhage: in 15 cases intraparenchymal (extending to the ventricular system in 2 cases), in 3 cases subarachnoid only, in 1 case intraventricular only. Two patients presented with increased intracranial pressure, in one case due to hydrocephalus; in one patients the AVM constituted an incidental discovery.

Angiographical features are presented in Table 1. The size of the AVM was measured by its volume, calculated as the product of the 3 diameters of the AVM (height, width, and length) multiplied by 0.52, according to the volume calculation recently presented in a paper by our group[21]. The extension of the draining system was evaluated through a 4-degree scale, as proposed in the above mentioned paper[21]. In one patient, the AVM was associated with a vertebral/PICA aneurysm.

For practical purposes – mainly regarding the choice of the surgical approach – a classification of cerebellar AVMs was adopted:

1) *Superior cerebellar AVMs*, involving the superior and anterior cerebellar surface, with feeders prevalently from the SCA and drainage through the precentral vein and vein of Galen (12 cases) (Fig.1);

2) *Inferior cerebellar AVMs*, involving the posterior and inferior cerebellar surface; these AVMs were fed primarily by the PICA and secondarily by the AICA, and their drainage was more often towards the straight sinus (6 cases);

3) *AVMs of the cerebello-pontine angle*, primarily fed by the AICA, with drainage towards the petrosal and lateral sinuses (3 cases) (Fig. 2);

4) *Holohemispheric AVMs*, involving a wide portion of the cerebellar hemispheres and with multiple often ectasic feeders (1 case).

Preoperative examination is summarized in Table 2. As regards modality of treatment, a direct microsurgical removal was performed in 18 cases (82%), while a combined treatment – consisting of staged preoperative embolization followed by surgical resection – was performed in 4 cases (18%) (Fig. 2); in Table 3, modality of treatment is plotted against AVM volume. To effect preoperative embolization,

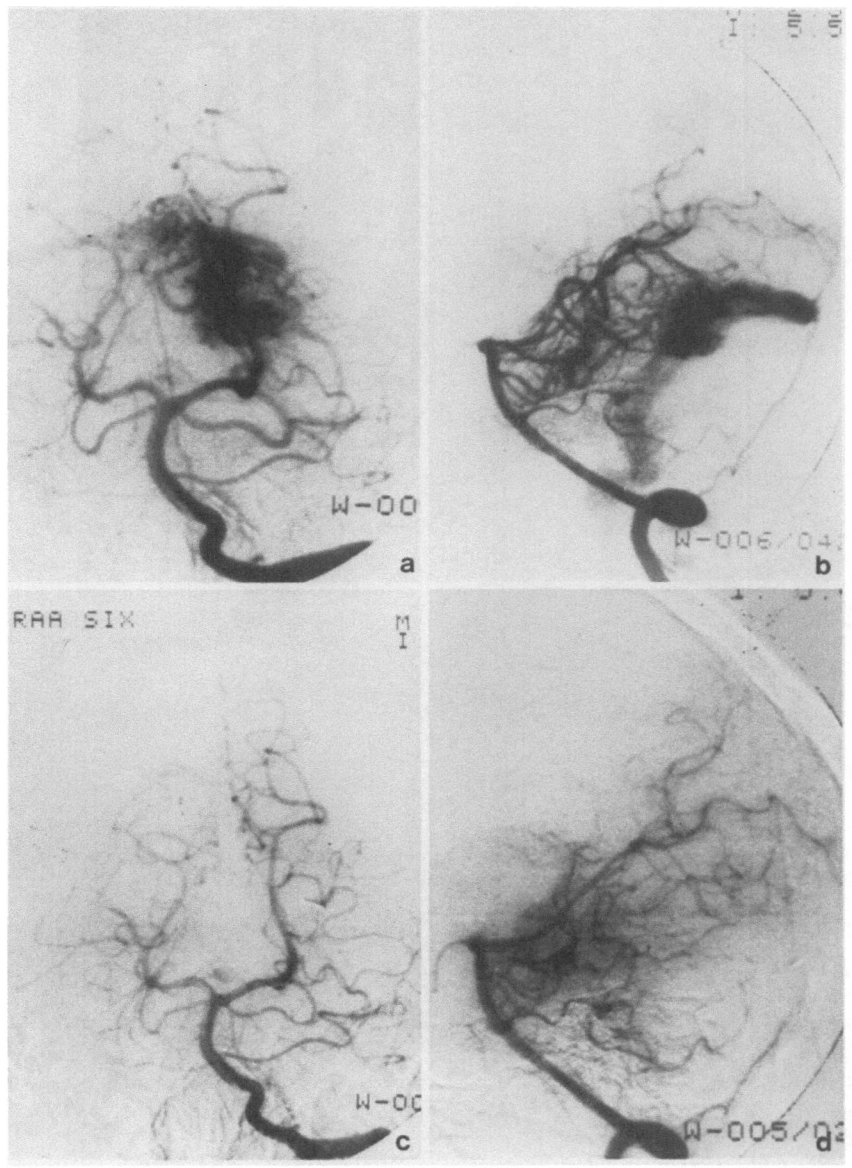

Fig. 1. (a, b) 18 year-old man with a left superior vermian-paravermian AVM (6 cm³); (c, d) postop. angiography. The patient developed transient postop. dysmetria, and was neurologically intact 3 months after surgery

selective embolization was adopted; details of the techniques employed are presented in other papers from our group[2,22].

20 patients were operated on in the sitting position, 2 in the prone position (one being a 5 year-old boy). As regards the surgical approach, all inferior cerebellar AVMs and a few superior cerebellar AVMs were operated through the standard suboccipital approach; the supracerebellar-infratentorial approach was used for most superior cerebellar AVMs, especially when they were located anteriorly; and the lateral retrosigmoid approach was used for cerebellopontine angle AVMs. Deep hypotension (with sodium nitroprusside) was adopted in 1 patient.

Results of treatment were related to intraoperative problems, postoperative complications, transient and permanent morbidity, and mortality.

Intraoperative and Postoperative Hyperemic Complications

Intraoperative hyperemic complications were considered to occur in patients with over 2000 ml of blood loss during surgery and in patients with paraventricular bleeding, i.e. long-lasting hemorrhages

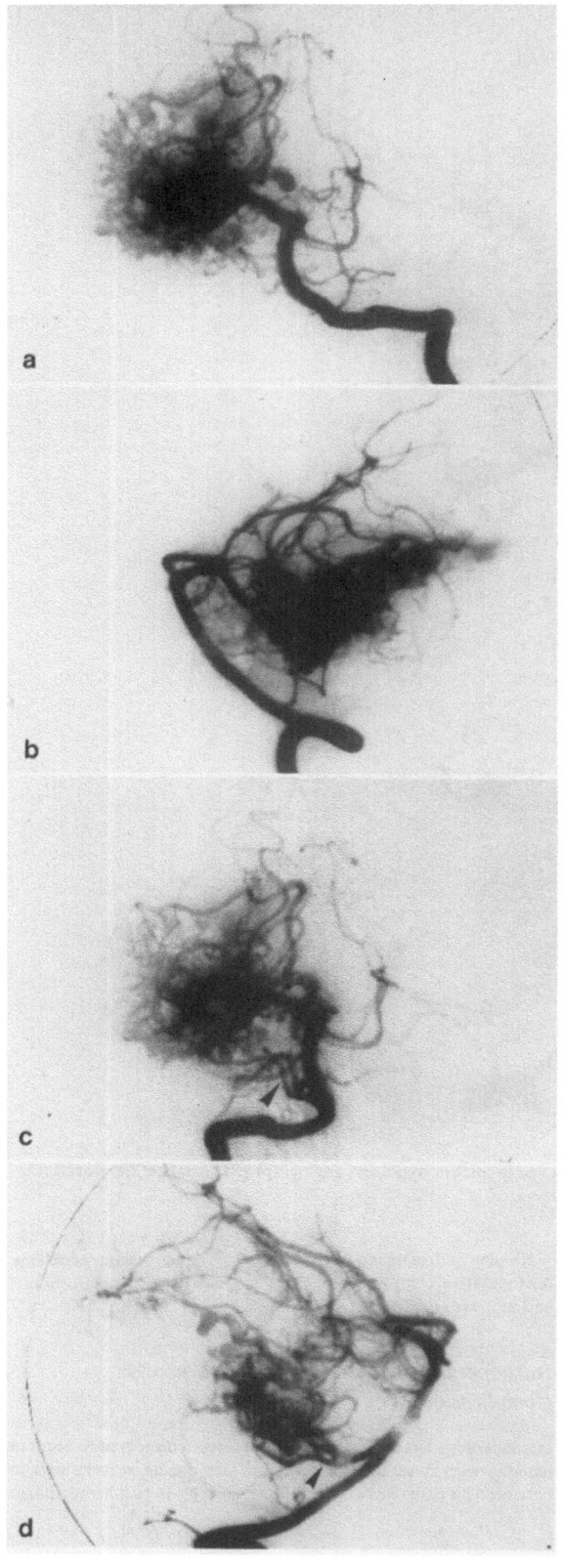

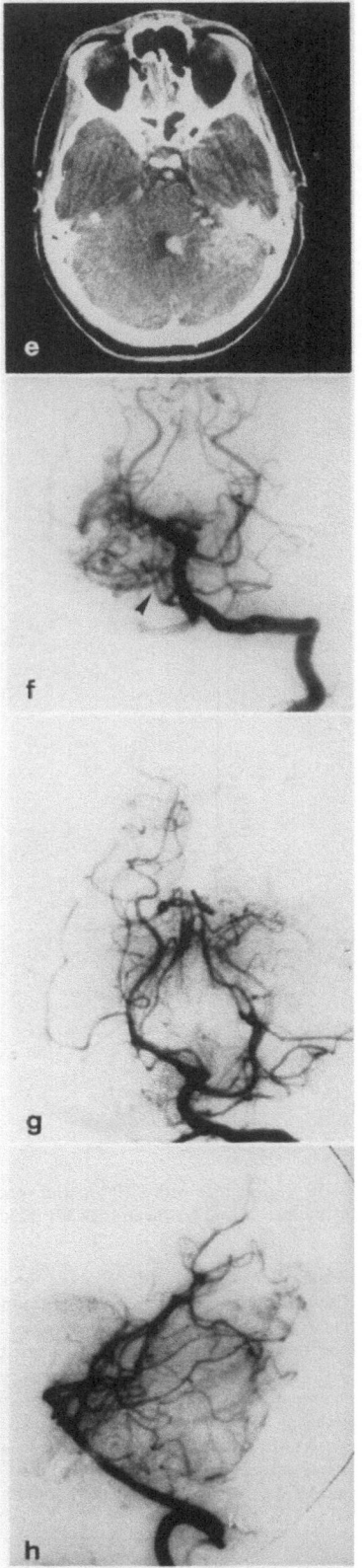

Table 1. *Angiographical Features*

AVM Volume			
	0–10 cm³	16	73%
	11–20 cm³	3	14%
	21–30 cm³	2	9%
	> 30 cm³	1	4%
Type of feeders			
	SCA	14	64%
	AICA	8	36%
	PICA	14	64%
	Dural	1	4%
Type of Drainage			
	superficial	15	68%
	deep (= towards vein of Galen)	7	32%
Draining system*			
	moderate (grade 1–2)	16	73%
	extensive (grade 3–4)	6	27%

* See Ref.[21].

Table 2. *Preoperative Examination*

No deficit	7	32%
Dysmetria/ataxia	12	55%
Hemiparesis	2	9%
Hypoesthesia	1	4%
Dysarthria	4	18%
Coma	2	9%

from small paraependymal[6,7] vessels. The main postoperative hyperemic complications considered were: a) cerebellar hematoma, and b) significant cerebellar edema.

Morbidity and Mortality

In the evaluation of morbidity, transient postoperative deficits were also considered. Permanent postoperative deficits were divided into:

Table 3. *Modality of Treatment*

AVM volume	Direct surgery		Combined treatment (embolization and surgery)	
0–10 cm³ (16 cases)	16	(100%)	–	
11–20 cm³ (3 cases)	1	(33%)	2	(67%)
> 20 cm³ (3 cases)	1	(33%)	2	(67%)
Total (22 cases)	18	(82%)	4	(18%)

a) old deficits (those present before surgery and improved or unchanged after surgery), and b) new deficits (those appearing after surgery or present before surgery, but clearly worsened after surgery). New permanent deficits were considered minor when they caused a moderate disability and major when they caused a severe disability according to the Glasgow Outcome Scale[13].

Results

During surgery, only 1 patient presented a severe blood loss, while 3 patients presented prolonged paraventricular bleeding; as shown by Table 4, intraoperative complications were never observed in patients with AVM volumes within 10 cm³.

As regards postop. hyperemic complications, 1 patient developed a postop. hemotoma (that was evacuated 2 days after surgery) and 1 patient significant cerebellar edema; postop. hyperemic complications were never observed in patients with AVM volumes within 10 cm³ (Table 4). Apart from hyperemic complications, an acute ventricular dilatation was observed in 2 patients (both submitted to CSF shunt later on)

Table 4. *Intraoperative and Postoperative Hyperemic Complications in Patients with Cerebellar AVMs*

Volume (cm³)	Intraoperative complications: severe hemorrhage		parav. bleeding		Postoperative complications: hematoma		edema	
0–10 (16 cases)	–		–		–		–	
11–20 (3 cases)	1	(33%)	1	(33%)	1	(33%)	–	
> 20 (3 cases)	–		2	(67%)	–		1	(33%)
Total (22 cases)	1	(4%)	3	(14%)	1	(4%)	1	(4%)

Fig. 2. (a, b) 34 year-old woman with a large right lateral ("c–p angle") AVM (24 cm³) fed by the rt. SCA. (c, d) The rt. AICA (arrow) – filling only from the rt. vertebral – also supplies the AVM. (e) CT scan, showing medial extension to the 4th ventricle. (f) Post-embolization left vertebral angiography, with decrease of AVM size and injection also of rt. AICA (arrow). (g, h) Postop. angiography. Postoperatively the patient developed severe rt. dysmetria and transient bilateral 6th nerve palsy; 6 months after surgery, she presented only mild rt. dysmetria

Table 5. *Morbidity and Mortality in Patients with Cerebellar AVMs*

Volume (cm³)	Transient deficit	New permanent deficit: minor		major	death
0–10 (16 cases)	10 (63%)	2	(12%)	–	–
11–20 (3 cases)	2 (67%)	1	(33%)	–	–
>20 (3 cases)	1 (33%)	2	(67%)	–	–
Total (22 cases)	13 (59%)	5	(23%)	–	–

and thrombosis of cerebral venous sinuses in one patient (who recovered completely following anticoagulation therapy).

As regards morbidity, transient deficits were commonly observed in our patients (59% of cases), independently from AVM volume; new minor deficits (dysmetria and/or ataxia) were observed in 23% of cases, showing a clear relation with AVM volume (67% of cases when AVM volume was over 20 cm³) (Table 5). Another 5 patients had already neurological deficits before surgery, which remained unchanged or improved after surgery. In summary, 12 patients were neurologically intact at follow-up and 10 patients showed minor postop. deficits (5 pre-existing and 5 new); no patient presented major deficits, and no patient died. Out of the 10 patients with minor deficits, 3 showed a minimal dysmetria, and 7 showed a moderate dysmetria and/or ataxia (with follow-up periods ranging from 1 year to 16 years).

Discussion

Anatomical Considerations

While removal of hemispheric cerebellar lesions can produce transient neurological deficits (dysmetria, ataxia, hypotonia, tremors, nystagmus), permanent deficits are frequently caused by removal of lesions involving the intrinsic nuclei and the cerebellar peduncles. Moreover, closure of thin proximal arteries can even lead to irreversible coma[8,9]. The "critical" vessels are:

a) direct or circumflex perforating branches originating from the PCA, SCA, AICA and PICA, and from the trunk of the basilar and vertebral arteries;

b) nutrient vessels originating mainly from the SCA, but also from the PICA (branches to the dentate nucleus) and the AICA (branches to the cerebellar peduncles).

It should be pointed out that perforating branches can feed also the postero-lateral surface of the brainstem, as the recurrent branches of the SCA to the quadrigeminal plate.

In infratentorial AVMs, the SCA is probably the most frequently involved artery[11,12]; less frequently involved is the AICA, which feeds mainly the cerebello-pontine angle, the antero-lateral surface of the cerebellum and the lateral recess of the 4th ventricle[18] passing through the foramen of Luschka. The third artery involved in the nutrition of infratentorial AVMs is the PICA, which supplies the inferior part of the cerebellar hemispheres, the 4th ventricle, and – partially – the dentate necleus[16]. Finally, dural branches from the occipital and vertebral arteries can feed these angiomas, whenever they involve the dura.

The venous drainage of infratentorial AVMs is complex, and frequently bilateral. Generally, the drainage is: a) towards the vein of Galen and the straight sinus, for superior lesions; b) towards the lateral sinus or the petrosal venous system, for infero-lateral lesions; c) towards the ponto-mesencephalic and petrosal veins, for lesions of the cerebello-pontine angle[17]. It should be pointed out that all of the infratentorial veins terminate as bridging veins, which should be carefully preserved[20].

Based on practical purposes, a classification of cerebellar AVMs has been proposed in this paper following the suggestion of Martin *et al.*, who divided cerebellar AVMs in superior, lateral (defined as "cerebello-pontine angle AVMs" in our series) and posterior (defined "inferior AVMs" in our series)[17]. Similarly to our classification, Yaşargil has divided cerebellar AVMs in superior, inferior, c-p angle and giant[27]. Subdivisions into hemispheric vs vermian AVMs have been made by various authors[9,24,27]; moreover the majority of authors has defined as "cerebello-pontine angle AVMs" those lesions that are located in the c-p angle cistern and involve the cerebellum only superficially[9,17,24], while we have enlarged this definition also to those AVMs that involve the lateral portion of the cerebellum (Fig. 2) (the so-called "flocculo-nodular AVMs" according to Drake)[9]. Our classification is meant to give an anatomical definition directly linked to the choice of the surgical approach and to the pattern of vascular supply.

Each of these types of AVMs can involve also the 4th ventricle and the intrinsic cerebellar nuclei (mainly the dentate nucleus). Some cerebellar AVMs are very extensive and do not fit into these 3 locations, due to wide involvement of the cerebellum. For these lesions we have adopted the term holohemispheric, already suggested by Drake[9].

Surgical Strategy

For cerebellar AVMs, some controversy still exists about positioning of the patient. In general: a) the sitting position can give technical advantages (especially decrease of venous tension and relaxation of cerebellum), but is linked with the risk of air embolism, particularly in the presence of very dilated veins; b) the prone position is rarely associated with a slack cerebellum, and presents the disadvantage of blood filling the operative field; c) the park-bench position requires particular experience and careful positioning, and can be associated to cerebellar swelling and venous engorgement[9]. While most authors agree that the sitting position is still the best[9,17,24,27], a reasonable compromise – especially for superiorly located cerebellar AVMs – is constituted by the so-called "Concorde" position (head more elevated than body and flexed anteriorly, with a tilt on one side), which reduces the disadvantages of the "classic" prone position[1].

As regards the surgical approach, we have favoured the standard (midline) suboccipital approach for the majority of our cases, reserving the supracerebellar-infratentorial approach or the lateral retrosigmoid approach to a few cases; so far, we have not used the subtemporal transtentorial[17] nor the occipital transtentorial[1,19,23] approaches. In general, the approach should be tailored to the location of the AVM, its size and its feeding and draining system.

Superior cerebellar AVMs can give considerable problems of exposure; the choice is between the infratentorial supracerebellar approach and the transtentorial (preferably occipital) approach. For superoanterior vermian-paravermian AVMs (with feeders only from the SCA and drainage to the vein of Galen) the best approach seems to be the transtentorial occipital, that gives an adequate exposure of the precerebellar space; for supero-lateral AVMs (with feeders from distal branches of the SCA and sometimes AICA, and drainage to the petrosal vein) the preferred approach is probably the infratentorial supracerebellar.

Inferior cerebellar AVMs can be conveniently approached through the standard midline suboccipital approach. It should be stressed that a deep extension of these AVMs can reach the 4th ventricle, which should be widely opened in order to control small feeding vessels. These angiomas are sometimes adherent to the lower cranial nerves; their dissection is however possible, generally without permanent consequences. The presence of feeders from the AICA – especially in the area of the 4th ventricle – should be carefully evaluated.

Cerebello-pontine angle AVMs can be conveniently approached through a lateral retrosigmoid approach. These lesions can be exposed as a c-p angle tumor, if they lay mainly in the cistern; when they extend to the inner portion of the cerebellum – towards the middle cerebellar peduncle and the 4th ventricle – the approach can be through a cortical incision. The exposure of the AICA in its post-meatal segment – at the level of the lateral recess – is fundamental when intraoperative hemorrhages occur; their control is difficult, and sometimes occlusion of the distal portion of AICA cannot be avoided (this maneuver is not linked with permanent deficits). When dissecting the AVM, a possible extension into the brainstem must be ruled out; small tufts of AVM – only superficially invading the brainstem – should be dissected and removed with extreme care. The use of a subtemporal transtentorial approach can be considered, whenever the origin of AICA is high on the basilar trunk.

Other Observations

As for the general surgical technique and the immediate postop. course, a few points are worth mention:

a) it is necessary to recognize the presence of collateral branches ("comb-like" arteries)[6,7] functional for important areas, especially in the distribution of the SCA;

b) some feeders can be hidden by large draining veins and should be adequately visualized[6,7];

c) a severe hemorrhage can occur in the area surrounding the 4th ventricle[9,17,27] and – if not satisfactorily handled with the bipolar[9] – it can require repeated tamponade;

d) at the end of the operation, hemostasis must be very carefully checked, by repeating the Valsalva maneuver[9];

e) after surgery, it is convenient to keep the patient in the sitting position for at least 24 hours, in order to avoid a dangerous increase in blood pressure, with the risk of postoperative hemorrhage[9].

The presence of a cerebellar hematoma associated with the AVM can constitute a considerable surgical problem; whenever it is possible, it is better to operate the patient in a chronic stage, when cerebellar edema is reduced or has subsided. The experience of a Co-operative Study on treatment of spontaneous posterior fossa hematomas[5] has allowed recognition of patients at risk for deterioration (on CT scan, hematoma with diameter over 3 cm, associated ventricular dilatation, shift of the 4th ventricle, intraventricular hemorrhage); in patients not at risk – according to CT scan findings – a waiting attitude seems a reasonable choice.

We strongly recommend postoperative angiography in order to prove the complete disappearance of the AVM. A frequently neglected area is the lateral recess of the 4th ventricle, where it is possible to leave small tufts fed by the AICA: the presence of a residual angioma entails a considerable risk of rebleeding[9].

Delayed venous thrombosis is a complication already pointed out by others before[17] and observed also in one of our cases; it is possibly due to the marked reduction of venous pressure and flow in posterior fossa occurring with the removal of the AVMs, especially after operations in the sitting position.

As shown by our results and by other series[17,24,27], surgical morbidity is relatively low for cerebellar AVMs; however the rate of hyperemic complications and postop. deficits is directly related to the size of the lesion, with high surgical risk over 20 cubic cm[21]. It is still uncertain if preop. embolization can reduce the risk of these complications in large cerebellar AVMs; the preliminary results presented to date[2,9,17,22,26] seem encouraging.

In the recent years, stereotactic radiosurgery has been proposed as an alternative approach to these lesions[3,4,25]; although the results reported are satisfactory – with minimal morbidity and nearly 80% obliteration rate at 2 years – a patient who is left with a residual AVM is still at risk of hemorrhage and cannot be considered as cured. Radiosurgery should probably be recommended when the AVM is very close to the brainstem; for all other cerebellar locations, direct surgery should still be considered the best choice.

In conclusion, direct microsurgical excision is advised for all cerebellar AVMs, especially considering the high risk of hemorrhage for untreated patients and the low surgical morbidity observed in our and in other clinical series; moreover – although experience with preoperative embolization of cerebellar AVMs is still limited – this adjunct seems a reasonable choice for the largest lesions.

References

1. Aoki N (1985) Combined occipital transtentorial and infratentorial supracerebellar approach in the Concorde position for the treatment of an arteriovenous malformation in the upper vermis: case report. Neurosurgery 17: 815–817
2. Benati A, Beltramello A, Colombari R, Maschio A, Perini S, Da Pian R, Pasqualin A, Scienza R, Rosta L, Piovan E, Scarpa A, Zamboni C (1989) Preoperative embolization of arteriovenous malformations with polylene threads: techniques with wing microcatheter and pathologic results. AJNR 10: 579–586
3. Bunge HJ, Chinela AB, Guevara JA, Antico JC, Lemme-Plaghos LA, Steiner L (1992) Radiosurgery in infratentorial arteriovenous malformations. In: Steiner L, Lindquist C, Forster D, Backlund EO (eds) Radiosurgery: baseline and trends. Raven, New York, pp 179–188
4. Colombo F, Benedetti A, Pozza F, Marchetti C, Chierego G (1989) Linear accelerator radiosurgery of cereberal arteriovenous malformations. Neurosurgery 24: 833–840
5. Da Pian R, Bazzan A, Pasqualin A (1984) Surgical versus medical treatment of spontaneous posterior fossa hematomas: a cooperative study on 205 cases. Neurol Res 6: 145–151
6. Da Pian R, Pasqualin A, Scienza R (1981) Microsurgical treatment of juxta-peduncular angiomas. Surg Neurol 17: 16–29
7. Da Pian R, Pasqualin A, Scienza R, Vivenza C (1980) Microsurgical treatment of ten arterio-venous malformations in critical areas of the cerebrum. J Microsurgery 1: 305–320
8. Drake CG (1975) Surgical removal of arteriovenous malformations from the brain stem and cerebellopontine angle. J Neurosurg 43: 661–670
9. Drake CG, Friedman AH, Peerless SJ (1986) Posterior fossa arterio-venous malformations. J Neurosurg 64: 1–10
10. Fults D, Kelly DL (1984) Natural history of arteriovenous malformations of the brain: a clinical study. Neurosurgery 15: 658–662
11. Hardy DG, Peace DA, Rhoton AL (1980) Microsurgical anatomy of the superior cerebellar artery. Neurosurgery 6: 10–28
12. Hoffman HB, Margolis MT, Newton TH (1974) The superior cerebellar artery. Section i. Normal gross and radiographic anatomy. In: Newton TH, Potts DG (eds) Radiology of the skull and brain: angiography, Vol 2, Book 2. Mosby, St Louis, pp 1809–1830
13. Jennett B, Bond M (1975) Assessment of outcome after severe brain damage. A practical scale. Lancet: 480–484
14. Laine E, Galibert P (1966) Aneurysmes arterio-veineux et cirsoides de la fosse posterieure. A propos de quarante observations. Reunion Franco-Belge de Neurochirurgie, Bruxelles, Juin 1966, pp 276–288
15. Lapras C (1975) Angiomas of cerebellum and brain stem. In: Pia HW, Gleave JRW, Grote E, Zierski J (eds) Cerebral angiomas. Advances in diagnosis and therapy, Springer, Berlin Heidelberg New York, pp 136–141
16. Lister JR, Rhoton AL, Matsushima T, Peace DA (1982) Microsurgical anatomy of the posterior inferior cerebellar artery. Neurosurgery, 10: 170–199
17. Martin NA, Stein BM, Wilson CB (1984) Arteriovenous malformations of the posterior fossa. In: Wilson CB, Stein BM (eds) Intracranial arteriovenous malformations. William and Wilkins, Baltimore, pp 209–221
18. Martin RG, Grant JL, Peace D, Theiss C, Rhoton AL (1980) Microsurgical relationship of the anterior inferior cerebellar artery and the facial-vestibulo-cochlear nerve complex. Neurosurgery 6: 483–507

19. Matsumura H, Makita Y, Sameda K, Kondo A (1977) Arteriovenous malformations in the posterior fossa. J Neurosurg 47: 50–56
20. Matsushima T, Rhoton AL, De Oliveira E, Peace D (1983) Microsurgical anatomy of the veins of the posterior fossa. J Neurosurg 59: 63–105
21. Pasqualin A, Barone G, Cioffi F, Rosta L, Scienza R, Da Pian R (1991) The relevance of anatomic and hemodynamic factors to a classification of cerebral arteriovenous malformations. Neurosurgery 28: 370–379
22. Pasqualin A, Scienza R, Cioffi F, Barone G, Benati A, Beltramello A, Da Pian R (1991) Treatment of cerebral arteriovenous malformations with a combination of preoperative embolization and surgery. Neurosurgery 29: 358–368
23. Salcman M, Nudelman RW, Bellis EH (1985) Arteriovenous malformations of the superior cerebellar artery: excision via an occipital transtentorial approach. Neurosurgery 17: 749–756
24. Samson D, Batjer H (1985) Arteriovenous malformations of the cerebellar vermis. Neurosurgery 16: 341–349
25. Steiner L (1984) Treatment of arteriovenous malformations by radiosurgery. In: Wilson CH, Stein B (eds) Intracranial arteriovenous malformations. William and Wilkins, Baltimore, pp 295–313
26. Terada T, Nakamura Y, Nakai K, Tsuura M, Nishiguchi T, Hayashi S, Kido T, Taki W, Iwata H, Komai N (1991) Embolization of arteriovenous malformations with peripheral aneurysms using ethylene vinyl alcohol copolymer. Report of three cases. J Neurosurg 75: 655–660
27. Yaşargil MG (1988) Infratentorial AVMs. In: Yaşargil MG (ed) Microneurosurgery, Vol III. Thieme, Stuttgart, pp 168–203

Correspondence: R. DaPian, M.D., Department of Neurosurgery, City Hospital, I-37126 Verona, Italy.

Embolization of Cerebral of AVMs

Overview of Embolic Materials and Clinical Use of EVAL

Y. Yonekawa, Y. Kaku, and **H. Iwata**[1]

Department of Neurosurgery, National Cardiovascular Center, Japan and [1]Department of Surgical Research, National Cardiovascular Center, Japan

Summary

Embolic materials available to-date are reviewed and classified. Characteristic properties of a newly developed embolic material, ethylene-vinyl-alcohol EVAL copolymer, along with experience of its clinical application are presented. Ease of its handling at the time of embolization and of operation are emphasized.

Keywords: Ethylene-vinyl-alcohol EVAL; embolic material; preoperative embolization.

Introduction

Recent advances in interventional neuroradiology have afforded new alternatives in the treatment of brain AVMs; particularly, the development of embolic materials and their delivery systems has facilitated the treatment of AVMs previously considered inoperable or marginally operable. This article is an overview of the embolic materials which have recently become available in the field of neurosurgery. In addition, we also describe our experience with 50 embolization procedures in 30 patients with AVM using the newly-developed embolic material, ethylene-vinyl-alcohol (EVAL) copolymer[9].

Embolic Materials

Embolic materials which have recently become available are listed in Fig. 1. Embolic materials are liquid or solid, and the latter can be biodegradable, such as gelatin, or non-biodegradable, such as formalized polyvinyl-alcohol (PVA). Liquid embolic materials consist of cyanoacrylate monomers and polymer solutions[3].

Solid Materials

The properties of biodegradable and non-biodegradable solid embolic materials are summarized in Tables 1, 2, and 3, respectively. Embolization with these particles is often used to occlude an arterial feeder proximal to the location of the nidus, following which surgery can be performed as soon as possible before a profuse collateral network (leptomeningeal, medullary, and dural) develops[5]. It is anticipated that the principal benefits of embolization with these particles will be decrease of blood loss associated with surgery and simplification of surgical approaches by occlusion of parts of the main feeding arteries of the AVM, which are difficult to access surgically[4,6].

Liquid Materials

Solidification of liquid materials can be obtained by polymerization of monomers or by diffusion of a solvent containing a polymer. Cyanoacrylate monomer is solidified by polymerization, while dimethyl sulfoxide (DMSO) solution containing EVAL and DMSO solution containing cellulose acetate are examples of polymer solutions which solidify by diffusion[3].

Upon contact with moisture or hydroxyl ions, cyanoacrylate monomeric units instantly solidify a polymer which is biodegradable, although its degradation rate is very low and slower than that of gelatin or collagen. Its N-butyl ester and iso-butyl ester of cyanoacrylate are also available. However this cyano-acrylate can cause adhesion of the catheter to the artery and sometimes polymerizes within the catheter, leading to incomplete injection of the embolizing material. In addition, polymerized cyanoacrylate forms a very hard mass, which is difficult to dissect and remove at the time of surgery[1,2,7,8].

Ethylene-Vinyl-Alcohol (EVAL) Copolymer

We have developed a new liquid embolic material, which is a mixture of ethylene-vinyl-alcohol (EVAL)

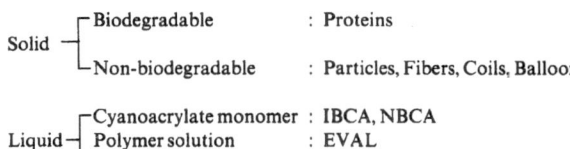

Fig. 1. Biomaterials for embolization

Table 1. *Biodegradable Polymers Used for Embolization*

Polymer	Examples
Proteins	collagen, gelatin
Polysaccharides	starch, chitin
Synthetic polymers	polyglycolide, polylactide

Table 2. *Non-Biodegradable Materials Used for Embolization*

Shape	Examples
Particles	formalized PVA, silicone
Fibers	polyester, silk
Coils	platinum, copper

Table 3. *Percent Compositions of EVAL Copolymers of Various Viscosities*

Material	Low viscosity	Medium viscosity	High viscosity
DMSO	27	27	27
EVAL	1	1.5	2
Metrizamide	7	7	7
Viscosity	16 cP	67 cP	116 cP

copolymer and metrizamide dissolved in DMSO[9]. The percent of composition of EVAL copolymers with various viscosities are summarized in Table 3. EVAL is a copolymer of polyethylene and polyvinyl alcohol, both of which are biocompatible polymers that have been used in implantation. Because polyethylene polymer is hydrophobic while polyvinyl alcohol polymer is hydrophilic, the copolymeric EVAL has both hydrophobic and hydrophilic properties. Upon contact with blood, the DMSO rapidly diffuses into the blood and forms a soft elastic sponge of EVAL copolymer that obstructs both the feeder and the nidus. In vitro experiments in which EVAL copolymer was injected into water through an 18-gauge needle, it formed a white gel-like droplet in about 3 seconds. In dogs, injection of EVAL copolymer into the renal artery

occluded vessels as small as 80 μm in diameter, and histological examination revealed no inflammatory reactions.

The advantages of EVAL copolymer as an embolic material are summarized as follows:

1) EVAL is of low viscosity and can be easily injected through the narrow lumen of a micro-catheter.

2) Since it is not adhesive, there is no risk of adhesion of the catheter to the vessels.

3) Because repeated injection through the same catheter without clogging under fluoroscopic guidance is possible, a sufficient volume of mixture can be delivered to the nidus.

4) Since EVAL copolymer forms a soft elastic sponge which can easily be compressed at the time of AVM dissection and easily shrunken at the time of electric coagulation, surgical excision options are increased.

However, although the non-adhesive property of the EVAL and DMSO mixture permits a safe removal of the micro-catheter, this property also increases the risk of unintended occlusion of a draining vein or venous outlet during the treatment of an AVM with considerable arterio-venous fistula area. If small amounts of the mixture are injected slowly and repeatedly under fluoroscopic guidance, this risk can be minimized.

Clinical Experience of Embolization Using EVAL Copolymer

Of 33 patients with brain AVM treated with endovascular embolization between April 1989 and April 1992, 30 underwent surgical removal subsequent to embolization. These patients included 13 females and 17 males, ranged in age from 5 to 58 years (mean age 31.5 years). These AVMs were Spetzler and Martin 2 Grade I, 2 Grade II, 8 Grade III, 7 Grade IV, and 11 Grade V.

Seventy-five to 100% obliteration of the AVM nidus was achieved with embolization in 9 patients (30%), 50% to 75% obliteration in 12 (40%), and less than 50% obliteration in 9 (30%).

There were no fatalities. In 3 patients (10%), rupture of feeding pedicles occurred during embolization. Two were treated conservatively without neurological deficit, and the remaining patient required surgical repair of the rupture site and developed mild hemiparesis. In 2 patients (6.7%), visual field deficit developed due to unintended occlusion of normal arteries. In 1 patient (3.3%), venous infarction occurred due to unintended occlusion of the venous outlet with embolizing material.

The morbidity rate related to surgical resection of the residual AVM was 6.7% (one patient with visual field defect and one with hemiparesis), and there was no post-surgical mortality.

Representative Case Reports

Case 1

A 29-year-old female experienced several episodes of scintillating scotoma and later developed a generalized convulsion. She was neurologically normal on admission. Angiogram revealed the presence of a medium-sized AVM in the left occipital lobe. To perform a functional test which revealed to be negative, we injected 50 mg of thiopental and 50 mg of lidocaine through a leak balloon catheter which had been introduced just proximal to the nidus, followed by 1.5 ml of EVAL mixture injected into the feeding pedicle. Almost complete obliteration of the nidus except its posterior part was achieved. This AVM was completely resected via a left occipital craniotomy 7 days after the embolization without any significant

blood loss; the patient showed no neurological deficit at the time of discharge. Photomicrographs of the resected EVAL-embolized AVM revealed partially organized thrombi among the EVAL sponges without any significant inflammatory infiltrates around the vessel wall.

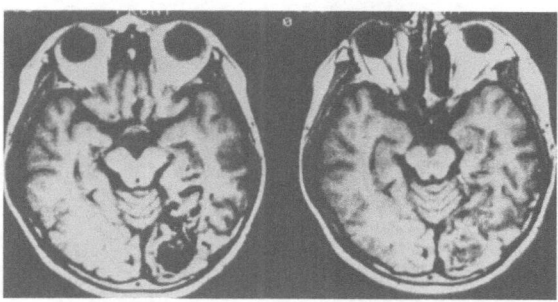

Fig. 3. Case 1. Left: MRI demonstrating the AVM in the occipital lobe as a flow-void area. Right: Post-embolization MRI demonstrating the embolized nidus as an area of isointensity

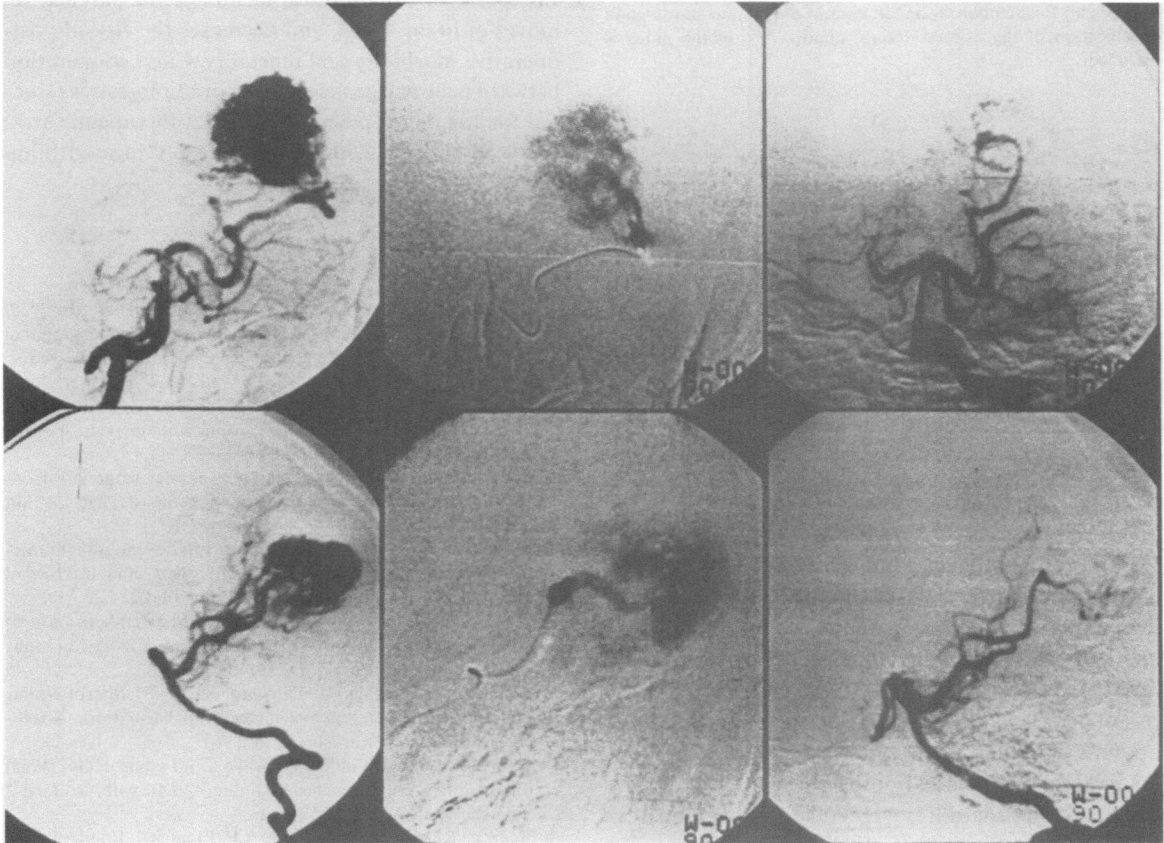

Fig. 2. Case 1. Left: Right vertebral angiogram demonstrating medium-sized AVM in the left occipital lobe; middle: Superselective angiogram; right: Post-embolization left vertebral angiogram demonstrating almost complete obliteration of the AVM

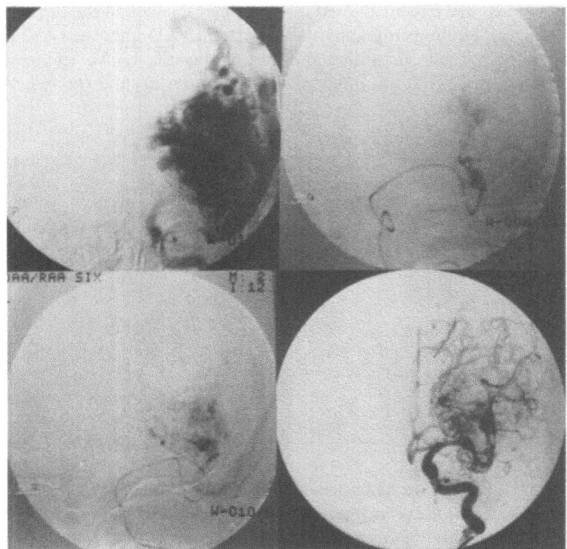

Fig. 4. Case 2. Upper left: Left carotid angiogram demonstrating a large high-flow AVM in the left parietal lobe with few normal vessels; lower right: Post-embolization left carotid angiogram shows good opacification of the normal vessels; almost 70% of the nidus is occluded

Case 2

A 28-year-old male whose intellectual function had gradually deteriorated suffered from frequent episodes of generalized convulsions. Angiogram revealed a large high flow AVM in the left fronto-parietal region with few normal vessels. Staged emboliztions were performed in this patient. A leak balloon catheter and Tracker 18 catheters were introduced into 6 feeding pedicles arising from left middle cerebral artery, and 0.7 ml to 1.8 ml of EVAL mixture was injected into each feeding pedicle after each functional test. Almost 2/3rds of the nidus could be occluded resulting in good opacification of normal vessels at angiography. The AVM was completely excised via staged left fronto-parietal craniotomy without neurological deficit.

Discussion

Despite recent advances in brain AVM embolization techniques and materials, complete obliteration of these lesions with embolization alone is not common and may be impossible in large and complicated AVM[11]. Evidence that partial obliteration reduces the risk of hemorrhage is lacking, and there are no follow-up data regarding the long-term presence of embolic materials in the brain[10]. For these reasons, we consider embolization procedures as preoperative treatment of AVM. The major purpose of performing preoperative embolization of brain AVM is to facilitate its surgical removal by decreasing blood loss, reducing the size of

components, and occluding the fistulous connections.

With respect to the material selected for preoperative embolization, the following properties are considered to be essential:

1) easily compressible at the time of AVM dissection (this is especially important in deeply located AVM);

2) easily dissectable from normal structures, hence relatively inert to adjacent structures; and

3) easily shrinkable at the time of electric coagulation.

In our clinical experience, EVAL copolymer mixture is superior to an acrylic agent in facilitating surgical resection, and comparable to an acrylic agent and far superior to a particulate embolic material in percent nidus occlusion.

Conclusion

Preoperative embolization facilitates the surgical removal of brain AVM, and decreases the risk of postoperative morbidity and mortality. Close cooperation between neurosurgeons and neuroradiologists is essential for the development of rational therapeutic strategies in patients with large or deeply located brain AVM.

References

1. Brothers MF, Kaufmann JCE, Fox AJ, Deveikis JP (1989) n-Butyl 2-Cyanoacrylate-substitute for IBCA in interventional neuroradiology: histopathologic and polymerization time studies. AJNR 10: 777–786
2. Debrun G, Vinuela F, Fox A, Drake CG (1982) Embolization of cerebral arteriovenous malformations with bucrylate. Experience in 46 cases. J Neurosurg 56: 615–627
3. Ikada Y (1992) Biomaterials in endovascular surgery. Fundamentals and future aspect. Neurosurgeons 11: 236–244 (in Japanese)
4. Lussenhop AJ, Rosa L (1984) Cerebral arteriovenous malformations. Indications for and results of surgery, and the role of intravascular techniques. J Neurosurg 60: 14–22
5. Lussenhop AJ, Spence WT (1960) Artificial embolization of cerebral arteries. Report of use in a case of arteriovenous malformation. JAMA 172: 1153–1155
6. Mullan S, Kawanaga H, Patronas NJ (1979) Microvascular embolization of cerebral arteriovenous malformations. A technical variation. J Neurosurg 51: 621–627
7. Pelz DM, Fox AJ, Vinuela F, Drake CG, Ferguson GG (1988) Preoperative embolization of brain AVMs with isobutyl-2 cyanoacrylate. AJNR 9: 757–764
8. Spetzler RF, Martin NA, Carter LP, Flom RA, Raudzens PA, Wilkinson E (1987) Surgical management of large AVM's by staged embolization and operative excision. J Neurosurg 67: 17–28

9. Taki W, Yonekawa Y, Iwata H, Uno A, Yamashita K, Amemiya H (1990) A new liquid material for embolization of arteriovenous malformations. AJNR 11: 163–168
10. Tseng YC, Tabata Y, Hyon SH, Ikada Y (1990) In vitro toxicity test of 2-cyanoacylate polymers by cell culture method. J Biomed Mat Res 24: 1355–1367
11. Vinuela F, Dion JE, Duckwiler G, Martin NA, Lylyk P, Fox A, Pelz D, Drake CG, Girvin JJ, Debrun G (1991) Combined endovascular embolization and surgery in the management of cerebral arteriovenous malformations: experience with 101 cases. J Neurosurg 75: 856–864

Correspondence: Yasuhiro Yonekawa, M.D., Neurochirurgische Klinik, Universitätsspital Zürich, Raemistrasse 100, CH-8091 Zürich, Switzerland.

Use of Ethanol in Preoperative AVM Embolization

P.D. Purdy, H.H. Batjer, T. Kopitnik, R. Risser and D. Samson

Department of Radiology, University of Texas Southwestern Medical Center, Dallas, Texas, U.S.A.

Summary

The selection of embolic materials for preoperative embolization is important in assurance of adequate occlusion with a low complication rate. Development of new microcatheters with smaller luminal diameters complicates that decision-making. We report here our experience with 33% ethanol (ETOH) solution in brain arteriovenous malformations (AVM).

This series consists of 23 separate embolization procedures in 19 patients with brain AVMs. All catheterizations and embolizations reported here were intracerebral branches of the anterior cerebral artery, middle cerebral artery, posterior cerebral artery, or basilar artery. Patients ranged in age from 3 to 65 years. Quantities of ETOH ranged from 0.1 cc to 1.2 cc.

Comparisons were performed between this group and our non-ETOH group for complications and angiographic results of embolization.

The angiographic results did not differ with ETOH use vs. use of only polyvinyl alcohol (PVA) and coils (p = 0.222). ETOH produced thrombosis in at least 1 fistulous connection which was too large for particles of PVA ranging up to 1.5 mm in diameter. Complications occurred in 4 out of 23 cases (17%), but the group was too small to achieve significance in its difference from our group with PVA and coils (6%) (p = 0.204).

ETOH can be used in conjunction with particulate embolization in brain AVMs. Its use requires caution, and only small aliquots are needed. It seems more hazardous than PVA plus coils, but statistical significance does not yet exist. It is a valuable adjunct in production of stasis under difficult circumstances.

Keywords: Ethanol; arteriovenous malformation; embolization.

Introduction

Over the past several years, many different embolic materials have been advocated for use in embolization of arteriovenous malformations. These include acrylic glue[1,5,6,9], PVA[8], platinum microcoils[4], silk suture material[3], and ETOH[2]. We present here our experience using ETOH in combination with other embolic materials in the preoperative embolization for AVMs and analyze our present complications and angiographic results with ETOH in comparison with other materials.

Material and Methods

Of 200 brain AVM embolizations performed at our institution, 158 have been via transfemoral catheterization. Of these, 144 were performed since 1987 and involved selective intracranial catheterization. Approximately 90%–95% of these were in a setting of preoperative embolization. Among these patients, 23 procedures in 19 patients involved the use of a 33% ETOH solution in combination with other embolic materials, either with or without the addition of microfibrillar collagen particles. The patients ranged in age from 3 to 65 years. Patients included 12 males and 7 females. AVMs ranged in size from 1–5 cm. Data was analyzed and compared against our data on non-ETOH embolizations for occurrence of complications and for angiographic results in those malformations in which superselective catheterization was performed and ETOH was or was not used.

Complications were scored as 0 for no neurologic complication, 1 for stroke, 2 for hemorrhage, or 3 for death. In all cases with fatal complication, fatality occurred as a result of hemorrhage. For statistical analysis purposes, any complication was rated as positive and scores of 0 were rated as negative. Angiographic outcome was scored as 1 for definite angiographic evidence of diminished perfusion to the malformation, 2 for probable but subtle evidence, or 3 for no evidence. For statistical analysis purposes, a score of 1 was counted as positive and any other score was counted as negative. Using the same scoring system for non-ETOH embolizations, the groups were compared using Fisher's Exact Test for differences in complication rate or angiographic outcome.

Results

Results are summarized in Table 1. Of 121 procedures performed without the use of ETOH, stroke or hemorrhage occurred in 9 (7%).

Of 23 procedures performed using ETOH, stroke or hemorrhage occurred in 4 (17%).

Angiographic results were rated as 1 in 21 of 23 embolizations using ETOH and as 2 in the other 2 embolizations.

Of the 121 embolizations performed without ETOH, 5 were not rated as to angiographic outcome. Thus, of the 116 that were rated, 103 were rated as 1, 10 were rated 2 and 3 were rated 3. Examination of embolic

Table 1. *Outcome and Complications*

	None	Outcome			Complications		
		1	2	3	1	2	3
ETOH, n = 23	0	21	2	0	1	3	0
No ETOH, n = 121	5	103	10	3	3	4	2
PVA + Coils only, n = 78	2	74	2	0	2	2	1

materials in this group reveals that of the 10 rated 2, 8 were performed prior to the time of the addition of micro-coils to our PVA use. Of those rated 3, none involved the combination of PVA plus microcoils. Thus, of 78 procedures recorded in which both PVA and coils were utilized, only 2 were recorded as an angiographic outcome rating of 2. Another 2 proce-dures in this group did not have an outcome rating

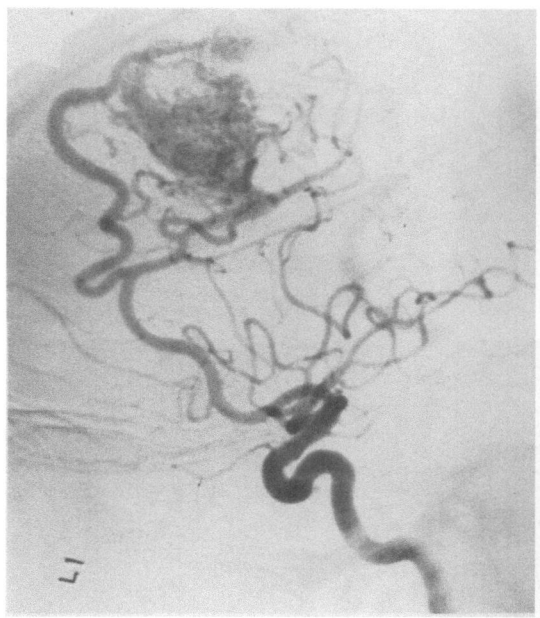

a

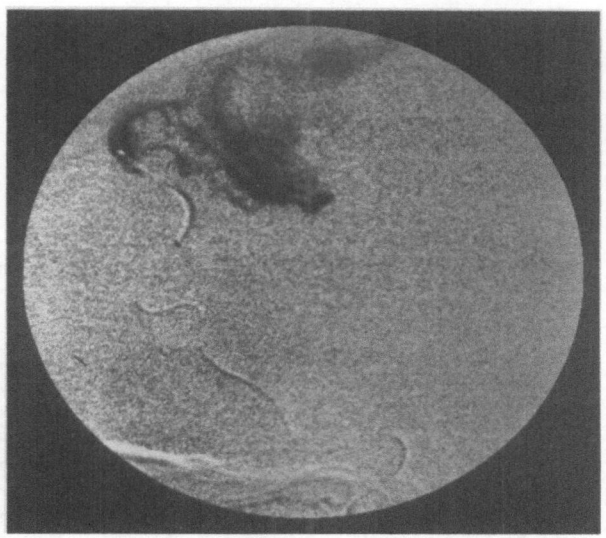

b

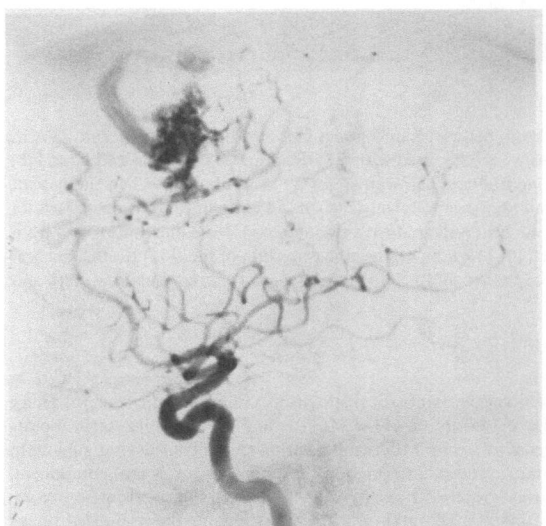

c

Fig. 1. (a) Lateral arteriogram of a left frontal AVM fed via branches of the anterior cerebral artery. Catheterization of a large callosomarginal artery feeding the malformation revealed a high flow fistula and necessitated the use of a very small catheter through which embolization with large particles or coils was not possible. (b) Catheter in position during embolization. (c) Angiogram at the end of the embolization shows occlusion of the majority of the malformation with small perforating vessels feeding it arising from the pericallosal artery. The embolization was conducted entirely using ETOH and 150–250 and 300–500 micron particles of PVA. The residual feeders were not felt to be important for embolization preoperatively. The patient subsequently underwent resection without development of neurologic deficit

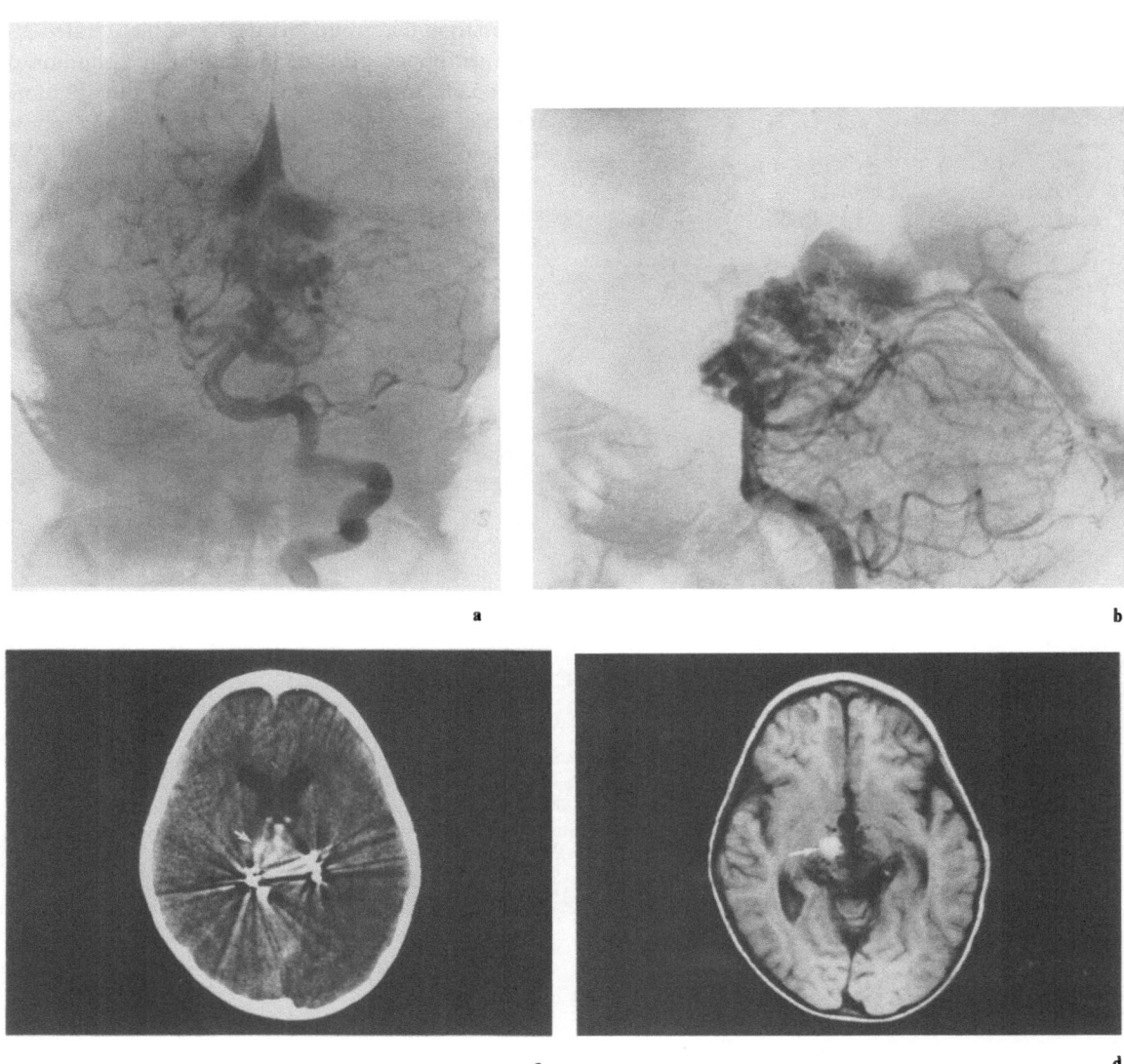

Fig. 2. (a) Three year-old male with bithalamic AVM extending to the midbrain peduncles underwent embolization with coils and PVA in addition to ETOH during 1 procedure. In the second procedure, some vessels were embolized with ETOH alone (A,B). AP (a) and lateral (b) arteriograms at the end of the embolization show the remaining AVM fed via multiple perforators. (c) CT scan obtained when the patient was noted to have a new third nerve palsy and to be slowly awakening from anesthesia following the second embolization. It demonstrates blood in the interpeduncular cistern, possibly extending into the cerebral peduncle on the patient's right (arrow). Note metallic artifact from the platinum coils placed bilaterally in the lateral posterior choroidal arteries. (d) MR scan verifies the extension of the clot into the cerebral peduncle (arrow). The patient's hospital course was complicated by hydrocephalus, and he slowly recovered to an ambulatory state and underwent radiosurgical therapy for his malformation

Fig. 3. A sixty-five year-old woman with a large posterior temporal AVM fed via the external carotid artery (ECA), middle cerebral artery (MCA), and posterior cerebral artery on that side. (a) Picture obtained during embolization of the MCA with PVA and coils. Arrow points to the tip of the Tracker catheter in the MCA. (b) Common carotid arteriogram following MCA embolization shows contrast hanging up in the MCA but continued rich perfusion via the ECA. (c, d) AP (c) and lateral (d) vertebral arteriogram shows posterior cerebral component. (e) AP view during embolization shows location of Tracker catheter (arrow). A total of 1.2 cc of 33% ethanol was injected in this vessel. (f) Lateral angiogram at termination of embolization shows significant reduction in malformation with coils occluding the embolized vessel. (g, h) The patient did well for 6 days, improving neurologically, but suffered a nearly fatal cerebral hemorrhage on the sixth postoperative day as she was preparing for discharge from the hospital. CT 5 days postoperatively (g) shows the AVM and multiple coils. CT on day 6 (h) shows large area of hemorrhage with transentorial herniation

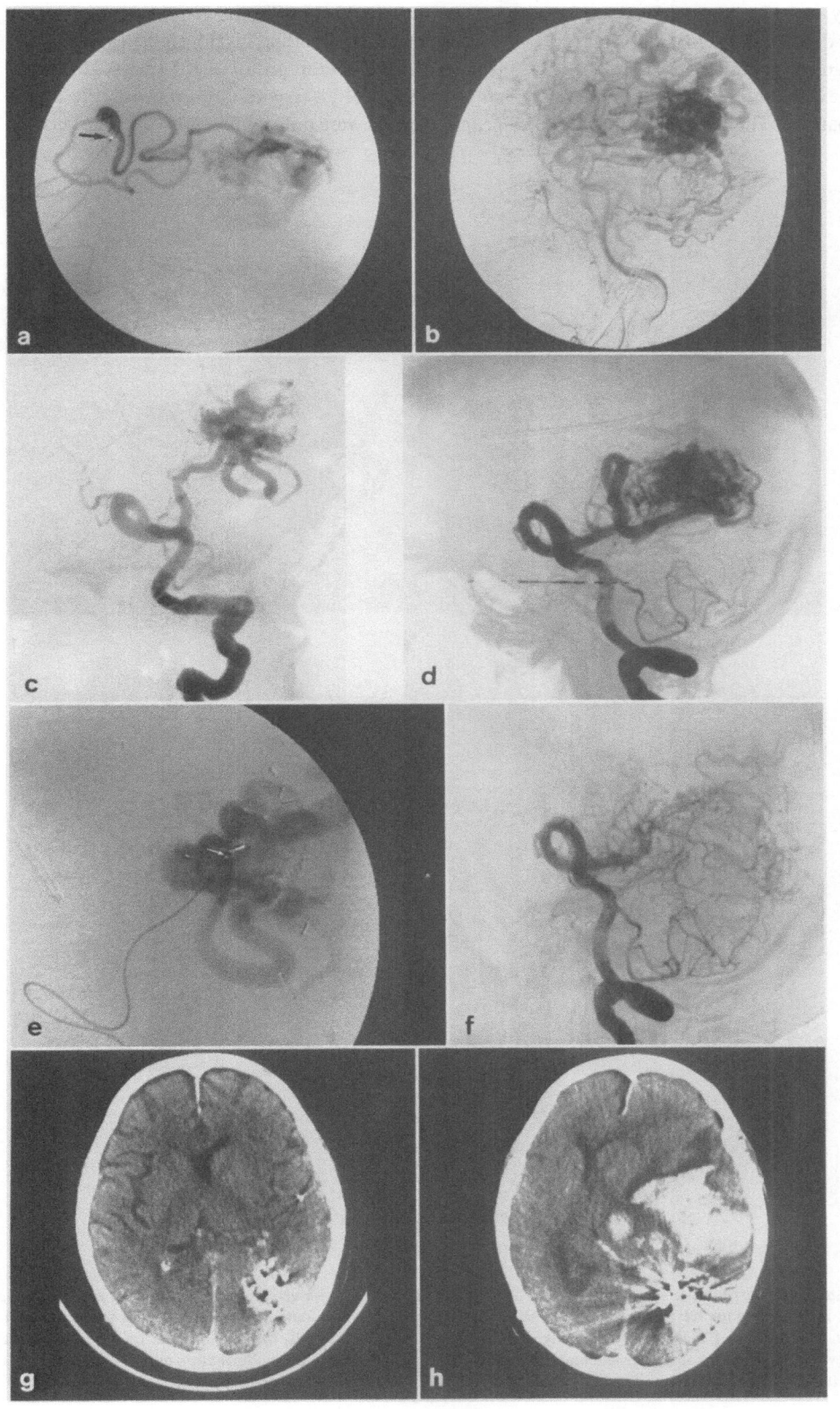

recorded. Additionally, for this group of 78, 2 strokes, 2 hemorrhages, and 1 death were recorded (total 6%). These overall results are summarized in Table 1.

Statistical analysis revealed no significant differences ($p < 0.05$) in any comparison. Though the complication rate with ETOH of 17% is disturbing, the group remains small enough that it is not statistically different from either the overall group of 121 ($p = 0.224$) or the smaller group of 78 ($p = 0.204$). Likewise, the angiographic results were not significantly different between

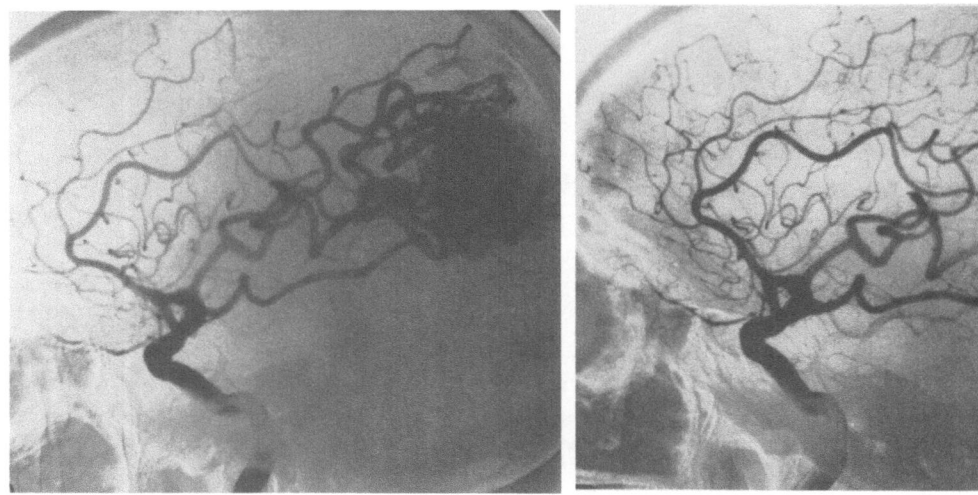

a   b

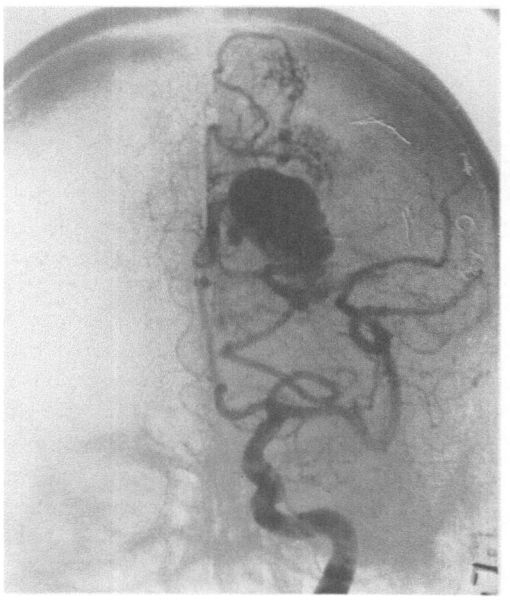

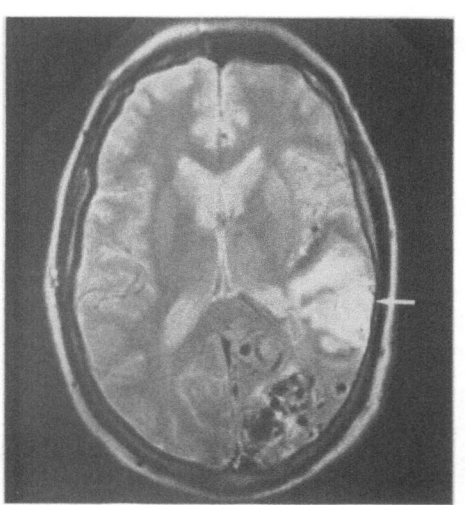

c   d

Fig. 4. (a) Lateral arteriogram of 61 year-old male shows parietal AVM fed by middle and posterior cerebral arteries. (b) After embolization, middle cerebral component is eliminated (c). AP view post-embolization shows elimination of middle cerebral artery component to better advantage. During injection of 0.2 cc 33% ETOH, artery abruptly occluded at the level of the coils, with rapid reflux on subsequent test injections. (d) The patient developed an anomic speech deficit, and MR shows high signal anterior to the malformation on T2-weighted images obtained post-embolization (arrow). Note also the lack of artifact from the coils, as the platinum produces no interference with MR (signal void)

the group of 78 and the ETOH group (p = 0.222). We have previously shown improved angiographic results when coils are used[8].

Discussion

Though the incidence of complications appears at first by this data to be higher in patients embolized with ETOH, the group remains too small to draw statistical conclusions as to differences, or they must be concluded not to be different. There are circumstances with significant fistulas in which it is helpful (Fig. 1). In 1 of the patients with hemorrhage, ETOH alone was used due to the small size of the feeding artery catheterized (Fig. 2). This may predispose toward a higher likelihood of hemorrhage due to the lack of blockage of the feeding vessel with a coil or other embolic device. In another patient who bled, another vascular territory was perfusing the malformation which was not embolized (Fig. 3). Thus, this may again lead to continued arterialization of the malformation and may be a factor increasing the probability of hemorrhage. Based on this data, particulate embolization may ultimately prove to be safer than embolization using ETOH. However, it is desirable to embolize the nidus of a malformation, and this cannot always be achieved with PVA particles, which sometimes wash through large fistulae. The use of coils for proximal occlusion will preclude embolization of the AVM nidus. Therefore, ETOH is sometimes helpful in these settings. It carries the advantage of penetration that is shared by acrylic glue, which also has benefit in these situations but which creates some rigidity in the malformation which may be a disadvantage for surgical retraction[7]. It is, however, highly toxic to the brain (Fig. 4). The complication rate with ETOH use must be weighed in the decision to employ it therapeutically.

Additionally, the solvent properties of ETOH may become apparent with some catheters. We noticed catheter perforations when using catheters with floppy, flow-directed tips. Though disturbing, these occurred distally and did not abort the embolic procedure. In fact, the perforations resulted in larger orifices in the catheters and permitted use of larger particles.

Acknowledgement

The authors thank Ms. Leslie Mihal for her assistance in the preparation of this manuscript.

References

1. Berenstein AB, Krall R, Choi IS (1989) Embolization with n-butyl cyanoacrylate in the management of CNS vascular lesions. AJNR 10: 883
2. Dion JE, Vinuela FV, Lylyk P, Lufkin R, Bentson J (1988) Ivalon-33% ethanol-avitene embolic mixture: clinical experience with neuroradiological endovascular therapy in 40 arteriovenous malformations. AJNR 9: 1029–1030
3. Eskridge JM, Hartling RP (1989) Preoperative embolization of brain AVMs using surgical silk and polyvinyl alcohol. AJNR 10: 882
4. Hilal SK, Khandji AG, Chi TL, Stein BM, Bello JA, Silver AJ (1988) Synthetic fiber-coated platinum coils successfully used for the endovascular treatment of arteriovenous malformations, aneurysms and direct arteriovenous fistulas of the CNS. AJNR 9: 1030
5. Kerber C (1975) Intracranial cyanoacrylate: a new catheter therapy for arteriovenous malformation. Invest Radiol 10: 536–537
6. Pelz DM, Fox AJ, Vinuela F, Drake CC, Ferguson GG (1988) Preoperative embolization of brain AVMs with isobutyl 2 cyanoacrylate. AJNR 9: 757–764
7. Purdy PD, Batjer HH, Risser RC, Samson DS (1992) Arteriovenous malformations of the brain: choosing embolic materials to enhance safety and ease of excision. J Neurosurg 77: 217–222
8. Purdy PD, Samson D, Batjer HH, Risser RC (1990) Preoperative embolization of cerebral arteriovenous malformations with polyvinyl alcohol particles: experience in 51 adults. AJNR 11: 501–510
9. Samson D, Ditmore QM, Beyer CW Jr (1981) Intravascular use of isobutyl 2-cyanoacrylate: part 1. Treatment of intracranial arteriovenous malformations. Neurosurgery 8: 43–51

Correspondence: Phillip D. Purdy, M.D., University of Texas Southwestern Medical Center at Dallas, 5323 Harry Hines Blvd., Dallas, TX 75235-8896, U.S.A.

Embolization of Cerebral AVMs with Polylene Threads: Technical Procedure, Results and Complications

A. Benati, S. Perini, A. Pasqualin[1], M.G. Pecoraro, A. Maschio, L. Rosta, E. Piovan, and **P. Zampieri**

Department of Neuroradiology and [1]Neurosurgery, City Hospital, Verona

Summary

In order to determine possible risk factors and to assess the value of polylene threads as particulate embolic agents for the treatment of brain AVMs, we reviewed our experience with this procedure. At present we utilize 1.5–2 mm long micro-emboli to occlude AVM nidus; they are inserted into a 22 gauge catheter needle (5 fragments for each needle) and then injected into the feeding vessel through a coaxial micro-catheter system. When AVM flow-rate is reduced, 2–3 cm long threads are injected through the same micro-catheter to complete the closure of the feeder. This double embolization, both of the nidus and of the afferent vessel is important in order to avoid bleeding inside the AVM, as a consequence of the stump pressure effect on the thin walled venules of the remaining portion of the nidus after embolization.

Embolization was performed in 108 patients: 71 of them (65%) underwent surgery; 14 (13%) radiosurgery; no other therapy was performed in 23 cases (21%). In all cases occlusion of the malformation and hemodynamic changes were carefully evaluated. A complete closure of the AVM was obtained in 3 cases only (2.5%); in the remaining 105 patients (97.5%), only an incomplete occlusion was observed, ranging from 5% to 70%, with average reduction of 37%.

Complications: hemorrhage was observed in 5 cases; it was less frequent (4,5%) but more severe than ischemia. It caused a transient neurological deficit in 2 cases, a permanent disability in 1 case and death in 2 patients. Ischemia was observed in 16 cases (15%) and caused a transient neurological deficit in 9 patients and permanent disability in 7 cases. A transient neurological deficit occurred in 11 patients. A permanent neurological deficit was observed in 8 cases (7.5%).

The overall complication rate was 19.5% (21/108); "stroke" rate (permanent deficit + death) 9% (10/108).

Clinical and angiographic results were evaluated in a follow-up period ranging from 1 to 4 years in 13 patients who didn't undergo surgical or radiosurgical therapy. Permanent occlusion of A-V malformation was never observed. In 6/13 cases a persistent reduction of AVM nidus was observed; in 11/13 cases occlusion of the feeders was stable. Re-bleeding occurred in a patient who had bled before embolization and in a patient who had never bled. No death occurred in this group of patients. No significant evaluation could be made on clinical follow-up, but severe headache markedly improved in 4/6 cases. Decrease in frequency of epileptic seizures was observed in 2/13 cases.

Keywords: Arteriovenous malformation; embolization; endovascular therapy, hemorrhage.

Introduction

Endovascular treatment of cerebral AVMs has been performed in our Department since 1983, using different procedures of embolization[1]. Our previous experience with balloon catheter systems and glue injection was not satisfactory, because of the risk of arterial rupture due to balloon inflation and difficult assessment of the proper polymerization time of cyanoacrylates (with consequent possible occlusion of the feeding arteries or drainage veins). Moreover occurrence of vasospasm due to catheter withdrawal was frequent. Pathologic findings in resected specimens often showed signs of angionecrosis related to the well-known hysto-toxicity of cyano-acrylates[6,16,18].

More satisfactory results were obtained using a particulate embolization technique based on selective injection of suture threads (polylene 3–0) into the feeders of the AVM[2]. This technique was frequently modified and refined during the last years according to the evaluation of angiographic, clinical and surgical results of the embolization and the incidence of complications.

In the first stage of our experience 2–3 cm long fragments of suture thread were injected directly into the feeding vessels of the malformation; afterwards, to avoid re-habitation of the A-V shunt by the neighbouring vessels, 2 mm long micro-emboli were injected more distally to occlude AVM nidus. At present, we occlude both the nidus and the afferent arteries (double embolization), possibly in each compartment of the malformation, in order to avoid any possible hemorrhagic complication during the treatment, and make recurrences less frequent.

The results of the embolization as pre-operative procedure in the surgically removable AVMs and its value as the sole therapeutic treatment of inaccessible

AVMs were previously reported[3,11]. Our recent experience of combined treatment of 75 AVMs is discussed elsewhere in this book.

The aim of the present report is to describe the technical procedure performed nowadays, to establish the value of this embolic agent, to assess the angiographic and clinical results and to determine any possible risk factors and the incidence of complications.

Technical Procedure

Our technique consists of a super-selective catheterization of the AVM feeders by means of a coaxial

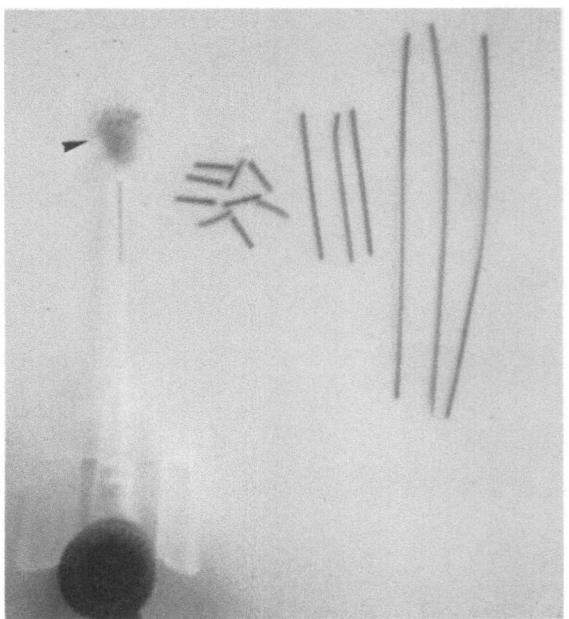

a

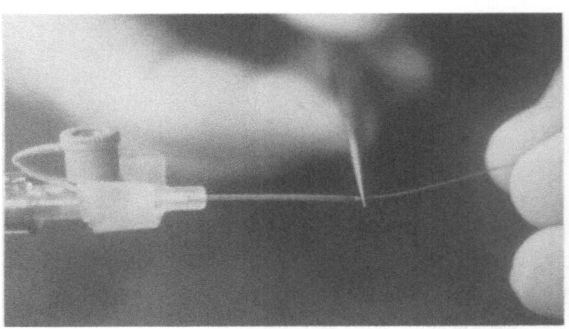

b

micro-catheter system. At present flow independent micro-catheters are preferred (Target therapeutics Tracker 18 Balt S Mag 3F/2F), but also flow directed micro-catheter (Ingenor Siltane 1.8F with enlarged tip) are successfully employed mainly for the catheterization of middle and posterior cerebral arteries that allow a good intravascular navigation.

Polyfilament polylene 3–0 (0.2 mm in diameter) is a suture thread commonly utilized in surgical rooms (Hammer-Ethicon). It can be cut in fragments of various length (from 1.5 mm to 2–3 cm or longer) according to the type of AVM and to the different stages of the embolization procedure (Fig. 1).

At present the procedure is performed as follows:

a. AVM Nidus Occlusion

We utilize 1.5–2 mm long micro-emboli that are inserted into a 22 gauge catheter-needle (Fig. 1. b, c). Five fragments are loaded inside each needle and then injected into the feeding vessel, through the coaxial micro-catheter system. Emboli are then discharged into the artery by 1.5–2 ml of saline. The polylene fragments break out into smaller micro-fibrils (Fig. 1a) which reach the nidus of the AVMs (Fig. 2b). A progressive embolization is achieved under continuous angiographic control and neurologic observation in the alert patient. Nidus occlusion is well demonstrated by angiography and MRI (Fig. 2a, Fig. 3).

The higher flow shunts are first occluded, followed by the slower-flow ones. When shunt flow is markedly reduced few threads deposit on the walls of the arterial pedicles, close to AVM nidus.

b. Feeder Occlusion

When AVM nidus is occluded, 2–3 cm long threads are injected through the same micro-catheter to complete-

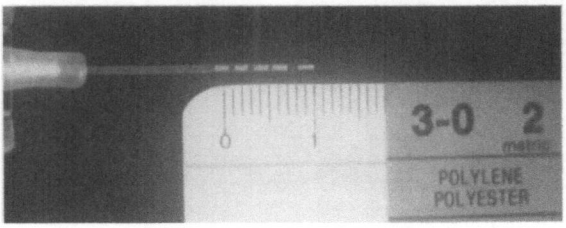

c

Fig. 1. (a) Polylene 3–0 suture threads are cut at various lengths as embolic agents. The fragments are 1.5 mm to 2–5 cm long. (b) Micro-emboli are inserted into a 22 G catheter-needle. (c) Every catheter needle is loaded with 5 micro-emboli. After injection the small polylene fragments break out into smaller micro-fibrils which can reach the AVM nidus (arrow)

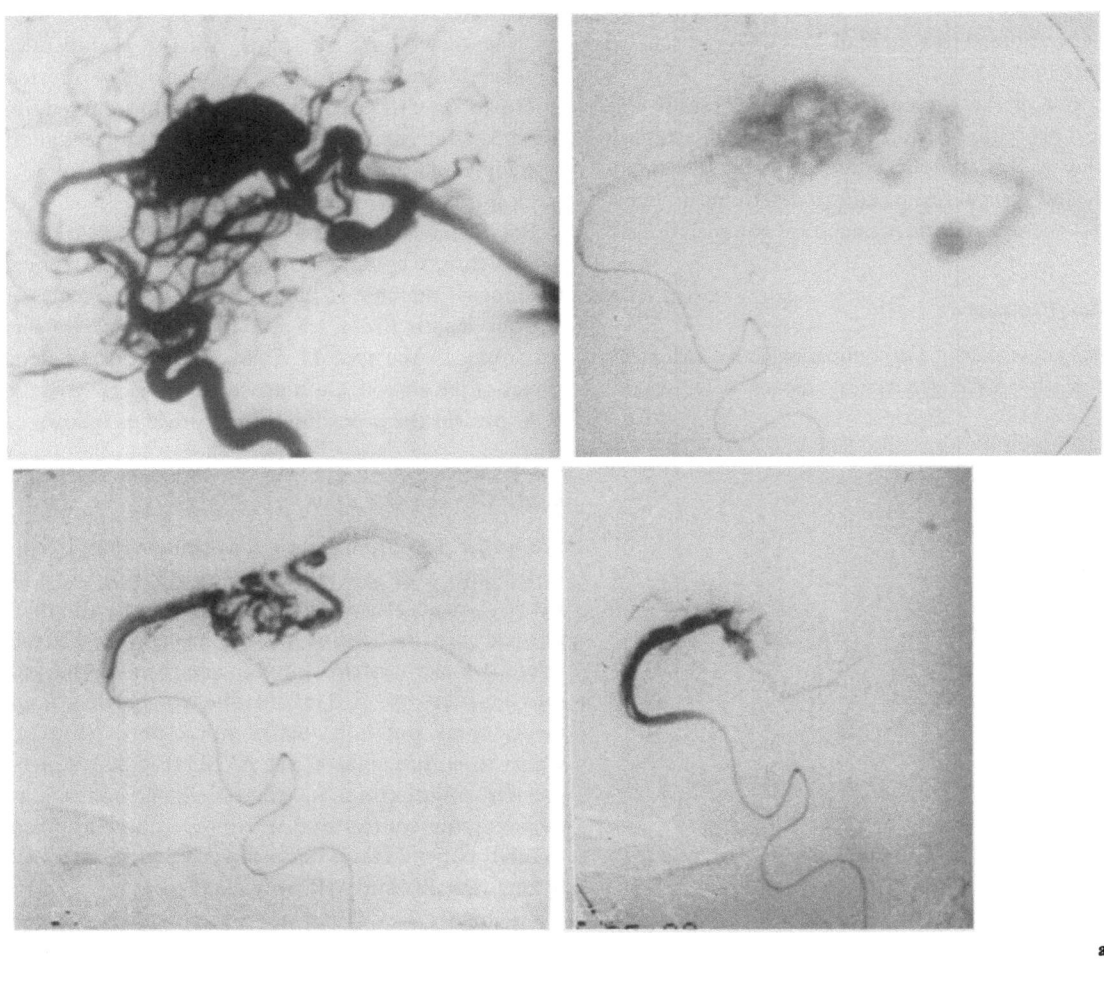

a

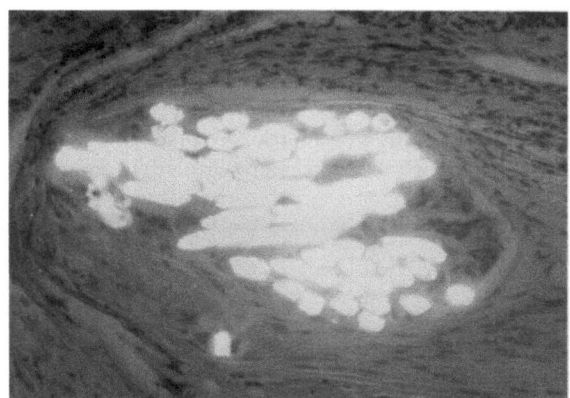

b

Fig. 2. Progressive obliteration of the AVM nidus during embolization of a callosal AVM (a). Micro-fibrils are well recognizable inside the nidus vessels at pathological examination (b)

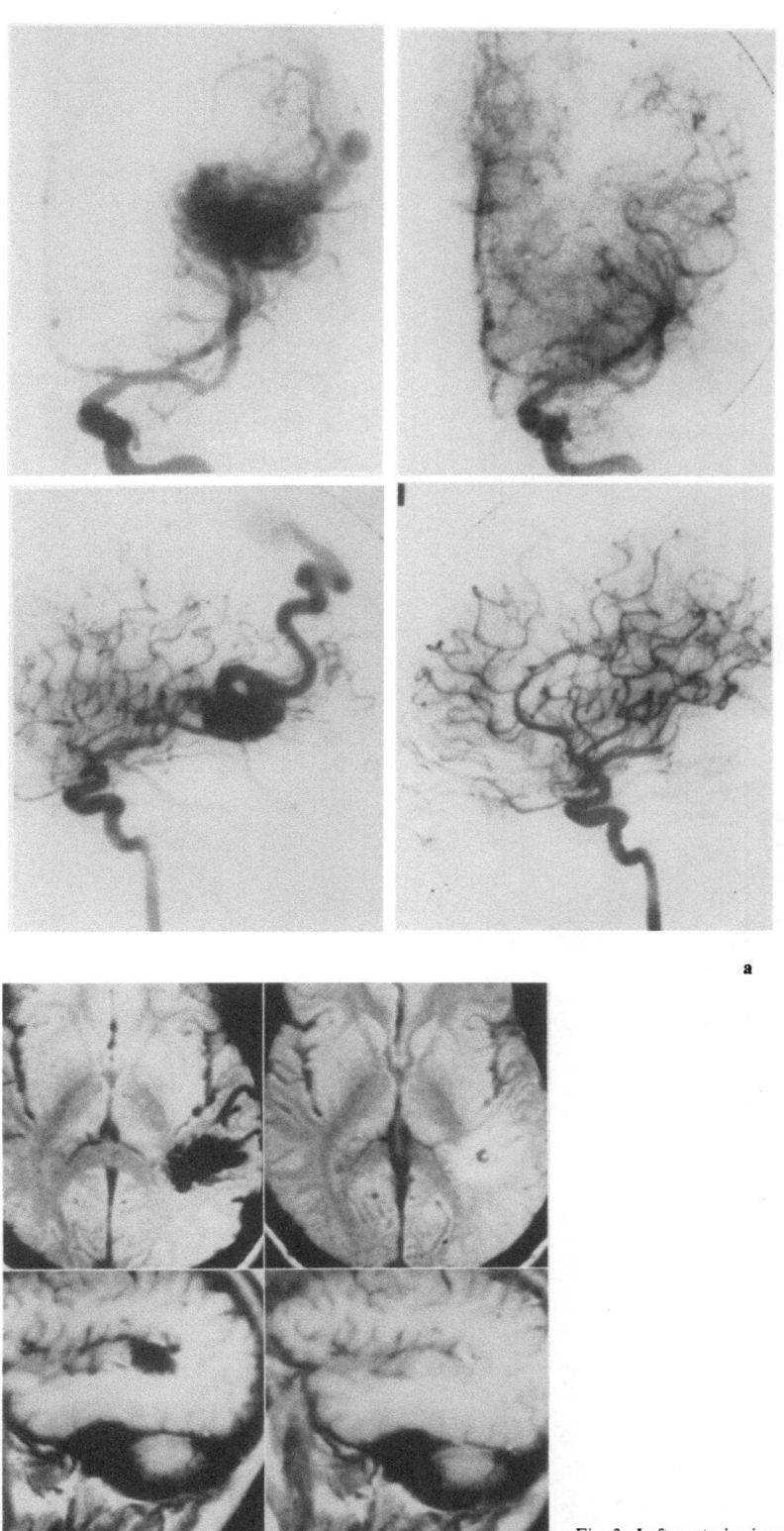

Fig. 3. Left posterior insular AVM before and after embolization. The occlusion of the nidus is well demonstrated on the angiograms (a) and on MR images (b)

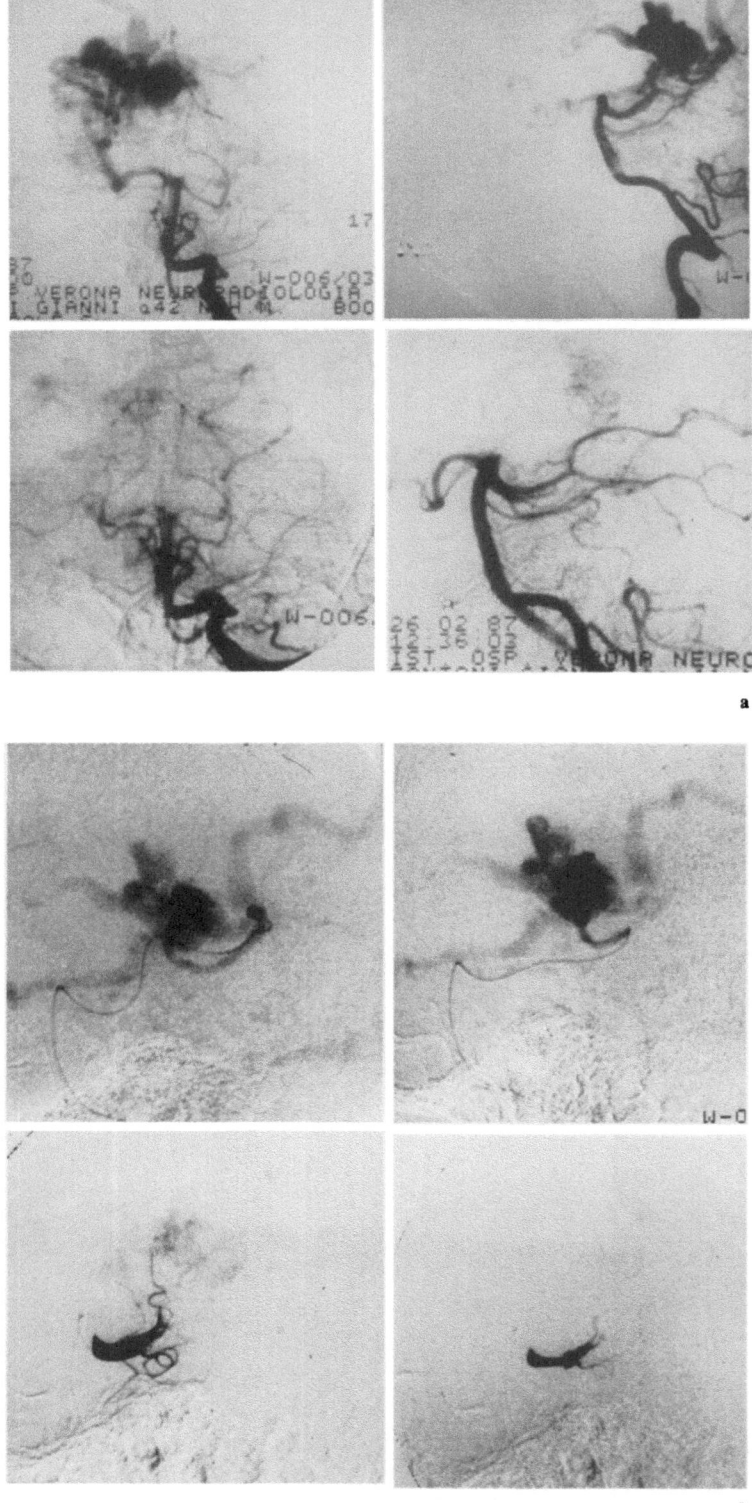

Fig. 4. (a) Right parasplenial AVM fed by posterior choroidal artery before (above) and after (below) embolization. (b) Stages of "double" embolization of the AVM nidus and feeder

ly occlude the feeder (Fig. 4). The handling of suture thread sometimes may be difficult; to shorten the procedure the fragments can be previously loaded into a 22 gauge catheter-needle and then injected through the micro-catheter.

This double embolization, both of the nidus and of the afferent vessel, is important in order to make AVM nidus occlusion more stable and to avoid bleeding inside the AVM, as a consequence of the stump-pressure effect on the thin walled venules of the remaining portion of the nidus after embolization.

Neither Amytal test nor evoked potentials were utilized during the procedure because the occlusion of a vascular feeder can be at no risk in many brain regions. Furthermore embolization may be needed also in critical or eloquent areas; in this case a particular care must then be taken during the procedure depending on the characteristic of the feeder, its catheterization and the flow-rate through the malformation. Once one feeder is embolized, the same micro-catheter can be moved to other feeders. In this way multiple pedicles can be embolized with the same micro-catheter.

Materials and Methods

From 1986 to 1992, 108 patients were treated in our Department by uni or multi staged embolization. Table 1 summarizes the clinical presentation of the patients; the mean age was 28.5 years, 16 patients were in pediatric age (15%).

The AVM was located in non critical brain areas in 58 cases and in 50 patients in critical areas: 15 in the rolandic and 11 in the speech area, 14 in the occipito-calcarine region, 5 in the basal ganglia, 3 in the cerebellar vermis or hemispheres and 2 in the corpus callosum. Five volume subgroups were identified: 0–10 cm^3 (13 cases, 12%); 11–20 cm^3 (31 cases, 28%), 21–30 cm^3 (27 cases, 25%), 31–50 cm^3 (25 cases, 23%) and > 50 cm^3 (12 cases, 11%). The volume calculation adopted is presented in a recent paper from our group[10].

Deep feeders (lenticulo-striate, thalamo-perforating, choroidal arteries, PICA and AICA) were present in 43 cases (40%) and were embolized in 21/43 patients.

Venous drainage was "extensive"[10] (multiple ectatic veins with or without huge venous dilatation or extensive hemispheric drainage) in 38 (35%) cases. Deep drainage (toward the vein of Galen) was present in 44 patients (40%).

Embolization was performed as a pre-operative procedure in 71 patients (65%). It was followed by radio-surgery in 14 cases (13%); no other therapy was performed in 23 (21%) cases (inaccessible AVMs). The criteria for pre-operative embolization were the following: a) high flow-AVMs as estimated at angiography and transcranial Doppler sonography; b) presence of ectatic feeders, in particular if poorly accessible to surgery; c) extensive venous drainage.

The main criteria for the definition of inaccessible AVMs treated by palliative embolization were the following: a) large malformations in critical site; b) patients age (pediatric or elderly); c) neurosurgeon's evaluation of risk of the operation; d) patient's consent to undergo the procedure.

Table 1. *Embolization of Cerebral AVMs with Polylene Threads: 108 Cases (1986–1992)*

Clinical symptoms	
Seizures	43 (45%)
Hemorrhage	20 (21%)
Headache	13 (13.5%)
Other	10 (10.5%)

M: 62, F: 46, age 10–47, mean 28.5.

Radiosurgery was carried out in patients with medium-small AVMs reduced to less than 10 cm^3, when deeply located within the nervous tissue. The occlusion of the A-V malformation was obtained in one or multiple sessions of embolization (1–6/mean 1.8 for patient) according to the number of feeders of the malformation and to its hemodynamic features and site.

In all cases occlusion of the malformation and hemodynamic changes were carefully evaluated. Complications were related to technical procedure, patient's age, AVM size and location, and anatomical and hemodynamic features.

In 13 patients, out of the 23 who received embolization as the sole therapeutic tool, it was possible to evaluate clinical and angiographic results during a follow-up period ranging from 1 to 4 years.

Results

A complete closure of the AVM was obtained in 3 cases only (2.5%); in the remaining 105 patients (97.5%) only an incomplete occlusion was observed, ranging from 5% to 70%, with an average reduction of 37%.

Table 2 shows that the best percentage of AVM reduction was observed in the first three volume subgroups (0–10, 11–20 and 21–30 cm^3) and decreased in large and huge AVMs (35 > 50 cm^3 in volume). In all cases however, morphological and hemodynamic changes, suggesting a decrease of blood flow-rate to the AVM and an improved flow to the normal brain, were present: a) reduced AVM nidus density; b) slowing of circulation time; c) decrease in size of the caliber of feeding vessels and venous drainage. The features of the hemodynamic assessment of these patients, when evaluated with Doppler sonography and rCBF testing, are reported elsewhere in this book.

Table 2. *Percent Reduction in Volume After Embolization According to Initial Volume*

Volume (cm^3)	Average	Vol. reduction: Min	Max
0–10 (13 cases)	50%	10%	100%
11–20 (31 cases)	40%	10%	100%
21–30 (27 cases)	40%	5%	70%
31–50 (25 cases)	30%	5%	60%
> 50 (12 cases)	25%	5%	60%

Table 3. *Complications of Brain AVM Embolization: 108 Cases (1986–1992)*

TD – motor-sensory impairment	5(4.5%)
– hemiparesis-aphasia	1(0.9%)
– dysphasia	2(1.8%)
– hemianopia	1(0.9%)
– amnesia	1(0.9%)
– deafness	1(0.9%)
	11(10%)
PD – motor impairment	5(4.5%)
– psychic disturbance	1(0.9%)
– hemianopia	2(1.8%)
	8(7.5%)
Death	2(1.8%)
Total	21(19.5%)

TD transient deficit; *PD* permanent deficit.

Complications

Table 3 summarizes the complications of brain AVMs embolization with polylene threads in our series of patients treated with this embolic material from 1986 to 1992.

Hemorrhage was observed in 5 cases; it was less frequent (4,5%) but more severe than ischemia. It caused a transient neurological deficit in 2 cases, a permanent disability in 1 case and death in 2 patients. *Ischemia* was observed in 16 cases (15%) and caused a transient neurological deficit in 9 patients and permanent disability in 7 patients. Hemorrhage was observed in patients treated by occlusion of the nidus only; it was never observed when double embolization of the nidus and of the feeder was achieved. Ischemia occurred more frequently when multistaged treatment was performed (16 cases) and when a previous incomplete surgical ablation with feeder occlusion was made. Both hemorrhage and ischemia occurred more frequently during embolization of deep AVM fed by deep arteries (13 cases, 62% of all complications).

In 2 cases complications were due to the technical procedure: in the first one a mild amnesia was caused by rupture of the ACA into the caudate nucleus during catheterization with a Tracker micro-catheter. In the second case a slight SAH occurred with mild headache persisting for three days and resolved with complete recovery without any clinical neurological deficit. No complication was observed when flow-directed micro-catheters were employed.

A *transient neurological deficit* occurred in 11 patients (10%). In 3 cases motor impairment was severe and abrupt in onset. In the first one (deep temporal AVM), a sudden hemiplegia was observed during the embolization of anterior choroidal artery; a complete recovery was seen within one hour. In the second patient (deep strio-thalamic AVM) a complete motor deficit was observed during embolization of MCA and posterior choroidal arteries. A complete recovery was obtained only 3 months later. In the remaining 8 cases symptoms were less severe with recovery in 1–2 days: deafness occured during AICA embolization. A *permanent neurological deficit* was observed in 8 cases (7.5%).

Motor impairment was always severe in onset, but fixed deficits were all compatible with a good performance. Persistent visual field deficit (2 cases) was easily tolerated by the patients in both cases (ipsilateral quadrantopsia). On the contrary a severe psychic disturbance represented a bad clinical outcome due to ischemia in one patient, following PCA embolization in a deep temporo-occipital AVM previously incompletely operated.

Death unfortunately occurred in 2 patients; in both cases a severe hemorrhagic complication was observed (Figs. 5 and 6).

No significant correlation between the angioarchitecture and the incidence of complications was observed.

The overall complication rate was 19.5% (21/108); "stroke" rate (permanent deficit + death) 9% (10/108). Table 4 shows the incidence of complications in relation to the different technical procedures performed from 1986 to 1988 and from 1989 to 1992, respectively. In our recent series all complication rates were lower but a significant difference was demonstrated only between the two "stroke" rates (15% versus 3.5%) attesting lower incidence of severe complications due to post-embolization hemorrhage obtained with "double embolization" of AVM nidus and feeder. No significative correlation between patient's age and incidence of complications was observed.

Follow-up: Table 5 summarizes clinical and angiographic results evaluated in a follow-up period ranging from 1 to 4 years, in 13 patients who didn't undergo surgical or radio-surgical therapy. Permanent occlusion of A-V malformation was never observed either with AVM nidus or double (feeder + nidus) embolization. In 6/13 cases a persistent reduction of AVM nidus was observed; in 11/13 cases occlusion of the feeders was stable. One re-bleeding occurred in a pa-

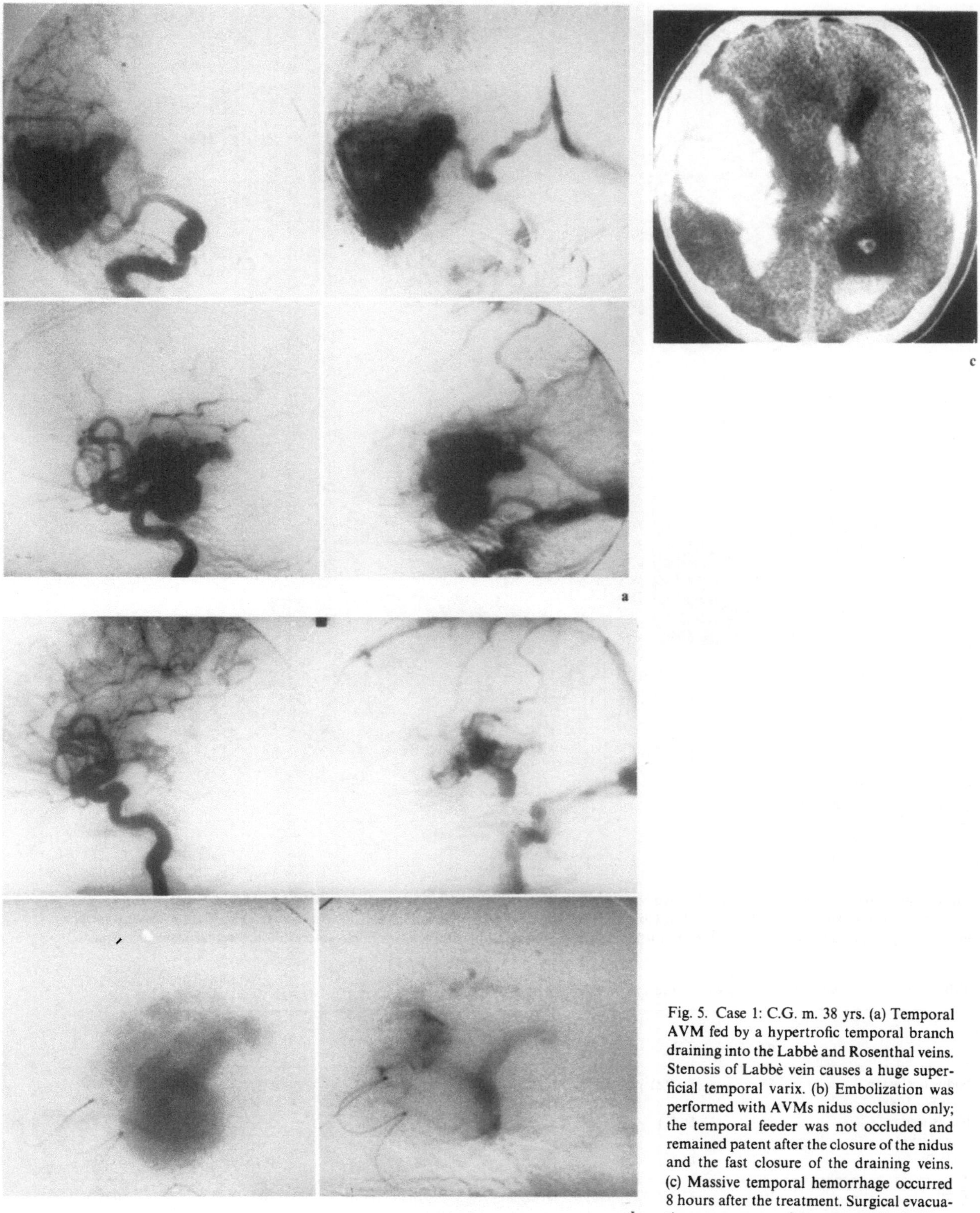

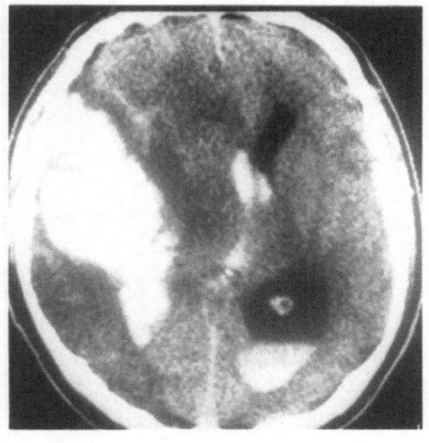

Fig. 5. Case 1: C.G. m. 38 yrs. (a) Temporal AVM fed by a hypertrofic temporal branch draining into the Labbè and Rosenthal veins. Stenosis of Labbè vein causes a huge superficial temporal varix. (b) Embolization was performed with AVMs nidus occlusion only; the temporal feeder was not occluded and remained patent after the closure of the nidus and the fast closure of the draining veins. (c) Massive temporal hemorrhage occurred 8 hours after the treatment. Surgical evacuation was unsuccessful to save patient's life

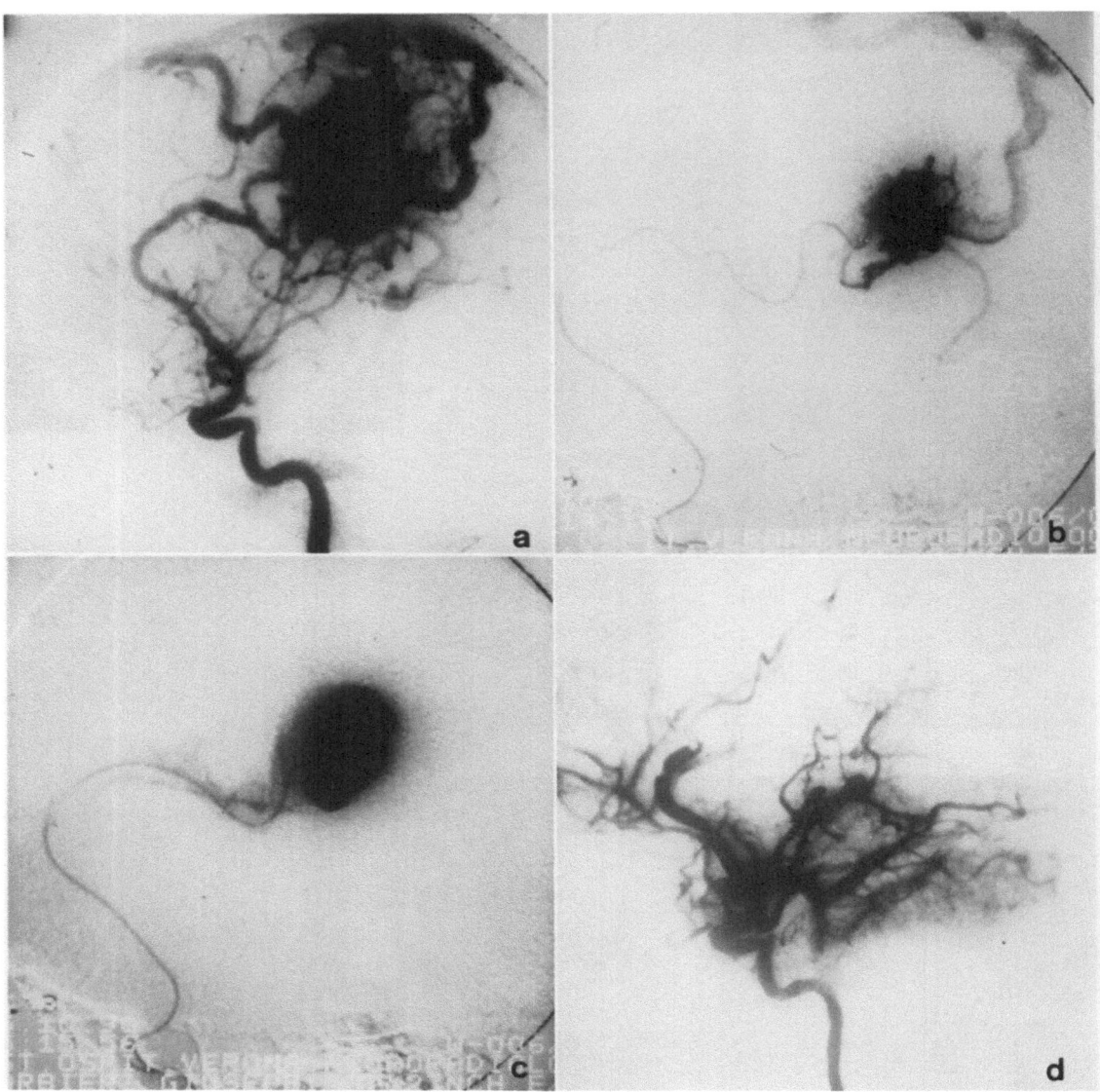

Fig. 6. Case 2: B.G. f. 23 yrs. (a) Callosal AVM fed by hypertrophic pericallosal artery with a large draining vein. (b) ACA feeder was catheterized and embolization was performed, causing fast closure of the draining vein with immediate hemorrhage. (c) The feeding vessel was then immediately occluded by polylene threads emboli (d) Hemorrhage stopped, but in the following days severe diffuse cerebral edema occurred

Table 4. *Complications of Brain AVMs Embolization: 108 Cases (1986–1992)*

	n	TD	PD	Death	Stroke rate	Overall c. rate
Nidus occlusion (1986–1988)	53	6(11%)	6(11%)	2(3.7%)	8(15%)	14(26.5%)
Nidus-feeder occlusion (1989–1992)	55	5(9%)	2(3.5%)	–	2(3.5%)	7(12.5%)
		ns	ns	ns	p < 0.04	ns
Total	108	11(10%)	8(6.5%)	2(1.8%)	10(9%)	21(19.5%)

Table 5. *Brain AVMs Treated by Embolization Only (13 Cases)* Follow-up 1–4 years

Angiographic and clinical cure	–
Nidus AVM reduction (40%–60%)	6/13 (46%)
Hemorrhage	1/13 (7.5%)
Re-bleeding	1/13 (7.5%)
Severe headache improvement	4/6
Seizures (decrease in frequency)	2/13

tient who bled before embolization and another in a patient who never bled. No death occurred in this group of patients.

The number of patients controlled is too low to make a comparison between bleeding, mortality rates and natural history. However our results confirm the expected rate[9] for the same period (4% per year and 1% per year respectively).

No significant evaluation could be made on clinical follow-up, but severe headache markedly improved in 4/6 cases. Decrease in frequency of epileptic seizures was observed in 2/13 cases.

Discussion

Endovascular procedures have markedly improved in the last period and now micro-catheters allow a good intravascular navigation but a valid and permanent embolic agent is not available; therefore a complete cure of all types of AVMs is not yet possible. Some interventionalists stress the value of liquid glues (n-isobutyl-cyanoacrylate) for the definitive "therapeutic embolization" of AVMs nidus[4,12,13]. However, also in these series a complete cure was obtained in a minority of cases of "small" malformations and revascularization of occluded nidus was frequently observed even though complete obliteration was previously achieved[5,15,19]. Therefore presurgical embolization still represents a more effective therapeutic tool which can reduce the hemodynamic effects of A-V cerebral shunt and allows a safer surgical intervention. Particulate embolization, better than liquid glues, allows a good ablation of the embolized AVM that remains soft under the surgeon's hands and can be more easily resected. The value of our pre-operative technique was previously reported and can be summarized as follows: a) polylene micro-fibrils can penetrate AVM nidus; b) they are highly hysto-compatible; c) multiple feeders

can be embolized through the same micro-catheter. Double embolization of both AVM nidus and feeder has markedly improved the morbidity and mortality rates of the procedure mainly avoiding the dangerous hemorrhagic complications due to stump pressure on the thin walled vessels of the malformation and breakthrough phenomenon.

In many centers PVA particles and platinum coils were successfully utilized for AVM nidus occlusion and feeder closure[14,17]. These embolic agents (Contour emboli) can quickly occlude the nidus of the malformation but can penetrate into the small functional branches originating from the same AVM feeder which are not evident if arterial steal is present. Polylene micro-emboli break-up into small micro-fibrils inside the feeding vessels and allow a progressive embolization which can prevent occlusion of the small functional branches that become evident at the angiographic controls during the procedure and which can be spared by the embolization. Platinum coils represent a good occlusion device for the feeding vessels, but their introduction is not without risk (pusher stiffness) and a reflux into normal arteries is possible[7,8]. Two–three cm long threads, on the contrary, reach the same goal without any danger of artery perforation.

In conclusion, our procedure represents a good therapeutic tool for presurgical intervention; it is not at high risk when a good catheterization of superficial feeder is obtained and when few feeders are occluded. The embolization of deep feeders is more risky mainly when AVM is located within the basal ganglia and if multiple pedicles were previously occluded. Revascularization of the AVM makes the value of this procedure controversial for the "therapeutic" embolization and complete cure of AVM malformation, mainly if large in volume and fed by deep vessels. Our results confirm the effectiveness of the method for palliative therapy of severe headache, mainly when embolization caused an important reduction of large venous superficial varices draining the AVM.

References

1. Benati A, Beltramello A, Maschio A, Perini S, Rosta L, Piovan E (1987) Endovascular treatment of intra-cranial AVMs. Combined embolization with a multi-purpose mobile-wing micro-catheter system. J Neuroradiology 14: 99–113
2. Benati A, Beltramello A, Colombari R, Maschio A, Perini S, Da Pian R, Pasqualin A, Scienza R, Rosta L, Piovan E, Scarpa A, Zamboni G (1989) Preoperative embolization of arteriovenous malformations with polylene threads: techniques with wing microcatheter and pathologic results. AJNR 10: 579–586

3. Benati A (1992) Interventional neuroradiology for treatment of inaccessible A-V malformations. Acta Neurochir (Wien) 118: 76–79

4. Berthelsen B, Lofgren J, Svendsen P (1990) Embolization of cerebral arteriovenous malformation with bucrylate. Acta Radiol 31: 1321

5. Fourier D, Terbrugge K, Rodesch G, Lasjaunias P (1990) Revascularization of brain arteriovenous malformation after embolization with bucrylate. Neuroradiology 32: 497–501

6. Fox AJ, Pelz DM, Lee DH (1990) Arteriovenous malformations of the brain: recent results of endovascular therapy. Radiology 177: 51–57

7. Morse SS, Clark RA, Puffenbarger A (1990) Platinum microcoils for therapeutic embolization: no neuroradiologic applications. AJR 155: 401–403

8. Nakstad PH, Bakke SJ, Hald JK (1992) Embolization of intracranial arteriovenous malformations and fistulas with polyvinyl alcohol particles and platinum fibre coils. Neuroradiology 34: 348–351

9. Ondra SL, Troupp H, George ED, Schwab K (1990) The natural history of symptomatic arteriovenous malformations of the brain: a 24 year follow-up assessment. J Neurosurg 73: 387–391

10. Pasqualin A, Barone G, *et al* (1991) The importance of some anatomical and haemodynamic factors for classification of cerebral arterio-venous malformations. Neurosurgery 28: 370–379

11. Pasqualin A, Scienza R, Cioffi F, Barone G, Benati A, Beltramello A, Da Pian R (1991) Treatment of cerebral arteriovenous malformations with a combination of preoperative embolization and surgery. Neurosurgery 29: 358–368

12. Pelz DM, Fox AJ, Vinuela F, Drake CC, Ferguson GG (1988) Preoperative embolization of brain AVMs with isobutyl-2-cyanoacrylate. AJNR 9: 757–764

13. Picard L, Moret J, Lepoire J (1984) Traitment endovasculaire des angiomes artério-veneux intracérébraux. J Neuroradiol 11: 9–28

14. Purdy PD, Samson D, Batjer HH, Risser RC (1990) Preoperative embolization of cerebral arteriovenous malformation with polyvinyl alcohol particles. AJNR 11: 501–510

15. Rao VR, Mandalam KR, Gupta AK, Kumpar S, Joseph S (1989) Dissolution of isobutyl-2-cyanoacrylate on long-term follow-up. AJNR 10: 135–141

16. Samson D (1986) Carcinogenic potential of isobutyl-2-cyanoacrylate. J Neurosurg 65: 571–572

17. Schumacher M, Horton JA (1991) Treatment of cerebral arteriovenous malformations with PVA. Results and analysis of complications. Neuroradiology 33: 101–105

18. Vinters HV, Galli KA, Lundie MJ, Kaufmann JCE (1985) The histotoxicity of cyanoacrylates. Review article. Neuroradiology 27: 279–291

19. Vinuela F, Fox AJ, Pelz D, Debrun G (1986) Angiographic follow-up of large cerebral AVMs incompletely embolized with isobutyl-2-cyanoacrylate. AJNR 7: 919–925

Correspondence: A. Benati, M.D., Department of Neuroradiology, City Hospital, I-37126 Verona, Italy.

Transcranial Doppler Sonography After Embolization and Staged Operation of AVMs and Balloon Occlusion of Carotid-Cavernous Sinus Fistula

R. Burger[1] and **W. Hassler**[2]

[1]Department of Neurosurgery, University of Würzburg and [2]Department of Neurosurgery, Municipal Clinic of Duisburg, Federal Republic of Germany

Summary

Transcranial Doppler sonography is a simple, noninvasive method for pre- and postoperative monitoring of altered cerebral hemodynamic conditions in AVMs and carotid-cavernous sinus fistulas. It's possible to verify successful treatment by embolization, operation or combined procedures in AVMs and occlusion of carotid-cavernous sinus fistulas by balloon occlusion. The hemodynamic adaptation in altered cerebrovascular systems seems to be less complicated by staged therapeutic procedures, as it occurs in patients with arteriovenous malformations; however staged procedures are only justified if the total complication rate does not exceed the side effects for each method.

No problems with adaptation of cerebral perfusion pressure exist in cases with an intact peripheral vascular system, as demonstrated in patients with CCSF. Neither transcranial doppler nor radiological or clinical signs of a normal pressure breakthrough phenomena were detectable in our series of 125 cases of vascular malformations.

Keywords: Transcranial Doppler; arteriovenous malformation; carotid; cavernous sinus fistula; embolization.

Introduction

Transcranial doppler sonography, a simple beside investigation for continous, noninvasive monitoring of flow velocities in basal cerebral arteries[1], is able to monitor hemodynamic influences of arteriovenous malformations (AVM) and carotid-cavernous sinus fistulas (CCSF) to the Circle of Willis. First it's possible to judge site-differences which should not be over 10%, second to calculate the pulsatility-index (PI) of flow spectra to imagine the peripheral stream resistance and third to study the vasomotor reactivity by hyperventilation or application of CO_2.

In comparison to the normal hemodynamic situation with autoregulated perfusion pressure, angiomas show several different characteristic qualities on TCD: High flow velocities, low pulsatility indices, which means low resistance flow and a disturbed vasomotor reactivity. The facility to monitor this characteristic changes in basal cerebral arteries depends on the size, distal or proximal location of angioma, number and length of angioma supplying arteries, as well as shunt volume and cross-sectional area of feeding arteries as described by Hassler and Burger[10,11,12]. Also the follow-up after treatment of AVMs by different modalities as superselective embolization, one stage or two staged operation, preoperative partial superselective embolization followed by total surgical excision and stereotactic radiosurgical elimination is possible. Hereby TCD shows the following typical changes: very low flow velocities, high stream resistance and recovery of CO_2 reactivity. The effect of the above mentioned different treatment modalities, especially the new procedure of embolization, to doppler flow spectra, the resulting treatment strategies and the hemodynamic changes after occlusion of carotid-cavernous sinus fistulas in comparison to changes in angiomas (normal pressure breakthrough phenomenon) will be discussed in this investigation.

Method and Patients

Doppler investigations were performed before and after operation of 125 angiomas, including 15 angiomas with staged treatment, and in 9 patients before and after occlusion of CCSF using a pulsed wave, range gated 2 Mhz Doppler (TC-64, EME, Germany). The following parameters were observed: first the time mean flow velocity (FVmean) of the Doppler spectrum and second, the pulsatility index (PI), a ratio between systolic, diastolic and mean flow velocity (systolic minus diastolic flow velocity divided by the mean flow velocity) as a parameter for estimating distal resistance in arterioles[7,13]. Normal values for FVmean have been reported by several authors elsewhere[2,3,8]. For the PI, Lindegaard et al.[13] described a mean value of 0.71 ± 0.1 in the middle cerebral artery (mean value $\pm$ standard deviation). Low peripheral resistance leads to a decreasing PI between 0.4 and 0.2[3,7].

In one patient with CCSF intraluminal arterial blood pressure was measured with a small pressure probe, inserted over the ballon catheter before ballon occlusion on both sides proximal to the fistula in the petrous portion of ICA (ICAp).

Results

A. Arteriovenous Malformations

Characteristic changes of flow velocity in TCD after operation, staged and combined procedures in angiomas will be demonstrated in some representative cases.

1. Two-Step Operation (Fig. 1)

This case represents the time course of flow velocity changes in a 30 year old woman with a left-sided angularis angioma, mainly supplied by MCA and partly supplied by PCA. Preoperative flow velocity mean in left MCA was 150 cm/s and 80 cm/s in the

PCA. The PI was decreased, and diastolic flow increased, a sign of low distal resistance. The contralateral MCA and PCA showed normal values. Immediately after the operation, the velocities in the left MCA and PCA were reduced, but the flow spectrum in the PCA showed again a low resistance flow. This indicated that the PCA was still acting as a feeding artery, supplying some remaining angioma.

Repeated angiography showed a remaining small feeder of left MCA and PCA. On the 11th day following the first operative stage, the PCA showed a compensatory increased flow velocity in comparison to the preoperative measurements, while the MCA increased only slightly. Decreasing flow velocities with increased PI were seen after the second operative stage in the left MCA and PCA. After the second operation, an increase in flow velocity was seen in the left MCA, which was presumed to be postoperative hyperemia. During this course of treatment, the contralateral flow velocities were unchanged.

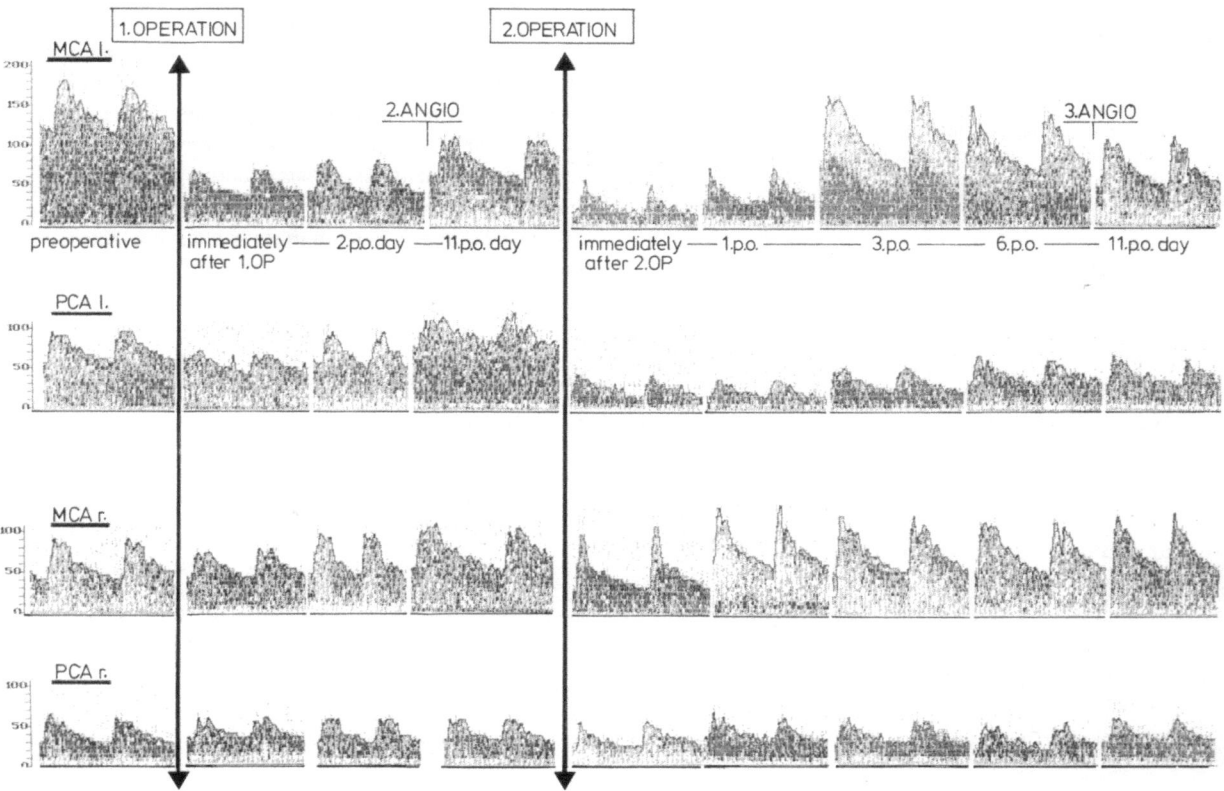

Fig. 1. Time course of flow velocities in TWO-STEP resection of a left angular angioma supplied mainly by the left middle cerebral artery and partly by the left posterior cerebral artery

2. Preoperative Embolization Followed by Surgical Excision (Figs. 2–4)

A 20 year old man presented with seizures from a left large posterior frontal angioma. The angioma was supplied by left MCA and ACA and through a steal effect via the precommunicating segment of the right ACA (Figs. 2 and 3). Before embolization, the MCA showed a flow velocity mean of 130 cm/s, the ACA A1 segment, 130 cm/s and the contralateral shunting A1 segment 86 cm/s. Only a slight decrease of distal resistance was found in the arteries. After the first stage of embolization of left ACA feeder, flow velocity decreased slightly from 130 to 112 cm/s. The flow velocity also decreased slightly to 80 cm/s in the opposite A1, indicating a reduced shunting from the opposite side. In the second stage, the anterior feeder of the right MCA was embolized. The flow velocity decreased from 150 to 136 cm/s because of a compensatory increase in supply from the posterior MCA feeder. After closing of the posterior MCA branch, further reduced flow velocities (94 cm/s) and increased PI values were measured in the left MCA, left ACA (86 cm/s) and right A1 segment (60 cm/s) and right MCA (40 cm/s). No explanation was found for decreased flow velocity in right-sided MCA. During the fourth and last stage, 53 days after the beginning of embolization, the anterior feeder was totally closed and the flow velocities in the left ACA decreased slightly to 70 cm/s and contralaterally to 64 cm/s. Angiographic investigation 3 months later showed a partially embolized angioma with increased flow velocities in left MCA (124 cm/s), and left ACA (78 cm/s). At this point surgical excision of the angioma was carried out (Fig. 4). After complete resection, the flow velocity diminished below normal values in both angioma feeders and in the right MCA. Distal resistance increased in the angioma feeders as sign of reestablished autoregulation. Between the 4th and 13th postoperative, a slight hyperemia was demonstrable, and flow velocities returned to normal values at the 16th day after resection of the angioma.

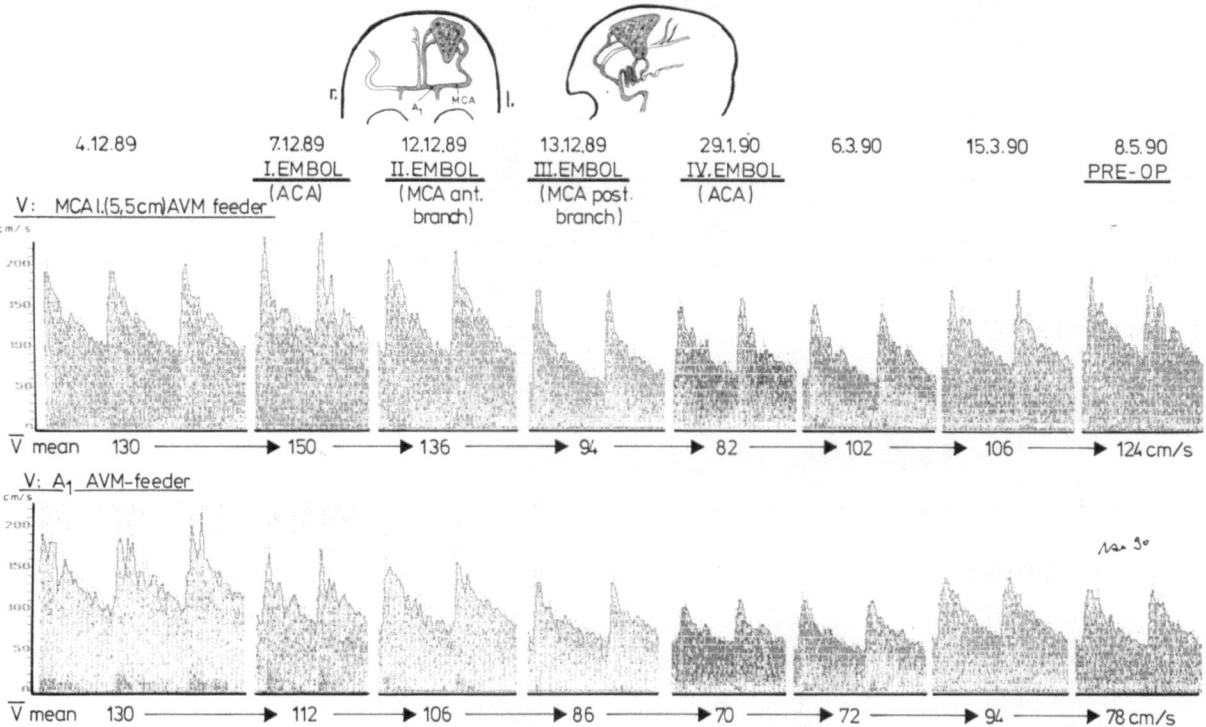

Fig. 2. Time course of flow velocities in the left middle cerebral artery and A1 feeder arteries before and after staged superselective embolization of a large left frontodorsal arteriovenous malformation and final excision

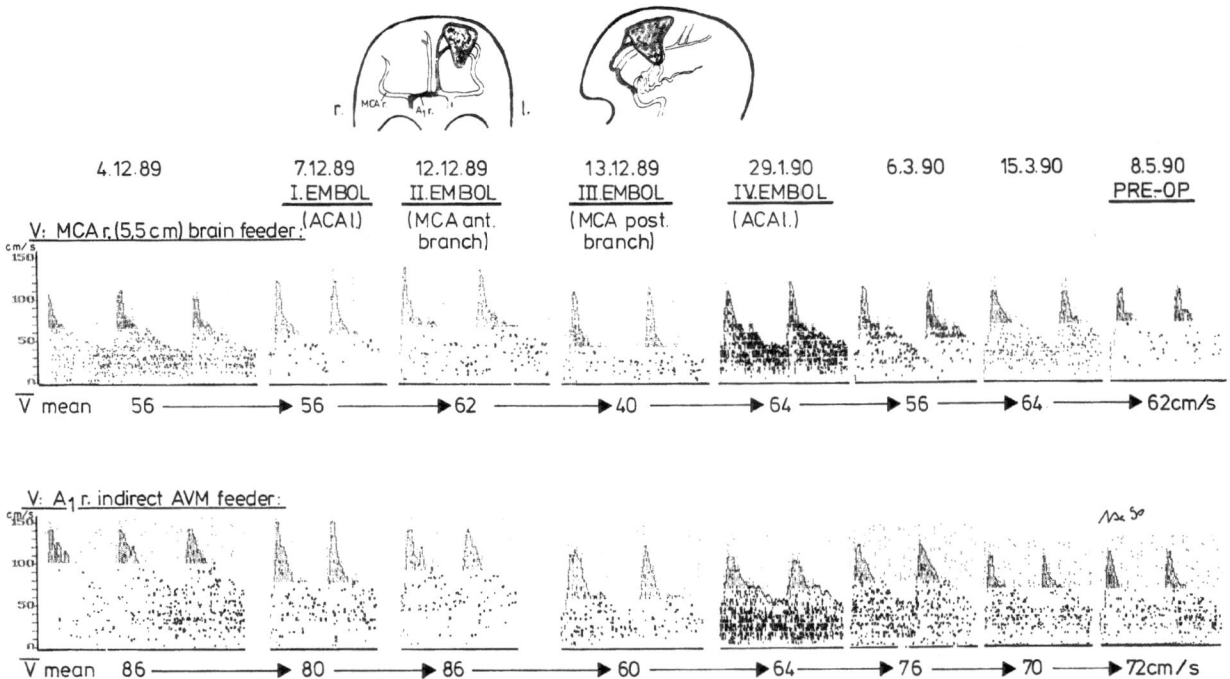

Fig. 3. Time course of flow velocities in the right middle cerebral artery and indirect arteriovenous malformation feeder artery A1 before and after staged superselective embolization of a large left fronto dorsal arteriovenous malformation and final excision

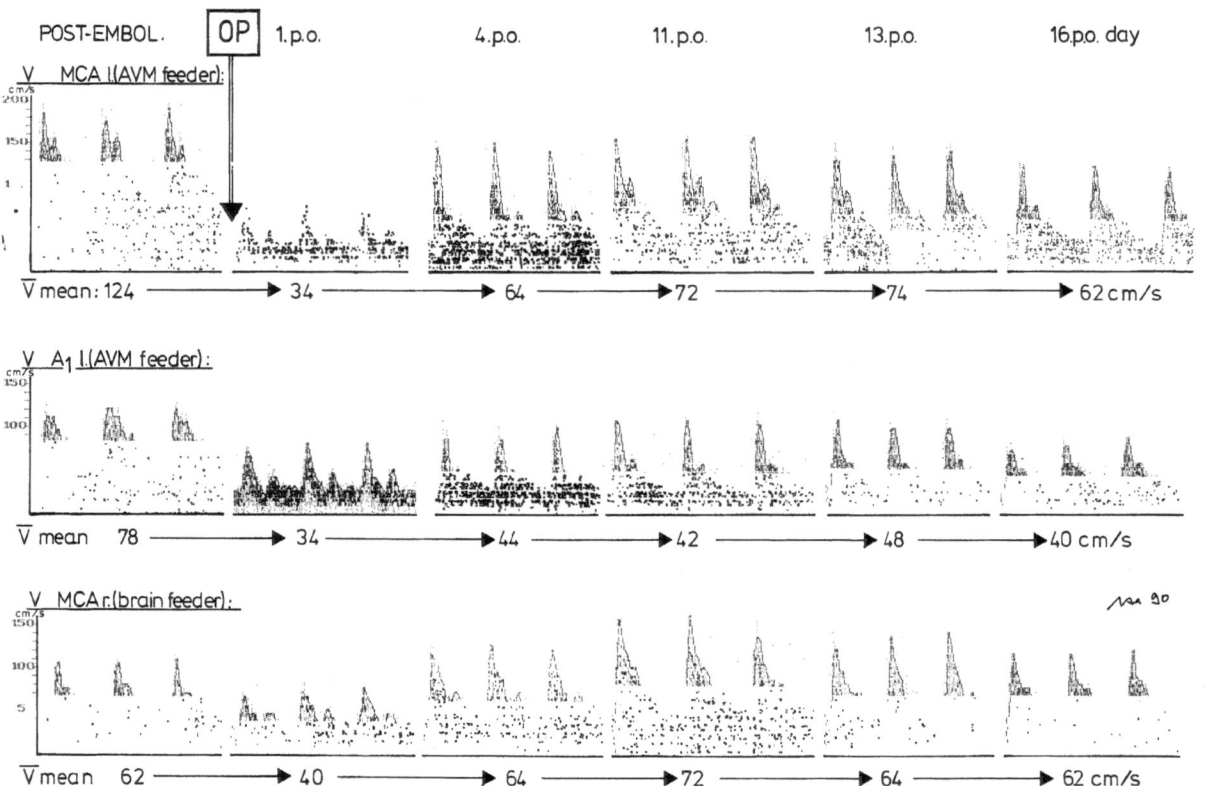

Fig. 4. Time course of flow velocities in the left middle cerebral artery and A1 feeder arteries and right middle cerebral artery after staged superselective embolization and excision of a large left frontodorsal arteriovenous malformation

3. Embolization Followed by Hemorrhage and Operative Removal

In another case (not illustrated) with a small left fronto-dorsal angioma supplied by the left MCA and A1 portion, flow velocities in TCD decreased clearly after three step embolization (once embolization of the left MCA feeder and several time of A1 feeder artery) and control angiography showed only a rest, but after the third embolization the patient suffered from a small hemorrhage so that the surgical excision was indicated. After operation flow velocities dropped clearly to sub-normal values with increased pulsatility indices and normalization of flow within six days from surgery.

B. Carotid-Cavernous Sinus Fistula

Since 1971 some authors have used CW-Doppler surveying influences of fistula flow to hemodynamic conditions in extracranial vessels[4,5,14,15]. Now TCD makes it possible to detect directly the severe hemodynamic changes in the Circle of Willis in patients with carotid-cavernous sinus fistulas (CCSF). Influences of "extracerebral" shunting to basal cerebral arteries and cerebral perfusion pressure and controll of successful occlusion of fistula by detachable balloons with regard to the hemodynamic adaptation are detectable. This will be demonstrated in a 24 year old woman suffering from a motorbicycle accident with traumatic left-sided CCSF. Investigations were done before, immediately after and in the days following occlusion of the fistula. Before occlusion additionally intraluminal pressure in the petrous portion of ICA (ICAp) proximal to the fistula was measured by a small pressure probe inserted through the balloon catheter.

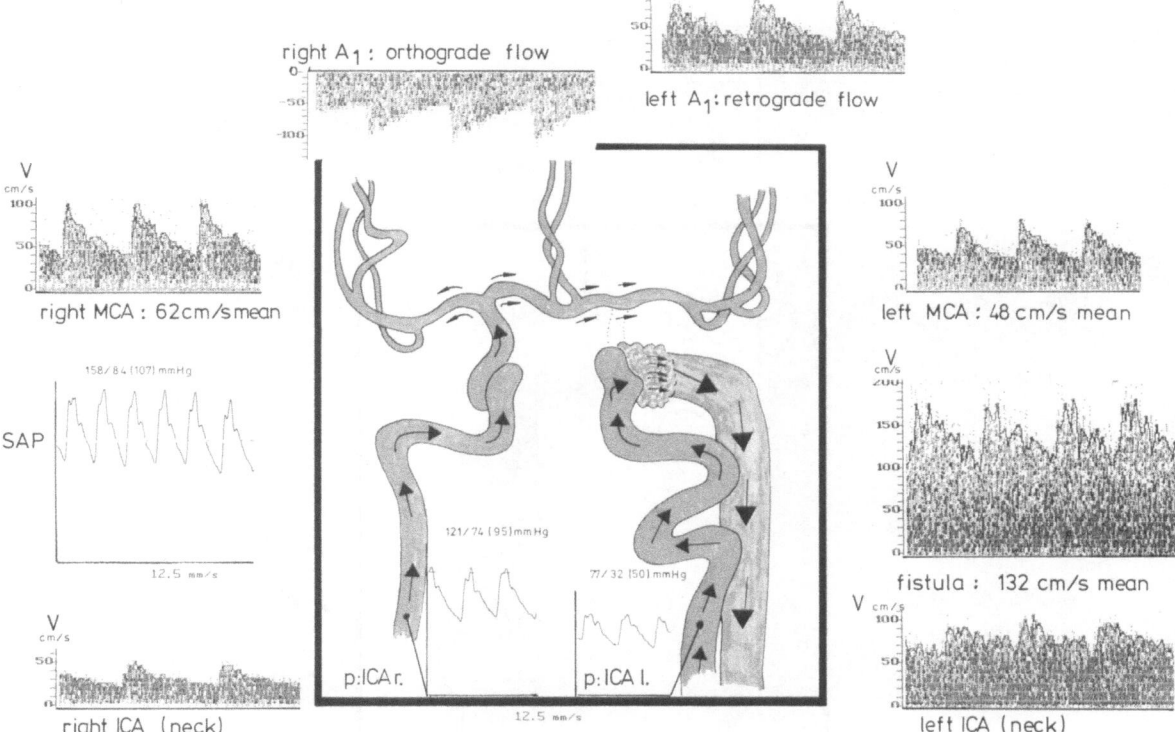

Fig. 5. Transcranial Doppler mean flow velocities (FVmean in cm/s) of basal cerebral arteries and extracranial portion of internal carotid arteries in the neck (ICAn) before occlusion of CCSF. The right MCA (FVmean = 62 cm/s) and the ICAn (FVmean = 35 cm/s) showed normal values, the right A1 a slightly increased flow velocity (FVmean = 65 cm/s) away from the probe, the left A1 (FVmean = 55 cm/s) a collateral flow towards the probe, the left MCA a decreased flow velocity (FVmean 48 cm/s), the left ICAn an increased flow velocity (FVmean = 75 cm/s) and directly at the point of fistula high flow velocities up to 132 cm/s. The vascular resistance is decreased in the left ICAn and directly at the fistula. By comparing the intraluminal mean arterial pressure (MAP) in the petrosal portion of both internal carotid arteries (ICAp), the left ICAp (MAP = 50 mmHg) showed a clearly lower intraluminal pressure than the right ICAp (MAP = 95 mmHg). *MCA* middle cerebral artery; *A1* A1 portion of anterior cerebral artery; *ICAn* neck portion of internal carotid artery; *ICAp* petrosal portion of internal carotid artery

1. Preocclusion Measurements

In Fig. 5 the right-sided ICA and MCA showed normal flow velocities with flow direction towards the probe, and the A1-portion a slightly increased flow velocity to 65 cm/s with direction away from the probe. On the fistula's side flow velocities in MCA were reduced to 48 cm/s and A1 showed a reversed flow towards the probe and the fistula as a sign of the present pathological situation. Accelerated flow velocities were measured in the left ICAn and directly at the fistula with a maximum FV mean over 132 cm/s. In both portions accelerated flow was combined with high end-diastolic flow velocites as a sign of low stream resistance. By comparing bilateral intraluminal mean arterial pressure in ICAp, pressure values of 50 mmHg proximal to fistula with regard to 95 mmHg on the opposite side appeared clearly reduced. On the left side the blood pressure curve also showed characteristics of low peripheral resistance which is a typical sign of flow proximal to a large carotid-cavernous sinus fistula.

2. Postocclusion Measurements

In Fig. 6 hemodynamic changes in the circle of Willis shortly after complete occlusion of the fistula can be demonstrated. The balloons were placed inside the fistula, so that the normal vascular anatomy was regained. Immediately after fistula occlusion flow velocities in A1-portions and MCA increased bilaterally with dominance on the left side, as a sign of a short hyperemia and hyperperfusion. Flow velocities in ICA were found in the normal range. The end-diastolic flow velocities in right and left MCA were slightly increased as a sign of reduced peripheral stream resistance in brain tissue. No fistula flow was detectable any more. Already after some minutes the flow velocities returned

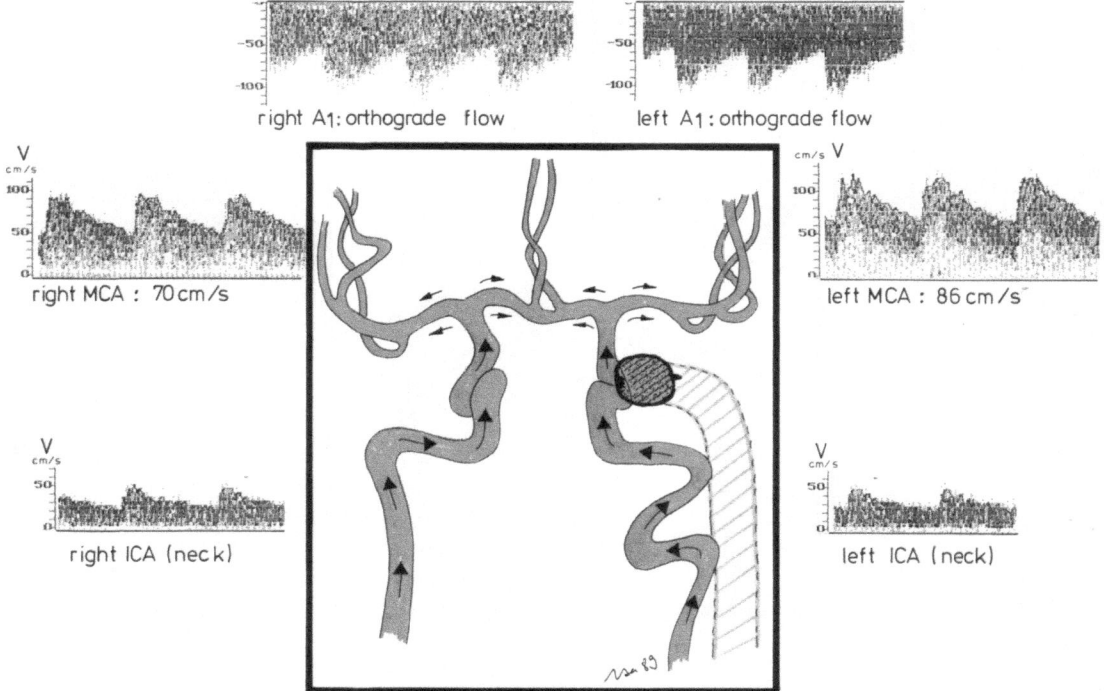

Fig. 6. Transcranial Doppler mean flow velocities (FVmean) of basal cerebral arteries and extracranial portion of internal carotid arteries in the neck (*ICAn*) after balloon occlusion of CCSF. Bilaterally mean flow velocities (FVmean) in ICAn (FVmean = 30 cm/s) showed normal values. FVmean in the right MCA (FVmean = 70 cm/s), the left MCA (FVmean = 86 cm/s) and the A1 portion of anterior cerebral artery on both sides (FVmean = 75 cm/s in the left A1; FVmean = 70 cm/s in the right A1) were slightly increased. After occlusion of fistula, collateral flow from right to left A1 portion returned back to physiological flow conditions with flow direction away from the probe in the left A1 portion. The vascular resistance in the left ICAn increased to normal values

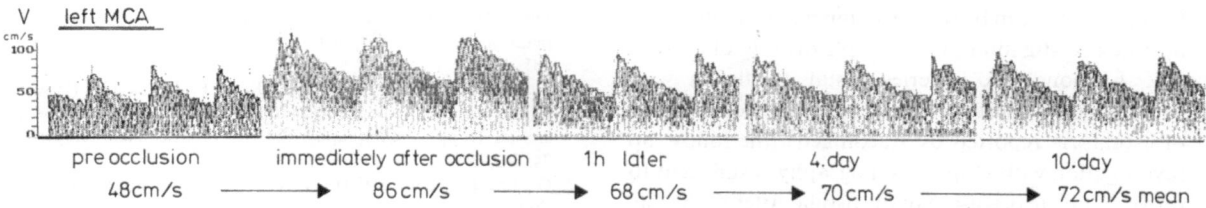

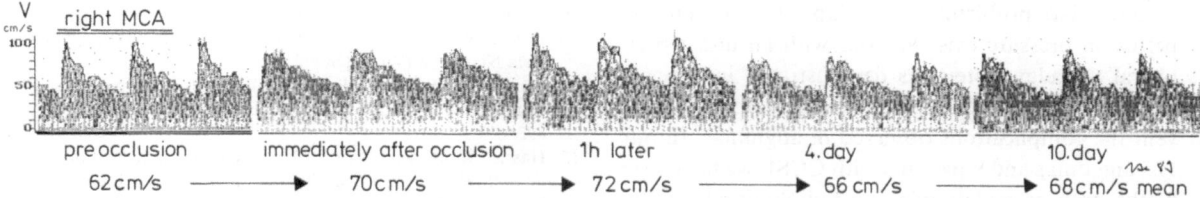

Fig. 7. Time course of mean flow velocities in both MCA before and after balloon occlusion of a left-sided CCSF. Compared to the right side, FVmean of the left MCA had decreased to 48 cm/s before occlusion of fistula. Immediately after intervention a slight hyperemia with dominance on the left side (right MCA = 70 cm/s, left MCA 86 cm/s) appeared. Normal values were already observed one hour later

to normal values, as shown by the measurement after one hour. No signs of longer lasting hyperemia were observed and a breakthrough phenomenon cannot be confirmed in this markedly changed hemodynamic situation. Successful obliteration of the fistula was documented by unchanged flow velocities in the following days (Fig. 7), as well as by angiography. Immediately after occlusion, the left-sided temporal pulsatile bruit and the pulsation of exophthalmos disappeared. Before leaving the hospital distended conjunctival veins and exophthalmos were reduced and the sixth nerve palsy remained stable. 10 months later a follow-up examination showed unchanged flow velocities in all basal cerebral arteries. Clinical symptoms of carotid-cavernous sinus fistula had totally disappeared.

Conclusion

A staged and combined procedure with superselective embolization, surgical excision and radiosurgery is safer for the marked hemodynamic adaptation after occlusion or operative removal of angioma. A combined strategy seems to avoid complications as bleeding or brain swelling, depending on an increased postoperative cerebral perfusion pressure. In our perioperative Doppler investigations[10,12], intraoperative measurements[11] and study of postoperative angiography[9] we have not observed a hemodynamic correlation for the breakthrough phenomenon. This theory described first by Spetzler[16] depends on morphological changes in the surrounding brain after angioma removal, especially swelling and bleeding complications. We think that these complications occur by operative mistake, venous thrombosis or passive pressure dependent reopenings of occluded vessels.

Staged procedures of different treatment modalities are only justified if the total complication rate does not exceed the individual complication rate of each method. In the future the side effects and influences of superselective embolization to the altered hemodynamic situation in AVMs have to be verified in larger series.

In patients with carotid-cavernous sinus fistula transcranial doppler allows also direct insonation of intracranial vessels[6] and of the pathological point. In the fistula supplying internal carotid artery at the neck we measured increased flow velocities with a decreased vascular resistance according to other authors[4,5,14,15]. In basal cerebral vessels we were able to discover an anterior collateral flow from the opposite side, a decreased flow velocity in left MCA as a sign of a "compensated" blood supply of the left hemisphere, and in this special case even a direct flow spectrum in the fistula. Especially before occlusion, influences of CCSF on cerebral hemodynamics are precisely detectable, and continous monitoring of flow velocity in distal arteries, mainly the ipsilateral MCA, is possible.

Complications can be recorded immediately after therapeutic investigations, for example drifting of detachable balloons into arteries distal to fistula with hemodynamic consequences, or incomplete occlusion of fistula. As reported by Buedingen[4], the follow up investigation with Doppler sonography is sufficient to prove complete occlusion of the fistula. After occlusion, we were able to demonstrate that flow velocities in both MCAs increased only for a short time above the normal level, returning to normal values after a few minutes. No problems with adaptation of cerebral perfusion pressure exist in cases with an intact peripheral vascular system, as demonstrated in patients with CCSF. The undisturbed autoregulation may prevent the complications observed in angiomas. In our 125 angiomas and 9 patients with CCSF we have seen neither transcranial doppler nor radiological hemodynamic signs of a normal pressure breakthrough phenomenon.

References

1. Aaslid R, Markwalder T-M, Nornes H (1982) Noninvasive transcranial Doppler ultrasound recording of flow velocities in basal cerebral arteries. J Neurosurg 57: 769–774
2. Aaslid R (1986) Transcranial Doppler sonography. Springer, Wien New York
3. Arnolds JA, von Reutern G (1986) Transcranial Doppler sonography. Examination technique and normal reference values. Ultrasound Med Biol 12: 115–123
4. Buedingen HJ, Gilsbach J, Von Reutern G-M (1978) Dopplersonographische Therapie- und Verlaufskontrolle einer Katheteroccludierten Cavernosus-Fistel. Arch Psychiat Nervenkr 226: 19–27
5. Diener HC, Voigt K, Dichgans J (1981) Diagnosis of intracranial malformations by Doppler sonography. Neurochirurgia 24: 185–191
6. Gomez CR, Gomez SM, Yoon K-W P, Kraus GE (1989) Evaluation and follow-up of carotid-cavernous fistulas by transcranial Doppler sonography: illustrative case. Neurosurgery 24: 749–751
7. Gosling RG, King DH (1974) Arterial assessment of Doppler shift ultrasound. Proc R Soc Med 67: 447–449
8. Harders A (1986) Neurological applications of transcranial Doppler sonography. Springer, Wien New York, pp 94–107
9. Hassler W, Gilsbach J, Gaitsch J (1983) Results and value of immediate postoperative angiography after operations for arteriovenous malformations. Neurochirugia 26: 146–148
10. Hassler W (1986) Hemodynamic aspects of cerebral angiomas Acta Neurochir (Wien) [Suppl] 37
11. Hassler W, Steimetz H (1987) Cerebral hemodynamics in angioma patients: an intraoperative study. J Neurosurg 67: 822–831
12. Hassler W, Burger R (1992) Arteriovenous malformations. In: Newell DW, Aaslid R (eds) Transcranial Doppler. Raven, New York, pp 123–135
13. Lindegaard K-F, Bakke SJ, Grolimund P, et al (1985) Carotid artery disease: assessment of intracranial hemodynamic pattern by noninvasive transcranial Doppler ultrasound. J Neurosurg 63: 890–898
14. Matjasko MJ, Williams JP, Fontanilla M (1975) Intraoperative use of Doppler to detect successful obliteration of carotid-cavernous fistulas. J Neurosurg 43: 634–636
15. Prolo DJ, Burres KP, Hanbery JW (1977) Balloon occlusion of carotid-cavernous fistula: introduction of a new catheter. Surg Neurol 7: 209–214
16. Spetzler RF, Wilson CB, Weinstein P, et al (1978) Normal perfusion pressure break-through theory. Clin Neurosurg 25: 651–672

Correspondence: R. Burger, M.D., Department of Neurosurgery, University of Würzburg, Josef-Schneider Str. 11, D-97080 Würzburg, Federal Republic of Germany.

Radiosurgery of Cerebral AVMs

Gamma Knife Radiosurgery in Cerebral Vascular Malformations

L. Steiner[1], C. Lindquist[2], B. Karlsson[2], W. Guo[2], and M. Steiner[1]

[1]Department of Neurological Surgery, University of Virginia, Health Service Center, Charlottesville, Virginia, U.S.A. and [2]Department of Neurosurgery, Karolinska Institute, Stockholm, Sweden

Summary

Following the description of the technique of Gamma Knife radiosurgery, a review of the results in vascular malformations is given. Maximal doses of 15–25 Gy with periphery doses of 10–62 Gy have been tested. With a dose of 25 Gy to the periphery of small AVMs, the incidence of total obliteration was 88%; in AVMs of moderate or large size, it was 78% respectively 50%.

Following repeated Gamma Knife surgery, total obliteration occurred in 83% of those patients who did not respond to the first treatment. Of 214 patients with combined endovascular and radiosurgical procedures two years follow-up angiography was available in only 32 cases. Total obliteration of the AVM occurred in 17 patients (53.1%). Of 25 small or moderately sized AV fistulae, 11 had 2 years follow-up angiography. Total obliteration occurred in 9 and subtotal obliteration in 1 case. Large multifistulae AVMs did not respond to radiosurgery. Of 8 carotid cavernous sinus fistulae, 4 had two years angiography follow-up. All 4 did obliterate. Of 16 cavernous angiomas partial regress occurred in 3 cases. There was one rebleed. In AVM vasogenic edema assessed on CT scan occurred in 10% and on MRI in 37%. Six percent of the patients had neurological deficits; however, these were permanent only in 3%. In repeated radiosurgery permanent deficits occurred in 6% of the cases. In long term in the majority of the patients pretreatment neurological deficits improved. Whether this improvement was related to the treatment or to the natural history of the disease remains open. Headache disappeared in up to 70% of the cases. Of 59 patients with seizures, 11 had no more seizures and didn't need anticonvulsant medication. Thirty became seizure free after the treatment; however, they continued with anticonvulsant medication. Findings by Kaplan Meier Life table estimates demonstrated 3.7% hemorrhage per year until 62 months after radiation. After this period the life curve ends in plateau which could be interpreted as proof of decrease of the risk of hemorrhage. Nevertheless this could be true only if it is observed in a large number of patients and for a long period of time. Our material did not fulfill this condition.

Keywords: Radiosurgery; Gamma Knife; vascular malformations; radiation induced vasogenic edema.

Introduction

Radiosurgery is a neurosurgical technique using ionizing beams instead of a knife or electrodes. By focusing the beams to the stereotactically localized intracranial target, a single high dose with steep gradient can be delivered to the target without craniotomy and with limited risk to the surrounding non target brain tissue. The instrument used is a neurosurgical tool and the term Gamma Knife was used for it by Leksell. The present review describes the method and the up-to-date results in vascular malformations.

Method

The Gamma Knife

The Gamma Knife[16,1] (Figs. 1, 2) consists of 1) the unit with the beam sources, 2) the collimators, 3) the treatment couch. Those, together with the stereotactic frame, and a computerized dose planning system provide an integrated radiosurgical tool.

The central body is built of thick cast iron and has a remote controlled shielded door which is opened and closed to allow the treatment couch with the patient in place, to move into treatment position, and to move out of the treatment space after the procedure has been carried out. The neurosurgeon can observe the patient on a screen at the control panel and communicate by a two-way intercom.

Two hundred and one Cobalt rods, each rod 20 mm in length and 1 mm in diameter, containing 12 to 20 cylinder-shaped pellets of Cobalt, are arrayed radially over a segment of sphere. The Gamma beams intersect in the center of the sphere (isocenter). The radiation emitted by a pellet is attenuated when it penetrates through other pellets. Therefore, the dose rate measured at the unit center point depends on the number and position of the Cobalt pellets and the sources in addition to the total activity. The total activity in the existing Gamma Unit is 6400 curies. The beams are individually collimated in a collimator system with two collimators in the central core of the machine and the collimator helmet attached to the treatment couch (Figs. 1, 2). The head of the patient is positioned in the collimator helmet by inserting the trunnions of the collimator helmet, in a sliding adjustable socket bearing of the Leksell base instrument (Figs. 3, 4). The socket bearing is set according to the Y and Z coordinates of the target (Fig. 3). The X coordinate is obtained by right to left adjustment of the trunnions (Fig. 4). Alignment between the collimators is controlled by micro switches. The beams are collimated towards the isocenter when the couch is in the treatment position; the 3 collimators are married and the beam channel becomes patent. The distribution of radiation around the

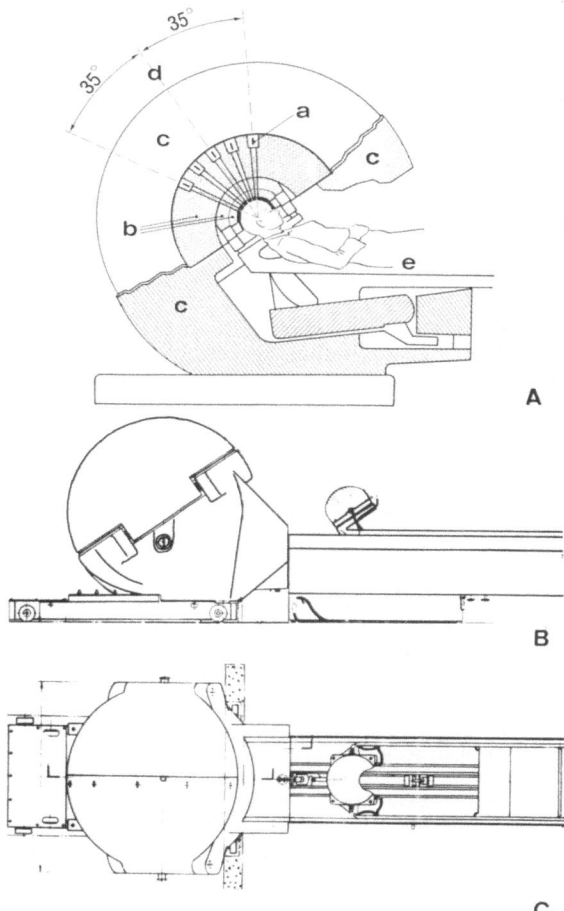

Fig. 1. (A, B, C) The Gamma Knife. Schematic drawing. *a* Cobalt source; *b* the collimator system; *c* shielding; *d* the center of the system; *e* remote controlled operating couch

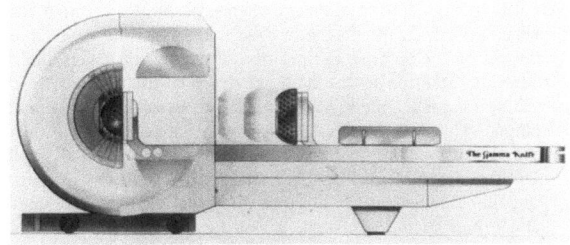

Fig. 2. Cross section of the Gamma Knife

unit center point is dependent on the size of the 201 orifices in the collimator system through which the beams have to pass. The standard collimator sizes are 4, 8, 14, and 18 mm. Using them, a tissue volume of 0.07 cc$_3$, 0.5 cc$_3$, 3 cc$_3$, and 6 cc$_3$, respectively receives 50% of the dose in the isocenter. The dose gradients are steep within the 90%, 70%, and 50% isodose configuration. Collimators can be used

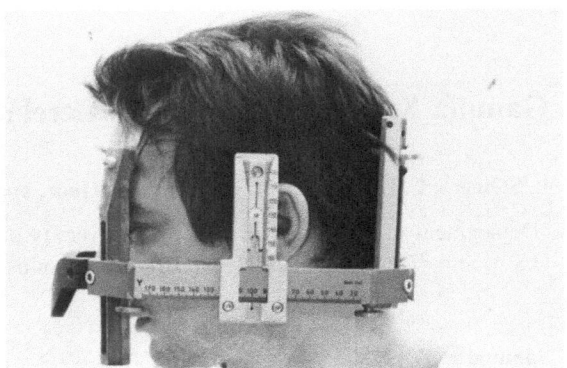

Fig. 3. Base ring with the socket bearing set according to the Y and Z coordinates of the target. The trunnions will be inserted in the socket bearings

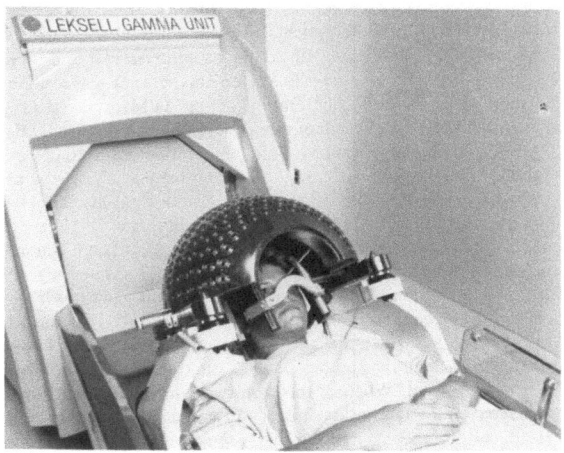

Fig. 4. The head of the patient is suspended in the collimator helmet by the trunnions inserted in the socket bearings

individually or combined and configurations of different size and shape can be obtained. To protect a particular eloquent brain structure close to the target, single beam channels can be plugged.

The Radiosurgical Procedure for Arteriovenous Malformations

The Target

As in open surgery, the aim in radiosurgery is to eliminate the nidus and to normalize the cerebral circulation. This should be achieved without damaging the nutrient arteries of the brain. However, in a number of cases in our series, the nidus was not totally included within an irradiation field considered optimal. Therefore, from the beginning, in our initial protocol the patients have been grouped according to the following:

1. The nidus is totally included in the 50% or higher periphery isodose.

2. The nidus is only partially included in the 50% or higher periphery isodose.

3. Only feeding vessels are included in the 50% or higher periphery isodose.

Only the first group is considered as receiving an optimal treatment. Radiation of the feeding vessels has led to the successful obliteration of the AVM in only a few cases but this doesn't mean that it could not work. The problem is that during the stereotactic treatment arteriogram not all feeding arteries are functional and therefore they are not visualized and hence not treated. If all feeding vessels would be radiated, the incidence of failure would be much lower. Even in a partially covered nidus we can obtain obliteration of the malformation if the embyrologically determined strategic sites of the pathologic shunts are included in the radiation field.

Pre- and Peri-Treatment Management

The patient is hospitalized the day before the treatment. An intravenous line is inserted on the ward and anti-convulsant medication is optimized, if required, by overload. A mild sedative such as Diazapam (10–20 mg) is given. In patients with vaso lability, Atropine 0.4 mg is given to block the vaso-vagal reflex.

Local anesthesia in adults is used. Even in children aged ten, general endotracheal anesthesia is not necessary, short intravenous sedation being used during the attachment of the base ring. In children under ten, general endotracheal anesthesia is used. The base ring[17] with the Leksell stereotactic coordinate frame is attached to the skull of the patient with aluminum screws or carbon fiber pins (Fig. 5) inserted in four shallow burr holes drilled 3 mm deep in the skull bone. The alignment of the base ring on the head should be

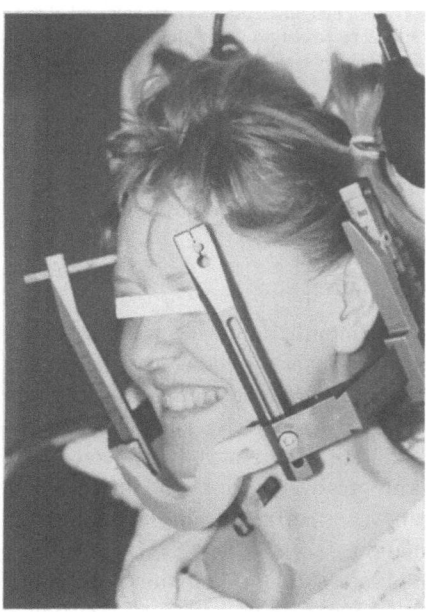

Fig. 5. Patient with "base ring" attached to the skull with carbon fiber pins inserted in shallow small holes drilled in the bone

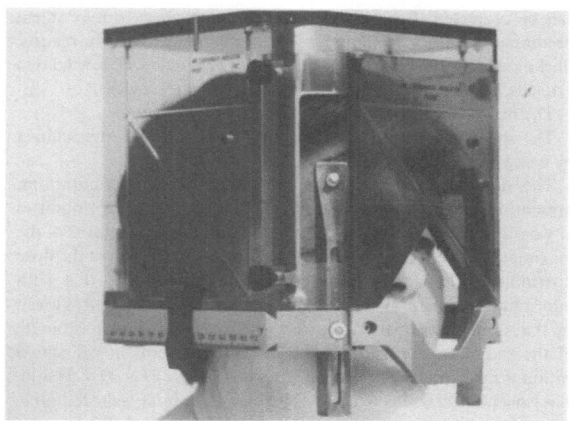

Fig. 6. Base ring with MR box for stereotactic MRI

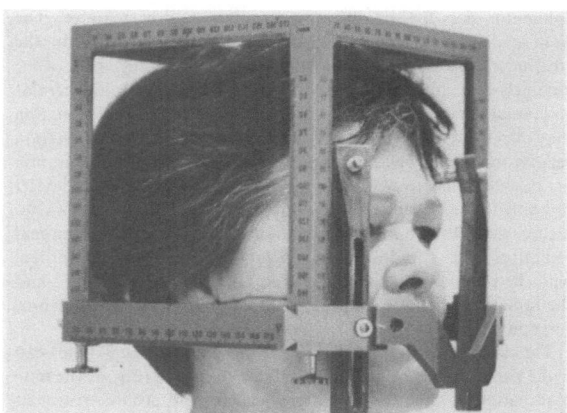

Fig. 7. Base ring with stereotactic frame for arteriography

carefully planned to avoid difficulties with suspending the head of the patient in the collimator helmet. If the target is close to the midline, the patient should be in the midline. If the target is laterally situated, the base ring should be shifted laterally with ear contralateral to the target close to the Y side bar of the respective side. Stereotactic CT or MRI (Fig. 6) and stereotactic arteriography (Fig. 7) are carried out with the base ring fixed in a frame holder attached to the angiography respectively MRI couch. A two plane rapid film sequence with three films per second is carried out. Depending on the location of the AVM and the available information from previous diagnostic angiograms, one to four vessels are injected. Substraction films with good visualization of the nidus and the scales of the stereotactic frame are required. A digital angiogram is also carried out. Replaying the sequences on the screen helps to define the nidus better. In selected cases, superselective catheterization of small distal-vessels gives additional information. A stereotactic MRI will not only improve the definition of the nidus, but in cases where the nidus is not visible clearly enough on one of the arteriogram views, the respective coordinate can be read from the MRI study. Additionally, the axial view of the MRI provides the third dimension, complementing the angiography that gives only coronal and sagittal planes. The distortion due to the field inhomogenity on MRI images can be corrected. By using the Siemens magnetom, this problem becomes negligible after shimming of the magnetic coils. The relative thickness of the image slices, chemical shift artifacts, and flow related artifacts are other potential pitfalls when using the MRI.

The magnification factor is obtained by digitization.

The coordinates of the targets are either digitized or determined by using a graphic method[2].

The dose planning program provides isodose configurations, presenting the distribution of radiation around the target point in any desired plane. Curves of the plot are given as percentages of the maximal dose delivered to the target. For the calculation of the dose distribution, the dose planning computer microvax is fed with information concerning the position of the target in the skull as given by the stereotactic coordinates and with data allowing an estimate of the radiation absorption. The dose distribution in calculated within a three dimensional matrix with a size of $31 \times 31 \times 31$ mm. The isocenters first selected from the stereotactic images are tentative and minor adjustments of their position may be needed. The steepest isodose gradient of the dose distribution, usually around the 50–90% isodose lines, should coincide with the periphery of the target. This may require several overlapping fields of radiation, each with a separate isocenter. To obtain optimal results, the use of different collimator sizes for the different isocenters may be required. The isodose distribution may also be changed by weighting. In the treatment of skull base lesions it can be useful to plug some of the channels so as to avoid unnecessary radiation to the brain stem or to cranial nerves. Changes in the position of the field of radiation may also be made by changing the incidence angle of the radiation relative to the skull base. When an appropriate isodose configuration is achieved it has to be superimposed on the angiogram and MRI not only in the isocenter planes, but in many planes of the AVM to assure that the whole malformation is included in an optimal radiation field. The dose planning provides a treatment protocol with the stereotactic coordinates from one or more isocenters, and the radiation time at each point of the dose decided by the neurosurgeon.

The coordinates are transferred to the base ring (Fig. 3). The head of the patient is positioned in the collimator helmet (Fig. 4), the time of radiation is set, and the treatment is started. Once the treatment is completed, the base ring is removed and the wounds from the attachment of the base ring are dressed with sterile cotton pads. Cortico-steroids are administered for twenty-four hours. The patient is allowed to eat immediately after the procedure and is discharged the day after the treatment.

Follow-up

At the start of the project, follow-up arteriography was repeated at three, six, nine, twelve, twenty-four, and sixty months after radiosurgery. Later when the postoperative course in pilot series was clarified, CT scanning without and with contrast medium was used for the early follow-up. With the advent of the MRI, either the latter or CT scanning was carried out to detect radiation induced changes in the normal neural tissue. If the AVM was visible on pre-treatment MRI or CT scan, these examinations were repeated every six months until the AVM was no longer visible. Then an arteriogram of good quality was mandatory. A digital angiography of good quality could be used as a final follow-up angiography.

In a group of thirty patients we did obtain a follow-up arteriogram five to eight years after the occlusion of the AVM had been demonstrated by an angiogram.

Clinical follow-up was continued every six months for those patients who still were not cured and once a year for the cured patients.

Material

Patient Population

Between April 1970 and August 1, 1992, 1800 patients with arteriovenous malformations referred from 34 countries have been treated by the authors 26, 27, 28, 29, 30, 31. One hundred twenty-one patients were treated for residual AVM following microsurgery. One hundred eighty-two patients had embolization of their AVM prior to radiosurgery.

Presenting symptoms were hemorrhage in 89% of the cases, seizures with or without hemorrhage in 8%, and minor or no symptoms in 3% of the cases.

The age of the patients ranged from three to seventy-six years. There were thirty-four children in age group 3–12 years and 170 teenagers in age group 13–17 years.

Parameters of the AVM

Seventy-three percent of the AVMs treated were located in deep or eloquent cerebral regions. The majority of the treated AVMs had a volume of less then 8cm^3. The largest treated AVM measured $60 \times 65 \times 60$ mm.

Treatment Variables

In 600 cases one isocenter was used; in 51 cases overlapping fields were used with two isocenters; in 383, three; in 115, four; in 25, five; in 9, six; in 3, seven; and 1 case, eight isocenters were used. The 14 mm collimator was most frequently used followed by the 8, the 18, and the 4 mm collimator in the named order.

Isodose levels of 50%, 70%, and 90% were used.

The rationale I had for the use of 50 Gy as maximum and 25 Gy as peripheral dose proved not to be pertinent. Nevertheless, the decision to use 25 Gy as a marginal dose was fortunate and at least in our material, it still seems to be the optimal dose. Maximum doses of 15–125 Gy and periphery doses of 10–62 Gy have been tested.

Results

Obliteration of the Malformation as Assessed on Angiogram

Arteriovenous Malformation

In the weeks and months following treatment only dynamic changes occur in the nidus and the feeding vessels as well as in the draining veins. The circulation time may decrease progressively. The caliber of the feeding arteries and of the drainage veins decreases in size. The nidus progressively shrinks and finally obliterates. As a result we see partial or subtotal obliteration of the malformation.

Subtotal obliteration, in our definition, is total disappearance of the nidus with persistence of early filling drainage vein. Only when, in addition to the total disappearance of the nidus, normalization of the efferent

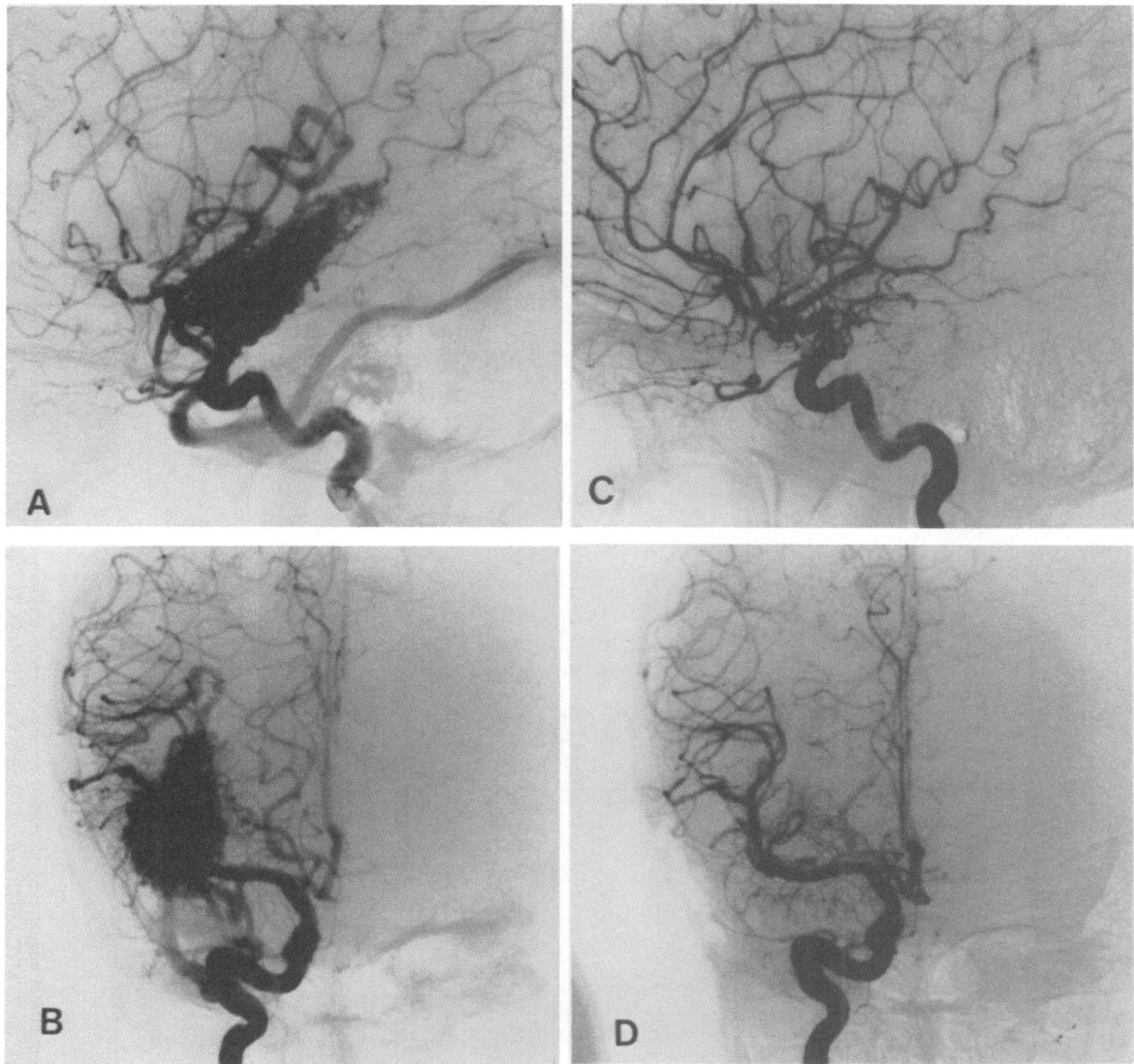

Fig. 8. (A) Lateral and (B) frontal views of a carotid angiogram visualizing an arteriovenous malformation in the left mediotemporal lobe in a eight year old boy who had a cerebral hemorrhage. The AVM is fed from the anterior choroidal and the posterior choroidal arteries. An MRI study revealed that the AVM involved also the lateral brain stem and posterior thalamus. One year following Gamma Knife surgery, on arteriography of both the left vertebral and left carotid arteries, the AVM no longer filled. (C) Lateral and (D) frontal views of the left carotid angiogram shows that the AVM did totally obliterate

and afferent vessels occurs, do we speak of a total obliteration; hence, a cure (Fig. 8).

Of 880 patients, 461 had a two years' angiographic follow-up. Three hundred sixty nine AVMs (80%) were totally obliterated within two years following the treatment. Obliteration of the AVM within one year following the treatment occurred in 230 of 360 cases (75.1%) cases. The process still continues after two

years and we have seen obliteration three to five years after the treatment.

If the results are related to the volume of the AVM, and to the peripheral dose delivered in 161 cases, the findings show that with a dose of at least 25 Gy to the periphery of an AVM no larger than 1 cm^3, the incidence of total obliteration was 88%: in AVM of 3 cm^3, 78%; in AVMs $4–8 \text{ cm}^3$ in size, 50% were obli-

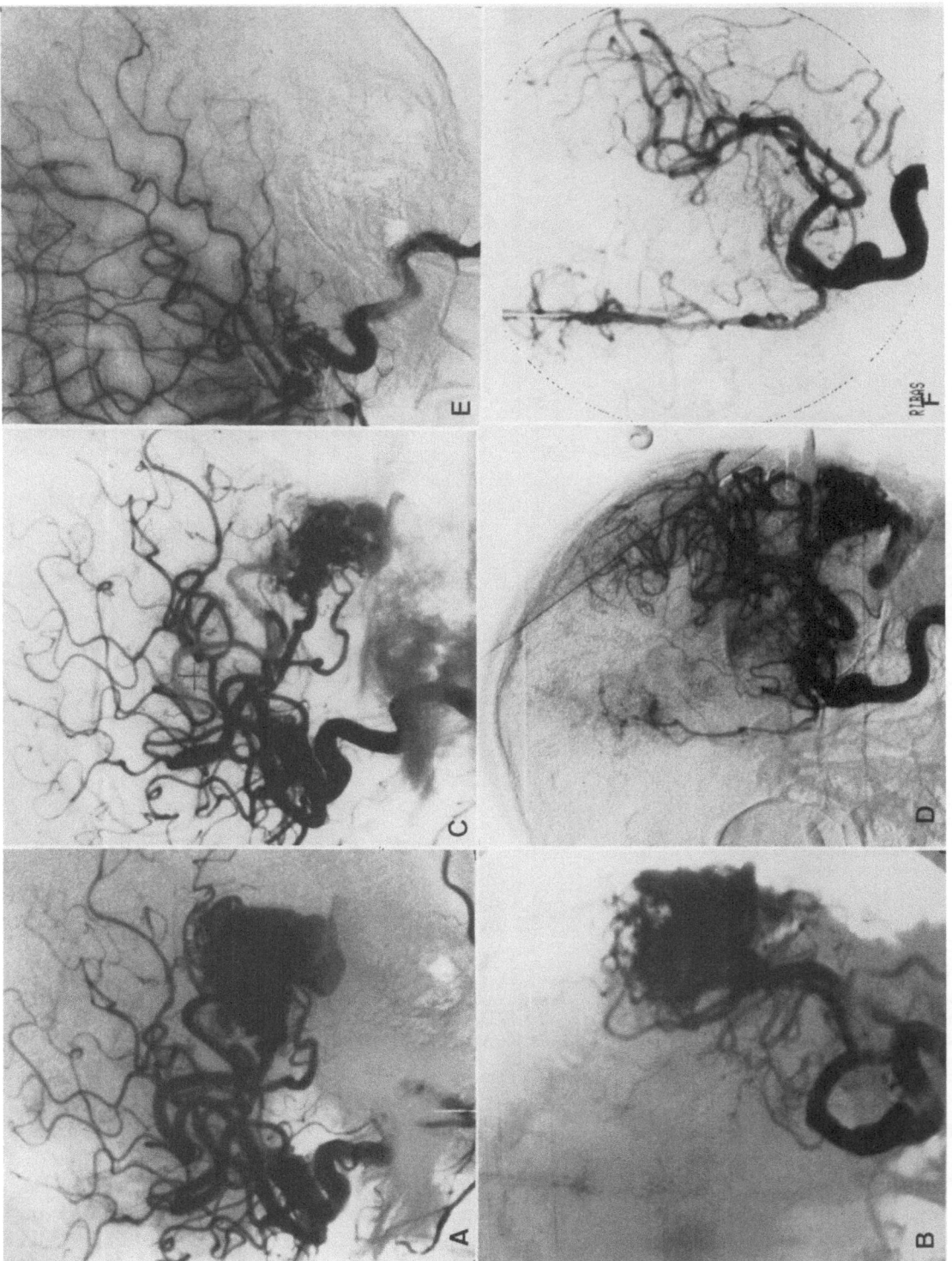

Fig. 9. (A) Lateral and (B) frontal views of a left carotid angiography visualizing an arteriovenous malformation in the left posterior temporal lobe. The size of the AVM was 37 × 30 × 25 mm. Embolization reduced the size of the AVM (C and D) and radiosurgery was carried out. Two years after the combined endovascular and radiosurgical treatment the AVM was totally obliterated. (E) lateral and (F) frontal views of a left carotid angiography

terated. With a peripheral dose of between 16–24-Gy studied in 101 cases, the incidence of total obliteration was 70% in the AVMs of 1–3 cm³ in size. In the group of AVMs measuring 4–8 cm³. 14 of 18 AVMs were obliterated (78%).

A total of 208 pediatric patients have been treated since 1970. Of the 208 patients in the series, 106 had a two years' follow-up arteriogram. Fifty-nine children have been treated since 1989. Hence, the majority have had no appropriate angiographic follow-up yet. Total obliteration occurred in 88 (83%) of the cases; subtotal obliteration in 5.8%; partial obliteration in 6.7%. In 2.9% no changes were observed. If we consider only the 97 patients who were optimally treated and had a two years' angiography study, the AVM obliterated in 85 cases (87.6%).

In 97 patients, radiosurgery was repeated when the AVM did not obliterate totally two or three years following the treatment. Two years' follow-up angiography is available in 40 cases and shows that 33 patients (83%) are cured.

Two hundred fourteen patients had embolization before radiosurgery. Two years' follow-up angiography is available in only 32 cases. Total obliteration (Fig. 9) of the AVM occurred in 17 patients (53.1%). If only the 23 optimally treated cases are considered, with total obliteration in 17 cases, the incidence of cure is 73.9%.

In the 30 cases with follow-up angiography 5 to 8 years after obliteration, no case of recanalization was observed.

Dural Arteriovenous Malformation Fistulae

Of 25 small or moderately sized fistulae over a stretch of 25 mm, eleven had two years' follow-up angiography. There were 3 total and 1 subtotal obliterations.

One patient had a rebleed one year following Gamma surgery; however, the AV fistula obliterated completely following a second treatment and the patient is without neurological deficits.

Of 8 large multifistulae malformations over a stretch larger than 25 mm no one obliterated. In 2 cases rebleed occurred, 1 lethal.

Of 3 dural AV fistulae associated with pial AVM, 1 obliterated.

Of 8 spontaneous carotid cavernous fistulae 4 obliterated. Four patients had not yet had follow-up.

Cryptic AV Malformations

Between 1983 and 1986 we treated with the Gamma Knife 16 cryptic vascular malformations. Five cases were infratentorial and 10 supratentorial. The follow-up of the cases was between 6–9 years. The maximal dose given was 50 Gy; the dose at the periphery of the malformation was 25 Gy.

Partial regress of the cavernous angioma as assessed on magnetic resonance and CT scan studies occurred in two cases at 15 and 35 months after radiosurgery. There were no visible changes on imaging in 13 cases. In one patient microsurgery was carried out five years following the Gamma Knife treatment and the histology of the specimen revealed that except for one still patent capillary, the malformation had been obliterated.

Thus, of 15 treated cavernous angiomas, 3 showed some degree of improvement which indicates favorable results in 20% of the treated cases. There was one rebleed.

In six cases, CT or MRI imaging revealed radiation-induced changes (40%). Four patient (26.6%) remained with permanent neurological deficits.

Venous Angioma

Between 1977 and 1991, we treated with the Gamma Knife 13 venous angiomas. In two cases cavernous angiomas were also present. In one case a distant arteriovenous malformation was also found. Two cases shared the venous drainage with an adjoining AVM. The treatment consisted in radiating the caput medusa and the convergence of the medullary veins.

The maximal target dose was 46±9 Gy (range 20–50 Gy) the periphery dose was 23± Gy (range 18–25 Gy). The duration of the clinical and angiography follow-up was 6–161 months. The same was true with MRI or CT scan. Complete obliteration of the venous angioma occurred in one case, partial obliteration in, no visible changes in 4, and pending result in 1 case.

During the follow-up period, 5 cases remained clinically unchanged and 1 case obtained improvement in seizure control. Two cases with bleeding as first symptom were free of rebleeding in the follow-up period. In 1 case both the venous angioma and the arteriovenous malformation were treated. Partial obliteration of both arteriovenous malformation and venous angioma was observed twenty-four months after radiosurgery. Four cases developed undue radiation effect at six, eight, twelve, and twenty-four months after radiosurgery respectively. In 1 case necrotic tissue resulted in increased intracranial pressure and necessitated extirpation six months after radiosurgery.

It is obvious that these results do not speak for using radiosurgery for venous malformations.

Arterial Aneurysms

Between 1972 and 1992, nine arterial aneurysms have been treated with the Gamma Knife. In 3 cases, the aneurysm was intranidal. In 5 cases, two years follow-up is available. Three of the five aneurysms were obliterated following radiosurgery. Two were unchanged.

One patient with symptomatic aneurysm refused surgery and therefore we decided to use the Gamma Knife. The aneurysm on the posterior communicating artery did obliterate one year after the treatment; however, even the parent vessel was occluded (Fig. 10). This didn't induce clinical symptoms.

Undue Effects

Changes in the non-target neural tissue were observed in 11% of the CT studies, and in 37% of the MRI studies. The latency between the treatment and the onset of radiation induced changes in the non target areas varied from 4–42 months (mean 9.9 months) and resolved between 1–29 months (mean 9.5 months) (Fig. 11).

Clinical Outcome

In 247 consecutive cases of AVMs treated by the Gamma Knife prior to January 1, 1984, the long term neurological outcome has been assessed[31]. Follow-up could be obtained in 239 of 247 cases (97%). Eleven of 239 patients had died. Recurrent hemorrhage was the cause of death in five patients. In the rest of 6 patients, death was unrelated to the AVM or to the treatment.

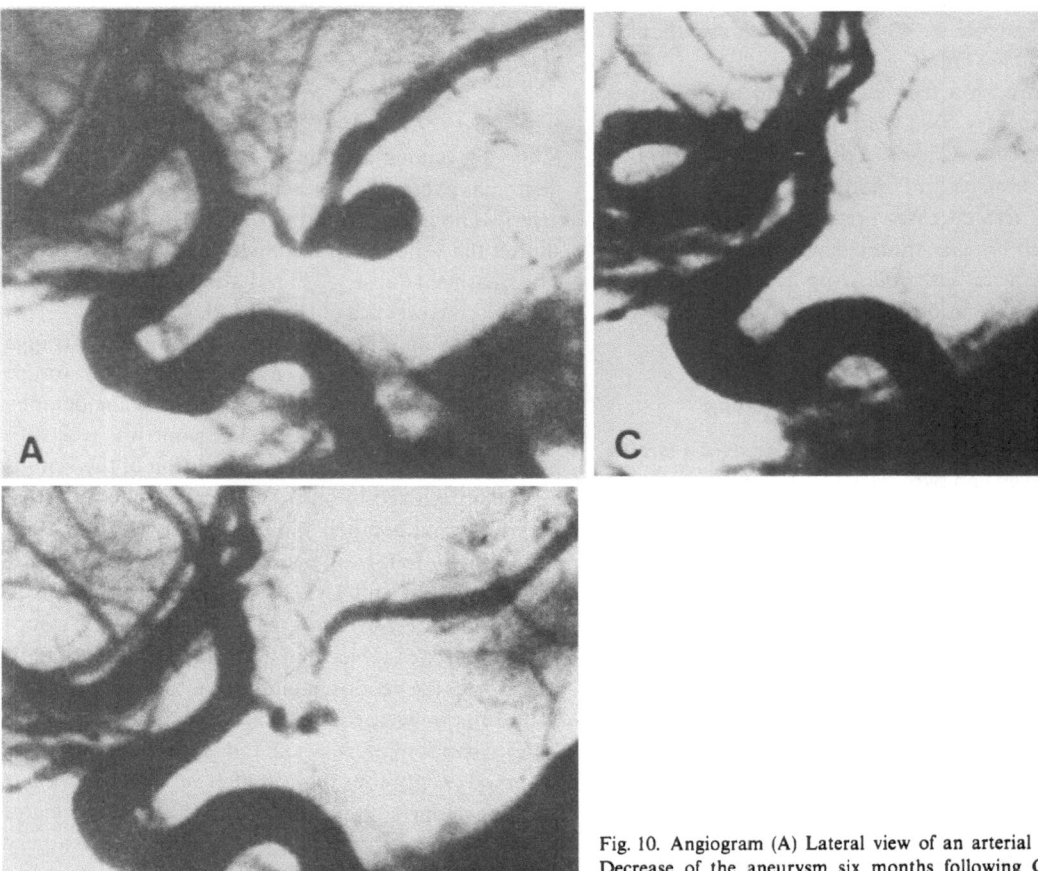

Fig. 10. Angiogram (A) Lateral view of an arterial aneurysm. (B) Decrease of the aneurysm six months following Gamma Knife Surgery. (C) Total obliteration of the aneurysm eleven months after treatment. Presumably due to inaccurate targeting the parent vessel was obliterated too. This caused no deterioration in the neurological condition of the patient

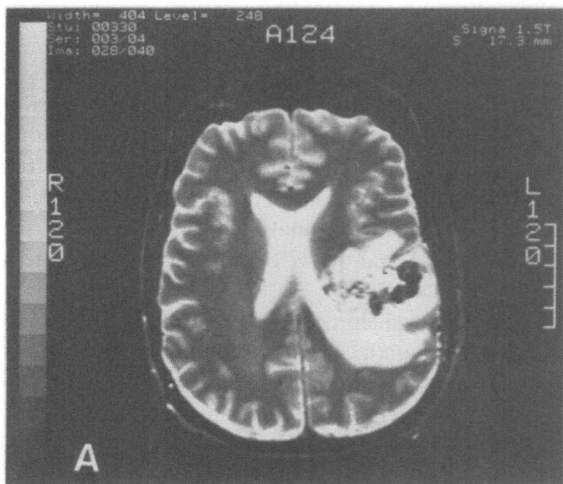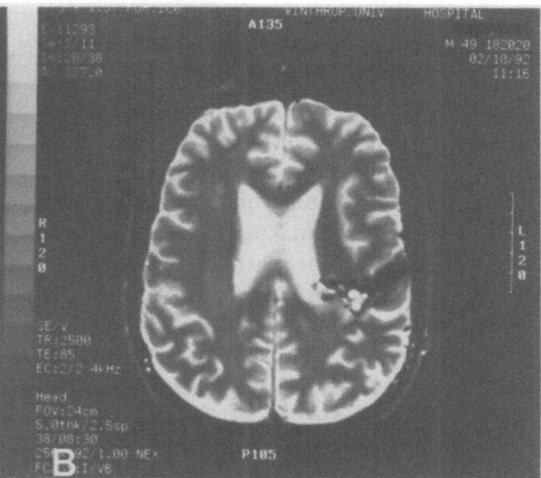

Fig. 11. MRI in a case of AVM demonstrating the course of the vasogenic edema following Gamma Knife Surgery. (A) Showing occurrence of vasogenic edema at four months following Gamma Knife surgery. (B) Resolution of the vasogenic edema eleven months after Gamma Knife surgery

Neurological Outcome

In the majority of the patients, pretreatment neurological deficits improved. Whether this improvement is related to the treatment or to the natural history of the disease remains open. The disappearance of chronic headache in up to 70% of the cases seems to have been related to radiosurgery.

Of 59 patients with seizures, 11 had no more seizures and didn't need anticonvulsant medication. Thirty patients became seizure-free after the treatment; however, they continued with anticonvulsant medication.

One hundred sixty-two patients were reported to have a full working capacity at the time of the follow-up. In 55 (31%) patients, this represented improvement in their condition prior to radiosurgery.

Eight patients with normal working capacity prior to treatment described themselves as occupationally handicapped after radiosurgery: in three cases following radiation-induced neurological deficits; in one case because of severe depression; and in another case because of chronic epilepsy.

One hundred fifty-eight (69%) patients were employed both prior to and following radiosurgery. In 16 instances, patients who were previously unemployed are now working. One patient with a traumatic arm injury, 4 patient who retired after treatment, and one who had a rebleed of the AVM, were unemployed at the time of the study.

Adverse Effects With Neurological Deficits

Six percent of the patients developed neurological deficits; however, only 3% the deficits were permanent.

In the group of AVMs treated twice, five percent developed permanent neurological deficits.

Mortality

As of May 1, 1986, 11 of the 239 patients for whom follow-up information was available had died. Recurrent hemorrhage was the cause of death in 5 patients, and 1 patient committed suicide because of intractable pain syndrome originating with his initial AVM rupture. The causes of death in the remaining five patients was unrelated to the AVM or to radiosurgery.

Discussion

History

It is not unusual that seminal ideas evolve in a border-line region between two disciplines like physics and mathematics, mathematics and chemistry.

Well aware of these for a creative mind fertile fields, Leksell explored them. As a result, he was the first to introduce the ultrasound in medicine and in 1951, he proposed the use of ionizing beams in neurosurgery, defining the technique as radiosurgery[15]. He realized that the scalpel is not necessarily the only possible physical agent for surgery in general and neurosurgery in particular, and he was convinced that is not the tool which defines a medical speciality but the patient and the mastering of the wealth of knowledge concerning the pathology, physiology, semiology, and management alternatives of the lesion. These provide the rationale for diagnosis, decision making, as well as management of the patients. It is obvious that a procedure doesn't become less neurosurgical just because it uses ionizing beams rather than a scalpel. Independent of its size, shape, or technical characteristics, the tool used for a neurosurgical patient remains a neurosurgical tool.

Following laboratory clinical investigations in order to define the advantages and drawbacks of different ionizing beams – photons, Gamma, heavy particles – the conclusion was drawn that a dedicated Co^{60} unit would be most appropriate for clinical use in neurosurgery.

At that time, Leksell's aim was to use the Gamma Knife for functional ailments – Parkinson's disease, pain, etc. and therefore, he wanted a discoid lesion to cut functional pathways. The first Gamma Knife was installed in Stockholm in 1968, and cancer patients with pain and a few Parkinson's disease patients were treated. Very soon it was realized that the new tool should be tried in the treatment of additional neurosurgical lesions. Steiner proposed the treatment of arteriovenous malformations, and in 1970 the first patient was selected. He suffered from chronic renal disease, high blood pressure, and had an arteriovenous malformation in the left temporal lobe. The nidus was too large to be covered with the isodose configurations provided by the available collimators and therefore its two feeding vessels were irradiated. Fifty Gy as maximum dose and 25 Gy as minimum dose were given. The decision for this dose was based, as it turned out, on false rationales; nevertheless, nineteen months later a follow-up angiography revealed that the malformation was totally obliterated[29].

The Gamma Knife was redesigned with collimators inducing spherical lesions more appropriate for tumors and vascular malformations and a second prototype was installed in the Department of Neurosurgery at the Karolinska Institute in 1970[16]. In 1977, at the First Neurosurgical World Congress, in San Paolo, Steiner presented the results in 30 cases of arteriovenous malformations[28]. More recently, the development of computerized treatment planning allowed to pinpoint a number of pitfalls and errors in previous treatments,

allowing a decrease in the incidence of failures and complications.

The introduction of the CT and MRI scan led to better assessment of the relationship between arteriovenous malformations and eloquent brain structures, to a more accurate definition of the nidus and to a dose planning, taking into consideration also the axial plane additionally to the coronal and sagittal plane of the lesion. The CT and the MRI changed also the pattern of the follow-up.

With the proliferation of the Gamma Knife Centers – 33 around the world – the number of the treated arteriovenous malformations with the Gamma Knife reached roughly 3000 of which 1800 were treated by the authors.

Radiobiology

Radiobiological data are scarce in radiosurgery, in general, and in radiosurgery for vascular malformations, in particular.

It is well established that radiation induces changes in small vessels in the skin[34], in larger pulmonary vessels[35] and in the human aorta[32]. The early changes consist of perivascular or endothelial cell swelling with increased nuclear basofilia, endothelial cell degeneration with necrosis, diapedesis of leukocytes into the interstitial space and increased colloids. Fissuring of the walls, spot hemorrhages, and thrombi may occur. The active fibroblastic activity increases and there is reparative proliferation of surviving endothelial cells with increased deposition of collagen in the media of vessel walls. The adventitia goes through a process of fibrosis. In the early phase the changes are slight and diffuse in small vessels; later they involve larger areas of the vessel walls. The proliferation of endothelial and medial cells, as well as of the subendothelial connective tissue increases progressively. Collagenous and hyalinic material deposits, together with the progressive reparative endothelial and medial thickening, lead to the fibrosis and occlusion of the pathological vessels of the arteriovenous malformation nidus. Total obliteration of medium sized vessels was demonstrated in a number of AVM specimen excised when only partial obliteration of the malformation following Gamma Knife treatment was achieved[26].

Interference with the oxygen supply is of little importance in radiosurgery. There are indications, however, that the vascular endothelium may be protected through injections of subhydril compounds, like cistamine, before irradiation[3]. Larson[13] suggests that the use of blood-born boronated macro-molecules or boronated substances with affinity for endothelial cells may serve as adjuvant neutron capture therapy in the radiosurgical treatment of larger arteriovenous malformations.

The important parameters that determine the radiation response for a given target structure, radiation quality, and dose distribution, are the absorbed radiation dose and perhaps the dose rate. The DNA is the main target in the cell. The initial chemical damage yields in base alterations, cross links within the DNA itself (or between DNA and a near-by protein) and DNA strand breaks[13].

Reparative processes due to enzyme systems may occur. The unrepaired or misrepaired double strand breaks are probably the main factor in the development of cell death with subsequent tissue changes of a wide gamut, from vasogenic edema to brain tissue necrosis. The cell populations that are likely to suffer first due to high dose irradiation are those with the highest rate of mitosis and subsequent cell loss. In healthy central nervous tissue subject to radiosurgery, two such critical subpopulations have been identified – endothelial cells and oligodendroglia[13]. Tumor tissue and vascular malformations often respond to a much lower dosage because of the higher proliferative activity of the pathological cell populations as compared with the healthy brain. Hall[9], and Nilsson et al.[20] demonstrated that dose survival curves can vary significantly even for cells of similar types. In radiosurgery, the response of any tissue, healthy or pathological, depends not only on the reproductive death of proliferative cells in critical cell populations but also on the extent to which repopulation occurs[13]. Demyeli-nation and white matter necrosis are caused by the loss of oligodendroglia, sometimes in combination with damage to endothelial cells and circulatory deficiencies. Depending on the volume irradiated, doses of 20 Gy or more are required to cause such alterations in the adult human brain. Evident neural degeneration in the gray matter requires slightly higher absorbed doses and is probably directly related to damaged endothelial cells and damage to the blood-brain-barrier system. There may be significant differences in the doses required. The effect of radiation on normal tissues is either acute, occurring within days or weeks, or late, taking many months or years to develop. In slowly proliferating cell populations in the brain, it takes very high doses to achieve an acute effect. With the possible exception of

acute vasogenic edema, that sometimes can be seen during the first weeks and months after irradiation, all undesired effects of radiation surgery are late. Demyelination and associated functional defects may occur many months and even years after irradiation[13].

Decision Making

Although, in short term, the arteriovenous malformation is a relatively benign lesion, in the long term an unfavorable natural history in untreated arteriovenous malformations is well documented[4,6-8,21]. Given the high risk for rebleed with a not negligible incidence of mortality and morbidity, the malformation should be eliminated.

Microsurgery[5,10,19,23-25] radiosurgery, embolization alone or combined should be decided, taking into consideration the natural history of the disease, the anticipated results of the available therapeutic alternatives, the patient's parameters, including: age; medical and neurological status; the presenting symptoms (hemorrhage, headache, epilepsy, or no symptoms); the variables of the AVM including its location, size, the number and flow pattern of feeding vessels; the presence of hematoma; the relationship of the malformation to surrounding brain structures; and possible results of blood flow and volume studies.

Rebleed

It has been contended that radiation of the AVM is by itself protective against AVM rupture[11,12].

In 432 patients treated between April 1970 and January 1986, there were 85 cases fulfilling the criterion given by Kjellberg[11,12]. The minimum dose of radiation received by the entire malformation should be 10 Gy; two years should have elapsed following the treatment.

Probability estimates were calculated using two methods: 1) the Person-Year method which calculates the risk from the total period of follow-up and 2) the Kaplan Meier Life Table which calculates the risk based on the time of follow-up to the event. The Person-Year method showed the risk for rebleed being comparable to that in the natural history of the disease. The findings by Kaplan Meier Life table estimates demonstrated increasing risk of nearly 3.7% per year until 62 months after radiation at which the last bleed occurred. The overall risk was 3.4% at 36 months; 7.2% at 48 months; and 11.2% at 62 months. Upper and lower bonds of the 95% confidence interval at 72 months were 4% and 18% respectively. Thus, within the limits of the Life Table estimates, radiosurgical treatment does not appear to confer any significant protection against repeated hemorrhages in the non-obliterated AVM in the first six years following the treatment. However, after this period the Life Table ends in a plateau which could be interpreted as proof of sustained decrease in the risk of hemorrhage in late follow-up.

There are serious arguments against such a conclusion from the Life Table. "Any conclusion based on the fine detail of the Life Table is likely to be wrong. A flat region on the right hand end of the Table does not imply that the real risk of death or other events such as bleeding among patients who are still alive is negligible, unless a large number of patients have trial times well into or beyond the flat region"[22].

The true risk of hemorrhage at sixty months in our series is likely (p = 0.91) to be between 4%–18% (rounded to the nearest integer). The upper bound of the 95% confidence interval for hemorrhage at the end of the observation is probably lower than 18% due to losses from the follow-up group. The 18%–20% rate at 96 months is also a possible but improbably value for hemorrhage at the end of the observation period and is consistent with a risk that is constant over the entire follow-up period. However, using a Poisson model of risk, a rate of hemorrhage as high as 1.2% per year would yield confidence limits including 0. To be sure, a lower rate may be explained by the fact that the majority of the AVMs may have been obliterated and thus the number of individuals at risk for bleeding was lower.

Cryptic Vascular Malformations

The still unknown natural history, the low incidence of documented favorable results, and the higher incidence of complication compared with arteriovenous malformations made us hesitant in using radiosurgery in cryptic vascular malformations. An additional argument for a moratorium in the treatment of theses cases is the fact that we lack a technique to monitor the results.

Arterial Aneurysms

This series, which demonstrates that arterial aneurysms can be obliterated by ionizing beams, is not offered as an argument to use radiosurgery in arterial aneurysm.

Arterial aneurysms should be eliminated by microsurgery since the risk for rebleed is high and the results of radiosurgery occur late, within 4–24 months. Concerning the non-ruptured asymptomatic aneurysm, the rationale for radiosurgery would seem more acceptable. However, considering the results of microsurgery with practically no mortality and very low morbidity in these cases, it is not probable that radiosurgery will ever have a role in the treatment of arterial aneurysms.

References

1. Berk H, Agarwal SK (1992) Physical aspects of radiosurgery with the Gamma Knife. In: Steiner L, Lindquist C, Forster D, Backlund E-O (eds) Radiosurgery. Baseline and trends. Raven, New York
2. Bergström M, Greitz T, Steiner L (1980) An approach to stereotaxic radiography. Acta Neurochir (Wien) 5: 157–165
3. Cerda H, Rosander K (1983) DNA damage in irradiated endothelial cells of the rat cerebral cortex. Protective action of cysteamine in vivo. Radiat Res 95: 317–326
4. Crawford PM, West CR, Chadwick DW, Shaw, MDM (1986) Arteriovenous malformations of the brain: natural history of unoperated patients. J Neurol Neurosurg Psychiatry 49: 1–10
5. DaPian R, Pasqualin A, Scienza R, Vivenza C (1980) Microsurgical treatment of ten arteriovenous malformations in critical areas of the cerebrum. J Microsurg 1: 305–320
6. Forster DMC, Steiner L, Hakanson S (1972) Arteriovenous malformations of the brain. A long-term clinical study. J Neurosurg 37: 562–570
7. Fults D, Kelly DL Jr (1984) Natural history of arteriovenous malformations of the brain: a clinical study. Neurosurgery 15: 658–662
8. Graf CJ, Perret GE, Torner JC (1983) Bleeding from cerebral arteriovenous malformations as part of their natural history. J Neurosurg 58: 331–337
9. Hall EJ, Marchese M, Hei TK, Zaider M (1988) Radiation response characteristics of human cells in vitro. Radiat Res 114: 415–424
10. Heros RC, Korosue K, Diebold PM (1990) Surgical excisions of cerebral arteriovenous malformations: late results. Neurosurgery 26: 570–578
11. Kjellberg RN (1988) Proton beam therapy for arteriovenous malformations of the brain. In: Schmidek HH, Sweet WH (eds) Operative neurosurgical techniques. Indications, methods, and results, 2nd Ed. Grune and Stratton, New York, pp 911–915
12. Kjellberg RN, Abe M (1988) Stereotactic Bragg peak proton beam therapy. In: Lunsford LD (ed) Modern stereotactic neurosurgery. Martinus Nijhoff, Boston, pp 463–470
13. Larsson B (1992) In: Steiner L, Lindquist C, Forster D, Backlund E-O (eds) Radiological fundamentals in radiology. Baseline and trends. Raven, New York
14. Leksell D (1987) Stereotactic radiosurgery. Neurol Res 9: 60–68
15. Leksell L (1951) The stereotaxic method and radiosurgery of the brain. Acta Chir Scand 102: 316–319
16. Leksell L (1971) Stereotaxic and radiosurgery: an operative system. Thomas, Springfield, Ill
17. Leksell L, Lindquist C, Adler JR, Leksell D, Jernberg B, Steiner L (1987) A new fixation device for the Leksell stereotaxic system: technical note. J Neurosurg 66: 626–629
18. Lindquist C, Guo W, Steiner L, Karlsson B (1993) Radiosurgery for venous angioma. J Neurosurg 78: 531–536

19. Malik GM Umansky F, Patel S, Ausman JI (1988) Microsurgical removal of arteriovenous malformations of the basal ganglia. Neurosurgery 23: 209–217
20. Nilsson S, Carlsson J, Larsson B (1980) Survival of irradiated glia and glioma cells studied with a new cloning technique. Int J Radiat Biol 37: 267–279
21. Ogilvy CS (1990) Radiation therapy for arteriovenous malformations: a review. Neurosurgery 26 (5): 725–735
22. Peto R, Pike MC, Armitage P, Breslow NE, Cox DR, Howard SV, Mantel N, McPherson K, Peto J, Smith PG (1976) Design and analysis of randomized clinical trials requiring prolonged observation of each patient. I. Introduction and design. Br J Cancer 34: 585–612
23. Solomon RA, Stein BM (1986) Management of arteriovenous malformations of the brain stem. J Neurosurg 64: 857–864
24. Spetzler RF, Martin NA, Carter LP, Flom RA, Raudzens PA, Wilkinson E (1987) Surgical management of large AVMs by staged embolization and operative excision. J Neurosurg 67: 17–28
25. Stein BM (1984) Arteriovenous malformations of the medial cerebral hemisphere and the limbic system. J Neurosurg 60: 23–31
26. Steiner L (1984) Radiosurgery in arteriovenous malformations in the brain. In: Wilson CB, Stein BM (eds) Intracranial arteriovenous malformations, current neurosurgical practice. Williams and Wilkins, Baltimore
27. Steiner L, Forster D, Leksell L, Meyerson BA, Boéthius J (1980) Gamma thalamotomy in intractable pain. Acta Neurochir (Wien) 52: 173–184
28. Steiner L, Greitz T, Leksell L, Noren G, Rähn T, Backlund E-O (1977) Radiosurgery in intracranial arteriovenous malformations. II. A follow-up study. Proceedings of the 6th International Congress of Neurological Surgeons. Excerpta Medica, Amsterdam
29. Steiner L, Leksell L, Greitz T, Forster DMC, Backlund EO (1972) Stereotaxic radiosurgery for cerebral arteriovenous malformations. Report of a case. Acta Chir Scand 138: 459–464
30. Steiner L, Lindquist C, Steiner M (1992) Radiosurgery in stroke. Stroke International 3: 8–16
31. Steiner L, Lindquist C, Adler JR, Torner JC, Alves W, Steiner M (1992) Clinical outcome of radiosurgery for cerebral arteriovenous malformations. J Neurosurg 77(1): 1–8
32. Thomas E, Forbus W (1959) Irradiation injury to the aorta and the lung. Arch Path 67: 256–263
33. Wilson CB, U HS, Domingue J (1979) Microsurgical treatment of intracranial vascular malformations. J Neurosurg 51: 446–454
34. Windholz F (1937) Zur Kenntnis der Blutgefäßveränderungen in Röntgebestrahlten Geweben. Strahlentherapie 59: 662–670
35. Wolbach SB (1909) The pathologic history of chronic x-ray dermatitis and early x-ray carcinoma. J Med Res 21: 415–449
36. Yasз'', ʁ⋏ ¢εɦ̃ɦ̃ɦ̃χ ʁˑᵛᵎˑ‡ɖ ʧ, ʋʋʋ mʤ ɬʧʁˑːˑ mʒˑʤ ə,ˑʲʲɖ ɹː ǳ'

Correspondence: L. Steiner, M.D., Ph.D., Department of Neurological Surgery, University of Virginia, Health Service Center P.O. Box 212, Charlottesville, VA 22908, U.S.A.

Combined Treatments for Cerebral AVMs

The Role of Embolization in the Surgical Resection of AVMs

B.M. Stein, J. Pile-Spellman, and **A. Kader**

Neurological Institute of the Columbia-Presbyterian Medical Center, New York, New York, U.S.A.

Summary

We have found embolization as a pre-operative adjuvant in the treatment of the medium to large AVMs of great benefit.

A review of the materials and brief resume of the different techniques of embolization is given. More recently we have done physiological monitoring before, during, and after embolization to help us in determining the course, frequency of embolization, and the value for surgery.

Specific cases are reviewed showing how embolization has been useful in blocking:

   1) deep aneurysms associated with AVMs,
   2) reducing the flow and turgor through malformations, and
   3) selectively interrupting deep, somewhat inaccessible feeders to AVMs.

A brief disscusion is given in terms of the usefulness or absence of usefulness in the technique of embolization to be followed by radiosurgery.

Keywords: Arteriovenous malformations; cerebral embolization; cerebrovascular; interventional neuroradiology; microneurosurgery.

Introduction

For approximately 20 years we have used various techniques of embolization in the management of large arteriovenous malformations of the brain[14,17]. In a series of 350 patients with arteriovenous malformations (AVMs), 30% over 5 cm/s in maximum diameter, virtually all of these had embolization as a preoperative adjuvant. In some of the medium sized AVMs measuring 3 to 5 cm/s, embolization was used sparingly to facilitate surgery. In other instances, embolization was used as a primary or the only treatment for large malformations considered inoperable so that they could be reduced in size. We were not certain in this latter group of lesions whether the partial reduction by embolization afforded any safety in terms of rebleeding. A longer-term follow up will be necessary to settle that issue. Therefore the primary purpose of this report is to discuss embolization as an adjuvant to surgery, making the surgical removal of these complicated large AVMs easier and safer.

Embolization has been used primarily to provide a graded reduction in the size of the AVM prior to final surgical obliteration. Past experience has indicated that too sudden obliteration of a large AVM may lead to a perfusion overload in the normal surrounding brain[1,2,13]. When a large number of high flow shunts existing close to the internal carotid circulation such as a large AVM of the frontal or temporal regions is suddenly obliterated, there may be hemorrhage in the surrounding otherwise normal brain tissue leading to the phenomenon called "perfusion pressure breakthrough"[13]. The reduction in the number of shunts, turgor and blood flow through the malformation by preoperative embolization makes surgery considerably easier in terms of dealing with the malformation at the time of microsurgical obliteration[4,6,11,12,17]. Furthermore, embolization can be used as a preoperative adjuvant to block deep feeders which may be inaccessible to the surgeon until later stages of the operation. Such feeders may be large in the case of the posterior cerebral artery or smaller, nevertheless with high flow, in the instance of choroidal, thalamoperforate, or lenticulostriate arteries (Fig. 1). All of these vessels play a significant role and add to the hazard of the resection of the AVM in its final stages.

While embolization procedures may be repeated innumerable times, any one time reduction in the malformation is limited and, even with multiple embolization, obliteration nearing completion is extremely rare. However, rather remarkable reduction in the angiographic appearance of the malformation may be obtained by either single- or multiple-stage embolization. It is difficult to predict which patients will respond best to embolization techniques. Generally speaking,

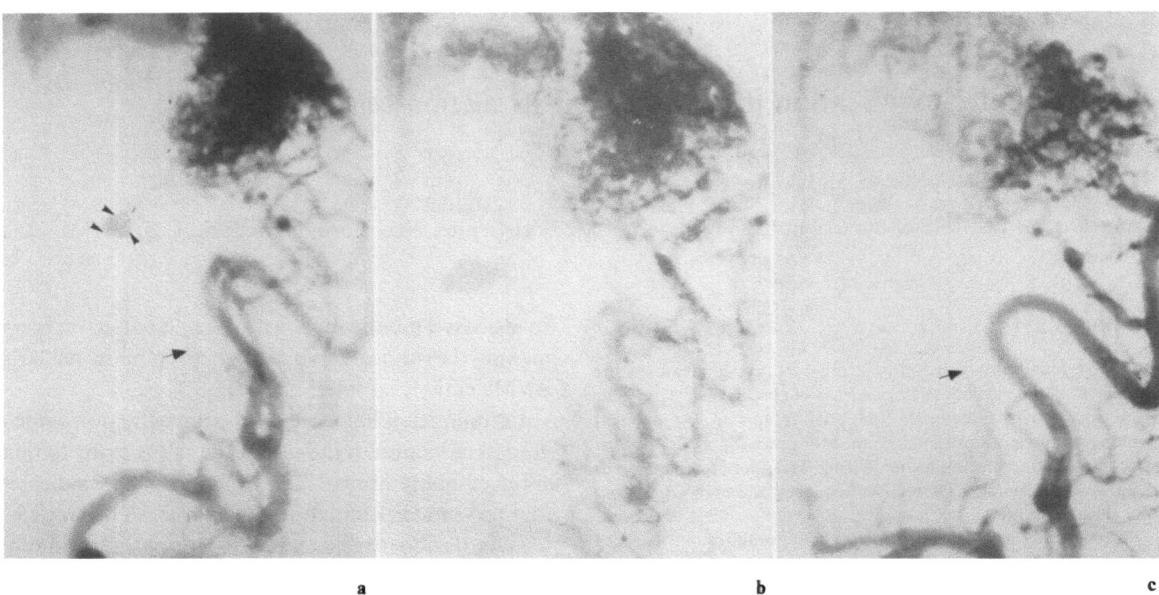

a   b   c

Fig. 1. (a) AP left carotid arteriogram showing deep aneurysm (arrowheads) supplied by a lenticulostriate artery (open arrowhead toward the apex of the AVM. (b) Same patient one week later with enlarging aneurysm. (c) Embolic occlusion of deep lenticulostriate artery via coil (arrow) with obliteration of the aneurysm

an arterial supply which is large and relatively short, without tortuosity, lends itself best to the intravascular techniques. To some extent, the result depends upon the evolution of intravascular techniques from rather primitive flow-directed techniques to ones where the embolic material can be placed directly into the malformation[18].

Evolution of Interventional/Intravascular Techniques

Early embolization procedurs were carried out through the use of particulate matter, specifically silastic and other pellets, injected quite proximal to the arteriovenous malformation, such as the internal carotid artery in the neck or the vertebral artery in the neck and carried to the malformation, flow-directed, relying entirely on the anatomy of the nutrient arteries as they travel toward the AVM[10]. There is a certain degree of predictability in the course of the emboli determined by the pre-embolic angiograms and the anatomy[18] (Fig. 2). However, pellets can go astery and occlude normal arteries due to the vicissitudes of the circulation and the pulse effect of the circulation. Fortunately, most of the people treated were young, collateral circulation developed rapidly, and the reduction of the actual shunt in the malformation encouraged the development of

collateral circulation (Fig. 3). Therefore, a "few" stray emboli generally produced no major neurological problems as long as major arteries were not occluded. As an offshoot of the embolization using pellets, balloon-guided techniques were utilized to force the silastic pellets into areas they would not otherwise travel when purely flow-directed[8,9]. For example, a balloon could be floated distal beyond the lenticulostriate arteries and then occlude the middle cerebral distal to these arteries, forcing the pellets to go at right angles into the lenticulostriate or other penetrating arteries, thereby occluding them (Fig. 4).

Moving beyond the era of pellet embolization, small particulate material such as polyvinyl alcohol particles were utilized in conjuction with flow-arresting platinum coils, the latter being quite small[8]. These coils have the advantage of reducing the flow into the AVM via the major arterial tributaries and thereby arresting the small particulate matter within the malformation, preventing it from overflowing and leaving via the venous phase (Fig. 5). However, this often resulted in the occlusion only of a major nutrient artery while leaving the nidus of the malformation open and able to establish rapid collateral circulation. This somewhat defied the basic aim of embolization to occlude the nidus primarily and thereby prevent the rapid estab-

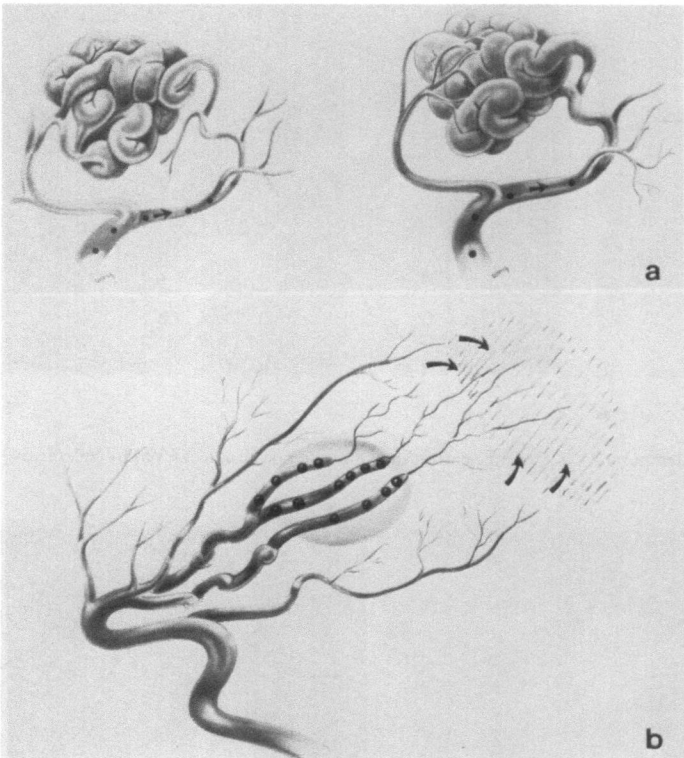
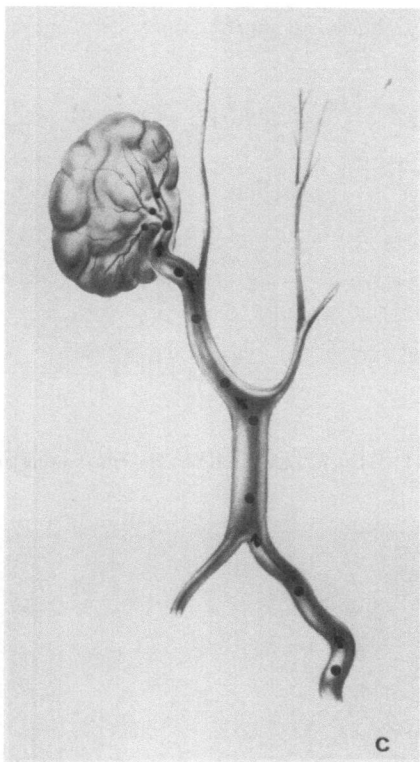

Fig. 2. (a) Drawing showing the effect of flow, arterial anatomy and size on the course of emboli. (b) Drawing of silastic emboli flow-directed via the vertebrobasilar system via the enlarged posterior cerebral to the AVM. (c) Drawing of graded occlusion of the middle cerebral artery branches that supply both the normal brain and AVM. By repeated embolizations and selective occlusion of these branches at the AVM a gradual development of collateral circulation protects the normal brain from infarction

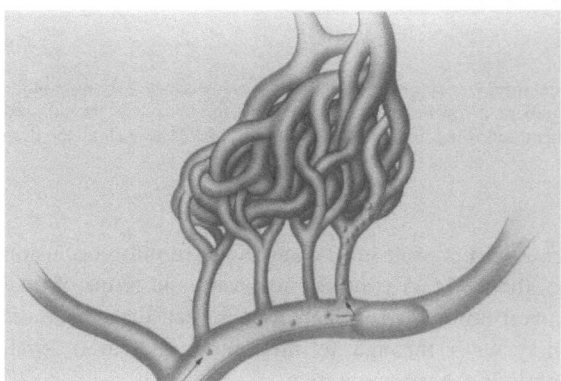

Fig. 3. Drawing demonstrating how a well-placed balloon can redirect silastic emboli at right angles into enlarged lenticulostriate arteries feeding an AVM

lishment of collateral circulation. The coils, however, were safe and rarely went astray. They appeared to have greatest usefulness in terms of occluding single penetrating arteries such as an enlarged lenticulostriate or choroidal artery feeding the deep apex of a malformation (Fig. 6). A single coil might well satisfy the desire to occlude such an artery. Coils of course were placed by small intravascular catheters.

The most sophisticated technique has been the infusion directly into the nidus via the nutrient artery of various congealing substances such as bucrylate[3,5,7,15,16]. The substance solidifies as it enters the bloodstream and is delivered at the origin of the AVM via the large nutrient arteries through a small intravascular catheter. This technique will allow access from multiple infusions of the various substances and appears to provide the

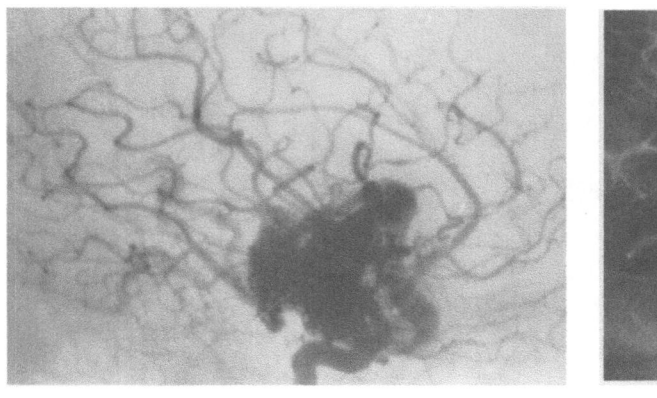 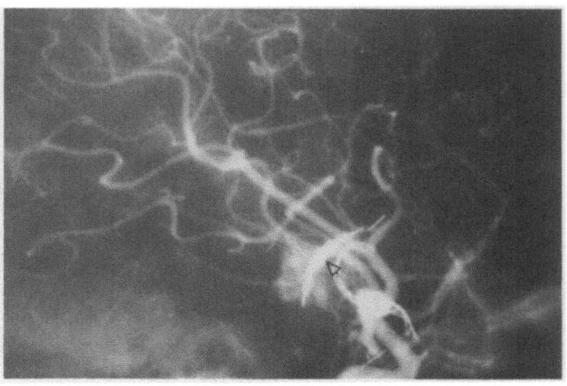

a   b

Fig. 4. (a) Lateral right carotid arteriogram showing large temporal AVM. (b) Same patient showing major occlusion of AVM by coils (arrow) and PVA

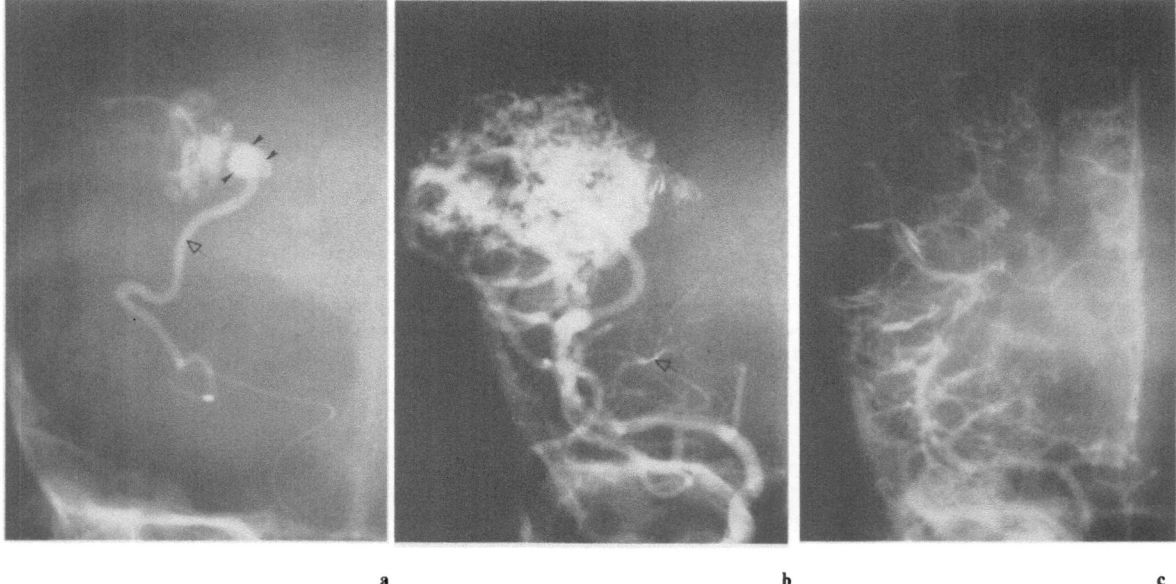

a   b   c

Fig. 5. (a) Right AP carotid arteriogram with selective catheterization of enlarged lenticulostriate artery (open arrow) feeding the apex of the AVM as well as an associated arterial aneurysm (arrowheads). (b) Same patient, arrow indicates selective occlusion by coils of the enlarged lenticulostriate artery and minimal filling of the aneurysm. (c) Same patient, following final embolization of the AVM as well as the deep lenticulostriate artery with coils and PVA

Table 1. *Summary AVM Operations*

Total operations	370
Mortality	1.0%
Excellent	92%
Good	6.0%
Poor	1.0%
Permanent/incomplete (large/inaccessible)	3.0%

most direct while most complete intra-nidus occlusion of the AVM. A concern, however, is in terms of flow arrest not being routinely used so that the substances may wash through to the venous system or even occlude the venous system.

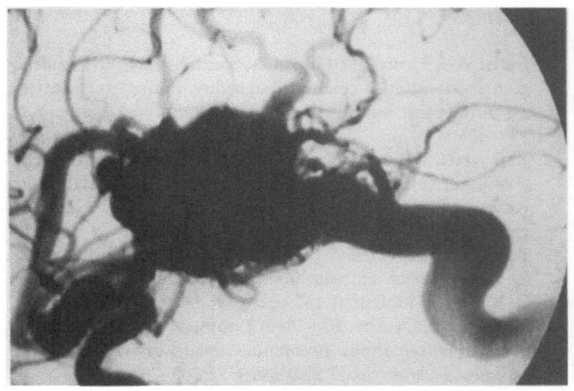
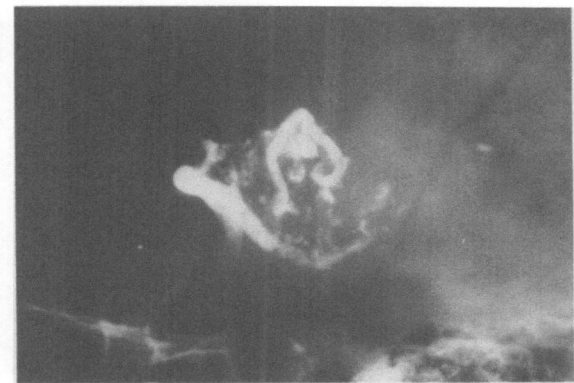

a

b

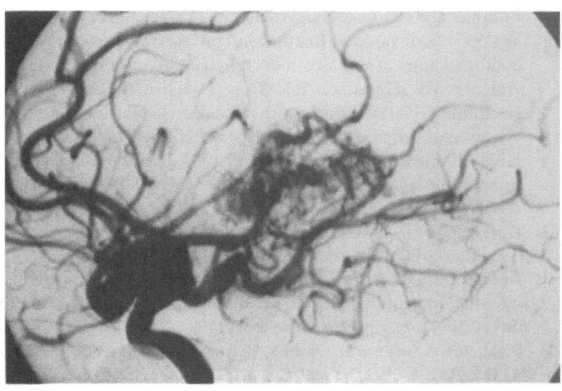

c

Fig. 6. (a) Right lateral carotid arteriogram showing a large temporal AVM with massive artery to venous shunting; (b) Bucrylate embolic material within the malformation delivered by a small intravascular catheter. (c) Same patient demonstrating the final result of embolization with bucrylate of the AVM

Table 2. AVM-Size (350 Patients)

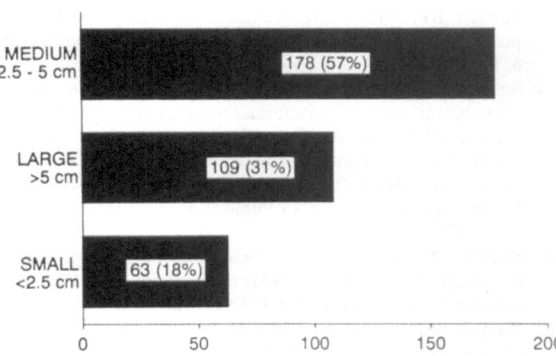

MEDIUM 2.5 - 5 cm   178 (57%)

LARGE >5 cm   109 (31%)

SMALL <2.5 cm   63 (18%)

0   50   100   150   200

Surgical Experiences

We have found that satisfactory preoperative embolization has made surgery definitively easier. Not only does the preoperative embolization help to avoid perfusion pressure breakthrough but it makes working on the malformation much easier. The interior occlusion that is created within the nidus will often prevent collaterals from reestablishing once the main nutrient artery has been occluded and this makes the access to the deeper portions of the AVM and the control of that area much easier. We generally wait four weeks after successful embolization to allow any edema, clinically silent infarction or ischemia to improve. We have not seen the overdevelopment of collateral circulation during that brief period. Working on the malformation creates a minor problem in that the substances do not allow us to collapse or compress the AVM during removal, rather they are firm, sometimes difficult to cut across, especially the coils, and cause us to use somewhat modified surgical techniques. Nevertheless, the benefit established by preoperative embolization far outweighs any difficulties that we might encounter because of the technique at the time of surgery. Accordingly, our surgical results for these large malformations

Table 3. *AVM-Outcome (370 Operations, 350 Patients)*

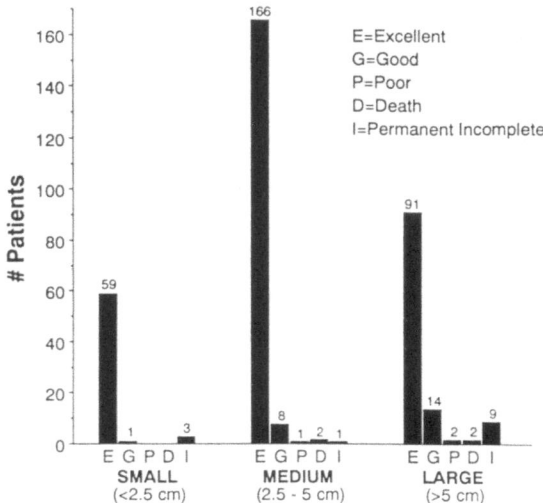

References

1. Batjer HH, Purdy PD, Giller CA, Samson DS (1989) Evidence of redistribution of cerebral blood flow during treatment for an intracranial arterioveous malformation. Neurosurgery 25: 599–605
2. Batjer HH, Devous MD, Sr, Seifert GB, Purdy PD, Bonte FJ (1989) Intracranial arteriovenous malformation: relationship between clinical factors and surgical complications. Neurosurgery 24: 75–79
3. Berenstein A, Kircheff II (1979) Catheter and material selection for transarterial embolization. I. Technical considerations. II. Materials. Radiology 132: 631–639
4. Cromwell LD, Harris BA (1980) Treatment of cerebral arteriovenous malformations. A combined neurosurgical and neuroradiological approach. J Neurosurg 52: 705–708
5. Debrun GM, Vinuela F, Fox A, Drake CG (1982) Embolization of cerebral arteriovenous malformations with bucrylate. Experience in 46 cases. J Neurosurg 56: 615–627
6. Fournier D, TerBrugge KG, Willinsky R, Lasjaunias P, Montanera W (1991) Endovascular treatment of intracerebral arteriovenous malformations: experience in 49 cases. J Neurosurg 75: 228–233
7. Halbach VV, Higashida RT, Yang P, Barnwells, Wilson CB, Hieshima GB (1988) Preoperative balloon occlusion of arteriovenous malformations. Neurosurgery 22: 303–308
8. Hilal SK, Sane P, Mawad ME, *et al* 1983 Therapeutic interventional radiologic procedures in neuroradiology. In: Abrams (ed) Abrams and angiography, 3rd Ed. Little, Brown, Boston, p 2223
9. Kerber CW (1980) Use of balloon catheters in the treatment of cranial arterial abnormalities. Stroke 11: 210–216
10. Luessenhop AJ, Rosa L (1984) Cerebral arteriovenous malformations. Indications for and results of surgery, and the role of intravascular techniques. J Neurosurg 60: 14–22
11. Pasqualin A, Scienza R, Cioffi F, Barone G, Benati A, Beltramello A, DA Pian R (1991) Treatment of cerebral arteriovenous malformation with a combination of preoperative embolization and surgery. Neurosurgery 29: 358–368
12. Spetzler RF, Martin NA, Carter P, Flom RA, Raudzens PA, Wilkinson E (1987) Surgical management of large AVMs by staged embolization and operative excision. J Neurosurg 67: 17–28
13. Spetzler RF, Wilson CB, Weinstein P, *et al* (1978) Normal perfusion pressure breakthrough theory. Clin Neurosurg 25: 651–672
14. Stein BM, Wolpert SM (1977) Surgical and embolic treatment of cerebral arteriovenous malformations. Surg Neurol 7: 359–369
15. Vinuela FV, Dion JE, Fox AJ, *et al* (1990) Interventional neuroradiology for intracranial arteriovenous malformations. In: Barrow DL (ed) Intracranial vascular malformations: Neurosurgical topics. AANS Publications Committee, Illinois, p 169–178
16. Vinuela FV, Fox AJ, Pelz D, Debrun G (1986) Angiographic follow-up of large cerebral AVMs incompletely embolized with isobutyl 2-cyanoacrylate. AJNR 7: 919–925
17. Wolpert SM, Stein BM (1975) Catheter embolization of intracranial arteriovenous malformations as an aid to surgical excision. Neuroradiology 10: 73–85
18. Wolpert SM, Stein BM (1979) Factors governing the course of emboli in the therapeutic embolization of cerebral arteriovenous malformations. Radiology 131(1): 125–131

with preoperative embolization have been excellent. In our opinion, it would have been impossible to operate with this degree of safety and excellent outcome without the technique of preoperative embolization.

Concerns and Complications

While embolization procedures carry approximately a 2% serious risk, there may be many temporary neurological deficits lasting a few weeks after successful embolization. These deficits being temporary, clear up and leave the patient with no residual. These deficits are somewhat dependent upon the various substances used and the technique of the particular interventional neuroradiologist. They are related primarily to inadvertent occlusion of normal arteries, to hemorrhage because of pressure overload in the malformation, especially if the venous outflow is occluded and in some instances to a "breaking up" of the configuration of the malformation after embolization of the nidus. This may leave patches of the malformation at the periphery. These are certainly difficult to target for radiosurgery, but not for surgery, since the whole mass even the occluded portion must be removed. This phenomenon does not present as great a problem as it would for the radiosurgery team.

Outcome

The overall outcome in the treatment of AVMs is presented in Table 1.

Correspondence: Bennett M. Stein, M.D., Neurological Surgery, College of Physicians and Surgeons of Columbia University, 710 West 168th Street, New York, NY 10032, U.S.A.

Further Experience in the Treatment of Cerebral Arteriovenous Malformations with Embolization Plus Surgery

R. Da Pian, A. Pasqualin, R. Scienza, G. Barone, S. Perini[1], and A. Benati[1]

Department of Neurosurgery and [1]Service of Neuroradiology, City Hospital, Verona, Italy

Summary

Seventy-five patients with cerebral arteriovenous malformations (AVMs) were treated with preoperative embolization followed by microsurgical resection. In 47 patients, the AVM was located in critical or eloquent areas; in 49 patients, AVM volume was over 20 cm³. Preoperatively, flow-directed embolization was performed in 11 early cases, and selective embolization with threads in the remaining 64 patients. The percentage of reduction of AVM volume averaged 37% after embolization. Eleven minor complications (transient neurological deficits, in 4 cases associated with ischemic areas and in 1 case with a small hemorrhage on CT scan) were observed after embolization; in one patient, a fatal intracranial hemorrhage occurred after embolization. When compared to flow-directed embolization, selective embolization was linked with decreased incidence of cerebral edema after surgery. When the percent reduction of AVM volume (after embolization) was 30% or more, the incidence of postoperative hematomas was significantly lower. There was no significant relation between timing of surgery after embolization and hyperemic complications or outcome. From a retrospective comparison of two groups of patients with similar AVM volumes (over 20 cm³) – those given combined treatment (n = 49) versus those treated by direct surgery only (n = 28) – intraoperative bleeding appeared to decrease in patients treated by embolization, and the incidence of postoperative edema was lower; moreover new major deficits and deaths were less frequent in patients treated by embolization. In conclusion, combined treatment with selective preoperative embolization and direct surgery may help the neurosurgeon in the treatment of large high-flow AVMs, reducing the risks connected with their surgical removal.

Keywords: Cerebral AVMs; embolization; hyperemic complications; AVM volume.

Introduction

The surgical treatment of large cerebral arteriovenous malformations (AVMs) is still subject to high risks[6,13,19,28] due to only marginally understood hemodynamic factors[2,9,15,19,22]. For these high-risk AVMs, preoperative endovascular procedures have been proposed[3,4,8,21,24] as an alternative to surgery only.

We have recently reported our preliminary experience with 49 patients treated with embolization followed by direct surgery[17]. The aim of this paper is to present our further experience with this treatment and to discuss the problems of this therapeutical approach.

Clinical Material and Methods

From 1983 to 1992, 75 patients with cerebral AVMs were treated in our Department with uni- or multi-staged embolization followed by radical removal of the lesion through a microsurgical approach. The mean age of the 75 patients submitted to preoperative embolization was 29.9 years (ranging from 14 to 58 years); there were 34 females and 41 males. Clinical history was presented by epilepsy only in 47 patients, hemorrhage only in 14 patients, epilepsy and hemorrhage in 5 patients; other clinical features (mainly headache) were present in 9 patients.

The AVM was located in 28 cases in supratentorial non-critical areas, in 4 cases in the cerebellum, and in 43 cases in supratentorial critical areas: 15 in the rolandic area, 10 in the visual cortex, 6 in the speech area, 5 in the insular cortex, and 7 in the limbic cortex. Deep feeders were observed in 35 cases, and one or more deep draining veins in 31 cases. According to the classification presented in a recent paper by our group, the draining system was moderate in 28 cases (single or multiple non-ectasic veins, with or without single ectasic vein), and extensive in 47 cases (multiple ectasic veins, or extensive hemispheric drainage)[16].

AVM size was measured through AVM volume, calculated as the product of the 3 AVM diameters (height, width, and length) multiplied by 0.52, according to the calculation recently presented by our group[16].

Embolization Procedures

As regards preoperative embolization, 2 modalities were adopted: a) free-flow embolization (in early cases), and b) selective embolization (in the majority of patients). In *free-flow embolization*, the embolic material was silastic sponge (Dow Corning, Midland, Michigan, USA), using the technique described by Mullan et al.[14]. Owing to the disadvantages of free-flow embolization (expecially lack of selectivity), this technique was abandoned in favour of selective embolization. For *selective embolization*, we have used flow-depen-

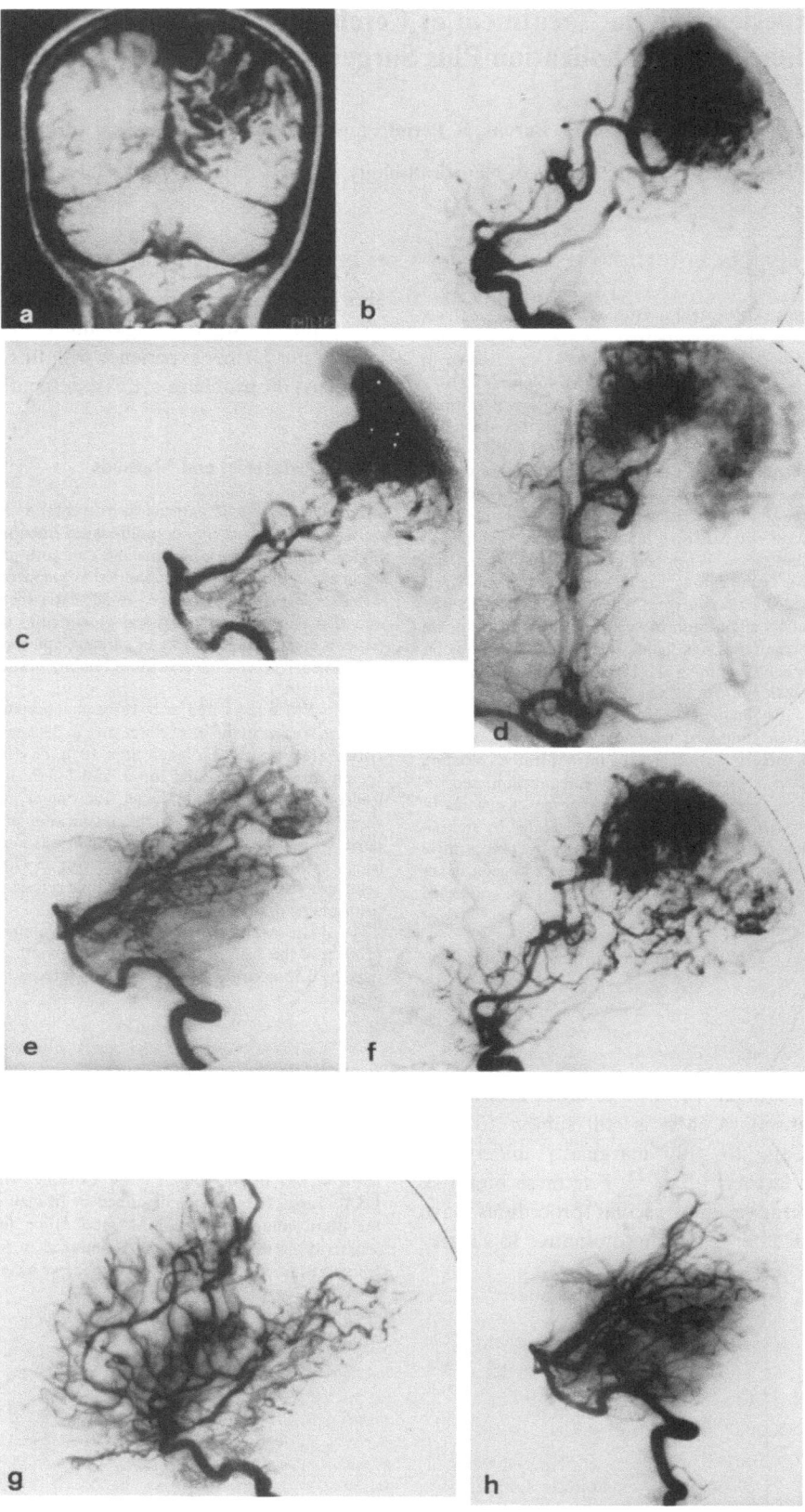

dent microcatheteres, the wing-microcatheter (Ingenor, Paris) or the Tracker flow-independent system (Target Therapeutics, Los Angeles). Most procedures were performed with our wing microcatheter[4]. As embolic agents, we primarily used polyfilament polylene 3–0 threads: at the beginning of the procedure, microemboli cut to a length of 1.5 −2 mm were discharged into the artery; when blood flow in the feeder was reduced by more than half, 2–3 cm threads were injected until complete closure of the feeder. Free-flow embolization was carried out in 11 patients (a total of 30 procedures), selective embolization in 60 patients (a total of 92 procedures), and both flow-directed and selective embolization in 4 patients (a total of 12 procedures). Only one procedure was performed in 28 patients (2 flow-directed and 26 selective), two procedures in 12 patients (3 flow-directed, 7 selective, and 2 combined), three procedures in 4 patients (2 flow-directed and 2 selective), and more than three procedures in 5 patients (3 flow-directed, and 2 combined).

Preoperative examination was negative in 57 patients; mild neurological deficits were present in 17 patients (hemianopia in 11, mild speech disturbances in 3, dysmetria in 3); one patient was in coma. Surgery was performed within 10 days from the last embolization in 19 patients, between 11 and 20 days in 15 patients, between 21 and 30 days in 11 patients, between 31 and 60 days in 12 patients and after 2 months in 18 patients (with slightly longer intervals in patients submitted to free-flow embolization). All patients underwent angiographically proven radical removal of the AVM through a microsurgical approach (Fig. 1). Deep controlled hypotension (around 60 mmHg of systolic blood pressure) induced by sodium nitroprusside – never exceeding the total dose of 10 μg/kg/min – was performed during surgery in 10 cases.

The efficacy of this combined treatment was evaluated by the rate of intraoperative and postoperative hyperemic complications, and by the morbidity and mortality rates. Moreover a clinical comparison was undertaken between two groups of patients with AVM volumes over 20 cm[3] admitted between 1977 and 1992: those treated by embolization before surgery (49 cases) and those who underwent only direct surgery (28 cases); based on a recent paper by our group[16], 20 cm[3] has been considered as the critical size for an AVM, with a significantly increased risk of hyperemic complications and with a significantly worse clinical outcome over this volume.

The chi-square test was used for statistical significance. Fisher's exact test was used when the sample size was too small for the chi-square test.

Results

Embolization

Angiographic obliteration of the AVM was never reached in this series of patients; the actual angiographical decrease in size ranged from 5% to 70% reduction of the previous volume, with an average reduction of 37% (Table 1). These changes were variably associated with dynamic changes, including: a) reduced density of the AVM; b) slowing of the circulation time; c) reduction

Table 1. *Percent Reduction in Volume After Embolization According to Initial AVM Volume*

Volume (cm³)	Average	Volume reduction: minimum	maximum
0–10 (6 cases)	− 27%	− 10%	− 50%
11–20 (21 cases)	− 40%	− 10%	− 70%
21–30 (23 cases)	− 41%	− 5%	− 70%
31–50 (20 cases)	− 30%	− 5%	− 55%
>50 (5 cases)	− 41%	− 5%	− 65%

in size of the feeding arteries; d) decreased caliber of the draining veins. Clear development of new collateral circulation adjacent to the AVM was observed in 11 patients; tiny networks of collateral vessels – mainly deep – were occasionally observed in a few other patients.

Immediately after embolization, 7 patients developed transient deficits (all after selective procedures): the CT scan was normal in 6 patients, and showed a small hemorrhage in 1 patient. Longer lasting deficits were observed in 4 patients (3 after selective procedures and 1 after free-flow embolization): all of these patients showed moderate ischemic areas on CT scan later on. Uncal herniation occurred in one patient treated with selective embolization and developing a large intracerebral hematoma a few hours after the procedure.

Complications of Surgery

During surgery, a severe blood loss (over 2000 ml) occurred in 13 patients, while paraventricular bleeding – i.e. long-lasting hemorrhages from small fragile vessels in the paraependymal area – occurred in 29 patients (Table 2). Postoperatively an intracerebral hematoma without ventricular shift was observed in 10 cases, cerebral edema with midline shift in 7 cases, and intracerebral hematoma with midline shift in 14 cases (Table 2); 7 patients underwent a second operation for evacuation of a large postoperative hematoma. Less

Fig. 1. (a) Coronal MRI of a 26 year-old woman with a very large left posterior parietal AVM (62 cm³); (b) ectatic feeders from lt. middle cerebral (MCA), and (c) from lt. posterior cerebral (PCA) arteries; (d) supply also from lt. anterior cerebral artery (ACA) injected from rt. internal carotid; (e) lt. vertebral angiography after embolization of PCA; (f) lt. carotid angiography after embolization of MCA; (g, h) postop. angiography. After surgery, the patient developed a complete rt. visual field deficit and transient dysphasia; 6 months later she still presented rt. hemianopia, without other disturbances

Table 2. *Intraoperative and Postoperative Complications According to AVM Volume (75 Patients)*

Volume (cm³)	Severe blood loss	Parav. bleeding	Postoperative hematoma: small	w/shift	Postop. edema
0–19 (26 c)	–	7 (27%)	3 (11%)	1 (4%)	1 (4%)
≥ 20 (49 c)	13 (36%)	22 (61%)	7 (14%)	13 (26%)	6 (12%)
Significance	p = 0.002	N.S.	N.S.	p = 0.01	N.S.
Total (75 c)	13 (17%)	29 (39%)	10 (20%)	14 (28%)	7 (9%)

frequently observed complications were distal ischemia (3 cases), scalp infection (2 cases), hydrocephalus (2 cases), brain abscess (1 case), cerebral venous thrombosis (1 case) and pneumonia (1 case).

When relating AVM volume with complications (Table 2), a severe blood loss was significantly more common with volumes over 20 cm³; large postoperative hematomas occurred rarely under 20 cm³, while they were observed in 26% of patients with an AVM volume over 20 cm³ (p = 0.01).

As regards type of preoperative embolization – considering only patients with AVMs over 20 cm³ – severe blood loss and expecially paraventricular bleeding occurred with similar incidence in patients submitted to selective versus flow-directed embolization (28% and 48% respectively after selective embolization, versus 27% and 45% respectively after flow-directed embolization). Postoperative cerebral edema was less frequent after selective embolization (8% versus 27%), while the incidence of a large hematoma was similar in

Table 3. *Intraoperative and Postoperative Complications According to Percent Reduction in Volume After Embolization (Only AVMs With Volume ≥ 20 cm³)*

Percent reduction	Severe blood loss	Parav. bleeding	Postoperative hematoma: small	w/shift	Postop. edema
0–29% (15 c)	5 (33%)	5 (43%)	1 (7%)	7 (47%)	—
30–49% (21 c)	6 (28%)	11 (52%)	4 (19%)	3 (14%)	4 (19%)
> 50% (13 c)	2 (15%)	6 (46%)	2 (15%)	3 (23%)	2 (15%)
Significance (0–29% vs ≥ 30%)	N.S.	N.S.	N.S.	p = 0.04	N.S.

Table 4. *Intraoperative and Postoperative Complications According to Interval From Last Embolization to Surgery (Only AVMs With Volume ≥ 20 cm³)*

Interval	Severe blood loss	Parav. bleeding	Postoperative hematoma: small	w/shift	Postop. edema
0–10 days (15 c)	3 (20%)	7 (47%)	2 (13%)	3 (20%)	2 (13%)
11–30 days (14 c)	6 (43%)	8 (57%)	2 (14%)	3 (43%)	2 (14%)
Over 30 days (20c)	4 (20%)	7 (35%)	3 (15%)	4 (20%)	2 (10%)
Significance (0–10 vs > 10)	N.S.	N.S.	N.S.	N.S.	N.S.

both groups (28% after flow-directed and 27% after selective embolization).

The observed relation between percent reduction of AVM volume (after embolization) and hyperemic complications is presented in Table 3: severe blood loss was progressively less frequent for increasing volume reductions, and large postop. hematomas were significantly less frequent (p = 0.04) when volume reduction was 30% or higher. A possible relation between timing of preoperative embolization and complications is evaluated in Table 4: severe blood loss was possibly more common in patients operated on between 11 and 30 days from the last embolization, while paraventricular bleeding was not timing-related; moreover, while postoperative cerebral edema did not show any relation with timing of embolization, large postop. hematomas were more frequent for patients operated on between 11 and 30 days from last embolization.

Clinical Outcome

27 patients exhibited transient postoperative deficits (disappearing before discharge in 9 cases and within 6 months from surgery in 18 cases). A complete recovery was observed in 41 cases (55%), a moderate disability in 24 cases (pre-existing to surgery in 9 cases), and a severe disability in 6 cases. 4 patients died: two from postoperative hematomas with midline shift, one from a post-embolization hematoma with midline shift, and one from a large brain abscess.

A relation between AVM volume and morbidity is presented in Table 5. In this and in the following tables, new permanent postoperative deficits were considered minor when causing a moderate disability, and major when causing a severe disability according to the Glasgow Outcome Scale[11] (none of our patients survived in a vegetative state). Transient deficits were unrelated to volume, while new permanent deficits were more frequent over 20 cm^3 (Table 5).

As regards type of preoperative embolization – considering only patients with AVM volume over 20 cm^3 - transient deficits were unrelated to type of embolization (34% after selective and 36% after flow-directed embolization), new minor deficits were observed in 18% of cases after flow-directed and in 26% of cases after selective embolization, new major deficits were observed in 9% of cases after flow directed and in 11% of cases after selective embolization; there was one death after selective embolization, and two deaths after flow-directed embolization.

Table 5. *Morbidity and Mortality According to AVM Volume (75 Patients)*

Volume (cm^3)	Transient deficit	New permanent deficit minor	major	Death
0–19 (26 cases)	10 (38%)	4 (15%)	1 (4%)	1 (4%)
≥ 20 (49 cases)	17 (35%)	11 (22%)	5 (10%)	3 (6%)
Significance	N.S.	N.S.		N.S.

Table. 6. *Morbidity and Mortality According to Percent Reduction in Volume After Embolization (Only AVMs With Volume ≥ 20cm^3)*

Percent reduction	Transient deficit	New permanent deficit minor	major	Death
0–29% (15 cases)	3 (20%)	2 (13%)	2 (13%)	1 (7%)
30–49% (21 cases)	9 (43%)	8 (38%)	1 (5%)	2 (9%)
≥ 50% (13 cases)	5 (38%)	1 (8%)	2 (15%)	–
Significance (0–29%) vs. ≥ 30%	N.S.	N.S.		N.S.

Table 7. *Morbidity and Mortality According to Interval from Last Embolization to Surgery (Only AVMs with Volume ≥ 20 cm^3)*

	Transient deficit	New permanent deficit minor	major	Death
0–10 days (15 cases)	4 (27%)	4 (27%)	2 (13%)	—
11–30 days (14 cases)	5 (36%)	2 (14%)	3 (21%)	2 (14%)
over 30 days (20 cases)	8 (40%)	5 (25%)	—	1 (5%)
Significance (0–10 vs. >10)	N.S.	N.S.		N.S.

The observed relation between percent reduction of AVM volume after embolization and clinical outcome is presented in Table 6: while transient deficits were not related to percent reduction of AVM volume, new permanent deficits were probably less common when volume reduction was 50% or higher; moreover, no death was observed for such volume reduction.

A possible relation between timing of preoperative embolization and clinical outcome is evaluated in Table 7: while transient deficits were probably less common in patients with shorter timing, permanent morbidity and mortality showed no relation with timing of preoperative embolization.

Clinical Comparison

When comparing two groups of patients – both with AVM volumes over 20 cm^3 – one submitted to preoperative embolization and the other to direct surgery – some anatomical risk factors were evaluated: as shown by Table 8, there was no significant difference in the incidence of these factors between the opposite groups. In Table 9, the rate of intraop. and postop. hyperemic complications was compared in the opposite groups: intraop. complications occurred less frequently in embolized patients, as well as postoperative edema. As for epilepsy, it was less common postoperatively after combined treatment (26% vs. 46%). In Table 10, clinical outcome was compared in the opposite groups: while transient deficits were more common in the embolized group, new major deficits and death were less frequently observed.

Table 10. *Combined Treatment Versus Surgery Only (AVM Volume ≥ 20 cm^3): Morbidity and Mortality*

	Transient deficit	New permanent deficit minor	major	Death
Combined treatment (49 cases)	17 (35%)	11 (22%)	5 (10%)	3 (6%)
Surgery only (28 cases)	7 (25%)	4 (14%)	5 (18%)	4 (14%)
Significance	N.S.	└─── N.S. ───┘		N.S.

Discussion

The rationale for submitting patients with cerebral AVMs to staged occlusion is mainly the risk of severe hyperemic complications following one-stage occlusion of large high-flow AVMs[6,13,19,28]; using a staged AVM occlusion, it is hoped that a progressive change in cerebral hemodynamics permits gradual redistribution of blood flow, thus avoiding the so-called normal perfusion pressure breakthrough (NPPB), first described by Spetzler *et al.* in 1978[22,28]. In our ex-

Table 8. *Combined Treatment Versus Surgery Only: Incidence of Risks Factors*

	Volume ≥ 30 cm^3	Eloquence	Deep feeders	Deep drainage	Drainage 3–4
Combined treatment (49 cases)	28 (57%)	34 (69%)	26 (53%)	19 (39%)	36 (73%)
Surgery only (28 cases)	12 (43%)	16 (57%)	19 (68%)	13 (46%)	18 (64%)
Significance	N.S.	N.S.	N.S.	N.S.	N.S.

Table 9. *Combined Treatment Versus Surgery Only (AVM Volume ≥ 20 cm^3): Intraoperative and Postoperative Complications*

	Severe blood loss	Parav. bleeding	Postoperative hematoma: small	w/shift	Postop. edema
Combined treatment (49 c)	13 (26%)	22 (45%)	7 (14%)	13 (26%)	5 (10%)
Surgery only (28 c)	11 (37%)	16 (57%)	2 (7%)	7 (25%)	7 (25%)
Significance	N.S.	N.S.	N.S.	N.S.	N.S.

perience hyperemic complications have shown a close relationship to AVM volumes over 20 cm[3], to the presence of deep feeders, to a large extension of venous drainage, and to high flow velocities (mean over 120 cm/sec) on transcranial Doppler sonography[16].

Although preoperative embolization is the most widespread modality of staged AVM occlusion, other methods have been suggested in order to avoid (or to reduce) hyperemic complications: a) preliminary surgical clipping or ligation of some feeders prior to surgery[1,13,19,28]; b) surgical resection in various stages[19,26,29]; c) preoperative selective balloon occlusion of AVM feeders[8]; d) intraoperative embolization prior to surgery[5,7,12,21,27]. As for a), b) and c) these methods have not gained wide-spread use, possibly for various drawbacks[23]; as for intraoperative embolization, it has been progressively replaced by endovascular navigation and superselective embolization[4,5,18,20].

Although preoperative embolization is not free from risks[5,14,20,27], selective embolization with small particles, mixtures, threads or coils[3,4,10,25] seems at present the best method, with a low rate of complications and still good reductions in size.

As regards the efficacy of preoperative embolization, we have observed only a trend towards reduction of hyperemic complications in embolized patients; it should be added that the number of comparable patients is still small, and many variables can influence the validity of embolization, such as type of embolization, timing of embolization, and particularly percent reduction of AVM volume after embolization. It is noteworthy that with preoperative embolization severe disability and mortality appear already decreased in our limited series of cases.

Apart from avoidance or reduction of hyperemic complications, another – although less important – reason for performing staged occlusion of an AVM is facilitation of the surgical procedure. At this regard, two points can be considered: a) decrease of bleeding, and b) facilitation of AVM dissection. Decrease of bleeding seems to occur in a large number of embolized AVMs, although not in all, according to our and other's experience[18,21]; amount of blood loss seems to be strictly related to presence or absence of deep feeders and to the degree of collateral circulation formed after embolization. In our clinical comparison a severe blood loss was less frequent after preoperative embolization (26% versus 39%) and the incidence of paraventricular bleeding was also decreased (45% versus 57%). Facilitation of dissection seems to be achieved only by

superselective embolization with coils[10], threads[4] or mixtures[25]; on the opposite, bucrylate embolization may create problems with surgical dissection – as stated by some authors[1,18,21] – and free-flow embolization often creates a diffuse lesion with poorly defined edges.

A major problem in preoperative embolization remains the choice of timing. If the operation is performed a few days after embolization, the danger of hyperemia during and after surgery cannot be excluded[24]; on the contrary, if the interval between embolization and surgery is long, development of collateral circulation[12,21,24] may cause major surgical problems. Recently, Stein has stated that the best timing of surgery is probably from one to two weeks after embolization[23], although our results indicate a slightly different timing.

For the future, we believe that selection of patients for preoperative embolization must be based not only on risk factors such as AVM volume, presence of deep feeders, extension of draining system and other angiographical criteria[16,21,28], but also on accurate hemodynamic testing with TCD and CBF methods[3,9,15,21]. Improvements in the technique of embolization are also needed, particularly to exclude deep feeders, to reach a higher percent of volume reduction with a still acceptable technique-related morbidity, and to avoid the development of new collateral circulation.

References

1. Andrews BT, Wilson CB (1987) Staged treatment of arteriovenous malformations of the brain. Neurosurgery 21: 314–323
2. Batjer HH, Devous MD, Meyer YJ, Purdy PD, Samson DS (1988) Cerebrovascular hemodynamics in arteriovenous malformation complicated by normal perfusion pressure breakthrough. Neurosurgery 22: 503–509
3. Batjer HH, Purdy PD, Giller CA, Samson DS (1988) Evidence of redistribution of cerebral blood flow during treatment for an intracranial arteriovenous malformation. Neurosurgery 25: 599–605
4. Benati A, Beltramello A, Colombari R, Maschio A, Perini S, Da Pian R, Pasqualin A, Scienza R, Rosta L, Piovan E, Scarpa A, Zamboni G (1989) Preoperative embolization of arteriovenous malformations with polylene threads: techniques with wing microcatheter and pathologic results. AJNR 10: 579–586
5. Debrun G, Vinuela F, Fox A, Drake CG (1982) Embolization of cerebral arteriovenous malformations with bucrylate. Experience in 46 cases. J Neurosurg 56: 615–627
6. Drake CG (1979) Cerebral arteriovenous malformations: considerations for and experience with surgical treatment in 166 cases. Clin Neurosurg 26: 145–208
7. Girvin JP, Fox AJ, Vinuela FV, Drake CG (1984) Intraoperative embolization of cerebral arteriovenous malformations in the awake patient. Clin Neurosurg 31: 188–247
8. Halbach VV, Higashida RT, Yang P, Barnwell S, Wilson CB,

Hieshima GB (1988) Preoperative balloon occlusion of arteriovenous malformations. Neurosurgery 22: 301–308

9. Hassler W (1986) Hemodynamic aspects of cerebral angiomas. Acta Neurochir (Wien) [Suppl] 37: 1–136

10. Hilal SK (1980) Treatment of intracranial aneurysms and arteriovenous malformations with preshaped thrombogenic coils. AJNR 11: 226

11. Jennett B, Bond M (1975) Assessment of outcome after severe brain damage. A practical scale. Lancet i: 480–484

12. Luessenhop AJ, Presper JH (1975) Surgical embolization of cerebral arteriovenous malformations through internal carotid and vertebral arteries. Long term results. J Neurosurg 42: 443–451

13. Mullan S, Brown FD, Patronas NJ (1979) Hyperemic and ischemic problems of surgical treatment of arteriovenous malformations. J Neurosurg 51: 757–764

14. Mullan S, Kawanaga H, Patronas NJ (1979) Microvascular embolization of cerebral arteriovenous malformations. A technical variation. J Neurosurg 51: 621–627

15. Okabe T, Meyer JS, Okayasu H, Harper R, Rose J, Grossman RG, Centeno R, Tachibana H, Lee YY (1983) Xenon-enhanced CT-CBF measurements in cerebral AVM's before and after excision. Contribution to pathogenesis and treatment. J Neurosurg 59: 21–31

16. Pasqualin A, Barone G, Cioffi F, Rosta L, Scienza R, Da Pian R (1991) The relevance of anatomic and hemodynamic factors to a classification of cerebral arterio-venous malformations. Neurosurgery 28: 370–379

17. Pasqualin A, Scienza R, Cioffi F, Barone G, Benati A, Beltramello A, Da Pian R (1991) Treatment of cerebral arteriovenous malformations with a combination of preoperative embolization and surgery. Neurosurgery 29: 358–368

18. Pelz DM, Fox AJ, Vinuela F, Drake CG, Ferguson GG (1988) Preoperative embolization of brain AVMs with isobutyl-2 cyanoacrylate. AJNR 9: 757–764

19. Pertuiset B, Ancri D, Sichez JP, Chauvin M, Guilly E, Metzger J, Gardeur D, Basset JY (1983) Radical surgery in cerebral AVM – Tactical procedures based upon hemodynamic factors. In: Krayenbuhl H (ed) Advances and technical standards in neurosurgery, Vol 10. Springer, Wien New York, pp 81–143

20. Rufenacht D, Merland JJ (1986) A new and original microcatheter system for hyperselective catheterization and endovascular treatment without risk of arterial rupture. J Neuroradiol 13: 44–54

21. Spetzler RF, Martin NA, Carter LP, Flom RA, Raudzens PA, Wilkinson E (1987) Surgical management of large AVM's by staged embolization and operative excision. J Neurosurg 67: 17–28

22. Spetzler RF, Wilson CB, Weinstein B, Mehdorn M, Townsend J, Telles D (1978) Normal perfusion pressure breakthrough theory. Clin Neurosurg 25: 651–672

23. Stein BM (1987) Comment on Andrews BT, Wilson CB: Staged treatment of arteriovenous malformations of the brain. Neurosurgery 21: 323

24. Stein BM, Wolpert SM (1977) Surgical and embolic treatment of cerebral arteriovenous malformations. Surg Neurol 7: 359–369

25. Taki W, Yonekawa Y, Iwata H, Uno A, Yamashita K, Amemiya H (1990) A new liquid material for embolization of arteriovenous malformations. AINR 11: 163–168

26. U HS (1985) Microsurgical excision of paraventricular arteriovenous malformations. Neurosurgery 16: 293–303

27. Vinuela F, Debrun GM, Fox AJ, Girvin JP, Peerless SJ (1983) Dominant hemisphere arteriovenous malformations: therapeutic embolization with isobutyl 2-cyanoacrylate. Am J Neuroradiol 4: 959–966

28. Wilson CB, U HS, Domingue J (1979) Microsurgical treatment of intracranial vascular malformations. J Neurosurg 51: 446–454

29. Yamada S, Brauer FS, Knierim DS (1990) Direct approach to arteriovenous malformations in functional areas of the cerebral hemisphere. J Neurosurg 72: 418–425

Correspondence: R. Da Pian, M.D., Department of Neurosurgery, City Hospital, I-37126 Verona, Italy.

The Team Approach to Combined Embolization and Resection of Arteriovenous Malformations

P.D. Purdy, H.H. Batjer, T. Kopitnik, and **D. Samson**

University of Texas Southwestern Medical Center at Dallas, Dallas, Texas, U.S.A.

Summary

In our series of patients undergoing preoperative embolization and subsequent resection of cerebral arteriovenous malformation (AVM), we have observed that close coordination between the neurosurgical and endovascular team members results in adaptation of approaches in both. The series consists of 200 embolizations in 139 patients with intracerebral AVMs. Of these, 97 underwent 144 procedures utilizing intracranial catheterization from a transfemoral approach. We reviewed this experience with regard to how the surgical approach is altered, the timing of surgery relative to the embolization, and the physical effect of embolic materials on the achievement of surgical resection.

Through preoperative conference regarding the surgical plan, vessels may be selected for embolization which maximize the benefit with the goal of embolizing vessels most inaccessible early during surgery. Following the embolization, the surgical approach may be altered on the basis of the result. Selection of embolic materials is affected by the planned ultimate treatment of the malformation. Specifically, acrylic glues may be better suited for primary embolic therapy and polyvinyl alcohol (PVA), due to improved compressibility and ease of sectioning when intravascular, may be better suited for preoperative therapy.

Therapy for AVMs is a multidisciplinary effort. Each specialty brings its own perspective and contribution to therapy, and coordination among members of a therapeutic team brings greater benefit to the patient than if components acted separately.

Keywords: Arteriovenous malformation; embolization.

Introduction

The preoperative embolization of AVMs has become the standard of surgical care in many if not most medium- or large-sized AVMs[1-5,8,10-12]. Studies comparing surgery with and without embolization do not exist in a controlled fashion, because the introduction of preoperative devascularization at various centers brought advantages so obvious that subsequent randomization was deemed inappropriate. These advantages included diminished blood loss and shorter surgical times. If conducted with the operative approach in mind, the interventional neuroradiologist may enhance the degree to which his efforts assist in the ultimate outcome. We present a discussion of certain principles that have evolved in our efforts during the past 12 years.

Material and Methods

Our series of AVMs embolized prior to surgery comprises 200 procedures in 139 patients. An additional 6 patients underwent embolization eleswhere and were subsequently operated on at our institution. Embolization via surgical exposure of feeding vessels and injection of isobutyl-cyanoacrylate (IBCA) was conducted in 42 procedures in 31 patients (Group 1). Thirteen patients underwent 14 procedures utilizing injection of particles of PVA into the internal carotid artery via an angiographic catheter (Group 2). The remaining 95 patients underwent 139 intracerebral catheterization procedures via a transfemoral approach. Embolic materials used alone or in combination during these procedures included PVA, platinum microcoils, 33% ethanol solution with and without microfibrillar collagen (Avitene) particles, and silk suture material. Approximately 95% of patients undergoing embolization subsequently underwent surgical resection. Materials and combinations thereof used during these procedures are summarized in Table 1.

The introduction of amytal testing in our practice has proven to be of statistically significant assistance in reduction of complication rates during embolization[7]. Amytal testing was performed in 76 procedures in 58 patients in this series following catheterization of their intracranial vessel but prior to embolization.

Based on the above experience, certain principles have emerged that guide embolic therapy. These are based, to some degree, on observations of principles of surgical therapy. To another degree, they are based on inherent principles of radiologic intervention. Though this series has been reported, in parts, in multiple publication[6,7,8,10], we present here a discussion of the principles of vascular selection, timing of surgery following embolization, and choice of embolic materials that have emerged as this experience was accumulated.

Results

In general, surgical resection of an AVM begins on the brain's surface and moves inward. Catheterization of a vessel feeding an AVM, on the other hand, begins

Table 1. *Embolic Materials Used (n = 200 Procedures)*

PVA	46
PVC + C	74
PVA + C + S	5
PVA + C + E	18
C	2
PVA + B	1
B	4
PVA + E	3
C + E	2
NR	3
IBCA	42

PVA polyvinyl alcohol; *C* platinum microcoils; *S* silk suture material; *E* 33% ethanol, with or without microfibrillar collagen added; *B* detachable balloons; *NR* not recorded, *IBCA* isobutyl cyanoacrylate. Data recorded per procedure, as opposed to per patient.

centrally and moves peripherally. These broad statements are, obviously, gross generalizations. However, they illustrate that fact that the part of the brain that is approached late during an AVM resection and is thus a source of bleeding throughout an operation is also the part of the brain which is oftern easiest to reach from an endovascular approach. For instance, an AVM in the occipital lobe fed by a large posterior cerebral artery might be difficult to resect de novo because the venous drainage cannot be retracted to clip the arterial feeders due to potential rupture. Therefore, the resection would involve tedious dissection of virgin arterial feeders if the malformation were not embolized. However, the endovascular approach allows relatively straightforward catheterization of posterior cerebral artery feeders with devascularization of the malformation. If there are middle cerebral artery collateral feeders extending around the occipital pole, these are very difficult to approach safely using endovascular techniques because of the long, tortuous intracranial course those vessels take to circumvent the occipital pole. However, these are the first vessels that are encountered during a surgical approach. Therefore, they are most easily dealt with at surgery. Thus, with preoperative embolization, the neurosurgeon now encounters the dominant residual feeders at the beginning of the resection and can largely devascularize the remaining nidus early in the operation. Discussion of the anticipated surgical plan may alter the embolic plan insofar as vessels may be prioritized in order to maximize the assistance to the surgeon during the resection.

A secondary advantage of devascularization preoperatively rests with the surgical margin that is achieved. In a setting of significant ongoing hemorrhage, the margins of the AVM are less distinct and must be approached more aggressively. Therefore, there is greater hazard in that setting of inclusion of normal brain tissue in the operative field. When the surgical bed is dry, margins are more distinct and easier to achieve conservatively.

Preoperative devascularization may also permit the brain surrounding the AVM to achieve a more normal physiologic state prior to resection. Though this is believed to offer some protection against postoperative complications such as normal perfusion pressure breakthrough bleeding, controlled series studying this are lacking. Though the ability of the surrounding brain to recover normal vascular responsiveness has been a rationale for delay following embolization prior to resection, the development of new collateral feeders will increase with increasing delays. Thus, there are arguments both for and against delay following embolization. In light of the conflicting arguments, timing decisions are often made to enhance convenience to the patient. However, findings of significant vascular steal from surrounding brain by an AVM on studies of cerebral blood flow may mitigate more strongly in favor of aggressive embolization and longer delay. In the absence of significant steal, we operate early.

Using the above principles, the neurosurgeon and interventional neuroradiologist can plan a surgical approach which offers the patient the best opportunity for limited morbidity from therapy. However, the tailoring of the embolic approach requires some knowledge of the anticipated surgical approach. Thus, if the surgeon would prefer to approach from the anterior aspect of the malformation, it may be most advantageous to embolize the posterior aspect of the malformation so that it will not be a source of ongoing hemorrhage throughout the resection. Conversely, if the embolizaton is easiest and safest from one approach, the operation may be altered such that the nonembolized vessels are surgically approached early during the procedure. Each malformation must be approached as an individual entity, and the treatment must be tailored to specific vascular anatomy. This is best achieved in a setting where the neurosurgeon and interventional neuroradiologist work closely together.

Another feature of preoperative devascularization is the introduction of foreign material into the blood vessel for purposes of occlusion. Though the statement is simplistic, if the material selected impedes the ability to subsequently conduct the resection, consideration of other materials should be made. Specifically, resection of a malformation involves not only dissection around the margins of the AVM, but also retraction of the malformation in order to expose the additional margins during the resection. If the embolic material creates too much rigidity within the malformation, this can cause the retraction to be more difficult and the malformation to be less mobile. This creates a circumstance in which the malformation acts more like a solid mass than like a pliable cluster of blood vessels. Thus, the retraction in essence pushes the malformation into adjacent brain tissue instead of compressing it. The effects of this are unknown, but the resection is made more difficult. This was our experience with IBCA, though we cannot comment on modified n-butyl-cyanoacrylate now used in some centers. This is also the effect created by platinum microcoils. However, if the nidus of coils is limited in size by the concurrent use of PVA sponge material, the addition of coils to provide proximal vascular occlusion assists in the overall angiographic effect and limitation of complications[6].

One advantage of liquid embolic agents is their ability to penetrate into the nidus of a malformation. By nidus obliteration, the embolization seems more thoroughly to limit intraoperative hemorrhage and collateral vascular development. We have observed small particles of PVA to achieve nidus embolization as well. Thus, selection of embolic materials can impact the degree to which nidus obliteration is achieved. Our approach currently is to begin with small particles (300–500 microns). If obliteration is ongoing, we continue with small particles. However, if after smaller particles are used for several milliliters no reduction in malformation is evident, larger particles are introduced (1–1.5 mm are the maximum commercially available size which can be routinely injected through a Tracker

Table 2. *Complications*

Material	No. of Procedures	Complications (%)
PVA + Coils (with or without silk)	78	5(6)
Ethanol (with or without PVA or coils)	23	4(17)

One procedure in PVA + coils group did not reflect complication result. Thus, n = 78 instead of 79. Statistical comparison between groups reveals p = 0.222 (Fisher's Exact Test). Complications included stroke, hemorrhage, or death and were scored as 0 or 1.

18 catheter). These achieve reduction in almost all malformations. Once definite reduction is observed, we will frequently move to smaller particles again to attempt to achieve occlusion of the nidus with the smallest possible particles. On occasion, fistulous flow carries even larger particles without devascularization. Ethanol will sometimes reduce the fistula and permit the particles to achieve obliteration. This may also be a setting particularly suited to glue. Though not statistically significant, the use of ethanol appears to have a higher complication rate than the use of PVA + coils (Table 2)[9].

Sometimes, catheterization at a fistula site is necessary with introduction of coils to occlude the fistula. Once the fistula is occluded, particles can again be used to embolize the surrounding nidus. We have found that angiographic effects are ultimately greater when the feeding vessel is occluded at the end of the embolization. This is generally done in our practice with the introduction of platinum microcoils in the feeding vessel.

Though we use amytal testing in nearly every embolization now, clinical trade-offs must sometimes be made. For instance, in a malformation near motor cortex, there have been occasions in which amytal testing produced a mild motor deficit but in which embolization was conducted anyway due to the anticipated surgical benefit of preoperative devascularization. In general, when such trade-offs are made, this is done in consultation between the neurosurgeon and neuroradiologist. This possibility is also discussed with patients prior to embolization. Likewise, in occipital lesions where introduction of a visual field cut is anticipated at least transiently during the postoperative state, the advantages achieved with embolization may justify increased risk of such a deficit from the embolization. Thus, the therapeutic team concept is important in understanding therapeutic goals and preventing misunderstandings and conflicts between the interventional neuroradiologist and neurosurgeon.

Discussion

As is true with any therapeutic circumstance, decisions regarding preoperative embolization of AVMs require trade-offs. On the negative side, additional procedures and risk are incurred, with associated additional expense. Considerations in decision-making include technical factors, neurologic risk without embolization, and combined risk of therapy. The neurologic risk of embolization must be factored into the overall therapeutic risk and is more acceptable in a setting where the surgical risk of neurologic deficit is also high. Consultation between the interventionist and surgeon prior to embolization and prior to surgery can maximize the benefit to surgery of embolization and optimize the surgical approach.

Acknowledgement

The authors thanks Ms. Leslie Mihal for her assistance in the preparation of this manuscript.

References

1. Berenstein AB, Krall R, Choi IS (1989) Embolization with n-butyl cyanoacrylate in the management of CNS vascular lesions. AJNR 10: 883
2. Dion JE, Vinuela FV, Lylyk P, Bentson J (1988) Ivalon-33% ethanol-avitene embolic mixture: clinical experience with neuroradiological endovascular therapy in 40 arteriovenous malformations. AJNR 9: 1029–1030
3. Eskridge JM, Hartling RP (1989) Preoperative embolization of brain AVMs using surgical silk and polyvinyl alcohol. AJNR 10: 882
4. Hilal SK, Khandji AG, Chi TL, Stein BM, Bello JA, Silver AJ (1988) Synthetic fiber-coated platinum coils successfully used for the endovascular treatment of arteriovenous malformations, aneurysms and direct arteriovenous fistulas of the CNS. AJNR 9: 1030
5. Pelz DM, Fox AJ, Vinuela F, Drake CC, Ferguson GG (1988) Preoperative embolization of brain AVMs with isobutyl-2 cyanoacrylate. AJNR 9: 757–764
6. Purdy PD, Batjer HH, Risser RC, Samson DS (1992) Arteriovenous malformations of the brain: choosing embolic materials to enhance safety and ease of excision. J Neurosurg 77: 217–222
7. Purdy PD, Batjer HH, Samson D, Risser RC, Bowman GW (1991) Intraarterial sodium amytal administration to guide pre-operative embolization of cerebral arteriovenous malformations. J Neurosurg Anes 3: 103–106
8. Purdy PD, Samson D, Batjer HH, Risser RC (1990) Preoperative embolization of cerebral arteriovenous malformations with polyvinyl alcohol particles: experience in 51 adults. AJNR 11: 501–510
9. Purdy PD, Batjer HH, Kopitnik T, Risser R, Samson D (1992) Use of ethanol in preoperative AVM embolization. Presented at the International Conference of New Trends in Management of Cerebrovascular Malformations, Verona, Italy, June 8–12
10. Samson D, Ditmore QM, Beyer CW Jr (1981) Intravascular use of isobutyl 2-cyanoacrylate. Part 1: treatment of intracranial arteriovenous malformations. Neurosurgery 8: 43–51
11. Scialfa G, Scotti G (1985) Superselective injection of polyvinyl alcohol microemboli for the treatment of cerebral arteriovenous malformations. AJNR 6: 957–960
12. Spetzler RF, Martin NA, Carter LP, Flom RA, Raudzens PA, Wilkinson E (1987) Surgical management of large AVMs by staged embolization and operative excision. J Neurosurg 67: 17–28

Correspondence: Phillip D. Purdy, M.D., Radiology, Neurology and Neurosurgery, The University of Texas Southwestern Medical Center at Dallas, 5323 Harry Hines Blvd., Dallas, TX 75235-8896, U.S.A.

Staged Occlusion of Arteriovenous Malformations

D.I. Levy, M.H. Khayata, and **R.F. Spetzler**

Division of Neurological Surgery, Barrow Neurological Institute, St. Joseph's Hospital and Medical Center, Phoenix, Arizona, U.S.A.

Summary

The surgical treatment of high-grade arteriovenous malformations (AVMs) is usually fraught with hemorrhagic problems and carries a significant risk. We have been able to lower the surgical risk by treating these lesions with preoperative and intraoperative embolization. Multiple embolization procedures may be needed, and these are often staged and combined with surgery, radiation therapy, or both. We have had good results utilizing a multidisciplinary approach to AVMs and recommend tailoring therapy to individual patients by incorporating these options into the treatment armamentarium.

Keywords: Arteriovenous malformation, cerebral; embolization; N butyl cyanoacrylate; radiosurgery; staged resection.

Introduction

The surgical treatment of arteriovenous malformations (AVMs) of the brain is designed to eliminate the risk of intracranial hemorrhage and neurologic deterioration. The decision to recommend surgery should be based on an objective comparison of the long-term risks presented by the untreated AVM with the more immediate surgical risk.

The Spetzler-Martin grading system[23,27] is used to assess the risk of surgical resection. This system incorporates the factors most important to the prediction of surgical risk: (a) size, (b) pattern of venous drainage, and (c) eloquence of the surrounding brain. A numerical value is assigned to each category and the sum, Grades I to V, is obtained. Grade I is the lowest and indicates small, easily accessible lesions with a low surgical risk. Grade V is the highest and represents the most difficult to resect. The technical difficulty of treating Grades II to V AVMs increases, as well as the morbidity and mortality associated with each. This topic is covered in depth in another chapter in this book.

The surgical management of high grade AVMs has been made easier by staged embolization[24]. Because these lesions are often surrounded by chronically ischemic brain due to AVM steal, the risk of normal perfusion pressure breakthrough is increased by complete excision or complete embolization in a single stage. We therefore recommend a staged embolization, resection, or both depending on the size and complexity of the lesion.

The surgical management of large AVMs has been associated with a high incidence of complications. In the literature, the combined mortality and serious morbidity for resection has approached 50%[2,11,29]. Using a management strategy of staged pre- and intraoperative embolization, surgical resection, or both, we have had good success in treating these lesions, with a 5% or lower rate of mortality or serious morbidity[24,27].

Grades I and II AVMs rarely require preoperative embolization. The surgical risk is low and there is rarely a justification to add the risks of embolization. The larger lesions (Grades III to V) present an enormous surgical challenge. Their removal is often facilitated by embolization, which minimizes intraoperative bleeding, a limiting factor for surgical excision of large AVMs.

Not every AVM needs treatment. The natural history of AVMs, as well as the status of an individual patient, requires consideration of conservative therapy. The patient's age, clinical presentation, and medical problems must be considered when assessing the need for invasive therapy[9]. Grade V AVMs are always large (> 6 cm), located in eloquent brain, and have a component of deep venous drainage that further complicates their excision. The decision to recommend surgery for such patients depends on the surgeon's previous operative experience. Currently, we recommend surgery, embolization, or both for Grade V AVMs when a patient has a fluctuating or progressive neurologic deficit in the distribution of the lesion or if repeated hemorrhage from the AVM is documented. It is of some comfort that large AVMs have lower pressures and are less likely to hemorrhage than smaller AVMs[22]. Therefore, in large AVMs in a person who is asymptomatic, invasive therapy is not needed as long as the AVM does not have an associated arterial aneurysm.

Natural History of Arteriovenous Malformations

The ongoing risk of a first hemorrhage from an AVM has been reported between 1% and 3% per year. The risk of recurrent hemorrhage is as high as 6% for the first year after a hemorrhage and 2% to 3.8%, thereafter[2,6,8,15]. The age range for the maximum incidence of hemorrhage appears to be between the ages of 11 and 35 years. Smaller AVMs appear to have a greater propensity to bleed than do larger malformations[10,22].

The risk of death associated with initial AVM rupture is about 10%, and the mortality rate appears to increase with each hemorrhage[10,20]. The incidence of neurologic deficits is about 50% for each hemorrhage[30]. In addition to the complications of intracranial hemorrhage, patients with AVMs face the risk of seizures, hydrocephalus, and the development of flow-related symptoms such as ischemic deficits from vascular steal or venous congestion.

Materials and Methods

The neurovascular team consists of a neurosurgeon, neuroradiologist, endovascular surgeon, neuroanesthesiologist, and support personnel. Extensive electroencephalographic studies and evoked potential monitoring are used in all cases, as is barbiturate anesthesia. Initial treatment of large AVMs usually consists of transfemoral embolization with Ivalon particles, Gelfoam®, or N-butyl cyanoacrylate glue (NBCA). The emboli are mixed with Ethiodol® for easy visualization. The emboli range from liquid to 290-micron particles that are injected as a slurry. In a recent protocol, we have been using NBCA or Avacryl® glue mixed with various quantities of Ethiodol®

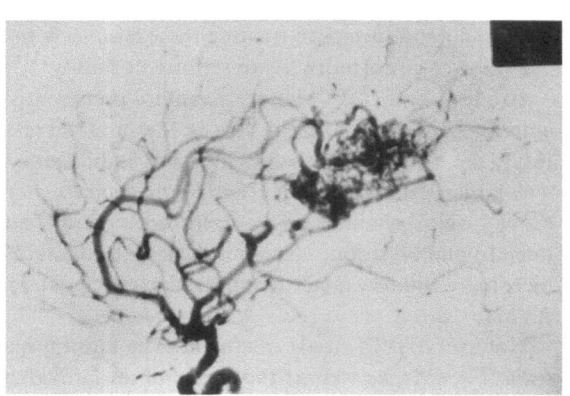
a

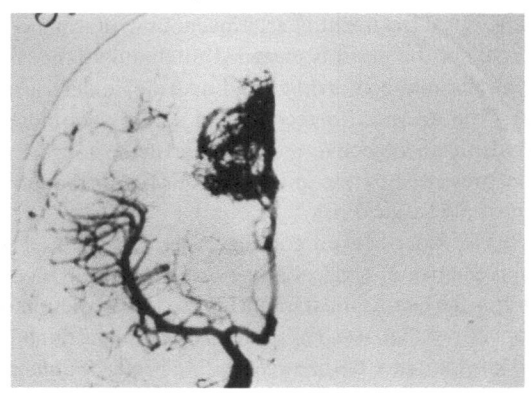
b

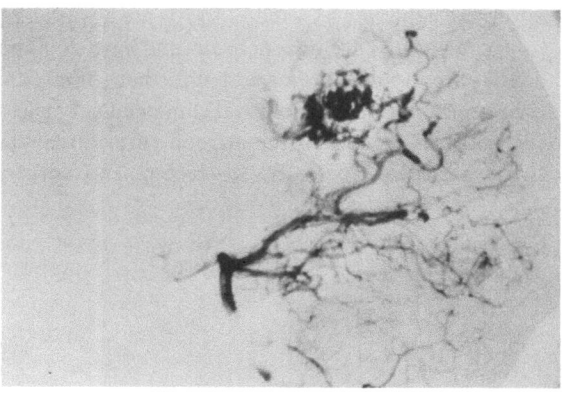
c

Fig. 1. Angiograms of a grade 4 arteriovenous malformation: (a) lateral right internal carotid artery (ICA) injection, (b) anteroposterior right ICA injection, and (c) lateral right vertebral injection

and Tantalum powder. This mixture has given satisfactory results. We have found that micro-operative endovascular embolization of AVMs has provided direct access to certain difficult vessels otherwise unreachable by the transfemoral approach and enables us to use larger diameter catheters. Consequently, larger amounts of glue can be injected more rapidly than would be afforded transfemorally. Depending on the result, further open embolization, transfemoral embolization, or surgical resection may be attempted in the next stage, targeting different feeders. One group of feeding vessels is usually embolized during each stage of treatment. A typical large AVM is fed by branches from the anterior, middle, and posterior cerebral arteries and would usually require a minimum of three separate embolization stages (Figs. 1, 2, and 3).

For intraoperative embolization procedures[27], the vessels should be isolated as close to the AVM nidus as possible. We routinely use a small needle (25–27 gauge) to puncture the vessel at the site of intended cannulation to measure intravascular pressures. Measurements are made with unobstructed flow and with proximal and distal vessel occlusion. These pressure measurements verify the arterial nature of the vessel and the direction of flow. The vessel is then cannulated with a 4-French Silastic catheter directed into the AVM. A short segment of the vessel is isolated and occluded proximally with temporary aneurysm clips, and the catheter is introduced through a small arteriotomy and secured with a silk tie. The catheter is secured to the craniotomy drape and to a Leyla bar with adhesive plastic strips to prevent accidental avulsion of the feeding artery. With the feeding vessel occluded proximally, digital subtraction angiography is performed to ascertain the extent of AVM filling. Proximal occlusion "flow control" of the feeding pedicles ensures that no reflux occurs in the normal vessel and that the glue mixture is not diluted. The portion of the AVM fed by the selected artery is flushed with 5% dextrose solution to enhance distal filling of the AVM and then embolized to complete its obliteration. The particles or glue is mixed with contrast material and injected under continuous fluoroscopic guidance in ideal "flow control" conditions. Digital subtraction angiography is repeated frequently to document the progress of the embolization.

After it has been embolized intraoperatively, the feeding vessel is typically ligated at the site of cannulation. Embolization increases intravascular pressure in the feeding vessel, and ligation prevents transmission of this elevated pressure to residual nonoccluded segments of the AVM. Permanent occlusion of the feeding vessel is

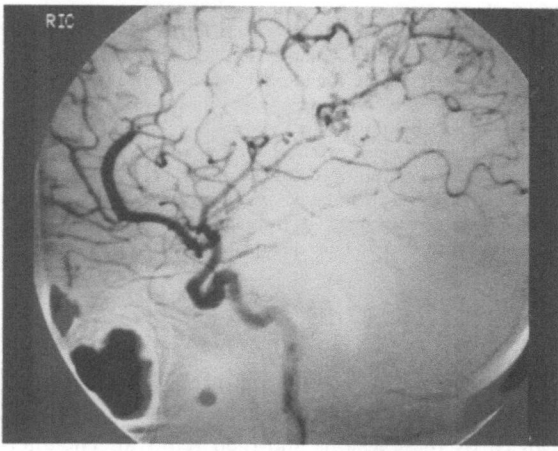

a

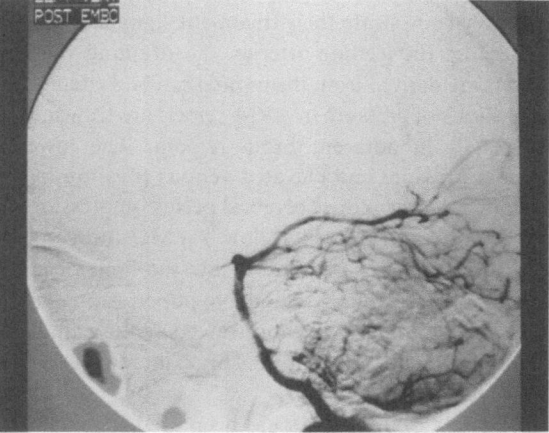

b

Fig. 3. (a, b) postembolization angiogram showing small residual arteriovenous malformation nidus fed by the anterior circulation. This patient underwent focused radiation for treatment of the residual lesion

an important factor in avoiding postembolization hemorrhage and is an advantage of intraoperative embolization compared to transfemoral techniques[16].

Surgical resection of these lesions is technically challenging even after embolization. Collateral filling, combined with the fragile nature of the deep venous structures, makes intraoperative hemorrhage common. Even after embolization, surgical resection has taken as long as 17 hours in grade V AVMs. Because of the expansive nature of these lesions, patient positioning and a generous craniotomy flap that exposes the lesion and feeding vessels are important for their safe resection. Surgery may be unnecessary in some lesions if they can be reduced to a small size by embolization. Treatment with focused radiation, such as LINAC or the gamma knife, can successfully obliterate a small residual nidus.

Over the past year we have treated approximately 50 arteriovenous malformations of the brain at our institution. Twenty-eight of these patients received transfemoral preoperative embolization prior

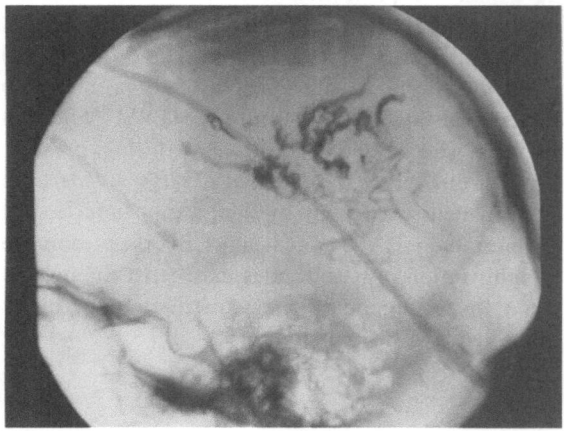

Fig. 2. Casts of embolic N-butyl cyanoacrylate after intraoperative and transfemoral embolization

to definitive treatment with surgical resection or radiosurgery. In ten cases the transfemoral embolization alone was not sufficient to make the arteriovenous malformation amenable to definitive treatment and these were therefore embolized by the intraoperative method. By combining these methods all 28 patients who received the transfemoral embolizations were amenable to definitive treatment using either radiosurgery or surgical resection.

There were four post-procedure hemorrhages, two transient neurological deficits that lasted less than one month, and four permanent neurological deficits (two with hemiparesis, one homonymous hemianopsia and one quadrantanopsia).

Discussion

Effective management of cerebral AVMs requires an understanding of the changes in cerebral hemodynamics caused by these lesions and their removal. The alterations in cerebral blood flow and perfusion pressure induced by these lesions may cause neurological deficits and may complicate their treatment significantly.

Because the feeding arteries and draining veins of AVMs are derived from the normal cerebral circulation, alterations of pressure in AVM vessels are transmitted to vessels in adjacent brain regions. The lowered arterial pressure and elevated venous pressure in the region of AVMs reduce cerebral perfusion pressure. In the vicinity of large high-flow AVMs, the cerebral perfusion pressure may fall below the limit of autoregulation, resulting in regional hypoperfusion[17,18,26]. This angiographically demonstrated situation amounts to a diversion flow from normal brain into the AVM – a "cerebral steal[7]".

A variety of techniques has been used to treat large AVMs[6,15,28, 29,32,33]. Surgical ligation of feeding arteries has been used as a preliminary step in excision of the malformation[32]. Because the low resistance system of the AVM is so hemodynamically attractive, however, collateral vessels replace the ligated arteries rapidly as a source of flow to the malformation[6,32]. AVMs have also been treated with flow-directed embolization:[12] silicone spheres are injected into the surgically exposed carotid or vertebral arteries. Further technical developments have permitted embolization through percutaneously introduced catheters. Excellent results have been reported using flow-directed embolization as a preliminary step to surgical excision of AVMs[16,28,33]. The spheres rarely occlude the nidus completely, however, and collateral vassels to the malformation maintain enough flow to present problems with hemostasis[33]. Indeed, Luessenhop and Rosa[11] have abandoned routine presurgical embolization of feeding arteries to avoid promoting the development of collateral supply

to the AVM from deep arteries that are less accessible surgically.

Several clinical groups have used a liquid embolic agent, isobutylcyanoacrylate (IBCA or Bucrylate®), both preoperatively (through steerable and flow-directed microcatheters) and intraoperatively as an adjunct to the surgical treatment of large AVMs[3,5,21]. Opinions about how effectively IBCA embolization facilitates AVM excision vary. Peerless[19] and Samson et al.[21] attribute no advantage to IBCA embolization as it is difficult to dissect the lesion from the brain. We share the concern about IBCA, especially for the treatment of large, deep malformations. The poorly compressible mass of the IBCA-embolized AVM may impair visualization and increase the difficulty of dissecting its deeper aspects. In our experience, the new polymer, NBCA, is largely free of these disadvantages. NBCA is a rubbery substance that can be manipulated, cut, and retracted safely. Its use transforms a bloody AVM operation into a comparatively dry, mass removal.

Ivalon spoge slurry or Avacryl® glue allows preferential obliteration of the AVM nidus, thereby decreasing the potential for collateral vessels to restore flow through the lesion.

External carotid artery (ECA) embolization must be monitored carefully to prevent inadvertent embolization of the brain from spontaneous opening of extrato intracranial anastomotic channels[25]. Several severe strokes have been attributed to ECA embolization[1].

In our series, all surgical procedures for selective embolization, feeding artery ligation, and AVM excision were performed under barbiturate anesthesia. We believe that the protection from temporary ischemia provided by barbiturates justifies their use[23,31,34]. Barbiturates also decrease cerebral blood flow (CBF) in normal vascular beds and may thus promote the preferential flow of emboli into the AVM[14]. Several patients who developed normal perfusion pressure breakthrough after the removal of large AVMs have been treated successfully by the prompt induction of barbiturate coma[4,13]. By reducing CBF, the preemptive administration of barbiturates may assist the normal brain to accommodate the redistribution of blood that attends AVM obliteration[29].

Conclusion

Many Grade V AVMs would once have been considered inoperable even though they induce ongoing neurologic damage. Today several options are avilable to help control and obliterate these challenging lesions. Transfemoral embolization, intraoperative embolization, and surgical resection all play an active role in the aggressive treatment of large AVMs. The stepwise reduction of flow through large AVMs afforded by staged embolization appears to minimize the risks of normal perfusion pressure breakthrough. The development of new types of embolization protocols with the introduction of new angiographic catheters has played a major role in transforming inoperable or high risk lesions into manageable lesions.

References

1. Ahn HS, Kerber CW, Deeb ZL (1980) Extra- to intracranial anastomoses in therapeutic embolization: recognition and role. AJNR 1: 71–75
2. Brown RD Jr, Wiebers DO, Forbes G, O'Fallon WM, Piepgras DG, Marsh WR, Maciunas RJ (1988) The natural history of unruptured intracranial arteriovenous malformations. J Neurosurg 68: 352–357
3. Cromwell LD, Harris AB (1980) Treatment of cerebral arteriovenous malformations: a combined neurosurgical and neuroradiological approach. J Neurosurg 52: 705–708
4. Day AL, Friedman WA, Sypert GW, Mickle JP (1982) Successful treatment of the normal perfusion pressure breakthrough syndrome. Neurosurgery 11: 625–630
5. Debrun G, Vinuela F, Fox A, Drake CG (1982) Embolization of cerebral arteriovenous malformations with bucrylate. J Neurosurg 56: 615–627
6. Drake CG (1979) Cerebral arteriovenous malformations: considerations for and experience with surgical treatment in 166 cases. Clin Neurosurg 26: 145–208
7. Feindel W, Perot P (1965) Red cerebral veins. A report on arteriovenous shunts in tumors and cerebral scars. J Neurosurg 22: 315–325
8. Fults D, Kelly DL Jr (1984) Natural history of arteriovenous malformations of the brain: a clinical study. Neurosurgery 15: 658–662
9. Golfinos JG, Wascher TM, Zabramski JM, Spetzler RF (1992) The management of unruptured intracranial vascular malformations. BNI Quarterly 8 (3): 2–11
10. Graf CJ, Perret GE, Torner JC (1983) Bleeding from cerebral arteriovenous malformations as part of their natural history. J Neurosurg 58: 331–337
11. Luessenhop AJ, Rosa L (1984) Cerebral arteriovenous malformations. Indications for and results of surgery, and the role of intravascular techniques. J Neurosurg 60: 14–22
12. Luessenhop AJ, Spence WT (1960) Artificial embolization of cerebral arteries. Report of use in a case of arteriovenous malformation. JAMA 172: 1153–1155
13. Marshall LF, U HS (1983) Treatment of massive intraoperative brain swelling. Neurosurgery 13: 412–414
14. Michenfelder JD, Milde JH, Sundt TM Jr (1976) Cerebral protection by barbiturate anesthesia. Use after middle cerebral artery occlusion in Java monkeys. Arch Neurol 33: 345–350
15. Mullan S, Brown FD, Patronas NJ (1979) Hyperemic and ischemic problems of surgical treatment of arteriovenous malformations. J Neurosurg 51: 757–764
16. Mullan S, Kawanaga H, Patronas NJ (1979) Microvascular embolization of cerebral arteriovenous malformations: a technical variation. J Neurosurg 51: 621–627
17. Nornes H (1984) Quantitation of altered hemodynamics. In: Wilson CB, Stein BM (eds) Intracranial arteriovenous malformations. Williams and Wilkins, Baltimore, pp 32–43
18. Nornes H, Grip A (1980) Hemodynamic aspects of cerebral arteriovenous malformations. J Neurosurg 53: 456–464
19. Peerless SJ (1982) Comments on Day AL, Friedman WA, Sypert GW, Meckle JP. Successful treatment of the normal perfusion pressure breakthrough syndrome. Neurosurgery 11: 629–630
20. Perret G, Nishioka H (1966) Report on the Cooperative Study of intracranial aneurysms and subarachnoid hemorrhage. Section VI. J Neurosurg 25: 467–490
21. Samson D, Ditmore QM, Beyer CW Jr (1981) Intravascular use of isobutyl 2-cyanoacrylate. Part 1: treatment of intracranial arteriovenous malformations. Neurosurgery 8: 43–51
22. Spetzler RF, Hargraves RW, McCormick PW, Zabramski JM, Flom RA, Zimmerman RS (1992) Relationship of perfusion pressure and size to risk of hemorrhage from arteriovenous malformations. J Neurosurg 76: 918–923
23. Spetzler RF, Martin NA (1986) A proposed grading system for arteriovenous malformations. J Neurosurg 65: 476–483
24. Spetzler RF, Martin NA, Carter LP, Flom RA, Raudzens PA, Wilkinson E (1987) Surgical management of large AVMs by staged embolization and operative excision. J Neurosurg 67: 17–28
25. Spetzler RF, Modic M, Bonstelle C (1980) Spontaneous opening of large occipital-vertebral artery anastomosis during embolization. Case report. J Neurosurg 53: 849–850
26. Spetzler RF, Selman WR (1984) Pathophysiology of cerebral ischemia accompanying arteriovenous malformations. In: Wilson CB, Stein BM (eds) Intracranial arteriovenous malformations. Williams and Wilkins, Baltimore, pp 24–31
27. Spetzler RF, Zabramski JM (1990) Grading and staged resection of cerebral arteriovenous malformations. Clin Neurosurg 36: 318–337
28. Stein BM, Wolpert SM (1980) Arteriovenous malformations of the brain. II: Current concepts and treatment. Arch Neurol 37: 69–75
29. U HS (1985) Microsurgical excision of paraventricular arteriovenous malformations. Neurosurgery 16: 293–303
30. Wilkins RH (1985) Natural history of intracranial vascular malformations: a review. Neurosurgery 16: 421–430
31. Wilkinson E, Spetzler RF, Carter LP, Raudzens PA (1985) Intraoperative barbiturate therapy during temporary vessel occlusion in man. In: Spetzler RF, Carter LP, Selman WR, Martin NA (eds) Cerebral revascularization for stroke. Thieme-Stratton, New York, pp 397–402
32. Wilson CB, U HS, Domingue J (1979) Microsurgical treatment of intracranial vascular malformations. J Neurosurg 51: 446–454
33. Wolpert SM, Stein BM (1975) Catheter embolization of intracranial arteriovenous malformations as an aid to surgical excision. Neuroradiology 10: 73–85
34. Yatsu FM (1983) Pharmacologic protection against ischemic brain damage. Neurol Clin 1: 37–53

Correspondence: c/o Editorial Office, Robert F. Spetzler, M.D., Barrow Neurological Institute, 350 W. Thomas Road, Phoenix, AZ 85013, U.S.A.

Outcome from Multimodality Treatment of Arteriovenous Malformations

A.R. Aspoas, A.D. Mendelow, J. Arrotegui, and **A. Gholkar**

Regional Neuroscience Centre, Newcastle General Hospital, Newcastle-upon-Tyne, U.K.

Summary

We report the outcome of 57 patients with Intracranial Arteriovenous Malformations (AVM) treated by a multimodality approach. The outcome correlates well with that predicted by the Spetzler Grading System in that all patients with grades 1 and 2 lesions remained independent. No deaths occurred in this series. The Spetzler Grading is useful for predicting the outcome of treatment and can be used when explaining risks to patients and their families.

Keywords: Arterioveneous malformation; grading; embolization; surgery.

Introduction

The management of Intracranial Arteriovenous Malformations (AVM) has improved with advances in surgical technique[10,14], neuroradiological equipment[10,15] and the development of stereoradiosurgery[8]. Since Spetzler and Martin (1986) produced their grading system[12] it has been possible to give accurate risks of operative morbidity and mortality[12]. The grading system is based on the size of AVM, presence of deep draining veins and the involvement of eloquent areas of brain. There is a range from 1 (a small lesion in a non-eloquent area, with only superficial draining veins) to 5.

The risks of surgery[3] can be weighed against the natural history of Intracranial AVMs[1,2,4,5,7,9]. All AVMs show histological evidence of haemorrhage, but in patients treated conservatively clinically significant haemorrhage[6] occurs in over 60% of patients within 20 years after the AVM has been diagnosed[1,2,5].

Clinical Material

A total of sixty five patients with intracranial AVMs were seen and only fifty seven have been treated. The sex distribution in the treated group was 26 males and 31 females, with a mean age of 34 years and a range of 4 to 66.

Presentation

The two commonest forms of presentation were epilepsy and haemorrhage. The majority of the lesions less than 6 cm presented with a bleed whilst those greater than 6 cm had an equal number presenting with seizures or haemorrhage.

Spetzler Grading

The grading of patients treated is listed below, with the middle three grades having the largest number of patients.

There were eight patients who had inoperable lesions (scored as grade 6 by Spetzler). One was a lesion 4 to 6 cm and the remaining 7 were greater than 6 cm, all involved eloquent areas and had a deep draining vein.

Treatment

The approach was multidisciplinary with the single objective of obliterating the malformation. If this is not achieved, there will be progressive collateral vascularization of the AVM, with unproven protection from future haemorrhage.

The small superficial lesions were treated using the standard microsurgical technique, whilst the larger AVMs had staged reduction in the blood supply with embolization prior to surgical excision. Normal perfusion pressure breakthrough was not seen using this approach[12]. Small deep seated lesions are treated with stereoradiosurgery, and some lesions were treated with all three modalities.

In the early phase embolization was performed by intraoperative catheterisation of the feeding vessel and the injection of particles (Ivalon Sponge). However with advances in neuroradiological techniques and the development of fine bore, flow guided catheters

Table 1. *Grading*

Grade	n
I	8
II	10
III	16
IV	15
V	8

Table 2. *Treatment*

Treatment	n
Surgery	27
Embolization and surgery	16
Embolization	6
Stereoradiosurgery	4
Surgery and stereoradiosurgery	2
Surgery, embolization and stereoradiosurgery	2
Total	57

Table 3. *Type of Preoperative Embolization in Combined Treatment*

Surgical embolization	10
Radiological embolization	5
Combination	1

Table 4. *Outcome of Fifty Seven Treated Patients*

Grade	GR	MD	SD	Total
I	7	1	0	8
II	8	2	0	10
III	11	4	1	16
IV	9	5	1	15
V	5	1	2	8
Total	40	13	4	57

GR good recovery; *MD* moderate disability; *SD* severe disability.

endovascular embolization via the femoral route was possible in the later series. A glue mixture (Isobutyl 2-cyanoacrylate) was used.

Patients treated with embolization by either method often had multiple procedures, the maximum being 6.

Management Outcome

There were no deaths in this group of treated patients and there were no patients left in the "persistent vegetative state". In grades I and II, all patients were independent, whilst in grades III, IV and V there were

Table 5. *Outcome of Combined Treatment of Embolization and Surgery*

	GR	MD
I	2	0
II	2	0
III	3	1
IV	3	3
V	2	0
Total	12	4

a total of four patients who had severe disability, that is to say were dependent on others for daily living.

All those patients treated with preoperative embolization and surgery (n = 16) became independent (four with moderate disability and twelve with good recovery) as shown in Table 5.

Discussion

Surgery is still the treatment of choice for small, superficial AVMs involving the non-eloquent areas of the brain. However with larger lesions involving eloquent areas a multidisciplinary treatment is required. Preoperative embolization aids surgical excision by, i) reducing the density of the AVM, ii) slowing the circulation time through the AVM, iii) reducing the size, iv) reducing the diameter of the draining veins, and v) restoring the surrounding cerebral circulation, preventing normal perfusion pressure break-through[13].

Embolization rarely obliterates the AVM completely[10]; in this study the AVMs in four patients were successfully treated endovascularly. Although the numbers are small there appears to be a trend with improved outcome of patients treated with a combination of preoperative embolization and surgery, which is confirmed by other authors[10,15].

Finally the Spetzler Grading System is a simple method using three radiological factors to grade patients, thereby replacing other complex systems which

Table 6. *Treatment Outcome*

Grade	No present study	No Spetzler study[12]	Independent present %	Independent Spetzler %
I	8	23	100	100
II	10	21	100	100
III	16	25	94	96
IV	15	15	94	93
V	8	16	75	88

require volume calculations of the lesion[11], assessment of rate of flow and degree of arterial steal. It can now be used to predict the outcome of multimodality treatment as the results of this study compare with others[12] (as illustrated in Table 6).

References

1. Brown DB, Wiebers DO, Forbes GS (1988) The natural history of unruptured intracranial arteriovenous malformations. J Neurosurg 68: 352–357
2. Brown DB, Wiebers DO, Forbes GS (1990) Unruptured intracranial aneurysms and arteriovenous malformations: frequency of intracranial haemorrhage and the relationship of lesions. J Neurosurg 73: 859–863
3. Celli P, Ferrante L, Palma L, Cavedon G (1984) Cerebral arteriovenous malformations in children. Clinical features and outcome to treatment in children and adults. Surg Neurol 22: 43–49
4. Crawford PM, West CR, Chadwick DW (1986) Arteriovenous malformation of the brain: natural history in unoperated patients. J Neurol Neurosurg Psychiatry 49: 1–10
5. Fults D, Kelly DL (1984) Natural history of arteriovenous malformations of the brain: a clinical study. Neurosurgery 15: 658–662
6. Graf CJ, Perret GE, Torner JC (1983) Bleeding from cerebral arteriovenous malformations as part of their natural history. J Neurosurg 58: 331–337
7. Jane JA, Kassell NF, Torner JC, Winn HR (1985) The natural history of aneurysms and arteriovenous malformations. J Neurosurg 62: 321–323
8. Lunsford LD, Kondziolka D, Flickinger JC, Bissonette DJ, Jungreis CA, Maitz AH, Horton JA, Coffey RJ (1991) Stereotactic radiosurgery for arteriovenous malformations of the brain. J Neurosurg 75: 512–524
9. Ondra SL, Troupp H, George ED, Schwab K (1990) The natural history of symptomatic arteriovenous malformations of the brain: a 24 years follow-up assessment. J Neurosurg 73: 387–391
10. Pasqualin A, Scienza R, Cioffi F, Barone G, Benati A, Beltramello A, Da Pian R (1991) Treatment of cerebral arteriovenous malformations with a combination of preoperative embolization and surgery. Neurosurgery 29: 358–368
11. Pasqualin A, Barone G, Rosta L, Scienza R, Da Pian R (1991) The relevance of anatomic and hemodynamic factors to a classification of cerebral arteriovenous malformations. Neurosurgery 28: 370–379
12. Spetzler RF, Martin NA (1986) A proposed grading system for arteriovenous malformations. J Neurosurg 65: 476–483
13. Spetzler RF, Martin NA, Carter LP (1987) Surgical management of large AVMs by staged embolization and operative excision. J Neurosurg 67: 17–28
14. Tew JM, Tobler WD (1986) Present status of lasers in neurosurgery. In: Advances and technical standards in Neurosurgery, Vol 13. Springer, Wien New York, pp 3–36
15. Vinuela F, Dion JE, Duckwiler G, Martin NA, Lylyk P, Fox A, Pelz D, Drake CG, Girvin JJ, Debrun G (1991) Combined endovascular embolization and surgery in the management of cerebral arteriovenous malformations: experience with 101 cases. J Neurosurg 75: 856–864

Correspondence: A.R. Aspoas, M.D., Regional Neuroscience Centre, Newcastle General Hospital, Westgate Road, Newcastle-upon-Tyne NE4 6BE, U.K.

Therapeutic Strategies for Brain AVMs. An Assessment of Benefits and Risks of Surgical and Endovascular Therapy

B. Richling, G. Bavinzski, A. Gruber, and **M. Killer**

Department of Neurosurgery, University of Vienna Medical School, Vienna, Austria

Summary

Therapy of brain AVMs is dominated by an assessment of risks rather than by a single therapy. A therapeutic concept deciding which therapy has to be applied to a certain AVM should not depend on local circumstances only. The ideal situation should offer surgical as well as endovascular therapy in high quality. This would allow the choice of therapy depending only on the morphological or clinical factors of each AVM.

A therapeutic concept is presented which is guided by an assessment of risks. The risk of natural history (dominated by the risk of hemorrhage) is assessed to the risk of therapy (surgical and/or endovascular). The decision tree allows a individual therapy adapted to the individual case.

Keywords: Brain AVMs; embolization; surgery; assessment of risks.

Introduction

Surgical, endovascular or the combination of both therapies seem to be accepted for the treatment of brain AVMs during the last years. But therapeutic concepts deciding which therapy has to be applied on a certain AVM or what kind of combination of therapies has to be performed vary from institute to institute. Depending on local circumstances, on the availability of endovascular treatment but also depending on the surgical routine and skill, different therapeutic strategies are used.

The presented therapeutic concept is the concept of an institution (Table 1) where both therapies are performed by the same people; where every decision to an endovascular step, every occlusion of an AVM-compartment is done by the ones who handle surgically the partially embolized AVM themselves.

A decision tree is presented allowing a therapeutic strategy for each individual AVM. This strategy follows the principle of assessing the risks of both therapies (surgical and/or endovascular) to the risk of natural history. The risk of endovascular surgery depends on factors like vascular architecture (i.e., the approachability by microcatheters) the flow pattern of the nidus and the skill of the endovascular surgeon. The surgical risk depends on the size and location of the AVM, the venous drainage and last but not least the skill of the surgeon. The risk of natural history is dominated by the risk of bleeding. This risk depends on a high degree on morphological factors like venous drainage pattern, ventricular location and associated aneurysms, and will be pointed out in the discussion.

Case Report 1

A 25 years old woman was admitted to the hospital presenting with cerebral fits of increasing frequency. Elevated dosage of anticonvulsant medications could not reduce the number and severity of the seizures. There was no evidence of bleeding in the history, neither was there any neurologic deficit. Angiography showed an interhemispheric AVM located in the gyrus cinguli with extension to the interhemispheric motor area and the fronto-parietal region (Fig. 1). This AVM was supplied by feeders of the anterior cerebral artery as well as by the middle cerebral artery. Multiple niduses of different feeders surrounded a high flow shunting center fed by a middle cerebral branch.

This AVM was embolized in 2 sessions. The first endovascular approach reached the feeders of the AcA; several compartments could be reached selectively with flow independent microguide-wire-supported microcatheters (Tracker 18). Due to the flow conditions in the different compartments (i.e., blocked flow or non-blocked

Table 1. *Clinical Material and Results Treatment of cerebral AVM's* $n = 199$

No. of patients embolized		152
No. of interventions	295	
Total occlusions	19	(17%)
Cases only operated		43
Embolization + OP	38	
Embolization + radiosurgery	21	
Morbidity	18	(9%)
Mortality	7	(3.5%)

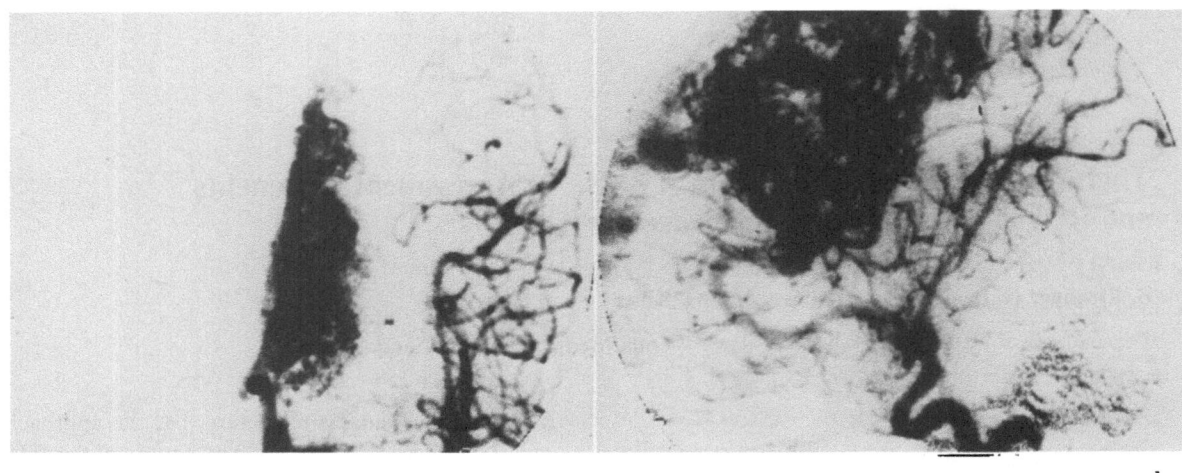

a   b

Fig. 1. (a) Left internal carotid artery angiogram shows the frontoparietal paramedian AVM. (b) Lateral view

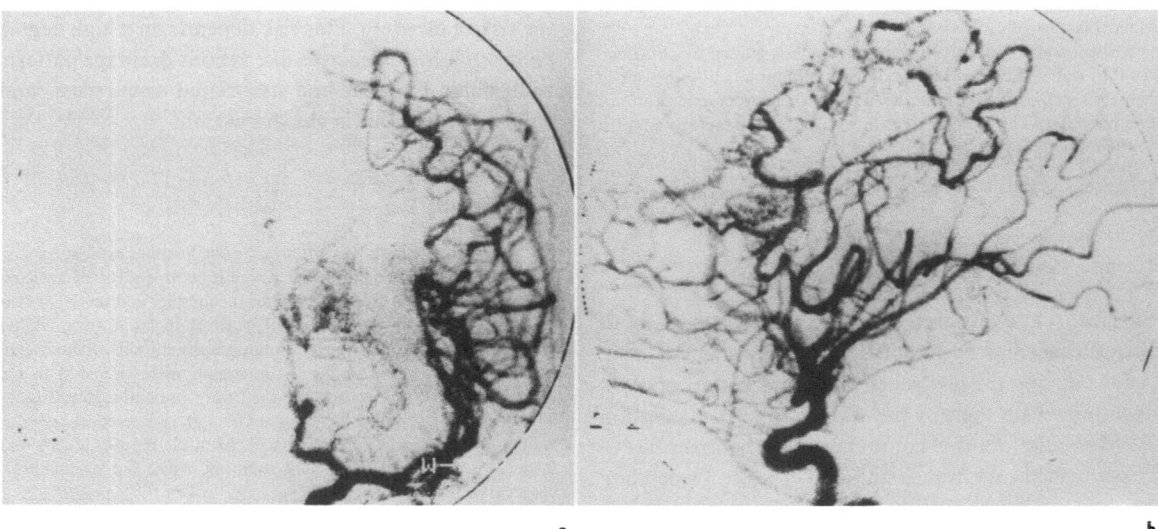

a   b

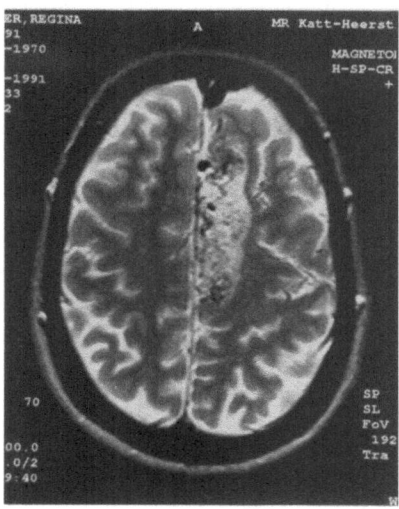

c

Fig. 2. (a, b) Angiographic result after 2 embolizations. (c) MRI-scan after 2 embolizations shows the partially thrombosed AVM

flow) different qualities of casting could be achieved. Some of the compartments could be casted solidly, others only by sprinkled parts of the Histoacryl/Lipiodol-mixture. In a second session approaches to the McA-territories were performed. After the tip of the microcatheter reached selective positions and angiographic studies in different views were performed, these compartments were casted. Here too some of the compartments could be casted solidly, others only partially. The result of the two endovascular sessions is shown in Fig. 2a. A partial but high degree embolization could be achieved resulting in a reasonable reduction of flow. The patient could be discharged 7 days after the embolization. The anticonvulsant medication could be reduced step by step. In the following 2 years there were no more cerebral fits, in spite of no anticonvulsant medication. The MRI-scan shows the result after 2 embolizations (Fig. 2b).

Case Report 2

A 15 year old boy was transferred from an outside hospital after several severe intraventricular bleedings. At time of admission the boy presented with a normal neurological status and consciousness. An examination of the coagulation factors showed a leak of factor VII. MRI and angiogram showed an AVM located in the splenium as well as in the right parasplenial and trigonal area (Figs. 3 and 4). Venous drainage consisted mainly of the vein of Galen.

The first endovascular access to the AcoA-territory led to selective approaches of the callosal part of the AVM. Several compartments were solidly or partially casted and finally an embolization of approximately 80% could be achieved. In a second endovascular session the compartments fed by the right posterior choroidal artery were entered. After selective angiographic studies, some of these compartments could be casted solidly, some of them partially. The result of the two endovascular sessions is shown in Fig. 5.

According to the strategy shown in Table 1 and especially according to the high risk of bleeding due to the chronic leak of factor VII, this boy had to undergo surgery. 6 days after the second embolization and after substitution of factor VII, a parieto-occipital bone flap was performed in prone position. By an interhemispheric approach the AVM could be resected totally without heavy bleeding. Surgical difficulty arose from multiple AV-shunts closed to the vein of Galen, not beeing embolized at the second session. Intraoperative angiography of the vertebral artery is shown in Fig. 6. The patient could be discharged 14 days after the operation to his home hospital without neurologic deficits.

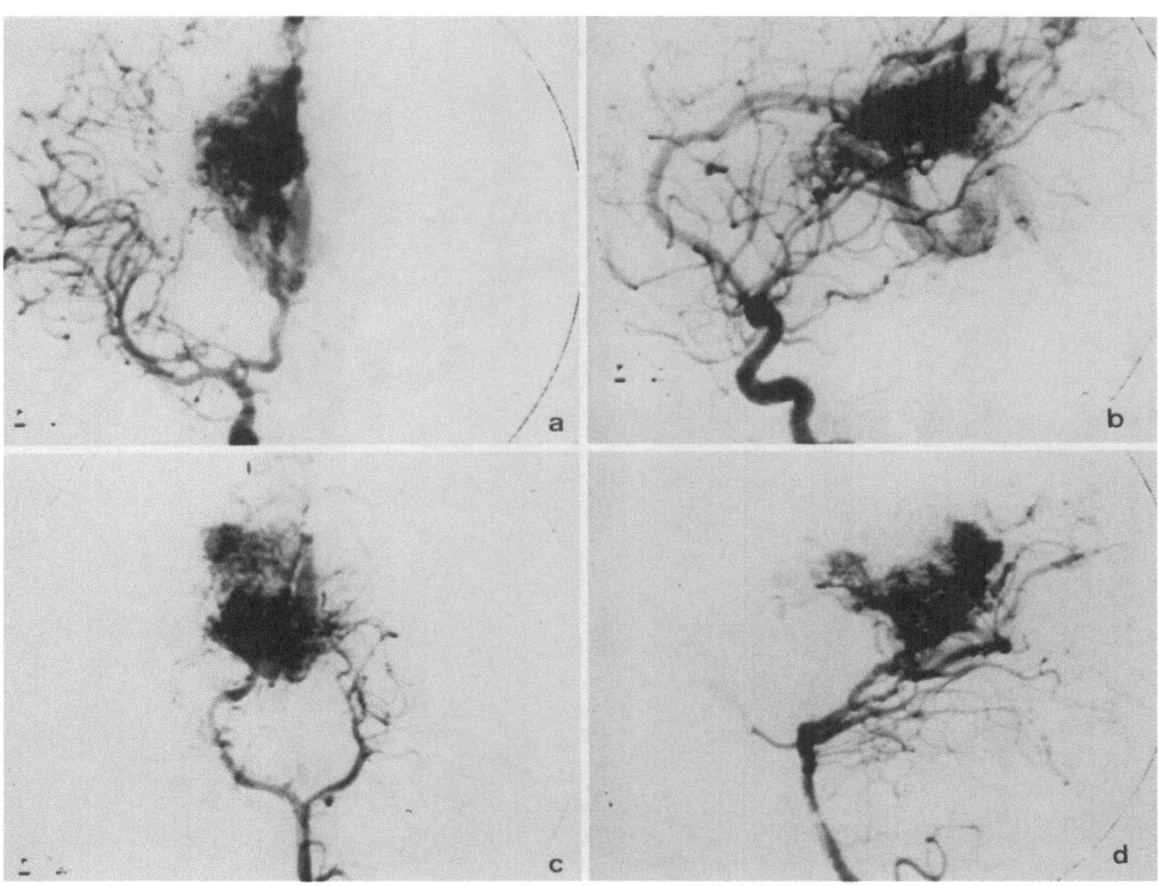

Fig. 3. (a) ap-view of the right internal carotid artery demonstrates the extension of the posterior callosal AVM. (b) Lateral view of the right internal carotid artery. (c, d) Angiography of the left vertebral artery (ap and lateral view)

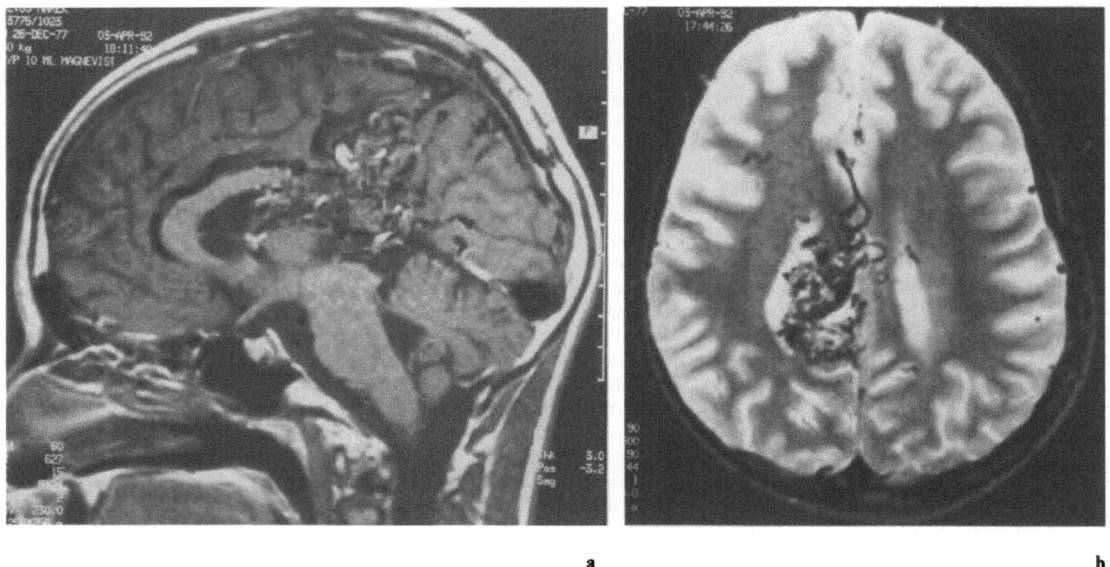

a   b

Fig. 4. (a) MRI-scan before endovascular and surgical treatment. Sagittal T1-weighted image shows the interhemispheric, callosal AVM with extension to the surface of the right pulvinar. (b) Axial T2-weighted image shows the paramedian extension of the AVM

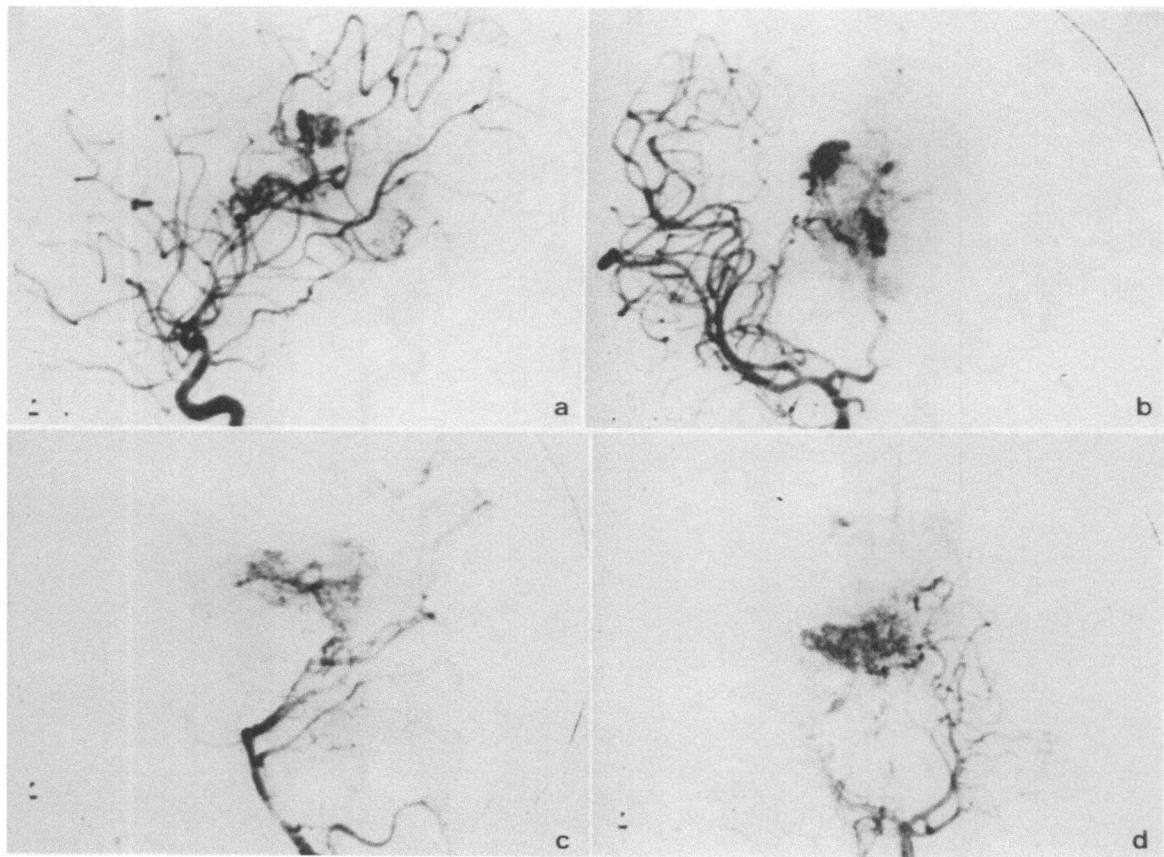

Fig. 5. Angio's after 2 embolizations: (a) After embolization from the territory of the right pericallosal artery, deep perforating feeders from M1 and the anterior choroidal artery remain. (b) Ap-view. (c) Verbtebral angiography shows the remaining part of the AVM supplied by feeders from the posterior choroidal arteries. (d) Vertebal angiography ap-view

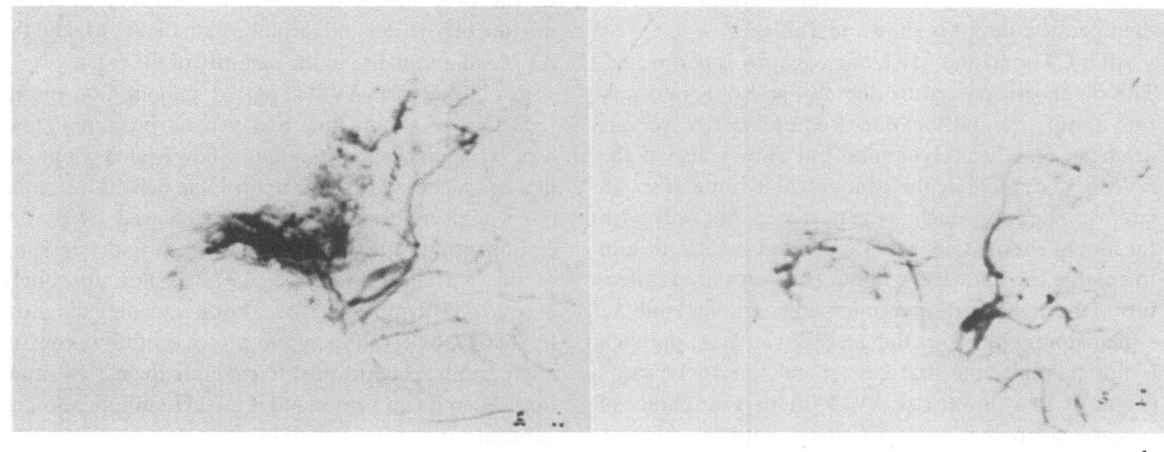

Fig. 6. (a) Intraoperative vertebral angiography before resection. (b) After resection of the AVM. Small niduses in the roof of the third ventricle were difficult to remove (lateral view)

Discussion

Therapy of brain AVMs should be guided by an assessment of risks. The risk of therapy has to be compared to the risk of natural history. The risk of therapy, i.e., the risk of endovascular or/and surgical treatment will be pointed out later on. The risk of natural history is dominated by the risk of hemorrhage. Many analysis have been performed to evaluate statistic data concerning the natural risk of bleeding[2,3,7,13,14]. During his lifetime, a patient with a brain AVM undergoes a bleeding risk of 40 to 60%. Concerning AVMs of the basal ganglia this risk comes up to 70 to 90% and approaches therefore to the risk of brain aneurysms[8,15,16].

The relationship between morphological (i.e., angiographic) findings and the rate of bleeding has been analyzed by several authors[1,4,9-12]. The highest statistical probability for a hemorrhage was found if 1. singular draining veins, 2. deep draining veins, 3. stenosis or impairment of venous drainage were present. Other predicting factors were intranidal or flowrelated aneurysms and ventricular or paraventricular location of the AVM. Albert et al.[1] point out that usually small AVMs are constituted by only 1 draining vein and therefore are prone to bleed more frequently than big AVMs having several draining veins.

AVMs with morphological factors predicting the risk of bleeding (further called "high risk AVMs") principally undergo an aggressive treatment with the aim of cure; other AVMs (further called "lower risk AVMs" presenting with headache, seizures or neurological deficits) undergo a step by step therapy adapted

Table 2. *Decision Tree Based on Different Natural Risks Included in the Concept*

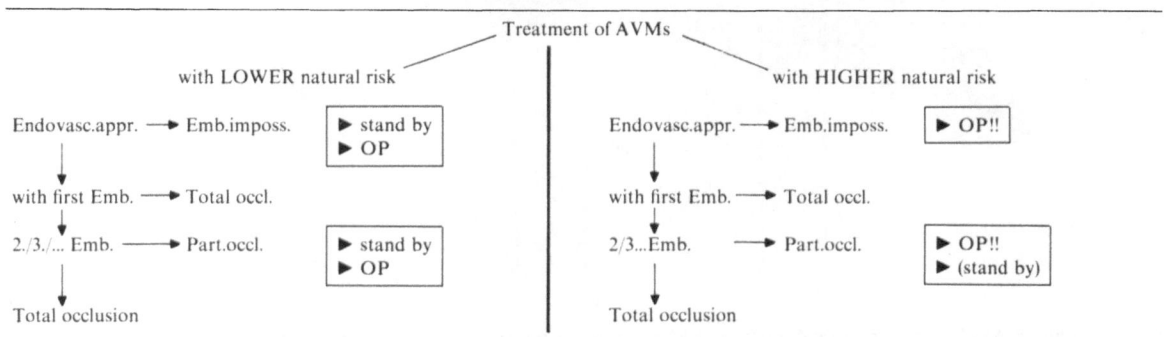

The radiosurgical therapy is not included in the concept.

to the effectiveness of treatment versus symptoms. This therapeutic concept is shown in Table 2.

After CT-scan and MRI, angiography is performed. This diagnostic procedure does not give only information about size and location, feeding arteries, venous drainage and hemodynamics, but shows also if the AVM is accessible by the endovascular route. If so, an endovascular approach is the next step, not only with the aim of endovascular therapy but also with the aim to enlarge the knowledge about the vascular architecture of the malformation by microangiographic studies.

If angiography shows that an endovascular approach is not possible, the first assessment has to be done (Table 2). In a "lower risk AVM" there is the choice of surgical extirpation or conservative treatment, whereas in "high risk AVMs" the malformation has to be extirpated whenever possible to prevent (further) bleeding.

If an endovascular approach is possible, this is performed before surgery with the aim of 1. total casting of the malformation, 2. partial preoperative embolization or 3. at least microangiographic studies.

The so-called "total occlusion" (Table 2) can only be compared to total surgical excision if the nidus is completely casted. A solid acrylic cast should (whenever possible) reach from the entrance of the nidus to the proximal draining vein. This is the only way of endovascular therapy promising a permanent result and cure.

The so-called "partial embolization" (Table 2) is more a functional than an angiographic term. An angiographically occluded AVM may be only partially embolized because of insufficient casting. Blocking of feeding

vessels or partial blocking of the nidus produces a mixture of particles and thrombosis in the AVM, and the AVM will recanalize in the majority of the cases.

For "lower risk AVMs" partial embolization means reduction of shunt, flow and venous pressure. These hemodynamic changes may reduce flow related symptoms like headache, seizures or neurologic deficit. If a satisfying clinical situation could be achieved by partial embolization (illustrative case 1) the surgical excision of the partially embolized AVM is not absolutely necessary. If symptoms reoccur or if screening diagnostics (TCD, MRI) show recent increase of flow, control angiography is performed to evaluate the actual situation. Then it can be decided if further embolization or surgical extirpation has to be done as a next step.

On "high risk AVMs" partial embolization can only be seen as a preoperative tool to facilitate and shorten the surgical extirpation (illustrative case 2). Although partial embolization reduces the pressure in the draining veins, it can not be guaranteed that the risk of rebleeding is diminished. An increase of bleeding risk by partial embolization is not to be expected as long as the venous draining pattern has not been changed by the embolization. A reduction in the number of draining veins by partial embolization however increases the risk of bleeding and requires urgent surgical extirpation.

If partial embolization is performed only by a "partial casting" (i.e., occlusion of feeding arteries, injection of particles or acrylic-drops into the nidus) recanalization is probable. This may occur by the

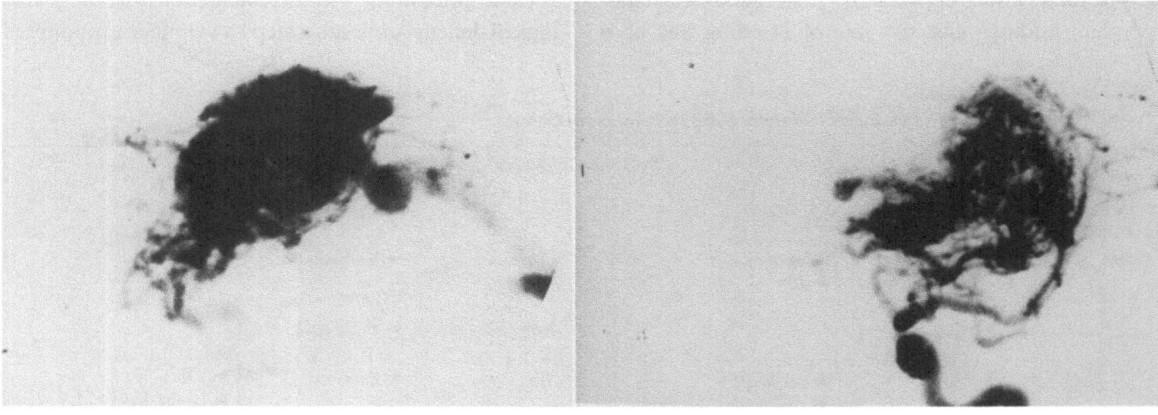

a   b

Fig. 7. A grade V AVM according to the Spetzler and Martin classification[17]. This AVM could only be partially embolized. (a) lateral view, left carotid angiography. (b) ap-view

reopening of occluded feeders but also by the creation of multiple capillary connections between the brain parenchyma and the AVM[5,6,18,19]. This situation makes a surgical procedure more difficult and increases the overall risk of treatment. If a partial embolization is done preoperatively, the time interval between the endovascular procedures and the operation should not exceed 2 to 4 weeks (illustrative case 2).

In the group of "high risk AVMs" only a few cases will be partially embolized and not operated afterwards. These are the rare cases (Fig. 7) where the AVM seems to be surgically inaccessible despite partial embolization: in other words the risk of surgery has been calculated to be higher than the risk of rebleeding. In these cases there is the hope that the reduction of flow and venous pressure will reduce the risk and frequency of bleedings.

An assessment of risks presupposes knowledge about the different risks. Even if we know about the influence of morphological factors like venous drainage and others on the risk of natural history, we are not able to predict exactly if a certain AVM is prone to bleed in the future or not. The risk of natural history therefore is only approximately known and this "approximate knowledge" has to be included in the individual decision. The risk of therapy depends primarily on the skill of the operator. This concerns the endovascular as well as the surgical procedure. Local, institutional circumstances will therefore always influence the risk of therapy, the assessment of risks and the final therapeutic decision.

Addendum

Since the presentation of this paper in June 1992 we have altered our strategy somewhat. With the advent of Gamma-knife-therapy we have the therapeutic option – especially for small AVMs – of radiosurgery. As it has been documented, small AVMs are more prone to bleed and the risk does not decrease after Gamma-knife-therapy. We have found radiosurgery to be of benefit either alone or in combination with endovascular therapy.

References

1. Albert P, Salgado H, Polaina M, Trujillo F, Ponce de Leaon A, Durand F (1990) A study on the venous drainage of 150 cerebral arteriovenous malformations as related to haemorrhagic risks and size of the lesion. Acta Neurochir (Wien) 103: 30–34
2. Andreussi L, Dhellemmes P (1990) Les malformations arterio-veineuses cerebrales, histoire naturelle-propositions therapeutiques. Agressologie 31(5): 237–239
3. Brown RD, Wiebers DO, Forbes G, O'Fallon WM, Piepgras DG, Marsh WR, Maciunas RJ (1988) The natural history of unruptured intracranial arteriovenous malformations. J Neurosurg 68: 352–357
4. Brown RD, Wiebers DO, Forbes GS (1990) Unruptured intracranial aneurysms and arteriovenous malformations: frequency of intracranial hemorrhage and relationship of lesions. J Neurosurg 73: 859–863
5. Fournier D, Terbrugge K, Rodesch G, Lasjaunias P (1990) Revascularization of brain arteriovenous malformations after embolization with brucrylate. Neuroradiology 32: 497–501
6. Germano IM, Davis RL, Wilson CB, Hieshima GB (1992) Histopathological follow-up study of 66 cerebral arteriovenous malformations after therapeutic embolization with polyvinyl alcohol. J Neurosurg 76: 607–614
7. Luessenhop AJ (1984) Natural history of cerebral arteriovenous malformations. In: Wilson CB, Stein BM (eds) Intracranial arteriovenous malformations. Williams and Wilkins, Baltimore, pp 12–23
8. Malik GH, Umansky F, Patel S, Ausman JI (1988) Microsurgical removal of arteriovenous malformations of the basal ganglia. Neurosurgery 23: 209–217
9. Marks MP, Lane B, Steinberg GK, Chang PJ (1990) Hemorrhage in intracerebral arteriovenous malformations: angiographic determinants. Radiology 176: 807–813
10. Marks PM, Lane B, Steinberg G, Chang P (1991) Vascular characteristics of intracranial arteriovenous malformations which correlate with symptoms of hemorrhage and steal. Neuroradiology [Suppl] 33: 184–186
11. Miyasaka Y, Yada K, Ohwada T, Kitahara T, Kurata A, Irikura K (1992) An analysis of the venous drainage system as a factor in hemorrhage from arteriovenous malformations. J Neurosurg 76: 239–243
12. Müller-Forell W, Valavanis A (1991) Neuroradiologische Exploration zerebraler arteriovenöser Gefäßmißbildungen. Radiologe 31: 269–273
13. Nagata S, Matsushima T, Fujii K, Takeshita I, Fukui M, Yasumori K (1991) Lateral ventricular arteriovenous malformations: natural history and surgical indications. Acta Neurochir (Wien) 112(1–2): 37–46
14. Ondra SL, Troupp H, George ED, Schwab K (1990) The natural history of symptomatic arteriovenous malformations of the brain: a 24-year follow-up assessment. J Neurosurg 73: 387–391
15. Shi YQ, Chen XC (1987) Surgical treatment of arteriovenous malformations of the striatothalamocapsular region. J Neurosurg 66: 352–356
16. Solomon RA, Stein BM (1987) Interhemispheric approach for the surgical removal of thalamocaudate arteriovenous malformations. J Neurosurg 66: 345–351
17. Spetzler RF, Martin NA (1988) A proposed grading system for arteriovenous malformations. J Neurosurg 85: 478–483
18. Tomashefski JF Jr., Cohen AM, Doershuk CF (1988) Longterm histopathologic follow-up of bronchial arteries after therapeutic embolization with polyvinyl alcohol (Ivalon) in patients with cystic fibrosis. Hum Pathol 19: 555–561
19. Vinters HV, Lundie MJ, Kaufmann JCE (1986) Long-term pathological follow-up of cerebral arteriovenous malformations treated by embolization with bucrylate. N Engl J Med 314: 477–483

Correspondence: B. Richling, M.D., Department of Neurosurgery, University of Vienna, Medical School, Waehringer Guertel 18–20, A-1090 Vienna , Austria.

Management of Critical Cavernous Malformations

Cavernous Malformations of the Brain Stem

M.G. Hamilton, T.M. Wascher, and **R.F. Spetzler**

Division of Neurological Surgery, Barrow Neurological Institute, Phoenix, Arizona, U.S.A.

Summary

Symptomatic cavernous malformations of the brain stem are uncommon, yet clinically dramatic. These lesions have a distinctive clinical presentation and clinical course, frequently causing severe, progressive neurologic impairment when left untreated. We have combined individualized case selection and surgical planning to treat 24 patients with symptomatic brain stem cavernous malformations. The selection of surgical approach was also individualized for each patient. Outcome was successful in 23 patients, all experiencing significant improvement in their neurological status compared to their preoperative state. One patient death occurred secondary to cerebellar infarction and aspiration pneumonia. These results indicate that with the use of proper selection criteria and surgical planning, patients with these lesions can be successfully surgically managed.

Keywords: Brain stem; cavernous angioma; cavernous malformation.

Introduction

Cavernous malformations have been reported to represent 8–15% of all intracranial vascular malformations, occurring in 0.1–0.5% of the general population[2,19,20,27,31]. Approximately 10–30% of all intracranial cavernous malformations are located within the brain stem and cerebellum and are more frequently symptomatic than their supratentorial counterparts[20]. Cavernous malformations comprise about 13% of all vascular malformations of the posterior fossa[22]. These congenital lesions exist in two forms: familial and sporadic cavernous malformations. As many as 50% of patients with cavernous malformations have a strong family history consistent with an autosomal dominant inheritance pattern, particularly in families of Hispanic descent[29,41].

Symptomatic cavernous malformations of the brain stem have a distinctive clinical presentation and clinical course that often causes severe neurological impairment when left untreated. This chapter discusses the clinical course, diagnosis, surgical indications, and the appropriate surgical management of cavernous malformations involving the brain stem.

Case Material and Results of Surgical Management

The aggressive surgical management of symptomatic cavernous malformations of the infratentorial space can provide favorable results[4,10,16,18,38,43]. Since 1985 the senior author (RFS) has operated on 70 intracranial cavernous malformations, of which 24 (34%) involved the brain stem. Operative indications for these 24 patients included: 1) progressive symptomatology, 2) superficial location of the malformation within the brain stem, and 3) an operative approach that could spare eloquent brain tissue[43].

The average age of these 15 female and 9 male patients was 38.4 ± 13.4 years (range, 14–71 years). Of the 24 patients, 20 (83%) described an acute onset of their symptomatology suggestive of an apopletic event. The neurological deficits at the time of surgery are delineated in Table 1. Nine of these patients had at least one additional lesion within the neuroaxis; six of these 9 patients had other family members with cavernous malformations in accordance with a familial inheritance pattern.

The location of the cavernous malformations and the surgical approaches employed to resect them are detailed in Table 2. The average size of the lesion in this series was 1.6 ± 1.1 cm (range, 0.4 – 4.0 cm). Two patients also had an associated venous malformation (Fig. 1) that required modification of the surgical approach in

Table 1. *Preoperative Neurological Signs and Symptoms in 24 Patients with Brain Stem Cavernous Malformations*

Sign and symptoms*	n	(%)
Facial pain/hypesthesia	13	(54.2)
Hemiparesis	11	(45.8)
Disorder of ocular motility	11	(45.8)
Severe headaches	10	(41.7)
Hemisensory deficit/dysesthesias	10	(41.7)
VII, VIII CN neuropathies	6	(25.0)
IX, X, XI, XII CN neuropathies	7	(29.2)
Ataxia, dysmetria	4	(16.7)
Parinaud's syndrome	2	(8.3)

*A patient may display more than one sign and/or symptom. *CN* cranial nerve.

Table 2. *Location and Surgical Approach Used in 24 Patients with Brain Stem Cavernous Malformations*

Location	n	(%)
Midbrain tectum	3	(12.5)
Supracerebellar infratentorial approach	2	
Occipital transtentorial approach	1	
Midbrain tegmentum	1	(4.2)
Combined approach		
Midbrain crura cerebri	1	(4.2)
Fronto-subtemporal transtentorial approach		
Pontomesencephalic junction	2	(8.3)
Supracerebellar infratentorial approach	1	
Fronto-subtemporal transtentorial approach	1	
Pontine tegmentum		
A) Midline	6	(2.5)
Suboccipital splitting of vermis		
B) Lateral	2	(8.3)
Combined petrosal approach		
Basis pontis	3	(12.5)
Subtemporal transtentorial approach	2	
Fronto-subtemporal transtentorial approach	1	
Pontomedullary junction	2	(8.3)
A) Combined approach	1	
B) Far lateral approach	1	
Medulla	2	(8.3)
Far lateral appraoch		
Cervicomedullary junction	2	(8.3)
Suboccipital approach + C1–C2 laminectomies		

Table 3. *Complications Related to Surgical Management of 24 Patients with Brain Stem Cavernous Malformations*

Complications	n	(%)
Transient		
Hemiparesis	5	(20.1)
Diplopia, disorder of ocular motility	4	(16.7)
VI, VII cranial nerve neuropathy	4	(16.7)
Hydrocephalus, shunt failure	3	(12.5)
Meningitis	2	(8.3)
Lower extremity deep venous thrombosis	2	(8.3)
Gait ataxia	1	(4.2)
IX, X, XI, XII cranial nerve neuropathies	2	(8.3)
Cerebrospinal fluid leak	1	(4.2)
Permanent		
Death (Cerebellar infarction/aspiration pneumonia	1	(4.2)
Dysmetria + internuclear ophthalmoplegia	2	(8.3)
Partial III cranial nerve neuropathy	1	(4.2)
Mild upper and lower extremity dysmetria	1	(4.2)
Mild internuclear ophthalmoplegia	1	(4.2)

one case. An arachnoid cyst and arteriovenous malformation, unrelated to the cavernous malformation, were observed in one patients each. Complete resection, as judged by intraoperative findings and postoperative MR imaging, was possible in 21 of the 24 cases (87.5%). The degree of resection in the remaining three cases was estimated between 90–95%. Histologic examination revealed acute or subacute thrombus in 67% and hemosiderin in 90% of the surgical specimens, thereby indicating the propensity of these lesions to undergo hemorrhage and rehemorrhage.

The median follow-up was 27 ± 22 months. Table 3 details the neurological deficits that appeared after or were exacerbated by surgery. Transient complications refer to neurological deficits that resolved completely. Overall, there was one death that was caused by aspiration pneumonia and cerebellar infarction 4 days after surgery. There was no major morbidity, and a permanent minor morbidity related to surgery occurred in 24% of surviving patients. At their last follow-up examination, all 23 of the surviving patients had experienced significant improvement in their neurological status compared to their preoperative state. These results indicate that symptomatic superficial cavernous malformations of the brain stem can undergo successful surgical treatment by combining individualized planning and case selection with appropriate surgical indications, approaches, and principles.

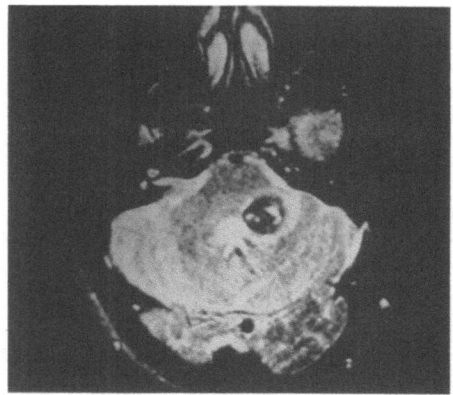 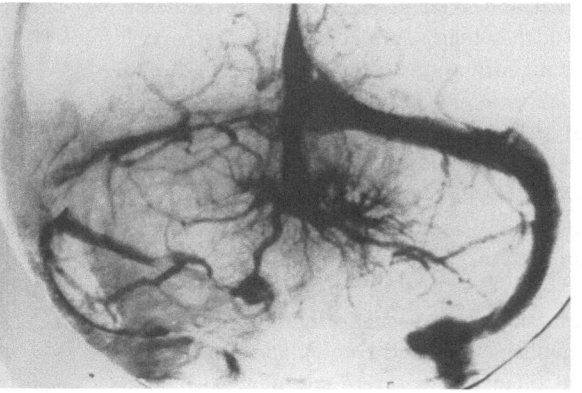

a   b

Fig. 1. (a) Axial, T2-weighted magnetic resonance image demonstrating a cavernous malformation located in the left posterolateral pons. (b) Venous phase of angiogram demonstrating dominant left transverse/sigmoid sinus and large centrally located venous malformation. To avoid affecting the venous malformation, the cavernous malformation was removed by a subtemporal transtentorial approach

Discussion

Clinical Presentation and Natural History

Cavernous malformations of the brain stem typically present in one of two ways: progressive neurological deficits caused by mass effect on adjacent brain stem tracts or nuclei or with the sequelae of hemorrhage. Because of their location, even small brain stem cavernous malformations can be associated with neurological deficits. As with other lesions in this region, neurological signs and symptoms can be predicted based on appropriate clinico-anatomic correlations. The most common signs and symptoms associated with brain stem cavernous malformations are facial pain or hypesthesia, hemiparesis and spasticity, hemisensory deficits and dysesthesia, disorders of ocular motility, and headache.

In contrast to arteriovenous malformations, cavernous malformations of the brain stem rarely bleed into the subarachnoid space or into the ventricular system[43]. This feature is a particularly useful characteristic for differentiating these lesions preoperatively from other causes of hemorrhage within the structures and spaces of the posterior fossa. More commonly, bleeding will occur into the sinusoidal space of the malformation itself, therefore resulting in acute enlargement. Significant hemorrhage into a cavernous malformation is, therefore, typically marked by acute onset of headache, vertigo, nausea, and vomiting associated with the new onset or exacerbation of existing neurological deficit occurring because of the acute change in mass within the brain stem.

The natural history of cavernous malformations has, until recently, been poorly understood. The widespread use of magnetic resonance (MR) imaging has allowed for a more careful examination of this issue. Supratentorial, nonfamilial cavernous malformations appear to hemorrhage at an annualized rate of 0.25–0.7%[31,42], while patients with familial cavernous malformations experience hemorrhage at a substantially higher annualized rate of 6.5% (1.1% per lesion year)[41]. In addition, MR imaging evidence suggests that these lesions are dynamic. Change is possible in both the number and size of lesions and in the MR imaging signal characteristics[26,43]. The appearance of new lesions may actually represent the growth of previously small lesions without symptomatic hemorrhage. The possible mechanisms of growth include either progressive ectasia of the vascular nidus or hemorrhage, microscopic or macroscopic, into the sinusoids of the malformation. Cavernous

malformations of the brain stem, once symptomatic, tend to pursue an aggressive, unrelenting clinical course marked by progressive neurological deterioration[4,31,43]. This downward spiral of neurological impairment may be interspersed with acute exacerbations, followed, in many cases, by some degree of neurological recovery.

Diagnostic Studies

The angiographic features of a cavernous malformation are entirely uncommon and nonspecific: the presence of an avascular region during the capillary phase, with or without mass effect, followed by the exhibition

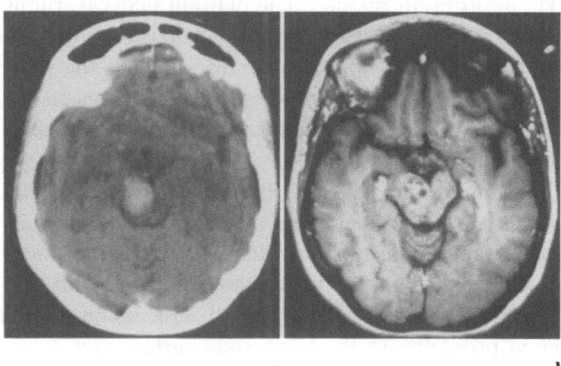

a   b

Fig. 2. (a) Unenhanced axial computed tomography (CT) of a right pontomesencephalic cavernous malformation that had recently hemorrhaged. (b) Corresponding axial, T1-weighted magnetic resonance image of the cavernous malformation identified on CT

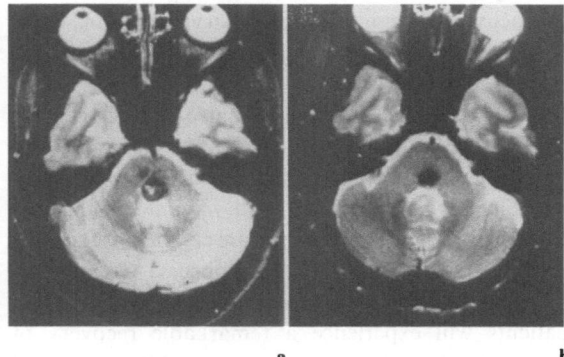

a   b

Fig. 3. (a) Axial, T2-weighted magnetic resonance (MR) image of a cavernous malformation located in the floor of the fourth ventricle in the pons. (b) Axial, T2-weighted postoperative MR image demonstrating complete removal of the lesion. This was accomplished via a suboccipital craniotomy with splitting of the vermis

of a dense venous pooling pattern[28,38]. Computed tomography (CT) improves detection ability only marginally, with the majority of cavernous malformations missed or misdiagnosed with routine enhanced CT imaging (Fig. 2). Only the advent of MR imaging established a technique as a gold standard for detecting cavernous malformations. Cavernous malformations have a highly characterisitc appearance on MR imaging. T2-weighted images reveal a reticulated core of mixed signal intensity surrounded by rim of decreased signal intensity (Fig. 3) that is related to the presence of hemosiderin deposits[28].

Surgical Indications

The appropriate management of brain stem cavernous malformations is safe excision, whenever technically possible. Several reports have documented the poor results that can occur when surgically accessible brain stem cavernous malformations are not treated aggressively[33,43].

Although the general physical and neurological status of the patient with a brain stem cavernous malformation must be considered, specific recommendations regarding the appropriate selection of possible surgical candidates can be offered: 1) the lesion should be in proximity to the brain stem surface and 2) the lesion should be accessible through a surgical approach that spares eloquent brain tissue. Each patient must be evaluated to determine if the deficits resulting from surgery outweigh the risks of expectant management. This last issue is of particular importance when deciding whether to operate upon a symptomatic lesion that is entirely surrounded by functional eloquent brain stem parenchyma. These lesions and asymptomatic brain stem cavernous malformations are usually best treated by close observation.

Specific recommendations can also be made regarding the appropriate time to wait after a brain stem cavernous malformation has hemorrhaged before intervening surgically. Patients with minimal posthemorrhage neurological dysfunction are candidates for early surgery. However, a different approach is required for patients who have an apoplectic event. Many patients will experience a remarkable recovery of neurological function after an ictus and it is beneficial to wait until their neurological status has become optimal before considering surgery.

General Principles of Preoperative and Intraoperative Management

The basis for successful management of brain stem cavernous malformations is the selection of the appropriate surgical approach that optimizes exposure of the lesion but minimizes distortion of the normal neurovascular relationships. There can be no error in localization of the lesion because there is no allowance for surgical exploration of the brain stem. A detailed knowledge of the normal anatomy of all structures associated with the brain stem is a prerequisite for undertaking a procedure of this type.

After localizing the lesion, the surgeion typically encounters a cavity containing a raspberry-like lesion composed of the vascular spaces of the malformation and the degradation products of prior hemorrhage. In contrast to supratentorial cavernous malformations, lesions located within the brain stem can be extremely adherent to the surrounding parenchyma[43]. Initial dissection should, if possible, concentrate upon circumferential separation of the malformation from the zone of surrounding gliosis before internal decompression of the lesion. This approach will devascularize the malformation, for despite the apparent lack of feeding vessels, bleeding can occasionally be quite brisk if the center of the malformation is entered before circumferential dissection[39].

The intracapsular contents are removed in a piecemeal fashion, and the remaining capsule is dissected from the brain stem and nerves. It is rarely advisable to attempt to deliver the intact malformation through a small opening. It is also crucial that all perforating arterial vessels be meticulously dissected free of the malformation and preserved.

As mentioned, a strong association exists between cavernous malformations and venous malformations. The concurrence of these lesions may be as high as 16%[30,43]. Interruption of a venous malformation can threaten the venous drainage of normal parenchyma and cause venous infarction[30]. Therefore, when a venous malformation coexists with a cavernous malformation, the surgical approach to the cavernous malformation must be tailored to preserve the venous drainage of the venous malformation.

Surgical Approaches to Brain Stem Cavernous Malformations

Suboccipital Approach

Lesions of the floor of the fourth ventricle (Fig. 3) and dorsal medulla are easily approached through a standard suboccipital craniotomy[3]. Intraoperative ultrasonography may be useful to guide dissection when the lesion is located within the cerebellar hemisphere and extends into the brain stem. With separation of the cerebellar tonsils or division of the vermis, midline posterior cavernous malformations as far rostral as the dorsal pontine tegmentum can be exposed safely. However, the suboccipital approach provides poor access to ventrally located lesions.

Infratentorial Supracerebellar Approach

The infratentorial supracerebellar approach was originally described by Krause and popularized by Stein[36,37]. The value of this approach is its ability to access malformations involving the tectum (Fig. 4) and pineal region without violation of normal brain parenchyma, while avoiding the deep venous system. The primary limitation of this approach is that it will not allow access to a malformation with significant superolateral extension above the tentorium.

Occipital Transtentorial Approach

The occipital transtentorial approach was originally described by Poppen and later modified by Jamieson[13,24]. This option allows exposure of the superior cerebel-

lar peduncles and vermis, the anterior medullary velum, the posterior third ventricle, the splenium, and the quadrigeminal plate. Compared to the infratentorial supracerebellar approach, this approach provides a broader exposure of the region on the tentorial incisura[26]. However, the occipital transtentorial approach may require retraction of the occipitoparietal lobe, resulting in sensory and visual field defects[37].

Far Lateral Approach

The far lateral approach was first elaborated by Heros[11] and modified by Spetzler[35] for the treatment of vertebrobasilar junction aneurysms. This technique provides an extremely flat approach to the clivus and anterior

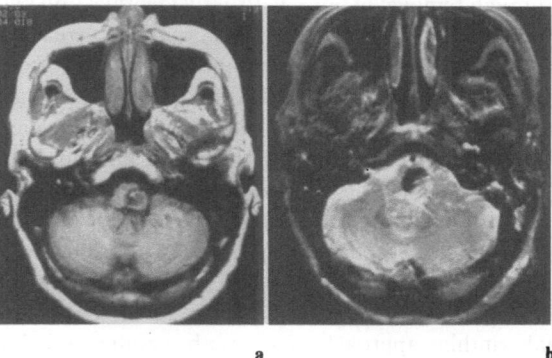

a   b

Fig. 5. (a) Axial, T1-weighted magnetic resonance (MR) image demonstrating a cavernous malformation located in the left lateral medulla. (b) Axial, T2-weighted postoperative MR image demonstrating complete removal of the lesion. This resection was accomplished via a far lateral approach

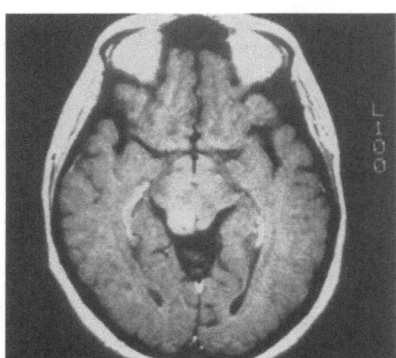

Fig. 4. Axial, T1-weighted magnetic resonance image demonstrating a cavernous malformation located in the right posterior midbrain. This lesion was completely removed by a supracerebellar, infratentorial approach

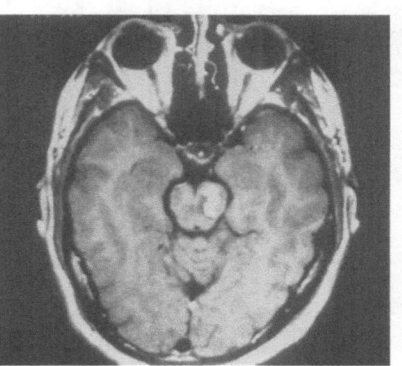

Fig. 6. Axial, T1-weighted magnetic resonance image demonstrating a cavernous malformation located in the left anterior midbrain. This lesion was completely removed by a fronto-subtemporal transtentorial approach

foramen magnum with exposure of the anterior and lateral medulla (Fig. 5), cervicomedullary junction, and associated structures. The critical anterolateral relationships of the inferior cranial nerves and the associated vasculature are exquisitely displayed with the far lateral approach, without retraction of any neurovascular structure.

Transtemporal Approaches

The transtemporal approaches are best suited for providing access to lesions in and around the internal auditory meatus. They are suitable for a patient who has lost serviceable hearing and has a cavernous malformation involving the pontomedullary junction. The principle of these exposures is to access the lesion through removal of bone, with early identification and preservation of the facial nerve, without cerebellar retraction. The translabyrinthine exposure shortens the exposure to the brain stem and provides adequate exposure of the anterolateral pontomedullary junction without brain retraction[5,15]. The translabyrinthine approach can be extended to the transcochlear approach[12] or the transotic approach[5] to expand the exposure and to permit access to the anterior pons. The primary disadvantages include hearing loss and temporary paralysis of the facial nerve if it is transposed. The translabyrinthine approaches can also be combined with a retrosigmoid approach to improve exposure of the lateral pontomedullary junction[8].

Frontotemporal/Subtemporal Transtentorial Approach

Cavernous malformations involving the anterior midbrain-interpeduncular fossa region can be approached adequately through a frontotemporal or a subtemporal craniotomy, as described by Yaargil[40]. This approach can be combined with wide splitting of the sylvian fissure, division of the tentorium[32], and extradural removal of the petrous apex[14] or posterior clinoid process[6]. Although these approaches require a certain degree of retraction, they do allow a direct delineation of the cranial nerves and associated vascular supply of the anterolateral brain stem (Fig. 6).

Combined Approaches

The limitations of exposure to a brain stem cavernous malformation with any of the preceding approaches can often be overcome by using a combination of these approaches. The combined petrosal approach, as first described by Malis[17], involves a combination of subtemporal, transtentorial, and retrosigmoid approaches with division of the sigmoid sinus. This combination provides excellent exposure to the upper two-thirds of the brain stem (Fig. 7), without retraction of neurovascular structures. Hearing and facial nerve function are typically spared[17]. The petrosal modification of this combined approach, as originally described by Al-Mefty[1], involves more extensive drilling of the tempo-

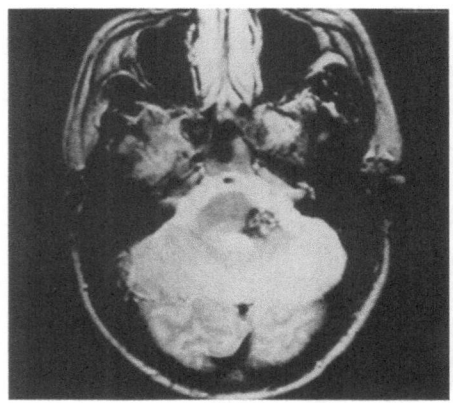
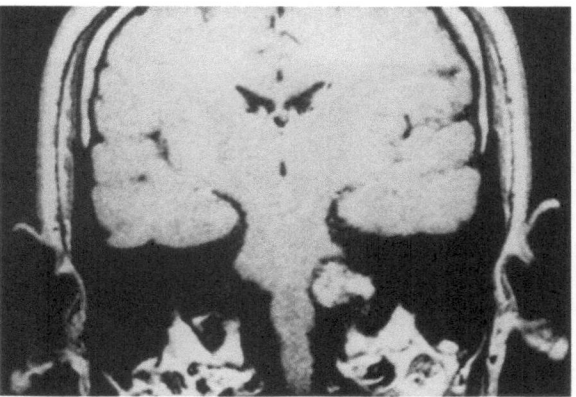

a   b

Fig. 7. (a) Axial, T2-weighted magnetic resonance (MR) image demonstrating a cavernous malformation located in the left middle cerebellar peduncle. (b) Coronal, T1-weighted MR image demonstrating the same lesion. This cavernous malformation was completely removed using a combined petrosal approach

ral petrous bone to permit a more direct and shorter line of sight to the anterolateral brain stem[34].

In addition, combined suboccipital-petrosal, retro-auricular and preauricular transpetrosal-transtentorial, anterior transpetrosal-transtentorial, and suboccipital-translabyrinthine approaches can be used to achieve access to brain stem cavernous malformations[7,9,14,34]. With the combination of the far lateral suboccipital, translabyrinthine, subtemporal, and transtentorial approaches (referred to as the *extensive combined* or the *far lateral-combined* approach), the entire anterior and lateral brain stem and craniovertebral junction and associated cranial nerves and vascular structures can be visualized (Spetzler, unpublished data).

Selection of the Appropriate Surgical Approach

The selection of the optimal surgical approach to a brain stem cavernous malformation requires the integration of a number of variables. In a given patient, the preexisting neurological condition; location of the lesion, both within the brain stem and in relation to the surface of the brain stem; size of the lesion (determined with high resolution, multiplanar or three-dimensional MR imaging); the presence of associated anomalies (venous malformation, arteriovenous malformation, bone defects); and the technical advantages and limitations of the previously described surgical approaches must all be weighed to determine whether surgical intervention is technically feasible, which approach is optimal, and if the potential surgical risks and neurological deficits would be acceptable to the patient.

References

1. Al-Mefty O, Fox JL, Smith RR (1988) Petrosal approach for petroclival meningiomas. Neurosurgery 22: 510–517
2. Curling OD Jr, Kelly DL Jr, Elster AD, Craven TE (1991) An analysis of the natural history of cavernous angiomas. J Neurosurg 75: 702–708
3. De Oliveira E, Rhoton AL Jr, Peace D (1985) Microsurgical anatomy of the region of the foramen magnum. Surg Neurol 24: 293–352
4. Fahlbusch R, Strauss C, Huk W, Rockelein G, Kompf D, Ruprecht KW (1990) Surgical removal of pontomesencephalic cavernous hemangiomas. Neurosurgery 26: 449–457
5. Fisch U, Mattox D (1988) Microsurgery of the skull base. Thieme, New York, pp 74–131, 546–577
6. Fujitsu K, Kuwabara T (1985) Zygomatic approach for lesions in the interpeduncular cistern. J Neurosurg 62: 340–343
7. Glasscock ME III, Gulya AJ, Pensak ML (1984) Surgery of the posterior fossa. Otolaryngol Clin North Am 17(3): 483–497
8. Glasscock ME III, Hays JW, Jackson CG, Steenerson RL (1978) A one-stage combined approach for the management of large cerebellopontine angle tumors. Laryngoscope 88: 1563–1576
9. Hakuba A, Nishimura S, Jang BJ (1988) A combined retroauricular and preauricular transpetrosal-transtentorial approach to clivus meningiomas. Surg Neurol 30: 108–116
10. Heffez DS, Zinreich SJ, Long DM (1990) Surgical resection of intrinsic brain stem lesions: an overview. Neurosurgery 27: 789–798
11. Heros RC (1986) Lateral suboccipital approach for vertebral and vertebrobasilar artery lesions. J Neurosurg 64: 559–562
12. House WF, Hitselberger WE (1976) The transcochlear approach to the skull base. Arch Otolaryngol 102: 334–342
13. Jamieson KG (1971) Excision of pineal tumors. J Neurosurg 35: 550–553
14. Kawase T, Shiobara R, Toya S (1991) Anterior transpetrosal-transtentorial approach for sphenopetroclival meningiomas: surgical method and results in 10 patients. Neurosurgery 28: 869–876
15. King TT, Morrison AW (1988) Translabyrinthine operation for the removal of acoustic nerve tumors. In: Schmidek HH, Sweet WH (eds) Operative neurosurgical techniques. Grune and Stratton, Orlando, pp 685–704
16. LeDoux MS, Aronin PA, Odrezin GT (1991) Surgically treated cavernous angiomas of the brain stem: report of two cases and review of the literature. Surg Neurol 35: 395–399
17. Malis LI (1985) Surgical resection of tumors of the skull base. In: Wilkins RH, Rengachary SS (eds) Neurosurgery. McGraw Hill, New York, pp 1011–1021
18. Mangiardi JR (1991) The surgical management of brainstem hematomas. Perspect Neurol Surg 2(1): 33–48
19. Martin NA, Wilson CB, Stein BM (1984) Venous and cavernous malformations. In: Wilson CB, Stein BM (eds) Intracranial arteriovenous malformations. Williams and Wilkins, Baltimore, pp 234–245
20. McCormick PC, Michelsen WJ (1990) Management of intracranial cavernous and venous malformations. In: Barrow DL (ed) Intracranial vascular malformations. American Association of Neurological Surgeons, Park Ridge, pp 197–217
21. McCormick WF (1969) Vascular disorders of nervous tissue: anomalies, malformations, and aneurysms, In: Bourne GH (ed) Structure and function of nervous tissue. Vol III, biochemistry and disease. Academic, New York, pp 537–596
22. McCormick WF, Hardam JM, Boulter TR (1968) Vascular malformations ("angiomas") of the brain, with special reference to those occurring in the posterior fossa. J Neurosurg 28: 241–251
23. Pendl G, Vorkapic P, Koniyama M (1990) Microsurgery of midbrain lesions. Neurosurgery 26: 641–648
24. Poppen JL (1966) The right occipital approach to a pinealoma. J Neurosurg 25: 706–710
25. Pozzati E, Giuliani G, Nuzzo G, Poppi M (1989) The growth of cerebral cavernous angiomas. Neurosurgery 25: 92–97
26. Reid WS, Clark WK (1978) Comparison of the infratentorial and transtentorial approaches to the pineal region. Neurosurgery 3: 1–8
27. Rigamonti D (1990) Natural history of cavernous malformations, capillary malformations (telangiectases), and venous malformations. In: Barrow DL (ed) Intracranial vascular malformations. Neurosurgical topics. American Association of Neurological Surgeons, Park Ridge, pp 45–51
28. Rigamonti D, Drayer BP, Johnson PC, Hadley MN, Zabramski J, Spetzler RF (1987) The MRI appearance of cavernous malformations (angiomas). J Neurosurg 67: 518–524
29. Rigamonti D, Hadley MN, Drayer BP, Johnson PC, Hoenig-Rigamonti K, Knight JT, Spetzler RF (1988) Cerebral cavernous malformations. Incidence and familial occurrence. N Engl J Med 319(6): 343–347
30. Rigamonti D, Spetzler RF (1988) The association of venous and

cavernous malformations. Report of four cases and discussion of the pathophysiological, diagnostic, therapeutic implications. Acta Neurochir (Wien) 92: 100–105

31. Robinson JR, Awad IA, Little JR (1991) Natural history of the cavernous angioma. J Neurosurg 75: 709–714
32. Rosomoff HL (1971) The subtemporal transtentorial approach to the cerebellopontine angle. Laryngoscope 81(9): 1448–1454
33. Simard JM, Garcia-Bengochea F, Ballinger WE, Mickle JP, Quisling RG (1986) Cavernous angiomas: a review of 126 collected and 12 new cases. Neurosurgery 18: 162–172
34. Spetzler RF, Daspit CP, Pappas CTE (1992) The combined supra- and infratentorial approach for lesions of the petrous and clival region: experience with 46 cases. J Neurosurg 76: 588–599
35. Spetzler RF, Grahm TW (1990) The far-lateral approach to the inferior clivus and the upper cervical region: technical note. BNI Quarterly 6(4): 35–38
36. Stein BM (1971) The infratentorial supracerebellar approach to pineal lesions. J Neurosurg 35: 197–202
37. Stein BM, Bruce JN, Fetell MR (1990) Surgical approaches to pineal tumors. In: Wilkins RH, Rengachary SS (eds) Neurosurgery update I. Diagnosis, operative technique, and neuro-oncology. McGraw Hill, New York, pp 389–398

38. Vaquero J, Carrillo R, Cabezudo J, Leunda G, Villoria F, Bravo G (1980) Cavernous angiomas of the pineal region. Report of two cases. J Neurosurg 53: 833–835
39. Yaşargil MG, Curcic M, Kis M, Teddy PJ, Valavanis A (1988) Microneurosurgery, IIIB. Thieme, New York
40. Yaşargil MG, Smith RD, Young PH, Teddy PJ (1984) Microneurosurgery I. Thieme, New York
41. Zabramski JM, Wascher TM, Johnson B, Golfinos J, Drayer B, Brown B, Spetzler RF (1994) The natural history of familial cavernous malformations: the results of an ongoing study. J Neurosurg (in press)
42. Zentner J, Hassler W, Gawehn J, Schroth G (1989) Intramedullary cavernous angiomas. Surg Neurol 31: 64–68
43. Zimmerman RS, Spetzler RF, Lee KS, Zabramski JM, Hargraves RW (1991) Cavernous malformations of the brain stem. J Neurosurg 75: 32–39

Correspondence: M.G. Hamilton, M.D., Division of Neurosurgery, Alberta Children's Hospital, 1820 Richmond Road, S.W., Calgary, Alberta T2T 5C7, Canada.

Cavernomas of the Basal Ganglia, Brain Stem and Spinal Cord. Surgical Strategy and Results

J.M. Gilsbach and **H. Bertalanffy**

Neurosurgical Department, Technical University (RWTH) Aachen, Federal Republic of Germany

Summary

Fourty-one surgically treated cavernomas of the basal ganglia and insula (15 cases), the midbrain (6 cases), the pons (12 cases), medulla oblongata (1 case) and spinal cord (7 cases) are presented. Surgical morbidity was mainly caused by lesions in the region of the approach if the cavernoma did not have contact to the pial or ventricular surface or by inadvertent occlusion of small perforating arteries or accompanying venous anomalies. The most problematic cases were basal ganglia cavernomas with surgically (vascular) induced capsular deficits. Four out of 5 patients with a fair to poor outcome due to surgical complications belonged to this group. The other had a midbrain cavernoma. The overall results (GOS) were good in 29 patients, fair in 8 and poor in 4. No patient died. Compared to the risky spontanous course, the calculable risk of surgical treatment can be accepted as one treatment principle.

Keywords: Cavernous angioma; deep seated; surgical treatment; results.

Introduction

The natural history of untreated cavernomas is not perfectly understood. Cavernomas bleed and rebleed in an unpredictable severity and period of time with a probability of 0.25–0.7% per year[3,12]. The aim of surgical treatment is the prevention of rebleeding. Additional aims can be the removal of an actual space-occupying hematoma or the mass effect by an enlarging cavernoma or the treatment of epileptic seizures by resection of surrounding gliotic tissue. The indication for surgery is dependent upon the expected surgical risk, that means mainly on the location and the accessibility of the cavernoma[1,22]. Published results on deep-seated or brain stem cavernomas are astonishingly good, especially if the lesion reached the surface of the brain[1,4,7,8–10,15,21]. Today symptomatic cavernomas with bleeding events are advised to be operated on if the surgical risk is acceptable. The main problem is however to predict the surgical morbidity for the individual patient. In order to elucidate the problem further, we reevaluated our series of cavernoma patients to find out which factors predict a good surgical outcome or morbidity.

Patients and Methods

Alltogether 41 patients were operated on deep seated cavernomas. The first 26 patients whose results were publised earlier[7] underwent the surgical procedure between 1983 and 1989 at the University Clinic of Freiburg when both authors worked there. The last 15 were treated between 1989 and March 1992 in Aachen since the serior author works there. Preoperatively all patients had a standard CT-scan and MR investigation as well as an angiography to visualize accompanying venous anomalies commonly described as venous angiomas. The choice of the approach was mainly based on the axial and coronal MR slices. Symptomatic cavernomas were operated upon if they contacted the pial or ventricular surface or if the covering brain substance was not thicker than approximately 2 mm and contained no functionally important tissue. No attempt was made to remove the yellowish surrounding gliotic tissue like in supratentorial cavernomas in order to remove the epileptic focus. Only the abnormal, mulberry-like vessels were progressively shrunk together with bipolar coagulation and finally removed. After poor results in the first cases due to occlusion of accompanying venous anomalies we strictly preserved large veins or additional venous angiomas which drained normal tissue and tried to preserve adherent small transit arteries.

In 12 out of 15 insular and basal ganglia cavernomas, reaching the gyri breves insulae or the gyrus longus insulae, a transsylvian approach was used. Out of them a pterional variant was used 4 times in lesions of the region of the amygdaloid body and the temporal peduncle. Only two cavernomas reached the brain surface at the intraventricular aspect of the thalamus. They were operated upon via an interhemispheric, transcallosal, transventricular route. In one the lesion was exposed using a subtemporal approach. The approach to 6 midbrain lesions was in all cases an infratentorial-supracerebellar one. For cavernomas in and near the midline the approach was chosen above the culmen cerebelli. For lateralized processes in the collicular or peduncular region a unilateral route above the quadrangular lobe was preferred. Eight of the 12 pontine cavernomas had close relationships to the floor of the 4th ventricle with or without a thin covering of ependyma. They were removed via a midline approach between the tonsil and uvula cerebelli in order to avoid splitting of the vermis. Four had lateralized surface relationships. They were approached via the cerebellopontine angle. In the one patient with a lesion in the olivar region an extreme lateral paracondylar approach[2] was used. Six out of 7 patients with spinal cord cavernomas underwent laminectomy and one hemilaminectomy. A lateral transmedullary approach was used in 5 patients because the malformation or the bleeding contacted the surface excentrically mostly in the dorsal root entry zone. In two a classical median myelotomy was used, because of a deep and median location of the cavernoma.

Retrospective analysis included a complete chart review and a follow-up 1 month to 4.5 years postoperatively.

Results

The results are detailed in Table 1. Eight out of 15 patients with basal ganglia and insular cavernomas had no or only transient surgically induced deficits. In 4 additional patients with the same cavernoma location, new or worsened deficits related to surgery were slight or moderate but permanent, a further 3 presented permanent and severe deficits. In 2 of these patients

long-lasting deficits were due to lesions of perforating arteries supplying the internal capsule and in two others the consequence of an occlusion of an accompanying venous drainage anomaly; the other 3 could be explained by direct lesions in the region of the approach, that means they were more or less inevitable. According to the Glasgow Outcome Scale (GOS) the overall result of this group was good in 8/15, fair in 5/15 and poor in 2/15. The morbidity was caused in all cases by surgery and not by the lesion itself.

The course after removal of 6 midbrain cavernomas was relatively benign. Five out of the 6 patients had a good result, one of them suffered temporary ataxia and hemihypesthesia due to local surgical irritation. One with a fair outcome due to persistent ataxia and dysarthria had an incompletely removed cavernoma which rebled and had to be reoperated.

Table 1

Name	Age	Location	Surgical approach	Clinical picture	Immediate new/ worsended p.o.deficits	Cause of new deficits	Outcome GOS
W, S, m	5	thalamus, capsula int.	interhemispheric transcallosal	slight hemiparesis	temporary hemiplegia	local rebleed, residual cavernoma	fair
W, G, f	36	basal ganglia	transsylvian	slight hemiparesis	hemiparesis worse, aphasia	direct internal capsular lesion	poor
M, C, f	25	insula/ capsula int.	transsylvian	fine motor impairment	temporary hemiplegia	arterial infarction, perforator lesion	fair
B, G, m	24	insula/ capsula int.	transsylvian	hemihypesthesia	severe hemiparesis, aphasia	venous infarction, venous anomaly	poor
S, P, m	30	thalamus/ peduncle	interhemispheric transcallosal	slight hemiparesis	hemiplegia, amnesia	venous infarction, thalamus	fair
K, B, f	31	insula, temporal peduncle	transsylvian	seizures	no	–	good
N, K, f	50	temporal peduncle	transsylvian	progressive hemiparesis	hemiparesis worse, temporary aphasia	direct capsular lesion	good
M, A, m	45	post. capsula int.	transsylvian	hemihypesthesia	no	–	good
S, B, m	42	insula	transsylvian	seizures, hemihypesthesia	no	–	good
S, I, f	42	insula/temp. ped.	transsylvian	seizures	no	–	good
M, M, f	55	insula	transsylvian	hemianopia	temporary hemiparesis, hemihypesthesia	direct capsular lesion	fair
K, O, m	49	insula/peduncle	subtemporal	hemianopia	hemianopia worse, temporary hemiparesis	direct irritation	good
P, K, f	63	insula	transsylvian	vertigo, no deficits	temporary hemihypesthesia	direct irritation	good
A, I, m	55	insula/ peduncle	pterional	slight hemiparesis	hemiplegia, aphasia	perforator lesion, infarction	fair
N, I, m	42	temp. peduncle/ gyrus parahip.	transsylvian	seizures, CN III incomplete	–	–	good
M, A, m	51	midbrain	infratentorial/ supracerebellar	ataxia, hemihypesthesia	ataxia worse, hemihypesthesia	direct irritation	good
S, I, m	33	colliculus inferior	infratentorial/ supracerebellar	hypesth V3, hemihypesthesia	no	–	good

Table 1 (continued)

Name	Age	Location	Surgical approach	Clinical picture	Immediate new/ worsended p.o.deficits	Cause of new deficits	Outcome GOS
O, R, m	28	quadrigeminal plate	infratentorial/ supracerebellar	hydrocephalus, shunt	no	–	good
O, R, m	13	quadrigeminal plate	infratentorial/ supracerebellar	hydrocephalus	no	–	good
L, R, f	38	quadrigeminal plate	infratentorial/ supracerebellar	hydrocephalus	no	–	good
H, E, f	47	midbrain	infratentorial/ supracerebellar	numbness, ataxia, dysarthria	ataxia, dysarthria worse	rebleed, residual cavernoma	fair
B, B, f	27	pons, lateral	cerebello-pontine angle	progressive hemiparesis, somnolence	CN V + VII	direct irritation	fair
L, R, m	39	inf. cerebellar peduncle	transventricular, 4th	ataxia, CN VI	no	–	good
S, K–H, m	56	pons, dorsal	transventricular, 4th	gait ataxia, CN III	temporary worsened ataxia	direct irritation	good
B, H, m	50	pons, dorsal	transventricular, 4th	–	no	–	good
L, S, m	6	pons, dorsal	transventricular, 4th	–	no	–	good
M, F, m	42	pons, lateral	transventricular, 4th	ataxia, diplopia	no	–	good
S, U, f	49	pons, brachium	cerebello-pontine angle	diplopia, gait ataxia	no	–	good
R, B, f	41	pons, lateral	cerebello-pontine angle	facial numbness	bil. ataxia, CN IV, VIII	direct lesion CN III, pons	good
S, M, m	30	pons, dorsal	transventricular, 4th	CN VII, VI, VIII III, hemiparesis	no	direct irritation	good
L, K, m	50	pons, dorsolateral	cerebello-pontine angle	hypesthesia trunk & face	temporary hypesthesia	direct irritation	good
K, S, m	13	pons	transventricular	diplopia, hemiparesis	temporary hemiparesis, CN VI, VII	direct lesion	good
R, S, f	53	pons, dorsal	transventricular, 4th	CN VII, VIII, IX, X, XI, ataxia, hemihypesthesia	paradoxical air embolism severe cerebral demage	–	poor
K, C, f	45	oliva	lateral paracondylar	CN III, dysarthria hemihypesthesia	CN IX + X	direct CN/nuclear lesion	good
A, B, m	50	C3/4	laminectomy, C3–5, lateral	hemiataxia, hemiparesis hemihypesthesia	–	–	fair
C, H, m	68	C1/2	laminectomy, C2, lateral	acute tetraplegia, respiratory insufficiency	–	–	poor
S, m	40	C1/2	laminectomy, C1/2/occiput	ataxia, tetraparesis	–	–	good
E, K–H, m	49	D11	laminectomy D11	progressive paraparesis hypesthesia	worsened ataxia	–	good
B, S, f	40	D10	laminectomy, D9–10, medial	rebleed, progressive paraparesis	hypesthesia worsened, ataxia	direct lesion	good
K, I, f	53	D1	hemilaminectomy, D2, lateral	progressive hemiparesis hypesthesia left leg	temporary worsening hemiparesis	direct irritation	good
V, H, f	30	D11/12	laminectomy, D11/12, lateral	hypesthesia, hemiparesis	hemihypesthesia, dorsal column deficits	direct lesion	good

Nine of the 12 patients with pontine cavernomas showed no, or only transient surgical morbidity. One suffered severe ischemic cerebral damage due to paradoxical air embolism during the surgical procedure in the sitting position. Two developed new deficits postoperatively due to local lesions. Altogether 11 had a good outcome and one a fair due to preexisting deficits. The only patient with a cavernoma of the medulla oblongata had a good outcome with persistent hoarseness probably due to a surgical lesion of the nucleus of the 10th cranial nerve.

Four of the 7 patients with spinal cord cavernomas did not offer new nor worsened postoperative deficits. In 2 slight dorsal column deficits could be observed postoperatively, and one had a temporary monoparesis.

Discussion

Indication

Easily accessible supratentorial cavernomas are normally recommended to be excised at least if they have become symptomatic. In principle this holds true also for deep-seated lesions, provided that they can be removed with an acceptable surgical risk, which should be lower than that of the spontaneous course. The risk of the natural course however is not fully understood. Nearly all cavernomas show evidence of hemorrhage, either microscopic or large[16] and some grow and become symptomatic due to a mass effect. The yearly bleeding risk is still not precisely known[16,19]. In the most recent papers on this topic it is calculated between 0.25 and 0.7 percent per person-year[3,12]. In brain stem cavernomas, a hemorrhage as well as a growing cavernoma mass can be much more deleterious than in hemispheric ones[7,12,16,21,22]. The factors which could enable us to calculate an individual risk like in arteriovenous malformations are, however, not clear.

The benefit of surgery includes the elimination of the bleeding risk and mass effect. That means the main risk of the natural course can be prevented and in addition some patients profit from the removal of the blood clot or the cavernoma mass. The surgical risk is however not seen unequivocally. Some authors judge it higher than that of the natural course and prefer a more conservative attitude, especially in benign clinical pictures[6,13] and if a layer of normal brain tissue is between cavernoma and pial surface[22]. The growing number of reports on operated deep seated cavernous malformations proves however, that surgery is accepted as one

treatment principle, expecially if the presumed operative risk is low or acceptable, that means in superficially located, symptomatic cavernomas[1,4,5,7,9,17,18,20-22]. With the available data and without prospective, possibly randomised series, it is, however, still impossible today to determine the individual surgical risk versus conservative management.

Technique

The 4 patients with arterial and venous infarctions in the internal capsule taught us to be extremely careful with vessels not belonging to the cavernoma. Especially transit or adherent perforating arteries in insular and basal ganglia cavernomas and in incidental venous angiomas posed problems. In the future, these problems can perhaps be avoided by a better microsurgical technique and an increased attention to additional venous "angiomas" during diagnostic and preoperative surgical planning. The presence or absence of anomalous draining veins should be excluded in all cases by a preoperative angiographic investigation, including the opacification of the veins. This problem is mentioned now more frequently in recent publications while it was more or less neglected in the first papers dealing with the surgical treatment of cavernomas[1,11,14,22]. The 20 patients with temporary or permanent local irritations or lesions of functionally important structures prove that the planning of the approach and the quality of dissection should be improved further. The risk of provoking new deficits or of worsening preexisting ones increases with the distance of the cavernoma to the brain surface. The thicker the substance to penetrate, the higher the risk. One of the disadvantages of those deep-seated, unvisible lesions is the lack of landmarks and information as to which functions are represented in the layer to be penetrated. The chance to destroy functionally important tissue around the cavernoma is low once the approach is open. The gliotic yellowish perifocal reactive scar tissue is relatively resistant to mechanical stimuli and prevents damage of the surrounding tissue[21,22]. The dissection of the mulberry vessels of the cavernoma is nearly bloodless and can easily be achieved by pure bipolar coagulation. Additional blunt or sharp dissection is often not necessary because the shrinkage is sufficient to separate the cavernoma from the brain tissue.

Conclusions

The relatively low incidence of permanent and severe deficits due to surgery shows that surgery in the brain stem, basal ganglia and medulla is principally possible with an acceptable surgical morbidity, provided the lesion reaches the surface and vascular accidents on adjacent vessels can be avoided.

References

1. Bertalanffy H, Gilsbach JM, Eggert H-R, Seeger W (1991) Microsurgery of deep-seated cavernous angiomas: report of 26 cases. Acta Neurochir (Wien) 108: 91–99
2. Bertalanffy H, Seeger W (1991) The dorsolateral, suboccipital, transcondylar approach to the lower clivus and anterior portion of the craniocervical junction. Neurosurgery 29: 815–821
3. Del Curling O, Kelly DL, Elster AD, Craven TE (1991) An analysis of the natural history of cavernous angiomas. J Neurosurg 75: 702–709
4. Fahlbusch R, Strauss C, Huk W, Röckelein G, Kömpf D, Ruprecht KW (1990) Surgical removal of pontomesencephalic cavernous hemangiomas. Neurosurgery 26: 449–457
5. Giombini S, Morello G (1978) Cavernous angiomas of the brain. Account for fourteen personal cases and review of the literature. Acta Neurochir (Wien) 40: 61–82
6. Kashiwagi S, van Loveren HR, Tew JM Jr (1990) Diagnosis and treatment of vascular brain-stem malformations. J Neurosurg 72: 27–34
7. Ledoux MS, Aronin PA, Odrezin GT (1991) Surgically treated cavernous angiomas of the brain stem: report of two cases and review of the literature. Surg Neurol 35: 395–399
8. Ogawa A, Katakura R, Yoshimoto T (1990) Third ventricle cavernous angioma: report of two cases. Surg Neurol 34: 414–420
9. Ondra SL, Doty JR, Mahla ME, George ED (1988) Surgical excision of a cavernous hemangioma of the rostral brain stem: case report. Neurosurgery 23: 490–493
10. Pozzatti E, Gaist G, Poppi M, Morrone B, Padovani R (1981) Microsurgical removal of paraventricular cavernous angiomas. J Neurosurg 55: 308–311
11. Rigamonti D, Spetzler RF (1988) The association of venous and cavernous malformations. Report of four cases and discussion of the pathophysiological, diagnostic, and therapeutic implications. Acta Neurochir (Wien) 92: 100–105
12. Robinson JR, Awad IA, Little JR (1991) Natural history of the cavernous angioma. J Neurosurg 75: 709–714
13. Roda JM, Alvarez F, Isla A (1990) Thalamic cavernous malformation: case report. J Neurosurg 72: 637–649
14. Sasaki O, Tanaka R, Koike T, Koide A, Koizumi T, Ogawa H (1991) Excision of cavernous angioma with preservation of coexisting angioma. J Neurosurg 75: 461–464
15. Seifert V, Gaab MR (1989) Laser-assisted microsurgical extirpation of a brain stem cavernoma: case report. Neurosurgery 25: 986–990
16. Simard JM, Garcia-Bengochera F, Ballinger WE Jr, Mickle JP, Quisling RG (1986) Cavernous angioma: a review of 126 collected and 12 new clinical cases. Neurosurgery 18: 162–172
17. Tatagiba M, Schönmayr R, Samii M (1991) Intraventricular cavernous angioma. A survey. Acta Neurochir (Wien) 110: 140–145
18. Vaquero J, Salazar, Martinez R, Martinez P, Bravo G (1987) Cavernomas of the central nervous system: clinical syndromes, CT scan diagnosis, and prognosis after surgical treatment in 25 cases. Acta Neurochir (Wien) 85: 29–33
19. Wilkins RH (1985) Natural history of intracranial vascular malformations. A review. Neurosurgery 16: 421–430
20. Yasargil MG (1988) Microneurosurgery, Vol IIIB. Thieme. Stuttgart pp 419–434
21. Yoshimoto T, Suzuki J (1986) Radical surgery on cavernous angioma of the brain stem. Surg Neurol 26: 72–78
22. Zimmermann RS, Spetzler RF, Lee KS, Zabramski JM, Hargraves RW (1991) Cavernous malformations of the brain stem. J Neurosurg 75: 32–39

Correspondence: J.M. Gilsbach, M.D., Neurosurgical Department, Technical University (RWTH) Aachen, D-52074 Aachen, Federal Republic of Germany.

Sellar and Parasellar Extra-Axial Cavernous Hemangiomas

D. Lombardi, F.B. Meyer[1], B.W. Scheithauer[2], M. Losa, and **M. Giovanelli Barilari**

Clinica Neurochirurgica, I.R.C.C.S. Ospedale S. Raffaele, Università di Milano, Italy
Department of [1]Neurosurgery and [2]Surgical Pathology, Mayo Clinic, Rochester, U.S.A.

Summary

Extra-axial cavernous hemangiomas involving the cavernous sinus in the sellar and parasellar region, are rare lesions previously associated with unacceptable surgical mortality and morbidity. Eight cases arising from the cavernous sinus, seven with endophytic growth and one esophytic, are analyzed according to clinical presentation, histology, surgical results and long-term follow-up.

Keywords: Sellar and parasellar lesion; cavernous hemangiomas; cavernous sinus; pituitary tumor.

Introduction

Extra-axial cavernous hemangiomas are rare vascular lesions considered distinct clinical entities from intra-parenchimal cavernous hemangiomas, despite similar pathological diagnosis[11]. Infact they differ in clinical presentation, radiological imaging[9], surgical mortality and morbidity[7]. There are approximately 22 published reports of attempted surgical resection of extra-axial cavernous hemangiomas in the middle fossa, achieving total removal only in 13.6% of the cases, with a perioperative mortality rate of 38%[1,5 – 7,10,12]. For this reason radiation therapy has been proposed as primary treatment[8,13].

In this report we analyze eight cases of cavernous hemangiomas involving the cavernous sinus collected reviewing the files of the Mayo Clinic, Rochester, Minnesota (U.S.A.)* and of the H.S. Raffaele, Milan (Italy).

Summary of Cases

Clinical Material

Between 1975 and 1991, eight patients, six female and two male, underwent surgery for extra-axial cavernous hemangiomas arising

---

* The Mayo clinic analyzed cases were pair of a previously published casistic regarding cavernous hemangiomas of the dural sinuses[4].

from the cavernous sinus, and extending in the sellar and parasellar region. Their clinical presentation is summarized in Table 1. Most symptoms and signs were due to compression and encasement of the cranial nerves by the tumor, in the cavernous sinus.

Two cases, in which the tumor was growing medially into the sellar region, presented with pure neuroendocrinological symptoms related to hypothalamic-pituitary deconnection.

Neuroradiological studies were not diagnostic in all cases. Five cases were misdiagnosed as meningiomas, two cases as pituitary adenomas and in the last case a IIIrd cranial nerve neurinoma was suspected. Rx skull in two cases, in which the tumor was growing medially toward the sella turcica showed eroded double floor sella. CT-scan, performed in all the cases showed an isodense lesion with marked enhancement after contrast administration. MRI, performed in four cases, showed an isodense mass in T1 with a peculiar hyperintensity in T2. MRI permitted a better definition of the intra-cavernous growth of the tumor but did not identify the vascular nature of the mass. Angiography, performed in 6 cases, demonstrated the encasement of the carotid artery with late capillary blush in 4 cases, and meningohypophiseal feeding arteries in 5 cases.

Histological Findings

Microscopically, each lesion consisted of endothelial-lined vascular spaces devoid of muscolature and possessing only a small quantity of poorly organized elastic tissue, varying from capillary to cavernous in dimension. Thrombosis with features of organization was apparent in five specimens; hemosiderin deposition was absent in all but two cases in which it was scant. In one case some large myelinated nerves were found lying adjacent to the dura. Dural attachment was clearly visible in four specimens in which the sinus dura appeared to represent a portion of the tumor capsule (Fig. 1).

Surgical Results

In seven cases the hemangioma appeared to arise within the cavernous sinus, causing expansion of the sinus with the dura forming the outer tumor capsule. In one case the tumor with sinus esophytic growth, was encasing the IIIrd cranial nerve at its entry in the cavernous sinus.

In five cases the tumor appeared as a dumbbell-shaped lesion both in the middle cranial fossa and in the cavernous sinus region, in two cases was growing medially toward the sellar region and in the case with sinus esophytic growth was presenting as a round mass in the middle cranial fossa.

Table 1. *Presenting Signs and Symptoms*

Headache	5
Diplopia	5
Facial numbness	3
Ptosis	3
Amenorrhea	2
Galactorrhea	2
Prolactin $> 80\mu g/l$	2
Symptoms associated with pregnancy	3

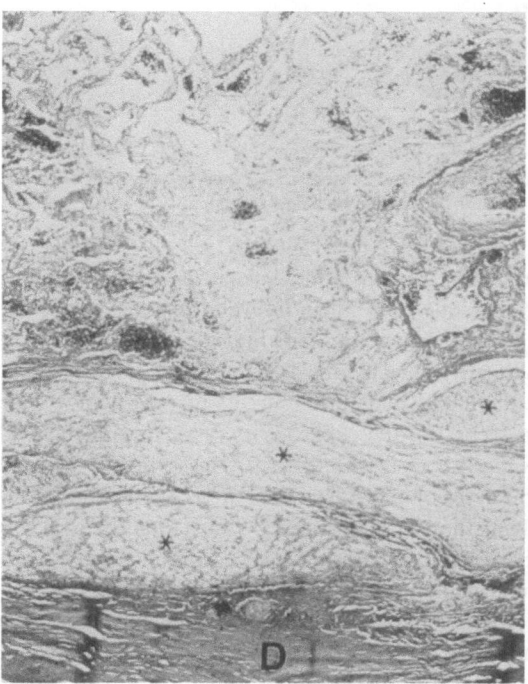

Fig. 1. This microphotograph shows the lesion lying within the cavernous sinus, in intimate contact with the dura (*D*) and several myelinated nerve fascicles which were presumably cranial nerve in origin

Successful tumor removal was achieved in five cases. In the remaining three patients only subtotal resection was obtained; a massive intra-operative hemorrhage in one case was the limiting factor. In the other two cases the preoperative diagnosis of pituitary adenoma led to a transsphenoidal approach which did not allow good cavernous sinus exposure and intraoperative bleeding control. In one of the three patients with subtotal tumor resection, post-operative radiation therapy was administered (4000 rad) and caused a reduction in lesion size by the 1-year follow-up examination.

In four cases successfull tumor removal was allowed by an accurate surgical planning: preoperative angiography with trial balloon occlusion of the internal carotid artery was helpful in determining the patients' ability to tolerate temporary carotid occlusion. The surgical approach to the cavernous sinus was performed with preservation of the neurovascular structures encased by the tumor

After a pterional craniotomy the lesser sphenoid wing including the anterior clinoid was removed extradurally with a high speed drill; the medial aspect of the greater sphenoid wing was also removed to expose both the carotid artery and the second division of the trigeminal nerve. After the dissection of the IInd, IIIrd and IVth cranial nerves and the interruption of the dural ring around the internal carotid artery the residual tumor removal was allowed through the cavernous sinus anteromedial and paramedial triangles[3].

In the case of the tumor with sinus esophytic growth, encasing the IIIrd cranial nerve at its entry in the cavernous sinus, a good exposure and total resection were allowed by a traditional pterional approach.

The most difficult aspect of tumor removal was hemostasis. The sources of hemorrhage were both the venous cavernous sinus and tumor arterial feeders (along with the anomalous microvascular component of the lesion). Early coagulation of the meningohypophyseal trunk facilitated hemostasis. However 2 to 8 units of transfusional blood were needed for hemodinamic stability.

There was no peri-operative mortality. In six cases there were no new post-operative neurological deficits and at long-term (5.5 years) follow-up examiniation significant recovery of preoperative deficits has occurred (Table 2). One patient experienced a new post-operative ophthalmoplegia which has slowly resolved, whereas another patient had increased numbness in the fifth nerve distribution.

Illustrative Case of a Cavernous Hemangioma Mimicking a Pituitary Adenoma

A 41 year old right-handed woman presented at another Hospital with 1-year history of irregular periods after her second pregnancy, persisting galactorrhea after lactation, and increased serum prolactin levels (80 µg/l). A demineralized sella turcica was noted on plain skull films. Computed tomography demonstrated a contrast-medium-enhanced mass (2 cm.) suggestive of a pituitary tumor. Bromocriptine therapy was started leading to a prompt decline of serum prolactin levels to < µg/l. A second CT scan, performed after 6 months of therapy with bromocriptine did not reveal any shrinkage of the tumor. After six months she experienced diplopia for 5 days and then total visual normalization. CT scan showed an increased size of the tumor (3 cm), with

Table 2. *Pre- and Post-operative Findings*

Cranial nerve deficit	Preoperative	Follow-up
2nd	1	0
3rd	4	3
4th	2	1
5th	3	4
6th	5	1
Amenorrhea	2	0
Galactorrhea	2	0

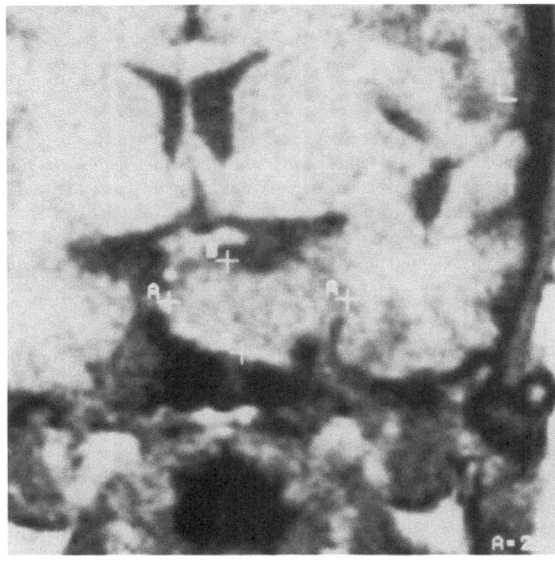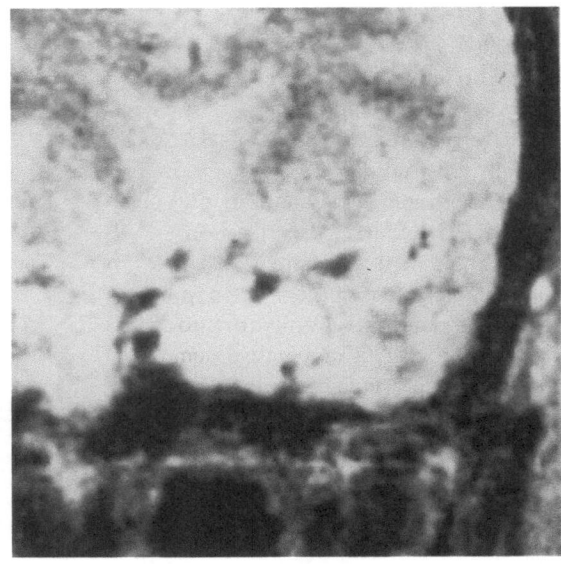

a   b

Fig. 2. This detailed MRI shows a cavernous hemangiomas growing medially toward the sellar region: the cavernous portion of the left carotid artery looks encased by the tumor. (a) The lesion appears isointense in T1, (b) and with a peculiar hyperintensity in T2

invasion of the cavernous sinus. MRI was consistent with a pituitary adenoma invading the cavernous sinus (Fig. 2). The patient, at this point, was referred to our Institution for further evaluation. Angiography did not demonstrate any pathological vascular abnormality. A presumptive diagnosis of a non functioning pituitary adenoma was done on the basis of neuroradiological studies, lack of tumor shrinkage during Bromocriptine treatment despite normalization of prolactine levels. Hyperprolactinemia at presentation was compatible with functional pituitary-hypo-thalamic deconnection. Transsphenoidal removal of the sellar lesion was advised. At operation, the most difficult aspect of tumor removal was hemostasis. The source of hemorrhage were the venous cavernous sinus and tumor arterial feeders along with the microangio-pathic component of the tumor. Particular attention was paid to obtain complete hemostasis after the partial removal.

The post-operative course was uneventful. Hyperprolactinemia, consequently to partial tumor decompression, normalized and menses resumed without bromocriptine therapy.

Discussion

Extra-axial cavernous hemangiomas of the sellar and parasellar region are rare lesion usually presenting

with mass effect, including headache and cranial nerve deficits[7] due to compression and encasement of the structures around and within the cavernous sinus. They are typically misdiagnosed preoperatively as meningiomas, and during surgery massive hemorrhage can occur. For these reasons successful tumor removal has rarely been reported[10,12]. In this series, we reported eight cases of extra-axial cavernous hemangiomas involving the cavernous sinus in which total removal was achieved in five cases after an accurate surgical planning including preoperative angiography with trial balloon occlusion to determine the patient's ability totolerate temporary carotid occlusion and proximal control of the internal carotid artery either in the neck or its intrapetrous course. Combined epidural and intradural approach[3] in four cases facilitated total resection and the preservation of the encased neurovascular structures. In the case of the tumor with esophytic growth, encasing the IIIrd cranial nerve at its entry in the cavernous sinus, a good exposure and total resection were allowed by a traditional pterional approach. In the remaining three cases only subtotal removal was achieved because of massive hemorrhage in one and the misdiagnosis of pituitary adenoma leading to transphenoidal surgery in two.

Beside the cases presenting with partial or typical cavernous sinus syndrome, presenting as a mass in the middle fossa or as a dumbbell-shaped lesion both in the middle cranial fossa and in the cavernous sinus region, orienting the surgeon to the pterional craniotomy that allow a better control of bleeding and of the encased structures, 25% of the analyzed cases, growing medially toward the sellar region, presented with pure neuroendocrinological symptoms, presumabaly due to hipothalamic-pituitary deconnection that added to a radiographic work-up compatible with pituitary adenoma induced the surgeon to a potentially lethal attempt to remove these tumors through a transphenoidal approach. Intraoperative hemorrhage due to both tumor and sinus bleeding was controlled, but is important to put more emphasis on the fact that the misdiagnosis with pituitary adenoma is even more dangerous than with meningiomas for the subsequent surgical planning, since some Authors[2] suggest the use of the transsphenoidal approach also when the invasive adenoma appears to involve the cavernous sinus.

Therefore we conclude that:

- the preoperative differential diagnosis with pituitary adenomas has to be considered before potentially lethal attempts to biopsy or remove these vascular tumors through a transsphenoidal approach,
- combined epidural and intradural approach to the cavernous sinus with early exposure of the neurovascular structures makes tumor removal possible with low morbidity,
- radiation therapy should be reserved as an adjunctive treatment after subtotal removal or as a primary treatment in elderly or debilitated patients.

References

1. Al-Mefty O (1989) Comment on Kudo T, Ueki S, Kobayashi H, Torigoe H, Tadokoro M (1989) Experience with ultrasonic surgical aspirator in a cavernous hemangioma of the cavernous sinus. Neurosurgery 24: 631
2. Buchfelder M, Falbusch R (1987) Transsphenoidal surgery of pituitary adenomas developed towards the cavernous sinus. In: Dolenc VV (ed) The cavernous sinus. Springer, Wien New York, pp 404–414
3. Dolenc V (1983) Direct microsurgical repair of intracavernous vascular lesions. J Neurosurg 58: 824–831
4. Meyer F.B, Lombardi D, Scheithauer B, Douglas AN (1990) Extra-axial cavernous hemangiomas involving the dural sinuses. J Neurosurg 73: 187–192
5. Mori K, Handa H, Gi H, Mori K (1980) Cavernomas in the middle fossa. Surg Neurol 14: 21–31
6. Namba S (1983) Extracerebral cavernous hemangioma of the middle cranial fossa. Surg Neurol 19: 379–388
7. Odake G, Tanaka K (1986) Cavernous hemangioma of the middle fossa. Case report and review of the literature. Neurol Med Chir 26: 58–67
8. Pàsztor E, Szabò G, Slowik WK, Zoltàn J (1964) Cavernous hemangioma of the base of the skull. Report of a case surgically treated. J Neurosurg 21: 582–585
9. Rigamonti D, Drayer BP, Johnson PC, Hadley MN, Zabramski J, Spetzler RF (1987) The MRI appearance of cavernous malformations (angiomas). J Neurosurg 67: 518–524
10. Rosenblum B, Rothman AS, Lanzieri C, Song S (1986) A cavernous sinus cavernous hemangioma: case report. J Neurosurg 65: 716–718
11. Russell DS, Rubinstein LJ (1989) Pathology of tumors of the nervous system, 5th Ed. Williams and Wilkins, Baltimore pp 730–736
12. Sawamura Y, de Tribolet N (1989) Cavernous hemangioma in the cavernous sinus: case report. Neurosurgery 26: 126–128
13. Shibata S, Mori K (1987) Effect of radiation therapy on extracerebral cavernous hemangioma in the middle fossa. Report of three cases. J Neurosurg 67: 919–922

Correspondence: D. Lombardi, M.D., Clinica Neurochirurgica, I.R.C.C.S. Ospedale S. Raffaele, Università di Milano, Via Olgettina 60, I-20132, Milano, Italy.

Intracranial Cavernous Angiomas: a Simple Method for Their Surgical Approach

F. Frank, A.P. Fabrizi, N. Acciarri, G. Piazza, R. Ricci[1], and G. Gaist

Division of Neurosurgery, [1]Neuroradiology Service, Bellaria Hospital, Bologna, Italy

Summary

Stereotactically aimed small craniotomies have been performed in 14 cases of cavernous angiomas that were either deep seated or located in highly functional areas. The method has been without risk both *quoad vitam* and *quoad valetudinem*. Epilepsy was the main presenting symptom of the patients and was cured in 21.4% of the cases. Seizures were reduced in 57.1% of the patients and were unchanged in the remaining 21.4%.

Keywords: Stereotactic guide; open-guided surgery; cavernous angiomas.

Introduction

Cavernous angiomas, or cavernomas, which are venous malformations, have a positive family history in 7% of the cases, and often give rise to either epileptic fits or cerebral hemorrhage. These lesions are only partially "benign", as they often restrain patients from performing their normal daily activities.

In a series of 74 patients with cavernomas that underwent surgery in our division of neurosurgery from 1980 to 1991, it was necessary to perform stereotactic localization in 14 of the cases in order to limit the damage to normal brain tissue and guide the ablation of small lesions, often under 1 centimeter in diameter (Fig. 1). The technique we employed to perform the stereotactic localization of the lesion and the craniotomy or craniectomy for its removal will be described.

Method and Results

Among the 74 patients that were operated for cerebral cavernomas, 14 cases are discussed for the particular surgical approach they underwent. These 14 patients harbored lesions that were either

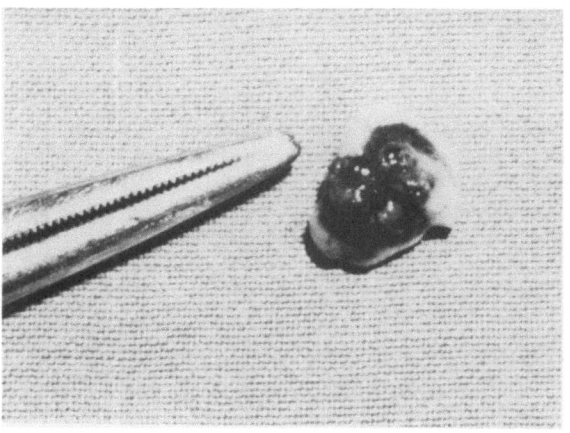

Fig. 1. Cavernoma (photo after removal)

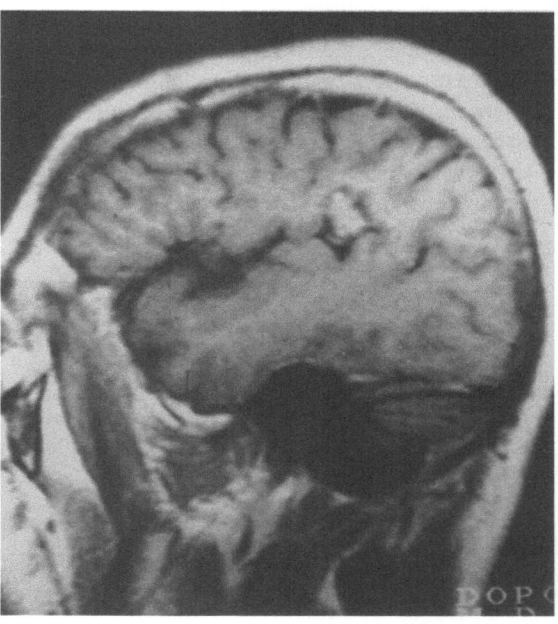

Fig. 2. MRI: lateral projection of a typical cavernoma. Small-sized malformation with surrounding perilesional ring sign of chronic old hemorrhage

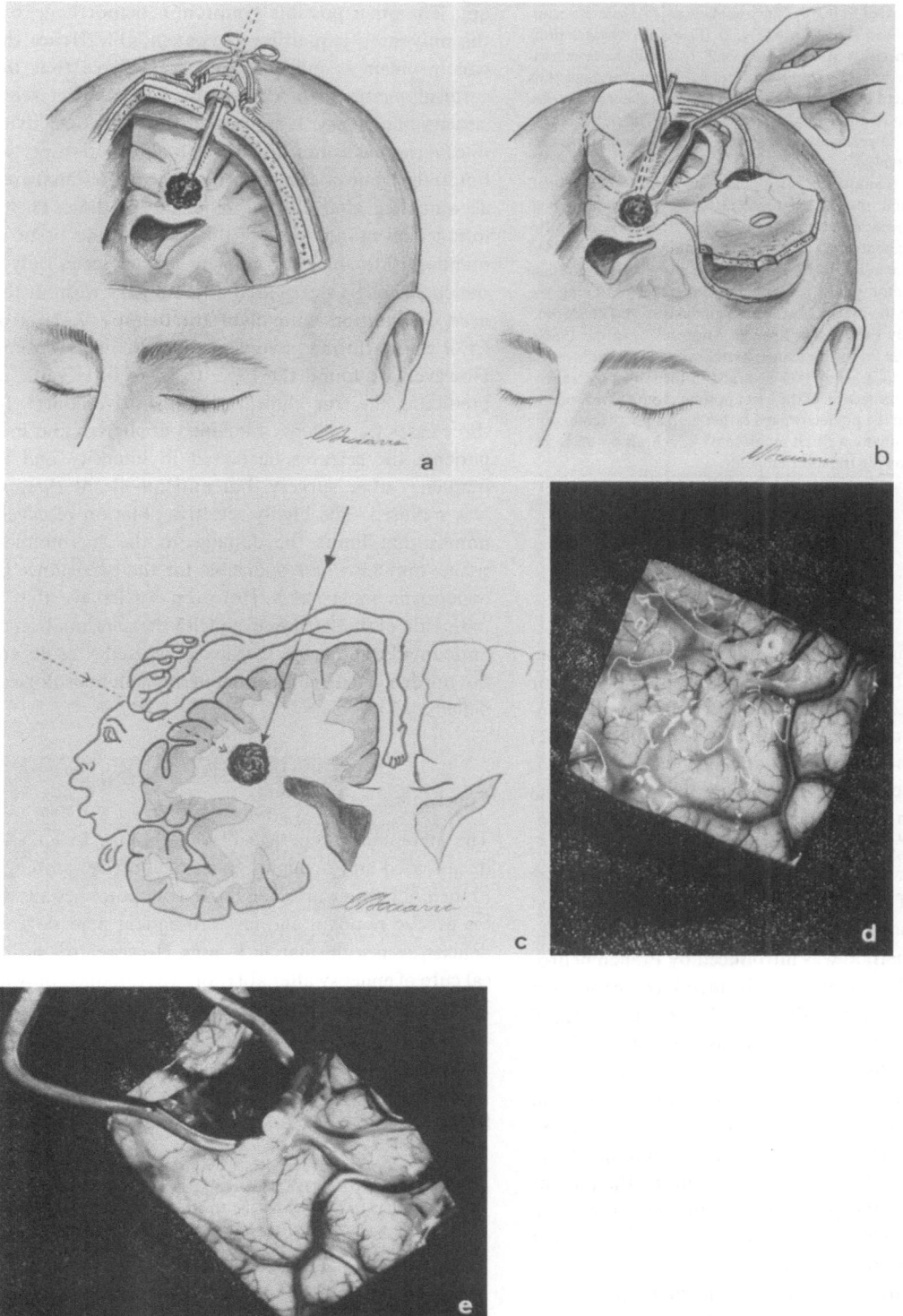

Fig. 3. (a–c) Artist's drawings of a–p and lateral views indicating the advantages of stereotactic open guided technique for cavernomas located in highly functional areas (rolandic lesion near Broca's area). The catheter guide is introducted paramedian to avoid damage to either speech or upper limb movements. (d,e) Intraoperative photographs showing the positioned catheter and the small cortical incision

deep-seated or located in highly functional areas. All these cavernomas were small-sized (1–1.5 cm.) (Fig. 2). Therefore, these lesions would have been either difficult to locate or could have caused damage in their removal by traditional means. The cavernomas thus treated were located in the following sites: seven in the frontal lobe, one in the thalamus, and six in the parietal lobe. The patients' age ranged from 4 to 54 years, and there was a sex prevalence for males (9 males and 5 females).

The operative technique or "open-guided surgery"[1–4,6–8] is aimed towards maximum sparing of cerebral tissue and neurological functions. The operation consists of two stages: the first being the stereotactic placement of a rubber catheter along a predetermined route reaching the lesion to be removed; the second stage consists in a small craniotomy which allows reaching and removing the cavernoma along the previously inserted guide (Fig. 3). The method was introduced by French and Spanish Authors[1,6,7] in the 1980's, and consists of the following stages: extracranial projection of the cavernoma onto a CT scout-view enlarged to the size of the stereotactic X-ray films[5]; selection of the best approach route; introduction of a catheter upon the predetermined target with a post-stereotactic CT control; and finally a small craniotomy which allows to resect the lesion by following the inserted guide.

Of the 14 operated patients two showed transient post-operative aphasia, and one presented a slight right hemiparesis persisting at one-year follow-up.

Discussion

Cavernous angiomas that are located in highly functional areas are those most frequently responsible for epilepsy. These lesions are also often located in rolandic and post-rolandic areas, and are very small on MRI (Fig. 2), and neurosurgeons approached these lesions with reluctance in the past. With the advent in the 1980's of open-guided surgery, promoted and sustained by Kelly[3,4], these lesions became surgically amenable with low risks *quoad valetudinem* and without risks *quoad vitam*. The Kelly method is highly sophisticated and totally computerized, but its cost is considerable.

A simpler method was introduced by French neurosurgeons[6,7] who stereotactically introduce a probe to a predetermined target; this is followed by a small craniotomy which permits to follow the probe all the way down to the lesion. Besides the lower cost, we believe that the French method is extremely useful and efficient. The so-called "*fil d'Arianne*" (as in Greek mythology) consents a precise programming of the surgical approach that is less harmful for the patient and at the same time precise in locating the cavernoma. A control CT before craniotomy has always indicated the exact location of the inserted guide.

According to the literature, the main presenting symptoms of patients affected with cavernous angiomas are usually focal seizures (at times generalized) which are often uncontrolled by anticonvulsant therapy. The other possible symptom is hemorrhage, but this only rarely jeopardises the patient's life. Hence, the true problem is epilepsy, and we believe that the surgical treatment of cavernoma is in a strict sense surgery of epilepsy. It seems that the epileptic activity of cavernomas is not due to the malformation per se, but to the hemosiderin deposits in the perilesional area accumulated after chronic repeated bleeding. Therefore, a perfect curettage of this surrounding tissue is mandatory to solve this ailment. In our series only 3 patients (21.4%) were cured after surgery without the need of addition anticonvulsant therapy. A control EEG was performed two years after the intervention. However, we found the EEG to be of little value in predicting the true clinical post-operative course. In three cases the epilepsy remained unaltered, and in 8 patients the seizures decreased in intensity and in frequency after surgery, but anticonvulsant therapy was required. The highly selective ablation of cavernomas that limits the damage to the surrounding tissue, may also be responsible for the persistance of epilepsy in most cases. However, we believe that a reduction of the seizures even with the continuation of anticonvulsant therapy is a success when the results are not burdened with subsequent permanent neurological deficits.

Conclusions

The stereotactic reperage of cavernomas located in deep-seated and/or highly functional areas combined to their ablation with small limited craniotomies allows for precise removal and few subsequent neurological deficits, even with rolandic lesions. However, the surgical cure of epilepsy after ablation was obtained only in 21% of the cases, and the seizures were reduced in another 57%.

References

1. Carrillo R, Garcia de Sola R, Gonzalez-Ojellon M, Garcià-Uria J, Bravo G (1986) Stereotactic localization and open microsurgical approach in the treatment of some intracranial deep arteriovenous malformations. Surg Neurol 25: 535–539
2. Hariz MI, Fodstad H (1987) Stereotactic localization of small subcortical brain tumors for open surgery. Surg Neurol 28: 345–350
3. Kelly PJ, Alker GJ Jr, Zoll JG (1982) A microstereotactic approach to deep-seated arteriovenous malformations. Surg Neurol 17: 260–262
4. Kelly PJ (1991) Tumor stereotaxis. Saunders, Philadelphia

5. Ruggiero G, Ricci R (1991) Proiezione extracranica di lesioni all'interno del cranio. Rivista di Neuroradiologia 4: 187–196

6. Sedan R, Peragut JC, Farnarier P, Derome P, Fabrizi A (1988) Guidage ste'r'eotaxique de certaines interventions a crane ouvert. Neurochirurgie 34: 97–101

7. Sedan R, Peragut JC, Fabrizi A (1989) Cavernomes et stéréotaxie. Neurochirurgie 35: 126–127

8. Sisti MB, Solomon RA, Stein BM (1991) Stereotactic craniotomy in the resection of small arteriovenous malformations. J Neurosurg 75: 40–44

Correspondence: Franco Frank, M.D., Division of Neurosurgery, Bellaria Hospital, Via Altura 3, I-40139 Bologna, Italy.

Auditory Evoked Responses and Blink Reflex in Brain-Stem Cavernous Angiomas. Report of 7 Cases

A. Talacchi, L. Cristofori, D. Garozzo, L. Deotto[1] and A. Bricolo

First Division of Neurosurgery and [1]Division of Neurology, University Hospital, Verona, Italy

Summary

Brain-stem auditory evoked responses (BAERs) and Blink Reflex (BR) were evaluated in 7 patients with brain-stem cavernous angiomas (CA). The average size of the lesions, measured by the maximum diameter as shown by magnetic resonance imaging (MRI), was 18 mm. Five lesions were located in the pons, 1 in the ponto-mesencephalic junction and 1 in the midbrain; 5 lied on the left side, 2 on the right. We compared the accuracy and sensitivity of the BAERs and BR methods with that of physical examination and of MRI. Both BAERs and BR seem sensitive tools in revealing brain-stem dysfunction. Of the two, BAERs are more specific for side and location (especially for lesions situated in the lower pons) and correlate with ear impairment, even if some lesions are silent since they do not involve the acoustic pathways. BR disclosed abnormalities of duration prevalently, but no typical patterns regarding location and clinical signs.

Keywords: Brain-stem auditory evoked response; blink reflex; cavernous angiomas; brain-stem.

Introduction

Brain-stem auditory evoked responses (BAERs) and blink reflex (BR) are considered sensitive tools either in detecting focal intrinsic brain-stem lesions or in the assessment of functional brain-stem impairment[5,12]. Therefore, both are used in the monitoring of silent and clinically manifest brain-stem lesions[1,7]. In this study seven patients with brain-stem cavernous angiomas (CA) were evaluated pre-operatively to investigate the possible correlation between the neurophysiological abnormalities, the location of the lesions and the neurological impairment.

Material and Methods

The pre-operative BAERs and BR studies of 7 consecutive patients treated at our institution for brain-stem CA were reviewed[2]. Among them 4 were males and 3 females; the average age was 37 years (ranging from 19 to 58 yrs.). Each patient was studied clinically and by CT, angiography and magnetic resonance imaging (MRI) with Gadolinium infusion. The radiological and clinical data were recorded within 9 days (on the average) from the data of neurophysiological testing. The measurement of the maximum diameter of the lesions was made from MRI images; the average size was 18 mm. Five CA were located in the pons (2 in the inferior third, 3 in the middle third), 1 in the ponto-mesencephalic junction and 1 in the midbrain; 5 were on the left side, 2 on the right. The location and the diameter of the lesion, and the clinical signs for each patient are reported in Table 1.

Both BAERs and BR were performed in 5 patients (in one patient they were made twice and each compared with the evolution of the clinical and radiological picture); 2 patients underwent only one test, BAERs and BR respectively.

The BR registration was performed using an OTE BASIS EPM electromyograph. BR were recorded from both orbicularis oculi muscles of the lower eyelids. The electric stimuli were applied on the first trigeminal branch emerging from the supraorbital foramen. They were delivered, after having reached the threshold, at a rate of 10 s, in order to avoid the so-called "habituation phenomenon". The stimulation was performed in two stages: during the first one, the analysing time lasted 100 m·s, during the second one it was 200 m.s. In both cases the sensibility was 200 mvolt and the frequency range was from 20 HZ to 20 kHZ. The direct retroauricolar stimulation of the facial nerve was performed in order to calculate its latency. The following were considered: the R1 latency, between the artificial stimulus and the first deflection of the R1 evoked response; the R2 dir and R2 cons latencies, between the artificial stimulus and the first deflection of the R2 evoked response; the R2 dir and R2 cons duration, between the first and the last evoked response.

BAERs were registered with monopolar surface electrodes in accordance with the 10–20 electrode system of the International EEG Federation. The different electrode was over M1 or M2, the indifferent electrode was over CZ and the earth electrode was placed over the left wrist. Left and right ears were tested separately and BAERs were recorded from each lobe ipsilateral to the side of the stimulation (70 db SL); the unstimulated ear was masked with 60 db white noise. At least two tracings were considered, each representing the mean of 2000 single responses elicited by each ear. TDH-39 p earphones were used; the auditory stimulator delivered 10 HZ clicks, each lasting 10 m·s. The resulting evoked response was amplified 16 times (ranging from 20 HZ to 500 HZ) and then filtered. The response had a 10 m·s duration, being the analysing time 1 m·s/div. The sensibility was 5 mvolt/div. The following parameters were considered: the absolute first peak latency; the differences between the ipsilateral I–III, III–V and I–V latencies. All of the cases (for both BAER and BR), which presented at least one of the considered parameters higher than the standard values of the control population (n = 30) examined at our institution, were considered abnormal. The differences were considered significant when values higher than 3 SD were found.

Results

BAERs were altered in 3 patients; BR disclosed abnormalities in 5 patients (Table 2).

As regards BAERs, they were pathologic always ipsilaterally to the lesion. In 2 out of 3 cases hypoacusia was present; the third case did not present auditory impairment, but the lesion was located just close to the exit of the 8th cranial nerve from the brain-stem. In the remaining 3 patients the CA lied outside the brain-stem acoustic pathways, always anteriorly (1 was located in the inferior third of the pons, the others in the ponto-mesencephalic junction and in the midbrain).

As regards BR, only 1 case was normal, while the others showed R2 alterations, simultaneously in the two components, R2 dir and R2 cons. Abnormalities were ipsilateral with respect to the side of the lesion, controlateral or bilateral; occurrence and side were independent from the location of the lesion and from the clinical signs.

Table 1. *Patient Data*

Patient	Age	Location of the lesion	Size (mm)	Clinical findings
C.C.	58	L pons inferior 1/3	11	L facial paresthesia, VI and VII CN deficits, R somatic paresthesia
P.A.	22	L pons middle 1/3	14	L VI CN deficit, bilat. hypoacusia, tinnitus, R somatic paresthesia
R.S.	53	R pons inferior 1/3	10	R VI CN deficit, L somatic motor deficit
P.F.	41	L pons middle 1/3	10	L facial paresthesia, VI and VII CN deficits
Z.D.	21	R pons middle 1/3	25	R VI, VII, VIII, XII CN deficits, L somatic motor deficit, nystagmus, ataxia
V.R.	44	L ponto-mes. junction	18	R V and VII CN deficits, L somatic motor deficit
M.P.	19	L midbrain	40	R III CN deficit, attention disturbance, R somatic motor deficit

L left; *R* right; *CN* cranial nerve.

Table 2. *Neurophysiological Assessment*

Patient		Blink reflex Ipsilateral R1	R2DIR	R2CONS	Controlateral R1	R2DIR	R2CONS	M Response IPS/CONTR	B.A.E.R. Ipsilateral I	I–III	III–V	I–V	Controlateral I	I–III	III–V	I–V
C.C.	L	11.4	27.7	28.2	11.0	28.0	28.9	3.61/1.88	1.57	2.29	*2.40*	*4.69*	1.54	2.05	1.40	3.45
	D		65.0	60.0		90.0	95.0									
P.A.I°	L	9.7	37.2	37.3	10.1	38.8	39.3	2.90/2.20	1.34	2.10	A	A	1.40	2.12	2.07	4.19
	D		34.0	36.6		36.8	42.0	2.36/2.20								
P.A.II°	L	9.1	31.8	28.2	9.6	32.4	32.2	2.36/2.20	1.34	2.04	2.25	4.27	1.54	2.00	2.08	4.08
	D		37.4	43.4		46.0	42.5									
R.S	L	*13.0*	31.1	29.1	10.6	32.6	28.6	—	—	—	—	—				
	D		84.8	80.8		38.5	42.5									
P.F.	L	9.9	34.8	32.0	9.0	36.5	35.0	2.90/2.12	1.33	2.26	2.20	4.46	1.37	2.15	2.17	4.32
	D		40.0	48.8		33.4	37.0									
Z.D	L	—			—		—	— —	1.40	A	A	A	1.42	2.33	1.79	4.12
V.R	L	10.6	25.2	29.0	10.0	29.0	27.0	3.40/2.40	1.57	1.60	2.07	3.67	1.54	1.84	2.09	3.93
	D		50.8	48.0	*80.5*	65.4										
M.P	L	11.3	32.8	34.6	12.7	34.1	33.8	A/2.60	1.58	2.32	2.03	4.35	1.57	2.24	1.98	4.22
	D		40.0	41.4	*92.4*	90.0										
Control	L	10.60	30.37	30.24	D 42.15	43.63		2.52 ± 0.36	1.50	2.10	1.85	3.96				
Population		± 0.78	± 2.76	± 2.64	± 3.72	± 3.95			± 0.10	± 0.11	± 0.12	± 0.16				

A absent; *L* latency; *D* duration; italic values are abnormal.

It is worth emphasizing that – as concerns BR – there was a prevalence of alterations of duration (4 cases) than of latency (1 case).

By combining of the two examinations (5 cases), in 3 cases the CA was not situated on the acoustic pathways, and the examinations resulted normal. Two lesions (1 in the ponto-mesencephalic junction and 1 in the midbrain) showed both controlateral delayed durations on BR, while the third lesion was associated with BAERs and BR examinations in the normal range. The remaining 2 cases were abnormal for both the studies.

One patient (P.A.) was submitted both to MRI and neurophysiological tests in the acute phases after clinical onset and at 3 weeks' interval. As the size of the CA was reduced, clinical symptoms and signs improved (tinnitus and somatic paresthesia). On BAERs, interpeak latency III–V reappeared and BR became normal, suggesting a good correlation among clinical/radiological findings and neurophysiological tests.

Discussion

According to our data and those of other authors[8,9,15], ipsilateral pathways play a dominant role in the generation of monoaurally evoked BAER components in man. Although human and animal anatomical studies – together with animal microelectrode studies – have concluded that the major functional part of the brainstem auditory system ascends controlateral to the ear stimulated, the majority of human pathophysiological correlations indicate that pathways ipsilateral to the active ear are responsible for the BAERs, except perhaps for wave V[3,14]. In fact the extensive but incomplete crossing of the auditory pathways at several brainstem levels complicates the generation of later components and their alteration by unilateral brain-stem lesions[4,13,17].

On the other side, an altered BR response does not mean that the reflex is mediated via pathways traversing the anatomic region involved by the lesion. In fact both components (R1 and R2) are multisynaptic responses subject to complex inhibitory and excitatory cerebral influences[6]. Moreover Rossi *et al.* noted that especially intrinsic lesions of the brain-stem could display quite different abnormal patterns[10].

In our series R1 latency was spared in all cases, while R2 did not seem to discriminate neither for location and side of the CA, nor for the neurological impairment of the 5th and the 7th cranial nerves. Nevertheless the number of cases is too small to draw any statement

on specific correlation between BR responses and anatomical/clinical factors. In fact the examination seems to be more often altered than BAERs in cases with brain-stem functional involvement due to CA. Both procedures have demonstrated a good sensitivity in revealing the direction of the clinical course in our patient who was studied twice after hemorrhage[13].

In conclusion, from the observation of a small series of CA of the brain-stem, BR seems to be more appropriate in the detection of brain-stem functional impairment than in the determination of 5th and 7th cranial nerve impairment, even if it does not give any specific information; the BAERs, on the contrary, seem to be slightly more suitable in the correlation with acoustic symptomatology and reflect – especially in the caudal pons – the side and the location of prevalent brainstem involvement.

References

1. Baum K, Scheuler W, Hegerl U, Girke W, Schorner W (1988) Detection of brainstem lesions in multiple sclerosis: comparison of brainstem auditory evoked potentials with nuclear magnetic resonance imaging. Acta Neurol Scand 77: 283–288
2. Bricolo A, Turazzi S, Cristofori L, Talacchi A (1991) Direct surgery for brainstem tumours. Acta Neurochir (Wien) [Suppl] 53: 148–158
3. Chiappa K (1983) Evoked potentials in clinical medicine. Raven, New York, pp 145–191
4. Chu N-S (1989) Brainstem auditory evoked potentials: correlation between CT midbrain-pontine lesion sites and abolition of wave V or the IV–V complex. J Neurol Sci 91: 165–177
5. Faught E, Oh SJ (1985) Brainstem auditory evoked responses in brainstem infarction. Stroke 16: 702–705
6. Fisher MA, Shahani BT, Young RR (1979) Assessing segmental excitability after acute rostral lesions: II. The blink reflex. Neurology 29: 45–50
7. Hammond SR, Yiannikas C (1987) The relevance of controlateral recordings and patient disability to assessment of brain-stem auditory evoked potential abnormalities in multiple sclerosis. Arch Neurol 44: 382–387
8. Markand ON, Farlow MR, Stevens JC, Edwards MK (1989) Brain-stem auditory evoked potential abnormalities with unilateral brain-stem lesions demonstrated by magnetic resonance-imaging. Arch Neurol 46: 295–299
9. Oh SJ, Kuba T, Soyer A, Choi IS, Bonikowski FP, Vitek J (1981) Lateralization of brainstem lesions by brainstem auditory evoked potentials. Neurology 31: 14–18
10. Rossi B, Buonaguidi R, Muratorio A, Tusini G (1979) Blink reflexes in posterior fossa lesions. J Neurol Neurosurg Psychiatry 42: 465–469
11. Scaioli V, Savoiardo M, Cimino C, Milanese C, Avanzini G (1989) Brainstem auditory evoked potential abnormalities and magnetic resonance imaging in posterior fossa lesions. Eur Neurol 29: 246–254
12. Starr A, Achor LJ (1975) Auditory brain stem responses in neurological disease. Arch Neurol 32: 761–768
13. Stockard JJ, Rossiter VS (1977) Clinical and pathologic cor-

relates of brain-stem auditory response abnormalities. Neurology 27: 316–325

14. Tsutsui T, Ohno M, Symon L, Wang A (1986) Combined measurement of brainstem auditory and somatosensory evoked potentials in a surgically treated brainstem hematoma. Surg Neurol 25: 575–581

15. York DH (1986) Correlation between a unilateral midbrain-pontine lesion and abnormalities of brain-stem auditory evoked potential. Electroencephalogr Clin Neurophysiol 65: 282–288

Correspondence: A. Talacchi, M.D., First Division of Neurosurgery, University Hospital, I-37126 Verona, Italy.

Management of Vein of Galen Malformations, Dural AVMs, Venous Angiomas

Endovascular Management of Vein of Galen Malformations

C.F. Dowd, V.V. Halbach, R.T. Higashida, K.W. Fraser, T.P. Smith, and G.B. Hieshima

Department of Radiology and Neurological Surgery, University of California, San Francisco Medical Center, San Francisco, California, U.S.A.

Summary

Vein of Galen malformations are congenital arteriovenous fistulas involving the fetal midline prosencephalic vein. In neonates, this entity presents as high-output congestive heart failure and is uniformly fatal in this population even with aggressive medical therapy. Endovascular management with staged embolization has become the treatment of choice, to diminish arteriovenous shunting thereby improving cardiac function and allowing definitive therapy at a later age.

We have treated 16 patients with vein of Galen malformations using endovascular techniques. A variety of transarterial and transvenous approaches were utilized. 8 of the 16 patients were angiographically cured. Four patients died despite embolization.

The early results of endovascular management of vein of Galen malformations, especially in the neonatal period, are encouraging, as the vast majority of these patients would otherwise succumb to cardiac failure early in the course of this disease.

Keywords: Embolization; endovascular therapy; interventional neuroradiology; vein of Galen malformation.

Introduction

Vein of Galen malformations are uncommon but often discussed pediatric vascular lesions. They represent abnormal arteriovenous shunts involving the midline fetal prosencephalic vein[6,12]. Symptoms vary depending on the age at presentation[1,7]: neonates generally present with severe congestive heart failure; infants with hydrocephalus, macrocephaly, or seizures; and older children with headaches.

Newborns with high output congestive heart failure are particularly refractive to therapy and the disease is almost uniformly fatal in this population[7,8] as the patients succumb to this high output left-to-right extracardiac shunt. We report our experience with endovascular therapy in a population of patients with vein of Galen malformations many of whom presented in the perinatal period with congestive heart failure.

Methods and Materials

Sixteen patients with vein of Galen malformations were treated by our group using a variety of endovascular techniques. 11 of the 16 patients presented either *in utero* (Fig. 1) or in the first week of life with high output congestive heart failure refractory to medical therapy, underscoring the selection bias toward the neonatal group in our patient population (Table 1). All other patients presented with hydrocephalus, hemorrhagic stroke, developmental delay and abnormal engorgement of facial veins as evidence for venous outflow restriction. All patients presented by age 3 months.

Our 16 patients underwent a total of 42 endovascular procedures. 10 of our 16 patients underwent the first embolization procedure within the first two weeks of life. Embolization was carried out by one of three endovascular routes. The transarterial route was considered the access of choice. A 4-French guiding catheter is placed, either transfemorally or via the umbilical artery, into the internal carotid or vertebral artery and a 2.2-French Tracker catheter (Target Therapeutics, Fremont, CA) is navigated as close to the fistula site as possible. Embolization materials include liquid adhesives (N-butyl cyanoacrylate), polyvinyl alcohol particles, silk suture segments, and platinum coils. When this route was precluded either by the small caliber of the feeding arteries in an infant or by the large number of arterial feeders, a transfemoral venous approach was utilized. A 4-French catheter was placed via the femoral vein and guided to the internal jugular vein. A Tracker catheter is then navigated through the transverse sinus, torcular, and falcine sinus to the region of the midline prosencephalic vein[12] (erroneously referred to as the vein of Galen) and in some cases, retrograde into the feeding arteries. The third approach utilizes a transtorcular route championed by Mickle and Quisling[11], whereby the neurosurgical team performs a small occipital craniotomy allowing passage of a 4-French guiding catheter. In some cases a short Tracker catheter is placed through this for embolization. In either the transfemoral venous or transtorcular routes, multiple platinum or steel coils, and

Table 1. *Vein of Galen Malformations-Patient Population*

Age	Symptom onset (no. patients)	1st Embolization (no. patients)
Birth–2 weeks	14	10
2 weeks–4 months	2	3
4 months–1 year	0	0
1 year–6 years	0	3

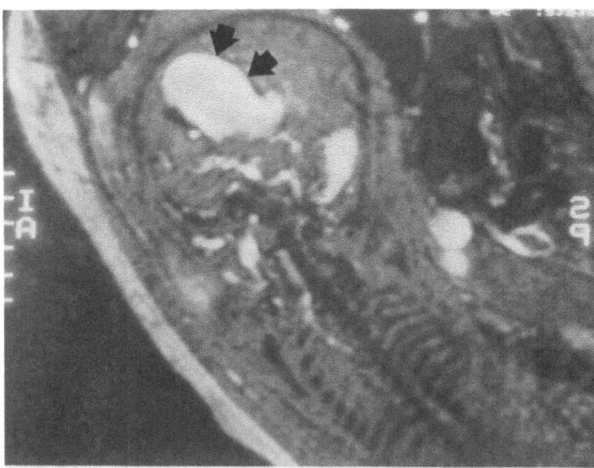
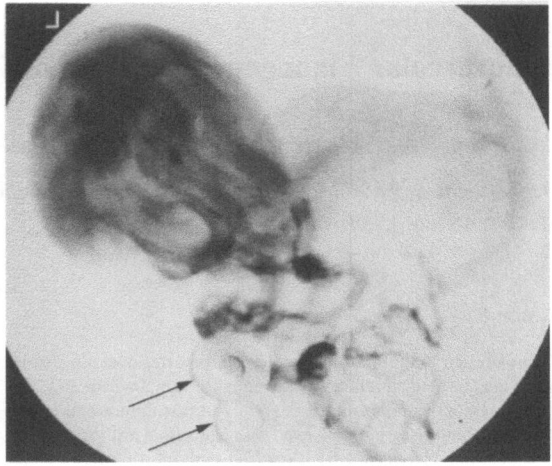

a   b

Fig. 1. Vein of Galen malformation, diagnosed in utero. (a) Obstetrical magnetic resonance imaging (MRI) scan at 36 weeks gestation. A vein of Galen malformations in evident (arrows) in this left anterior oblique projection of the fetus. (b) Left vertebral arteriogram, lateral projection, at 2 hours of life, performed via umbilical artery catheterization, confirms large vein of Galen malformation and correlates well with in utero MRI scan. A planned delivery by Cesarian section allowed the patient to be treated immediately. Despite multiple embolizations, the patient died of severe heart failure. Note one-centimeter markers (arrows) to allow sizing of arteries and varix

sometimes silk sutures, are the embolic materials of choice. In all cases pre- and postembolization control angiograms are obtained.

Results

Of our 16 patients, we have achieved angiographic cure in 8 by endovascular means (Figs. 2 and 3). Of these 8 angiographic cures, 3 patients are entirely normal neurologically, 4 exhibit mild neurological deficits and one patient demonstrates significant neurological deficits.

Four of the 16 patients showed significantly decreased arteriovenous shunting on the last post-embolization control angiogram. Of these 4, three are neurologically normal. One of these 3 demonstrates mild residual cardiac failure and one has significant neurological deficits one year after the last embolization.

Four patients died in this series. All died within the first several weeks of life from severe high output congestive heart failure and in these patients the combination of aggressive medical management and endovascular therapy could not reverse the course of the cardiac decompensation.

Among the 42 procedures, there were 5 endovascular complications. Four perforations were identified, 2 were asymptomatic, and one required placement of a ventriculostomy. This patient recovered well. All perforations were sealed using platinum coils. Additionally, a coil was lost in one patient on the venous side, and an atrial septal defect allowed passage of this platinum coil to the left heart and subsequently to the left internal carotid artery. This patient died soon thereafter from cardiac decompensation.

Discussion

Vein of Galen malformations, although relatively unusual, have generated much discussion in the literature. Yaşargil[13] and others[6] have put forth classification

▶

Fig. 2. 4 month-old with macrocephaly. (a) mid-sagittal MRI scan shows vein of Galen malformation with dilated midline prosencephalic vein. (b) and (c) Left common carotid (b) and left vertebral (c) arteriograms, lateral projections, confirms presence of vein of Galen malformation supplied by chorodial and pericallosal arteries. (d) and (e) Posterior choroidal arteriograms, lateral projections, before (d) and after (e) platinum coil embolization. No further arteriovenous (a–v) shunting is seen post-embolization. Note reflux of contrast into pericallosal feeder (e, arrow). (f) Left vertebral control arteriogram, lateral projection, at age 10 months, shows residual a–v shunting through a second choroidal artery (arrow). (g) Choroidal arteriogram, lateral projection, prior to platinum coil embolization. (h) and (i) Post-embolization left vertebral arteriograms, lateral (h) and Townes (i) projections, show no residual a–v shunting. (j) post-embolization left common carotid arteriogram, lateral projection, confirms angiographic cure. Patient is neurologically normal at age 26 months

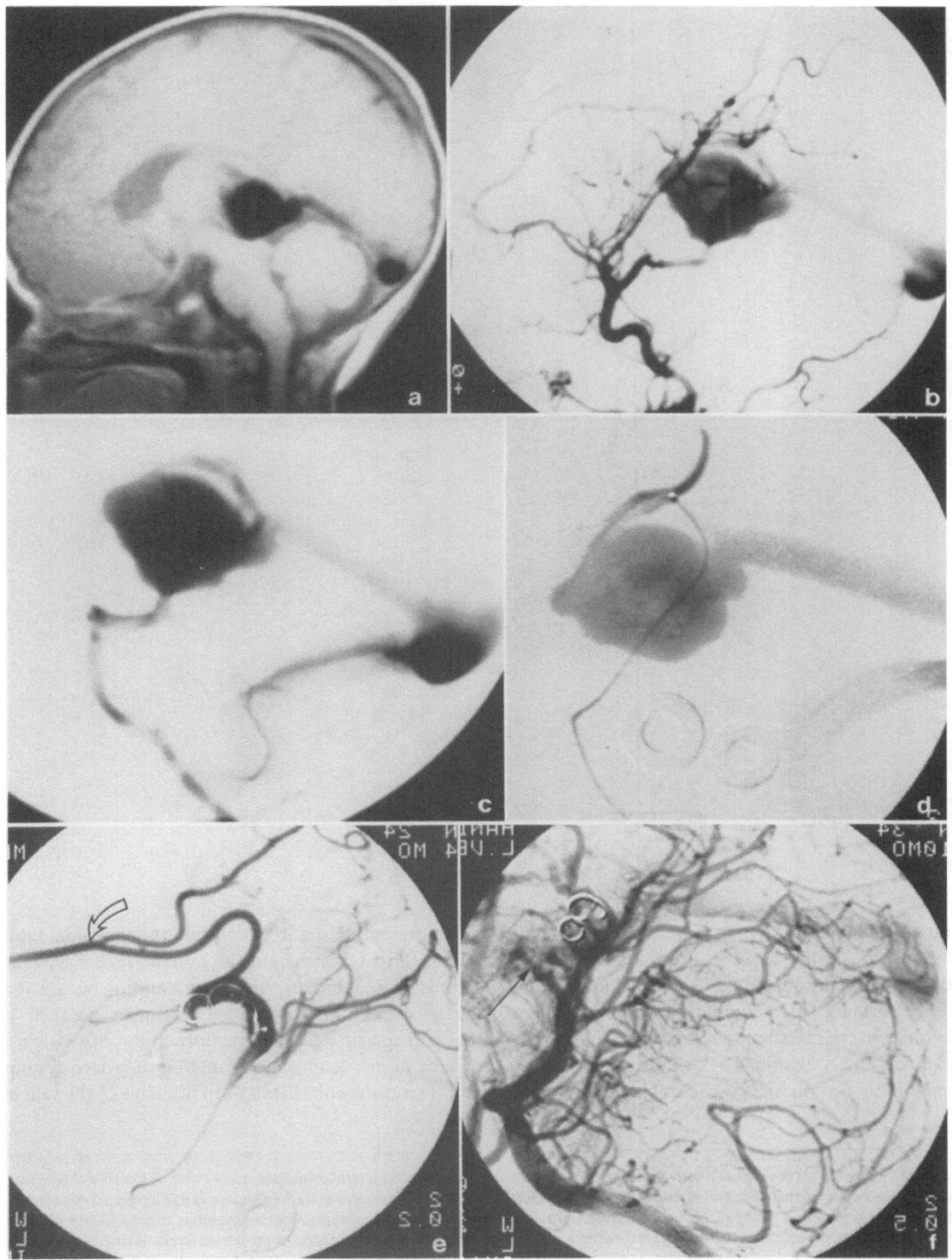

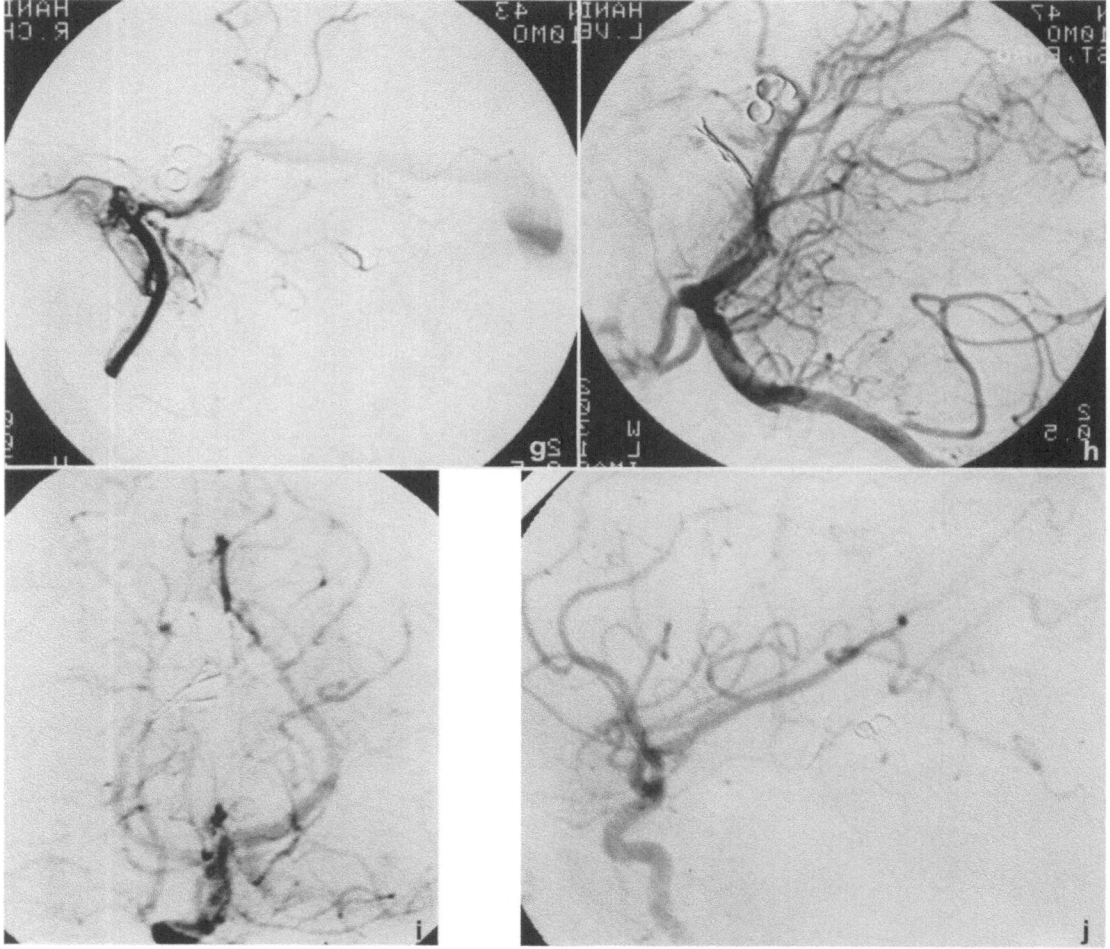

Fig. 2 (*continued*)

schemes to differentiate types of vein of Galen malformations. Basically, these malformations can be
devided into the choroidal type, usually demonstrating
multiple choroidal, thalamoperforator and pericallos-
sal feeding arteries and presenting as neonates; the
mural type, usually identified as a single arteriovenous
connection to the midline prosencephalic vein and

often presenting slightly later than the choroidal type;
and a third type wherein the midline prosencephalic
vein is dilated, but arteriovenous shunting occurs at a
distance from this structure. This third type, then, is
not a true vein of Galen malformation, but either a
nearby arteriovenous malformation or a deep venous
dural arteriovenous fistula with drainage to the vein of

Fig. 3. 2 week-old with congestive heart failure. (a) right internal carotid arteriogram, lateral projection, shows vein of Galen malformation
draining to falcine sinus. (b) left vertebral arteriogram, lateral projection, during transtorcular coil embolization at age 23 days. Transtorcular
catheter (arrows) is seen as a filling defect in the falcine sinus. Transarterial approach would not allow adequate distal catheter position.
(c) plain skull film, lateral projection, during transtorcular embolization. (d) right common carotid control angiogram, lateral projection, at
age 6 months, shows residual arteriovenous (a–v) shunting. (e) midline prosencephalic venogram, lateral projection, prior to further coil
embolization. Microcatheter was placed from a transfemoral access. Catheter tip is at the anterosuperior aspect of the varix (arrow), where
embolization commenced. (f) right common carotid post-embolization angiogram, lateral projection, shows no residual a–v shunting. Child
is 3 years 6 months old and demonstrates minimal right leg weakness only

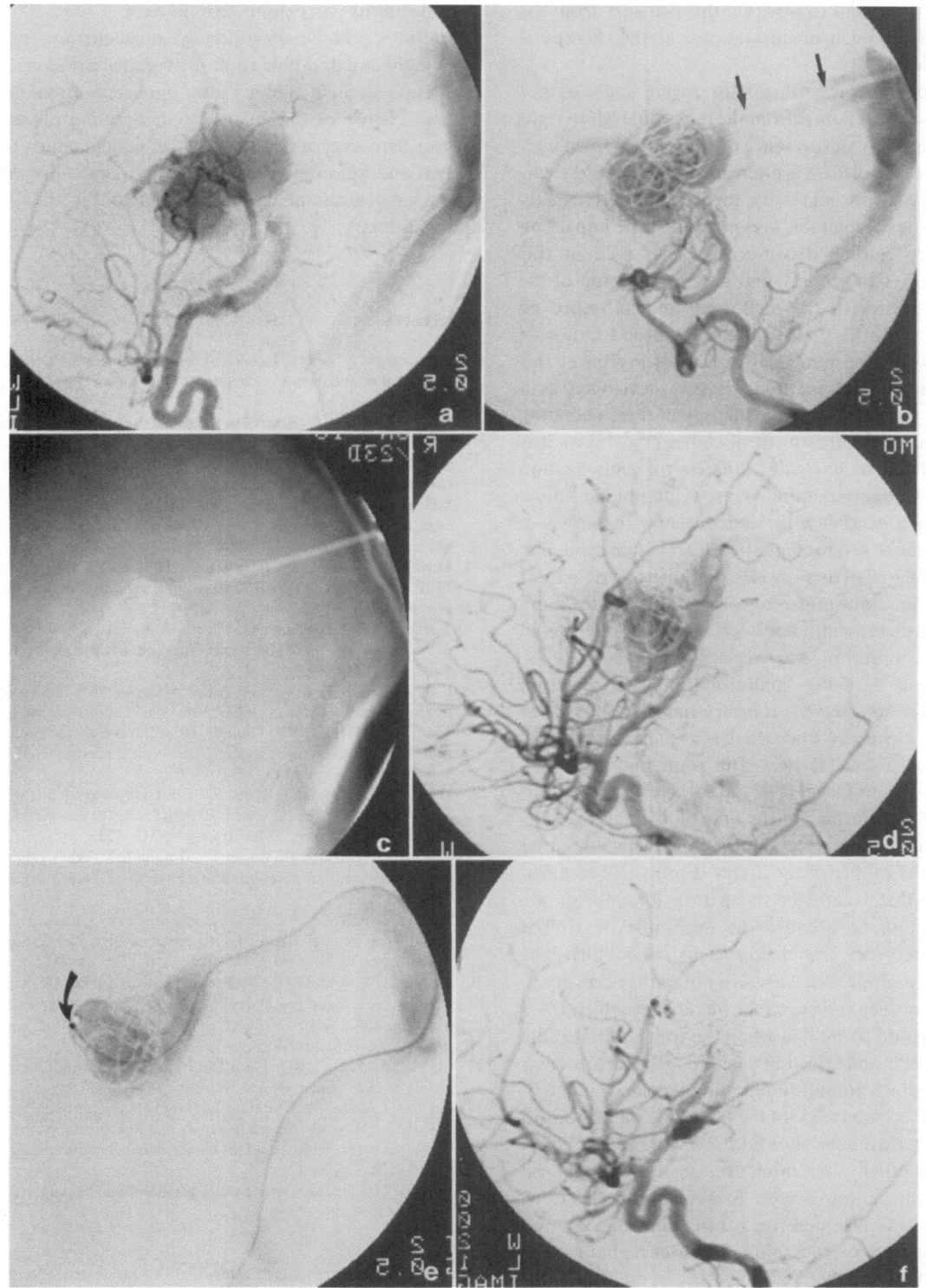

Galen. It is crucial to separate this category from the true vein of Galen malformations, as the therapy is quite different.

In neonates presenting with severe high output congestive heart failure from the functional left to right shunt caused by the presence of the vein of Galen malformation, the disease is uniformly fatal without treatment. Even with aggressive medical therapy usually including lasix, digitalis, and pressors, little impact on the severe cardiac decompensation is seen in this population. Craniotomy and surgical clipping of the feeding arteries to the malformation has improved survival very little[3,5,7] because of the deep location of the malformation and relative lack of myelin at this age. Endovascular methods, largely developed as a response to lack of effective therapy in these neonates, have become the treatment of choice[3-6,9-11]. As it is most difficult to navigate catheters for embolization through small arteries and veins, we do not consider a patient as a candidate for endovascular therapy as a neonate unless severe congestive heart failure is present. In fact, the goal of therapy is to diminish arteriovenous shunting to allow improved cardiac function for more definitive therapy at a later age, and most often serial staged embolizations are necessary.

The vein of Galen malformation is a spectrum disease. We consider the transarterial route the access of choice, especially when there is a single (mural type) or only few arterial feeders. This route may be undertaken via the umbilical artery, if catheterization of this structure is performed at the time of birth allowing its use. Transarterial access may be precluded either because the caliber of the artery is too small to allow adequate distal catheter navigation for appropriate embolization, or because the multitude of arterial feeders precludes embolizing each individually. The transvenous approach was born out of the necessity to identify another endovascular method by which these patients could be treated when the transarterial route failed. Mickle and Quisling[11] devised the transtorcular route by which embolic coils could be placed immediately on the venous side of the fistulous connections to reduce arteriovenous shunting. We[4] and others[2] have developed other transvenous accesses, both by femoral and jugular venous access, to accomplish the same goal. We have also described transvenous access and catheterization of the midline prosencephalic vein, with retrograde catheterization of the feeding artery for embolization[4] which we feel is a particularly effective method of embolization, as the feeding artery can be occluded at its entry point into the vein.

The early preliminary results are most encouraging. With eight angiographic cures in 16 patients, it is clear that endovascular therapy has impacted upon the natural history of this otherwise devastating disease process. However, a large number of patients must be treated and followed to adulthood to assess fully the final neurological and cardiac sequelae of this disease and its therapy.

References

1. Amacher AL, Shillito J (1973) The syndromes and surgical treatment of aneurysms of the great vein of Galen. J Neurosurg 39: 89–98
2. Casasco A, Lylyk P, Hodes JE, Kohan G, Aymard A, Merland J-J (1991) Percutaneous transvenous catheterization and embolization of vein of Galen aneurysms. Neurosurgery 28: 260–266
3. Ciricillo SF, Edwards MSB, Schmidt KG, Hieshima GB, Silverman NH, Higashida RT, Halbach VV (1990) Interventional neuroradiological management of vein of Galen malformations in the neonate. Neurosurgery 27: 22–28
4. Dowd CF, Halbach VV, Barnwell SL, Higashida RT, Edwards MSB, Hieshima GB (1990) Transfemoral venous embolization of vein of Galen malformations. AJNR 11: 643–648
5. Edwards MSB, Hieshima G, Higashida R, Halbach V (1988) Management of vein of Galen malformations in the neonate. Int Pediatr 3: 184–188
6. Garcia-Monaco R, Lasjaunias P, Berenstein A (1992) Therapeutic management of vein of Galen aneurysmal malformations. In: Vinuela F, Halbach VV, Dion JE (eds) Interventional neuroradiology: endovascular therapy of the central nervous system. Raven, New York, pp 113–127
7. Hoffman HJ, Chuang S, Hendrick EB, Humphreys RP (1982) Aneurysms of the vein of Galen. Experience at the Hospital for Sick Children, Toronto. J Neurosurg 57: 316–322
8. Johnston IH, Whittle IR, Besser M, Morgan MK (1987) Vein of Galen malformation: diagnosis and management. Neurosurgery 20: 747–758
9. Lasjaunias P, Rodesch G, Pruvost P, Laroche FG, Landrieu P (1989) Treatment of vein of Galen aneurysmal malformation. J Neurosurg 70: 746–750
10. Lasjaunias P, Rodesch G, TerBrugge K, Pruvost Ph, Devicter D, Comoy J, Landrieu P (1989) Vein of Galen aneurysmal malformations: report of 36 cases treated between 1982 and 1988. Acta Neurochir (Wien) 99: 26–37
11. Mickle JP, Quisling RG (1986) The transtorcular embolization of vein of Galen aneurysms. J Neurosurg 64: 731–735
12. Raybaud CA, Strother CM, Hald JK (1989) Aneurysms of the vein of Galen: embryologic considerations and anatomical features relating to the pathogenesis of the malformation. Neuroradiology 31: 109–128
13. Yaşargil MG (1988) Microneurosurgery, Vol 3B. Thieme, New York, pp 353–357

Correspondence: Christopher F. Dowd, M.D., Department of Radiology and Neurological Surgery, University of California San Francisco Medical Center, 505 Parnassus Avenue, Room L-352, San Francisco, California 94143-0628, U.S.A.

Dural Arteriovenous Fistulas: the Role of Endovascular Therapy

C.F. Dowd, V.V. Halbach, R.T. Higashida, T.P. Smith, K.W. Fraser, and **G.B. Hieshima**

Departments of Radiology and Neurological Surgery, University of California, San Francisco Medical Centre, San Francisco, California, U.S.A.

Summary

Dural arteriovenous fistulas present with a variety of signs and symptoms depending on the location of the shunt and on the pattern of venous drainage. We have treated a total of 221 dural fistulas using a variety of endovascular and surgical techniques, sometimes in combination. Cavernous sinus fistulas, most often presenting with visual symptoms, can be treated by transvenous coil embolization, and cure has been achieved in 101 of 117 patients. Transverse-sigmoid sinus fistulas can present with pulsatile tinnitus or intracerebral hemorrhage depending on venous drainage pattern. Cure has been achieved in 42 of 66 patients. Fistulas in a variety of other locations, including superior sagittal sinus, inferior petrosal sinus, deep venous system, and anterior cranial fossa have also been encountered. As dural fistulas encompass a wide clinical spectrum from benign to dangerous, invasive therapy must be tailored to the risk of non-treatment in any specific case. Endovascular therapy provides a primary therapeutic option in these patients.

Keywords: Dural arteriovenous fistula; embolization; endovascular therapy; interventional neuroradiology.

Introduction

Dural arteriovenous fistulas (DAVFs) are acquired arteriovenous shunts in the dura mater most often within the wall of a major dural sinus. These fistulas are classified by the name of the sinus or by the anatomical location where the arteriovenous connections occur. Patients present with a wide spectrum of symptoms depending on the location of the fistula and on the pattern of venous drainage [1-13,17,20]. We have treated a total of 221 DAVFs using a variety of endovascular techniques, sometimes in conjunction with surgery[1], located in the cavernous, transverse-sigmoid, superior sagittal, inferior petrosal, and deep venous sinuses as well as in the anterior cranial fossa.

Methods and Materials

A total of 221 patients with DAVFs were identified (Table 1). The majority of DAVFs involved the cavernous (117 patients) or trans-verse-sigmoid (66 patients) sinuses. Symptoms depended on DAVF location and on the venous drainage pattern.

Cavernous sinus DAVFs most often present with pulsatile tinnitus, and proptosis and chemosis from retrograde arterialized venous drainage in the superior and inferior ophthalmic veins. More ominous presenting signs and symptoms, including diminished visual acuity from impaired retinal perfusion or neurological deficits and intracranial hemorrhage from retrograde venous drainage to cortical veins, are less common. Compliant patients without cortical drainage, significant common carotid bifurcation atherosclerosis, rapid loss of visual acuity or an underlying hypercoagulable state are candidates for carotid-jugular compression therapy in which the contralateral hand is used to compress the common carotid artery and jugular vein for a period not to exceed 30 seconds several times per hour. This theoretically reduces arterial inflow and raises venous pressure in order to promote thrombosis.

Transverse-sigmoid DAVFs most commonly present with pulsatile tinnitus, especially if the fistula is located in proximity to the temporal bone and middle ear cavity. Headaches may be localized to the region of the fistula or generalized. The pattern of venous drainage is an important factor affecting clinical presentation as neurological deficits are often associated with DAVFs exhibiting abnormal venous drainage to the cortical veins, which can result in venous hypertension, infarction, or hemorrhage.

Petrosal DAVFs are similar in presentation to cavernous DAVFs because venous drainage may involve the ophthalmic veins or jugular system. Deep venous sinus and anterior cranial fossa (ethmoidal) DAVFs most commonly present with intracranial, subarachnoid, or subdural hemorrhage because of the presence of cortical or parenchymal venous drainage and resulting venous hypertension.

Table 1. *Dural Arteriovenous Fistula Locations*

Location	No. of patients
Cavernous sinus	117
Transverse-sigmoid sinus	66
Superior sagittal sinus	10
Deep venous sinus	9
Anterior cranial fossa	8
Inferior petrosal sinus	6
Torcular herophili	3
Craniocervical junction	2
Total	221

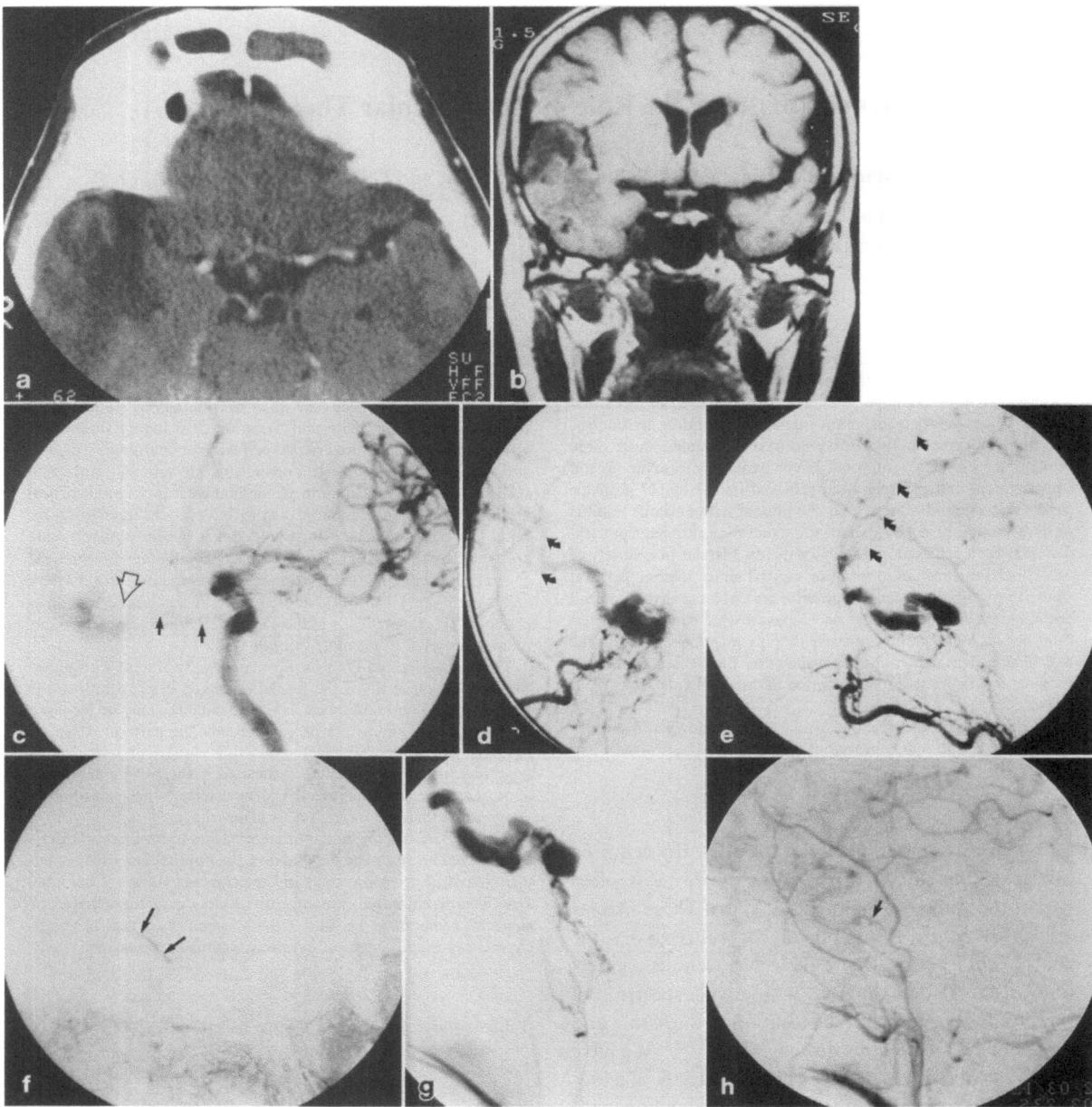

Fig. 1. High-risk cavernous sinus DAVF. 70 year-old woman with headaches and chemosis of the right eye. (a) Transaxial computed tomography (CT) scan with intravenous contrast shows right temporal lobe edema. (b) Coronal magnetic resonance (MRI) scan (TR) 600/TE 20) confirms dramatic right temporal lobe edema and/or infarction. (c) Left internal carotid (ICA) arteriogram, frontal projection, shows right cavernous sinus DAVF (open arrow) supplied by branch of left meningohypophyseal trunk (closed arrows). (d) and (e) Right external carotid (ECA) arteriogram, frontal (d), and lateral (e) projections, confirms cavernous sinus DAVF supplied by ascending pharyngeal, meningeal, and foramen rotundum branches. Retrograde drainage via sphenoparietal sinus into cortical veins (arrows) is responsible for temporal lobe edema. (f) Right ECA arteriogram, lateral projection (delayed venous phase of 2E) shows opacification of posterior superior ophthalmic vein (arrows) demonstrating near-static flow. This finding explains the patient's eye symptoms. (g) Right ascending pharyngeal arteriogram, lateral projection, shows abundant fistula supply. Because we were unable to access the cavernous sinus via a transvenous route, liquid adhesive embolization was performed from this position after a negative provocative lidocaine test. (h) Right ECA arteriogram, lateral projection, post-embolization, shows minimal static opacification of the posterior cavernous sinus at the fistula site (arrow) without cortical venous drainage. Contrast reflux into ICA is seen. Control arteriogram performed 2 months later confirmed angiographic cure

Transarterial embolization is carried out from a transfemoral access by superselective catheterization of the appropriate artery using a Tracker catheter (Target Therapeutics, Fremont, California). Embolic agents include polyvinyl alcohol (PVA) particles and liquid adhesives (N-butyl cyanoacrylate).

Transvenous embolization is carried out from a transfemoral access by superselective catheterization of the appropriate vein using a Tracker catheter. This most often involves cavernous sinus catheterization via the inferior petrosal sinus or catheterization of the transverse-sigmoid sinuses via the internal jugular vein. Embolic agents include platinum or steel coils (Cook, inc., Bloomington, Indiana) and custom-cut segments of 4.0 silk suture.

Results

Two hundred twenty-one patients with a variety of DAVFs were treated by a combination of endovascular therapy (transarterial, transvenous, or via direct operative access) and surgery.

Cavernous sinus DAVFs are treated according to duration and severity of symptoms, and whether cortical venous drainage is present. Cure was achieved in 101 of 117 patients with cavernous sinus DAVFs.

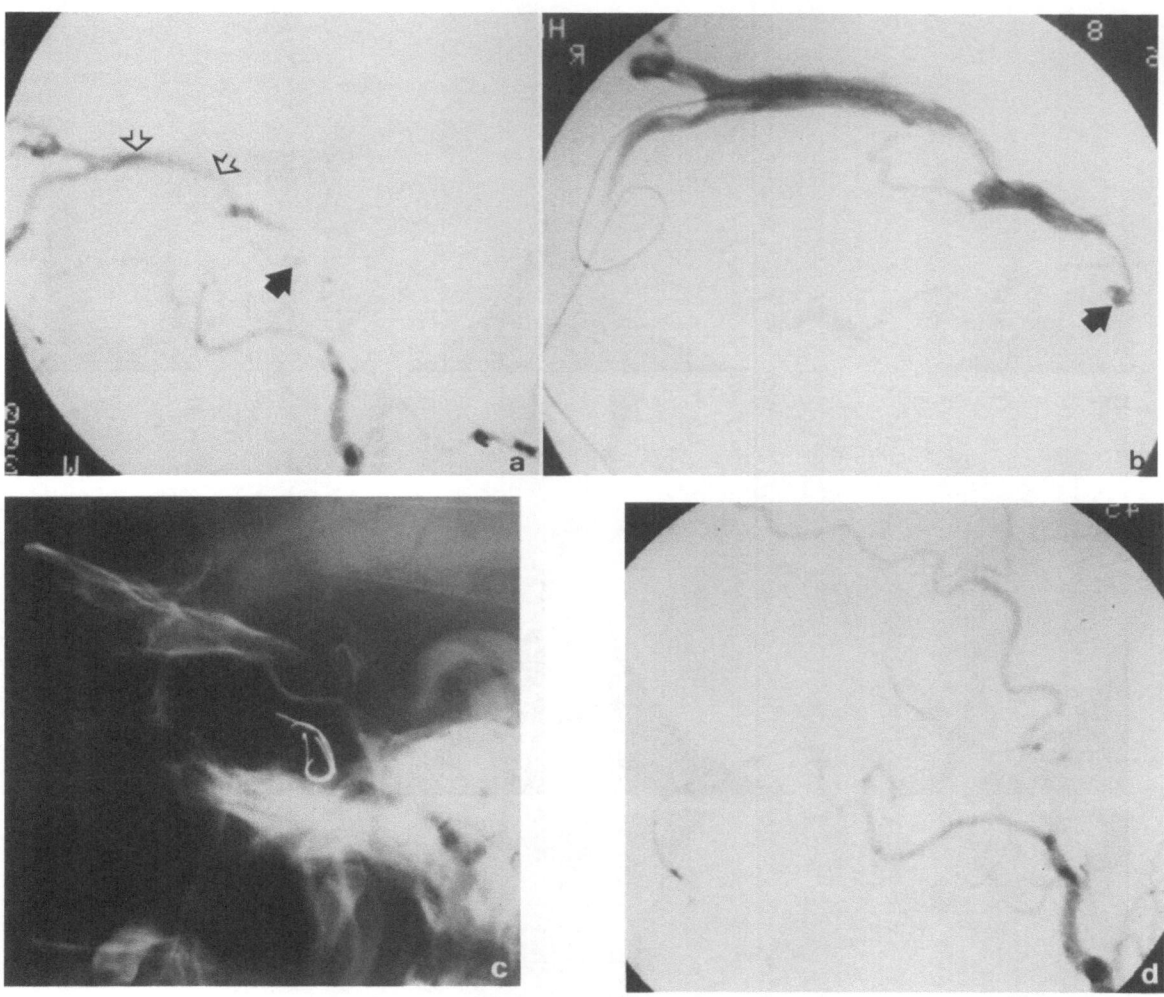

Fig. 2. Cavernous sinus DAVF. 58 year-old man with proptosis and chemosis for six months. (a) Right external carotid (ECA) arteriogram, lateral projection, shows DAVF of the cavernous sinus supplied by accessory meningeal and foramen rotundum branches draining only to the superior ophthalmic vein (SOV) (open arrows). The fistula site is delineated (closed arrow). (b) Right superior ophthalmic venogram, lateral projection, prior to coil embolization. Microcatheter has been navigated from a transfemoral access through the external jugular and angular veins to the SOV. Catheter tip is at the fistula site (arrow). (c) Plain skull film, lateral projection, shows multiple platinum coils at the fistula site. (d) Right ECA arteriogram, lateral projection, after transvenous coil embolization, shows no residual fistula. Within weeks the patients symptoms had resolved completely

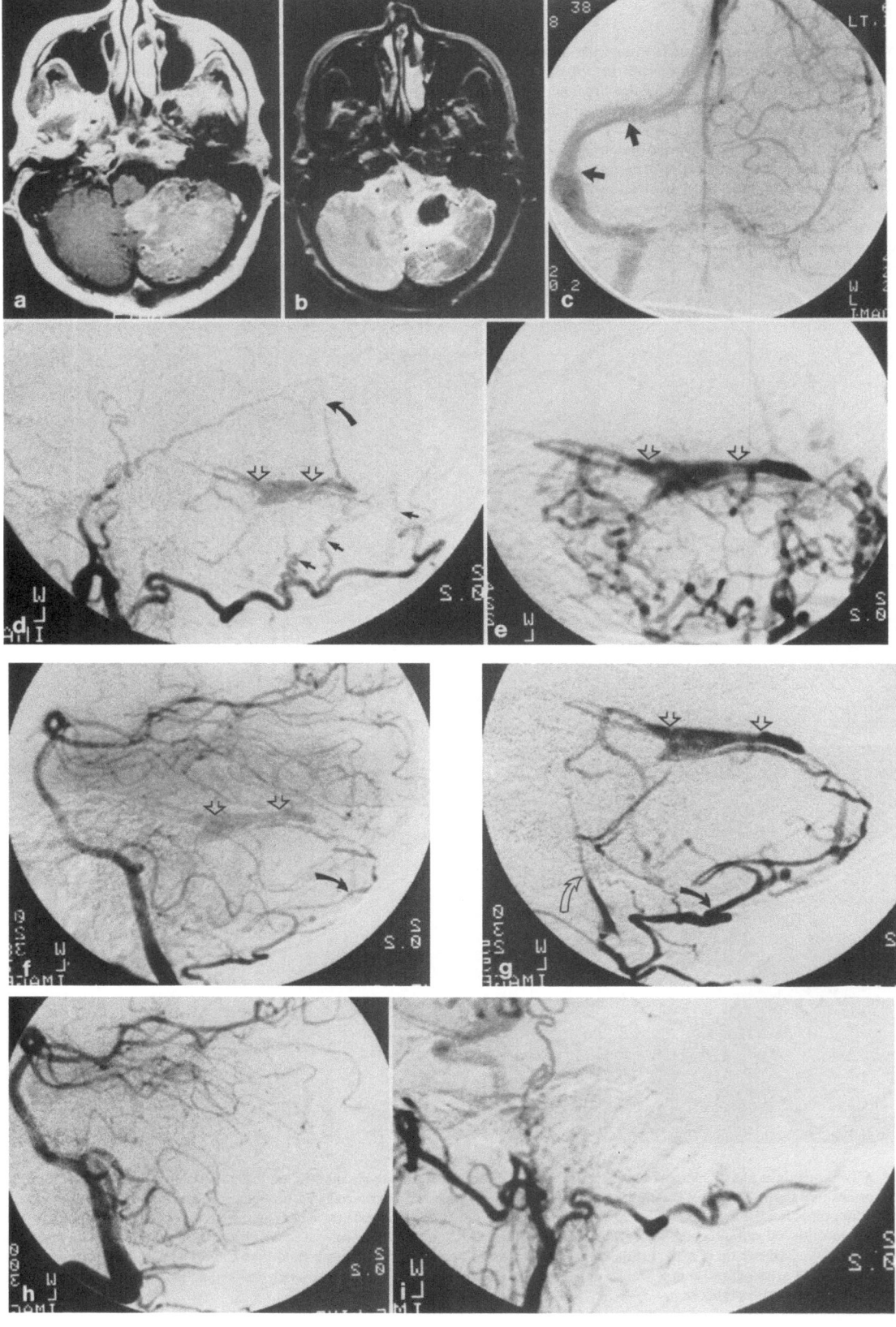

Eighteen of 53 patients with cavernous DAVFs who undertook carotid-jugular compression therapy were cured without other forms of therapy. There were no complications. Subselective catheterization and embolization of external carotid feeding branches, either with particulate emboli or liquid adhesives (Fig. 1), resulted in clinical cure or improvement in symptoms of 35 of 45 patients in whom this therapy was used. It was difficult to achieve angiographic cure in some patients because of the large number of arterial inputs necessitating catheterization and embolization of each one. Transvenous embolization has become our endovascular therapy of choice in patients who fail carotid-jugular compression therapy by achieving catheterization of the cavernous sinus via the inferior petrosal sinus in most cases, or rarely via the superior ophthalmic vein (Fig. 2). Forty-four of 54 patients in whom this endovascular method was used were cured after deposition of multiple platinum coils in the cavernous sinus.

Therapeutic options for treatment of transverse-sigmoid sinus DAVFs depend entirely on the routes of venous drainage. Cure was achieved in 42 of 66 patients. In low risk fistulas, the involved sinus is patent and the flow antegrade. Low risk fistulas can be followed clinically assuming the patient can tolerate the pulsatile tinnitus. Transarterial embolization, either with liquid adhesives or particles, can reduce the arterial supply and achieve cure in some cases (13 of 26 patients). Transvenous embolization with platinum or steel coils may provide a cure if the involved sinus appears abnormal and demonstrates diverted venous drainage (high-risk DAVF), and if this sinus can be catheterized. Alternatively, craniotomy and surgical access to the transverse or sigmoid sinus can permit such coil embolization as well. Eleven of 20 patients treated by transvenous coil embolization were cured. In addition to surgical access for coil embolization, craniotomy and surgical coagulation of the fistula site preceded by transarterial particulate embolization (Fig. 3) has achieved cure in 15 of 17 patients.

Anterior cranial fossa DAVFs, commonly termed "ethmoidal" DAVFs because of the arterial supply from anterior and posterior ethmoidal branches of the ophthalmic arteries, are treated by craniotomy and surgical coagulation, as safe arterial or venous access to this location is usually not achievable. Cure was achieved surgically in 8 of 8 patients. Likewise, deep venous DAVFs have been treated by a combination of transarterial particulate embolization followed by either surgical coagulation/obliteration of the fistula site or surgical access for liquid adhesive embolization. Cure was achieved in all 9 patients with one postoperative death. Aggressive therapy is warranted because of the risk of stroke and hemorrhage in these fistulas. Superior sagittal sinus DAVFs were likewise treated by a combination of pre-operative embolization and either surgical exploration as access for liquid adhesive embolization or as definitive surgical obliteration. Cure was achieved in 10 of 10 patients, with one surgical complication.

Discussion

The features of a DAVF which direct treatment are a) the location of the fistula and b) the venous drainage pattern[13]. DAVFs are dynamic lesions which run the spectrum from benign diseases in the absence of cortical

Fig. 3. Complex transverse sinus DAVF. 68 year-old woman with several month history of dizziness and nausea with acute worsening, new left facial numbness and mild weakness, and gait instability with falling to the left. (a) gadolinium-DTPA-enhanced transaxial MRI scan (TR 600/TE 20), performed after symptom onset but before acute worsening, shows left cerebellar hemisphere swelling and enhancement, with several foci of signal void representing abnormal vessels. No discreet arteriovenous malformation nidus is seen. (b) Transaxial MRI scan (TR 2800/TE 80), performed in the same plane as A several days after abrupt symptom worsening, shows a new left cerebellar hemorrhage. A central dark area (deoxyhemoglobin) is surrounded by high-signal edema. (c) Left internal carotid artery (ICA) arteriogram, frontal view, venous phase, shows absent normal venous drainage to the left transverse sinus with opacification of the right transverse sinus (arrows) only. (d) Arterial, and E, magnified venous phases of a left external carotid (ECA) arteriogram, lateral views, show a transverse sinus DAVF supplied by several transmas-toid perforating branches (d, small arrows) of the occipital artery and by posterior division of the middle meningeal artery (d, curved arrow). These feeding arteries were catheterized superselectively and embolized. The isolated segment of left transverse sinus (open arrows) drains only to multiple cerebellar veins (e), and demonstra-tes no normal antegrade venous drainage. (f) Left vertebral arteriogram, lateral view, also shows the DAVF (open arrows) supplied by posterior meningeal artery (curved arrow). (g) Selective left posterior meningeal arteriogram (closed curved arrow), lateral view, opacifies the affected isolated left transverse sinus (open arrows). Note contrast reflux into left vertebral artery (curved open arrow). The microcatheter was navigated to a more distal position in the posterior meningeal artery prior to embolization to avoid reflux of embolic material into the vertebral artery. (h) Left vertebral, and (i) left ECA arteriograms, lateral views, after embolization of occipital, middle meningeal, and posterior meningeal artery supply, show no residual DAVF. The patient subsequently underwent craniotomy and resection of the affected transverse sinus to remove the possibility of future recanalization of the DAVF. She has recovered fully from her hemorrhage

venous drainage, visual loss[18], or elevated intracranial pressure, to dangerous, in the presence of venous sinus restriction and aberrant cortical venous drainage, placing the patient at significant risk for cerebral infarction or hemorrhage. Initially, a DAVF may drain entirely into the affected venous sinus in an antegrade fashion. Over time, because of high flow or pressure, this venous drainage pathway may become inadequate if venous stenosis or occlusion develops and in such cases the venous drainage may be reversed to other dural sinus pathways or into cortical/parenchymal veins. Such a phenomenon is an indication for urgent therapy[6].

Selection of appropriate therapy is tailored to the degree of risk associated with the DAVF. Some fistulas may undergo spontaneous regression without therapy or even following diagnostic angiography. Another form of conservative treatment is carotid-jugular compression therapy, which can be especially useful in cavernous sinus DAVFs[14]. In the absence of cortical venous drainage, significant common carotid bifurcation atherosclerosis, and rapid loss of visual acuity, this therapy can result in static blood flow at the site of the fistula due to a combination of reduced arterial inflow and venous outflow.

Transarterial endovascular approaches require navigation of microcatheters through feeding arteries as close to the fistula site as possible. As the goal of therapy is obliteration of the fistula site, proximal artery occlusion will only encourage collateral fistula supply and preclude future use of this artery as an access to the fistula. Liquid adhesive agents are most effective when there is low risk of embolizing normal dural arteries because of diminished rate of recanalization. Particulate embolic material (PVA) is technically easier to use however, and despite greater possibility of recanalization, may be selected when there is increased risk of normal artery embolization. Transarterial embolization is coupled with pretherapeutic provocative testing with 2% cardiac lidocane to identify supply to normal cranial nerves[15]. Transarterial therapy is also useful when a surgical procedure is planned as definitive therapy, for the purposes of diminishing arteriovenous shunting preoperatively.

Transvenous catheterization embolization of the fistula site may be efficacious when DAVFs remain patent despite transarterial therapy or when a DAVF has inadequate arterial access. DAVFs involving the cavernous sinus are particularly well suited for this technique[8], and this has become our treatment of choice in this lesion. From a transfemoral venous access, a microcatheter is navigated through the internal jugular vein and inferior petrosal sinus to the cavernous sinus, allowing platinum coil or silk suture embolization. A transfemoral approach via the external jugular vein and superior ophthalmic vein may also allow cavernous sinus access when the inferior petrosal sinus cannot be traversed. This therapy has also been useful in transverse-sigmoid sinus dural fistulas[10] when the sinus appears diseased angiographically and does not provide significant normal venous outflow. This sinus can be packed with a series of platinum or steel coils under these circumstances either by transfemoral venous route or craniotomy and direct surgical access of this area. Care must be maintained to avoid obstructing outflow of the vein of Labbe when it flows in a normal antegrade direction. A normal transverse sinus with antegrade flow in the absence of cortical venous drainage should not be considered for this technique.

In some cases, craniotomy and surgical obliteration of the DAVF may be necessary. This is especially true in anterior cranial fossa (ethmoidal) DAVFs[12,16] which most commonly present with intracranial hemorrhage, because of the lack of safe arterial or venous access routes for endovascular therapy. This is also true in deep venous sinus DAVFs[11] and in high risk transverse-sigmoid DAVFs[19].

In conclusion, we have had experience with 221 patients with a variety of dural arteriovenous fistulas. Our experience indicates that endovascular techniques have become a mainstay of therapy in this disease process and that a continued collaboration among interventional neuroradiologists, neurosurgeons, ophthalmologists, neurologists, and skull base surgeons will allow development of improved therapeutic techniques.

References

1. Barnwell SL, Halbach VV, Higashida RT, Hieshima GB, Wilson CB (1989) Complex dural arteriovenous fistulas: results of a new combined neurosurgical and interventional neuroradiology treatment in 16 patients. J Neurosurg 7: 352–358
2. Barnwell SL, Halbach VV, Dowd CF, Higashida RT, Hieshima GB (1990) Dural fistulas involving the inferior petrosal sinus: angiographic findings in six patients. AJNR 11 (3): 511–517
3. DeMarco JK, Dillon W, Halbach VV, Tsuruda JS (1990) Dural arteriovenous fistulas: evaluation with MR imaging. Radiology 175: 193–199
4. Halbach VV, Higashida RT, Hieshima GB, Goto K, Norman D, Newton TH (1987) Dural fistulas involving the transverse and sigmoid sinuses: results of treatment in 28 patients. Radiology 163: 443–447

5. Halbach VV, Higashida RT, Hieshima GB, Reicher M, Norman D, Newton TH (1987) Dural fistulas involving the cavernous sinus: results of treatment in 30 patients. Radiology 163: 437–442

6. Halbach VV, Hieshima GB, Higashida RT, Reicher M (1987) Carotid-cavernous fistulas: indications for urgent therapy. AJNR 8: 627–633

7. Halbach VV, Higashida RT, Hieshima GB, Cahan L, Rosenblum M (1988) Treatment of dural arteriovenous malformations involving the superior sagittal sinus. AJNR 9: 337–343

8. Halbach VV, Higashida RT, Hieshima GB, Hardin CW, Pribram H (1989) Transvenous embolization of dural fistulas involving the cavernous sinus. AJNR 10: 377–384

9. Halbach VV, Higashida RT, Hieshima GB, Hardin CW (1989) Embolization of the dural branches arising from the cavernous internal carotid artery. AJNR 10: 143–150

10. Halbach VV, Higashida RT, Hieshima GB, Mehringer CM, Hardin CW (1989) Transvenous embolization of dural fistulas involving the transverse and sigmoid sinuses. AJNR 10: 385–392

11. Halbach VV, Higashida RT, Hieshima GB, Wilson CW (1989) Treatment of dural fistulas involving the deep cerebral venous system. AJNR 10: 393–399

12. Halbach VV, Higashida RT, Hieshima GB, Wilson CW, Barnwell SL, Dowd CF (1990) Dural arteriovenous fistulas supplied by ethmoidal arteries. Neurosurgery 26(5): 816–823

13. Halbach VV, Higashida RT, Hieshima GB, Dowd CF (1992) Endovascular therapy of dural fistulas. In: Vinuela F, Halbach VV, Dion JE (eds) Interventional neuroradiology: endovascular therapy of the central nervous system. Raven, New York, pp 29–50

14. Higashida RT, et al (1986) Closure of carotid cavernous sinus fistula by external compression of the carotid artery and jugular vein. Acta Radiol [Suppl] 369: 591–593

15. Horton JA, Kerber CW (1986) Lidocaine injection into the external carotid branches: provocative test to preserve cranial nerve function in therapeutic embolization. AJNR 7: 105–108

16. Kobayashi H, Hayashi M, Noguchi Y, Tsuji T, Handa Y, Caner HH (1988) Dural arteriovenous malformations in the anterior cranial fossa. Surg Neurol 30(5): 396–401

17. Picard L, Bracard S, Mallet J, Per A, Glaccobe HL, Roland J (1987) Spontaneous dural arteriovenous fistulas. Semin Intervent Radiol 4: 219–240

18. Sanders MD, Hoyt WF (1969) Hypoxic ocular sequelae of carotid-cavernous fistulae. Br J Ophthalmol 53: 82–97

19. Sundt TM, Piepgras DG (1983) The surgical approach to arteriovenous malformations of the lateral and sigmoid dural sinuses. J Neurosurg 59: 32–39

20. Vinuela F, Fox AJ, Debrun GM, Peerless SJ, Drake CG (1984) Spontaneous carotid cavernous fistulas: clinical, radiological, and therapeutic considerations. Experience with 20 cases. J Neurosurg 60(5): 976–984

Correspondence: Christopher F. Dowd, M.D., Department of Radiology and Neurological Surgery, University of California San Francisco Medical Center, 505 Parnassus Avenue, Room L-352, San Francisco, California 94143-0628, U.S.A.

Treatment of 23 Dural AVMs Located at the Transverse and Sigmoid Sinuses

J. Hernesniemi[1], **T. Saari**[2], and **M. Puranen**[2]

Departments of [1]Neurosurgery and [2]Radiology (Neuroradiology), University Hospital of Kuopio, Kuopio, Finland

Summary

Dural arteriovenous malformations (DAVM) located at the transverse and sigmoid sinuses are rare acquired lesions. Results and complications of mainly direct surgery are reviewed in 23 patients with primary lesions. There were 18 excellent, three good and one poor result (from diminished vision preceding surgery). One patient died suddenly due to sinus thrombosis one week after surgery. Three patients had venous hemorrhagic infarction in the tributaries of the vein of Labbe. To avoid recurrences, direct surgery is still needed.

Keywords: Arteriovenous malformation; dural arteriovenous malformation; lateral and sigmoid sinuses; operative approach.

Introduction

Dural arteriovenous malformations (DAVM) are rare lesions even in their commonest location in the posterior fossa. Their surgical treatment was described by Hugosson, Sundt and Piepgras, the latter describing 41 cases from the Mayo Clinics in a time period of 13 years[4,12,13]. In recent years we have had the opportunity to diagnose and treat several of these lesions with the described, but rather seldomly published surgical method[4,12-13]. This experience in a small defined area shows that these lesions might be more common than expected.

Patients and Methods

This study is based on 23 patients treated for a posterior fossa dural AVM located at transverse and sigmoid sinuses at the University Hospital of Kuopio, Finland from 1981 to V/1992. Twenty-one patients were treated during the last five years. At the same time 1100 patients with cerebral aneurysms and 100 with cerebral AVMs were treated – all patients coming from eastern Finland (population 870,000).

The mean age of the patients was 53.2 years, range 15–80 years. Fourteen patients were females. Nearly all lesions (18) were located on the left; in a few cases contralateral small feeders were noted. One fistula mainly located at the confluens sinuum is included to show all

possible complications of surgery (this 26 year-old patient died from sinus thrombosis after uneventful surgery). No case had had previous direct or endovascular surgery. The most common symptom and finding was a bruit (Table 1). All patients had a preoperative CT and angiograms, in most instances studies of both carotids and one vertebral artery were made. It is difficult to categorize these cases by measuring the DAVMs; however 16 patients had undisputably large lesions (diameter more than two inches and multiple feeders from the external and internal carotid arteries and vertebral muscle branches, Fig. 1). Highest number of feeders was usually seen in the corner between the lateral and sigmoid sinuses; the majority of the feeders were derived from the occipital artery. Sinus occlusion was seen frequently as a part of the disease. Five DAVMs were medium-sized, between one and two inches in diameter and with several feeders, and two were small with "one" feeder. In very few cases was any history of sinus thrombosis or other undiagnosed episode detected; in general we agree that these lesions are acquired.

Surgery

All patients were operated on by the first author; pre-operative and operative embolization were performed mainly by Saari and Puranen. Four early cases were treated by a combination of ligation of the external carotid arteries and perioperative open embolization of the external carotid artery feeders with gelfoam or glue and eventual lateral suboccipital craniotomy (two cases). Fifteen patients were treated by lateral subocci-pital craniotomy as described by Hugosson and Sundt[4,]

Table 1. *Symptoms in 23 Patients with Dural AVMs at the Transverse and Sigmoid Sinuses*

Bruit as main symptom	22
Severe bruit	18
Moderate bruit	4
Headache	14
Cardiac symptoms	5
Hemiparesis or dysphasia	2
Impaired vision	1
Epilepsy or mental deficit	0

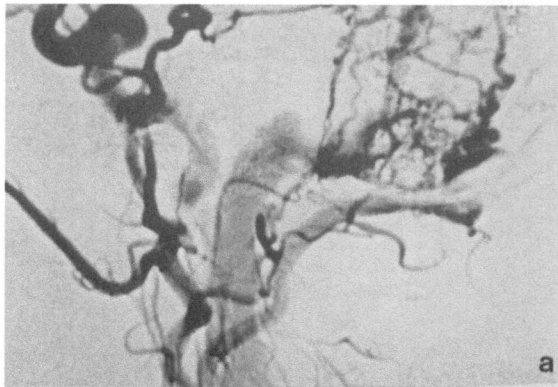

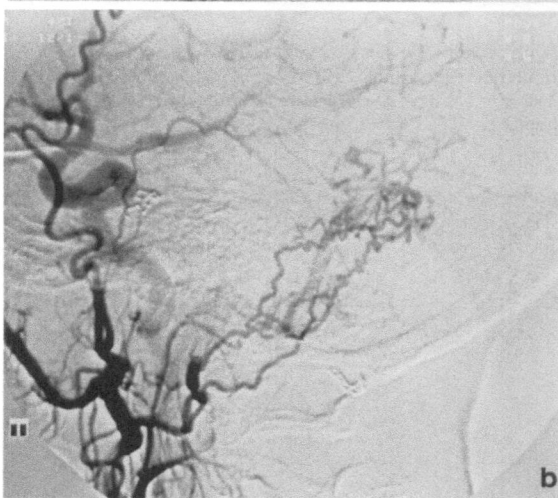

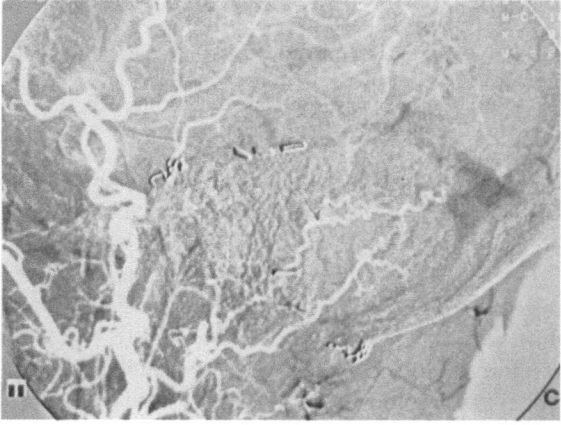

Fig. 1. (a–c) Lateral angiograms in a large right-sided dural AVM at the transverse and sigmois sinuses in a 44-years-old female with a severe bruit as the only symptom: preoperatively. (a) after embolization with coils and glue (b), and after direct surgery with total occlusion (c)

[12,13]. In 8 of these cases preoperative embolization was used. Four cases were treated by embolization alone with one total occlusion; in two of these further embolization or direct surgery is planned (one aged patient with partial occlusion died from unrelated heart failure).

All patients with direct surgery were operated on in the park bench position. Moderate hypotension (80–100 mmHg systolic) was maintained during the operation. Mannitol infusion was given routinely. Lumbar drainage was used in most cases, as it was felt easier to ligate the sinus with the extra space achieved by lumbar drainage and/or evacuation of cerebrospinal fluid under microscopic control from the cerebellar basal cisterns. A question mark or slightly curved incision was used in smaller DAVMs, and a single layer flap was turned. Enlarged occipital and posterior auricular arteries were cut and coagulated with heavy bipolar coagulation. A muscle incision was made in the neck by cutting current, and again bleedings were bipolarly coagulated. Bone bleedings were treated by heavy monopolar coagulation or bone wax. A lateral suboccipital bone flap with 4–5 burr holes was made. Burr holes were heavily waxed if bleeding occurred, and a Gigli saw or craniotome was used to cut the medial portions. The lateral parts were cut by drilling the bone away as far laterally as possible, as described by Yaşargil[14]. Dry drilling with a large diamond burr under the microscope is extremely useful for reducing bony bleeding by the high temperature produced. The bone flap was quickly elevated and wet tamponade was held in place, and all the dural bleeders were secured by heavy bipolar coagulation. Eventual sinus bleeding(s) were treated initially with Oxycel® tamponade. At least in this step, the microscope was positioned and used during the extirpation period. In the case of epidural bleeding, several tacking sutures were used.

The sinus was ligated in the medial part of the craniotomy. Preoperatively the vein of Labbé or other draining veins were carefully studied in angiograms. An attempt was made to preserve the vein of Labbé in all cases. Resection proceeded in the manner described by Sundt: in the corner, several arterial feeders were found, and heavy bipolar coagulation and removal of the bone by dry drilling were necessary. Finally, the lateral portion was removed. The sinus was stopped with oxidized cellulose, large muscle pieces and/or tissue glue, and clipped with large Weck clips or sutured. No dural substitutes were used. In several cases tacking sutures played an important part in the otherwise routine closure, due to the high vascularity of the dura mater. Postoperatively hypotension at moderate levels was used during the first days in intensive care. All patients except one (refused after one reoperation and bone flap removal) had postoperative control angiograms.

Results

The results can be seen in Tables 2–4.

Of the 17(15 + 2) patients treated with direct surgery, three had postoperative venous hemorrhagic infarction (Fig. 2): two patients made good recoveries but in one case recraniotomy was needed, resulting in dysphasia and a field deficit (moderate disability). One perioperative huge epidural hematoma outside the operative area was evacuated immediately as a continuation of the first procedure (Fig. 3). The patient already had bilateral dilated pupils, but was conscious immediately after evacuation of the huge epidural hematoma in the supratentorial region on the same side. Difficulties were encountered in stopping the bleeding from abnormal dural vessels. This case had had preoperative embolization under heparin treatment, and the patient was operated on in the same day.

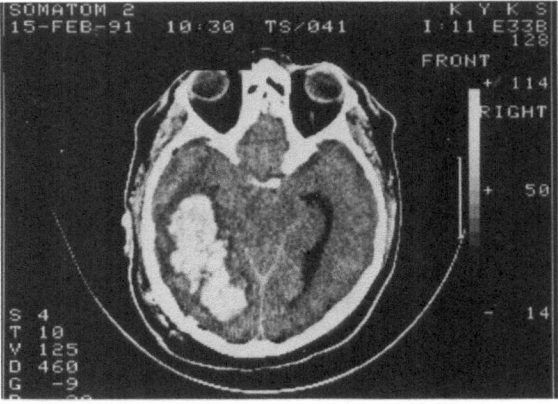

Fig. 2. A huge left-sided venous hemorrhagic infarction at the tributaries of the vein of Labbé in 44-years-old male on the second postoperative day. A recraniotomy resulted in field deficit and dysphasia

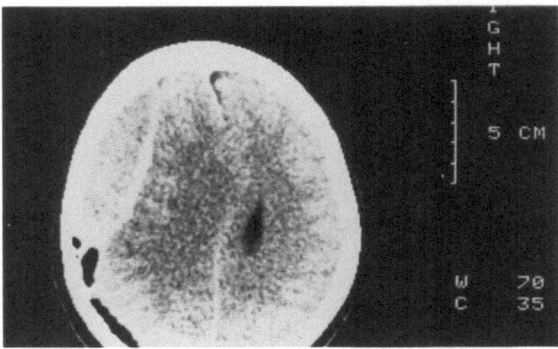

Fig. 3. A perioperative extradural hematoma outside the operative area in a 54-years-old female. The patient had fixed dilated pupils; an immediate new craniotomy resulted in moderate disability

Table 2. *Mode of Treatment in 23 Dural AVMs at the Transverse and Sigmoid Sinuses*

Multiple ligation of feeders	2
Multiple ligation of feeders and subsequent craniotomy	2
Craniotomy	15
(with preoperative embolization)	8
Embolization alone	4

Table 3. *Total Occlusion Rate in 23 Patients with Dural AVMs at the Transverse and Sigmoid Sinuses*

Craniotomy	14/15
Multiple ligation and subsequent craniotomy	2/2
Embolization	1/4
Multiple ligation	1/2

Table 4. *Outcome in 23 Patients with Dural AVMs at the Transverse and Sigmoid Sinuses (Glasgow Outcome Scale[5])*

Good recovery	18
Moderate disability (all caused by surgery)	3
Severe disability (preoperative defict)	1
Dead	1

This patient had 3700 ml of bleeding; otherwise bleeding has not been a problem as all other cases had bleeding of less than 850 ml.

One patient already mentioned died one week after operation on the day of planned discharge to home, due to confluens sinus thrombosis. In 18 cases the result was excellent, in three cases good and in one case poor, as the patient already had diminished vision preoperatively. All patients had their bruits terminated but peculiarly other disturbing noises not objectively demonstrable were heard. Most patients went back to work. Total occlusion of the lesion was achieved in 16 of 17 cases with direct surgery (Table 3). One patient had contralateral carotid cave aneurysm, which was ligated without problems.

Discussion

Our experience is similar to that of the Mayo Clinic 12–13. Some experience in cerebrovascular surgery is needed, and especially rather rapid operative technique is recommended. The mobile microscope has been extremely useful during removal of these lesions, in contrast to the opinion of Sundt. Bleedings during opening of the skull can be treated very effectively, and the bleeding points in dura and bone can be located more easily and handled better under good illumination and magnification, a finding not different from aneurysm or tumour surgery. In fact we think the rareness of bleeding problems is due to the use of the microscope. Preoperatively the fate of the healthy sinus and the vein of Labbé has to be observed very closely.

The vein of Labbé is the most vulnerable point in this surgical strategy. The consequences of obstruction of the vein of Labbé are extremely severe and may result in permanent deficits, the risk being increased by the mostly left-sided presentation. A partial resection of the transverse sinus is recommended in the presence of a prominent v. of Labbé to preserve the flow. Endovascular therapy alone or in combination with direct surgery are the methods of choice before surgery. A long-term follow-up of the patients with endovascular occlusion is still lacking; a rather rapid recurrence in two of our cases warns us not to rely too heavily on embolization alone. Anastomosis between the external carotid and vertebral arteries by muscle branches may result in fatalities when endovascular methods are used.

Therapeutic Recommendations

Endovascular surgery may provide definitive treatment in small and medium-sized dural AVMs and has to be used in aged or otherwise fragile patients. In large lesions direct surgery is needed; preoperative embolization seems to be helpful.

References

1. Aminoff MJ (1973) Vascular anomalies in the intracranial dura mater. Brain 96: 601–612
2. Handa J, Yoneda S, Handa H (1975) Venous sinus occlusion with a dural arteriovenous malformation of the posterior fossa. Surg Neurol 4: 433–437
3. Houser OW, Baker Jr HL, Rhoton Jr AL, (1972) Intracranial dural arteriovenous malformations. Radiology 105: 55–64
4. Hugosson R, Bergström K (1974) Surgical treatment of dural arteriovenous malformation in the region of the sigmoid sinus. J Neurol Neurosurg Psychiatry 37: 97–101
5. Jennet B, Bond M (1975) Assessment of outcome after severe brain damage. A practical scale. Lancet i: 480–484
6. Kosnik EJ, Hunt WE, Miller CA (1974) Dural arteriovenous malformations. J Neurosurg 40: 322–329
7. Kuehner A, Krastel A, Stoll W (1976) Arteriovenous malformations of the transverse dural sinus. J Neurosurg 45: 12–19
8. Lamas E, Lobato RD, Esparza J, Escudero (1977) Dural posterior fossa AVM producing raised sagittal sinus pressure. Case report. J Neurosurg 46: 804–810
9. Magidson MA, Weinberg PE (1976) Spontaneous closure of a dural arteriovenous malformation. Surg Neurol 6: 107–110
10. Newton TH, Cronqvist S (1969) Involvement of dural arteries in intracranial arteriovenous malformations. Radiology 93: 1071–1078
11. Nicola GC, Nizzoli V (1968) Dural arteriovenous malformations of the posterior fossa. J Neurol Neurosurg Psychiatry 31: 514–519
12. Obrador S, Soto M, Silvela J (1975) Clinical syndromes of arteriovenous malformations of the transverse-sigmoid sinus. J Neurol Neurosurg Psychiatry 38: 436–451
13. Sundt TM Jr, Piepgras DG (1983) The surgical approach to arteriovenous malformations of the lateral and sigmoid dural sinuses. J Neurosurg 59: 32–39
14. Sundt TM Jr, Piepgras DG, Forbes GS (1988) The surgical approach to arteriovenous malformations of the lateral and sigmoid dural sinuses. In: Schmidek HH, Sweet WH (eds) Operative neurosurgical techniques, Vol II. Saunders, Philadelphia, pp 855–862
15. Yaşargil MG (1986) Microneurosurgery in 4 volumes, Vol 1. Thieme Stuttgart, pp 238–241

Correspondence: Juha Hernesniemi, M.D., Department of Neurosurgery, University Hospital of Kuopio, SF-70210 Kuopio, Finland.

Diagnosis and Management of Venous Angiomas

J.M. Zabramski, R.F. Spetzler, and **D. Rigamonti**

Division of Neurological Surgery, Barrow Neurological Institute, Phoenix, Arizona, U.S.A.

Summary

Cerebral vascular malformations are congenital abnormalities that affect from 1% to 5% of the population. They are typically divided into four types: 1) arteriovenous malformations (AVMs); 2) venous malformations; 3) cavernous malformations; and 4) telangiectases.

Venous malformations are by far the most common cerebral vascular malformation identified on pathologic studies outnumbering AVMs by a ratio of approximately 6:1. The fact that the majority of venous malformations are asymptomatic explains their relative rarity in surgical pathology reviews. On gross examination, venous malformations are characterized by the presence of a tuft of medullary veins that converge into a single enlarged central trunk that may drain superficially, or into the deep venous system.

Microscopically, they are composed of multiple venous channels with normal histological architecture. One or more central draining veins is usually enlarged and occasionally may reach varicose proportions. The enlarged central branches may show evidence of thickening and hyalinization. The vascular channels of venous malformations are usually separated by normal-appearing neural parenchyma. Gliosis or evidence of degenerative changes occurs infrequently, and when present, is focal. They are generally benign lesions without a potential for either microscopic or massive hemorrhage, and may simply represent an anomalous venous drainage pattern rather than a vascular malformation in the usual sense of the word. When hemorrhage does occur in association with a venous malformation, the clinician should be suspicious of the presence of an angiographically occult vascular lesion.

We have found a strong association between venous malformations and cavernous malformations. In our experience at the BNI, six patients have presented with hemorrhage and angiographic evidence of a venous malformation. One patient underwent surgery, and a hematoma was found to be related to an unsuspected cavernous malformation. In the remaining five patients, evaluation with MRI demonstrated findings consistent with a coexisting cavernous malformation, verified surgically in four patients. We recommend that patients with "symptomatic" venous malformation undergo high-field strength MRI to rule out other underlying pathology. When symptomatic hemorrhage is present, the surgeon is well advised to evacuate the hematoma, search for other pathology and avoid the temptation to resect the venous malformation. Resection of venous malformations has been associated with catastrophic infarction, presumably from sudden interruption of the cerebral venous drainage carried by the malformation.

Keywords: Cerebral vascular malformations; venous malformations; cavernous malformations; surgical management.

Introduction

Cerebral vascular malformations are congenital abnormalities that affect form 1% to 5% of the population. They are typically divided into four types: 1) arteriovenous malformations (AVMs); 2) venous malformations; 3) cavernous malformations; and 4) telangiectases.

Venous malformations are by far the most common cerebral vascular malformation identified on pathologic studies. In an unselected autopsy series of more than 5,000 patients, McCormick found that 270 patients (4.7%) harbored vascular malformations (Table 1). Venous malformations composed 64% of the identified lesions, followed by capillary telangiectases (18%), AVMs (11%), and cavernous malformations (7%). The fact that most venous malformations are asymptomatic explains their relative rarity in reviews of surgical pathology. When symptoms are present in a patient with a venous angioma, a careful search, including the use of magnetic resonance imaging (MRI), will often reveal other more clinically significant pathology[19].

These lesions are rarely associated with hemorrhage. In such cases, we have found a strong association

Table 1. *Vascular Malformations in 270 Patients Results of 5754 Consecutive Autopsies*

Type of vascular malformation	Number of patients
Venous malformation	173
Capillary telangiectases	50
Arteriovenous malformations	30
Cavernous malformations	19

Adapted from McCormick WF (1984) Pathology of vascular malformations of the brain. In: Wilson CB, Stein BM (eds) Intracranial arteriovenous malformations. Baltimore, Williams and Wilkins, pp 44–63

between venous angiomas and cavernous malformations[17]. When the two lesions coexist, the cavernous malformation is the most likely source of hemorrhage. The pathology, diagnosis, and management of venous angiomas are discussed.

Pathology

On gross examination, venous malformations are characterized by the presence of a tuft of medullary veins that converge into a single enlarged central trunk.

Microscopically, they are composed of multiple venous channels with normal histological architecture[10]. One or more central draining veins are usually enlarged and occasionally may reach varicose proportions. The enlarged central branches may show evidence of thickening and hyalinization. The vascular channels of venous malformations are usually separated by neural parenchyma that appear normal. Gliosis or evidence of degenerative changes is infrequent, and when present, focal. Gross or microscopic evidence of hemorrhage is rare.

Diagnostic Studies

The angiographic appearance of venous malformations is pathognomonic. Enlarged medullary veins converge in a radial pattern on a central draining trunk that drains either to the superficial system or, less commonly, to the deep venous system (Fig. 1). In our experience, the angiogram always demonstrates this *caput medusa* appearance with normal arterial and capillary phases. The presence of an early draining vein should always raise suspicion of an AVM.

The computed tomography (CT) appearance of venous malformations has been described by numerous authors [1,3,5,8,12,20,21,23]. The most commonly reported finding is a linear or curvilinear enhancement after the administration of contrast. A nodular hyperdense area on nonenhanced studies has also been reported. Mass effect and edema are rare and suggest that other pathology is present.

In a series of 30 patients from our institution, Rigamonti et al.[19] reported that precontrast-enhanced CT scans suggested the presence of an abnormal vascular structure in 55% of cases. Contrast-enhanced CT scans were positive in 96% of cases, revealing the typical linear enhancement in 86% of patients and globular enhancement in 8%. CT was negative in only one patient (4%).

More recently, MRI has been used to diagnosis venous malformations[2,4,7,18,21]. MRI has the advantage of not requiring the administration of contrast to detect venous angiomas.

The typical appearance of the venous malformation on T1- and T2-weighted images is a linear hypointense vascular void[18]. Mass effect and edema are rare. An area of increased signal intensity on a T2-weighted

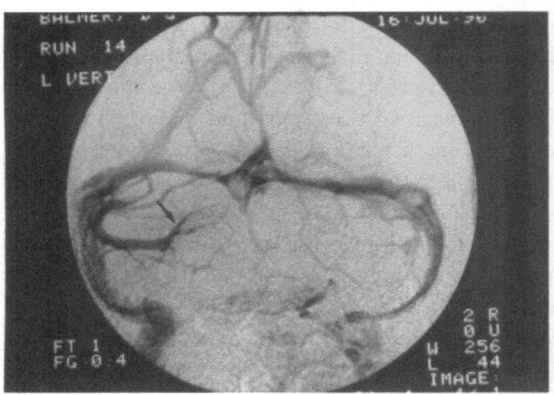
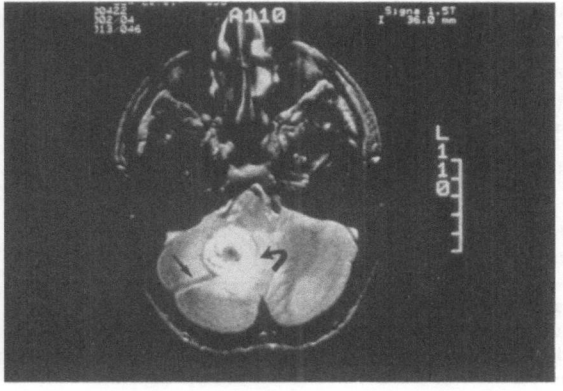

a   b

Fig. 1. (a) Anterior-posterior view of left vertebral artery angiogram, demonstrating a typical caput medusa appearance of a venous malformation in the right cerebellum. (b) T1-weighted magnetic resonance image in the same patient demonstrating the typical linear flow-void associated with venous malformation (straight arrow) in combination with an area of mixed signal intensity (curved arrows) consistent with hemorrhage into a cavernous malformation. At surgery, the diagnosis of cavernous malformation was confirmed. The patient underwent evacuation of the hematoma and resection of the cavernous malformation without complication

image was seen in one of our patients who later died of glioblastoma and in another patient who presented with stroke. In five patients, an area of mixed signal intensity consistent with cavernous malformation (Fig. 1) was seen and confirmed by surgical pathology in four[17].

Clinical Presentation

Cerebral venous malformations have been reported to cause epilepsy, progressive neurologic deficits, and hemorrhage[3,13,16,17]. Frequently convulsions have been associated with venous malformations[1,6,13,22]. A positive correlation, however, between the location of the angioma and the electroencephalographic seizure focus is unusual.

The most frequent complaint leading to diagnosis of venous malformation is headache. In our series, 67% of patients complained of headache (Table 2). The second most common complaint was nausea and vomiting in 13% of patients. Seizures, psychiatric disturbances, amenorrhea, and symptoms of focal cerebral ischemia each had presenting complaints in 7% of patients. When the lesions were located in the supratentorial compartment (60% of patients), the venous angioma was most often considered incidental to the complaints. In patients with posterior fossa venous malformations, the symptoms were more often consistent with the location of the lesion[3,6,15,16]. In our series, 12 patients had cerebellar venous malformations. Among these patients, 67% had symptoms referable to the posterior fossa, including four patients who presented with episodes of gait ataxia, three with diplopia, two with numbness, and one each with dysphagia and decreased hearing[19]. In two of these patients, the symptoms were associated with evidence of hemorrhage from an associated cavernous malformation. although neurologic deficits were more frequent with posterior fossa lesions, 33% of the patients in our series with cerebellar venous malformations presented with headache only.

The incidence of hemorrhage from venous malformations is unclear. Hemorrhage appears more in cerebellar lesions – more than two dozen cases are reported in the literature[5,8,11,14,15,20,24,25]. Operative intervention has been recommended in the management of hemorrhagic lesions[9,14]. Operative resection of a venous malformation, however, may interrupt the venous drainage from the surrounding normal brain, precipitating acute venous engorgement, swelling, and infarction, with devastating consequences.

When hemorrhage is associated with a venous malformation, the clinician should be suspicious of the presence of an angiographically occult vascular lesion. We have found a strong association between venous malformations and cavernous malformations[17].

In our experience, six patients have presented with hemorrhage and angiographic evidence of a venous malformation. Early in our experience, one patient with hemorrhage and a cerebellar venous angioma underwent surgery. Intraoperatively, the hematoma was found to be related to an unsuspected cavernous malformation. After the hematoma was evacuated and the cavernous malformation was resected, attempted removal of the venous malformation led to acute swelling that necessitated partial resection of the cerebellar hemisphere. In the remaining five patients, evaluation with MRI demonstrated findings consistent with a coexisting cavernous malformation (Fig. 1). Four of these five patients underwent surgery with pathologic confirmation of cavernous malformation as the source of hemorrhage. In the remaining patient, MRI evaluation for a 15-year history of partial-complex seizures revealed a deep cavernous malformation centered in the left external capsule-putamen region, spreading into the left temporal lobe. Two linear areas of signal flow void were demonstrated immediately adjacent to the rim of the cavernous malformation. Angiography confirmed the presence of a venous malformation. Because the lesion was located in eloquent cortex, surgery was not recommended. During follow-up this patient has remained stable, with good control of his seizures.

Conclusion

Venous malformations are typically benign lesions. They likely represent an anomalous venous drainage

Table 2. *Clinical Presentation of Venous Malformations (N = 30 Patients)*

Headache	67%
Nausea/vomitig	13%
Gait ataxia	13%
Diplopia	10%
Focal cerebral ischemia	7%
Seizures	7%
Psychiatric	7%
Amenorrhea	7%
Dysphagia	3%
Decreased hearing	3%

pattern rather than true vascular malformations in the usual sense.

We recommend that patients with "symptomatic" venous malformations undergo high-field strength MRI to rule out other underlying pathology. When symptomatic hemorrhage is present, the surgeon is well advised to evacuate the hematoma, to search for other pathology, and to avoid the temptation to resect the venous malformation.

References

1. Agnoli AL, Hildebrandt G (1985) Cerebral venous angiomas. Acta Neurochir (Wien) 78: 4–12
2. Augustyn GT, Scott JA, Olson E, Gilmor RL, Edwards MK, (1985) Cerebral venous angiomas: MR imaging. Radiology 156: 391–395
3. Beatty RM, Zervas NT (1983) Stereotactic aspiration of a brain stem hematoma. Neurosurgery 13: 204–207
4. Cammarata C, Hans JS, Haaga JR, Alfidi RJ, Kaufman B (1985) Cerebral venous angiomas imaged by MR. Radiology 155: 639–643
5. Hacker DA, Latchaw RE, Chou SN, et al (1981) Case report. Bilateral cerebellar venous angioma. J Comput Assist Tomogr 5: 424–426
6. Jellinger K (1975) The morphology of centrally-situated angiomas. In: Pia HW, Gleave JRW, Grote E, et al (eds) Cerebral angiomas: advances in diagnosis and therapy. Springer, Wien New York, pp 9–18
7. Lee BCP, Herzberg L, Zimmerman RD, Deck MDF (1985) MR imaging of cerebral vascular malformations. AJNR 6: 863–870
8. Maehara T, Tasaka A (1978) Cerebral venous angioma: computed tomography and angiographic diagnosis. Neuroradiology 16: 296–298
9. Malik GM, Morgan JK, Boulos RS, Ausman JI (1988) Venous angiomas: an underestimated cause of intracranial hemorrhage. Surg Neurol 30: 350–358
10. McCormick WF (1984) Pathology of vascular malformations of the brain. In: Wilson CB, Stein BM (eds) Intracranial arteriovenous malformations. Williams and Wilkins, Baltimore, pp 44–63
11. McCormick WF, Hardman JM, Boutler TR (1968) Vascular malformations (angiomas) of the brain with special reference to those occurring in the posterior fossa. J Neurosurg 28: 241–245
12. Michels LG, Bentson JR, Winter J (1977) Computed tomography of cerebral venous angiomas. J Comput Assist Tomogr 1: 49–154
13. Mishikawa J, Maehara T (1978) CT scan. Cerebral vascular disease, venous angioma. Igaku No Ayumi 104: 137–138
14. Moritake K, Handa H, Mori K, Ishikawa M, Morimoto M, Takebe Y (1980) Venous angiomas of the brain. Surg Neurol 14: 95–105
15. Numaguchi Y, Kitamura K, Fukui M, Ikeda J, Hasuo K, Kishikawa T, Okudera T, Uemura K, Matsuura K (1982) Intracranial venous angiomas. Surg Neurol 18: 193–202
16. Partain CL, Guinto FC, Scatliff JH (1979) Cerebral venous angioma: correlation of radionuclide brain scan, transmission computed tomography and angiography. J Nucl Med 20: 1166–1169
17. Rigamonti D, Spetzler RF (1988) The association of venous and cavernous malformations. Report of four cases and discussion of the pathophysiological, diagnostic, and therapeutic implications. Acta Neurochir (Wien) 92: 100–105
18. Rigamonti D, Spetzler RF, Drayer BP, Boyanowski WH, Hodak J, Rigamonti KH, Plenge K, Powers M, Rekate H (1988) Appearance of venous malformations on magnetic resonance imaging. J Neurosurg 69: 535–539
19. Rigamonti D, Spetzler RF, Medina M, Rigamonti K, Geckle DS, Pappas C (1990) Cerebral venous malformations. J Neurosurg 73: 560–564
20. Rothfus WE, Albright LA, Casey KF, Latchaw RE, Roppolo HMN (1984) Cerebellar venous angioma: "benign" entity? AJNR 5: 61–66
21. Scott JA, Augustyn GT, Gilmor RL, Maeley J Jr, Olson EW (1985) Magnetic resonance imaging of a venous angioma. AJNR 6: 284–286
22. Suganuma Y, Oie K, Tanigawa K Matsushima Y, Inaba Y (1978) A case of cerebral venous angioma. Neurol Surg 6: 77–83
23. Valavanis A, Wellauer J, Yaşargil MG (1983) The radiological diagnosis of cerebral venous angioma: cerebral angiography and computed tomography. Neuroradiology 24: 193–199
24. Wendling LR, Moore JS Jr, Kieffer SA, Goldberg HI, Latchaw RE (1976) Intracerebral venous angioma. Radiology 119: 141–147
25. Wolf PA, Rosman NP, New PFJ (1967) Multiple small cryptic venous angiomas of the brain mimicking cerebral metastasis. A clinical, pathological, and angiographic study. Neurology 17: 491–501

Correspondence: c/o Editorial Office, Joseph M. Zabramski, M.D., Barrow Neurological Institute, 350 West Thomas Road, Phoenix, AZ 85013-4496, U.S.A.

Management of Venous Angiomas of the Brain

S. Gilman and **G.M. Malik**

Department of Neurological Surgery, Henry Ford Hospital, Detroit, Michigan, U.S.A.

Summary

Venous angioma (V.A.) is a well recognized cerebral vascular malformation; however, studies over the past 25 years provide conflicting data as to their true clinical importance and risk of hemorrhage. Most of the studies base their conclusions solely on angiographically proven cases. Though angiography provides definitive diagnosis, it has become obvious that appropriate MRI and possibly CT evaluations are sufficiently accurate. Following a previous series of 21 patients with angiographical diagnosis only (years 1975–1987), since July 1987, 38 patients at our institution have had V.A. diagnosed by angiography, 28 of whom had prior MRI studies. MRI failed to diagnose V.A. in only one of 24 cases where hemorrhage was absent. In four cases, hemorrhage precluded the exact diagnosis. In addition, 65 MRIs and 50 contrast enhanced CT scans have strongly suggested the diagnosis of V.A. raising the total to 155 lesions. Overall, the hemorrhage rate was 5.8% with nine proven bleeds without findings suggestive of cavernous angioma. Looking only at those cases proven angiographically, the rate was 22.5%. Only six of the remaining cases who had not hemorrhaged were felt to be symptomatic from their lesion. This review reaffirms our previous findings that V.A. has the propensity for bleeding; however, the actual incidence would seem to be lower than previously suggested when based solely on angiographically proven cases.

Keywords: Venous angioma; angiography; MRI; hemorrhage.

Introduction

Russell and Rubenstein classify cerebrovascular malformations into four familiar categories: AVM, cavernous angioma, capillary telangiectasia and venous angioma[10]. Until McCormack and Sarwar did a prospective pathological study on 4,069 brains, it was thought that venous angioma was the rarest of these lesions[12]. Having uncovered that some 63% of cerebral vascular malformations were, in fact, venous angiomas, it has become apparent that, quite possibly, they are the most common.

Venous angiomas consist of a focal collection of dilated medullary veins arranged in a radial fashion which converge upon a central dilated draining trunk. Its first description was by Duret in 1874 who noted their transcerebral course and intracerebral anasto-moses[2]. Normal parenchymatous brain tissue intervenes between these anomalous veins. These malformations of the venous circulation convey the characteristic angiographic appearance of the so-called caput medusae, in reference to its resemblance of the snake covered head of the mythical gorgon medusa (Fig. 1).

Theories regarding the etiology of the venous angioma are varied. Saito and Kobayashi believe that during during embryogenesis some accident occurs in the formation of the medullary veins and the venous angioma is formed in compensation[11]. Others, however, believe that the abnormal drainage pattern represents developmental fetal circulation which has persisted into adulthood or which has been reactivated secondary to prior vascular occlusion or other alteration of venous drainage[13]. Lasjunais feels they constitute simply an extreme anatomical variation based on the hemodynamic equilibrium between the superficial and deep drainage systems of the brain[3].

Histologically, the venous angiomas are composed of dilated medullary veins dispersed about unaltered white matter. These veins have no internal elastic lamina and only rarely scattered elastic fibers and muscle cells. Although others, such as Huang *et al.* have described transitional forms with small feeding hypertrophic arterial components, microscopically they consist entirely of veins[3].

The venous drainage of most venous angiomas is towards the superficial venous system, but occasionally the deep, subependymal system is involved in the venous drainage. After review of 58 angiograms of venous angioma, Valvanis found that nearly 70% drained exclusively into the superficial venous system, while 22% drained exclusively into the deep, subependymal system and 8.6% into both[14].

The variability of drainage patterns in venous angiomas is explained by the anatomy of medullary veins, which consist of two discreet groups. The superficial

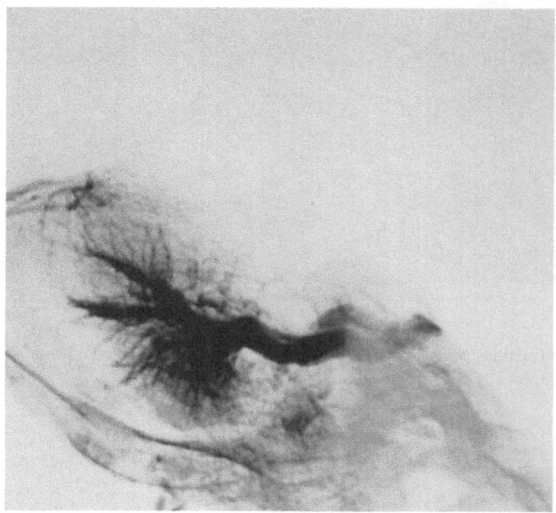

Fig. 1. Lateral angiographic view of posterior fossa venous angioma demonstrating classic caput medusa

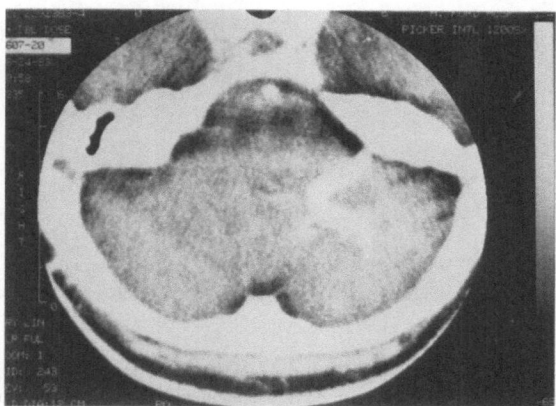

Fig. 2. Axial contrast enhanced CT illustrating large posterior fossa venous angioma

group consists of veins which begin juxtacortically, are short and run though the cortex to join the pial veins. The deep group of medullary veins are longer in their course and converge towards the lateral ventricles, finally draining into the subependymal venous system. There also exists anastomotic or transcerebral veins, which normally connect the two groups of medullary veins or run directly from the pial to the subependymal veins. The drainage pattern of venous angiomas thus depends on the location of the lesion in the white matter and the type of medullary veins involved. In fact, Valvanis has classified venous angiomas based on the drainage pattern into: 1. Juxtacortical, 2. Subcortical, 3. Paraventricular[14].

Clinical Series

Amongst controversy surrounding the natural history and significance of the venous angioma, Malik and Morgan reported their experience from our institution. From 1975 to 1987, cerebral angiography performed at Henry Ford Hospital revealed 23 venous angiomas in 21 patients. Nine of these patients presented to us with intracranial hemorrhage. There were seven men and fourteen women with an average age at diagnosis of 38 years. Eleven of the lesions were supratentorial, predominantly in the frontal lobes. All but one of these drained into the superficial venous system, most into the superior sagittal sinus. There were twelve infratentorial lesions, half of which drained from the cerebellar hemispheres. The others drained from either the vermis or the brain stem. Ten of the twelve infratentorial lesions drained into the transverse sinus, while two drained into the vein of Galen. Estimates of the average diameter of the radial array of the medullary veins were made, but correlation between size and hemorrhage could not be established[5] (Fig. 2).

CT scanning was helpful in localizing the venous angioma in 80% of the cases by finding either a nodular area of increased density or a linear/curvilinear transcortical draining vein[5]. Yaşargil similarly reported that 87% of venous angiomas can be detected and localized by contrast enhanced CT[14].

Of the 21 patients with angiographically proven venous angiomas, eleven were felt to have unassociated symptoms and the venous angioma was an incidental finding. Ten patients, however, became surgical candidates – nine for hemorrhage associated with the venous angioma and one for intractable seizures whose EEG focus correlated well with the location of the lesion. Two of the nine who presented with hemorrhage had documented prior hemorrhage[5].

It was therefore concluded that hemorrhage from cerebral venous angioma was not as uncommon as once thought as a full 43% of angiographically confirmed venous angiomas were found to have bled. Those who had bled or were clinically symptomatic from the lesion were deemed good surgical candidates for evacuation of the clot and/or resection of the lesion. Once a venous angioma has bled, presumably, it has declared its inherent weakness and recurrent hemorrhage is likely[5].

Undoubtedly, venous angioma found by angiography is biased in selecting patients generally quite ill or in some way symptomatic. These are the patients who are known to have or are suspected to have bled. It has become apparent over the last several years with growing MRI capabilities that MRI is very sensitive in detecting venous angiomas of the brain, particularly with the addition of contrast enhancement or with special pulse sequences geared towards evaluating the vasculature of the brain (Fig. 3a–c). Recent studies report up to 96% sensitivity[15]. Since July of 1987, 38 more cerebral angiograms at Henry Ford Hospital have disclosed venous angiomas, nine of which have bled. Of these 38 patients, 28 had MRI performed prior to angiography. Of these, the presence of venous angioma was strongly suggested in 23 cases (Fig. 4a–d). In four of the remaining five studies, hemorrhage precluded a definitive diagnosis and angiography was suggested. In only one of the twenty-eight angiographically confirmed cases did MRI fail to suggest the diagnosis of venous angioma. In this particular case, the lesion was not seen until a second angiogram was performed. In all cases, either gadolinium enhanced images or gradient recall images were obtained (Fig. 5a and b). MRI with gadolinium enhancement or gradient recall images since July of 1987 have uncovered another 65 patients with highly suspected venous angioma, all without evidence of prior

a b c

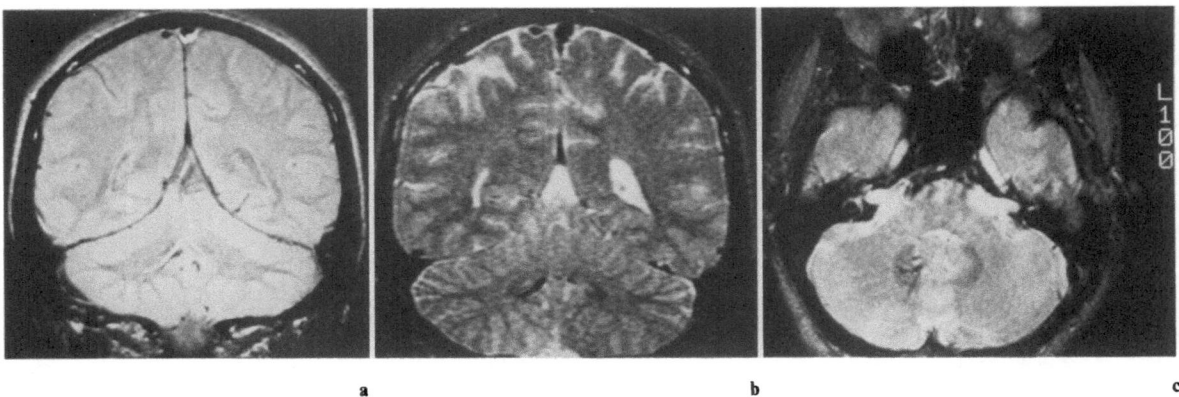

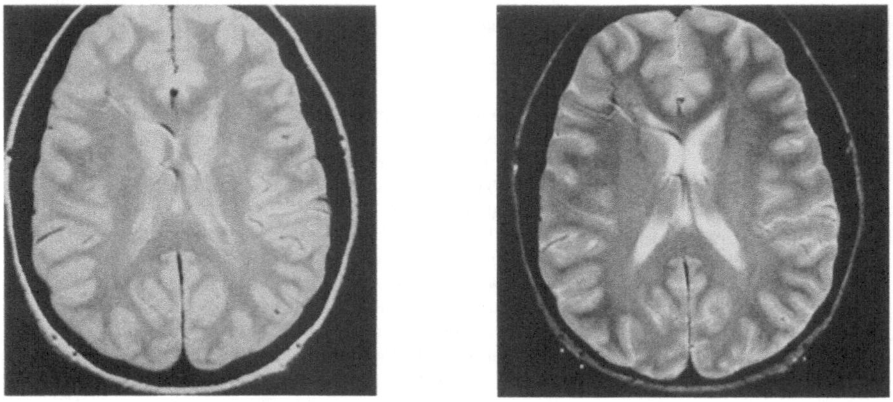

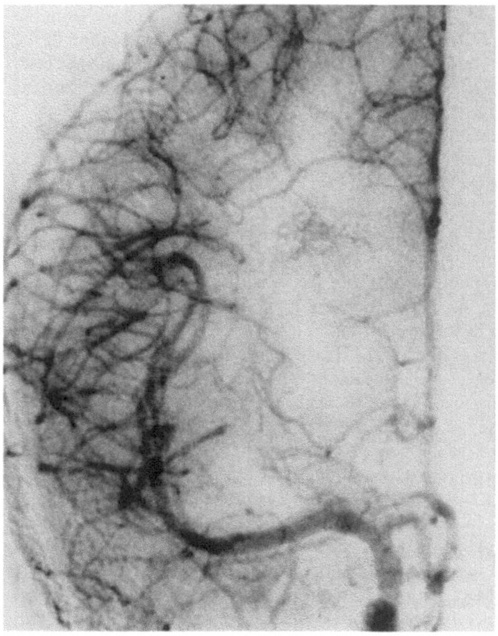

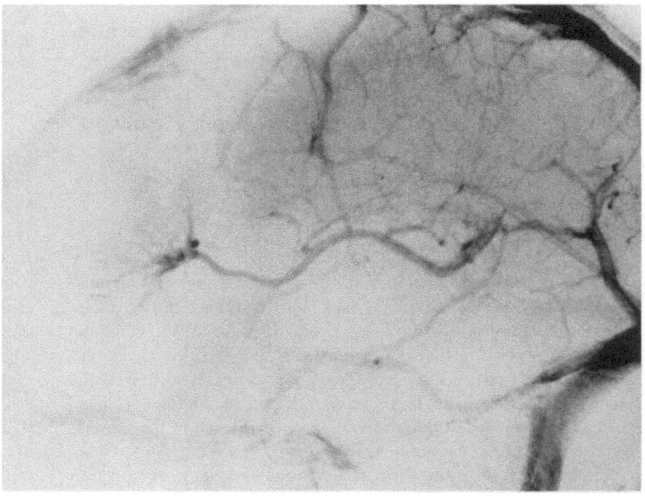

Fig. 3. (a) Coronal T_1 weighted image demonstrating deep posterior fossa paravermian venous angioma. (b) Same lesion, T_2 weighted coronal image. (c) Same lesion, proton density axial image. Venous angioma angiographically confirmed

a b

d

c

hemorrhage. None have undergone cerebral angiography. Only a small portion of these patients ever received neurosurgical consultation. If MRI is nearly 100% sensitive in detecting venous angioma, as recent studies suggest, then 9 out of 104 venous angiomas diagnosed at Henry Ford Hospital since July of 1987 have hemorrhage at some time (8.3%).

Another 50 patients who received only contrast enhanced CT scans of the head since July of 1987 have been diagnosed as harboring a venous angioma. Diagnosis by CT was in accordance with the characteristic patterns including: 1. Homogeneously enhancing round area noted in the white matter. 2. Linear, transcerebral enhancement. 3. Combined linear and round enhancement[11] (Fig.

6a and b). For various reasons, follow-up MRI or angiography was not obtained on these patients as most of them never came to the attention of the neurosurgery service. In total then, 38 angiograms, 65 MRIs and 50 contrast enhanced CTs have strongly suggested the presence of cerebral venous angioma at Henry Ford Hospital since July of 1987, for a total of 155 lesions. With nine bleeds in this series, the total hemorrhage rate was 5.8%.

Of the recent 38 patients who had angiographic confirmation (all of whom were seen by a neurosurgeon), 15 were felt to be symptomatic. Nine patients had sustained hemorrhage in the region of the venous angioma. Another six patients had symptoms referable to the lesion, but had never bled. Two patients had mild dysmetria on the

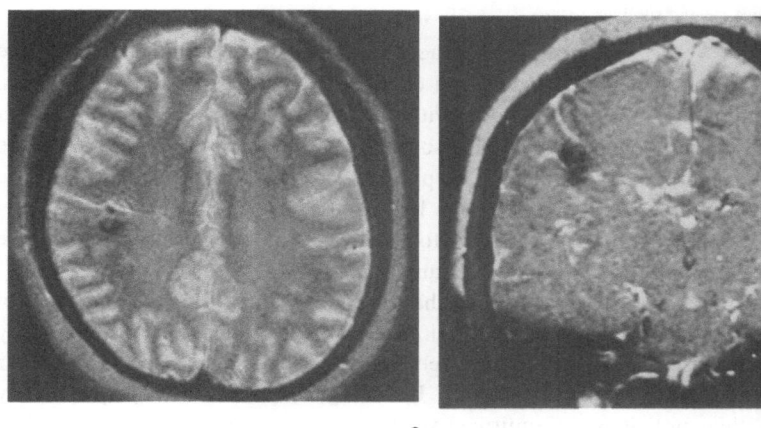

Fig. 5. (a) T_2 weighted axial image demonstrating juxtacortical draining vein with associated hemorrhage from angiographically confirmed venous angioma. (b) Coronal gradient recall image of same lesion demonstrating venous angioma with associated hemorrhage

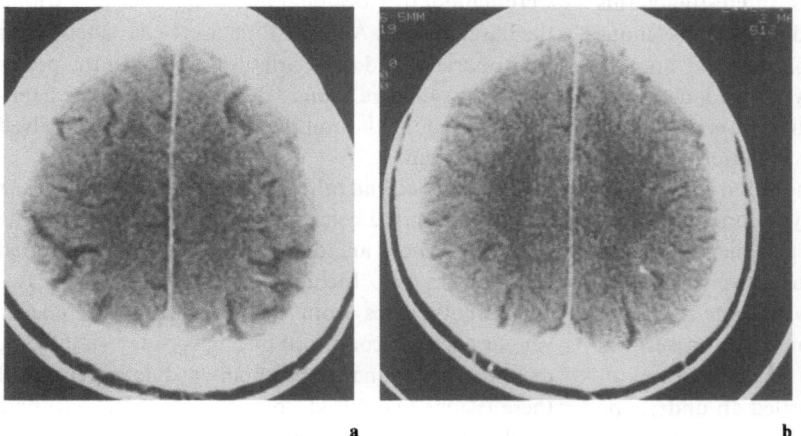

Fig. 6. (a) Contrast enhanced axial CT image demonstrating round pattern of enhancement of angiographically proven venous angioma. (b) Same lesion, axial contrast enhanced image demonstrating linear enhancement

Fig. 4. (a) Axial proton density MR image demonstrating typical appearance of deep white matter frontal venous angioma. (b) Axial T_2 weighted image of same lesion. (c) AP angiographic image of same lesion in the early venous phase. (d) Lateral image in late venous phase clearly demonstrating caput medusa converging on the internal cerebral vein via the septal vein

same side of their cerebellar lesion, two patients had persistent frontal headache ipsilateral to their lesion, and another two patients had seizure foci by EEG which correlated well with the location of the lesion. With regard to the 65 cases picked up by MRI and the 50 cases found by contrast enhanced CT scans, we can only presume one of two things after review of the charts. Either the primary care physician or the consulting neurologist was not convinced that the location of the lesion fit the patient's symptoms or symptoms could be well controlled without the need for surgical consultation. A small percentage of these patients were seen in neurosurgical consultation; however, none were deemed candidates for surgery or angiography. In most, there was poor correlation between symptoms and location of the lesion. Hence, the fact that 15 out of 38 (39%) of the patients angiogrammed were in some way symptomatic from the lesion reflects a very strong bias in the patients we see and surely is not representative of the true incidence of hemorrhage.

Discussion

Literature concerning the venous angioma is replete with contrasting reports regarding symptomatology of these patients. Some claim a high correlation between symptomatology and location of the lesion, while others claim only a small minority have symptoms referable to the lesion[1]. Unfortunately, most of these studies included only patients with angiographically confirmed lesions, which is not reflective of the actual incidence. But even if we are to consider only the cases proven angiographically, more often than not, it is difficult to definitively ascribe one's symptoms to this lesion barring hemorrhage. While cases of epilepsy with good EEG correlation exist, this is the exception more than the rule. Recently, Rigamonti et al. presented their series of 30 venous angiomas. Interestingly, this was the first study in which the diagnosis of venous angioma was not dependent upon cerebral angiography. Of their 30 patients, only 25 had definitive angiography. Nineteen of their patients were found by MRI. In that study, a poor correlation between symptomatology and location of the lesion was found[8]. However, of those felt to be truly symptomatic, lesions in the cerebellum had the highest chance of having related symptoms. Four out of their twelve patients with cerebellar lesions presented with acute cerebellar dysfunction. Only two of those underwent a surgical procedure, both for evacuation of cerebellar hematomas. Pathology in both cases revealed an underlying cavernous angioma along with the venous angioma. The source of the hemorrhage was actually felt to be the cavernous angioma[8].

In our own experience of 21 previous and 38 more recent patients with angiographically confirmed venous angioma (total of 59), only three patients were found to have an associated cavernous angioma. Two were in

the parietal lobes and one in the cerebellum. Including the 65 cases diagnosed by MRI only 3 out of 124 had an associated cavernous angioma. In each of these three cases, the patient was believed to be symptomatic from the cavernous angioma. Two of the three underwent resection with pathological confirmation, the other was lost to follow-up. In one of the two surgical cases, the preoperative MRI disclosed only the venous angioma. At surgery, however, the hemorrhage, while in the same general region of the venous angioma, was clearly associated with the cavernous angioma. Of the 19 patients who underwent resection of venous angioma or evacuation of hematoma, none revealed the presence of cavernous angioma histologically. Thus, we agree with Rigamonti et al. that venous angioma may be associated with cavernous angioma; but the incidence appears to be quite infrequent. In the case where both lesions are suspected to be present, however, symptomatology is more than likely due to the cavernous angioma.

It is felt that the most frequent sites of occurrence of venous angiomas are the frontal lobes supratentorially and the cerebellum infratentorially[9]. This parallels our experience. Including our cases of angiographically confirmed venous angioma and those detected solely by MRI, a total of 127 venous angiomas have been found. Seventy-three venous angiomas were supratentorial (59.3%) while 54 were infratentorial (40.7%). Supratentorially, 32 were frontal, 23 were parietal, 4 were temporal, 1 occipital and 9 were located within the basal ganglia. Another three were characterized as frontoparietal and one parieto-occipital. In the posterior fossa, 49 were found within the cerebellar hemispheres or along the midline vermis. Only five involved the brain stem.

Rofthus et al. and others believe that there may exist a difference in the behavior and natural history of the cerebellar venous angiomas compared to those located supratentorially[9]. Including four of their own cases and twenty cases from the literature of cerebellar venous angioma confirmed by angiography, pathology, or both, they found that as many as fifteen percent of these lesions may bleed, sometimes with catastrophic results. They add that though there is a three to one predominance of supratentorial versus infratentorial venous angiomas, almost half of the cases reported in the literature to have bled were in the posterior fossa. Thus, they conclude that venous angiomas in this location may, in fact, have natural history similar to that of AVM[9].

In our own series of 59 patients with 63 angiographically and/or pathologically confirmed venous angiomas, 11 of the 38 supratentorial lesions had bled (29%), and 7 out of 25 infratentorial lesions had bled (28%). When adding the patients whose venous angiomas were diagnosed by MRI, the totals are as follows: 11 out of 73 supratentorial lesions have bled (15%) and 7 out of 54 (13%) infratentorial lesions have bled, a roughly equal distribution. Furthermore, we have found the ratio of supratentorial to infratentorial lesions to be approximately 1.35:1, a rather significant difference from prior literature. Therefore, while the results of posterior fossa hemorrhage may certainly be catastrophic, as it may be from any cause, a higher propensity to bleed than those supratentorially is not supported by our data. Interestingly, four out of our five cases of venous angioma involving the brain stem have bled, three recurrently.

In analyzing the issue of sex predominance, we previously found a tendency for women to be more susceptible to hemorrhage, although the overall numbers were too low to be significant. We noted that six of the nine hemorrhages occurred in women[5]. However, the study included 7 men and 14 women. Pooling the 59 patients confirmed by angiography since 1975, there have been 24 men and 35 women. Of the 24 men, 7 have bled; and of the 35 women, 11 have bled. Again, roughly equal ratios and no clear sexual predominance. This only reflects our slightly higher incidence of venous angiomas in women than men.

Our current understanding of the natural history of these lesions is based on incomplete data. Although McCormack and Sarwar declared that venous angiomas were clearly the most common cerebrovascular malformations found at autopsy, literature dealing with these lesions is surprisingly scarce. This is, in part, because without angiography there has been a great reluctance to make a definitive diagnosis. We believe that this is what is precluding our ability to make informed decisions regarding the natural history and treatment of these lesions.

With the power of current diagnostic tools and radiographic imaging, we are finally coming to see what McCormack and Sarwar saw when they prospectively analyzed 4,069 brains for presence of cerebrovascular malformation. A full 63% of the vascular anomalies of the brain found in their series were confirmed to be venous angioma[12]. Very recent studies on MR imaging of cerebrovascular malformations boast impressive results in localizing and characterizing

venous angiomas with the use of gadolinium enhancement and special pulse sequences. Wilms et al. found that 27 out of 28 angiographic or surgically confirmed cases could be seen with gadolinium enhanced MRI images[15]. We experienced similar results in our series with hemorrhage being the major inhibitor of diagnosis. Anyone with hemorrhage into the brain without an underlying reason or set of risk factors, however, would certainly come to cerebral angiography anyhow.

From what we have found, one can see how greatly the statistics change when one selects out small groups to study. When considering only angiographic or surgically proven cases, the numbers are impressive for the incidence of hemorrhage from these lesions. However, these numbers are biased such that reasonable conclusions cannot be drawn.

Surely, anyone who has hemorrhaged from venous angioma or any other cause ought to be fully studied and probably have some sort of surgical procedure performed, whether that be to relieve mass effect, make a diagnosis or resect the offending lesion. In the case of venous angiomas, many authors have cautioned that no operation ought to be undertaken without full and complete knowledge of the entire venous system, for oftentimes these enlarged transcerebral veins are the only means of outflow from a particular region of the brain[6]. This appears to be especially true within the posterior fossa as inadvertent interruption of such a structure may cause fatal venous infarction or malignant swelling. Thus, any patient known to have hemorrhage at some time from a venous angioma should undergo cerebral angiography even if asymptomatic at the time. It has been our experience that once a venous angioma has bled, rebleeding is not at all uncommon. In Morgan's series of nine patients treated previously for hemorrhage, two had ruptured in the past[5]. Since his report, in which only four patients underwent complete resection, one of the five patients who had only partial resection has rebled. Of the nine cases studied since 1987, one patient presented to us with a history of prior bleed. This patient had undergone resection of a brain stem clot several years prior for this and then underwent proton beam radiation therapy. He recently presented to us, two years after another hemorrhage. In this regard, MRI is helpful as well. It can detect areas of subacute and chronic hemorrhages by the presence of methemoglobin. A decision to go ahead with cerebral angiography is then easily made.

Contrast enhanced CT scanning has also been reported by several authors to be some 80 to 87%

sensitive in the diagnosis of venous angioma[14]. In cases where the diagnosis meets with criteria described earlier, we advocate follow-up with MRI with gadolinium or special pulse sequences designed to highlight the vessels of the brain such as the gradient recall images. If MRI reveals the same, the diagnosis of venous angioma is reasonable and nothing further ought to be done unless there is a suspicion that other vascular malformations are in the differential diagnosis or there is evidence of methemoglobin.

Although we have no current information as to the annual rate of hemorrhage of venous angiomas as we do with aneurysms or arteriovenous malformations, the low incidence of rupture along with the potential hazards associated with interrupting anomalous venous drainage leads us to believe that barring exceptional circumstances these lesions are probably best left alone.

References

1. Angoli AL, Hildebrandt G (1985) Cerebral venous angiomas. Acta Neurochir (Wien) 78: 4–12
2. Duret H (1874) Recherches anatomiques sur la circulation de l'encephale. Arch Physiol Norm Pathol 6: 316–353
3. Huang YP, Robbins A, Patel SC, et al (1984) Cerebral venous malformations (and a new classification of cerebral vascular malformations). In: Kapp JP, Schmidek HH (eds) The cerebral venous system and its disorders. Grune and Stratton, New York pp 373–474
4. Lasjaunais P, Burrows P, Planet C (1986) Developmental venous anomalies (DVA): The so-called venous angioma. Neurosurg Rev 9: 233–244
5. Malik GM, Morgan JK, Boulos RS, Ausman JI (1988) Venous angiomas: an underestimated cause of intracranial hemorrhage. Surg Neurol 30: 350–358
6. Nishizaki T, Tamaki N. Matsumoto S, Fujita S (1986) Consideration of the operative indications for posterior fossa venous angiomas. Surg Neurol 25: 441–445
7. Namaguchi Y, Kitamura K, Fukui M, Ikeda J, Hasuo K, Kishikawa T, Okudera I, Uemura K, Matsuura K (1982) Intracranial venous angiomas. Surg Neurol 17: 193–202
8. Rigamonti D, Spetzler RF, Medina M, Rigamonti K, Geekle D, Pappas C (1990) Cerebral venous malformations. J Neurosurgery 73: 560–564
9. Rofthus WE, Albright AL, Casey KF, Latchaw RE, Roppolo HMN (1984) Cerebellar venous angioma: "benign" entity? AJNR 5: 61–66
10. Russell DS, Rubenstein LJ (1959) Pathology of tumors of the nervous system. Edward Arnold, London pp 72–94
11. Saito Y, Kobayashi N (1981) Cerebral venous angioma: clinical evaluation and possible etiology. Radiology 139: 87–94
12. Sarwar M, McCormick WF (1978) Intracerebral venous angioma. Arch Neurol 35: 323–325
13. Toro VE, Geyer CA, Sherman JL, Parisi JE, Brantley MJ (1988) Cerebral venous angiomas: MR findings. J Comp Asst Tomogr 12 (6): 935–940
14. Valvanis A, Wellauer J, Yaşargil MG (1983) The radiological diagnosis of cerebral venous angioma: cerebral angiography and computed tomography. Neuroradiology 24: 193–199
15. Wilms G, Demaerel P, Marchal G, Baert AL, Plets C (1991) Gadolinium-enhanced MR imaging of cerebral venous angiomas with emphasis on their drainage. J Comp Assist Tomogr 15 (2): 199–206

Correspondence: G.H. Malik, M.D., Department of Neurological Surgery, Henry Ford Hospital, 2799 West Grand Blvd., Detroit, MI 48202, U.S.A.

Subject Index

Advances and Technical Standards in Neurosurgery

This series, sponsored by the European Association of Neurosurgical Societies, has already become a classic. In general, one volume is published per year.

The Advances section presents fields of neuro-surgery and related areas in which important recent progress has been made.

The Technical Standards section features detailed descript of standard procedures to assist young neurosurgeons in their post-graduate training. The contributions are written by experienced clinicians and are reviewed by all members of the Editorial Board.

Volume 21

1994. 69 figures. Approx. 250 pages.
Cloth approx. DM 200,–, approx. öS 1400,–
ISBN 3-211-82482-0

Advances:

G.J. Pilkington, P.L. Lantos: Biological Markers for Tumours of the Brain.
C. Daumas-Duport: Histoprognosis of Gliomas.
F. Cohadon: Brain Protection.

Technical Standards:

S.F. Ciricillo, M.L. Rosenblum: Aids and the Neurosurgeon. An Update.
M. Choux, et.al.: The Surgery of Spinal Dysraphism Lesions.
P. Cosyns, et.al.: Functional Stereotactic Neurosurgery for Psychiatric Disorders. An Experience in Belgium and The Netherlands.

Volume 20

1993. 96 figures. XIII, 308 pages.
Cloth DM 240,–, öS 1680,–
ISBN 3-211-82383-2

Advances:

R.D. Lobato: Post-traumatic Brain Swelling.
K.-F. Lindegaard, W. Sorteberg, and H. Nornes: Transcranial Doppler in Neurosurgery.
A.E. Harding: Clinical and Molecular Neurogenetics in Neurosurgery.

Technical Standards:

B. Williams: Surgery for Hindbrain Related Syringomyelia.
J.-F. Hirsch and E. Hoppe-Hirsch: Medulloblastoma.
F. Resche, J.P. Moisan, J. Mantoura, A.de Kersaint-Gilly, M.J. Andre, I. Perrin-Resche,
D. Menegalli-Boggelli, Y. Lajat, and S. Richard: Haemangioblastoma, Haemangioblastomatosis, and von Hippel-Lindau Disease.

Prices are subject to change without notice

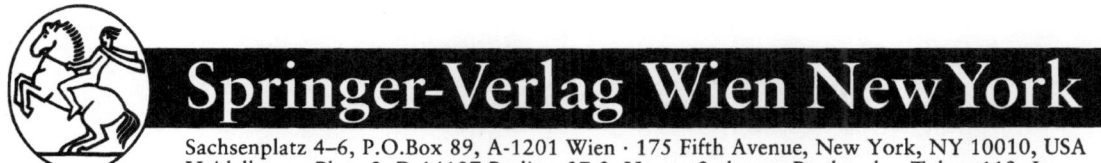

Springer-Verlag Wien New York

Sachsenplatz 4–6, P.O.Box 89, A-1201 Wien · 175 Fifth Avenue, New York, NY 10010, USA
Heidelberger Platz 3, D-14197 Berlin · 37-3, Hongo 3-chome, Bunkyo-ku, Tokyo 113, Japan

U. Ito, A. Baethmann, K.-A. Hossmann, T. Kuroiwa,
A. Marmarou, H.-J. Reulen, K. Takakura (eds.)

Brain Edema IX

1994. 281 figs. XV, 590 pages.
Cloth DM 330,–, öS 2310,–
Reduced price for subscribers to "Acta Neurochirurgica":
Cloth DM 297,–, öS 2079,–
ISBN 3-211-82532-0
(Acta Neurochirurgica / Supplementum 60)

This volume is an up-to-date report on progress in the understanding of brain edema,
with a spectrum reaching from most recent molecularbiological findings to respective
clinical developments. Major topics deal with (a) the blood-parenchymal cell border
under normal and pathological conditions causing brain edema, (b) neuronglial interactions and their disturbances in tissue damage, (c) formation, propagation and resolution of brain edema, and finally (d) treatment of vasogenic and cytotoxic brain
edema. In the basic science approaches emphasis is given to newly discovered mole-
cules, such as vascular endothelial growth factor, which might control permeability of
the blood-brain barrier, e.g. in brain tumors. The complex issue of mediator compounds of secondary brain damage is further developed as to its manyfold involvement, for example in barrier dysfunction, cell swelling, disturbances of the microcirculation, and others. The report further contains comprehensive assessments of
edema pathophysiology by advanced technologies, such as in-situ hybridization on
the one hand side or NMR-diffusion imaging on the other. Novel forms of treatment
acquiring increasing specificity represent a central focus.

Prices are subject to change without notice

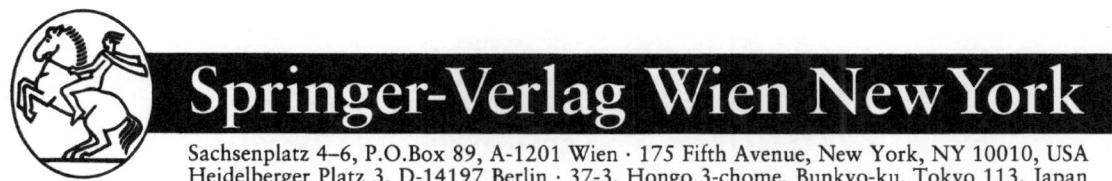

Springer-Verlag Wien New York

Sachsenplatz 4–6, P.O.Box 89, A-1201 Wien · 175 Fifth Avenue, New York, NY 10010, USA
Heidelberger Platz 3, D-14197 Berlin · 37-3, Hongo 3-chome, Bunkyo-ku, Tokyo 113, Japan